PEDIATRIC NEUROLOGY

PRINCIPLES AND PRACTICE

SECOND EDITION

VOLUME ONE

KENNETH F. SWAIMAN, M.D.

Professor of Neurology
Professor of Pediatrics
Director, Division of Pediatric Neurology
University of Minnesota Medical School
Minneapolis, Minnesota

with 530 illustrations

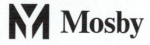

St. Louis Baltimore Boston Chicago London Madrid Philadelphia Sydney Toronto

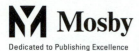

Editor: Stephanie Manning
Developmental Editors: Elaine Steinborn, Carolyn Malik
Assistant Editor: Jo Salway
Project Manager: Carol Sullivan Wiseman
Production Editor: Diana Lyn Laulainen
Editing Assistant: Jennifer J. Byington
Designer: Betty Schulz
Manufacturing Supervisor: Kathy Grone

SECOND EDITION
Copyright © 1994 by Mosby–Year Book, Inc.

Previous edition copyrighted 1989.

Printed in the United States of America

Composition by Graphic World, Inc.
Printing/binding by Maple-Vail Book Manufacturing Group

Mosby–Year Book, Inc.
11830 Westline Industrial Drive
St. Louis, Missouri 63146

Library of Congress Cataloging in Publication Data
Pediatric neurology: principles and practice / [edited by] Kenneth F. Swaiman. — 2nd ed.
    p.   cm.
  Includes bibliographical references and index.
  ISBN 0-8016-6695-3
  1. Pediatric neurology.   I. Swaiman, Kenneth F.
  [DNLM: 1. Nervous System Diseases — in infancy & childhood.   WS
340 P3713 1993]
RJ486.P336 1993
618.92'8 — dc20
DNLM/DLC
for Library of Congress   93-25352
                                  CIP

95 96 97 / 9 8 7 6 5 4 3 2

Contributors

Gary M. Abrams, M.D.

Associate Professor of Clinical Neurology
Columbia University
New York, New York
Medical Director/Chief of Neurology
Helen Hayes Hospital
West Haverstraw, New York

Stephen Ashwal, M.D.

Professor, Pediatrics and Neurology
Loma Linda University School of Medicine
Loma Linda, California

Bruce O. Berg, M.D.

Professor of Neurology and Pediatrics
Director, Child Neurology
University of California Medical Center
San Francisco, California

Peter H. Berman, M.D.

Professor of Pediatrics and Neurology
University of Pennsylvania School of Medicine
Director, Division of Neurology
Children's Hospital of Philadelphia
Philadelphia, Pennsylvania

Galen N. Breningstall, M.D.

Pediatric Subspecialties (Neurology)
Park Nicollet Medical Center
Minneapolis, Minnesota

William F. Chandler, M.D.

Professor, Section of Neurosurgery
Department of Surgery
University of Michigan Medical Center
Ann Arbor, Michigan

Raymond W.M. Chun, M.D.

Professor, Emeritus
University of Wisconsin School of Medicine
Professor, Department of Neurology and Pediatrics
University of Wisconsin Center for Health Sciences
Madison, Wisconsin

James Cloyd, Pharm D.

Professor and Head
Department of Pharmacy Practice
College of Pharmacy
University of Minnesota
Clinical Pharmacist
Minnesota Comprehensive Epilepsy Program
Minneapolis, Minnesota

Michael E. Cohen, M.D.

Chairman, Department of Neurology
Professor of Neurology and Pediatrics
State University of New York at Buffalo
Chief, Division of Child Neurology
Children's Hospital of Buffalo
Buffalo, New York

Carl J. Crosley, M.D.

Associate Professor of Neurology and Pediatrics
Vice Chairman, Department of Neurology
SUNY Health Science Center at Syracuse
Syracuse, New York

William DeMyer, M.D.

Section of Child Neurology
James Whitcomb Riley Hospital for Children
Indianapolis, Indiana

Salvatore Di Mauro, M.D.

Lucy G. Moses Professor of Neurology
Columbia-Presbyterian Medical Center
New York, New York

Darryl C. De Vivo, M.D.

Director of Pediatric Neurology
Departments of Neurology and Pediatrics
The Presbyterian Hospital in the City of New York
Sidney Carter Professor of Neurology
Professor of Pediatrics
Departments of Neurology and Pediatrics
College of Physicians and Surgeons
Columbia University
New York, New York

William B. Dobyns, M.D.

Associate Professor of Neurology and Pediatrics
Division of Pediatric Neurology
University of Minnesota Medical School
Minneapolis, Minnesota

Fritz E. Dreifuss, M.B., F.R.C.P., F.R.A.C.P.

Professor of Neurology
University of Virginia Health Sciences Center
Charlottesville, Virginia

Patricia K. Duffner, M.D.

Professor of Neurology and Pediatrics
State University of New York at Buffalo
Associate Chief
Division of Child Neurology
Children's Hospital of Buffalo
Buffalo, New York

Paul R. Dyken, M.D.

Professor and Chairman of Neurology
University of South Alabama
College of Medicine
Mobile, Alabama

Owen B. Evans, M.D.

Professor and Chairman
Department of Pediatrics
University at Mississippi Medical Center
Jackson, Mississippi

Lydia Eviatar, M.D.

Associate Professor of Pediatrics and Neurology
A. Einstein College of Medicine
Bronx, New York
Chief, Pediatric Neurology
Schneider Children's Hospital of Long Island Jewish Medical Center
New Hyde Park, New York

Gerald M. Fenichel, M.D.

Professor of Neurology and Pediatrics
Chairman, Department of Neurology
Vanderbilt University Medical Center
Nashville, Tennessee

Marvin A. Fishman, M.D.

Professor of Pediatrics and Neurology
Baylor College of Medicine
Chief, Neurology Service
Texas Children's Hospital
Houston, Texas

Bhuwan P. Garg, M.D.

Associate Professor of Neurology
Department of Neurology
Indiana University School of Medicine
Director, Pediatric Neurology
James Whitcomb Riley Hospital for Children
Indianapolis, Indiana

Herbert E. Gilmore, M.D.

Assistant Professor of Pediatrics
Tufts University School of Medicine
Division of Pediatric Neurology
Children's Hospital
Baystate Medical Center
Springfield, Massachusetts

Gerald S. Golden, M.D.

Adjunct Professor of Neurology
University of Pennsylvania
Vice President
Division of Medical School Liaison
Medical Board of Medical Examiners
Philadelphia, Pennsylvania

Alan Hill, M.D., Ph.D.

Professor and Head
Department of Neurology
Department of Pediatrics
University of British Columbia
Head, Division of Neurology
British Columbia's Children's Hospital
Vancouver, British Columbia, Canada

Deborah G. Hirtz, M.D.

Developmental Neurology Branch
National Institute of Neurological Disorders and Stroke
National Institutes of Health
Bethesda, Maryland

Ronald I. Jacobson, M.D.

Assistant Clinical Professor of Pediatrics
New York Medical College
Attending Pediatric Neurology
Westchester County Medical Center
Valhalla, New York

Robert L. Kriel, M.D.

Professor
Departments of Neurology, Pediatrics, and Pharmacy Practice
School of Medicine and College of Pharmacy
University of Minnesota
Pediatric Neurologist
Hennepin County Medical Center
Minneapolis, Minnesota
Pediatric Neurologist
Gillette Children's Hospital
St. Paul, Minnesota

Bernard G. Lemieux, M.D., F.A.A.P., D.A.B.P., F.R.C.P.(C), S.C.P.Q.

Professor of Neurology, Pediatrics, and Genetics
Department of Pediatrics
Centre Hospitalier Universitaire de Sherbrooke
Child Neurologist
Centre Hospitalier Universitaire de Sherbrooke
Sherbrooke, Quebec, Canada

Lawrence A. Lockman, M.D.

Associate Professor of Neurology and Pediatrics
Division of Pediatric Neurology
University of Minnesota Medical School
Minneapolis, Minnesota

Keith Meloff, M.D., F.R.C.P.(C)

Consultant Neurologist
Hugh MacMillan Rehabilitation Center
Visiting Lecturer
Department of Rehabilitation Medicine
University of Toronto
Toronto, Ontario, Canada
Consultant Neurologist
Timmins and District Hospital
Timmins, Ontario, Canada
Associate Medical Director
CIBA, Canada
Mississauga, Ontario, Canada

Hugo Moser, M.D.

Professor of Pediatrics and Neurology
Kennedy Krieger Institute
Johns Hopkins University School of Medicine
Director, Center for Research on Mental Retardation and Related Aspects of
  Human Development
Baltimore, Maryland

Sakkubai Naidu, M.D.

Associate Professor of Neurology and Pediatrics
Johns Hopkins University School of Medicine
Director, Neurogenetics Unit
Kennedy Krieger Institute
Baltimore, Maryland

Karin B. Nelson, M.D.

Acting Chief, Neuroepidemiology Branch
National Institute of Neurological Disorders and Stroke
National Institutes of Health
Bethesda, Maryland

Michael J. Painter, M.D.

Professor of Neurology and Pediatrics
University of Pittsburgh School of Medicine
Chief, Division of Child Neurology
Children's Hospital of Pittsburgh
Pittsburgh, Pennsylvania

Arthur L. Prensky, M.D.

Allen P. and Josephine B. Green Professor of Pediatric Neurology
Washington University School of Medicine
Pediatrician and Neurologist
St. Louis Children's Hospital
St. Louis, Missouri

Isabelle Rapin, M.D.

Professor, Neurology and Pediatrics
Albert Einstein College of Medicine
Bronx, New York

N. Paul Rosman, M.D.

Professor of Pediatrics and Neurology
Tufts University School of Medicine
Chief, Division of Pediatric Neurology
Floating Hospital for Children
Director, Center for Children with Special Needs
New England Medical Center
Boston, Massachusetts

A. David Rothner, M.D.

Chief, Section of Pediatric Neurology
The Cleveland Clinic
Cleveland, Ohio

Barry S. Russman, M.D.

Professor of Pediatrics and Neurology
University of Connecticut Medical School
Chief, Pediatric Neurology
Newington Children's Hospital
Newington, Connecticut

Robert S. Rust, M.A., M.D.

Chief, Section of Child Neurology
Departments of Neurology and Pediatrics
University of Wisconsin Hospital and Clinics
Madison, Wisconsin

Mark S. Scher, M.D.

Associate Professor of Pediatrics, Neurology, and Psychiatry
University of Pittsburgh, School of Medicine
Director, Developmental Neurophysiology Laboratory
Magee-Womens Hospital
Pittsburgh, Pennsylvania

Sanford Schneider, M.D.

Professor, Pediatrics and Neurology
Loma Linda University School of Medicine
Head, Division of Child Neurology
Loma Linda University Medical Center
Loma Linda, California

Bennett A. Shaywitz, M.D.

Chief, Pediatric Neurology
Professor of Pediatrics, Neurology, and Child Study Center
Yale University School of Medicine
New Haven, Connecticut

Sally E. Shaywitz, M.D.

Professor of Pediatrics and Child Study Center
Department of Pediatrics
Yale University School of Medicine
New Haven, Connecticut

Phyllis K. Sher, M.D.

Associate Professor of Neurology and Pediatrics
University of Minnesota Medical School
Division of Pediatric Neurology
Minneapolis, Minnesota

Stephen A. Smith, M.D.

Assistant Professor of Neurology and Pediatrics
Division of Pediatric Neurology
Hennepin County Medical Center
University of Minnesota Medical School
Minneapolis, Minnesota

Russell D. Snyder, M.D.

Professor of Neurology and Pediatrics
University of New Mexico Medical Center
University of New Mexico Hospital
Albuquerque, New Mexico

Kenneth F. Swaiman

Preface to the first edition

It is concurrently tiring, humiliating, and intellectually revitalizing to compile a book containing the essence of the information that embraces one's life work and professional preoccupation. For me, there is a certain moth-to-the-flame phenomenon that cannot be resisted; therefore this new book has been produced.

Pediatric neurology has come of age since my initial interest and subsequent immersion in the field. Concentrated attention to the details of brain development and function has brought much progress and understanding. Studies of disease processes by dedicated and intelligent individuals accompanied by a cascade of new technology (e.g., neuroimaging techniques, positron emission tomography, DNA probes, synthesis of gene products, sophisticated lipid chemistry) has propelled the field forward. The simultaneous increase of knowledge and capability of pediatric neurologists and others who diagnose and treat children with nervous system dysfunction has been extremely gratifying.

Although once within the realm of honest delusion of a seemingly sane (but unrealistic) devotee of the field, it is no longer possible to believe that a single individual can fathom, much less explore, the enumerable rivulets that coalesce to form the river of knowledge that currently is pediatric neurology. Streams of information in certain areas sometimes peacefully meander for years; suddenly, when knowledge of previously obscure areas is advanced and the newly gained information becomes central to understanding basic pathophysiologic entities, a once small stream gains momentum and abruptly flows with torrential force.

This text is an attempt to gather the most important aspects of current pediatric neurology and display them in a comprehensible manner. The task, although consuming great energies and concentration, cannot be accomplished completely because new conditions are described daily.

The advancement of the field necessitated that preparation of this text keep pace with current knowledge and present new and valuable techniques. My colleagues and I have made every effort to discharge this responsibility. Because of continuous scientific progress, controversies are extant in some areas for varying periods; wherever possible, these areas of conflict are indicated.

This book is divided into four unequal parts. Part I contains a discussion of the historic and clinical examination. Part II contains information concerning laboratory examination. Chapters relating to the symptom complexes that often reflect the chief complaints of neurologically impaired children compose Part III. Part IV provides detailed discussion of various neurologic diseases that afflict children.

Although every precaution has been taken to avoid error, bias, and prejudice, inevitably some of these demons have become embedded in the text. The editor assumes full responsibility for these indiscretions.

It is my fervent hope that the reader will find this book informative and stimulating and that the contents will provide an introduction to the understanding of many of the conditions that remain mysterious and poorly explained.

Kenneth F. Swaiman, M.D.
Autumn, 1988

Preface to the second edition

There is exhilaration at considering old information in the context of new ideas, advances, and revelations. Although time passes quickly, the whirlwind of scientific advances accelerates at an even more astonishing rate. Pediatric neurology continues to be in the forefront of pediatric focus because of the many inherited conditions manifested by our patients. In some respects, we are at an awkward juncture. Genetic mapping and DNA studies are providing us with clues to many conditions and explanations of phenotypic variation. Nevertheless we do not know the precise nature of many gene products. The knowledge of the means of introduction into affected humans of absent proteins or their nucleic acid precursors has not yet reached a significant stage of implementation.

Certain conditions that were not known or only vaguely appreciated have become mainstays of pediatric neurologic evaluation. Mitochondrial encephalomyopathies, peroxisomal diseases, and migrational disorders have assumed an important niche in our consideration of unexplained pediatric neurologic disease. Higher cortical function is rapidly assuming its rightful scientific place in child neurology.

The vast body of knowledge that constitutes child neurology is reflected in the subsequent narrative. The anatomic, physiologic, and biochemical underpinnings of the discipline in conjunction with the maturing developmental base continue to provide a never ending challenge.

It is a difficult task to meld the knowledge and writing styles of the many contributors to this text. Every attempt has been made to provide reasonable uniformity among the chapters. Great effort has been made to produce a book that accurately reflects the current state of the field, but some areas are controversial or in rapid stages of evolution and changing concepts and facts are inevitable. We have attempted to prevent premature judgments and to elaborate on these particulars.

As in the previous edition, this work is divided into four distinct parts. Part I includes discussion of the historic and clinical examination. Part II details information concerning laboratory examination. Symptoms and signs that often comprise chief complaints of neurologically involved children compose Part III. Part IV provides thorough discussion of various neurologic conditions that afflict children.

No text of this magnitude is without blemish. The editor assumes responsibility for all errors, biases, and prejudices that have found their way into these pages.

I earnestly desire that you will find these volumes educational, stimulating, and occasionally provocative.

Kenneth F. Swaiman, M.D.
Autumn, 1993

Acknowledgments

I have a feeling of accomplishment mixed with relief when publication day nears. Both general and personal words of appreciation are in order. I wish to extend my ongoing appreciation to the Chivas Brothers of Aberdeen, Scotland who have provided precious moments of tranquil evening contemplation, seemingly inspired perception, and determination to begin and continue during times of certified frenzy and frustration.

The book reflects the expertise, dedication, and writing ability of the many contributors who share their knowledge with the reader and me in these volumes.

Without doubt the prolonged task of writing and editing this book could not have been accomplished without the industry and understanding of others. I am indebted to them.

Julie Wildgen was of inestimable help in the long editing process of the many pages of galleys. Martin Finch once again has produced new illustrations of precision that provide instruction while displaying his obvious artistic talent. Cathy Muchow provided the managerial skills to track and manage flow of manuscripts, galleys, and page proofs and the avalanche of phone calls attendant to compilation of this work.

The staff at Mosby has been encouraging, patient, and skillful; it is fitting that I thank Elaine Steinborn, Carolyn Malik, and Diana Laulainen for their proficiencies and forbearance during this long process of publication.

A small group of individuals has borne the personal consequences of my prolonged efforts. I wish to thank my wife Phyllis for her continuing support and patience, as well as for her talented assistance in developing the cover design. I am grateful to my colleagues who have been understanding during my periods of inelastic fixation.

Finally, I would like to acknowledge the many readers of the first edition who have provided valuable suggestions in addition to numerous compliments that help make this project worthwhile.

Kenneth F. Swaiman, M.D.

Contents

Part One

Clinical Evaluation

may provide helpful information. At times, unfortunately, adults who participate in the session may not be objective or capable of accuracy. Conversely, the experienced clinician often finds it unwise to disregard caretakers' comments, even though the comments are somewhat unusual or incompatible with the clinician's diagnostic bent.

The features associated with the chief complaint compose the history of the present illness. The questioning should provide an incisive interaction between parents (or patient) and clinician and should be directed at formulating the differential diagnosis. This portion of the communication process requires skill and perseverance. An all-inclusive neurologic history is impossible; that which makes the history meaningful and complete may be the seemingly trivial information that is not readily recalled or divulged. The accomplished clinician must uncover this information by directed and specific inquiry.

The chief complaint should trigger the process of differential diagnosis in the examiner's thinking, which begins as a listing of the disease conditions that could cause the chief complaint at the child's age. The following three specific questions should be answered, if possible, in the history of the present illness: (1) is the process acute or insidious; (2) is it focal or generalized; and (3) is it progressive or static?

The order in which disease findings develop and the precise time of onset of symptoms and signs may be critical factors in the process of accurate diagnosis. The presence of repeated episodes or associated phenomena should be determined. Detailed questions should be asked of the caretakers and child to elucidate the facts.

Sequelae of traumatic events develop over a period of minutes to a day (Figure 1-1). Although the clinical manifestations of cerebrovascular events normally develop over minutes to hours, the underlying process may be longstanding; therefore acute onset of vascular symptoms may be the result of a subacute or chronic process. Infectious processes, electrolyte imbalances, and toxic processes (endogenous or exogenous) usually reach their zenith within a day to several days. Degenerative diseases, inborn metabolic conditions, and neoplastic conditions usually progress insidiously over weeks or months.

Based on the chronologic aspects of the history the clinician should ask questions related to the most likely pathologic processes. Thus, for example, when the history suggests a subacute process, the clinician should probe for characteristics associated with an infectious process (e.g., exposure to a known infectious source, recent infection, vomiting, diarrhea, or fever) or with specific toxins (e.g., over-the-counter medications, prescribed medications, insecticides, or other toxins found around the home).

Evaluation of whether a condition is focal or generalized is embedded in the neurologic diagnostic process. A focal neurologic lesion is not necessarily one that causes focal manifestations but is one that can be related to dysfunction in a circumscribed neuroanatomic location. For example, a focal lesion in the brainstem may cause ipsilateral cranial nerve difficulty and contralateral corticospinal tract involvement. If the difficulties are not focal within this definition, they usually result from a generalized process or from several lesions (multifocal). Neoplastic and vascular diseases frequently result in focal processes; occasionally trauma results in such abnormalities. Generalized or multifocal conditions are usually associated with degenerative, congenital, metabolic, or toxic abnormalities.

The clinician must always attempt to determine whether the condition is progressive or static. Documentation of increasing loss of normal function or an increase in any symptoms, including pain, is essential.

Questions should be crafted to obtain evidence that the child is no longer capable of acts that were previously performed. This information is essential to the diagnosis of progressive disease, which is usually preceded by a period of normal development. Occasionally, previous formal neurologic and psychometric evaluations may be available. Documentation may be forthcoming from family photographs, family video tapes, or baby books.

Conditions that are static or improve spontaneously are usually the result of traumatic episodes, congenital abnormalities, acute toxicity, or resolving infection.

A detailed developmental history is often the best means of substantiating whether a condition is progressive or static. The history should include a log of motor milestones and should contain specific information regarding motor, language, and adaptive-social behavior. The Denver Developmental Screening Test [Frankenburg and Dodds, 1967], the revised form [Frankenburg et al., 1981], the Denver II screening test (Figure 1-2) [Frankenburg et al., 1992], or other developmental surveys allow a more precise approach to the determination of whether gains or losses of skills have occurred and aid in the decision as to whether a process is progressive or static.

The Denver Developmental Screening Test (DDST) has undergone a major revision and restandardization and is now available as the Denver II. The DDST II will undoubtedly replace the older versions of the DDST.

Standardization testing for the Denver II included evaluating each item to determine if significant differences existed between subpopulations. These subpopulations included gender, ethnic group (black, white, or Hispanic), maternal education (less than 12 grades completed or more than 12 grades completed), and place of residence (rural, semirural, or urban).

The Denver II differs from the DDST in the selected

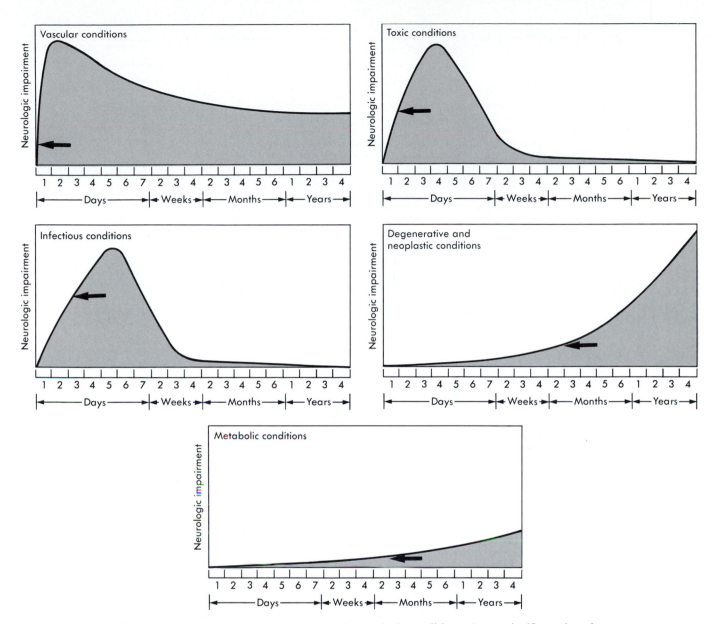

Figure 1-1 Patterns of onset and course of neurologic conditions. Arrow signifies point of clinical recognition. (Modified from Baker AB. Outline of clinical neurology. Dubuque, Iowa: William C. Brown, 1958.)

items, test form, and interpretation. The total number of items has been increased from 105 to 125, most of the new items are in the language section; items that were judged as difficult to administer or interpret have been modified or eliminated. The technical manual should be consulted if a delay is identified because it may be caused by sociocultural differences.

The test form for the Denver II resembles the DDST in the vertical placement of items. Key Denver items have been eliminated so that the age scale coincides with the American Academy of Pediatrics' suggested schedule for health maintenance exams to facilitate the Denver II's use during these visits. The norms for the

distribution bars have been in accordance with the new standardization data. A valuable addition to the front of the form is a checklist for documentation of the child's behavior during testing.

Scoring and interpretation changes have also been made. If a child is able to perform an item to the right of the age line, performance is designated an *advance*. If the child passes or fails an item between the 25th and 75th lines, performance is designated an *OK*. If the child fails an item from the 75th to the 90th lines, performance is designated as a *caution*. If the child is unable to pass an item to the left of the age line, performance is designated as a *delay*. Sufficient items should be admin-

Text continued on p. 8.

DIRECTIONS

DATE

NAME

BIRTHDATE

HOSP. NO.

1. Try to get child to smile by smiling, talking or waving to him. Do not touch him.
2. When child is playing with toy, pull it away from him. Pass if he resists.
3. Child does not have to be able to tie shoes or button in the back.
4. Move yarn slowly in an arc from one side to the other, about 6" above child's face. Pass if eyes follow 90° to midline. (Past midline; 180°)
5. Pass if child grasps rattle when it is touched to the backs or tips of fingers.
6. Pass if child continues to look where yarn disappeared or tries to see where it went. Yarn should be dropped quickly from sight from tester's hand without arm movement.
7. Pass if child picks up raisin with any part of thumb and a finger.
8. Pass if child picks up raisin with the ends of thumb and index finger using an over hand approach.

9. Pass any enclosed form. Fail continuous round motions.

10. Which line is longer? (Not bigger.) Turn paper upside down and repeat. (3/3 or 5/6)

11. Pass any crossing lines.

12. Have child copy first. If failed, demonstrate

When giving items 9, 11 and 12, do not name the forms. Do not demonstrate 9 and 11.

13. When scoring, each pair (2 arms, 2 legs, etc.) counts as one part.
14. Point to picture and have child name it. (No credit is given for sounds only.)

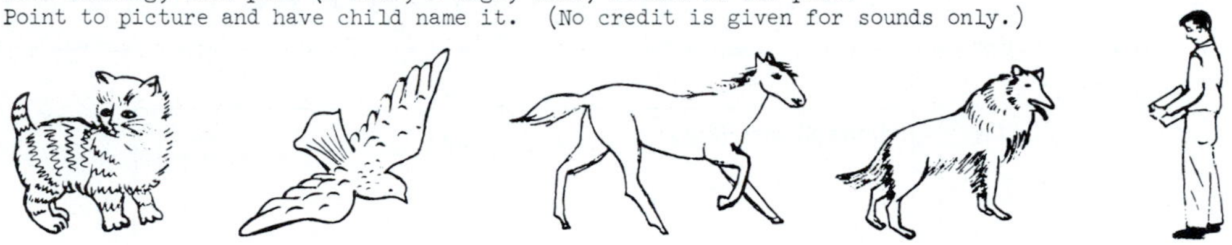

15. Tell child to: Give block to Mommie; put block on table; put block on floor. Pass 2 of 3. (Do not help child by pointing, moving head or eyes.)
16. Ask child: What do you do when you are cold? ..hungry? ..tired? Pass 2 of 3.
17. Tell child to: Put block on table; under table; in front of chair, behind chair. Pass 3 of 4. (Do not help child by pointing, moving head or eyes.)
18. Ask child: If fire is hot, ice is ?; Mother is a woman, Dad is a ?; a horse is big, a mouse is ?. Pass 2 of 3.
19. Ask child: What is a ball? ..lake? ..desk? ..house? ..banana? ..curtain? ..ceiling? ..hedge? ..pavement? Pass if defined in terms of use, shape, what it is made of or general category (such as banana is fruit, not just yellow). Pass 6 of 9.
20. Ask child: What is a spoon made of? ..a shoe made of? ..a door made of? (No other objects may be substituted.) Pass 3 of 3.
21. When placed on stomach, child lifts chest off table with support of forearms and/or hands.
22. When child is on back, grasp his hands and pull him to sitting. Pass if head does not hang back.
23. Child may use wall or rail only, not person. May not crawl.
24. Child must throw ball overhand 3 feet to within arm's reach of tester.
25. Child must perform standing broad jump over width of test sheet. (8-1/2 inches)
26. Tell child to walk forward, ⌒⌒⌒⌒→ heel within 1 inch of toe. Tester may demonstrate. Child must walk 4 consecutive steps, 2 out of 3 trials.
27. Bounce ball to child who should stand 3 feet away from tester. Child must catch ball with hands, not arms, 2 out of 3 trials.
28. Tell child to walk backward, ←⌒⌒⌒⌒ toe within 1 inch of heel. Tester may demonstrate. Child must walk 4 consecutive steps, 2 out of 3 trials.

DATE AND BEHAVIORAL OBSERVATIONS (how child feels at time of test, relation to tester, attention span, verbal behavior, self-confidence, etc,):

Figure 1-2 Denver Developmental Screening Test (Denver II) directions. (From Frankenburg WK, et al. Pediatrics 1992; 89:91.)

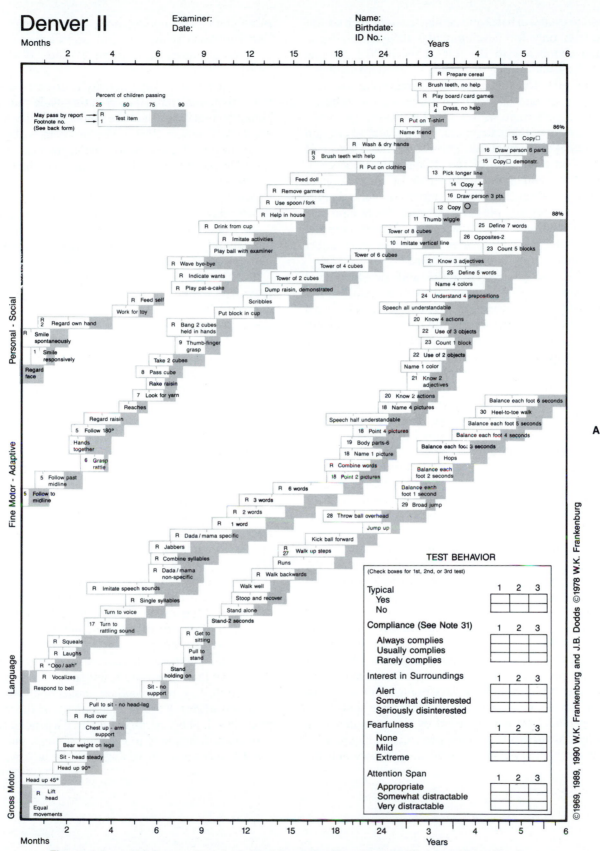

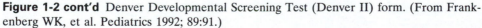

Figure 1-2 cont'd Denver Developmental Screening Test (Denver II) form. (From Frankenberg WK, et al. Pediatrics 1992; 89:91.)

istered to establish basal and ceiling levels in each sector. To screen only for developmental delays, only items located completely to the left of the child's age line should be administered. Retesting is recommended in 1 to 3 months for performance scored as a caution. Retesting for one or more delays, as well as refusals, should be performed within 1 to 2 weeks.

It is essential that examiners, parents/caretakers, and educational personnel recognize that the Denver II provides an evaluation of the child's current developmental level and is not a predictor of future rate of development or eventual maximum attainment. Abnormalities in more complex and abstract functioning may not be recognizable until a later age. Alteration in the child's biologic or environmental status may affect developmental rate and achievement.

The review of past medical and developmental histories is an essential component of a good history-taking session. Information should be sought from records and from questioning the mother about health problems and diseases that occurred during pregnancy and about medications, including over-the-counter preparations, that the mother received. It is important to record both the expected date of delivery and the actual date of delivery. Review of birth records and hospital records, including those of the mother, may reveal information concerning difficulties with pregnancy and problems in the perinatal period. It is important to determine the status of the newborn infant. Information concerning Apgar scores, depression of activity, neonatal seizures, and hypotonia, as well as information about whether tracheal intubation and ventilatory support was needed should be sought.

The clinician should ask specific questions regarding the age of attainment of developmental landmarks and should make every attempt to discern whether the child is delayed in many areas of development or has developed normally in some areas but not in others.

It should be remembered that children who have normal motor development but also have hearing impairment may have delayed speech. On the other hand, the presence of neuromuscular disease may cause obvious retardation of motor development but may allow normal development of social and language skills.

A specific form may be used by the examiner as a guideline to the history-taking procedure (Figure 1-3). There are many systems for recording history and the subsequent examination; none is exceedingly popular. The problem-oriented–record approach continues to be used in many institutions [Weed, 1970; Walker, 1976].

The question of hyperactivity is often at the core of the caretakers' complaint. A rating scale may be completed by teachers to aid the clinician in diagnosis (Figure 1-4) [Connors, 1969]. The problem is discussed in detail in Chapter 60. School behavior can also be assessed by parents/caretakers, as shown in the box on pgs. 14 and 15.

Many children are involved in some planned day activity, day care, or school program after the age of 2 or 3 years. A questionnaire, as in Figure 1-5, can be devised that will allow supervisory personnel to record intellectual, motor, and emotional characteristics.

It is essential that an adequate family history be recorded. Ages of siblings (including those who have died and those aborted), parents, grandparents, uncles, and aunts should be available. It is particularly helpful to gain details of the health history of dead siblings and relatives because familial conditions that might otherwise go undiscovered are often revealed.

Questions concerning neurologic diseases initially should be specific; then more generalized questions should be asked because parents may not understand the more specific approach. The presence of epilepsy, cerebral palsy, deafness, mental retardation, movement disorders, blindness, ataxia, weakness, and/or progressive intellectual and motor deterioration must be determined. Less specific names, such as fainting spells, nervous breakdowns, strokes, and palsies, may strike a responsive cord. It is imperative that the clinician ask if any family members suffer from the same problems that afflict the patient.

It should be remembered that autosomal-dominant traits may be present in successive generations, although the degree of expressivity may vary. Autosomal-recessive traits will often not manifest in successive generations but may be present in siblings. Consanguinity must be considered when autosomal recessive disease is part of the differential diagnosis. X-linked recessive conditions are manifest in male siblings, male first cousins, and maternal uncles. Careful questioning of the mother, if possible, is highly desirable. Finally, if a genetic condition is suspected, it is wise to examine siblings, parents, and other family members to augment the history.

Text continued on p. 17.

GENERAL HISTORY FORM

PREGNANCY

Gestation data

Birth date _____

Expected date _____

Birth weight _____

Birth occipito-
frontal circumference
(from old records) _____

Medication taken by mother (check each one taken)

Vitamins _____

Iron _____

Calcium _____

Hormones _____

Weight reduction
medication _____

Diuretics _____

Contraceptives _____

Sedatives, tranquilizers _____

Antiepileptics _____

Other _____

Illnesses (record month of pregnancy in which illness occurred)

Colds, flu, etc. _____

Kidney, bladder infection _____

Rubella (German measles) _____

Rashes _____

Other infectious
diseases _____

Exposures to
infectious diseases _____

Diabetes _____

Kidney disease _____

Surgery _____

Radiographs and/or scans _____

Other (explain) _____

_____

Labor and delivery

Breech or unusual
presentation _____

Forceps use _____

Delay in respira-
tion or cry (Apgar
scores if available) _____

Was oxygen adminis-
tration necessary? _____

Type of anesthesia
employed for mother _____

_____

Newborn period

Jaundice _____

Cyanosis _____

Infection _____

Seizures _____

Anemia _____

Other _____

_____

Medications administered _____

_____

Home from hospital in _____ days

DEVELOPMENT (indicate month skill attained)

Smiled _____

Laughed out loud _____

First words _____

Put words together
(e.g., "Daddy, bye-bye") _____

Complete sentences _____

Rolled over _____

Sat without support _____

Crawled _____

Pulled to standing _____

Walked around
furniture _____

Walked unassisted _____

Rode tricycle _____

ILLNESSES

Hospitalizations

Age: _____   Reason: _____

_____

Age: _____   Reason: _____

_____

Age: _____   Reason: _____

_____

Operations

Age: _____   Reason: _____

_____

Age: _____   Reason: _____

_____

Injuries

Age: _____   Reason: _____

_____

Age: _____   Reason: _____

Figure 1-3 General history form that can be used for obtaining medical history, developmental history, and family history of children with neurologic problems. (Courtesy Division of Pediatric Neurology, University of Minnesota Medical School.)

Continued.

Teacher Questionnaire—School Behavioral Assessment

Pupil's name _____ **Date** _____

Teacher: Please place a checkmark in the appropriate column for each item. Choose the degree of activity that best describes the child's behavior.

Observation	Degree of activity			
	Not at all	**Rarely**	**Fairly often**	**Very often**
Classroom behavior				
Constantly fidgets				
Hums and makes other odd noises				
Demands must be met immediately— easily frustrated				
Coordination poor				
Restless or overactive				
Excitable, impulsive				
Inattentive, easily distracted				
Fails to finish things started—short attention span				
Overly sensitive				
Overly serious or sad				
Daydreams				
Sullen or sulky				
Cries often and easily				
Disturbs other children				
Quarrelsome				
Mood changes quickly and drastically				
Obnoxious behavior				
Destructive				
Steals				
Lies				
Temper outbursts, explosive and unpredictable behavior				
Childish and immature				
Easily frustrated in efforts				
Difficulty in learning				

Figure 1-4 Teacher questionnaire for behavioral assessment. Modified from Connors CK. Am J Psychiatr 1967; 126:884.

Teacher Questionnaire—School Behavioral Assessment—cont'd

Pupil's name _____ **Date** _____

Teacher: Please place a checkmark in the appropriate column for each item. Choose the degree of activity that best describes the child's behavior.

	Degree of activity			
Observation	**Not at all**	**Rarely**	**Fairly often**	**Very often**
Group participation				
Isolates self from other children				
Seems unaccepted by group				
Seems easily led				
No sense of fair play				
Seems to lack leadership				
Does not get along with opposite sex				
Does not get along with same sex				
Teases other children or interferes with their activities				
Denies mistakes and blames others				
Attitude toward authority				
Submissive				
Defiant				
Impudent				
Shy				
Fearful				
Excessive demands for teacher's attention				
Stubborn				
Overly anxious to please				
Uncooperative				
Attendance problem				

Figure 1-4 cont'd For legend see opposite page.

Parents/Caretaker Questionnaire — School Behavioral Assessment

Pupil's name _____ Date _____

School Performance

Have teachers expressed concern about your child's learning?   Yes ___ No ___

If yes, please list the grade at which concern was expressed and the subject(s) of concern.

Grade   **Subject(s)**

Have teachers expressed concern about your child's behavior?   Yes ___ No ___

If yes, please list the grade at which concern was expressed and the behavior of concern.

Grade   **Behavior(s)**

Have teachers expressed concern about your child's relationships with other children?   Yes ___ No ___

If yes, please list the grade at which concern was expressed and the nature of the concern.

Grade   **Problem**

Has your child repeated any grades?   Yes ___ No ___

If yes, what grade(s) was repeated and what reason(s) were given?

Has your child received special education services?   Yes ___ No ___

If yes, please list the grade and type of service provided. Services in schools include: Chapter 1 or Title 1 support; Learning Disabilities; Emotional Behavioral Disorder; Physical and Other Health Impairment; Mildly Mentally Handicapped; Trainable Mentally Handicapped; Adaptive Physical Education; Speech and Language; Occupational Therapy; and Physical Therapy.

Grade   **Service**

Courtesy Division of Pediatric Neurology, University of Minnesota Medical School.

Continued.

Parents/Caretaker Questionnaire — School Behavioral Assessment — cont'd

Current Behavior

Please indicate how often your child engages in the following behaviors:

	Never or Seldom	Occasionally	Very often or always
Expresses fears	_____	_____	_____
Daydreams	_____	_____	_____
Loses belongings	_____	_____	_____
Has difficulty finishing what he/she begins	_____	_____	_____
Fails to follow directions	_____	_____	_____
Forgets	_____	_____	_____
Has mood swings	_____	_____	_____
Has difficulty sitting still	_____	_____	_____
Lies	_____	_____	_____
Is fascinated with fire	_____	_____	_____
Appears clumsy	_____	_____	_____
Stutters	_____	_____	_____
Is verbally aggressive	_____	_____	_____
Is physically aggressive	_____	_____	_____
Has difficulty falling asleep	_____	_____	_____
Has nightmares or sleepwalking	_____	_____	_____
Has difficulty making or keeping friends	_____	_____	_____
Seems unaffected by discipline	_____	_____	_____

SCHOOL REPORT

This report is confidential and for our use only

I.   Identifying information

Name _____ Birthdate _____ Grade _____

Address _____

School _____ School phone _____

School address _____

Teacher _____ Principal _____

Retention _____

II. Child's school history (please attach a transcript of grades, results of any achievement tests, including results of IQ tests, and previous psychologic and/or speech evaluations)

III. Special characteristics (check all that apply under each category)

Reading level	Above grade ☐	Average ☐	Slightly below ☐	Severe difficulty ☐
Motivation	Intense ☐	Average ☐	Indifferent ☐	Resistant ☐
Behavior	Aggressive ☐	Average ☐	Shy ☐	Withdrawn ☐
Attention	Absorbed ☐	Attentive ☐	Needs urging ☐	Easily distracted ☐
Relationship to authority figures	Too deferent ☐	Coopera-tive ☐	Sometimes rebels ☐	Defiant ☐
Relationship with peers	Well liked by all ☐	Normal ☐	One or two friends ☐	Isolated ☐
Achievement	"Over-achiever" ☐	Up to ability ☐	Sporadic ☐	Severe problems ☐
Attendance	Never misses ☐	Normal absence ☐	Frequent absence ☐	Extended absence ☐
Eyesight		Normal ☐	Question-able ☐	Visual defect ☐
Hearing		Normal ☐	Question-able ☐	Hearing loss ☐
Motor coordination	Excellent ☐	Average for age ☐	Poor ☐	Handicapped (describe) ☐
Speech	No problem ☐		Minor difficulty ☐	Severe difficulty ☐

Figure 1-5 School information form that can be used to obtain child's school history from school, day care center, or day activity center. (Courtesy Division of Pediatric Neurology, University of Minnesota Medical School.)

SCHOOL REPORT—cont'd

Other health problems (specify) _____
_____

Special help given	Remedial reading	Speech therapy	Special education	Tutoring	Other
	☐	☐	☐	☐	☐

IV. Briefly give your impression of the child's behavior in school: any examples or anecdotes would be appreciated _____
_____
_____
_____

V. Attitude towards school _____

Attitude towards peers _____

Attitude towards self _____

Attitude towards teacher _____

VI. Are there any problems that you think need special attention? Yes ☐ No ☐ (please describe in detail) _____
_____
_____

VII. What do you like best about this child? _____

What do his or her classmates like best? _____

VIII. What do you think can be done to help the child overcome his or her current difficulties? What resources are available in the school, school district, or community? _____
_____

IX. What is your impression of the home environment of the child (stimulating, average, detrimental)? Describe any specific features that you think may be important. _____
_____

X. What is the relationship between school personnel and the child's parents? _____

Signature _____
Title _____
Date _____

Figure 1-5 cont'd For legend see opposite page.

REFERENCES

Baker AB. Outline of clinical neurology. Dubuque, Iowa: William C. Brown, 1958.

Connors CK. A teacher rating scale for use in drug studies with children. Am J Psychiatry 1969; 126:152.

Frankenburg WK, Dodds JB. Denver developmental screening test. J Pediatr 1967; 71:181.

Frankenburg WK, Fandal AW, Sciarillo W, et al. The newly abbreviated and revised Denver Developmental Screening Test. J Pediatr 1981; 99:995.

Frankenburg WK, Dodds JB, Archer P, et al. The Denver II: a major revision and restandardization of the Denver developmental screening test. Pediatrics 1992; 89:91.

Walker HK. The problem-oriented medical system. JAMA 1976; 236:2397.

Weed LL. Medical records, medical education, and patient care. The problem-oriented record as a basic tool. Chicago: Year Book Medical, 1970.

2

Neurologic Examination of the Older Child

Kenneth F. Swaiman

The next four chapters are devoted to the neurologic examination of children. The material is organized on the basis of age for convenience of presentation; however, detailed discussion of the conventional neurologic examination of children is provided in this chapter, including evaluation of the cranial nerves.

Examination of a child older than 2 years of age should be as informal as possible while maintaining a basic flow pattern to permit complete evaluation. The older child has acquired a large repertory of skills since infancy (see box on p. 20). Many neurologic functions of children between the ages of 2 and 4 years are examined in the same manner as those under 2 years of age. As is the case with younger children, patients between 2 and 4 years of age may be most comfortable sitting on the parent's lap. Observation and play techniques are essential means of monitoring intellectual and motor function. The examiner should be equipped with small toys, dolls, and pictures with which to interest the child and provide for more ease of interaction.

After 4 years of age, the components of the neurologic examination are more conventional and routine, and by adolescence the examination is much the same as the adult examination.

OBSERVATION

Much can be learned by observation during the history-taking session. Older children will sit in a chair or perform tasks, such as reading or drawing, with crayons or colored pencils. If the child participates actively in the history-taking procedure, the child's understanding and contribution to the session allow the examiner to make judgments about the child's intellectual skills. Additionally, the child's language skills can be assessed. Problems with stuttering, dysarthria, nasal speech, dysphonia, and problems of articulation will be manifest. This session will also provide an additional opportunity to evaluate facial movements. Head nodding, lip tremors, eye blinking, and staring may be evidence of epilepsy. Movement disorders involving the face, such as chorea or tic, as well as other movement disorders involving the neck, limbs, and trunk, may be noticeable (e.g., athetosis, chorea, dystonia, myoclonus, tics, and spasms).

This portion of the examination also provides an opportunity to assess the child's behavior. Impulsivity, short attention span, and relative dependence may be manifest. The child may be unable to sit or play quietly. Distractibility may be evident in response to minor external stimuli. Parent-child interaction may also be observed during this time. The parent may threaten or use physical force or obsequiously cajole the child. The child's response may be inappropriate.

The following questions must be answered. Does the child respond positively to the parent's interaction? Does the child attempt to manipulate the parent? Is the response transient or persistent? Is the parent's attitude one of caring or hostility?

SCREENING GROSS MOTOR FUNCTION

Beginning sometime between 4 and 6 years of age, most children of normal intelligence will participate in a screening motor examination. The child should stand before the examiner and allow the examiner to demonstrate the desired motor acts. The child should be asked to hop in place on each foot (first one then the other), tandem walk forward and backward, toe walk, and heel walk. The child is asked to rise from a squatting position. The child is then asked to stand with the feet close together, eyes closed, and arms and hands outstretched. This maneuver allows for simultaneous assessment of the Romberg sign and adventitious movements, particularly of the face, arms, and hands. The child is then

---

Emerging Patterns of Behavior from 1 to 5 Years of Age

---

15 Months

Motor:	Walks alone; crawls up stairs
Adaptive:	Makes tower of two cubes; makes a line with crayon; inserts pellet in bottle
Language:	Jargon: follows simple commands; may name a familiar object (ball)
Social:	Indicates some desires or needs by pointing; hugs parents

18 Months

Motor:	Runs stiffly; sits on small chair; walks up stairs with one hand held; explores drawers and waste baskets
Adaptive:	Piles three cubes; imitates scribbling; imitates vertical stroke; dumps pellet from bottle
Language:	10 words (average); names pictures; identifies one or more parts of body
Social:	Feeds self; seeks help when in trouble; may complain when wet or soiled; kisses parents with pucker

24 Months

Motor:	Runs well; walks up and down stairs, one step at a time; opens doors; climbs on furniture
Adaptive:	Tower of six cubes; circular scribbling; imitates horizontal stroke; folds paper once imitatively
Language:	Puts three words together (subject, verb, object)
Social:	Handles spoon well; often tells immediate experiences; helps to undress; listens to stories with pictures

30 Months

Motor:	Jumps
Adaptive:	Tower of eight cubes; makes vertical and horizontal strokes but generally will not join them to make a cross; imitates circular stroke, forming closed figure
Language:	Refers to self by pronoun "I"; knows full name
Social:	Helps put things away; pretends in play

36 Months

Motor:	Goes up stairs alternating feet; rides tricycle; stands momentarily on one foot
Adaptive:	Tower of nine cubes; imitates construction of "bridge" of three cubes; copies a circle; imitates a cross
Language:	Knows age and sex; counts three objects correctly; repeats three numbers or a sentence of six syllables
Social:	Plays simple games (in "parallel" with other children); helps in dressing (unbuttons clothing and puts on shoes); washes hands

48 Months

Motor:	Hops on one foot; throws ball overhand; uses scissors to cut out pictures; climbs well
Adaptive:	Copies bridge from model; imitates construction of "gate" of five cubes; copies cross and square; draws a man with two to four parts besides head; names longer of two lines
Language:	Counts four pennies accurately; tells a story
Social:	Plays with several children with beginning of social interaction and role-playing; goes to toilet alone

60 Months

Motor:	Skips
Adaptive:	Draws triangle from copy; names heavier of two weights
Language:	Names 4 colors; repeats sentences of 10 syllables; counts 10 pennies correctly
Social:	Dresses and undresses; asks questions about meaning of words; domestic role-playing

---

Modified from Behrman RE, et al. Nelson textbook of pediatrics, 14th ed. Philadelphia: WB Saunders, 1992.

asked to perform finger-to-nose movements with the eyes closed and finger-to-finger-to-nose movements with the eyes open.

After this rapid screening procedure the examiner can begin a more detailed and systematic evaluation, bearing in mind any suggested abnormalities evident during the screening process.

DEEP TENDON REFLEXES (MUSCLE STRETCH REFLEXES)

Deep tendon reflexes are readily elicited by conventional means with a reflex hammer while the child is sitting quietly. If the child is crying or overtly resists, the examiner should postpone this portion of the examination. The child may be reassured if the examiner taps the brachioradialis reflex of the caretaker or the examiner. Deep tendon reflexes customarily examined include the biceps, triceps, brachioradialis, patellar, and Achilles reflexes. Each tendon reflex is mediated at a specific spinal segmental level or levels (Table 2-1) [Haymaker and Woodhall, 1962; Hollinshead, 1969]. Hyperactive reflexes or a clonic response to tapping of the reflex results from corticospinal dysfunction. Hyperreflexia may also be signaled by an abnormal "spread" of responses, which includes contraction of muscle groups that usually do not contract when a reflex is being elicited (e.g., crossed thigh adductor or finger flexor reflexes). Although bilateral brisk reflex response may be normal, particularly when only one reflex is involved, unilateral hyperreflexia virtually always signals a pathologic process.

Hyporeflexia may be associated with lower motor unit involvement (e.g., anterior horn cell disease, peripheral neuropathy, or myopathy). However, hyporeflexia may occasionally be found with central depression, poor central control of the gamma-loop (central hypotonia), or involvement of the posterior root (intramedullary or extramedullary). With anterior horn cell involvement (e.g., infantile spinal muscular atrophy or Kugelberg-Welander disease), the patellar reflexes are greatly diminished or absent early because the cells subserving

the proximal muscles of the legs are profoundly involved first. Sensory involvement, particularly peripheral, is often detectable in the presence of neuropathies. Similarly, the distal deep tendon reflexes tend to be involved earlier and to a greater degree. Reflexes may be normal early in the course of certain myopathies, including the muscular dystrophies, and absent later.

Cerebellar disease generally decreases muscle tone and may decrease tendon reflexes because of gamma-loop responsiveness. Enhancement of tendon reflex response when reflexes are seemingly absent can be promoted by having the child squeeze an object such as a block or ball or perform the more traditional Jendrassik maneuver (hooking the fingers together while flexed and then attempting to pull them apart).

OTHER REFLEXES

A plantar (flexor) toe sign response is normal in children. Impairment of corticospinal tract function leads to extensor responses. The Babinski reflex is elicited by firm, steady, slow stroking from posterior to anterior of the lateral margin of the sole with an object such as a key or a smooth, broken tongue blade. The stimulus should not be painful. A positive (plantar) response is a slow, tonic hyperextension of the great toe. This response is the constant and necessary feature of a positive response. The other four toes may also hyperextend or they may slowly spread apart (fanning).

Flicking the patient's nail (second or third finger) downward with the examiner's nail (the Hoffmann reflex) results in flexion of the distal phalanx of the thumb. No response or a muted response may occur in normal children; a brisk or asymmetric response occurs in the presence of corticospinal tract involvement.

Abdominal reflexes are obtained by stroking the abdomen from lateral to medial with strokes beginning just above the umbilicus, lateral to the umbilicus, and just below the umbilicus directed toward the umbilicus. Unilateral absence of the reflex usually is associated with acquired corticospinal dysfunction.

The cremasteric reflex is elicited in males by stroking the inner aspects of the thigh in a caudal-rostral direction and observing the contraction of the scrotum. The reflex is normally present and symmetric. Absence or asymmetry also indicates corticospinal tract involvement.

Developmental reflexes are discussed in Chapter 3.

CEREBELLAR FUNCTION

Head tilt may be associated with tumors of the cerebellum. The tilt is usually ipsilateral to the involved cerebellar hemisphere, but exceptions are common. Herniation of the cerebellar tonsils through the foramen magnum secondary to increased intracranial pressure may cause head tilt; therefore neoplasms that induce

Table 2-1 Muscle stretch (tendon) reflexes

Reflex	Nerve	Segmental level
Biceps	Musculocutaneous	C_5, C_6
Brachioradialis	Radial	C_5, C_6
Gastrocnemius and soleus (ankle jerk)	Tibial	L_5, S_1, S_2
Hamstring	Sciatic	L_4, L_5, S_1, S_2
Jaw	Trigeminal	Pons
Quadriceps (knee jerk)	Femoral	L_2-L_4
Triceps	Radial	C_6, C_8

increased intracranial pressure, other than those of the cerebellum, may cause head tilt. Cerebellar function is also evaluated during testing of station and gait (see Chapter 17). Cerebellar dysfunction is usually associated with hypotonia.

Tremor in cerebellar disease occurs with action (intention). Cerebellar function is assessed in a number of ways. Handpatting (alternating pronation and supination of the hand on the thigh while the other hand remains stationary on the other thigh) is a good method for assessing dysdiadochokinesis. The maneuver is repeated with each hand separately to assess the presence of mirror movements (synkinesis). Other tests that monitor cerebellar integrity include repetitive finger-tapping (thumb to forefinger), foot-tapping, and finger-to-nose, finger-to-finger (examiner's)-to-nose, and heel-to-knee-to-shin stroking. These rapid movements are an index of cerebellar function when limb strength and sensation are intact. Breaks in rhythm and nonfluidity of movement, suggestive of cerebellar dysfunction, are evident during this phase of the examination.

CRANIAL NERVE EXAMINATION

In older children the cranial nerve examination may be performed in an orderly fashion, beginning with the first cranial nerve and testing through the twelfth. Examination of infants and younger children usually requires some modification of the sequence and may need some ingenious improvisation of the procedure, according to the abilities of interaction and willingness on the part of the child. As is the case with all examinations of infants and young children, the less-threatening portions of the examination should be performed first.

Olfactory nerve (cranial nerve I)

Olfactory nerve function is rarely impaired in childhood. Cranial nerve I can be evaluated by having the child smell pleasant aromas (e.g., chocolate, vanilla, or peppermint) through each nostril while the other is manually occluded. Olfactory sensation is intact if the child appreciates a change in odor; precise identification is unnecessary. Anosmia occurs most commonly in children with upper respiratory infections or after head trauma, often occipital. Neoplasms in the inferior frontal lobe or cribriform plate regions can cause anosmia. Unilateral anosmia is more worrisome than bilateral anosmia because of the possibility of a unilateral neoplasm.

Optic nerve (cranial nerve II)

Examination of cranial nerve II, the optic nerve, is one of the critical portions of the neurologic examination because of the long anterior-to-posterior span of the visual pathways within the brain. Formal visual acuity testing is possible with a Snellen chart or a "near card" in older children. Visual acuity and visual field testing should be performed in an appropriately lit room. The visual test objects should be easily visible and without glare. On occasion, when subtle changes are being investigated, it is efficacious to hold the visual field test object against a background of less contrast, thus increasing the difficulty of identification.

Function can be difficult to evaluate in the very young child. Gross vision can be assessed in children younger than 3 or 4 years of age by their ability to recognize familiar items of varying sizes, shapes, and colors. Beyond 4 years of age, the *E* test is useful. The child is taught to recognize the *E* and to discern the direction in which the three "arms" are pointing and point a finger accordingly. Most older children can be taught the essentials of the test in less than a minute. During the acuity evaluation, E's of different sizes, rotated in different directions, are presented to the child.

For each eye, the visual field (range of vision) is assessed by confrontation with an object that is moved from a temporal to nasal direction along radii of the field. A small (3 mm) white or red test object or toy can be used. A modification of the same procedure can be used for double simultaneous testing by moving two test objects or penlights simultaneously from the temporal to the nasal fields then from the superior and inferior portions of the temporal and nasal fields while the child looks directly at the examiner's nose. Finger counting can be used if acuity is grossly distorted. In cases of extreme impairment, perception of a rapidly moving finger can be used.

Visual acuity is rarely affected by papilledema until there is scarring of the nerve head. This lack of acuity change is in marked contrast to the early loss of visual activity that accompanies inflammation of the optic nerve.

The optic disc (optic nerve head) of the older child is sharply defined and often salmon-colored, which differs from the pale gray color of the disc of an infant. In the presence of a deep cup in the optic disc the color may appear pale, but the pallor is localized to the center of the disc. The pallor of optic atrophy is both central and peripheral and is accompanied by a decreased number of arterioles in the disc margins. Most commonly, papilledema is associated with elevation of the optic disc, distended veins, and lack of venous pulsations. Hemorrhages may surround the disc. Before papilledema is obvious, there may be blurring of the nasal disc margins and hyperemia of the nerve head.

Pupils should be observed in light that allows the pupils to remain mildly mydriatic. The diameter, the regularity of contour, and responsivity of the pupils to light should be examined. The upper lid is usually at the margin of the pupil. In Horner syndrome, impairment of the sympathetic pathway results in a miotic pupil, mild ptosis, and defective sweating over the ipsilateral side of the face (see Figure 4-2). Dragging a finger over the child's forehead may aid in the recognition of anhidrosis. The fixed, dilated pupil usually is associated with other signs of oculomotor nerve dysfunction and may signal cerebellar tonsillar herniation.

The presence or absence of the pupillary light reflex differentiates between peripheral and cortical blindness. Lesions of the anterior visual pathway (i.e., retina to lateral geniculate body) result in the interruption of the afferent limb of the pupillary light reflex producing absent or decreased reflex. Anterior visual pathway interruption can cause amblyopia in one eye. In this situation the pupil fails to constrict when stimulated with direct light; however, the consensual pupillary response (the response when the other eye is illuminated) is intact. Varying degrees of visual loss may modify this phenomenon so that the full response to direct stimulation is delayed, but the consensual reflex is brisk. The deficient pupillary reflex is revealed by alternately aiming a light source toward one eye, then the other. In the eye with decreased vision, consensual pupillary constriction is greater than the response to direct light stimulation (Marcus Gunn pupil); furthermore, the pupil of the affected eye may dilate slightly during direct stimulation.

Oculomotor, trochlear, and abducens nerves (cranial nerves III, IV, and VI)

The oculomotor, trochlear, and abducens cranial nerves control extraocular motor movements; obviously, these nerves must operate synchronously or diplopia ensues.

Cranial nerve III innervates the superior, inferior, and medial recti, the inferior oblique, and the eyelid elevator (levator palpebra superioris). Cranial nerves IV and VI innervate the superior oblique muscle and the lateral rectus muscle, respectively. Unfortunately, for purposes of understanding, the function of extraocular muscles depends somewhat on the direction of gaze. In short the lateral and medial recti are abductors and adductors of the globe, respectively. The superior rectus and inferior oblique are elevators, and the inferior rectus and superior oblique are depressors. The oblique muscles act in the vertical plane while an eye is adducted. The recti muscles serve this function when an eye is abducted (Figure 2-1). When directed forward (primary position), the oblique muscles effect torsion around the antero-posterior axis (rotation) of the globes [Cogan, 1966]. The eye position that results from paralysis of each eye muscle is listed in Table 2-2.

In *heterophorias* (also termed *phorias*), both globes are directed normally on near or far objects during fixation; however, one or both deviate when one eye is occluded while the other eye fixes. Forcing fixation of the uncovered eye by alternately covering each eye confirms the diagnosis of heterophorias. This predisposition may be evident when the child is febrile or fatigued. Exophoria is a predisposition to divergence, whereas esophoria is a predisposition to convergence.

Eye deviations detectable during binocular vision are *heterotropias* (also termed *tropias*). Adduction tropias are esotropias; abduction tropias are exotropias. Tropias are most often caused by compromised extraocular muscle innervation. Extraocular palsies can frequently be detected by observation of eye movements. A red glass is placed in front of an eye and a focused, relatively intense white light is aimed at the eyes from various visual fields while the child fixes on the light. A merged, solitary red-white image is perceived when extraocular movements are normal; however, when muscle paresis is present, the child reports a separation of the red and white images when looking in the direction of action of the affected muscle. The farthest peripheral image is the one perceived by the abnormal eye; this eye can be identified by the color of the image. Minimal extraocular muscle palsies may be heralded by delayed eye movement to the appropriate final position. Volitional turning of the head accompanies paresis of the lateral rectus muscle to forstall diplopia; the head is deviated toward the paretic muscle, and the eyes are directed ahead. In superior oblique or superior rectus muscle palsies, tilting of the head toward the shoulder opposite the side of the paretic eye muscle occurs.

Extraocular muscle dysfunction is associated with many conditions that affect the brainstem, nerves, neuromuscular junction, or muscles. Among the diseases are ophthalmoplegic migraine, cavernous sinus thrombosis, brainstem glioma, myasthenia gravis, and congenital myopathy. Cranial nerve VI function may be impaired by increased intracranial pressure (ICP), irrespective of cause. Squint, usually esotropia, often accompanies decreased visual acuity in infants and young children [Smith, 1967].

Ptosis and extraocular muscle paralysis accompany dysfunction of cranial nerve III. Ptosis resulting from oculomotor nerve compromise is usually more pronounced than is the malposition of the lid associated with Horner syndrome. This symptom is of great diagnostic aid because the lid does not significantly elevate when the patient is asked to look up. Complete oculomotor nerve paralysis, although uncommon, causes the eye to position downward and outward. Poor adduction and elevation are also evident (Figure 2-2).

Version eye positioning may accompany either irritative or destructive brainstem lesions and cerebral hemispheral lesions. In destructive brainstem conditions the conjugate eye movement (version) deviation is toward the opposite side. Destructive cerebral hemi-

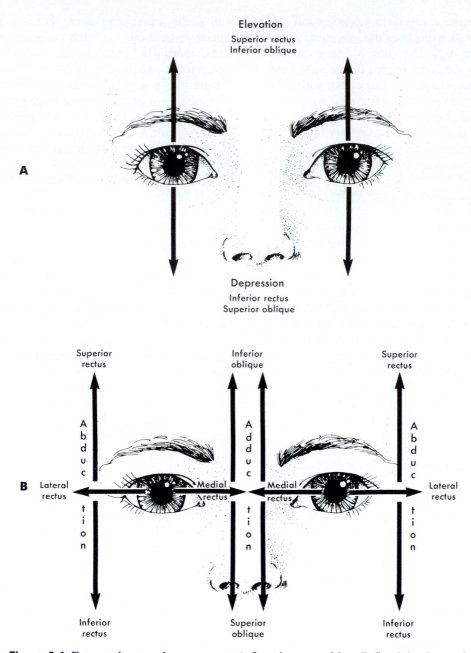

Figure 2-1 Extraocular muscle movement. **A,** In primary position. **B,** In abduction and adduction. (Courtesy Division of Pediatric Neurology, University of Minnesota Medical School.)

spheral lesions will cause the eyes to deviate toward the side of the lesion; conversely, an irritative cerebral hemispheral lesion causes the eyes to turn away from the side of the lesion.

Eye-movement deviations of the binocular disconjugate (nonparallel) type secondary to brainstem dysfunction also occur in children. Vertical gaze paresis results from dysfunction of the tectal area of the midbrain. Patients with a pineal tumor or hydrocephalus are unable to elevate the eyes for upward gaze.

Brainstem lesions, especially those in the midbrain or pons, may disrupt the medial longitudinal fasciculus

Table 2-2 Extraocular muscle paralysis

Paretic muscle	Cranial nerve	Eye deviation
Inferior oblique	III	Down and out
Inferior rectus	III	Up and in
Lateral rectus	VI	Medial
Medial rectus	III	Lateral
Superior oblique	IV	Upward and outward (head tilted)
Superior rectus	III	Down and in

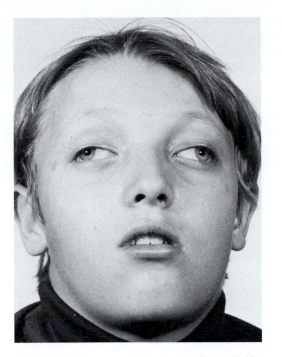

Figure 2-2 Oculomotor nerve paralysis, bilateral. (Courtesy Division of Pediatric Neurology, University of Minnesota Medical School.)

(MLF). The resultant impairment of conjugate eye movement is referred to as an *internuclear ophthalmoplegia*. These lesions engender weakness of medial rectus muscle contraction of the adducting eye, which is accompanied by a monocular nystagmus in the abducting eye. Occasionally, paresis of lateral rectus muscle movement in the abducting eye may occur. Medial longitudinal fasciculus involvement may be unilateral or bilateral and may be associated with hemoglobinopathies, demyelinating disease, or brainstem vascular disease [Cogan, 1966].

Internal ophthalmoplegia consists of a fully dilated pupil that is unreactive to light or accommodation. Extraocular muscle function is normal when each muscle is tested separately. The oculomotor nerve, nucleus, or ciliary ganglion may be sites of involvement.

External ophthalmoplegia results in ptosis and paralysis of all extraocular muscles. Pupillary reactivity is normal. This pattern of involvement may accompany myasthenia gravis, hyperthyroidism, ocular myopathy, Möbius syndrome, tumors or vascular lesions of the brainstem, Wernicke disease, botulism, and lead intoxication.

Opticokinetic nystagmus (OKN) is a useful test in evaluating the eye movements of children. A drum or tape with stripes or figures is slowly rotated or drawn before the child's eyes in both horizontal and vertical directions. With fixation, the child should visually track the object in the direction the tape is being drawn, with a rapid, rhythmic movement (refixation) of the eyes in

the reverse direction to enable fixation on the next figure or stripe. Absence of such a response may result from failure of fixation, amaurosis, or disturbed saccadic eye movements.

The child who appears clinically blind because of a conversion reaction will exhibit a normal opticokinetic nystagmus response. Children who manifest congenital nystagmus and have an opticokinetic nystagmus response in the vertical plane will likely have adequate functional sight. Absence of opticokinetic nystagmus in the presence of congenital nystagmus heralds reduced visual acuity. If asymmetry of opticokinetic nystagmus response is evident, lateral lesions in the posterior half of the cerebral hemisphere are extant. The lesion is on the side that manifests reduced or absent opticokinetic nystagmus reactivity. The area of involvement is generally in the posterotemporal, parietal, or occipital areas. Hemianopic field defects may be present.

Spontaneous nystagmus—involuntary oscillatory movements of the eye—may be horizontal, vertical, or rotary; a patient can exhibit all three types. The movements may consist of a slow and fast phase, thus giving rise to the term *jerk nystagmus*. However, the phases may be of equal duration and amplitude, thus appearing pendular.

Nystagmus, especially vertical nystagmus, is most commonly induced by medications (e.g., barbiturates, phenytoin, carbamazepine). Such nystagmus often has a jerk component and is usually most prominent in the direction of gaze. Vertical nystagmus that is not associated with medications indicates brainstem dysfunction. Horizontal nystagmus indicates dysfunction of the cerebellum or brainstem vestibular system components; the nystagmus is coarser (i.e., the amplitude of movements greater) when the direction of gaze is toward the side of the lesion. A rare condition, seesaw nystagmus, is characterized by dysconjugate (alternating) movement of the eyes, which move upward and downward in a seesaw motion. This type nystagmus accompanies lesions in the region of the optic chiasm (see Chapter 49).

Trigeminal nerve (cranial nerve V)

Cranial nerve V, the trigeminal nerve, has both motor and sensory functions.

The motor division of the trigeminal nerve innervates the masticatory muscles—masseter, pterygoid, and temporalis. Temporalis muscle atrophy manifests as scalloping of the temporal fossa. The masseter muscle bulk may be assessed by palpation while the patient firmly closes the jaw. Pterygoid muscle strength is evaluated by having the patient open the mouth and "slide" the jaw from one side to the other while the examiner resists movements with the hand so as to assess muscle strength. The jaw reflex is elicited when the examiner places a finger on the patient's chin while the mouth is slightly open and taps the finger so as to stretch the masticatory muscles. A rapid muscle contraction with closure of the mouth is the reflex response. This stretch reflex receives both its afferent and efferent nerve control from cranial nerve V; the segmental level is located in the midpons. The expected reflex reaction is absent with motor nucleus and peripheral trigeminal nerve compromise. Conversely, this reflex is overactive in the presence of supranuclear lesions; rarely, jaw clonus may be evident. Because of weakness of the ipsilateral pterygoid muscles, unilateral impairment of the trigeminal nerve causes deviation of the jaw toward the side of the lesion.

Cranial nerve V is also responsible for sensations of the face (Figure 2-3) and the anterior half of the scalp. Brainstem compromise can affect clearly delineated laminar sensory deficits; however, mapping of such deficits is difficult in children. The corneal reflex, provided its sensory limb by the trigeminal nerve, may be diminished or absent after trauma, in cerebellopontine angle tumors, in brainstem tumors, or in childhood mesenchymal diseases.

Facial nerve (cranial nerve VII)

Taste sensation over the anterior two thirds of the tongue, secretory fibers (parasympathetic) innervating the lacrimal and salivary glands, and innervation of all facial muscles are accomplished by cranial nerve VII.

Complete motor dysfunction on one side of the face ensues when the cranial nerve VII pathway is disrupted in the nucleus, pons, or peripheral nerve. The patient is unable to move the forehead upward, close the eye forcefully, or elevate the corner of the mouth on the side of the affected nerve (Figures 2-4 and 2-5).

In contradistinction, central (supranuclear) facial nerve impairment produces only paresis of the muscles involving the lower face, with resultant drooping of the angle of the mouth, disappearance or diminution of the nasal labial fold, and increased palpebral fissure. The muscles of the forehead, which are innervated bilaterally, are unaffected. The cardiofacial syndrome is a congenital weakness that causes failure of depression of the angle of the mouth and is unrelated to facial nerve palsy [Nelson and Eng, 1972].

Taste sensation in the anterior two thirds of the tongue is in part subserved by the chorda tympani nerve, which traverses the path of the facial nerve for a short distance. Testing of taste sensation is difficult. Evaluation of taste requires that the patient extend the tongue and that the examiner hold the tip of the tongue with a piece of gauze and place salty, sweet, acid, and sour and bitter materials, usually represented by salt, sugar, vinegar, and quinine, on the anterior portion of the tongue. The patient's tongue must remain outside of the mouth until the test is completed. An older patient should be able to identify each substance.

Auditory nerve (cranial nerve VIII)

Function and evaluation of cranial nerve VIII is discussed in detail in Chapters 21, 22, and 61. Although cranial nerve VIII is known as the auditory nerve, it has both an auditory and a vestibular function. Gross auditory impairment may be suspected during the history-taking session while the child is in the room. The child may not respond directly to questions or to

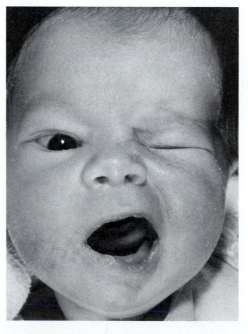

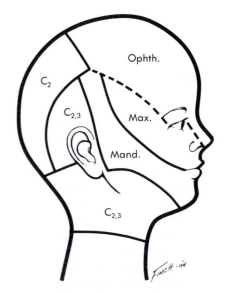

Figure 2-3 Facial sensation supplied by the trigeminal nerve. (Courtesy Division of Pediatric Neurology, University of Minnesota Medical School.)

Figure 2-4 Facial paralysis, peripheral type, right. (Courtesy Division of Pediatric Neurology, University of Minnesota Medical School.)

directions from the parents. More specific testing with whispered language, the ticking of a watch, a party noisemaker, or a tuning fork may be used to gain more information.

Patients who fail to develop speech or who have slow speech development, as well as those who have difficulty with fluency and articulation, should be suspected of having hearing impairment. Older children can cooperate with formal audiometric testing. Formal audiometric testing may not be possible in younger infants, but brainstem auditory-evoked potentials may provide the necessary information concerning hearing impairment and the level of the dysfunction within the nervous system.

Both clinical history and caloric testing can be used for gross assessment of vestibular function. More complex evaluation should be undertaken if the screening tests or the complaint indicates a need for more detailed assessment. Complaint of nausea, ataxia, vertigo, or unexplained vomiting, singly or in combination, may indicate both labyrinthine and vestibular pathologic origins. Caloric testing can be performed with relative ease. While the patient is in the supine position, the head is flexed at 30 degrees. Ice water, 10 ml, is injected over a period of 30 seconds into one external auditory canal at a time. The conscious patient develops coarse nystagmus towards the ipsilateral ear; no eye deviation occurs. If the patient has some degree of obtundation, there is a modification of the response. The eyes become tonically deviated ipsilaterally, with accompanying nystagmus occurring contralaterally. If the patient is comatose, cold water stimulation usually causes tonic devia-

tion ipsilaterally and no nystagmus. If the coma is profound, no eye changes occur. Multiple examinations will provide some objective monitoring of changes in the level of consciousness.

Glossopharyngeal and vagus nerves (cranial nerves IX and X)

Examination of the larynx, pharynx, and palate will provide most of the desired information concerning the function of cranial nerves IX and X. Unilateral paresis of the soft palate causes an ipsilateral droop even when the patient is expelling air through the open mouth or gagging in response to a tongue blade. Bilateral involvement causes a flaccid, soft palate bilaterally. With bilateral paresis, the voice becomes nasal and regurgitation of fluids occurs during drinking. During evaluation of swallowing the child should be asked to swallow up to 10 times to determine not only the efficacy of swallowing but also stamina. The examiner can evaluate the difficulty and the relative movements of the hyoid during the evaluation.

The gag reflex is mediated through cranial nerve IX and is elicited by touching the posterior pharyngeal mucosa with the tongue blade. Normal individuals may have absence or seemingly disproportionately violent response; therefore assessing the importance of changes in the gag reflex is difficult in the absence of other findings. Although the larynx can be studied under direct or indirect laryngoscopy, the presence of stridor, hoarseness, or dystonia suggests the need for more detailed examination of brainstem and cranial nerve IX integrity.

Spinal accessory nerve (cranial nerve XI)

Cranial nerve XI provides innervation for the trapezius and sternocleidomastoid muscles. (It is noteworthy that cranial nerve XI comprises some fibers from C_1 and C_2, as well as from the motor nucleus in the brainstem and is thus unique, combining both brainstem and cervical cord origins.) The trapezius muscles are assessed when the patient is asked to shrug the shoulders against resistance placed by the examiner. Atrophy of the muscle, as well as a drooping of the shoulder, provides further information on the status of the trapezius. The sternocleidomastoid muscle is tested by exerting resistance against the child's head while the child attempts rotation to one side. It should be remembered that weakness of the sternocleidomastoid muscle results in inability to rotate the head to the contralateral side. Muscle bulk of the sternocleidomastoid muscle is readily palpable and is readily visible in the presence of moderate-to-severe atrophy. Congenital or acquired lesions in the area of the foramen magnum most commonly cause difficulties of cranial nerve XI.

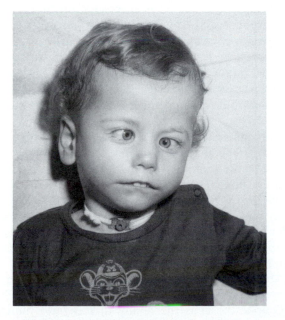

Figure 2-5 Möbius syndrome manifested by bilateral cranial nerve VI and VII palsy.

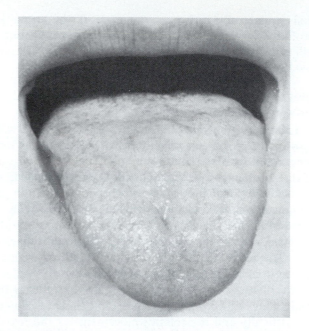

Figure 2-6 Fasciculation of the tongue, especially of the right lateral border, in a patient with group 2 Werdnig-Hoffman disease. (Courtesy Division of Pediatric Neurology, University of Minnesota Medical School.)

Hypoglossal nerve (cranial nerve XII)

The tongue muscle is the primary responsibility of cranial nerve XII. Atrophy and fasciculation of the tongue occur when the ipsilateral hypoglossal nucleus or hypoglossal nerve is involved. The protruded tongue deviates toward the involved side. The child cannot push the tongue against the cheek of the unaffected side. Speech may be muffled or dysarthric. Bilateral involvement of hypoglossal nuclei or cranial nerve XII may be severely incapacitating. The tongue muscle will be markedly atrophied, and fasciculations of the tongue may be very prominent (Figure 2-6). The patient may be unable to protrude the tongue beyond the lips, and there is marked dysarthria with unintelligibility of speech. Although chewing and swallowing are somewhat affected by unilateral tongue weakness, bilateral involvement results in gross difficulty.

Cranial nerve XII dysfunction may result from supranuclear bulbar palsy secondary to unilateral or bilateral corticospinal tract involvement. Although the signs and symptoms may resemble those of involvement of the hypoglossal nucleus or nerve, lower motor unit signs such as fasciculations and atrophy are absent. Certain movement disorders, particularly dystonia, may interfere with normal tongue movements and confound the examiner.

SENSORY SYSTEM

Cooperation of the patient is paramount to the success of the sensory examination in children. Vibration sense and joint and position sense are usually easily tested in all four limbs.

Touch may be assessed by a single stimulus or by double simultaneous stimulation of two skin areas. The latter tests extinction of perception over an involved area. Testing should include areas of the face, trunk, and limbs.

The ability to localize the area of contact of a tactile stimulus, topagnosis, is monitored by touching the patient, whose eyes are closed, on the face, arm, hand, leg, or foot with the examiner's finger or a cotton swab; the child is asked to point to or verbally identify the area. The loss of ability to localize the stimulus is associated with cortical, parietal lobe dysfunction.

In a more sophisticated test the patient is touched on two parts of the body simultaneously (double simultaneous stimulation test). *Extinction* is the term used to denote failure of the child to perceive both stimuli. The contralateral parietal lobe to the side on which the unidentified stimulus was applied is the site of dysfunction.

Pain, as tested with pinprick, must be assessed gently, rapidly, and in a nonthreatening and playful manner.

Testing for segmental sensory level during childhood is, at times, an essential portion of the examination. Because the patient must be attentive and cooperative, the examination often must be repeated for corroboration.

Segmental sensory innervations of the arm and leg are illustrated in Figures 2-7, 2-8, and 2-9 [Keegan and Garrett, 1948]. The nipples are at approximately the T_5 level and the umbilicus at the T_{10} level.

Cortical sensory function can be tested in the older child. So-called cortical sensory functions require attentiveness and cooperation and involve complex processing. Because the tests are primarily of parietal lobe function, testing of these functions assumes and requires intact sensory neurologic pathways from the diverse cutaneous specialized nerve endings, muscles, and joints and subsequent connections with the parietal lobe.

Stereognosis is the recognition of familiar objects by touch. After the patient closes the eyes, objects are placed by the examiner in one of the child's hands and then the other. The patient should recognize the objects by size, texture, and form. Objects may include a button, safety pin, or key. Coins are particularly useful because older patients can be asked to differentiate among them. The patient must be able to manipulate the objects freely with the fingers and palms.

Absence of stereognosis is astereognosis. Astereognosis usually results from lesions of the parietal lobe.

Graphesthesia is the ability to recognize numbers, letters, or other readily identifiable symbols traced on the skin. It is necessary to ascertain that the child is

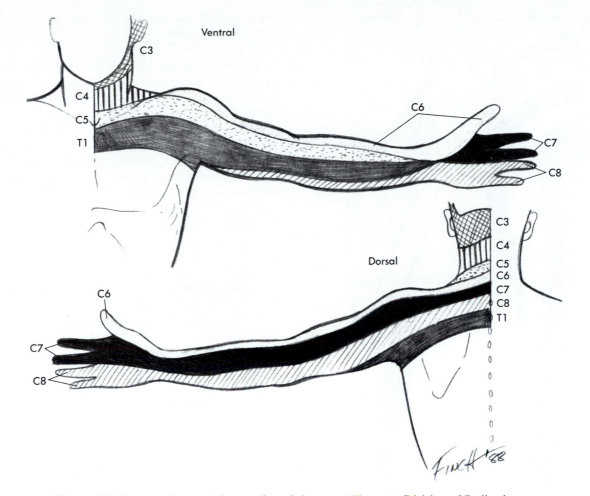

Figure 2-7 Segmental sensory innervation of the arm. (Courtesy Division of Pediatric Neurology, University of Minnesota Medical School; after Keegan JJ, Garrett FD. Anat Rec 1948; 102:409.)

capable of identifying the symbols. This ability can be determined best by tracing the symbols in a preliminary trial while the child's eyes are open. When the patient's eyes are closed, the figures are traced over the palm or forearm. Failure to identify the symbols is termed *dysgraphesthesia*. By 8 years of age most children are able to correctly identify all single digits.

The ability to distinguish between closely approximated stimulation at two points is two-point discrimination. The minimal distance between two simultaneous points of stimulation is determined. Normal findings for children ages 2 to 12 years have been reported [Cope and Antony, 1992]. Testing of this modality is frequently performed over the fingertips. Differences in perception over homologous areas on both sides are sought. Absence or impairment of two-point discrimination results from parietal lobe dysfunction.

SKELETAL MUSCLES

Tone, bulk, and strength of the skeletal muscles should be determined during this portion of the examination. The segmental innervation of the trunk muscles and the extremities and the motor functions of the spinal nerves are listed in Tables 2-3, 2-4, and 2-5.

The strength of limb muscles, when possible, is assessed by testing the child's ability to counteract resistance imposed by the examiner on proximal and distal muscle groups or individual muscles.

Muscle testing (adapted from Baker [1958]).

The skeletal muscles selected below are responsible for primary movements (see Table 2-6). Frequently, more than one muscle will participate in the movement. For this reason, while testing the selected muscles, the examiner should observe and palpate surrounding muscles to detect any substitution of action of other muscles.

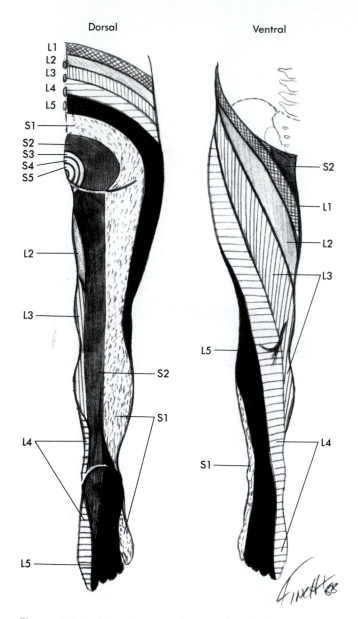

Dorsal   Ventral

Figure 2-8 Segmental sensory innervation of the leg. (Courtesy Division of Pediatric Neurology, University of Minnesota Medical School; after Keegan JJ, Garrett FD. Anat Rec 1948; 102:409.)

The following scoring system is useful for recording muscle power*:

5- Normal power
4- Inability to maintain position against moderate resistance
3- Inability to maintain position against slight resistance or gravity
2- Active movement with gravity eliminated

*Adapted from Medical Research Council, War Memorandum No. 7. Aids to the investigation of peripheral nerve injuries. 2nd ed. London: His Majesty's Stationery Office, 1943. (Reprinted 1960.)

1- Trace of contraction
0- No contraction

While testing for muscle function, it is most convenient for the patient to maintain a fixed position against force. The examiner can assess the strength of various muscles by instituting the action of the antagonist. This strategy obviates the necessity of providing new directions for each muscle tested and simplifies the procedure for both patient and examiner. The fixed positions depicted in Figure 2-10, p. 40, will be used routinely and will be referred to by the following letters:

Position A. The arm is adducted, the forearm flexed at the elbow, and the wrist across the xiphoid process.

Position B. The child lies on the back with the lower extremity flexed at 90 degrees at the hip and knee. The examiner should support the lower limb at the ankle.

Position C. The child lies on the back with the leg and foot in normal extension.

Whenever the weakness of any muscle group prevents the use of any of these positions, then substitute positions should be improvised.

Unfortunately, while examining young children, problems with cooperation or coordination may make it impossible to evaluate maximal strength; furthermore, only gross testing may be possible, during which various functions are tested by utilizing game-playing or gross maneuvers, such as the "wheelbarrow" maneuver.

Arm and shoulder strength can also be assessed by using functional operations. The child is asked to lean against a wall with the legs placed a foot or two from the wall edge and the arms outstretched with the palms against the wall. Strength of the shoulder girdle and arm extension can be evaluated. Winging of the scapulas will also be evident. Alternatively the child can be placed on the floor and asked to "wheelbarrow" (i.e., walk on the hands) while the examiner holds the child's feet. The child should be placed on the floor and asked to rise without aid. The normal child will spring erect. The child with weakness of the hip extensors will engage in the Gowers' maneuver and literally climb up the legs and push off into the erect position (Figure 2-11, see p. 40).

During examination of gait, the examiner must be aware of the presence of normal associated movements of the arms, circumduction of the legs, footdrop, unusual positions of the feet, and waddling. The presence of a limp may also be evident.

Muscle bulk is evaluated by gentle palpation and observation. Abnormalities include atrophy and fasciculations that accompany anterior horn cell disease and muscle hypertrophy, particularly of the gastrocnemius and deltoid muscles associated with Duchenne muscular dystrophy and other dystrophies, as well as myotonia congenita. Muscle tenderness, nerve tenderness, and nerve hypertrophy can also be assessed by palpation.

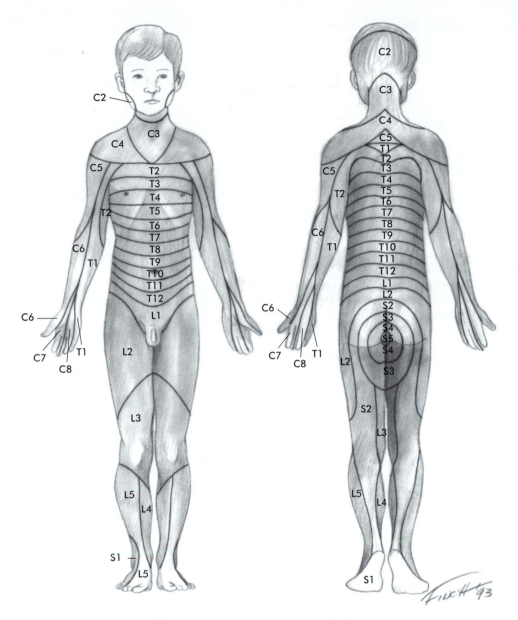

Figure 2-9 Radicular cutaneous fields.

Myotonia can be elicited by tapping over the thenar eminence and deltoid muscles. Tapping the tongue should be performed at the end of the examination and only when other elements of the history or examination make this evaluation essential. Tapping individual muscles with the reflex hammer elicits the myotatic reflex, which may be useful in the detection of myopathy because the reflex is absent in myopathies.

Muscle tone is evaluated when the child is relaxed so that resistance to passive movement can be monitored. Aside from passive movement of limbs at joints, the examiner also assesses the extensibility of muscles by shaking the limbs and determining the range of motion.

Tone may be decreased in the presence of cerebellar disease and anterior horn cell disease. Tone may be increased because of the rigidity associated with basal ganglia disease and spasticity associated with corticospinal tract dysfunction.

GAIT

The evaluation of gait is discussed in detail in Chapter 17, but a brief outline is presented here. The child should be asked to walk back and forth normally, preferably in a corridor, and up and down steps. The examiner should observe whether the gait is wide- or narrow-based, whether there is symmetric reciprocal movements of the arms, and whether the legs and feet move in a symmetric and normal fashion. The child should also be asked to run because running exaggerates neurologic impairment. Flexion or extension of an arm with subsequent

Text continued on p. 40.

Table 2-3 Motor functions of the spinal nerves*

Nerves	Muscles	Function
A. Cervical plexus (C_1-C_4)	Deep cervical	Flexion, extension, and rotation of the neck
Cervical	Scalene	Elevation of the ribs (inspiration)
Phrenic	Diaphragm	Inspiration
B. Brachial plexus (C_5-T_1)		
Anterior thoracic	Pectorales major and minor	Adduction and depression of the arm downward and medially
Long thoracic	Serratus anterior	Fixation of scapula on raising the arm
Dorsal scapular	Levator scapulae	Elevation of scapula
	Rhomboid	Drawing the scapula upward and inward
Suprascapular	Supraspinatus	Elevation and outward rotation of the arm
	Infraspinatus	Outward rotation of the arm
Subscapular	Latissimus dorsi ⎫ Teres major ⎭	Inward rotation and adduction of the arm toward the back
	Subscapularis	Inward rotation of the arm
Axillary	Deltoid	Raising of arm to the horizontal
	Teres minor	Outward rotation of the arm
Musculocuta- neous	Biceps brachii	Flexiona and supination of the forearm
	Coracobrachialis	Elevation and adduction of the arm
	Brachialis	Flexion of the forearm
Median	Flexor carpi radialis	Flexion and radial deviation of the hand
	Palmaris longus	Flexion of the hand
	Flexor digitorium sublimis	Flexion of the middle phalanges of second through fifth fingers
	Flexor pollicis longus	Flexion of the distal phalanx of the thumb
	Flexor digitorum profundus (radial half)	Flexion of the distal phalanges of second and third fingers
	Pronator quadratus	Pronation
	Pronator teres	Pronation
	Abductor pollicis brevis	Abduction of metacarpus I at right angles to plam
	Flexor pollicis brevis	Flexion of proximal phalanx of thumb
	Lumbricals I, II, III	Flexion of the proximal phalanges and extension of the other phalanges of first, second, and third fingers
	Opponens pollicis brevis	Opposition of metacarpus I
Ulnar	Flexor carpi ulnaris	Flexion and ulnar deviation of the hand
	Flexor digitorum profundus (ulnar half)	Flexion of distal phalanges of fourth and fifth fingers
	Adductor pollicis	Adduction of metacarpus I
	Hypothenar	Abduction, opposition, flexion of the little finger
	Lumbricals III, IV	Flexion of the first phalanx and extension of the other phalanges of fourth and fifth fingers
	Interossei	Same action as preceding. Also spreading apart of fingers and bringing them together.
Radial	Triceps brachii	Extension of the forearm
	Brachioradialis	Flexion of the forearm
	Extensor carpi radialis	Extension and radial flexion of the hand
	Extensor digitorum communis	Extension of proximal phalanges of second through fifth fingers
	Extensor digiti quinti propius	Extension of the proximal phalanx of the little finger

From Haymaker W. Bing's local diagnosis in neurological diseases. 15th ed. St. Louis: Mosby, 1969.
*Various muscles may receive still other nerve supplies than those mentioned. The following are the principal accessory nerve supplies: the *brachial muscle* receives fibers from the radial nerve; the *flexor digitorum sublimis*, from the ulnar; the *adductor pollicis*, from the median; the *pectineus*, from the femoral; the *adductor magnus*, from the tibial.

Table 2-3 Motor functions of the spinal nerves* — cont'd

Nerves	Muscles	Function
Radial — cont'd	Extensor carpi ulnaris	Extension and ulnar deviation of the hand
	Supinator	Supination of the forearm
	Abductor pollicis longus	Abduction of metacarpus I
	Extensor pollicis brevis	Extension of the proximal phalanx of the thumb
	Extensor pollicis longus	Abduction of first metacarpus and extension of the distal phalanges of the thumb
	Extensor indicis proprius	Extension of the proximal phalanx of the index finger
C. Thoracic nerves		
Thoracic	Thoracic and abdominal	Elevation of the ribs, expiration, abdominal compression, etc.
D. Lumbar plexus (T_{12}-L_4)		
Femoral	Iliopsoas	Flexion of the leg at the hip
	Sartorius	Inward rotation of the leg together with flexion of the upper and lower leg
	Quadriceps femoris	Extension of the lower leg
Obturator	Pectineus	
	Adductor longus	
	Adductor brevis	Adduction of the leg
	Adductor magnus	
	Gracilis	
	Obturator externus	Adduction and outward rotation of the leg
E. Sacral plexus (L_5-S_5)		
Superior gluteal	Gluteus medius	Abduction and inward rotation of the leg, also under certain circumstances, an outward rotation
	Gluteus minimus	
	Tensor fasciae latae	Flexion of the leg at the hip
	Piriformis	Outward rotation of the leg
	Gluteus maximus	Extension of leg at the hip
Inferior gluteal		
Sciatic	Obturator internus	
	Gemelli	Outward rotation of the leg
	Quadratus femoris	
	Biceps femoris	
	Semitendinosus	Flexion of the leg at the hip
	Semimembranosus	
(1) Peroneal	Tibialis anterior	Dorsiflexion and supination of the foot
(a) Deep	Extensor digitorum longus	Extension of the toes
	Extensor hallucis brevis	Extension of the great toe
(b) Superficial	Peroneus	Pronation of the foot
(2) Tibialis	Gastrocnemius	
	Soleus	Plantar flexion of the foot
	Tibialis posterior	Adduction of the foot
	Flexor digitorum longus	Flexion of the distal phalanges II through V
	Flexor hallucis longus	Flexion of distal phalanx I
	Flexor digitorum brevis	Flexion of middle phalanges II through V
	Flexor hallucis brevis	Flexion of middle phalanx I
	Plantar	Spreading and bringing together and flexion of the proximal phalanges of the toes
Pudendal	Perineal and sphincters	Closure of sphincters of the pelvic organs. Also participation in the sexual act. Contraction of pelvic floor.

Table 2-4 Segmental innervation of muscles of extremities

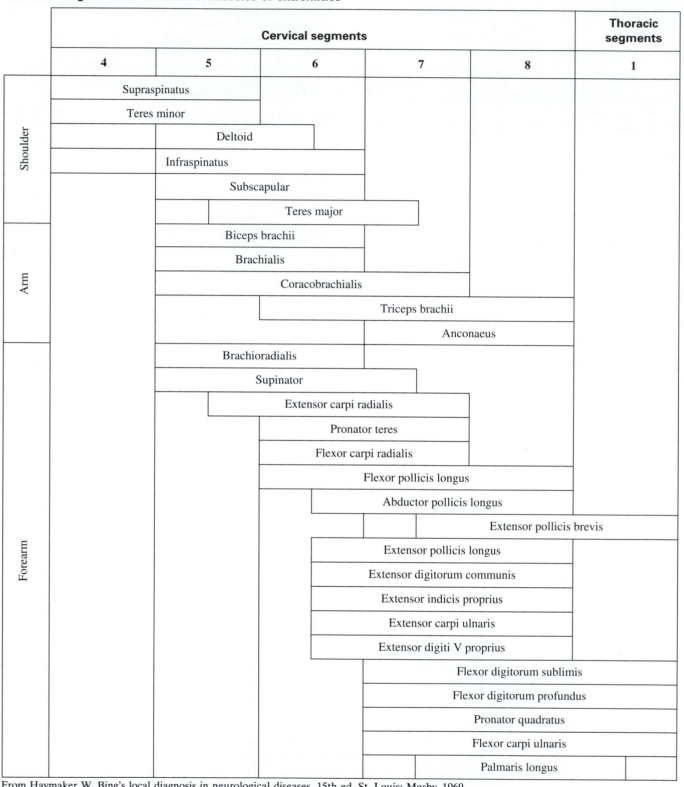

Region	Muscle	4	5	6	7	8	T1
		Cervical segments					**Thoracic segments**
Shoulder	Supraspinatus	■	■				
Shoulder	Teres minor	■	■				
Shoulder	Deltoid		■	■			
Shoulder	Infraspinatus		■	■			
Shoulder	Subscapular		■	■			
Shoulder	Teres major		■	■	■		
Arm	Biceps brachii		■	■			
Arm	Brachialis		■	■			
Arm	Coracobrachialis		■	■	■		
Arm	Triceps brachii			■	■	■	
Arm	Anconaeus				■	■	
Forearm	Brachioradialis		■	■			
Forearm	Supinator		■	■	■		
Forearm	Extensor carpi radialis		■	■	■		
Forearm	Pronator teres			■	■		
Forearm	Flexor carpi radialis			■	■		
Forearm	Flexor pollicis longus			■	■	■	
Forearm	Abductor pollicis longus			■	■	■	
Forearm	Extensor pollicis brevis				■	■	■
Forearm	Extensor pollicis longus			■	■	■	
Forearm	Extensor digitorum communis			■	■	■	
Forearm	Extensor indicis proprius			■	■	■	
Forearm	Extensor carpi ulnaris			■	■	■	
Forearm	Extensor digiti V proprius			■	■	■	
Forearm	Flexor digitorum sublimis				■	■	■
Forearm	Flexor digitorum profundus				■	■	■
Forearm	Pronator quadratus				■	■	■
Forearm	Flexor carpi ulnaris				■	■	■
Forearm	Palmaris longus				■	■	■

From Haymaker W. Bing's local diagnosis in neurological diseases. 15th ed. St. Louis: Mosby, 1969.

Table 2-4 Segmental innervation of muscles of extremities—cont'd

Region	Muscle	Thoracic T12	Lumbar L1	L2	L3	L4	L5	Sacral S1	S2	S3
Hip	Illiopsoas	●	●	●	●					
Hip	Tensor fasciae latae					●	●	●		
Hip	Gluteus medius					●	●	●		
Hip	Gluteus minimus					●	●	●		
Hip	Quadratus femoris					●	●	●		
Hip	Gemellus inferior					●	●	●		
Hip	Gemellus superior						●	●	●	
Hip	Gluteus maximus						●	●	●	
Hip	Obturator internus						●	●	●	
Hip	Piriformis							●	●	
Thigh	Sartorius			●	●					
Thigh	Pectineus			●	●					
Thigh	Adductor longus			●	●					
Thigh	Quadriceps femoris			●	●	●				
Thigh	Gracilis			●	●	●				
Thigh	Adductor brevis			●	●	●				
Thigh	Obturator externus				●	●				
Thigh	Adductor magnus				●	●				
Thigh	Adductor minimus				●	●				
Thigh	Articularis genu				●	●				
Thigh	Semitendinosus					●	●	●	●	
Thigh	Semimembranosus					●	●	●	●	
Thigh	Biceps femoris						●	●	●	●
Leg	Tibialis anterior					●	●			
Leg	Extensor hallucis longus					●	●	●		
Leg	Popliteus					●	●	●		
Leg	Plantaris					●	●	●		
Leg	Extensor digitorum longus					●	●	●	●	
Leg	Soleus						●	●	●	

Continued.

Table 2-4 Segmental innervation of muscles of extremities—cont'd

	Cervical segments				Thoracic segments	
Hand	4	5	6	7	8	1
Abductor pollicis brevis				X	X	X
Flexor pollicis brevis				X	X	X
Oppenens pollicis			X	X		
Flexor digiti V					X	X
Opponens digiti V					X	X
Adductor pollicis					X	X
Palmaris brevis					X	X
Abductor digiti V					X	X
Lumbricals					X	X
Interossei					X	X

	Thoracic segments	Lumbar segments					Sacral segments		
Leg—cont'd / Foot	12	1	2	3	4	5	1	2	3
Gastrocnemius						X	X	X	
Peroneus longus						X	X		
Peroneus brevis						X	X		
Tibialis posterior						X	X		
Flexor digitorum longus						X	X	X	
Flexor hallucis longus						X	X	X	
Extensor hallucis brevis					X	X			
Extensor digits brevis					X	X	X		
Flexor digiti brevis						X	X		
Abductor hallucis						X	X		
Flexor hallucis brevis						X	X	X	
Lumbricals						X	X	X	
Adductor hallucis							X	X	
Abductor digiti V							X	X	
Flexor digiti V brevis							X	X	
Opponens digiti V							X	X	
Quadratus plantae							X	X	
Interossei							X	X	

Table 2-5 Segmental innervation of the trunk muscles

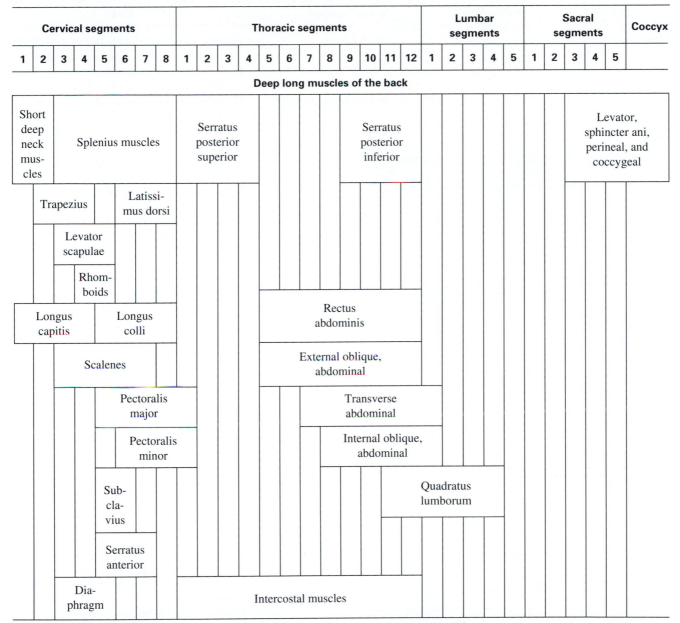

From Haymaker W. Bing's local diagnosis in neurological diseases. 15th ed. St. Louis: Mosby, 1969.

Table 2-6 Muscle testing (Use in conjunction with Figure 2-10)

Muscle	Innervation	Normal function	Test
Supraspinatus	C_4-C_5	Initiates arm abduction	Holding the patient at his or her side, have the patient attempt to abduct the limb
Deltoid	C_5-C_6	Abduction of arm between 15 and 90 degrees	Have the patient maintain abduction of arm at 45 degrees against resistance
Lower trapezius	C_2-C_4	Elevation of arm above shoulder	Have patient maintain elevation of arm above the shoulder against resistance
Serratus	C_5-C_7	Fixes the medial border of the scapula	Using the position A, apply pressure in axis of the humerus
Infraspinatus	C_5	External rotation of the arm	Using position A, apply downward pressure on forearm
Subscapularis and teres major	C_5-C_8	Internal rotation of the arm	Using position A, pull the wrist away from the body
Pectoral and latissimus dorsi	C_5-C_8	Adduction of the arm	Using position A, abduct the arm in the midaxillary line
Brachioradialis	C_5-C_6 radial	Flexion of elbow	Using position A (forearm must be pronated), push downward at the wrist
Biceps	C_5-C_6 musculo-cutaneous	Flexion of elbow	Using position A but with forearm supinated, push downward at wrist
Triceps	C_7-C_8	Extends forearm	Using position A, push upward at wrist
Pronators	C_6-C_7	Pronates forearm	Using position A, rotate forearm so that the upper border of the hand turns outward
Supinators	C_5-C_6	Supinates forearm	Using position A, rotate the forearm so that the upper border of the hand turns inward
Flexors of wrist	C_7-median/ulnar		Using position A but with hand supinated, push down on the palmar surface of the hand
Extensors of wrist	C_7-radial		Using position A but with hand pronated, push down on the dorsal surface of the hand
Extensors of the digits	C_7-radial		Using position A but with hand pronated, push down on the first phalanx of each digit
Flexors of fingers (grip)	C_8-T_1 median/ulnar		Using position A, have patient squeeze hard
Adductor of thumb	T_1-ulnar		Using position A with thumb adducted, pull upward on the thumb
Opponens thumb	T_1-median		Using position A with hand supinated, have patient resist the separation of the tip of the little finger from the tip of the extended thumb
Interossei	T_1-ulnar	Extends fingers	Using position A but with hand supinated and fingers spread apart, attempt to approximate the fingers

Table 2-6 Muscle testing (Use in conjunction with Figure 2-10)—cont'd

Muscle	Innervation	Normal function	Test
Back muscles		Extends the back	Use position C, place hand beneath patient's back and have the patient arch the back
Abdominal muscles		Contracts the abdominal wall	With patient in supine position, place hand on patient's abdomen and have patient attempt to rise from a recumbent position
Intercostal muscles		Raises the rib cage	With patient in supine position, observe action of intercostals on deep inspiration; observe excursion and observe for asymmetry of excursion of chest
Diaphragm	C_4	Participates in respiration and facilitates coughing	Have patient cough and observe the epigastric impulse
Iliopsoas	L_2 femoral	Flexion of hip on abdomen	Using position B, place hand above knee and push downward
Adductors of hip	L_2-L_3 obturator	Adducts leg at the hip	Using position B, place hand on the medial surface of the thigh and push outward
Gluteus medius and minimus	L_4-L_5	Abduction of leg at the hip	Using position B, place hand on outer aspect of thigh and push inward
Quadriceps	L_3 femoral	Extension of the knee	Using position B, attempt to further flex the leg at knee
Hamstrings	S_1-S_2 sciatic	Flexors of the knee	Using position B, attempt to extend the leg at the knee
Tibialis anticus	L_4 peroneal	Dorsiflexion of the foot	Using position C, place hand on the dorsal surface of the foot and push in a plantar direction
Triceps surae	L_5-S_2 tibial	Plantar flexion of the foot	Using position C, place hand on ball of foot and push in the direction of the patient
Posterior tibial	L_4 tibial	Inverts the foot	Using position C, grasp the foot at the arch and rotate so that the plantar surface of the foot turns outward
Peroneals	L_5 peroneal	Everts the foot	Using position C, grasp the foot at the arch and rotate so that the plantar surface turns inward
Dorsiflexors of toes	S_1 peroneal		Using position C, push in a plantar direction against the dorsal surface of the toes
Plantar-flexors of toes	S_2 tibial		Using position C, place hand on the plantar surface of the toes and push in the direction of the patient
Gluteus maximus	S_1-S_2	Extension of the leg at the hip	With patient lying on the side and with the lower limbs maintained in normal extension, place hand on back of thigh and push forward

3

Neurologic Examination After the Newborn Period Until 2 Years of Age

Kenneth F. Swaiman

Maturation of physiologic processes and anatomic structures of the developing central and peripheral nervous systems is concomitantly associated with the systematic acquisition of skills and responses. Adequate neurologic assessment depends on comparing the results of the infant's examination with established norms (Table 3-1) [Gesell and Amatruda, 1956; Illingsworth, 1972]. (The reader is advised to review Chapter 2 to permit maximum understanding of the material in this chapter.)

It is critical that the infant remain calm and cooperative for the longest possible time during the examination; therefore the least intrusive portions of the examination should be performed first.

APPROACH TO THE EVALUATION

Experienced examiners develop individual approaches to and sequences for the evaluation. Most schemes embody much of the following material. Although arbitrary, examination of the infant can be subdivided into stages.

Observation occupies most of the first stage. Some observations will have been made during the history-taking session. The parents should undress the child except for the undershirt, underwear and plastic pants, or diaper. The child should remain on the parent's lap. At first the clinician should continue questioning the parents about pertinent aspects of the history. Usually the child becomes reassured that the clinician is well-meaning. Observation allows limited assessment of cranial nerve function, unusual facies, gross structural deformities (including those of the head and neck), symmetry of strength and movements of the extremities, and unusual posturing.

At the beginning of the second stage, while the child remains on the parent's lap, examination of the head, deep tendon reflexes, muscle tone, superficial and deep sensation, gross response to sound, and visual fields can be evaluated. Examination of the toe signs can be performed.

The parent is then asked to undress the child completely, and the child is placed on a table. During this segment of the examination, more interactive assessment of muscle function and further developmental assessment of the developmental reflexes, traction response, parachute response, and sitting and standing abilities take place. The sensory examination is best performed at this time.

The third stage may require assistance from a parent or assistant. At this time, examination of the abdomen, genitalia, back, and anal area is accomplished. Examination of the mouth, tongue, and sternocleidomastoid muscles should also be performed. If previously deferred, measurement of the occipitofrontal circumference (OFC) is mandatory. At this point the fundi and ears are examined.

At the beginning of the fourth stage of the examination, the child is placed on the floor so that assessment of crawling, walking, and running can be accomplished.

EVALUATION OF THE PATIENT

Details of each stage of the evaluation are provided next.

Stage 1

Stage 1 of the evaluation should be performed with an ease in approach. In particular the examiner should avoid quick movements or display of instruments that

Table 3-1 Child development from 2 months through 2 years*

2 months	9 to 10 months
Keeps hands predominantly fisted	Sits well without support, pulls self to sit
Lifts head up for several seconds while prone	Stands holding on
Startles to loud noise	Waves "bye-bye"
Follows with eyes and head over 90-degree arc	Drinks from cup with assistance
Smiles responsively	
Begins to vocalize single sounds	**11 to 12 months**
	Walks with assistance
3 months	Uses pincer grasp
Occasionally holds hands fisted	Uses two to four words with meaning
Lifts head up above body plane and holds position	Creeps well
Holds an object briefly when placed in hand	Assists in dressing
Turns head toward object, fixes and follows fully in all	Understands a few simple commands
directions with eyes	
Smiles and vocalizes when talked to	**13 to 15 months**
Watches own hands, stares at faces	Walks by self—falls easily
Laughs	Says several words, uses jargon
	Scribbles with crayon
4 months	Points to things wanted
Holds head steady while in sitting position	
Reaches for an object, grasps it, brings it to mouth	**18 months**
Turns head in direction of sound	Climbs stairs with assistance, climbs up on chair
Smiles spontaneously	Throws ball
	Builds two-to four-block tower
5 to 6 months	Feeds self
Lifts head while supine	Takes off clothes
Rolls from prone to supine	Points to two to three body parts
Lifts head and chest up in prone position	Uses many intelligible words
Exhibits no head lag	
Transfers object from hand to hand	**24 months**
Babbles	Runs, walks up and down stairs alone (both feet per
Sits with support	step)
Localizes direction of sound	Speaks in two- to three-word sentences
	Turns single pages of book
7 to 8 months	Builds four- to six-block tower
Sits in tripod fashion without support	Kicks ball
Stands briefly with support	Uses pronouns "you," "me," "I"
Bangs object on table	
Reaches out for people	
Mouths all objects	
Says "da-da," "ba-ba"	

*Data from Illingworth RS. The development of the infant and young child. 5th ed. Baltimore: Williams & Wilkins 1972; Knobloch H, Stevens F, Malone AF. Manual of developmental diagnosis. New York: Harper & Row, 1980; Frankenburg WK, Sciarillo W, Burgess D. J Pediatr 1981; 99:995.

could be interpreted as threatening. Smiling at the infant and speaking in soft and reassuring tones are highly effective. The child should sit on the parent's lap and face the examiner. It is preferable that the child be placed in this position during the history-taking session so that familiarity with the examiner, the room, and the clinician is developed.

Observations made of the child while in this position during the initial conversation may provide much information to the skilled examiner. The sequence of examination should be flexible and should be determined by the child's comfort and temperament and by the natural postures and positions assumed by the child. Flexibility on the part of the examiner may be the key to a successful session. Nevertheless, a reasonably complete examination should be performed. The clinician must not lose sight of the need for all pertinent data to be collected. Above all, it is imperative that the physician systematically conduct that portion of the examination related to the chief complaint.

The examiner must be highly sensitive to the child's mood and defer those parts of the examination that appear to upset the child until last.

The clinician should make judgments concerning the

facial and extraocular movements and the asymmetry and character of limb movements. Additionally, the child's state of alertness, awareness of surroundings, and affect should be evident. The child's vocalization should be age-appropriate.

Head. The examination of the head must be performed systematically. Observation of asymmetry, indentations, and protuberances should be performed. Evaluation of all the cranial sutures and associated fontanels can be performed by gentle palpation. The dimensions of the anterior fontanel should be carefully recorded [Popich and Smith, 1972]. The examiner should determine by observation and palpation the presence of suture synostosis, suture separation, bulging fontanel, frontal bossing, and unusual shapes of the head, including trigonocephaly, marked dolichocephaly or brachycephaly, or plagiocephaly.

If the child is comfortable the occipitofrontal circumference should be measured. If the child becomes agitated from placement of the tape measure, the measurement should be deferred until later (stage 3). The largest measured circumference should be recorded and plotted on a graph of normal data. (When hydrocephalus is suspected in the early months of life, ultrasonography, CT, or MRI should be performed.) Simultaneously, unusual masses under the scalp and gross asymmetries of the skull should be sought.

The cranium is auscultated for the presence of unusual intracranial bruits. However, intracranial bruits occur commonly in childhood, and cautious interpretation is advised. Asymmetric bruits and those that can be suppressed by carotid artery suppression are frequently pathologic.

If possible, the tension of the anterior fontanel should be evaluated when the child is held in an upright position. The size of the anterior fontanel varies [Popich and Smith, 1972]. The anterior fontanel pulsates in unison with the heart beat, becomes fuller or bulging when the child cries, and may be full in disease states in which there is increased intracranial pressure. The posterior fontanel usually admits only a finger at time of birth and generally is not palpable by 2 months of age.

Other fontanels are usually difficult to palpate readily except in pathologic states. Occasionally accessory fontanels may be found along the suture, particularly the sagittal sutures. They usually are benign abnormalities.

The examiner should auscultate the infant's skull. However, caution is indicated because intracranial bruits are frequently normal, although abnormalities, such as vein of Galen malformations, produce extremely loud bruits. The vein of Galen malformation is associated with increasing frontal circumference, high-input cardiac failure, and distress while the infant is in the supine position. Seizures may also be present.

Ultrasound examinations of the newborn cranial vault may provide much information concerning the presence of hemorrhage, ventricular size, and amplitude of cerebral pulsations. At times the use of transillumination with a flashlight may suggest the presence of a fluid compartment within the brain or over the cortical mantle. Such findings are present in hydranencephaly, porencephaly, subdural effusions, caput succedaneum, hydrocephalus, and infiltrated intravenous sites.

Cranial nerves. Examination of cranial nerve function can be performed primarily through observation. More details concerning examination of each cranial nerve can be found in Chapter 2.

Using bright objects facilitates the assessment of extraocular muscle movements. Nystagmus and strabismus may be detected during this portion of the examination. If a cooperative child appears uninterested in bright objects, the possibility that a visual defect or an underlying intellectual defect is present must be considered. Rolling movements of the eyes and dysconjugate gaze suggest gross visual impairment. Double simultaneous stimulation, that is, bringing two bright objects into different visual fields (one in each temporal area) simultaneously, will normally cause the child to look from one object to the other. Failure to take notice of one object may indicate homonymous hemianopsia. A tape with repetitive bars or objects should be drawn horizontally and then vertically across the child's field of vision. Lack of opticokinetic response results from lack of visual fixation or from gross impairment of vision. Unusual transient deviations of the eyes may occur in the first year of life [Echenne and Rivier, 1992].

A beam from a small flashlight should be directed at each eye to allow evaluation of pupillary responses, anisocoria, and the red retinal reflex. The examiner should initially direct the light beam at the child's hand or abdomen so that the child is aware of the safety of the procedure.

The presence of abnormalities, such as symmetry of the palpebral fissures, the relative size of the two globes, the angulation of the eyes when compared with other facial components and with the ears, cataracts, conjunctival telangiectases, colobomas of the iris, ptosis, proptosis, and malformed or eccentrically placed pupils, can be determined at this time. Additionally, hair color, patterning distribution, and texture should be assessed.

During the entire examination the examiner should observe the child's facial movements closely. Smiling at the child, tickling the child, or making unusual noises or facial grimaces will often cause the child to smile or laugh, allowing observation of the nasolabial folds. The presence of facial weakness secondary to central or peripheral cranial nerve VII dysfunction should be determined. Widening of the ipsilateral palpebral fissure often accompanies facial nerve weakness. It is essential

reserved until late in the examination; careless use of the pin will destroy rapport with the patient. The child may cry or make short, whimpering sounds.

Decreased muscle bulk may not be appreciated because of the large amount of subcutaneous fat. Therefore muscle atrophy may be undetected. The examiner should be careful to palpate muscle mass beneath the fat and not misinterpret the subcutaneous tissue as muscle.

The skin of the infant is observed for obvious areas of abnormality that may suggest certain conditions, including neuroectodermal diseases. Examination of the spine may indicate the presence of scoliosis, sinus tracts, scars, dimples, and hemangiomas. Unusual skin lesions or hair growth over the spine suggests the presence of an underlying mesodermal defect, including diastematomyelia. The spine should be palpated along its entire course for defects.

Abdominal and cremasteric reflexes are present at birth. The abdominal reflex is elicited by stroking the skin of the upper, middle, and lower portions of the abdomen. Each stroke elicits a muscle contraction mediated by a different group of thoracic and lumbar nerves. The response results in the retraction of the umbilicus toward the stimulated side. The various spinal cord segmental levels involved in the reflex arc range from T_8 to T_{12}.

The cremasteric reflex is elicited by stroking the inner thigh, beginning 3 to 5 cm below the inguinal crease. The cremasteric reflex results in an elevation of the testicles because of contraction of the overlying smooth muscles. The cremasteric reflexes are mediated by spinal nerves L_1 and L_2.

Stage 2

For stage 2 of the evaluation the child should be placed on a table with the parent standing close by for reassurance to the child and assistance, if necessary, to the examiner. Motor evaluation can be performed on an examining table or on a larger carpeted surface. By 3 months of age the infant holds the head and chest off the table while in the prone position. Good head control while sitting with support is evident by 4 months of age. The child should be able to sit without support and maintain adequate balance by 8 to 9 months of age. Unassisted assumption of the sitting position should occur by 10 months of age. The child should crawl by 10 months, pull to a standing position by 10 months, and creep by 11 months. The child should walk with support by 12 months and without support by 13 to 14 months. Lack of these abilities should be evaluated in concert with other findings.

Trunk, shoulder, and pelvic girdle tone and strength should be evaluated further. The child is held in both vertical and horizontal suspension and observed. A hypotonic child, when held in a horizontal suspension, will often droop over the examiner's arm [Paine, 1960]. In vertical suspension the child may slide through the examiner's hands. The child may be unable to maintain a standing posture when the feet are placed on the table surface. Increased tone, or hypertonicity, usually the result of spasticity, may manifest by a backward curve of the extended head, neck, and back while in horizontal suspension. The legs may be extended and may "scissor" while the child is in vertical suspension, and the child may stand on the toes when the feet are allowed to touch the table (Figure 3-4).

Developmental reflexes.   The developmental reflexes are patterned responses that are achieved by certain ages. General development of the nervous system can be assessed by eliciting these reflexes. Occasionally they may have localizing value, but usually they do not. The abnormalities may be the continued presence of a reflex that should have dissipated, absence or poor manifestation of the expected response, or a response that is not symmetric. These reflexes are listed in Table 3-2 [Paine, 1960]. Although the Moro reflex may be demonstrated by several maneuvers, essentially, the position of the head in relation to the trunk must be altered in the supine position. Eliciting this reflex is usually performed while the child is in the supine position; the head is lifted off the padded examining table and then allowed to fall approximately 30 degrees

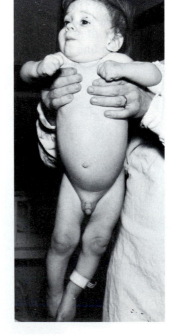

Figure 3-4 Extended legs, scissoring, toe stance, and fisting in an infant with spastic quadriplegia. (Courtesy Division of Pediatric Neurology, University of Minnesota Medical School.)

in relation to the trunk [Parmelee, 1964]. The examiner should allow the head to fall onto his or her hand. The expected response is extension and abduction of the arms and extension of the fingers. This posturing is followed by adduction of the arms at the shoulder. The child often emits a cry (Figure 3-5).

An abnormality in the Moro reflex does not signify a specific area of involvement but rather a diffuse process, usually depression of the CNS. Generalized weakness or severe spasticity may also cause limitation of the Moro reflex. If the Moro reflex is asymmetric, motor abnormalities, such as Erb's or Klumpke's brachial plexis palsies or fractures of the humerus or clavicle [Dekaban, 1970], should be considered. Spastic hemiplegia may also result in an asymmetric Moro reflex. Although the Moro reflex is usually present in children up to 5 or 6 months of age, the manifestation of the reflex changes with maturation. By 2 months of age the Moro reflex is

Table 3-2 Developmental reflexes

Reflex	Appearance age	Disappearance age
Adductor spread of knee jerk	Birth	7 to 8 months
Landau reflex	10 months	24 months
Moro	Birth	5 to 6 months
Palmar grasp	Birth	6 months
Parachute	8 to 9 months	Persists
Plantar grasp	Birth	9 to 10 months
Rooting	Birth	3 months
Tonic neck response	Birth	5 to 6 months
Truncal incurvation	Birth	1 to 2 months

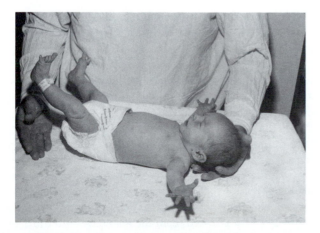

Figure 3-5 The Moro response to rapid extension of the neck in a 2-day-old infant. The abduction phase of arm movement is illustrated. A cry usually accompanies the response. The leg position is variable.

incomplete. The usual pattern is that the adduction phase is greatly attenuated.

The tonic neck reflex reaches a peak at 2 months of age but may be present in the neonatal period. The reflex gradually diminishes and is absent by 6 months of age. To elicit the reflex, the head is turned to one side while the child is supine and the shoulders fixed. The arm and leg on the side toward which the face is turned extend, and the arm and leg on the opposite side flex. The degree of response varies widely but is usually symmetric. In any event a normal infant will not remain in the reflex position when the reflex is elicited. If the struggling infant does not break the reflex response, the response is abnormal. The response should not be present beyond 6 months of age [Paine et al., 1964]. A unilateral reflex may indicate a lesion in the hemisphere opposite the direction in which the face is turned. The same consideration holds true if the response is obligate or persists beyond the expected age. The weak child may also have an abnormal response secondary to central or peripheral motor unit involvement. Sitting or standing is impaired when an overactive tonic neck reflex is present. Athetoid and spastic infants may also have an exaggerated response.

An object or the examiner's finger is placed in the palm of the infant's hand to elicit the palmar grasp reflex. The child has an involuntary flexion response and grasps the object. This reflex subsides by 3 to 6 months of age, and voluntary grasping is evident. The obligatory involuntary grasp reflex may persist and often indicates infantile hemiplegia [Paine, 1964].

To elicit the Landau reflex, the infant is held prone in horizontal suspension by the examiner. The examiner flexes the infant's head. Flexion of the legs and trunk is the normal response. This response is present in the majority of infants by 5 months of age and absent by 2 years of age [Cupps et al., 1976]. Virtually all normal infants have a positive Landau response by 10 months of age. When held in horizontal suspension, 55% of infants spontaneously elevate their heads above the horizontal plane by age 5 months and 95% by 6 months [Paine et al., 1964].

The placing reflex response can be demonstrated by holding the upright infant in a manner that causes the dorsi of the infant's feet to touch the underside of a table top. The infant will flex the legs at the hip and knees so that contact with the underside of the surface ceases.

One of the most useful maneuvers is the traction response. The response is elicited while the infant is lying supine. The examiner grasps each hand of the infant and pulls the infant gently and slowly, allowing the infant to assist, to a sitting position. Marked head lag with little resistance to the examiner's pulling efforts is present in the newborn period (Figure 3-6). After a month or so, when the child comes forward, the infant's

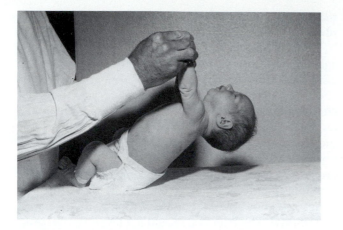

Figure 3-6 The traction maneuver causes little response in a 2-day-old infant. There is little or no perceptible flexion of the neck or the arms at the elbows.

head comes forward with neck flexion, and then transiently is extended at the neck. Usually by age 3 to 5 months of age at the latest, the infant is able to pull against the examiner with arm flexion at the elbow, hold the head and trunk in a straight line, and otherwise actively participate while the examiner pulls the infant to the upright position. No head lag is observed and little or no forward motion of the head occurs as the child reaches the upright position. Asymmetry should signal a neurologic difficulty. A traction response in which the infant is brought to a sitting position only transiently followed by rapid assumption of a standing position because the legs are extended at the hips and knees is suggestive of the presence of corticospinal tract difficulty bilaterally.

A valuable measure of vestibular function in the newborn can be obtained by holding the infant in a supine position; the feet are closest to the examiner. The examiner, with the infant lying on the arm, rotates in one direction and then reverses direction. The eyes of the infant will deviate in the direction of rotation accompanied by intermittent nystagmus to the opposite side. Extraocular movements may also be assessed during this maneuver.

It is essential that the examiner take into account the overall pattern of developmental responses. An abnormality of one reflex does not indicate significant neurologic abnormality. There are other developmental reflexes, but those discussed here appear to be the most often evaluated and the most useful.

Stage 3

Examination of the optic fundi should be performed with the infant supine on the table, on the parent's lap, or at times held over the parent's shoulder with the infant's head held tightly to the parent's head. Abnormalities of the fundi, including vascular changes, abnor-

malities of the optic disc, retinal changes, and abnormalities of the lens and media should be sought. Mydriatic agents are rarely needed, although sometimes both mydriatic agents and sedation are necessary. During the first few months of life the optic discs may be somewhat gray. This normal finding should not be confused with optic atrophy. Changes in the retina include chorioretinitis and retinitis pigmentosa. The discs may be hypoplastic or swollen.

The general portion of the examination follows. The presence of hepatosplenomegaly should be determined because many storage diseases, which also affect brain, may be the cause of organ enlargement. The anal sphincter should be examined for tone and the presence of an anal cutaneous reflex. Congenital anomalies of the genitalia should also be sought.

The remainder of the general examination, particularly the intrusive aspects, such as evaluating the auditory meati, tympanic membranes, mouth, and teeth, should be performed at this time.

Stage 4

If the child crawls, stands, or walks, the child should be placed on the floor. If the child crawls, the floor should be carpeted or a suitable pad should be provided. The child should be encouraged to crawl, walk, or run by rolling a ball across the room or sliding an object such as a block across the floor. Waddling, footdrop, limp, or ataxia may be evident. The manner in which the child stoops and bends to retrieve a ball or block may show premature hand dominance, athetosis, tremor, or weakness of the legs. The child should be observed when arising from the floor to a standing position to determine the presence of Gowers maneuver (see Figure 2-11).

The clinician should make every attempt to evaluate the child's gait to determine the presence of hemiparesis or ataxia (Chapter 17).

Unlike in the examination of adults, the testing of individual muscle groups in infants is usually impracticable. Nevertheless, both evaluation of spontaneous movements and use of some specific maneuvers (e.g., traction response, wheelbarrow maneuver, arising from the floor) will provide information about spasticity, weakness, and incoordination.

As is the case at all stages of childhood, a comparison of the examination findings must be made with expected norms.

Arm and shoulder strength can also be assessed using functional techniques depending on the level of development. The child is asked to lean against a wall with the legs placed a foot or two from the wall edge and the arms outstretched with the palms against the wall. Strength of the shoulder girdle and arm extension can be evaluated. Winging of the scapulas will also be evident. Alternatively, the child can be placed on the floor and asked to

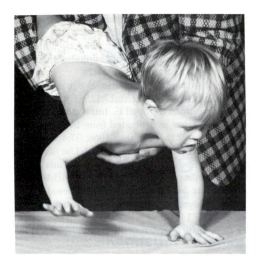

Figure 3-7 Abnormal parachute response. (Courtesy Division of Pediatric Neurology, University of Minnesota Medical School.)

"wheelbarrow" while the examiner holds the child's feet. Strength of the shoulder girdle and arms can be assessed by the parachute response, which in older children should lead into the wheelbarrow maneuver (Figure 3-7). Again, formal individual muscle testing can be used in the older child whenever necessary.

The sensory examination is difficult and is usually limited to rather gross evaluation of touch and pain; however, it can be accomplished with persistence and patience. Examination of touch, position sense, and vibration sense should be performed first. When a tuning fork is placed on the appropriate bony prominence, a look of surprise, usually of bemusement, appears. Evaluation of pain should be performed last and only after the examiner demonstrates to the child the method that will be used.

The child should be asked to stand in one place with the feet together and then asked to close the eyes to be evaluated for Romberg sign. The examiner should observe the child for titubation of the head, nystagmus, and dysmetria while reaching for objects. Finger-to-nose and finger-to-finger-to-nose tests while the eyes are closed are frequently accomplished in children older than the age of 3. The heel-to-shin test is frequently possible in children older than the age of 4. Depending on the maturity and abilities of the older infant, many of the maneuvers suggested in Chapter 2 for the child are applicable.

Further examination of muscle strength can be accomplished by using the parachute response; the examiner holds the child in the prone position over an examining table and thrusts the patient toward the table surface. A fully developed response at 8 months of age consists of arm extension and extension of the wrists, allowing the palms of the hands to make contact with the

table. The infant will support body weight with arms and shoulders. Each arm and shoulder can be tested individually if the opposite arm is pulled from the table by the examiner, forcing the child to support a majority of body weight on one arm and shoulder. A somewhat older infant may be induced to wheelbarrow and move forward on the hands, further demonstrating arm and shoulder strength. The child should be invited to crawl.

Assessment of the deep tendon reflexes is best performed with the child in a parent's or assistant's lap. The biceps response in most infants is difficult to elicit, but the triceps and brachyradialis reflexes are usually present. Patellar tendon and Achilles tendon responses are normally present and easy to elicit. Toe signs can be evaluated as in older children.

General considerations

Throughout the examination the clinician should evaluate the child's alertness, interest in the surroundings, and ability to learn during the examination. The child's speech pattern should also be assessed. By 15 months of age the child should have 2 to 6 spoken words, and by 18 months, 2 to 20 words. Short phrases consisting of 2 or 3 words are usually part of the child's repertoire by 21 to 24 months. By 2 years of age most children have a vocabulary of up to 50 words. Using specific scales to evaluate intelligence and development levels is of some help, but may not be altogether reliable. It is therefore important that the examiner become proficient in informal means of assessing these characteristics.

REFERENCES

Cupps C, Plescia MG, Houser C. The Landau reaction: a clinical and electromyographic analysis. Dev Med Child Neurol 1976; 18:41.

Dekaban A. Examination. In: Dekaban A, ed. Neurology of early childhood. Baltimore: Williams & Wilkins, 1970.

Dodge PR. Neurologic history and examination. In: Farmer TW, ed. Pediatric neurology. New York: Paul B. Hoeber, Medical Book Department of Harper & Brothers, 1964.

Echenne B, Rivier E. Benign paroxysmal tonic upward gaze. Pediatr Neurol 1992; 8:154.

Gesell A, Amatruda CS. Developmental diagnosis. New York: Paul B. Hoeber, Medical Books Department of Harper & Brothers, 1956.

Hogan GR, Milligan JE. The plantar reflex of the newborn. N Engl J Med 1971; 285:502.

Illingsworth RS. The development of the infant and young child, 5th ed. Baltimore: Williams & Wilkins, 1972.

Paine RS. Neurologic examination of infants and children. Pediatr Clin North Am 1960; 7:41.

Paine RS, Brazelton TB, Donovan DE. Evolution of postural reflexes in normal infants and in the presence of chronic brain syndromes. Neurology 1964; 14:1036.

Parmelee AH Jr. A critical evaluation of the Moro reflex. Pediatrics 1964; 33:773.

Popich GA, Smith DW. Fontanels: range of normal size. J Pediatr 1972; 80:749.

SOME NOTES ON TECHNIQUES OF ASSESSMENT OF NEUROLOGIC CRITERIA

POSTURE: Observed with infant quiet and in supine position. Score 0: Arms and legs extended; 1: beginning of flexion of hips and knees, arms extended; 2: stronger flexion of legs, arms extended; 3: arms slightly flexed, legs flexed and abducted; 4: full flexion of arms and legs.

SQUARE WINDOW: The hand is flexed on the forearm between the thumb and index finger of the examiner. Enough pressure is applied to get as full a flexion as possible, and the angle between the hypothenar eminence and the ventral aspect of the forearm is measured and graded according to diagram. (Care is taken not to rotate the infant's wrist while doing this maneuver.)

ANKLE DORSIFLEXION: The foot is dorsiflexed onto the anterior aspect of the leg, with the examiner's thumb on the sole of the foot and other fingers behind the leg. Enough pressure is applied to get as full flexion as possible, and the angle between the dorsum of the foot and the anterior aspect of the leg is measured.

ARM RECOIL: With the infant in the supine position the forearms are first flexed for 5 seconds, then fully extended by pulling on the hands, and then released. The sign is fully positive if the arms return briskly to full flexion (Score 2). If the arms return to incomplete flexion or the response is sluggish it is graded as Score 1. If they remain extended or are only followed by random movements the score is 0.

LEG RECOIL: With the infant supine, the hips and knees are fully flexed for 5 seconds, then extended by traction on the feet, and released. A maximal response is one of full flexion of the hips and knees (Score 2). A partial flexion scores 1, and minimal or no movement scores 0.

B

POPLITEAL ANGLE: With the infant supine and his pelvis flat on the examining couch, the thigh is held in the knee-chest position by the examiner's left index finger and thumb supporting the knee. The leg is then extended by gentle pressure from the examiner's right index finger behind the ankle and the popliteal angle is measured.

HEEL TO EAR MANEUVER: With the baby supine, draw the baby's foot as near to the head as it will go without forcing it. Observe the distance between the foot and the head as well as the degree of extension at the knee. Grade according to diagram. Note that the knee is left free and may draw down alongside the abdomen.

SCARF SIGN: With the baby supine, take the infant's hand and try to put it around the neck and as far posteriorly as possible around the opposite shoulder. Assist this maneuver by lifting the elbow across the body. See how far the elbow will go across and grade according to illustrations. Score 0: Elbow reaches opposite axillary line; 1: Elbow between midline and opposite axillary line; 2: Elbow reaches midline; 3: Elbow will not reach midline.

HEAD LAG: With the baby lying supine, grasp the hands (or the arms if a very small infant) and pull him slowly towards the sitting position. Observe the position of the head in relation to the trunk and grade accordingly. In a small infant the head may initially be supported by one hand. Score 0: Complete lag; 1: Partial head control; 2: Able to maintain head in line with body; 3: Brings head anterior to body.

VENTRAL SUSPENSION: The infant is suspended in the prone position, with examiner's hand under the infant's chest (one hand in a small infant, two in a large infant). Observe the degree of extension of the back and the amount of flexion of the arms and legs. Also note the relation of the head to the trunk. Grade according to diagrams.

If score differs on the two sides, take the mean.

Figure 5-1 cont'd For legend see p. 63.

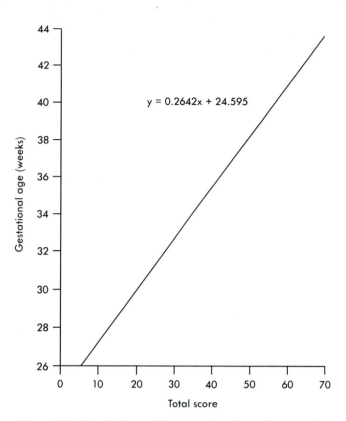

$$y = 0.2642x + 24.595$$

Figure 5-2 Graph for reading gestational age from total score. (Redrawn from Dubowitz LMS, Dubowitz V, Goldberg C. J Pediatr 1970; 77:1.)

evaluation was based on 10 neurologic and 11 external (e.g., skin texture, breast size, ear form) characteristics. The external evaluation was adapted from Farr et al. [1966a; 1966b]. The scoring scheme is detailed in Figures 5-1 and 5-2, as well as in Table 5-2 [Dubowitz et al., 1970].

Deep tendon reflex assessment

The assessment of deep tendon reflexes in preterm infants can be of value in the presence of many conditions (e.g., spinal cord anomalies, peripheral nerve injuries, congenital myopathies, infantile spinal muscular atrophy). A standard method of deep tendon reflex examination for preterm infants has been proposed [Kuban et al., 1986]. The methods of elicitation are listed in Table 5-3 and depicted in Figure 5-3 [Kuban et al., 1986]. In a study of preterm infants greater than 27 weeks postconceptional age the pectoralis major reflex was elicited in all, regardless of maturity. In 98% of the infants with greater than 33 weeks' gestation the achilles, patellar, biceps, thigh adductors, and brachioradialis reflexes were obtained. It is noteworthy that the infants with less than 33 weeks' gestation had decreased elicitation rates for patellar and bicep reflexes and had overall decreases in reflex intensity when compared with

their older counterparts. For all infants in the study, the following tendon reflexes were found to be present in decreasing order: finger flexors, jaw, crossed adductors, and triceps. Contrary to conventional wisdom, head position had no effect on the reflexes [Kuban et al., 1986].

Body attitude

During maturation, preterm infants adopt typical postures that correspond to gestational age. These postures have been charted and are very useful for evaluation of gestational age [Dubowitz et al., 1970; Dubowitz and Dubowitz, 1981].

Muscle tone

Assessment of muscle tone in the preterm infant is requisite to completion of a good neurologic evaluation [Amiel-Tison, 1968; Saint-Anne Dargassies, 1966]. The muscle tone of small-for-date infants differs from that of infants with only a short gestation.

At 26 to 28 weeks' gestation, the infant is extremely hypotonic. When held by the examiner in vertical suspension, the infant will not extend his or her head, limbs, or trunk (Figure 5-4). The change from the hypotonia of the preterm infant to the flexion posture of the term infant is manifest first in the legs and then in the arms and head. At 34 weeks' gestation, the infant lies in the frogleg position while supine; the legs are flexed at the hip and knee, but the arms remain extended and relatively hypotonic (Figure 5-5).

Measurement of various limb angles offers some objective evidence for the degree of tone. The popliteal angle, measured by maximum extension of the leg at the knee with the hip fully flexed, decreases from 180 degrees at 28 weeks (Figure 5-6) to less than 90 degrees at term. Similarly, the adductor angle of the hip and dorsiflexion angle of the foot diminish to almost 0 degrees at term (Figure 5-7).

During the traction maneuver, the head lags considerably with little resistance until after 30 weeks' gestation. The head extensors develop gradually, followed by the flexors. By 38 weeks, the head follows the trunk, is maintained briefly, and then falls forward when the infant is pulled from a supine to a sitting position during the traction maneuver.

In small preterm infants the scarf sign, which is elicited by folding the arm across the chest toward the opposite shoulder, is present if the elbow reaches the opposite shoulder (Figure 5-8). It is noteworthy that in term infants the elbow cannot be brought beyond the midline.

The extreme hypotonia of preterm infants permits the legs to be flexed at the hip so that the heel can be passively brought to the side of the face (heel-to-ear maneuver). Understandably, this positioning is re-

Table 5-2 Scoring system for external criteria

External sign	Score*				
	0	1	2	3	4
Edema	Obvious edema of hands and feet; pitting over tibia	No obvious edema of hands and feet; pitting over tibia	No edema		
Skin texture	Very thin, gelatinous	Thin and smooth	Smooth; medium thickness; rash or superficial peeling	Slight thickening; superficial cracking and peeling especially of hands and feet	Thick and parchment like; superficial or deep cracking
Skin color	Dark red	Uniformly pink	Pale pink; variable over body	Pale; only pink over ears, lips, palms, or soles	
Skin opacity (trunk)	Numerous veins and venules clearly seen, especially over abdomen	Veins and tributaries seen	A few large vessels clearly seen over abdomen	A few large vessels seen indistinctly over abdomen	No blood vessels seen
Lanugo (over back)	No lanugo	Abundant; long and thick over whole back	Hair thinning especially over lower back	Small amount of lanugo and bald areas	At least half of back devoid of lanugo
Plantar creases	No skin creases	Faint red marks over anterior half of sole	Definite red marks over > anterior half; indentatons over < anterior third	Indentations over > anterior third	Definite deep indentations over > anterior third
Nipple formation	Nipple barely visible; no areola	Nipple well defined; areola smooth and flat, diameter < 0.75 cm	Areola stippled, edge not raised, diameter < 0.75 cm	Areola stippled, edge raised, diameter > 0.75 cm	
Breast size	No breast tissue palpable	Breast tissue on one or both sides, < 0.5 cm diameter	Breast tissue both sides; one or both 0.5 to 1.0 cm	Breast tissue both sides; one or both > 1 cm	
Ear form	Pinna flat and shapeless, little or no incurving of edge	Incurving of part of edge of pinna	Partial incurving whole of upper pinna	Well-defined incurving whole of upper pinna	
Ear firmness	Pinna soft, easily folded, no recoil	Pinna soft, easily folded, slow recoil	Cartilage to edge of pinna, but soft in places, ready recoil	Pinna firm, cartilage to edge; instant recoil	
Genitals					
Male	Neither testis in scrotum	At least one testis high in scrotum	At least one testis right down		
Female (with hips half abducted)	Labia majora widely separated, labia minora protruding	Labia majora almost cover labia minora	Labia majora completely cover labia minora		

From Dubowitz LMS, Dubowitz V, Goldberg C. J Pediatr 1970; 77:1.
*If score differs on two sides, take the mean.

Table 5-3 Deep tendon reflexes evaluated in premature babies

Deep tendon reflexes	Innervation	Technique of elicitation
Jaw	Cranial nerves V and VII	The point of the finger is placed over the chin so that the jaw is slightly open. The hammer strikes the index finger tip.
Pectoralis major	Predominantly C_7 and C_8, lateral pectoral nerve	The examiner's index finger is firmly placed in a caudad (or cephalad) direction onto the axilla over the pectoralis major.
Biceps	C_5 and C_6, musculocutaneous nerve	The examiner's index finger is placed onto the biceps tendon in the superomedial aspect of the antecubital fossa with the arm flexed at the elbow.
Brachioradialis	C_5, C_6, radial nerve	The tendon of the muscle is struck directly over the distal third of the radius while slowly flexing and extending the arm.
Triceps	C_7, C_8, radial nerve	The examiner's finger is placed over the triceps tendon at its distal aspect proximal to the elbow. The triceps tendon also may be struck directly while flexing and extending the arm.
Finger flexors	C_8, T_1, median nerve	The examiner's finger is placed horizontally across the base of the infant's fingers to elicit a partial grasp. The examiner's finger is then struck.
Patellar	L_3, L_4, femoral nerve	The reflex hammer strikes examiner's finger placed across the patellar tendon, or the latter is struck directly while flexing and extending the leg at the knee.
Thigh adductors and crossed adductors	L_3, L_4, obturator nerve	The examiner's index finger to be struck is placed diagonally across the medial aspect at the knee (thigh adductor) with the little finger placed on the contralateral leg to maintain a 45- to 60-degree angle (crossed adductor).
Achilles	L_5, S_1, tibial nerve	The examiner's finger to be struck is placed horizontally across the plantar aspect of the infant's foot, which is partially dorsiflexed.

From Kuban KCK, Skouteli HN, Urion DK, et al. Pediatr Neurol 1986; 2:266.

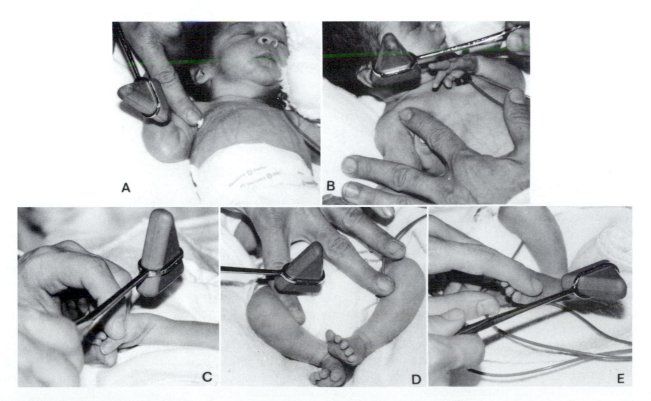

Figure 5-3 Elicitation of deep-tendon reflexes in a premature infant of 32 weeks' gestation. **A** and **B,** Pectoralis major; **C,** brachioradialis; **D,** thigh adductors and crossed adductors; and **E,** Achilles. (From Kuban KCK, Skouteli HN, Urion DK, et al. Pediatr Neurol 1986; 2:226.)

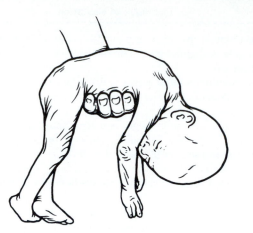

Figure 5-4 Premature baby, 30 weeks' gestation. Note the hypotonic posture with lack of extension of the spine and head and lack of flexion of the extremities.

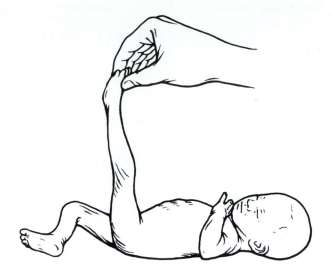

Figure 5-6 The popliteal angle is 180 degrees in a 30 weeks' gestation premature infant.

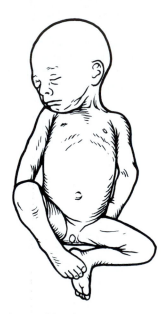

Figure 5-5 Frogleg position in a premature infant of 31 weeks gestation, 2 weeks' after birth.

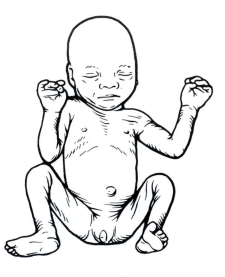

Figure 5-7 A premature infant of 30 weeks' gestation. The adductor angle of the thighs is almost 180 degrees.

stricted in the older infant because of increasing tone (Figure 5-9).

Tone may also be monitored while postural and righting reflexes are assessed. During the stepping maneuver, the 28-week preterm infant will not support weight (Figure 5-10). However, over the next few weeks there is gradual support of weight, and by 34 weeks a good supporting response is present. Tremors and even clonic movements are manifest in the small preterm infant but are not normally discernible after 32 weeks' gestation. Stretching movements of the limbs are common in small preterm infants while they are awake but somewhat less common during sleep. These movements may spread to include the trunk and head.

Cranial nerves

Some features of the preterm infant examination are different than features of the older infant's examination. Head position is unpredictable in the small preterm infant, but, by 35 weeks' gestation, there is a preference for the head to be held to the right. By 39 weeks' gestation the head is held to the right approximately 80% of the time while the infant is at rest [Gardner et al., 1977].

The small preterm infant may cry in response to provocation [Fenichel, 1978], but crying often occurs when the infant is unprovoked. By 36 to 37 weeks' gestation, the cry is more vigorous, frequent, persistent, and is easily elicited by noxious stimuli.

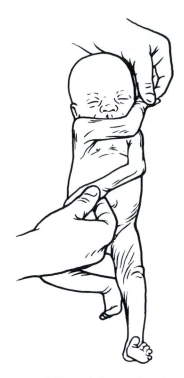

Figure 5-8 Infant of 32 weeks' gestation showing "scarf sign," with the elbow approximating the opposite shoulder.

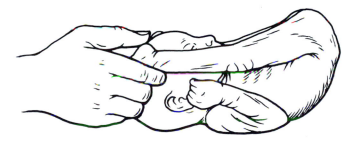

Figure 5-9 Diminished tone in the very small 30 weeks' gestation premature infant allows the heels to reach the head easily. The pelvis should be flat on the table.

The pupillary light reflex is absent before 29 to 30 weeks, and in the resting state the infant's pupils are usually meiotic. The reflex becomes progressively evident and is mature by 32 weeks.

Although they may forcefully close their eyes when a bright light is directed toward them, infants of 28 weeks' gestation or less will not turn in the direction of the light. By using a large target (a large red ball, hoop, or a handful of yarn), visual fixation and even rudimentary scanning and tracking may be evident in infants of 31 to 32 weeks' gestation [Hack et al., 1976]. Associated with this, there may be widening of the palpebral fissure. By 36 to 38 weeks' gestation, the infant rotates the head toward a light and closes the eyes forcefully when a strong light stimulus is presented.

The doll's eye reflex is elicited in the 28- to 32-week

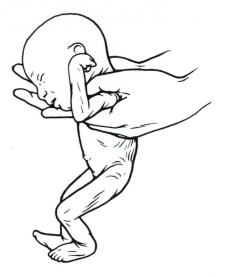

Figure 5-10 Premature infant of 30 weeks' gestation supports his weight briefly. Toe-walking may be evident.

preterm infant who has no compromise of consciousness. The ease of eliciting a response is enhanced because infants do not visually fixate. Later (by 36 weeks' gestation), this response is not elicited in the normal infant.

Developmental reflexes

Observation and description of the major reflex changes peculiar to the preterm infant have been undertaken by many authors [Amiel-Tison, 1968; Lubchenco, 1970; Saint-Anne Dargassies, 1966; Fenichel, 1985] (Table 5-4).

The rooting and sucking reflexes in small preterm infants are perfunctory but become vigorous by 34 weeks. The Moro reflex, first present in fragmentary form at 24 weeks, is well developed by 28 weeks, although it fatigues easily and lacks a complete adduction phase. Not until 38 weeks' gestation is the entire response characteristic of the term infant observed.

At 28 weeks, the grasp reflex is evident just in the fingers; by 32 weeks the palm and fingers participate. Slightly later contraction of the muscles of the shoulder girdle and elbows occurs during the traction maneuver when the infant is pulled from a supine to a sitting position.

The tonic reflex is elicited by turning of the head to one side. The arm on the side to which the head is turned extends and the other arm flexes. The legs may follow suit, but the response is often absent or subtle. This "fencing" position often can be elicited in the 35-week preterm infant.

The crossed-extensor reflex is obtained by stroking the sole of one foot while holding the leg firmly in extension. The response occurs in the opposite leg and comprises rapid flexion at the hips and knees with

Table 5-4 Neurologic maturation

Function	26 weeks	30 weeks	34 weeks	38 weeks
Resting posture	Flexion of arms Flexion or extension of legs	Flexion of arms Flexion or extension of legs	Flexion of all limbs	Flexion of all limbs
Arousal	Unable to maintain	Maintain briefly	Remain awake	Remain awake
Rooting	Absent	Long latency	Present	Present
Sucking	Absent	Long latency	Weak	Vigorous
Pupillary reflex	Absent	Variable	Present	Present
Traction	No response	No response	Head lag	Mild head lag
Moro	No response	Extension; no adduction	Adduction variable	Complete
Withdrawal	Absent	Withdrawal only	Crossed extension	Crossed extension

From Fenichel GM. The neurological consultation. In: Fenichel GM, ed. Neonatal neurology. 2nd ed. New York: Churchill Livingstone, 1985.

attendant withdrawal, followed by extension, adduction, and fanning of the toes. The complete response, elicited at about 36 weeks, is informative when asymmetric. Otherwise, it only establishes that some degree of primitive function is present.

The stepping response (automatic walking) can be induced by resting the infant's soles on a mattress and rocking the infant gently from one foot to the other and is usually present by 37 weeks' gestation.

This procedure usually initiates a walking sequence, which is facilitated by the examiner supporting the infant's weight and tilting the infant forward. The preterm infant usually walks on his or her toes, whereas the term infant uses a heel-to-toe sequence. The response is manifest at 32 to 34 weeks' gestation.

Ongoing neurologic examinations of the preterm infant are most important for the assessment of development and neurologic status. When the preterm infant reaches the equivalent of 40 weeks' gestation, the neurologic examination's results are not the same as those of a term newborn [Illingworth, 1972]. The preterm infant continues toe-walking and, even at 40 weeks', manifests relative hypotonia, incomplete dorsiflexion of the foot, and a greater popliteal angle when compared with the term newborn. Because the preterm infant at 40 weeks' gestation lies with relatively less elevation of the pelvis, the prone-body profile is flatter than that of the term newborn (Figure 5-11).

ASSESSMENT OF HEAD GROWTH PATTERNS

It is essential to measure and plot growth data to facilitate early detection of abnormal patterns. The shape of the head changes markedly with growth in preterm infants. The ratio of anteroposterior diameter to biparietal diameter increases rapidly in preterm infants during the first few months of life [Baum and Searls, 1971].

There are known differences between the extrauterine body growth patterns of preterm infants and the extrauterine body growth patterns of the term infant

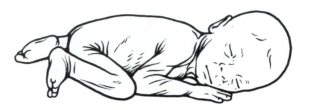

Figure 5-11 Prone 32-week premature infant. Hips are abducted, and pelvis is low.

[Babson et al., 1970; Gardner and Pearson, 1971; Lubchenco et al., 1966; Usher and McLean, 1969]. The occipitofrontal circumference of preterm infants often shrinks during the first few days of life. Expected patterns of extrauterine head growth are reasonably well documented, making diagnosis of hydrocephalus or microcephaly in the preterm infant possible. It is essential that frequent serial occipitofrontal circumference measurements be obtained to allow early diagnosis. A standard plotting curve must be used to monitor head growth in the preterm infant. A useful standard plot is depicted in Figure 5-12 [Babson and Benda, 1976]. Conventional symptoms and signs of hydrocephalus are not immediately evident even though the presence of ventricular dilatation is documented with imaging techniques [Korobkin, 1975; Volpe et al., 1977].

The presence of certain characteristics should alert the clinician to the presence of hydrocephalus [Sher, 1982], such as full fontanel with separation of the cranial sutures, abnormally high rate of occipitofrontal circumference increase, frontal bossing, scaphocephaly, and increased ratio of head size to body length.

The preterm infant's state of health is a major determinant of head growth [Sher and Brown, 1975a; 1975b]. Mean occipitofrontal circumferences for small and large, healthy, preterm infants, as well as sick infants, are graphed [Sher and Brown, 1975a] for comparison with the data of O'Neill [1961]. Irrespective of gestational age, sick infants were designated as those who

GROWTH RECORD FOR INFANTS
in relation to
GESTATIONAL AGE AND FETAL AND INFANT NORMS
(combined sexes)

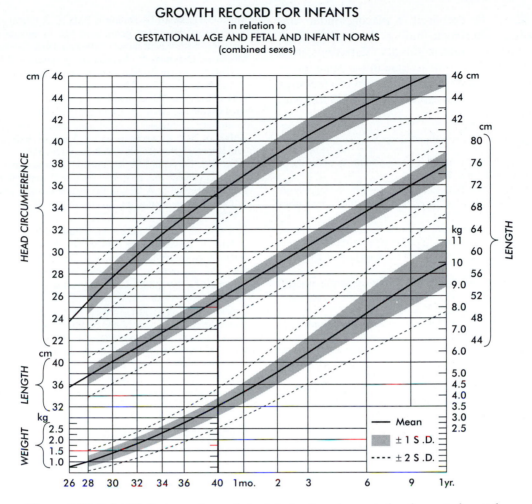

Figure 5-12 A fetal-infant growth graph for infants of varying gestational ages to be used for plotting growth from birth until 1 year of age after "term" has been reached.   From Babson SB, Benda GI. J Pediatr 1989; 89:814-20.

were maintained with mechanical ventilation and intravenous therapy for varying lengths of time up to 2 weeks [Sher and Brown, 1975a; 1975b]. Infants with easily correctable metabolic abnormalities or minimal degrees of hyperbilirubinemia not requiring exchange transfusion were excluded from the sick group.

On the basis of that study [Sher and Brown, 1975a; 1975b] some conclusions are possible [Sher, 1982]:

The rate of occipitofrontal circumference increase in the healthy preterm infant is approximately double (1.1 cm/week) that of the term infant in the first and second months after delivery.

The rate of occipitofrontal circumference in the healthy preterm infant is approximately equal (0.5 cm/week) to that of the term infant in the third and fourth months.

The average rate of occipitofrontal circumference for ill preterm infants is 0.25 cm/week for the first 3 months.

Preterm infants with a short gestation have more rapid rates of occipitofrontal circumference increase than those infants with longer gestation.

Preterm infants with rates of occipitofrontal circumference increase greater than the expected rate should be evaluated for the presence of hydrocephalus.

Preterm infants who are healthy and who fail to achieve the least expected rate of occipitofrontal circumference increase may have intrinsic brain disease.

When comparisons are made based on postconceptional age, the occipitofrontal circumference of preterm infants is greater than that of the term infant, at least for the first 5 postnatal months [Fujimura et al., 1977]. The maximum velocity of head growth in healthy, preterm infants with good caloric intake occurs shortly postpartum and decreases thereafter.

The prognosis for normal development of low birth weight infants is much better since the advent of focused obstetrical practices related to the preterm infant and neonatal intensive care units [Hutson et al., 1986; Kitchen and Murton, 1985]. The clinician must be cognizant of the normal, rapid rate of head growth and avoid unnecessary procedures designed to diagnose hydrocephalus.

Caution should be exercised in placing undue emphasis on isolated neurologic findings that deviate from expected findings in preterm infants. Variations from infant to infant and from time to time in the same infant are common. The infant's general pattern of responses should weigh heavily in the assessment of CNS integrity at any one moment.

REFERENCES

Amiel-Tison C. Neurologic evaluation of the maturity of newborn infants. Arch Dis Child 1968; 43:89.

Babson SC, Behrman RE, Lessel R. Fetal growth: liveborn birth weights for gestational age of white middle class infants. Pediatrics 1970; 45:937.

Babson SG, Benda GI. Growth graphs for the clinical assessment of infants of varying gestational age. J Pediatr 1976; 89:814.

Baum JD, Searls D. Head shape and size of newborn infants. Dev Med Child Neurol 1971; 13:576.

Cruz-Martinez A, Ferrer MT, Martin MJ. Motor conduction velocity and H-reflex in prematures with very short gestational age. Electromyogr Clin Neurophysiol 1983; 23:13.

Dubowitz L, Dubowitz V, Goldberg C. Clinical assessment of gestational age in the newborn infant. J Pediatr 1970; 77:1.

Dubowitz L, Dubowitz V. The neurological assessment. In: Dubowitz L, Dubowitz V, eds. The neurological assessment of the preterm and full-term newborn infant. Clin Dev Med 1981; 79:35.

Dubowitz W, Whittaker GF, Brown BH, et al. Nerve conduction velocity: an index of neurological maturity of the newborn infant. Dev Med Child Neurol 1968; 10:741.

Farr V, Kerridge DF, Mitchell RG. The definition of some external characteristics used in the assessment of gestational age in the newborn infant. Dev Med Child Neurol 1966a; 8:507.

Farr W, Kerridge DF, Mitchell RG. The value of some external characteristics in the assessment of gestational age at birth. Dev Med Child Neurol 1966b; 8:657.

Fenichel GM. Neurological assessment of the 25 to 30 week premature infant. Ann Neurol 1978; 4:92.

Fenichel GM. The neurological consultation. In: Fenichel GM, ed. Neonatal neurology, 2nd ed. New York: Churchill Livingstone, 1985.

Fujimura M, Seryu JI. Velocity of head growth during the prenatal period. Arch Dis Child 1977; 52:105.

Gardner D, Pearson J. A growth chart for premature and other infants. Arch Dis Child 1971; 46:783.

Gardner J, et al. Development of postural asymmetry in premature human infants. Dev Psychobiol 1977; 10:471.

Hack M, Mostow A, Miranda SB. Development of attention in preterm infants. Pediatrics 1976; 58:669.

Hutson JM, Driscoll JM, Fox HE, et al. The effect of obstetric management on neonatal mortality and morbidity for infants weighing 700-1000 grams. Am J Perinatol 1986; 3:255.

Illingworth RS. The development of the infant and young child. 5th ed, Baltimore: Williams & Wilkins, 1972.

Kitchen WH, Murton LJ. Survival rates of infants with birth weights between 501 and 1,000 gm: improvement by excluding certain categories of cases. Am J Dis Child 1985; 139:470.

Korobkin R. The relationship between head circumference and the development of communicating hydrocephalus following intraventricular hemorrhage. Pediatrics 1975; 56:74.

Kuban KCK, Skouteli HN, Urion DK, et al. Deep tendon reflexes in premature infants. Pediatr Neurol 1986; 2:266.

Lubchenco LO. Assessment of gestational age and development at birth. Pediatr Clin North Am 1970; 17:125.

Lubchenco LO, Hansman M, Boyd E. Intrauterine growth in length and head circumference as estimated from live births at gestational ages from 26 to 42 weeks. Pediatrics 1966; 37:403.

Miller G, Heckmatt JZ, Dubowitz LMS, et al. Use of nerve conduction velocity to determine gestational age in infants at risk and in very-low-birth-weight infants. J Pediatr 1983; 103:109.

Moosa A, Dubowitz V. Assessment of gestational age in newborn infants: nerve conduction velocity versus maturity score. Dev Med Child Neurol 1972; 14:290.

O'Neill E. Normal head growth and prediction of head size in infantile hydrocephalus. Arch Dis Child 1961; 36:241.

Saint-Anne Dargassies S. Neurologic maturation of the premature infant of 28 to 41 weeks' gestational age. In: Falkner F, ed. Human development. Philadelphia: WB Saunders, 1966.

Scher MS, Barmada MA. Estimation of gestational age by electrographic, clinical, and anatomic criteria. Pediatr Neurol 1987; 3:256.

Sher PK, Brown S. A longitudinal study of head growth in preterm infants. I. Normal rates of head growth. Dev Med Child Neurol 1975a; 17:705.

Sher PK, Brown S. A longitudinal study of head growth in preterm infants. II. Differentiation between "catch-up" head growth and early infantile hydrocephalus. Dev Med Child Neurol 1975b; 17:711.

Sher PK. Neurologic examination of the premature infant. In: Swaiman KF, Wright FS, eds. The practice of pediatric neurology. St. Louis: Mosby, 1982.

Usher R, McLean F. Intrauterine growth of liveborn caucasian infants at sea level: standard obtained from infants born between 24 and 44 weeks' gestation. J Pediatr 1969; 74:901.

Volpe JJ. Neurology of the newborn, 2nd ed. Philadelphia: WB Saunders, 1987.

Volpe JJ, Pasternak JF, Allan WC. Ventricular dilation preceding rapid head growth following neonatal intracranial hemorrhage. Am J Dis Child 1977; 131:1212.

SUGGESTED READINGS

Bacola E, et al. Perinatal and environmental factors in late neurogenic sequelae. I. Infants having birth weights under 1,500 grams. Am J Dis Child 1966a; 112:359.

Bacola E, et al. Perinatal and environmental factors in late neuro-genic sequelae. II. Infants having birth weights from 1,500 to 2,500 grams. Am J Dis Child 1966b; 112:369.

Critchley EM. The neurological examination of neonates. J Neurol Sci 1968; 7:427.

Crosse VM. The premature baby, 4th ed. London: J & A Churchill, 1957.

Cruise MO. A longitudinal study of the growth of low birth weight infants. I. Velocity and distance growth, birth to 3 years. Pediatrics 1973; 51:620.

Dekaban A. Examination. In: Dekaban A, ed. Neurology of early childhood. Baltimore: Williams & Wilkins, 1970.

Dodge PR. Neurologic history and examination. In: Farmer TW, ed. Pediatric neurology. New York: Harper & Brothers, 1964.

Dubowitz W, Whittaker GF, Brown BH, et al. Nerve conduction velocity: an index of neurological maturity of the newborn infant. Dev Med Child Neurol 1968; 10:741.

Farr V, Kerridge DF, Mitchell RG. The value of some external characteristics in the assessment of gestational age at birth. Dev Med Child Neurol 1966; 8:657.

Rawlings G, Reynolds EOR, Stewart A, et al. Changing prognosis for infants of very low birth weight. Lancet 1971; 1:516.

Robinson RJ. Assessment of gestational age by neurologic examination. Arch Dis Child 1966; 41:437.

Saint-Anne Dargassies S. Long-term neurological follow-up study of 286 truly premature infants. Dev Med Child Neurol 1977; 19:462.

Volpe JJ. The neurological examination: normal and abnormal features. Neurology of the newborn, 2nd ed. In: Markowitz M, ed. Major problems in clinical pediatrics, vol 22. Philadelphia: WB Saunders, 1987.

Part Two

Laboratory Evaluation

6

Pediatric Electroencephalography and Evoked Potentials

Mark S. Scher

Clinical neurophysiologic studies are an integral part of the diagnostic evaluation of the pediatric patient with suspected CNS dysfunction. EEG and evoked potential analyses comprise most of these diagnostic tests. The pediatric neurologist must acquire an understanding of the clinical relevance of these studies. It is vital that neurologists appreciate the importance of proper instrumentation and recording technique to obtain a reliable pediatric EEG study, either in the setting of the EEG laboratory or at the child's bedside.

The first section of this discussion acquaints those with limited experience in EEG with the techniques of recording and with interpretation of electrocortical phenomena unique to the child. The neurologist must appreciate how to apply EEG studies to the evaluation of the child in the context of a specific clinical situation. Both changes in age and state of arousal of the patient emphasize the broad limits of normality, as outlined in the second section of this discussion. The third section describes examples of abnormal EEG patterns in the context of common pediatric neurologic disorders [Hrakovy, 1990]. The final section is devoted to computer applications for the analysis of spontaneous EEG and evoked potential data.

The neurologist must understand the analytic steps involved in interpreting EEG or evoked potential studies. Proper application ultimately requires the following two essential elements of teaching beyond the scope of this brief discussion: (1) presentation of multiple examples of the same neurophysiologic phenomena and (2) use of both typical and atypical clinical situations in which common and complex electrographic patterns are noted. Several excellent reviews can supplement this discussion and assist the physician with the evaluation of patients who exhibit these phenomena [Hrakovy, 1990; Werner, 1991; Cracco, 1986; Blume,

1982; Tharp, 1981; Niedermeyer, 1987; and Lopes da Silva, 1981].

Proper application of EEG and evoked potentials necessitates an understanding of the limitations and benefits of these studies. These tests only supplement proper history-taking and physical examination techniques, which comprise the clinical diagnostic process. Overinterpretation of data without consideration of the clinical situation must be avoided. The neurologist must always exercise clinical judgment in the context of the individual patient before relying on the results of any laboratory test.

INSTRUMENTATION AND RECORDING TECHNIQUES

Each channel on the EEG measures the electropotential difference between two points on the scalp under the assigned electrodes. Ten electrodes are required as a minimum number for adequate EEG recordings [American EEG Society Guidelines, 1986]. A greater area of cerebral activity can be measured with more channels of EEG. EEG laboratories devoted to pediatric studies should use 16 to 24 channels. In the neonate, it may be more practical to apply fewer electrodes, as will be discussed below. The International 10-20 System of electrode placement is the standard method of electrode application and routinely requires the placement of 22 electrodes on the head. The basis of the 10-20 system begins with measurements of the following four standard points on the head: the nasion, inion, and left and right preauricular points [Holmes, 1987]. The electrodes are spaced at either 10% or 20% of the total distance between pairs of skull landmarks. These scalp locations correspond to anatomic landmarks. The electrode names correspond to the underlying brain regions over which they are positioned. Electrodes with odd numbers correspond to regions in the left hemisphere, whereas even numbers refer to the areas in the right hemisphere. Midline electrodes have a zero ("z") as a suffix. Additional electrodes may be used to localize electrical activity. Readjustment of the electrode placements may be required for preterm neonates and for patients with skull deformities.

Silver-silver chloride electrodes are the most commonly used electrode. Application to the scalp is achieved with either paste or collodion. Needle electrodes are no longer recommended. A qualified, well-trained electrodiagnostic technologist is critical to ensure proper application, particularly with the child. Careful but rapid placement of electrodes is obviously helpful to the success of the study. The *electrode arrays,* or *montages,* refer to the combination of electrodes examined at any particular point in time. There are principally two types of channel relationships. Bipolar recordings measure electrocortical activity between two active brain areas. Referential recordings compare a reference, or neutral electrode, with an active electrode. The neutral electrode is usually placed on the ear or mastoid. Another common referential montage is the average referential recording. Activity from all available electrodes is averaged and compared with any one electrode.

There are both advantages and disadvantages with each recording technique. For instance, bipolar recordings permit better localization of electrographic phenomena, whereas referential recordings better display EEG patterns that have widespread distribution. The technologist should perform each recording using a variety of montages. Both important maturational patterns and abnormal features in pediatric EEG can be best displayed using multiple montage displays.

Polarity-localization

Proper use of electrode placement and montage choice allows accurate comparisons between homologous brain regions. In this way the neurologist can localize EEG data on an anatomic basis and can also standardize regional or hemispheric findings over multiple EEG recordings. An understanding of the principles of polarity is essential to use the localization technique.

The inputs of the two electrodes for one EEG channel are generated by two differential amplifiers, termed *input terminal one* and *input terminal two.* With a differential amplifier, the output is proportional to the voltage difference between these two input terminals. The direction of the pen deflection depends on differences in polarity of this voltage difference. By convention, when input terminal one is relatively more negative, there is an upward deflection in the pen. Other

possibilities follow, such as a downward deflection if input terminal one is relatively more positive. The reverse situation pertains to input terminal two; therefore when input terminal two is relatively more negative, there is a downward deflection [Cooper et al., 1980].

An EEG waveform in a particular location is assumed to arise from an electrical dipole within the brain. This hypothetic dipole arises from a group of neurons whose dendritic processes are oriented perpendicular to the scalp. An electrical field is represented on the scalp, with the maximum voltage potential near the center and decreasing levels of voltage denoted by concentric rings that successively enlarge from this central point. Most abnormal electrographic potentials are represented by a dipole with the negative end toward the surface and the positive end inward. Depending on the particular orientation of the dipole in relation to the surface, its field representation on the scalp has different shapes. On occasion in pediatric EEGs, surface positive waveforms are noted, such as the positive sharp waves in newborn recordings and the dipole represented on the scalp in patients with rolandic epilepsy.

Given the common practice of comparing groups of electrodes in a linear fashion, the amplitude and polarity expressed for each electrode in a bipolar recording may demonstrate a phase reversal in adjacent electrodes. This reversal is represented by a simultaneous pen deflection in opposite directions in two adjacent bipolar channels. By this technique the electroencephalographer can localize focal EEG phenomena as long as sources of artifact are not suspected. For accurate localization, two linear electrode arrays at right angles to each other should intersect through the region to be examined. This technique can effectively localize most waveforms that are considered to have vertical dipoles in relation to the scalp.

Instrumental control settings

Each EEG recording must clearly indicate all instrumental settings at the beginning of the study. Any adjustments in sensitivity, paper speed, or filter settings must be marked. Calibration signals should both begin and conclude the recordings to indicate to the electroencephalographer how the amplifier and pen-writing apparatus respond to all instrumental settings.

Sensitivity settings

Sensitivity settings should begin with the standard 7 μV/mm position and be adjusted accordingly throughout the record. Lower sensitivities (i.e., ≥ 10) are used for higher amplitude signals in which the pens block and do not reflect maximum amplitude. Higher sensitivities (< 7 μV/mm) are needed when lower amplitude signals do not cause sufficient pen deflection.

Filter settings

Both high- and low-frequency filters are required to allow accurate representation of the appropriate range of frequency-specific waveforms of cerebral origin. Adjustment of these filters should be made judiciously so that genuine brain-generated activities are not eliminated along with undesirable, noncerebral artifactual signals. High-frequency filters are set at a standard 70 Hz so as not to blunt the appearance of fast frequencies, including abnormal spike-and-sharp waves. On an exceptional basis, lower settings may be needed when excessive fast-frequency artifacts exist, such as 60-cycle interference from other electrical devices. Lower frequency filter settings, commonly referred to as *time constants*, routinely vary between 0.3 and 0.1. For situations when slow-frequency waveforms need to be analyzed or eliminated, longer or shorter time constants, respectively, can be chosen. This procedure is particularly important in EEG recordings of neonates and young infants, in whom slower frequency activities need to be clearly represented.

Paper speed

The conventional 30 mm/sec paper speed is selected unless specific clinical situations require that the paper record be compressed or elongated to examine better the electrical phenomena. Slower speeds are recommended for newborn recordings and polysomnographic sessions, in which slowly occurring activity can be compressed for easier analysis. Faster speeds can assist occasionally in identifying 60-cycle interference and in distinguishing muscle potentials from spikes of cerebral origin.

Physiologic noncerebral channels

Important information can be derived from recording muscle movement, respiratory activity, eye movement, and cardiac activity. These monitors can assist in defining specific portions of the sleep cycle. Noncerebral physiologic observations, such as respiratory pauses or cardiac arrhythmias, may have relevance to the clinical problem that prompted the request for an EEG study. Sleep state–dependent apnea and congenital heart block are two clinical situations in which noncerebral physiologic monitoring can be crucial to the diagnosis. Finally, important sources of artifact can be more readily identified and eliminated by using noncerebral monitors; thus cerebral activity can be more accurately displayed.

Artifact recognition

As with adults [Brenner, 1981; Richey and Norman, 1976], physiologic and nonphysiologic artifacts must be properly identified in pediatric recordings because either may interfere with the interpretation of cerebral activity. The following three basic forms of artifacts have been classified: instrumental, external, and physiologic. Accurate descriptions by the technologist can assist the neurologist in the diagnosis of a neurologic disorder in adults [Klass and Reiher, 1965], children [Blume, 1982], and neonates [Scher, 1985] (Figure 6-1). Such artifacts may help define normal and abnormal sleep and waking behavior. The technologist should not only try to identify the source of any artifacts but initially reproduce them and then attempt to eliminate those artifacts that were identified during the recording.

Recording setting

The pediatric EEG laboratory should be within easy access to both inpatients and outpatients. Technologists must be able to travel rapidly to areas within the medical facility, to perform portable EEG studies in the emergency room, intensive care unit, or the patient's hospital room.

To obtain quality recordings, effort must be made to elicit the child's most cooperative behavior. A well-illuminated, neatly organized room with a friendly decor will assist in preparing the child. Ample time should be arranged for proper electrode application and recording. It is highly recommended to obtain unmedicated, awake, drowsy, and natural sleep recordings on all children. Despite the special challenge provided by the infant and young toddler, it is possible to obtain quality tracings without the use of sedative medications.

Approximately 1% of children may require sedation. Chloral hydrate, 50 to 80 mg/kg, is most commonly used and should only be administered to a child who has not been recently fed. Psychotropic or sedative drugs should be avoided because they produce more profound behavioral and EEG effects. Infant recordings should be obtained around a scheduled feeding or naptime. At least 90 minutes should be scheduled for electrode application, EEG recording, and clean-up. With some exceptions, the parents' presence during the recording session should be discouraged. The technologist should accurately record the pertinent clinical history of the child that explains the reason for obtaining the EEG study. Information from parents and/or the medical record should include the child's age; gestational and postconceptional ages should be included for a neonatal patient. The physician who ordered the study should be identified, and the written request for an EEG study should clearly state the clinical problem that prompted the EEG request.

Notations by the technologist of the recording conditions must include the state of arousal and cooperation of the patient. Skull defects, vital signs, pertinent laboratory studies, and medications should be listed because each may affect the technical recording and clinical correlation of the EEG recording. For instance,

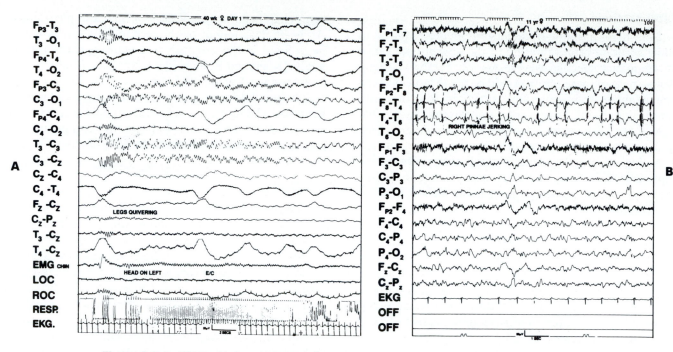

Figure 6-1 A, EEG of infant of 40 weeks' gestation, 1 day after birth, with severe asphyxia secondary to a ruptured vilamentous cord with exsanguination. Background activity is markedly suppressed with superimposed physiologic artifact from excessive tremulousness. Readjustment of the patient's head lessened this artifact. **B,** An 11-year-old girl with brainstem encephalitis. On neurologic examination the right pinnae displayed myoclonic movements. Myogenic potentials on EEG (in the region of the right temporal area, T_4) represent the segmental myoclonus noted on examination. (**A** from Scher MS. Am J EEG Technol 1985; 25:257). (**B** Courtesy Dr. P. Crumrine, Pittsburgh, Pennsylvania).

a cephalohematoma, hypothermic state, or barbituate overdose may all attenuate the EEG activity on a regional or bihemispheric distribution but have dramatically different clinical interpretations.

Frequent and accurate annotations by the technologist must describe changes in state throughout the spontaneous and activation portions of the record. Passive or active eye opening and closure are essential, and repositioning of the patient may be required to eliminate or minimize artifacts. Most importantly, consensual validation of suspicious cerebral activity with an encephalographer must always be a high priority.

NEUROPHYSIOLOGIC BASIS FOR ELECTROENCEPHALOGRAPHY

Electrical activity generated by the brain can be classified in three broad categories. Spontaneous and evoked electrical activity detected on the scalp as oscillatory potentials are primarily discussed in this section. Electrical potentials generated by single neurons recorded by microelectrodes are only briefly mentioned in the context of an overall discussion of the neurophysiologic basis of EEG. Informative reviews of the neurophysics of electrical fields in the brain are available in other reference sources [Nunez, 1981; Niedermeyer and Lopes da Silva, 1981; Pedley and Traub, 1990].

The central problem for the neurologist is how to relate scalp potentials to underlying physiologic processes. It is an empirical observation that scalp potentials are expressed as an admixture of frequency-dependent waveforms that are characterized by temporal and spatial characteristics. Those potentials depend on the nature and location of current sources within the brain that have both electrical and geometric properties specific to the size and shape of the scalp, skull, and underlying brain substance. This concept is crucial to both understanding maturational patterns and appreciating the neurophysiologic substrate of CNS dysfunction in children. The major source of these oscillating potentials measured on the scalp is synaptic activity.

A more limited contribution to the scalp-derived potential comes from the action potential of the neuron itself. To fully appreciate how synaptic potentials are generated on the scalp, the neurologist must acquire an understanding of the intracellular and extracellular ionic environment of the neuron. The neuronal cell contains fluid restricted by a cylindric membrane that limits the movement of ions in and out of the cell. Because the axon and dendrites are connected to the cell body, the same ionic flux pertains to these structures. The restriction in ionic movement results in a resting voltage potential difference, with high concentration of sodium and chloride outside of the cell, whereas potassium is concentrated within the neuron. A sodium-potassium pumping system maintains these concentration gradients, with a resting potential of approximately -80 μV.

In the production of an action potential a rapid depolarization of the membrane occurs with a transient increase in sodium permeability, matched by an equal but opposite outflow of potassium. Subsequently, the gradual decrease in sodium conduction and the outflow of potassium leads to repolarization.

The depolarization, or action, potential travels down the axon to synaptic clefts where chemical transmitters are released. Presynaptic membrane release of neurotransmitters begins the process of cell-to-cell communication, with activation of the postsynaptic membrane by either depolarization or hyperpolarization. Depolarization by specific neurotransmitters similarly causes an inward flux of sodium, creating a voltage gradient that is termed the *excitatory postsynaptic potential*. Hyperpolarization by other neurotransmitters cause an outward flow of sodium, contributing to an *inhibitory postsynaptic potential*. The summation of excitatory postsynaptic potentials and inhibitory postsynaptic potentials within a region involving a number of synapses determines the degree of postsynaptic membrane depolarization or hyperpolarization. If excitatory postsynaptic potentials predominate, depolarization will lead to an action potential. If inhibitory postsynaptic potentials predominate, hyperpolarization will follow, preventing the occurrence of an action potential. Although synaptic potentials are lower voltage than action potentials, their longer time course and larger membrane surface area contribute primarily to scalp-detected EEG activity.

During the excitatory postsynaptic potential or inhibitory postsynaptic potential there is a current flow in a loop orientation with opposite polarities at each end of the axonal or dendritic processes of the cell. Because most neurons are oriented radially to the cortical surface, these current flows follow a radial direction in and out as detected by surface electrodes. The polarity, as recorded on the surface, reflects an excitatory or inhibitory current flow, depending on the nature of the summated synaptic potentials and on the site of the synapse. Virtually all electrical activity recorded on the scalp is generated by current flow across the synaptic membranes of cortical neurons. Subcortical activity does not substantially contribute to the generation of current flow and electric fields. Rather, diencephalic structures, such as the thalamus, exert a modulatory effect on cortical rhythms, such as the regulation of the dominant alpha rhythm, and on the appearance and rhythmicity of sleep spindles.

Neurophysiologic basis of abnormal electrical patterns

A number of electrical patterns appear to correlate with specific clinicopathologic situations in adults and children. In general, epileptiform and nonepileptiform abnormalities are subdivided, with presumably different neurophysiologic and/or neuropathologic substrates. The following discussion briefly outlines selected experimental findings that help explain certain abnormal patterns relevant to pediatric and adult EEGs, which are then addressed in a later section.

Interictal spike discharges, the hallmark of the epileptic neuron in experimental models of epilepsy, involve a specific type of membrane depolarization, referred to as a *paroxysmal depolarization shift*. There are general similarities between the neuronal events underlying this interictal epileptogenetic process [Jeffreys, 1990]. In hippocampal and neocortical slice recordings taken after penicillin application [Ayala et al., 1973], high-voltage discharges appear in the EEG that are associated with an intracellularly recorded paroxysmal depolarization shift. These phenomena appear in the intracellular recordings on both experimental animals and human cortices. The depolarization is of relatively high voltage (10 to 15 μV) and long duration (100 to 200 ms) and is associated with a burst of spike discharges. The event produces a train of action potentials that conduct away from the neuron along the axon. The interictal paroxysmal depolarization shift is then followed by a period of hyperpolarization. Over time, this depolarization can summate to form a prolonged depolarization with a persistent loss of hyperpolarization, recorded on the surface as continuous spike discharges coinciding with the tonic phase of a generated tonic-clonic seizure. Subsequently, large inhibitory potentials occur alternately with recurrent rhythmic depolarization, which coincides with the clonic phase of the seizure. Despite the higher threshold to achieve depolarization and the longer refractory period noted in immature animals [Prince and Gutnick, 1972], an understanding of paroxysmal depolarization shift is crucial to an appreciation of maturational aspects of epileptogenesis.

Based on these experimental observations, several possible explanations are proposed to explain the mechanism by which the normal neuronal activities convert to those of abnormal interictal discharges [Prince, 1985]. One mechanism involves intrinsic membrane abnormalities that promote burst-generating properties in individual neurons by an imbalance of calcium and sodium ionic movements [Schwartzkroin and Prince, 1978]. Another mechanism involves the loss of inhibition by a group of neurons because of the absence of an inhibitory neurotransmitter, gamma-aminobutyric acid (GABA) [Prince, 1985]. Finally, a third mechanism of summated excitatory postsynaptic potentials helps explain how large groups of neurons generate depolarization shifts [Prince, 1978].

These proposed mechanisms unfortunately do not necessarily explain the transformation from an interictal to an ictal event. Therefore other mechanisms have been proposed based on further experimental studies, including changes in the ionic microenvironment that result in enhanced neuronal excitability, axonal burst generation, and cholinergic alteration of neuronal properties [Prince, 1985].

Metabolic factors related to glucose or electrolyte imbalance or noncerebral factors, such as trauma or fever, may all facilitate the onset of seizures, particularly in children. Further biochemical and anatomic alterations within a seizure may further promote seizure generation by neuronal destruction or glial proliferation [Aird et al., 1984].

Abnormal suppression or slowing of EEG activity

Besides the presence of spike- or sharp-wave discharges for the diagnoses of seizure disorders, other types of abnormal EEG patterns coincide with different neuropathologic substrates [Daly et al., 1990]. Unfortunately, little information exists to correlate altered neuronal properties, such as the mechanisms discussed for epileptogenesis. Rather, clinical interpretations of the following EEG patterns are mostly empirically based on correlative neuropathology.

Local suppression or absence of background rhythmic activity is a strong indication of brain dysfunction, irrespective of age or location in the brain. Complete absence of activity usually implies cortical necrosis in close proximity to the surface [Goldensohn, 1979a, 1979b]. However, incomplete depression of background activity is the more common situation. Asymmetric suppression of frontal beta activity, central rhythms, dominant alpha activity, or sleep spindles in association with polymorphic delta waves strongly indicate a destructive process in the brain underlying those electrodes [Arfel and Fischgold, 1961] (Figure 6-2, *A*). EEGs of neonates showing asymmetric background activities usually suggest that the brain lesion is in the attenuated location [Scher and Tharp, 1982].

Continuous polymorphic delta waves constitutes a category of EEG abnormality that may suggest a

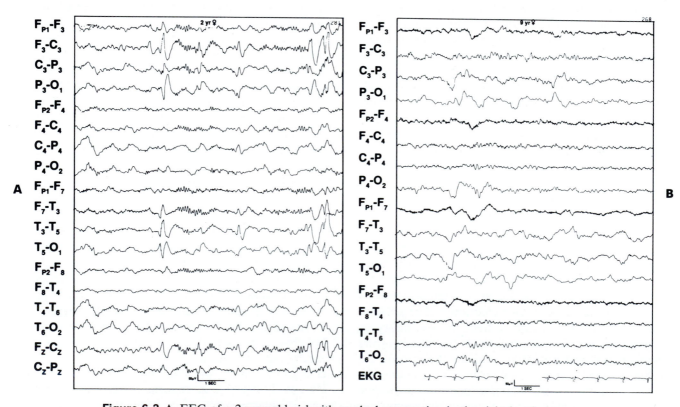

Figure 6-2 A, EEG of a 2-year-old girl with marked attenuation in the right hemisphere, both above and below the sylvian fissure. Absence of vertex waves and suppression of sleep spindles seen. Extensive right hemisphere encephalomalacia documented on imaging studies. **B,** EEG of a 9-year-old girl with slowing in the left posterior quadrant. Arteriovenous malformation in the left hemisphere was noted on imaging studies.

structural brain lesion on either an acquired or congenital basis (Figure 6-2, *B*). Irregular delta waves between 0.5 to 2.5 Hz do not react to eye opening, arousal, or sleep. Correlations with brain lesions in animals [Gloor et al., 1968] and in humans at autopsy have been described [Rhee et al., 1975]. Focal slowing may imply focal destructive lesions of white matter on a congenital, vascular, neoplastic, or infectious basis. Polymorphic delta waves can commonly appear immediately after a seizure of focal onset and with reversible conditions, such as migraine [Hockaday and Whitty, 1969], both common occurrences in children. The combination of bilateral synchronous rhythmic discharges and polymorphic delta waves occur in diffuse encephalopathies involving white and gray matter. Certain brain regions are more likely to express polymorphic delta waves, such as the frontal, temporal, and occipital areas. The association of background rhythm depression and polymorphic delta waves makes the likelihood of destructive lesions quite high, especially tumors. Parasagittal and parietal lesions often are associated with attentuation of rhythms or prominent theta rhythms.

Intermittent rhythmic delta activity is another category of nonepileptiform abnormality with a variety of neuropathologic correlates. Runs of sinusoidal 2.5 Hz are generally reactive to eye opening, hyperventilation,

or arousal. Two distinct distributions of rhythmic delta over the scalp have been identified. Frontal intermittent delta activity (Figure 6-3, *A*) and occipital rhythmic delta activity (Figure 6-3, *B*) generally indicate modification of cortically generated EEG by midline subcortical structures. The thalamus, reticular-activating system, and midbrain can contribute to the dysfunction between subcortical gray matter and cortical neurons [Daly, 1975]. These two types of rhythmic delta activity are largely age-related. Frontal intermittent delta activity is usually noted in adult patients, whereas occipital rhythmic delta activity is found mainly in children. Intermittent rhythmic delta activity does not necessarily indicate that the major pathologic condition is in that region. Both occipital rhythmic delta activity and frontal intermittent delta activity have been documented in 53% of 145 children with posterior fossa tumors [Martinius et al., 1968]. As a rule, it has little localizing value in supratentorial masses, although it may be accentuated on the side of a tumor [Hess, 1975]. It is crucial to remember that intermittent rhythmic delta activity is nonspecific and can also be noted with systemic metabolic disorders, increased intracranial pressure, encephalitis, and trauma.

Epileptiform discharges can be found in combination with slowing as an indication of a structural process.

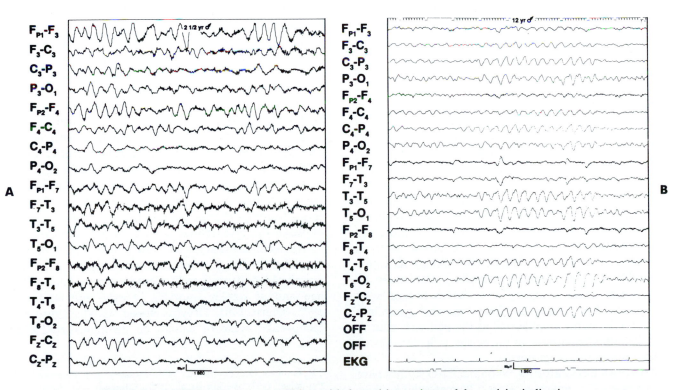

Figure 6-3 A, EEG of a 2½-year-old boy with frontal intermittent delta activity indicative of a diffuse encephalopathy on a hypoxic-ischemic basis. **B,** EEG recording of a 12-year-old boy with a predominantly occipital intermittent rhythmic delta activity indicative of a diffuse encephalopathy on a metabolic basis.

Focal discharges during a seizure have better localizing value than interictal spikes [Hess, 1975]. In general, slow-growing neoplasms, such as oligodendrogliomas or astrocytomas, produce more epileptiform activity than rapidly growing tumors [Kershman, 1949]. Spike discharges are more common after surgery, such as with meningiomas, but neurologists are advised to exercise extreme caution concerning the presence of spike discharges as reliable guidelines to localization of destructive lesions. At present, imaging studies are far more reliable laboratory guides.

SIGNIFICANCE OF NORMAL VARIATION IN EEG: MATURATIONAL PATTERNS
Guidelines for interpretation

EEG analysis requires a systematic, orderly process in which a series of steps are followed and a proper interpretation is reached [Hrakovy, 1990]. The rhythmicity of spontaneous EEG signals gives a continuous admixture of scalp-generated oscillatory potentials. EEG frequencies are classified into the following four band ranges: delta activity is less than 4 Hz; theta activity is less than 8 Hz; alpha activity is 8 to 13 Hz; and beta activity is greater than 13 Hz. In general the amplitude of EEG activity is inversely proportional to frequency.

Specifically, for pediatric EEGs, the amount of slow activity decreases with increasing age, and the persistence and frequency of slow activity vary in different regions. Not only is it important to appreciate the presence and degree of expression of frequencies in various regions at different ages, but other parameters, such as waveform, manner of occurrence (e.g., random, continuous), and amplitude, are essential to visual analysis. By this cumulative analysis, using a list of parameters of EEG activity [Hrakovy, 1990], the neurologist can attempt to assign normal or abnormal clinical significance to the EEG pattern. Critical information regarding both age and state of the patient affects the ability of the neurologist to judge normality in the EEG record. It may require several EEG recordings and the persistence or resolution of abnormal electrical activity relative to the state of the patient to assess normality properly. Several recordings also allow an appreciation of the ontogeny, or evolution, of significant age-specific EEG patterns. These general guidelines must be repeatedly emphasized as the pediatric neurologist acquires an appreciation of the rich diversity of normal maturational patterns.

Newborn EEG patterns. Neonatal EEG studies have been reported for nearly 40 years [Okamato and Kirikae, 1951]. Pioneering investigations by several independent researchers have all contributed information concerning the developmental neurophysiology of the immature brain.* Some of these studies predate the development of the tertiary care neonatal intensive care unit, and thus the neurologist using EEG had an understandably limited role in the diagnostic assessment and clinical care of the sick neonate.

More recently, improvement in the recording equipment and standardization of the recording techniques have become available in the modern neonatal intensive care unit setting. An internationally accepted system of electrode placement adapted for the neonate and young infant permits standardization of recordings between laboratories [American EEG Society, 1986]. The development of 16-channel and 21-channel EEG machines with improved filtering systems and electrode construction minimizes environmental and physiologic sources of artifacts. Synchronized video EEG studies permit more accurate comparison between electrographic and behavioral changes in the assessment of seizures, movement disorders, and sleep cycles [Scher, 1987a].

Several fundamental principles for neonatal EEGs serve as an introduction to an understanding of its chief clinical application. There are expected changes in the scalp-generated EEG patterns for neonates of different gestational ages. The experienced encephalographer can approximate the electrical maturity within 2 weeks of the gestational age.† Changing electrical patterns reflect the postconceptional age of the neonate independent of birth weight. Maturation of the neonate's sleep-wake behavior follows maturation of the CNS and is independent of the birth weight [Schulte et al., 1971]. Preterm neonates, when corrected to term postconceptional age, should have similar EEG patterns and sleep behavior as term, appropriate-for-gestational-age newborns.

Detailed electrographic and anatomic correlations that compare sulcal-gyral development with evolving electrical patterns have been compared with clinical information concerned with gestational maturity [Scher, 1987d] (Figures 6-4 and 6-5). Out of 25 infants, 23 had maturational agreement within 2 weeks between electrical patterns and sulcal-gyral measurements of the inferior frontal, superior temporal, and calcarine gyri and between the cytoarchitecture of various brain regions.

Regional changes in electrical activity clearly occur in the EEG of the premature neonate when recordings are obtained after 24 to 25 weeks estimated gestational age and at weekly intervals [Torres and Anderson, 1985; Tharp, 1981; Dreyfus-Brisac, 1979] (Figure 6-6). Sleep-wake behavior cannot be distinguished for pa-

---

* References Dreyfus-Brisac, 1955; Hrakovy and Petersen, 1964; Parmelee, 1967; Werner et al, 1977; Ellingson and Peters, 1980; Lombroso, 1980; Tharp, 1981; Torres and Anderson, 1985; Prechtl et al, 1969; Anders et al, 1971; Watanabe, 1972a.

†References Dreyfus-Brisac et al, 1955; Parmelee, 1967; Tharp, 1981b; Dreyfus-Brisac, 1979.

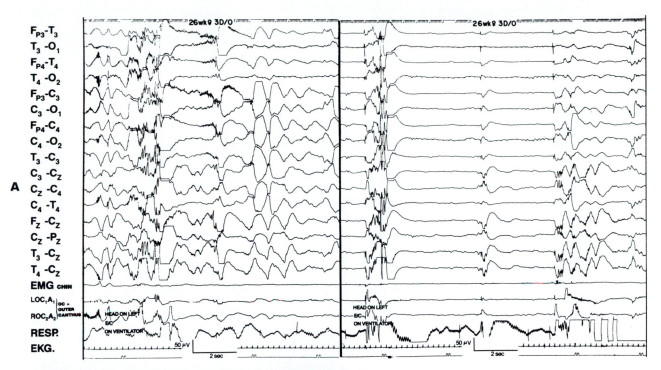

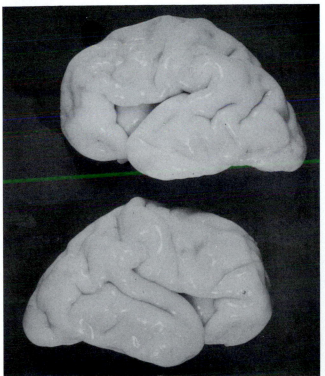

Figure 6-4 A, Two EEG tracings of a 26 weeks' gestation, 3-day-old girl. First frame demonstrates generalized theta and delta slowing with prominent vertex central slow activity. Note the bitemporal attenuation. In the second frame, synchronous interburst intervals of less than 40 seconds in duration are demonstrated, as well as delta brush patterns in the vertex region. **B,** Lateral view of brain of patient in **A.** Underdeveloped frontal and temporal lobes with insula clearly visible. Immature sulcation pattern, especially the rolandic, calcarine, and superior temporal sulci. (From Scher MS and Ahdab-Barmada M. Pediatr Neurol 1987; 3:256.)

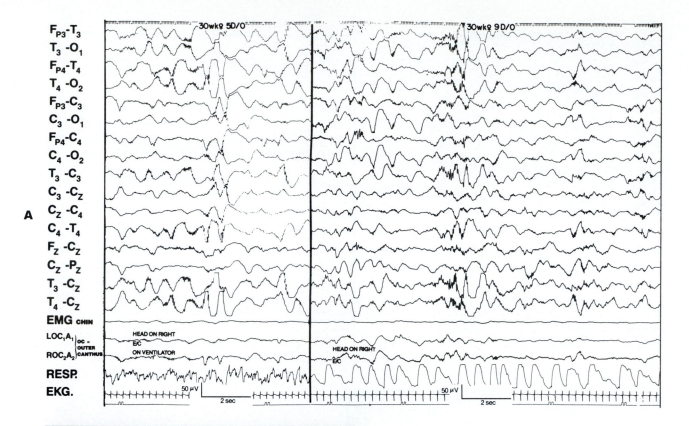

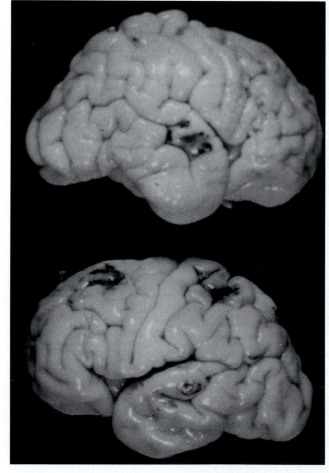

Figure 6-5 A, Two samples of EEG of a 30 weeks' gestation, 5-day-old girl. In the first frame a greater degree of spontaneous, continuous EEG activity noted, with temporal delta and delta brush patterns. In the second frame, occipital delta and delta brush patterns noted. **B,** Lateral view of brain for patient described in **A.** Greater degree of sulcation evident. Note the more complete elaboration of the rolandic, superior temporal, and calcarine sulci. (From Scher MS and Ahdab-Barmada M. Pediatr Neurol 1987; 3:256).

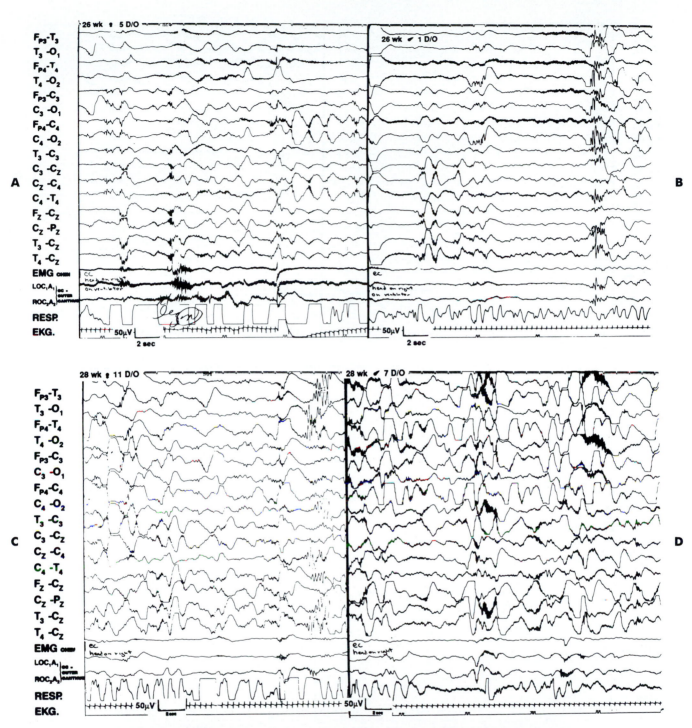

Figure 6-6 A, A 26 weeks' gestation, 5-day-old girl. Relatively continuous background of slow and fast frequencies. Rhythmic central delta is noted with superimposed delta brushes in the same region. Asymmetric/asynchronous occipital delta activity is also noted. Prominent temporal attenuation is also seen. Myoclonic movement is indicated (*arrow*). **B,** A 26 weeks' gestation, 1-day-old boy. Discontinuous background activity consisting of central and vertex delta slow activity with superimposed delta brushes. Diffuse theta bursts with occasional occipital theta bursts are also noted. **C,** A 28 weeks' gestation, 11-day-old girl (postconceptional age, 29.5 weeks). Largely continuous background activity with predominant delta slowing. More active temporal activity including prominent temporal theta bursts. Delta brushes are seen in the occipital and vertex regions as well. **D,** A 26 weeks' gestation, 7-day-old boy (postconceptional age, 29 weeks). Rhythmic occipital delta in different head regions with prominent temporal delta brushes. Periodic breathing is noted in the respiratory channel.

Continued.

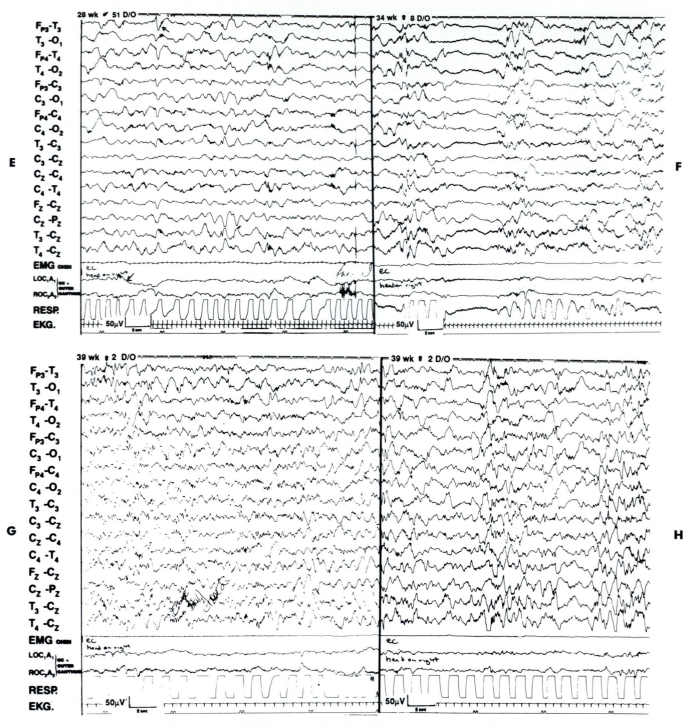

Figure 6-6, cont'd E, A 28 weeks' gestation, 51-day-old boy (postconceptional age, 35 weeks). Continuous background activity that is appropriate lower amplitude for the corrected age. This activity consists of fast frequencies with delta brushes in multiple head regions. An isolated frontal sharp wave is present, as well as rapid eye movements. **F,** A 34 weeks' gestation, 8-day-old girl (postconceptional age, 35 weeks). Discontinuous background with age-appropriate short interburst intervals. Rhythmic occipital delta with good interhemispheric synchrony. Periodic breathing noted in the respiratory channel. **G,** A 39-weeks' gestation, 2-day-old girl. High voltage slow wave (HVS) pattern of quiet sleep with scattered sharp waves particularly in the temporal regions. Regular respirations with no movements are noted in the polygraphic channels. **H,** A 39 weeks' gestation, 2-day-old girl. Tracé alternant pattern of quiet sleep with synchronous high-amplitude bursts with age-appropriate brief interbursts intervals and a well-developed background. Agreement with the polygraphic criteria of sleep for respirations and movements.

tients less than 30 weeks of age, but other hemispheric or regional patterns demonstrate predictable evolving characteristics.

Ontogeny of EEG features. The description of evolving EEG sleep patterns in the asymptomatic, presumably healthy preterm infant has been the subject of many excellent reviews [Hrachovy, 1990; Lombroso, 1985; Tharp, 1981; Pope et al., 1991; Scher, 1993a, 1993b; Torres et al., 1985]. Improvements in neonatal intensive care, however, require periodic revisions to include more premature neonates [Anderson et al. 1985; Torres et al. 1985]. These revisions are particularly relevant for the early premature infant less than 32 weeks' gestation in whom tremendous improvements in survival rates have occurred over the last decade. It is always important to verify which EEG-sleep patterns are within the range of normal only after systematic neurodevelopmental assessment of such children.

Regional and hemispheric EEG patterns for preterm and term neonates are described next, arbitrarily assigned within specific gestational age ranges. Temporal, spatial, and state organization of the EEG recordings that comprise the cerebral activity during each age range are highlighted with appropriate illustrations.

Gestational age of less than 28 weeks. Neonates with a gestational age of less than 28 weeks who fall below the limits of viability may not survive long enough to receive even one EEG recording. However, useful information is now available to characterize the neurophysiologic profile of these very premature neonates who survive. An undifferentiated EEG sleep profile is typically observed with no distinctive features noted between waking or sleep portions. The record is largely discontinuous, with short periods of continuous EEG activity that may last for as long as 1 minute. Patterns of motility alternate between segmental myoclonic movements of the face or body to more generalized myoclonic and tonic posturing either in an axial or appendicular distribution.

A pattern of alternating active and sleep periods in preterm infants is characterized as discontinuity or tracé discontinu [Dreyfus-Brisac, 1968; Ellingson, 1964; Tharp, 1981]. Most recently, Anderson et al. [1985] found that 60% of EEG recordings consisted of discontinuity. These same authors found that the average interburst interval during this age range was between 8 and 16 seconds, with the longest interburst intervals being between 15 and 88 seconds. Similar ranges for the duration of interburst intervals have been found by other authors [Benda et al., 1989; Connell et al., 1987; Eyre et al., 1988; Hughes et al., 1983, 1987]. This finding is in sharp contrast to earlier descriptions of interburst intervals as long as 2 minutes in duration [Lombroso, 1985]. Such a difference may be, in part, based on the medical condition of the neonate at the time of the recording and/or the lack of information concerning long-term follow-up.

Activity predominates in the vertex, central, and occipital regions. Bitemporal attenuation is common [Scher et al., 1987] and may reflect, in part, intrahemispheric asynchrony. Underdevelopment of the inferior frontal and superior temporal gyri may also help explain the relative quiescence of activity in this brain region.

EEG activity consists of mixed frequencies, predominated by delta activity in the parasagittal and occipital regions. Occipital delta is either isolated to one or two waveforms and is rarely longer than 5 to 6 seconds in duration or rhythm in nature. Faster frequencies in the theta, alpha, and beta ranges are also intermixed in multiple head regions. Diffuse theta bursts are commonly seen either during continuous or discontinuous periods.

Beta/delta complexes are transient patterns that identify premature neonates of varying conceptional ages. This pattern is the principal regional electrographic feature of the preterm infant. Random or briefly rhythmic 0.3 to 1.5 Hz delta activity of 50 to 250 μV [Hrachovy et al., 1990] has superimposed bursts of low-to-moderate–amplitude faster frequencies with a frequency range of 10 to 20 Hz. The amplitude of such activity on bipolar recordings rarely exceeds 60 to 75 μV. Historically, various terms have been applied to such complexes, including *spindle delta bursts*, *brushes*, *spindlelike fast waves*, and *ripples of prematurity*. These complexes can be readily seen as early as 24 to 26 weeks, largely in the central and midline regions, as well as the occipital regions.

Runs of monorhythmic alpha and/or theta activity are seen independent of delta brushes principally in the occipital regions in the neonate less than 28 weeks' gestation. This transient pattern has recently been described in more detail [Hughes et al., 1990] and can last for 6 to 10 seconds in either an asynchronous or asymmetric manner. Such activity should be distinguished from the more diffuse bursts of moderate-to-high–amplitude theta that commonly are noted at this degree of prematurity (see Figure 6-5).

Intrahemispheric and interhemispheric synchrony have been variably described by different authors. Lombroso described synchronous bursts as morphologically similar bursts of activity appearing within 1.5 seconds. He estimated that synchronous periods ranged from only 50% of all periods of activity at 31 to 32 weeks to 100% at 40 to 43 weeks postconceptional age with a midpoint of 70% to 85% at 35 to 36 weeks' postconceptional age [Lombroso, 1989, 1985]. This finding is in sharp contrast to Anderson's observations [Anderson, 1985] that interhemispheric synchrony had a mean of 93% for 1-minute epochs at 27 weeks' postconceptional age with a mean of 94% at 29 to 32 weeks' postconceptional age.

One must consider that a high degree of intrahemispheric synchrony already exists in the premature infant less than 30 weeks' gestation. However, it is also reasonable to consider that more epochs of asynchrony occur as the distance from the midline increases, given the rapid brain growth beyond 30 weeks' postconceptional age. Rapid growth of temporal and parietal structures in particular may contribute to more frequent episodes of asynchrony [Hrachovy et al., 1990]. In addition, measures of asynchrony must include not only information about postconceptional age but also EEG state. Asynchrony should be assessed for all background rhythms [Tharp, 1981] and not only bursts during discontinuous epochs [Anderson et al., 1985; Lombroso, 1985].

Gestational age of 28 to 31 weeks. Cyclic organization of state remains largely undifferentiated [Lombroso, 1989, 1985]. However, periods of body and eye movements are more distinctively associated with irregular respirations during continuous periods of EEG.

Discontinuous epochs still predominate but decrease in duration as compared with the very premature neonate of less than 28 weeks' postconceptional age. Interbursts become progressively briefer with a dramatic increase in low-to-moderate–amplitude faster rhythms primarily in the theta range.

By 32 weeks' postconceptional age, the degree of discontinuity has decreased to 45% of the record [Anderson et al., 1985]. Dreyfus-Brisac [1970] found an alternating pattern in 24% of records at 32 to 34 weeks' gestation. The average interburst intervals at 29 to 31 weeks' postconceptional age ranged between 5 and 14 and 4 and 11 seconds, respectively, with means of 9 and 7 seconds; whereas the longest interburst periods for these two postconceptional age groups were found to be between 16 to 57 and 6 to 41 seconds with means of 36 and 20 seconds, respectively.

Monorhythmic occipital delta is now quite abundant at 28 to 31 weeks with durations that are greater than 30 seconds.

Delta brush patterns continue to be abundant, involving not only the vertex and central regions but also the occipital and temporal regions [Watanabe, 1972a]. It may, at times, be difficult to differentiate delta brushes in the temporal region, particularly because of superimposition with temporal theta bursts.

Another useful developmental marker is the appearance of rhythmic 4.5 to 6 Hz activity occurring independently and synchronously in each midtemporal region. Although this activity is noted at less than 28 weeks' postconceptional age, it is expressed maximally between 28 and 32 weeks' postconceptional age. Historically, this feature has been described as "temporal sawtooth waves" [Werner et al., 1991]. Amplitudes range from roughly 20 to 200 μV; with maturation, these bursts may reach the alpha frequency. In a recent study of 436 infants [Hughes et al., 1987] a parabolic polynomial

function has described the age incidence of temporal theta activity, strongly reflecting the pattern as a maturational landmark. Temporal theta can obtain a maximum incidence of 36% at 29 to 30 weeks, after which it diminishes rapidly. At 32 weeks, only 12% of the record exhibits this pattern [Anderson et al., 1985]. This rhythmic theta activity should be distinguished from repetitive sharp activity in the theta range seen at near-term and term ages in the midline and rolandic regions, particularly during the quiet sleep segment.

The clinical significance of sharp-wave transients in healthy, preterm infants has been poorly documented at early preterm ages. Regional patterns associated with maturation must be considered before assigning spike or sharp-wave criteria to a transient waveform. Sharply contoured delta brushes and temporal or occipital theta bursts may appear epileptiform without clearly satisfying morphologic criteria of an epileptiform discharge (see Figure 6-9, *A*).

Sporadic multifocal spikes and sharp waves can be seen at any gestational age [Ellingson, 1964; Harris 1970; Monod et al., 1960; Parmelee et al., 1968; Samson-Dollfus, 1955; Torres et al., 1985; Werner et al., 1991], but few studies include preterm infants less than 32 weeks' estimated gestational age. Anderson et al. [1985] studied the incidence and location of spikes and sharp waves in 33 preterm infants, 27 to 32 weeks' estimated gestational age. Both features were infrequent, with spikes less common than sharp waves. Both morphologies were most abundant in frontal and temporal regions, with frequency increasing from 27 to 32 weeks. Central sharp waves decreased in number over this same time period, whereas occipital and vertex discharges had the lowest incidence. Unfortunately, only 55% of infants were verified as normal on follow-up at 6 to 8 months of age. Larger preterm populations with longer periods of neurodevelopmental follow-up are needed before assigning clinical significance to sharp waves in asymptomatic preterm infants.

Gestational age of 32 to 34 weeks. Body and eye movements take on a more phasic rather than tonic pattern. There is better differentiation between continuous sleep associated with active sleep and quiet or non-rapid eye movement sleep segments. Few movements, except for buccolingual movements and occasional myoclonic jerks [Curzi-Dascalova et al., 1988], occur during the more discontinuous segments. Variable respirations persist, but short periods of regular respirations are present during discontinuous portions of the recording.

EEG background is more continuous with cyclic periods of tracé discontinu. Synchronous delta frequencies of varying amplitude still predominate, interrupted by random inactive periods. Faster frequencies, also of variable amplitudes, are also present and are represented by the faster component of a delta brush pattern.

Regional patterns (i.e., brushes, theta bursts) predominate the rolandic and occipital regions, as well as the temporal and midline regions.

The most characteristic feature at this age range is the notable increase in multifocal sharp waves (see next section) and the appearance of reactivity to stimulation, characterized by transient periods of attenuation of background physiologically different from the quiescent epochs during tracé discontinu.

Sharply contoured activity predominates in the temporal and central regions, with positive temporal sharp waves frequently seen in synchronous or independently occurring runs. The sharp activity in the central regions is more likely negative in polarity and should be carefully distinguished from physiologic artifacts that can occur because of fontanel pulsation or ventilatory excursions. Positive temporal sharp waves need to be differentiated from pathologic-rolandic and vertex-positive sharp waves that are seen in the sick neonate with either intraventricular hemorrhage or periventricular leuko-malacia [Scher, 1991].

Reactivity to stimulation appears in this gestational age range. Nonspecific EEG changes are induced by tactile or painful stimulation, usually with an abrupt attenuation or desynchronization of background, which can be difficult to distinguish from low-amplitude quiescent periods until later in gestational maturity, when one can more readily distinguish between active and quiet sleep. Uncommonly, bursts of higher amplitude delta activity may also characterize the reactivity periods. It is unknown whether these are the precursors of more discrete arousal patterns, such as K complexes and hypersynchronous delta that are seen at older ages.

Reactivity to photic stimulation has recently been studied more systematically [Anderson, 1985]. Responses to photic stimulation clearly are seen in the EEG of the early premature infant [Ellingson, 1958]. Responses to isolated flashes have a prominent, negative-wave component. Ellingson [1960] described the later positive component occurring with maturation, with decreasing latency in proportion to increasing postconceptional age [Ellingson, 1958]. In contrast to isolated flashes, repetitive flashes or photic driving has also been investigated by several authors, but such responses are difficult to detect in the EEG of the neonate [Ellingson, 1960, 1964]. Only between 4% and 5% of premature and term infants exhibit photic driving with a wide range of flicker frequencies. Anderson and Torres [1985] found that even early premature infants between 27 to 32 weeks exhibit driving in 64% of 34 neonates when the frequencies are limited to 2 to 10 flashes per second. Some authors have claimed that these driving responses are more readily seen in the premature infant because of the more continuous, higher amplitude mixture of background frequencies [Monod, 1977].

Responses to other forms of sensory stimulation, such as auditory or painful stimulation have been the object of less attention in both the premature and the term neonate. Monod and Garma [1971] investigated behavioral and physiologic responses to auditory clicks in the premature neonate. These authors found vertex spikes in response to auditory clicks in neonates at 32 to 34 weeks' postconceptional age, which is in contrast to a less distinctive response with more mature ages. Sudden, loud auditory stimuli more effectively produce EEG changes than visual [Ellingson, 1958] or tactile [Dreyfus-Brisac, 1957] stimuli. Such periods of desynchronization have been postulated to be associated with the psycho-physiologic property of habituation and may represent electrographic representation of perceptual memory and discriminatory functions of the neonate [Anderson, 1985].

Gestational age of 34 to 37 weeks. Cyclic alterations between wakefulness and sleep, as well as longer periods of continuous periods of EEG, predominate during this age range. More concordant segments between cerebral and noncerebral signals resemble active and quiet sleep of the term infant. For instance, motility patterns take on a distinctive phasic quality that predominates during active sleep. An absence of motility except for generalized myoclonic and facial movements is seen during quiet sleep. Myogenic activity measured at the chin characteristically remains low during the periods of active sleep, and higher and more phasic activity occurs during quiet sleep. The cyclic nature of the active and quiet sleep periods still lacks the well-defined 30 to 70 minute cycle seen in the term infant.

Electrographic components of the EEG sleep cycle in this gestational age range show a predominance of continuous EEG activity comprised of mixed delta and theta wave activity usually lower in amplitude (20 to 100 μV) than at younger gestational ages. Low-amplitude faster rhythms of alpha and beta activity are more prominent, with the remaining delta brushes present primarily in the temporal and occipital regions. Brushes also appear more commonly during quiet than active sleep.

Frontal sharp transients of 50 to 150 μV are predominantly noted at 34 to 35 weeks' gestation but may be seen at earlier gestational ages. Historically, these waveforms were termed *encoches frontales* [Monod et al., 1960] and popularly identified as *frontal sharp transients* [Hrakovy et al., 1964] as well as *pointes lents diphasiques frontales* [Arfel et al., 1977; Monod et al., 1960]. These sharp waves usually have an initial surface positive component followed by a negative component but are also associated with rhythmic, sharply contoured, frontal delta activity [Goldie et al., 1971] and can occasionally be high amplitude (250 μV).

In contrast, fewer multifocal sharp transients occur

and, as with more preterm neonates, are sometimes difficult to distinguish from the intermixed background theta or beta background frequencies.

The discontinuous quality of the EEG sleep tracing during this postconceptional age range indicates the appearance of a tracé alternant rather than a tracé discontinu pattern noted in younger premature infants. Quiescent periods now consist of more activity that may exceed 15 mV/ml, with a greater mixture of low-amplitude faster rhythms.

Gestational age of 38 to 42 weeks. Electrographic/polygraphic patterns are fully elaborated during this age range. Alternating periods of wakefulness and sleep, as well as cyclic changes between four segments of sleep state, can be identified. Two active sleep and quiet EEG patterns comprise this cycle, with a length varying from 30 to 70 minutes, and are associated with the presence or absence of rapid eye movements, body movements, autonomic signs, and arousal episodes.

Although conventional wisdom dictates that only the term and near-term infant possess such an organized EEG sleep cycle, concordance among specific EEG and polygraphic parameters has been described in the preterm infant as early as 30 weeks' gestation [Curzi-Dascalova et al., 1988]. A developmental match between cerebral and noncerebral physiologic parameters fundamentally reflects the coordination of specific neural systems within the maturing system. There indeed may be a more established order of state in the premature infant that has not been readily recognized by visual analysis techniques. A rudimentary cycle may be more easily detected in the premature neonate by more quantitative techniques [Scher et al., 1990].

The EEG sleep organization of the term neonate has traditionally been considered to be similar for a premature infant who has matured to a term age as compared with the appropriate-for-gestational-age term neonate. Two active sleep segments occupy 50% of the sleep time of the term infant and are comprised of mixed frequency pattern and a low-voltage irregular pattern that begin and end the sleep cycle, respectively. Quiet sleep segments are situated in between and consist of high-voltage slow and tracé alternant segments, and make up 35% to 40% of the cycle. Transitional or indeterminate segments during which discordance between EEG and polygraphic criteria of sleep state is defined, make up 10% to 15% of the cycle. The mixed frequency active sleep pattern comprises moderate-amplitude delta and lower- amplitude theta, alpha, and beta range activities. This EEG background can also be identified in the waking neonate.

The low-voltage regular pattern is characterized by continuous, low-amplitude admixture of frequencies (15 to 30 mV), mostly in the theta and beta ranges. Considerable amounts of alpha activity are intermixed both posteriorly and anteriorly. This pattern can be seen during wakefulness and active sleep. Two quiet sleep segments, high-voltage slow and tracé alternant, occupy the second and third positions in this idealized EEG sleep cycle. The high-voltage slow pattern comprises diffuse, continuous, high-amplitude 50 to 150 mV delta activity, intermixed with theta and beta range activity of lower amplitude. The high-voltage slow segment is quite brief (4% to 6% of the cycle) and is rapidly replaced by the tracé alternant pattern. The tracé alternant segment comprises a discontinuous tracing of high-amplitude bursts of slow activity in the delta and theta range, alternating with lower amplitude faster frequencies in sharp waves seen synchronously over both hemispheres.

Frontal sharp waves may be abundant especially during quiet sleep. These waveforms are bilateral and synchronous but also can be asymmetric. Frontal sharp waves are seen less often during active and indeterminate sleep segments and are least likely to be noted during low-voltage regular active sleep [Arfel et al., 1977; Statz et al., 1982]. During sleep, frontal sharp transients are noted until the beginning of the second month of life [Ellingson et al., 1980; Werner et al., 1991].

As with preterm infants, the clinical significance of spikes and sharp waves in asymptomatic term neonatal populations remains controversial. Most groups do not have adequate follow-up data or were selected based on clinical problems. Clancy et al. [1985] identified 69 healthy infants who had an acute, life-threatening event (i.e., near-miss SIDS). Analyses of 10 minutes of active sleep documented more frequent sharp waves in near-term than term infants. Temporal sharp waves were more abundant than centrally located discharges, persisting until 45 weeks' postconceptional age and disappearing by 50 weeks' postconceptional age.

Karbowski [1980] studied 1-hour sleep recordings in 82 term, healthy newborns without subsequent follow-up. He found that 81% had predominately right centrotemporal sharp waves, with an average interval of 3 minutes and 47 seconds. Only 12% had predominately left central waves, with an average interval of 15 minutes. All discharges were noted primarily in indeterminate sleep.

As a final illustration, Statz et al. [1982] followed 24 term healthy infants 9 to 12 months of age after obtaining a neonatal sleep recording. They noted sporadic, multifocal, nonrepetitive discharges during quiet sleep in all infants; only 25% of infants had discharges during active sleep. The parietal region had the most abundant discharges, with intervals between 38 seconds and 25 minutes.

Clearly, the clinical significance of spikes and sharp waves that appear in both preterm and term neonatal recordings needs further investigation. As recently emphasized [Karbowski et al., 1980], sporadic sharp waves may be either normal or abnormal, depending on the clinical context, the EEG background activity, location, morphology, and postconceptional age. Unless discharges are repetitive, periodic, or positive in polarity, pathologic significance should be cautiously assigned.

Central sharp-wave transients and rhythmic, sharply contoured theta found in the parasagittal and vertex regions are also visualized. This midline pattern is rhythmic and has a spindlelike appearance [Hayakawa et al., 1987]. It is unknown whether this rhythmic activity is rudimentary sleep spindle activity that will appear at 2 to 4 months of age.

Delta brush patterns are occasionally noted during the quiet sleep segment but are rare and isolated primarily to the temporal and occipital regions.

As described, synchrony should be 100% during sleep of the term neonate. Transient asymmetries, mainly in the temporal regions, can be observed, particularly during the initial minutes of quiet sleep [Challamel et al., 1984; O'Brien et al., 1987].

Ontogeny of EEG sleep by the end of the neonatal period (i.e., 28 days after a term birth) has been systematically investigated by only a few researchers [Beckwith et al., 1986; Ellingson et al., 1980; Lombroso et al., 1979]. Gradual disappearance of tracé alternant by 3 to 6 weeks after a term birth has been described. Change of rapid eye movement and active sleep onset to quiet sleep onset have also been described. Sleep spindles commonly noted at 2 to 4 months of age may be seen as early as 4 to 6 weeks of age, and frontal sharp waves are normally noted 3 to 4 weeks after birth.

Although no significant differences can be distinguished between the maturational criteria at 1 month in preterm as compared with term infants, some slight differences have been noted which comprise elements of sleep architecture. Longer bursts during tracé alternant, early sleep spindle appearance, more immature patterns at term, better phase stability, and specific frequency bands are described [Joseph et al., 1976]. Behavioral criteria of sleep are also different between the two groups [Watt et al., 1985], suggesting that sleep organization of the preterm neonate to term and beyond is not entirely equivalent to the term newborn.

Normal EEG patterns in infancy through adolescence

Waking patterns. Although sleep patterns predominate in the newborn, a greater variability in state develops during infancy, which prepares the child for sustained periods of wakefulness. Therefore waking EEG patterns are the first part of the discussion of normal EEG patterns in childhood. Emphasis is placed on specific patterns that have relevance for clinical applications.

One of the fundamental characteristics of the waking EEG is the dominant background activity. Berger [1932] initially described how the dominant frequency increased as age advanced during childhood. By 3 to 4 months of age, a discernible occipitoparietal rhythm of 3 to 4 Hz is noted (Figure 6-7, *A*). The activity approximates 5 Hz by 6 months and increases to 6 to 7 Hz by 9 to 18 months of age (Figure 6-7, *B*). The 6 to 7 Hz frequency remains fairly stable until 2 years of age when it will vary between 7 to 8 Hz. By 3 years of age the dominant waking rhythm of childhood is within the alpha range in 82% of children [Eeg-Oloffsson, 1971; Peterson and Eeg-Olofsson, 1971] (Figure 6-7, *C*). The mean frequency is 9 Hz by 7 years of age and 10 Hz by 15 years of age (Figure 6-7, *D*).

Certain modifications in the waking dominant activity have been observed under different conditions. Passive eye closure causes the dominant rhythm to become better developed, whereas eye opening clearly attentuates the activity. This phenomenon will become initially apparent at 5 to 6 months of age [Kellaway and Peterson, 1964]. The dominant rhythm may slow by 1 to 2 Hz during the drowsy state, sometimes accompanied by a lessening of associated muscle artifact.

The amplitude, asymmetry, and locus of the dominant rhythm also changes with increasing age. Higher amplitudes are seen at younger ages, with maximum amplitudes at 6 to 9 years that subsequently decline during adolescence. Asymmetry of this activity can be expected with higher amplitude on the right in 20% of children, although differences of 50% or greater must be considered with suspicion. No correlation to hand dominance has been demonstrated. About 70% of adults and 95% of children will have an occipital location to the dominant rhythm, but at least 3 independent alpha rhythms can be recorded over the scalp-occipital, temporal, and central regions [Kellaway, 1979], which may differ in frequency as much as 2 Hz. More anterior expression of the dominant rhythm becomes evident during adulthood.

Mu rhythm. The mu, or central, rhythm commonly is 9 ± 2 Hz, and should not be confused with the central dominant rhythm of 7 to 9 Hz noted in infants. Although the mu rhythm is only noted in less than 5% of children younger than 4 years of age, it can be observed in 18% of children between 8 to 16 years of age and is somewhat more frequently observed in females. It can be blocked by movement of the opposite limb rather than eye opening. Although the mu rhythm might frequently appear asymmetrically and alternately in either hemisphere, a persistent asymmetry suggests a structural lesion on the attentuated side or irritation on the predominant side (e.g., after head injury).

Beta activity. Three distinctive band ranges are described for beta-range frequencies in waking EEGs of children [Hrakovy, 1990]. Limited diagnostic use can be

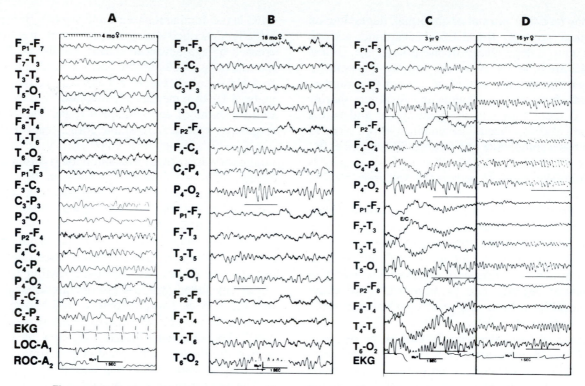

Figure 6-7 Posterior dominant rhythms (*line markings*) at four different ages during childhood while the patient was awake with eyes closed. **A,** Four Hz dominant rhythm seen at 4 months of age. **B,** Dominant rhythm of 6 to 7 Hz at 16 months of age. **C,** Dominant rhythm of 9 Hz at 3 years of age. **D,** Dominant rhythm of 10 to 12 Hz that is well regulated in a 16-year-old adolescent.

applied to the overall description of fast activity. Beta activity range of 18 to 25 Hz is most commonly encountered, with 14 to 16 and 35 to 40 Hz ranges less frequently noted. Symmetric distribution over each anterior head region is usually observed. Asymmetries of as much as 30% to 40% can be encountered without the presence of a structural lesion. Important diagnostic conclusions can be assigned if reduction in beta activity greater than 50% is noted, especially when associated with delta or theta slowing in the same head region. On the other hand, prominent scalp edema can also attenuate the high-frequency EEG signals in the absence of cerebral pathologic conditions. Symmetric prominence of beta activity is commonly encountered in certain sedative medications, especially in the barbiturate or benzodiazepine classes of drugs. Skull defects can contribute to an asymmetric exaggeration of beta activity over the bony defect [Cobb et al., 1979], although it usually has little clinical relevance.

Theta and delta slowing. Theta rhythms are commonly encountered in the frontocentral regions and are usually related to drowsiness or heightened emotional states. Although in the past theta rhythms have been associated with a variety of clinical conditions, including epilepsy, their common occurrence is now better appreciated as a normal variant [Hrakovy, 1990].

Posterior slow waves located in the parietooccipital regions, commonly referred to as *posterior slow waves of youth,* constitute the most frequently observed normal delta slow activity in the waking EEG record of children (Figure 6-8). Commonly located in the occipitoparietal or occipitotemporal regions is a 2.5 to 4.5 Hz monorythmic or polymorphic delta wave with an amplitude less than 100 μV [Aird and Gastaut, 1959]. Superimposed alpha activity is also observed with these delta waves, which can have either symmetric or asymmetric occurrence. The neurologist should view an asymmetry greater than 50% between regions with suspicion. It will block with eye opening and disappear with the alpha rhythm during drowsiness. Rarely noted before 2 years of age, it has maximum expression between 8 and 14 years, especially in females. Approximately 25% of normal children will have this pattern [Eeg-Oloffsson, 1971]. The distinction between this pattern and other abnormal slow-wave activity should be based on complexity of the waveform, persistence, symmetry, and amplitude, all in the context of closed-head injury, hypoxia, or other encephalitides.

Lambda waves. Lambda waveforms can be observed in normal patients while they are viewing a well-illuminated picture of complex design. Sharply con-

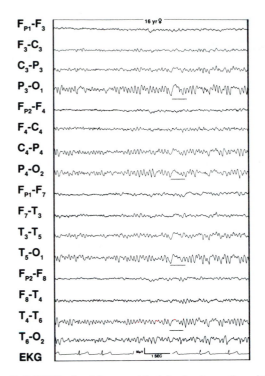

Figure 6-8 EEG of a 16-year-old girl who is awake with eyes closed. A biooccipital posterior slow wave of youth noted (*line marking*).

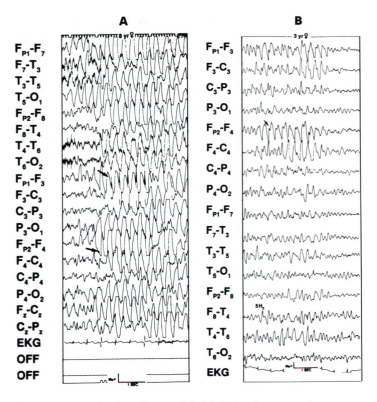

Figure 6-9 EEG of an 8-year-old girl during hyperventilation. *Arrows* indicate notching of the high-amplitude slow activity in the absence of epileptiform discharges. **B,** EEG of a 9-year-old girl during drowsy, light sleep. Notched, high-amplitude delta activity is seen (*arrow*) in the absence of epileptiform discharges.

toured occipital transients with a prominent surface-positive phase lasting 75 to 150 msec are described, although an extremely sharp appearance may cause suspicion. Eye closure or darkening of the room will eliminate lambda waves, whereas occipital spike discharges will persist. These transients are noted in young infants and can be observed occasionally in neonates [Tharp, 1986].

Hyperventilatory response. Historically, a response to hyperventilation was considered evidence of brain abnormality in children [Lindsley and Cutts, 1940]. However, it has now become commonplace to observe prominent high-amplitude slowing in normal children, maximum in expression between 8 to 12 years [Peterson and Eeg-Olofsson, 1971] and persisting into adulthood. A greater degree of response has been associated with lower blood glucose or carbon dioxide concentrations.

Proper testing procedure requires 3 to 5 minutes of overbreathing by the child to elicit the response. Careful notation of artifact and an anticipation of spikelike high-amplitude sharp waves are emphasized [Hrakovy, 1990; Blume, 1982]. Superimposed faster frequencies may appear to be spike discharges, are followed by slow waves during hyperventilation, and are commonly over-interpreted as an abnormal finding (Figure 6-9, *A*). Only the appearance of clearly defined abnormal spike complexes or focal, lateralizing findings are to be interpreted as abnormal.

Photostimulation. Although not as helpful as hyperven-

tilation and sleep, photostimulation may produce a variety of electrographic phenomena that can be useful to the neurologist. It is suggested to use a strobe light with 500,000-foot by 2,000,000-foot candles of intensity at a distance of 12 inches from the face and at multiple flash frequencies. Both occipital and parietal channels should be included, with one channel recording the output signal from the light source.

Two artifacts should always be anticipated. The photoelectric effect usually appears in the frontopolar electrodes and is caused by high resistance or defective grounding of these electrodes. Simply shielding these electrodes from the light source may be sufficient to determine if it is present. A second artifact results from the photomyoclonic effect. Muscle contractions, usually around the anterotemporal, frontal, and frontopolar electrodes, are recorded in response to the light flashes.

Taking these possible sources of artifact into consideration, the normal phenomenon anticipated is a sharp surface-positive waveform, maximal in the parietal and occipital electrodes, which matches the flash frequency (Figure 6-10, *A*). Photostimulation might induce drowsiness, including a normal sharp-wave phenomenon

pathways, as documented by fetal ultrasonography [Prechtl, 1984; Robertson, 1982, 1987], differences in motility behavior in preterm infants may signify altered brain development in an extrauterine environment.

Infant/childhood sleep. With maturation, the infant's ultradian sleep cycle lengthens to 75 to 90 minutes. It is composed of one rapid eye movement (or active) sleep segment that follows four non-rapid eye movement (or quiet sleep) segments. Regional EEG patterns occur within these sleep segments, which are important for neurologists to learn to identify.

Vertex waves and sleep spindles. The transitional state of drowsiness is sometimes referred to as *stage 1* of sleep and may include sharp-wave discharges that are maximal in amplitude over the vertex and central region. Commonly, symmetric central diphasic waveforms become better expressed and more abundant during *stage 2* sleep, which coincides with the appearance of sleep spindles. These waveforms usually have an initial surface-negative wave, followed by a surface-positive phase. The onset of vertex waves can be between 2 and 5 months of age and can appear asymmetric, particularly at younger ages. If this asymmetry exceeds 20%, the neurologist must consider the presence of a lesion on the attenuated side (see Figure 6-2, *A*). Also, excessively asynchronous appearance of vertex waves has been associated with either increased intracranial pressure or structural midline defects, such as agenesis of the corpus callosum [Kellaway, 1979].

Sleep spindles primarily define stage 2 of sleep and are not clearly expressed until 3 to 4 months of age. Synchrony is gradually achieved with increasing age, and most spindles are bilaterally synchronous by 18 months (Figure 6-11, *A*). The waveform of sleep spindles in infants differs from that of older patients. The duration of spindles ranges from 1.5 to 1.8 seconds at 4 to 6 months. At this age, they frequently reach 4 to 6 seconds, which subsequently shortens to 0.5 second by 25 to 54 months [Tanguay et al., 1975].

Spindles lasting as long as 4 to 6 seconds are frequently observed in infants younger than 1 year of age, but "extreme" spindles have been described in neurologically abnormal children of older ages (Figure 6-11, *B*). The common frequency range is 13 to 14 Hz, but slower spindle frequencies of 10 to 12 Hz are also noted in about 5% of children older than 5 years. Spindle density is highest at 3 to 9 months and at a minimum at 27 to 54 months [Kellaway, 1952]. Faster bursts of 18 to 22 Hz may resemble spindles but are usually associated with medications, such as benzodiazepines and barbituates.

Occipital sharp transients. Two types of sharp transients can occur in the occipital region during sleep. Posterior sharp transients of sleep are surface-positive, checkmark-like waveforms, which usually occur in runs

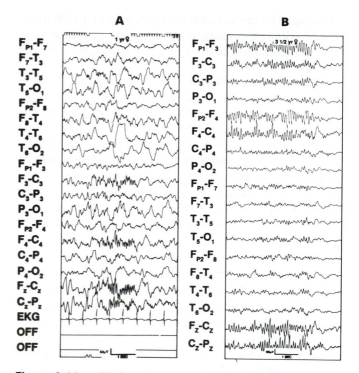

Figure 6-11 A, EEG of a 1-year-old girl with symmetric sleep spindles also noted in the vertex region. Well-developed frequency amplitude gradient is also present. **B,** EEG of a 3½-year-old girl with developmental delay and cerebral palsy during sleep showing "extreme" spindling in the absence of a frequency amplitude gradient.

of 4 to 5 Hz but may occur singly. Although appearing asymmetrically, these waveforms are bilaterally synchronous.

Although posterior sharp transients of sleep can appear between 4 and 5 years of age, they are most commonly encountered during the early sleep of young adults 15 to 35 years of age [Vignaendra and Matthews, 1974] (Figure 6-12, *C*).

The other form of occipital transients in children also appears during drowsiness, with either a cone-shaped configuration or a diphasic sharp wave resembling a vertex transient [Kellaway, 1979].

Frequency distribution during sleep. As described, more pronounced beta activity can be noted during drowsiness. As stage 2 sleep emerges, a definite frequency and amplitude gradient can be appreciated between the anterior and posterior head regions. Higher frequency, lower amplitude activity predominates in anterior head regions, with the converse situation occurring in posterior head regions. With deeper sleep, this gradient is less well defined. Its absence or poor organization have been noted in children with developmental delay [Slater, 1979] (see Figure 6-11, *B*).

Arousal patterns. Infants younger than 2 months of age have only a diminution of background amplitude with

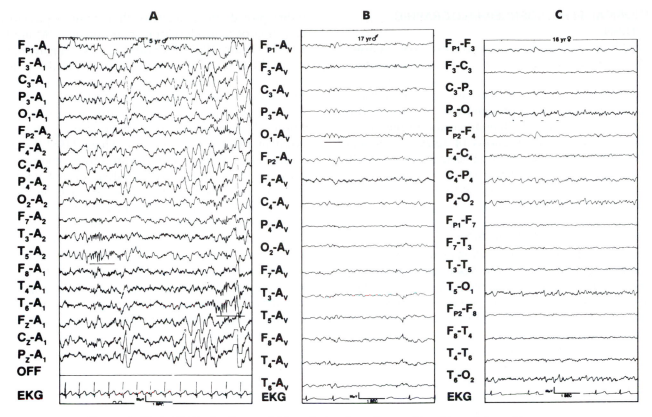

Figure 6-12 A, EEG of a 5-year-old boy during drowsiness with a 14- and 6-positive sharp-wave pattern noted in the right temporal region. **B,** EEG of a 17-year-old boy during drowsiness, with a 6 per second phantom spike-wave pattern seen over the left hemisphere. **C,** A 16-year-old girl with bioccipital posterior occipital sharp transients seen during drowsiness. (**B** Courtesy Dr. P. Crumrine, Pittsburgh, Pennsylvania.)

arousal. By 2 to 3 months of age, diphasic slow waves accompany this desynchronization and may merge with delta waves by 5 months of age. With further arousal, 4 to 8 Hz rhythmic waveforms are noted diffusely or in the frontocentral regions, last for several seconds, and disappear by 4 years of age. More monorhythmic 4 to 5 Hz activity may persist into young adulthood and can be seen in 40% of children 10 to 14 years of age [Gibbs and Gibbs, 1950]. Postarousal hypersynchrony of 2.5 to 3.5 Hz appears frontally and more posteriorly with further arousals. Such changes may cease at any time, and the recording revert to the previous sleep pattern.

Patterns of uncertain significance. This discussion of normal EEG concludes with a consideration of patterns that can be more readily confused with epileptiform phenomena. It is necessary for the neurologist to anticipate the appearance of these normal patterns and appreciate the historical significance of their proposed association with various medical conditions.

The most commonly encountered pattern is the 14-and-6 positive spike discharge (Figure 6-12, *A*). Although initially assigned clinical significance, this pattern has subsequently been noted in several control populations [Lombroso et al., 1966]. These surface-positive waveforms appear in the posterotemporal regions or adjacent areas during sleep, with a 60- to 70-μV-comb-shaped configuration and lasting as long as 3 seconds. It is best noted with a referential montage and has a peak incidence during adolescence.

The 6 Hz spike-wave complexes are less common waveforms, having maximal amplitude in the centroparietal regions. Historically considered clinically important in patients with headache and autonomic symptoms, it can be seen in normal controls, especially adolescents [Gibbs and Gibbs, 1964]. These complexes can be induced by diphenhydramine in 30% of normal volunteers [Tharp, 1966] (Figure 6-12, *B*).

Small, sharp spikes and psychomotor variants are uncommonly noted in young children but rarely have a relationship with clinical syndromes. Indeed, small, sharp spikes are higher in incidence in a normal population, rather than in a patient population [White et al., 1977; Gibbs et al., 1963], and psychomotor variant patterns are described in as many normal, asymptomatic individuals as in study patients.

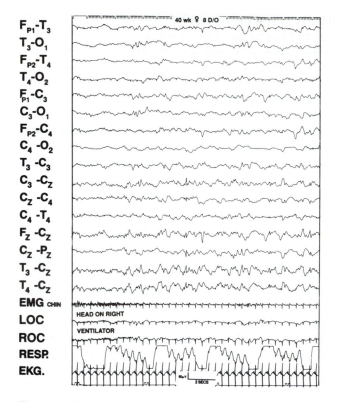

Figure 6-16 EEG of a 40 weeks' gestation, 8-day-old girl with an atypical low-to-moderate voltage invariant pattern after severe intracranial hemorrhage.

Table 6-1 Major electroencephalographic abnormalities*

	Near-term and term infants† (36 to 41 or more weeks)	Preterm infants‡ (30 to 36 weeks)
Inactive§	X	X
Burst suppression	X	X
Slow	X	X
Low-voltage‖	X	
Monorhythmic	X	
No spatial/temporal organization	X	
Asymmetry	X	X (>50%)
Interhemispheric asynchrony	X	X
Abnormal superimposed patterns	X	
Focal spikes	X	X
Seizures	X	X

*Modified from Scher MS. Cerebral neurophysiological assessment of the high-risk neonate. In: Guthrie RD, ed. Recent advances in neonatal care. Clinics in critical care medicine. New York: Churchill Livingstone, 1987.
†Monod N, Pajot N, Guidasci S. Electroencephalogr Clin Neurophysiol 1972; 32:529.
‡Tharp BR, Cukier F, Monod N. Electroencephalogr Clin Neurophysiol 1981; 51:219.
§Below 5 μV or isoelectric, 0.5 to 1 Hz.
‖Maximal 25 μV.

side of the injury [Scher and Tharp, 1982]. The attenuation disappeared in 20% of these EEGs within 3 weeks, without asymmetry in subsequent records, whereas increased slowing of the background developed in the same region or hemisphere on subsequent records for other patients. Because of the high association of cerebral lesions with these lateralized or parasagittal EEG abnormalities, the clinician is strongly advised to obtain cranial imaging studies for accurate anatomic localization. Aso et al. [1989] found that hemispheric asymmetry and/or focal attenuation was associated with significant brain pathology in both term and preterm patients.

Transient asymmetries have also been described in asymptomatic neonates [Challamel et al., 1984; O'Brien, 1987] noted during the initial portion of quiet sleep. Judgment must be used before proceeding to imaging procedures to assess such patients for structural lesions.

Neonatal seizures. Despite the urgency to reach a prompt diagnosis of seizures in the newborn, several unique features of this condition impede timely recognition and treatment. The varied and less organized clinical expression of neonatal seizures makes the diagnosis more difficult [Harris and Tizard, 1970; Rose and Lombroso, 1970; Dreyfus-Brisac and Monod, 1964; Volpe, 1987]. Accepted clinical criteria [Volpe, 1987]

may not always distinguish seizure movements from pathologic nonseizure movements. New classifications are being developed [Mizrahi and Kellaway, 1984b] that will improve the clinical accuracy of the observer. Technologies utilizing prolonged EEG or synchronized EEG-video monitoring sessions will more likely dominate the diagnosis of clinical and electrographic seizures [Mizrahi, 1984b; Scher, 1989].

Several neonates may have seizures that go undetected unless the EEG study is used. Some of these patients are pharmacologically paralyzed for ventilatory care [Tharp and Laboyrie, 1983], whereas others fail to demonstrate clinical seizures despite the appearance of electrographic seizures in the absence of a paralytic agent [Coen et al., 1982].

EEG seizures are recognized by the electroencephalographer based on the evolution in discharges that can be clearly distinguished from the background and are not related to artifact. The frequency of these discharges is usually in the slow range, with a variety of waveforms. The evolution of discharges implies a gradual change in the locus, amplitude, waveform, and/or distribution. The arbitrary definition for the minimum duration of a seizure is 10 seconds, with the average duration being 2 to 5 minutes for either term or preterm neonates, unless

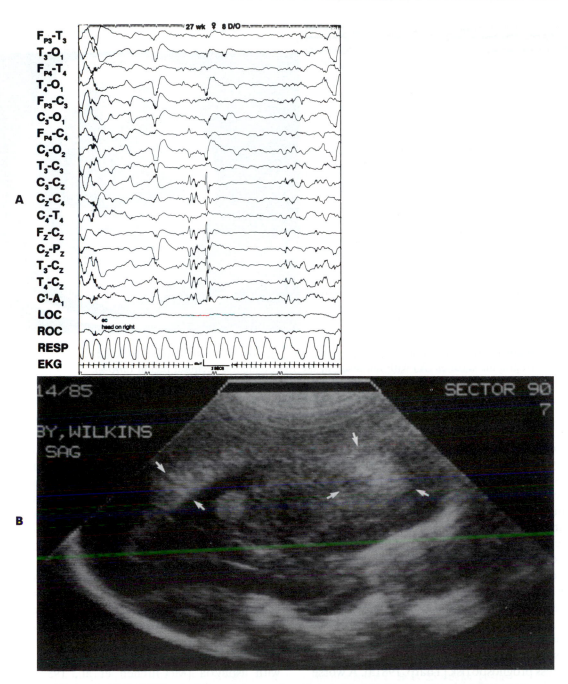

Figure 6-17 A, EEG of a 27 weeks' gestation, 8-day-old girl with prominent midline (C_2) positive sharp wave, also seen in an adjacent electrode (C_1). **B,** Cranial ultrasound of same patient, with prominent periventricular echodensities (*arrows*). (From Scher MS, et al. J Child Neurol 1988; 3:135.)

status epilepticus is noted [Clancy et al., 1987; Scher et al., 1993]. Clinical ictal activity may accompany the electrical seizure (Figure 6-19, *A* and *B*). Only a few patterns are associated with a particular clinical presentation. For example, alpha-range rhythms have been associated with respiratory disturbances, such as apnea, as the clinical correlate appearing with an electrographic seizure [Watanabe et al., 1977]. Five categories of

clinical seizure types have been described [Volpe, 1987] and may be associated with any number of EEG seizure patterns. Focal or multifocal EEG seizures can be observed, and generalized discharges are seen rarely. The rare occurrence of a clinical seizure without a coincident EEG accompaniment has been described (Figure 6-19, *C*) [Watanabe et al., 1977]. Although one explanation is that there is a nonseizure movement

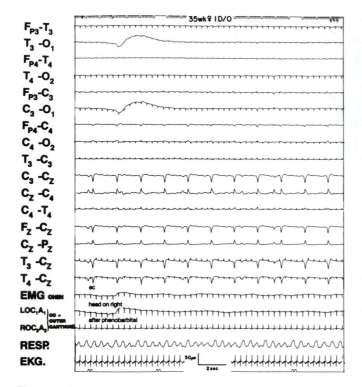

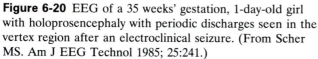

Figure 6-20 EEG of a 35 weeks' gestation, 1-day-old girl with holoprosencephaly with periodic discharges seen in the vertex region after an electroclinical seizure. (From Scher MS. Am J EEG Technol 1985; 25:241.)

impression by the documentation of interictal epileptiform abnormalities. Because it is uncommon to either witness a clinical seizure or confirm electrical seizures during the EEG recording, the neurologist must primarily rely on an accurate historical description of the questionable event. There are instances, however, when the history is unclear, and one or multiple EEG studies may be helpful.

Among a variety of EEG patterns, certain features have been associated with patients with seizure disorders; these features are commonly referred to as *epileptiform* [Zivin and Ajmone-Marsan, 1968]. Epileptiform waveforms include spikes, sharp waves, spike-and-wave, sharp-and-slow-wave, and multiple spikes. The sharp wave has a waveform that is characteristically negative in polarity, with a duration of 70 to 200 msec. This finding is contrasted with the spike morphology, which is of shorter duration and sharper morphology (between 20 and 70 msec). The slow-wave complex that may accompany either waveform is generally between 1 to 5 Hz [Maulsby, 1971; Kooi, 1966].

These epileptiform features are not necessarily associated with clinical seizures. One study found 2.7% of 743 normal children had epileptiform EEG activity. This percentage increased to 8.7% during sleep [Eeg-Oloffsson, 1971]. Also, certain forms of genetic epilepsy

have asymptomatic family members with abnormal EEG discharges [Doose et al., 1969]. Conversely, patients with well-documented seizures may have normal EEGs, particularly children who are younger than 2 years of age [Scher, 1986]. Only 56% of patients with seizures in one study [Ajmone-Marsan and Zivin, 1970] had epileptiform activity on the first EEG.

Generalized epileptiform patterns

Spike (polyspike)-and-wave pattern. The most frequently encountered pattern of the spike-and-wave pattern is bilaterally synchronous single or polyspike discharges, followed by rhythmic slow waves (Figure 6-21, *A*). Both features are surface negative, and these discharges can be 100 to 200 msec long. Discharges in certain regions, such as the frontal areas, appear slightly before the generalized burst or are maximally expressed in one particular location. One may see fragments of the spike-and-wave pattern, depending on the selected montage or sensitivity setting resulting from the cancellation effect of bipolar recordings or the low amplitude of the complex, respectively. The highest frequency of the discharges is at the onset of seizures (3 to 6 Hz), with slowing to 2.5 to 4 Hz during the seizure. Augmentation of the discharges can be seen with hyperventilation [Dalby, 1969] and non-rapid eye movement sleep, although the spike-and-wave can become slower and more complex in morphology during sleep. Two nonspecific phenomena are often associated with generalized spike-and-wave, consisting of either bursts of 2 to 4 Hz rhythmic waves or more monorhythmic occipital delta.

The most significant clinical correlation is that patients with this pattern have a strong association with a generalized seizure disorder. Although it can be noted in patients without clinical seizures, most patients demonstrate a history of generalized motor or absence seizures. Generalized 3-Hz spike-and-wave discharges with absence seizures make up 10% of all patients with the absence description [Penry et al., 1975]. A motor accompaniment is noted in 90% of patients [Penry et al., 1975; Doose et al., 1973], and 14% have myoclonic seizures [Dalby, 1969]. The reaction time to an auditory stimulus is slowed during the occurrence of the spike-and-wave complex [Browne et al., 1974].

Patients can "outgrow" these discharges, as evidenced by longitudinal studies between 5 and 14 years that suggest age penetrance of the clinical seizure with or without the EEG abnormality [Metrakos and Metrakos, 1974]. Up to 50% of adolescents develop generalized motor seizures. If spike-and-wave discharge is the only abnormality on the EEG, the incidence of other neurologic deficits is low.

Photostimulation may elicit a spike-and-wave discharge (see Figure 6-10, *B*) but can only support the evidence for seizures suggested by clinical history. This

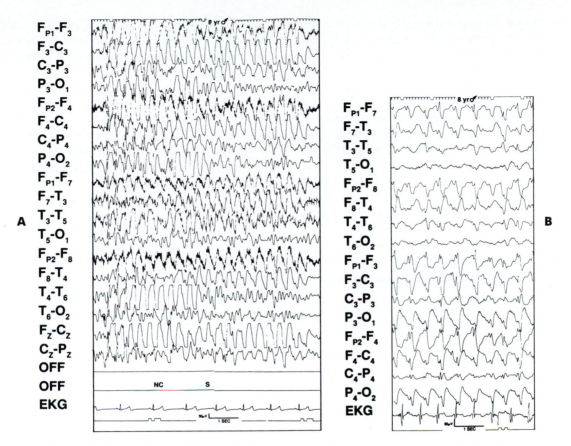

Figure 6-21 A, A 9-year-old boy with 3-per-second spike-and-wave discharges in the absence of clinical signs. **B,** An 8-year-old boy with sharp-and-slow-wave complex. The patient demonstrated mental retardation.

pattern also appears in 3.4% of normal controls [Doose, 1969] and in 20% of siblings of patients with photoparoxysmal seizures who have never had clinical seizures. Only 10% of these siblings had clinical seizures. A prolonged response that outlasts the stimulus is the strongest indication of a seizure disorder [Reilly and Peters, 1973], but there is an age-dependent expression of this abnormal pattern between 5 and 15 years. This pattern is most easily elicited with a 10 to 16 flash per second frequency. Patients on dialysis, with electrolyte disturbances, or exhibiting withdrawal from drugs, such as barbiturates and alcohol, are more susceptible to photoparoxysmal responses with or without clinical accompaniment.

Sharp-and-slow-wave complex. The sharp-and-slow-wave complex pattern consists of a sharp wave of negative polarity lasting 100 to 200 msec and slow waves lasting 350 to 400 msec in a frequency of 1 to 2 Hz (Figure 6-21, *B*). Although diffusely distributed over the scalp in most patients, it may be asymmetric or confined to either anterior or posterior quadrants. This waveform is augmented only during sleep and can be associated with sudden desynchronization of the record, which is

associated with a burst of beta activity termed an *electrodecremental response*. Although the highest incidence of sharp-and-slow-wave complex is between 1 and 5 years of age, it is also noted well into adulthood. Hypsarrhythmia can precede the sharp-and-slow-wave complex during the first year of life.

Of clinical seizures with sharp-and-slow-wave complex, 90% are tonic [Blume et al., 1973], and these seizures are resistant to therapy, persisting at least 15 years after beginning treatment [Markand, 1977]. Other types of clinical seizures can also occur, depending on the age of onset; tonic seizures at 16 months, absence seizures at 32 months, myoclonic seizures at 39 months, and tonic-clonic seizures after 43 months [Chevrie and Aicardi, 1972].

Mental subnormality is noted in 30% of patients at diagnosis. When seizures are present before 2 years of age and are caused by CNS disease, the child will more likely exhibit delayed development. The clinical and EEG syndrome that includes the three features of seizures, mental subnormality, and sharp-and-slow-wave complex is termed the *Lennox-Gastaut syndrome* [Lennox, 1945; Gastaut, 1966].

Hypsarrhythmia. Hypsarrhythmia is the most common interictal EEG pattern associated with infantile spasms. The most common clinical description is a sudden, symmetric, tonic muscle contraction producing flexion/extension of the trunk and extremities, although a variety of movement patterns have been described [Hrakovy, 1990]. The EEG pattern is a chaotic mixture of high-amplitude slow waves, multifocal spikes, and intrahemispheric/interhemispheric asynchrony (Figure 6-22). This EEG pattern is generally noted between 3 months and 5 years of age and can be preceded by a burst-suppression or low-voltage invariant pattern in the newborn period. Hypsarrhythmia can also be preceded by a normal EEG [Jeavons and Bower, 1974].

During a spasm, an electrodecremental response interrupts the high-amplitude slowing by a sudden diminution of all activity with a duration of 1 second to 1 minute.

The role of EEG is limited to diagnosis only, with no reliable correlation with etiologic cause, course, or prognosis, including mental development.

Generalized periodic discharges. Generalized periodic discharges are distinguished from bilateral synchronous spike-and-wave discharges by the broader waveforms in the context of a periodic quality. This pattern is noted with two clinical situations: Creutzfeldt-Jakob disease in adults and subacute sclerosing panencephalitis in children.

The periodic complexes in subacute sclerosing panencephalitis appear at 1- to 3-second intervals [Celesia, 1973] but have no relationship with the clinical progression of the disease. Similarly, there is no relationship between the myoclonic movements and these discharges. The periodic discharges may first arise from a normal background and may initially be noted only during sleep.

Secondary bilateral synchrony. Penfield and Jasper [1946] originally described bilateral discharges that resulted from the initial excitation of postulated subcortical or unilateral discharges. This concept has been adopted in the diagnostic procedures related to the evaluation for the surgical treatment of epilepsies. Such an approach attempts to excise surgically the dominant focal epileptic focus in a patient who has been refractory to anticonvulsant therapy alone. The amytal or metrazol test may abolish the bilateral discharges if a carotid injection is performed into the hemisphere responsible for generating the primary discharge [Gloor et al., 1976]. In children an intravenous pentobarbital injection has been alternately suggested [Lombroso and Erba, 1970]. By locating the dominant epileptic focus, surgical excision of this abnormal tissue will presumably abolish most or all of the bilateral discharges and allow complete or improved control with anticonvulsant drugs.

Focal epileptiform patterns. The incidence of focal spike discharges in the normal population (1.5% of 1000 children) has already been stressed [Peterson and Eeg-Olofsson, 1971]. Spike discharges in symptomatic patients should be correlated with the clinical context in which the discharges are noted. Focal spikes are noted in children with cerebral palsy in the absence of clinical seizures; however, the presence of focal spikes in children younger than 2 years of age implies severe neurologic impairment. The spike foci on a single EEG examination is not a reliable indicator of structural brain lesions because the location of the spike discharges on subsequent EEG studies may be relocated to two or more different foci [Trojaborg, 1968]. With these facts in mind, the neurologist should consider certain electroclinical syndromes associated with focal or multifocal spike foci in children.

Rolandic spikes. Rolandic spikes are associated with the most common genetic epilepsy of childhood. High-amplitude spike-and-slow waves are prominently noted singly or in runs in the central and midtemporal regions (Figure 6-23, *A*). Shifting laterality is noted in the same or subsequent EEG studies, and these focal discharges may be associated with generalized spike-and-wave discharges in 5% of children. The EEG background activity is otherwise normal, and certain patients have

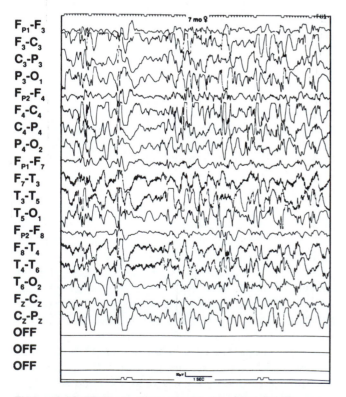

Figure 6-22 EEG of a 7-month-old girl with infantile spasms demonstrating a hypsarrhythmic pattern consisting of high-amplitude disorganized slow activity, intermixed spike-and-slow-wave discharges, and an electrodecremental response.

rolandic spikes that appear only during sleep, commonly during non–rapid eye movement sleep [Beaumanoir et al., 1974; Dalla Bernardina and Beghini, 1976]. An unusual polarity relationship is associated with the discharges, consisting of a simultaneous negative and positive phase-reversal in two different locations of the spike discharge, which may represent a horizontal rather than a more common vertical dipole and is associated with abnormal EEG activity.

This genetic epilepsy is clinically expressed in an age-dependent manner between 3 and 14 years of age; it is rarely noted beyond adolescence. Commonly, a nocturnal seizure is observed, with focal motor phenomena usually involving the face; buccolingual involvement and salivation are evident. Generalized seizures also frequently occur. Despite the familial aspect of this epilepsy, 13% of family members may demonstrate rolandic spikes without clinical seizures [Heijel et al., 1975].

Temporal spikes and sharp waves. Although not associated with a distinctive epileptic syndrome, temporal spike discharges must be distinguished from the spikes associated with rolandic epilepsy. The electroencephalogra-

pher can ascertain a difference by determining if there is a more limited temporal location to the spike without the expression of a dipole as described previously (Figure 6-23, *B*).

According to a study by Eeg-Oloffsson [1971], temporal spikes are rarely seen in normal children (2 out of 743 patients) but are frequently seen in epileptic patients (92% of 666), including children with complex partial seizures [Currie et al., 1971].

Complex partial seizures commonly begin during childhood [Falconer, 1971; Ounsted et al., 1966], and anatomic abnormalities have been noted in some of these patients. Static lesions, such as mesial temporal sclerosis, hippocampal herniation, or hamartoma, have all been described [Earle et al., 1953; Falconer and Taylor, 1968], and several of these patients also demonstrate homonoymous hemianopsia or quadrantanopsia on visual field testing, presumably caused by perinatal occlusion of the posterior cerebral artery [Remillard et al., 1974].

Multiple independent spike foci. Patients with spike discharges in at least three noncontiguous electrode positions are considered to have multiple independent spike

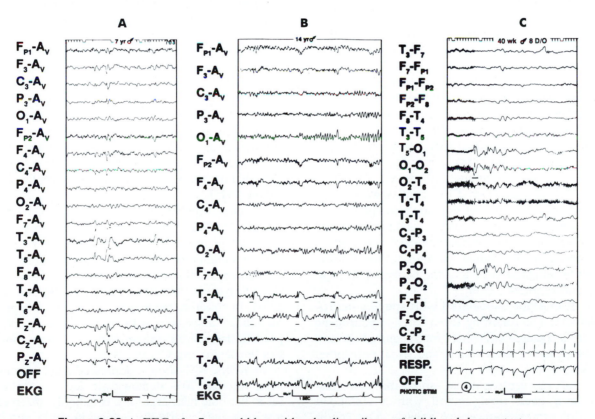

Figure 6-23 A, EEG of a 7-year-old boy with rolandic epilepsy of childhood demonstrating a horizontal dipole of sharp-wave discharges. Note the upward negative deflection simultaneous to the positive downward deflection of the discharge. **B,** EEG of a 14-year-old boy with complex partial seizures demonstrating frequent repetitive temporal spikes. **C,** Forty weeks' gestation, 8-day-old boy after hypoxic-ischemic insult, who showed photic-induced occipital spikes at slow flash frequencies.

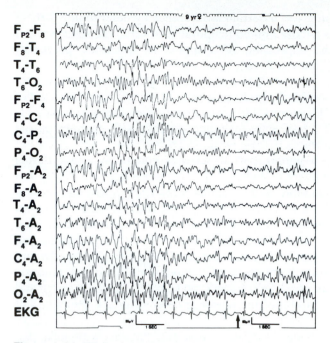

Figure 6-24 EEG of a 9-year-old girl with a mixed seizure disorder with multifocal sharp waves.

foci (Figure 6-24). No patients in a normal population have this pattern [Eeg-Oloffsson, 1971], whereas 63 of 1500 patients with EEG recordings [Blume, 1978] do. Of these patients, 90% had clinical seizures; 80% of the seizures were generalized motor seizures. Although 66% of patients have subnormal intelligence, the neurologist can anticipate normal cognitive abilities if there are few spike discharges with a normal EEG background. Sleep can augment spikes and activate new foci, but hyperventilation or photic stimulation cannot. Of these patients, 25% had previous EEG studies with either hypsarrhythmia or sharp-and-slow-wave complex. Etiologic possibilities for this pattern include perinatal insults, CNS infections, neurocutaneous syndromes, degenerative disease, trauma, or anoxia. No etiologic cause can be assigned in 29% of the patients [Noriega-Sanchez and Markand, 1976].

Spike discharges associated with specific neurologic defects. The following three types of neurologic deficits are associated with spike foci: acquired aphasia of childhood, motor dysfunction, and visual perceptual difficulties.

Temporal or centroparietal spike-and-wave discharges have been rarely noted with a childhood condition of expressive-receptive aphasia. This condition develops in previously normal children between 3 and 8 years of age [Worster-Drought, 1971; Shoumaker et al., 1974], and the aphasia can precede the onset of seizures by several years [Landau and Kleffner, 1957]. Long-term follow-up studies have also documented

resolution of seizures in most of these patients, but treatment has no effect on asphasia, which disappears partially or completely over a period of years [Mantovani and Landau, 1980].

Some children have demonstrated evidence of motor difficulties with central spike discharges on their EEG studies [Lairy and Harrison, 1968]. No clinical seizure manifestations have been observed. Subsequent reports have now corroborated and supplemented these earlier findings [Shewmon et al., 1988].

Occipital spikes have been observed in children with visuoperceptual and oculomotor abnormalities [Kellaway et al., 1955] (Figure 6-23, C). Seizures were also noted in 54% of 318 children with occipital spikes [Smith and Kellaway, 1964], and most had seizures before 1 year of age. Generalized motor seizures are the most common type, and only 9% reported ictal manifestations that were visual in nature. Only 34% of patients with ocular difficulties and occipital spikes have clinical seizures, but only 2 of 743 normal children have occipital foci [Eeg-Oloffsson, 1971].

Periodic discharges. Generalized periodic discharges and neonatal periodic patterns have already been discussed. The present description pertains to the EEG phenomenon that consists of repetitive stereotypic focal discharges that remain lateralized with a duration of either at least 10 minutes or 20% of the recording time. The waveform morphologies can be varied and are collectively referred to as *periodic lateralized epileptiform discharges* [Chatrian et al., 1964]. This phenomenon represents either an acute or a subacute process in adults or children; usually a brain lesion, such as infarction, contusion, or cerebritis, can be identified. Periodic discharges in the temporal region may suggest an encephalitic process caused by a herpetic infection [Elian, 1975].

Biphasic or polyphasic discharges of 100 to 200 msec and 100 to 200 μV are noted and have a frequency of 1 to 2 Hz (Figure 6-25). These discharges persist for a limited number of days or weeks in adults and are replaced by focal polymorphic delta slowing. Multifocal periodic patterns can also occur [Dela Paz and Brenner, 1981]. In children, more subacute or chronic processes have been associated with either focal or multifocal periodic lateralized epileptiform discharge abnormalities [PeBenito and Cracco, 1979].

In adults, 90% show a depressed level of consciousness, whereas 70% demonstrate focal neurologic defects. Periodic discharges are commonly observed after a seizure, particularly if it is focal in onset, and 80% of these patients have frequent seizures [Sternberg et al., 1972]. An unusual seizure disorder in children has been described, consisting of agitation and confusion [Tharp, 1972], in which periodic discharges in the frontal regions are noted when the patient is either awake or asleep.

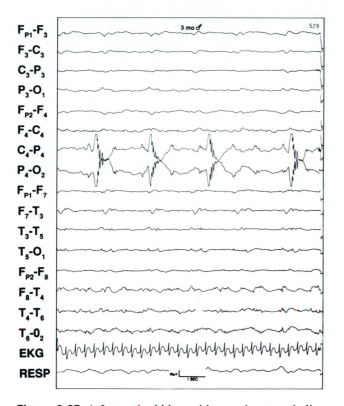

Figure 6-25 A 3-month-old boy with prominent periodic discharges in the right parietal region. The patient had an ischemic cerebrovascular lesion in the distribution of the posterior cerebral artery.

Abnormal nonepileptiform patterns

Besides the value of EEG in the diagnosis of epilepsy and focal cerebral disease, this laboratory tool can be useful in evaluating patients with medical conditions that directly or indirectly disturb cerebral function. This diagnostic category includes diffuse encephalopathies, which usually correlate with alterations in a patient's mentation or level of consciousness. In general an EEG is obtained as an indicator of cerebral dysfunction and as a measure of severity of the disturbance.

The most common change consists of slowing of the background rhythms, with varying degrees of severity, which will range from slowing of the dominant rhythm to generalized delta slowing, or suppression of all EEG activity. The slower the frequency, the more severe the abnormality. An asymmetry of slowing or focal slowing superimposed on diffuse bihemispheric slowing indicates more localized disturbances in addition to diffuse abnormalities. Clearly, polymorphic rhythmic slowing unreactive to afferent stimuli indicates severe cerebral dysfunction.

As indicated in the section on the neurophysiologic basis of EEG, an intermittent rhythmic slowing that attenuates with eye opening or arousal suggests a projected rhythm from presumably diencephalic or subcortical structures.

ROLE OF PEDIATRIC EEG IN SPECIFIC NEUROLOGIC SITUATIONS

This concluding section on pediatric EEG consists of a general overview of EEG patterns associated with specific neurologic conditions encountered during childhood. It should be emphasized that nonepileptiform abnormalities are frequently noted with a diverse group of clinical diagnoses and can assist in either the diagnosis or prognosis of a dynamic disease process.

Febrile seizures

Depending on the timing of the EEG study relative to a seizure during a febrile illness, abnormalities can be noted. These findings, however, are unlikely to have clinical value if observed within hours or days of the febrile seizure. Two situations when an EEG study can be useful during this early period include a suspected focal brain lesion or a continuing subclinical seizure in a patient who has failed to regain full consciousness within an expected interval [Blume, 1982].

In a sequential study of patients with uncomplicated febrile seizures, 33% will have prominent delta activity either diffusely or over the posterior head regions. This activity resolves within 2 weeks and has no prognostic significance [Frantzen et al., 1968]. Furthermore, of 218 patients in the study, the documentation of 42 patients with bisynchronous spike-and-wave discharges and of 19 patients with focal spikes also failed to predict either the recurrence of febrile seizures or the occurrence of later nonfebrile seizures. Only crucial historical information of antecedent neurologic difficulties, such as a focal seizure, prolonged duration (i.e., > 15 min), abnormal examination findings, or family history of seizures, have predictive value for later epilepsy [Nelson and Ellenberg, 1983].

Head trauma

As with adults, the degree of EEG abnormality in children after blunt trauma is in proportion with the severity of the insult. However, the magnitude of the EEG abnormalities in children may exceed the clinical severity more often than occurs in adults. The most striking acute change is in the posterior delta rhythm [Silverman, 1962]. The persistence of abnormalities, such as posterior slowing, may suggest subsequent functional difficulties [Mizrahi and Hrakovy, 1984a].

Headaches

By comparison, clinical judgment is more reliable than EEG to determine the etiologic cause of a headache syndrome in children. However, there is a high percentage of EEG abnormalities in children with headache associated with either migraine syndromes [Prensky and Sommer, 1979] or seizure disorders. Focal delta waves have been described with complicated migraine and a hemiplegic description [Slatter, 1968]. Epileptiform abnormalities together with headache complaints are noted in a substantial number of children with a prodromal or ictal headache component associated with a seizure disorder.

Prognosis after hypoxic-ischemic insults

With either hypoxia or ischemia, progressive EEG changes begin with slowing of the dominant rhythm, followed by the emergence of theta and delta slowing, and finally the suppression of all background activity. This information can be useful, particularly when provided by serial studies in the comatose patient.

Two reports suggest serial EEG evaluations as an adjunct to clinical assessment. Pampiglione and Harden [1968] and Seshia et al. [1979] found that certain EEG findings help to predict outcome. Normal EEG activity suggests a favorable outlook, whereas delta slowing requires follow-up studies before prognostic statements can be affirmed. Low-voltage, invariant EEG background activity, suppression-burst activity, or electrocerebral silence all strongly suggest an unfavorable outcome. Less frequently, diffusely distributed monorhythmic activity (i.e., alpha or spindle waveforms) also suggests a poor prognosis for clinical recovery in patients with altered levels of consciousness.

Determination of brain death

Unlike adults, the current criteria for brain death do not easily apply to all ages of children. Published guidelines [Task Force, 1987] suggest clinical and laboratory examination procedures for the child. As with adults, this report emphasizes clinical history and physical examination criteria. Several age-dependent observation periods are recommended, at which times both clinical examination and EEG studies can be obtained. Because the EEG may not always agree with the clinical assessment of irreversible coma, EEG is only a confirmatory study. With complete absence of brainstem functions, residual low-amplitude EEG activity may persist on rare occasions. Electrocortical silence will more likely result on subsequent EEGs, or the patient will deteriorate progressively and then die as a result of cardiopulmonary failure [Ashwal and Schneider, 1987]. Other ancillary studies evaluating cerebral blood flow may be helpful. These difficulties can be compounded by hypothermia or sedative medication, situations that can erroneously contribute to a low-amplitude or isoelectric tracing.

The neurologist must carefully adhere to the EEG guidelines for the confirmation of brain death [American EEG Society Guidelines, 1986] to avoid potential interpretive error.

CNS infections

With an encephalitic process, EEG changes are principally rhythmic or arrhythmic slowing. As previously described for herpes encephalitis, focal or lateralizing findings may also be seen nonspecifically with many kinds of encephalitides. EEG can also help monitor for seizures that are subtle or purely electrical.

With meningitis, acute EEG changes resemble those noted with encephalitis. Given the different neuropathologic complications of meningitis, such as subdural effusion, empyema, or cerebritis, EEG may suggest the presence of these lesions with the appearance of lateralizing EEG findings.

Degenerative diseases

Most degenerative diseases diffusely affect cerebral function and cause generalized changes on EEG. EEG may help to narrow the diagnostic possibilities given the child's age, symptoms, course, and neurologic findings. In general, gray matter disease is considered when bilaterally synchronous paroxysms occur, referable to cortical or subcortical gray matter disease, whereas white matter disease has been associated with diffuse, high-amplitude slowing, of either a continuous or an intermittent pattern. On occasion, the EEG abnormality may facilitate the suspicion of a diagnostic category of degenerative disease in an otherwise healthy patient [Blume, 1982].

In certain instances, specific EEG patterns are noted with types of degenerative diseases. Patients with neuronal-ceroid lipofuscinosis may first exhibit high-amplitude polyspikes over the posterior head region in response to slow rates of flash stimuli [Pampiglione and Harden, 1973]. GM_2 gangliosidosis in certain patients may be associated with stimulus-sensitive myoclonus with periodic or multifocal sharp waves [Morrell and Torres, 1960], as can be seen on EEGs of newborns with a variety of inherited metabolic diseases [Mises et al., 1977], such as with glycine encephalopathy (Figure 6-26). Conditions in older patients in which stimulus-sensitive myoclonus can be associated with EEG abnormalities include familial myoclonic epilepsy [Blume, 1982] and cherry-red spot myoclonus syndrome [Engel et al., 1977]. EEG findings with subacute sclerosing panencephalitis have already been discussed.

Reye syndrome

Although deeper stages of coma in patients with Reye syndrome parallel EEG deterioration [Aoki and Lombroso, 1973], these two aspects do not have a temporal relationship. However, given the increasing use of pharmacologic paralysis for ventilatory care, EEG remains useful as a guide to the level of encephalopathy, related to either increased intracranial pressure [Kindt et al., 1975] or to the short-chain fatty acid levels [Trauner et al., 1977].

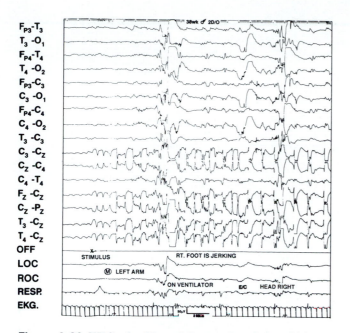

Figure 6-26 EEG of a 38 weeks' gestation, 2-day-old boy with glycine encephalopathy. Stimulus-induced electroclinical seizure noted (X) with clonic movement of the right lower extremity and coincident electrographic seizures in primarily the vertex region. (From Scher MS, et al. Neuropediatrics 1986; 17:137.)

Nonepileptic paroxysmal disorders

Two clinical situations exemplify how the EEG can support this category of paroxysmal disorders. Syncope and, more specifically, breath-holding episodes may resemble clinical seizures. The absence of epileptiform activity while the episode is precipitated during a recording session will support this diagnosis. The associated electrocardiographic changes coincident with the episode may allow further subclassification of the type of episode [Gastaut, 1968].

Psychogenic seizures should be suspected when there is no diffuse slowing or alteration of background disturbances when an EEG is obtained within 24 hours after a suspected, generalized motor seizure. In addition, the coincident occurrence of repetitive behavioral changes in the absence of epileptiform activity strongly suggests, although it does not prove, that psychogenic seizures may be present, even in the context of a well-established seizure disorder of cerebral origin.

Computer analyses of electrographic data. Using computers, automated analyses of electrographic information can assist in the interpretation of analog EEG recordings. Although traditional methods of visual analysis are qualitative and can be subjective, computer analyses process more information efficiently and quantitatively. Prolonged studies over many hours to days can be performed with little loss in accuracy. The presentation of electrographic data to the electroencephalographer is more efficiently presented using computer display methods [Gotman, 1990]. Computer analyses can never replace the decision-making strengths of an experienced electroencephalographer, especially with respect to artifact identification and pattern recognition. Computers should only be an important adjunct to the visual analysis process.

It is suggested that the reader consult supplementary texts to obtain an understanding of the basic methods of computer EEG analysis, including spectral analysis, digital filtering, transient pattern detection, multiple channel analysis and signal averaging [Gotman, 1990; Weitkunat, 1991]. Application of computer techniques concerning spontaneous EEG sleep and evoked potential analyses is discussed next as examples of how computer analyses can be applied to clinical neurophysiologic data.

Computer strategies for EEG sleep analyses. Computer analyses of EEG sleep better define the complicated relationships between cerebral and noncerebral physiologic activity. Automated techniques for such analyses have been applied to both adult and pediatric populations and only recently to neonatal populations. Most techniques rely on conventional methods of spectral analysis that assume *stationary* of neurophysiologic signals (i.e., a predictable sine-cosine wave to represent physiologic data). Nonstationarity characterizes many neurophysiological phenomena, and algorithms are available for appropriate investigation [Weinkunat, 1991]. Ideally, a computer system is needed that can compare behavioral and electrographic components of sleep in a manner that preserves the integrity of continuous signals over time, while simultaneously investigating the time- and frequency-dependent relationships among signals that compose the rhythmicity of EEG sleep cycles [Scher et al., 1990]. Through graphic displays of the digitized data, such as in Figure 6-27, one can detect patterns of sleep organization, as expressed by spectral content, autonomic behavior, or motility during specific states of sleep, compared with the visual score of sleep.

Other applications of computer analyses include the detection of transient electrographic or behavioral events, such as seizure activity or arousals, which may be applicable to the clinical situations of seizure detection or assessment of encephalopathic states.

EVOKED POTENTIAL ANALYSIS

An evoked potential is the electrographic response of the brain to an environmental stimulus. Each evoked potential is represented by a sequence of waves, the amplitudes and latencies of which represent both conduction and neuronal processing of sensory information through the CNS. Stimulus evoked potentials have been used to assess auditory, visual, and somatosensory function. These techniques involve computer averaging

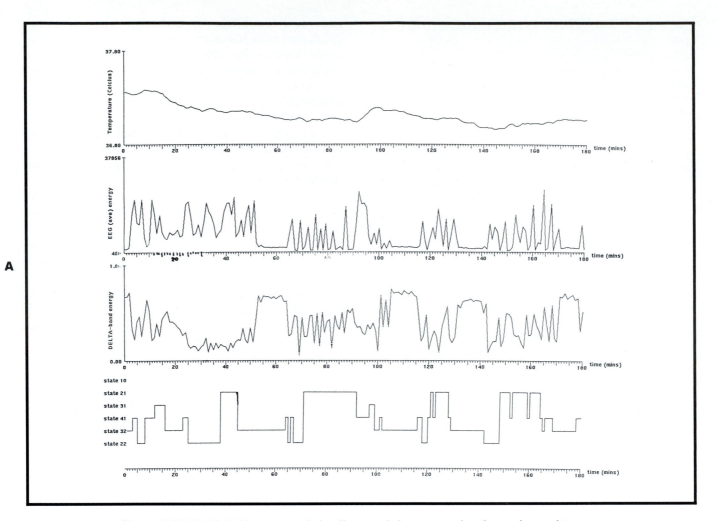

Figure 6-27 Multiple histograms of visually scored sleep states, band energies, and temperature in the neonate (**A**) and infant (**B**). In the neonatal recording, high delta energy values are present during quiet sleep (state 32). Other states are defined as follows: State 10 = awake, state 21, 22 = active sleep, state 31, 32 = quiet sleep, and state 41 = indeterminate sleep. For the infant recording, note the high-delta and low-alpha and -beta values during stage IV non–rapid eye movement sleep.

of the electrical potentials evoked by auditory, visual, or somatosensory stimulus. Scalp-recorded evoked potentials are much less apparent on paper records than are spontaneous EEGs, and the averaging technique allows the summation of numerous evoked potentials to be time-locked to the sensory stimuli. All random activity that is not stimulus-related will cancel itself over time.

Individual component waves are identified by polarity convention, usually depicted by upward negativity, and either their peak latency in milliseconds after the stimulus or their numerical order in the evoked potential complex.

The major portion of this section pertains to the descriptions of early components that occur within the first 50 msec after the stimulus. Intermediate compo-

nents (up to 200 msec) are then briefly discussed. More detailed descriptions are also available.*

Auditory-evoked potentials

Since the demonstration by Jewett and Ramano [1972] that brainstem activity can be reproducibly recorded from the scalp, subsequent studies have solidified the concept that the series of waves constituting the auditory brainstem response are localized primarily in anatomically separate areas along the auditory pathway in the brainstem.

Auditory-evoked potentials can be elicited by brief click stimuli delivered to each ear at a rate of 5 to 30 per

*References Cracco and Cracco, 1986; Spehlmann, 1985; Mizrahi and Dorfman, 1980; Dorfman et al., 1980.

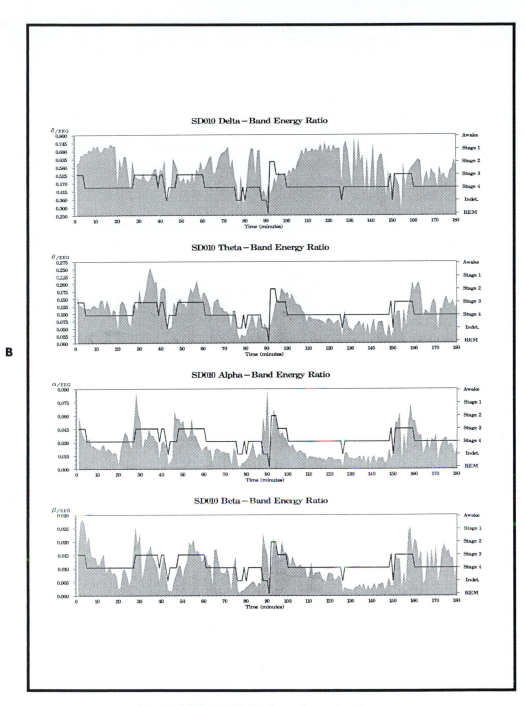

Figure 6-27 cont'd For legend see opposite page.

second, and the responses are recorded with a single pair of scalp electrodes, often on the vertex. Seven positive waveforms are postulated to be generated from these stimuli. The first wave corresponds to the auditory nerve itself, although the fifth positive wave is the most easily measurable response, generated at or near the inferior colliculus.

Attempts have been made to define maturational changes in brainstem responsivity in terms of auditory-evoked potential [Despland, 1985]. The following generalizations are suggested: (1) the waveform and amplitude of components depend on chronologic age, with increasing amplitudes over time; (2) although the peripheral transmission reflected by wave 1 matures before the subsequent waves representing central transmission, latencies do not reach adult values until 12 to 18 months; (3) the threshold for auditory responsivity is lower than that obtained by auditory cortical events or behavioral testing, and is similar to that in adults; and (4) different waveform components become more distinct at slower rates of stimulation, until 1 month of age.

Given these maturational guidelines, clinical applications of auditory-evoked potentials can be judiciously applied to the evaluation of children suspected of either hearing impairment or neurologic dysfunction. A report of the Joint Committee on Infant Hearing adopted by the American Academy of Pediatrics [Salamy, 1984] has identified newborns at risk for hearing loss. Principal clinical situations include asphyxia, hyperbilirubinemia, intracranial hemorrhage, and developmental disorders. Such infants require close auditory and neurodevelopmental follow-up care. Auditory-evoked potentials can be a powerful tool for testing the integrity of the brainstem, especially in the comatose neonate or in the infant receiving neuromuscular blockade. One illustrative example demonstrates prolonged intraaxial latencies for the auditory-evoked potentials in a comatose infant with nonketotic hyperglycinemia (Figure 6-28). Spongy leukodystrophy was noted on gross and microscopic examination of the brain and involved all myelinated traits, including structures subserving the auditory pathway [Scher et al., 1986].

Auditory-evoked potentials are most useful through-out childhood for the diagnosis of demyelinating diseases, extramedullary and intramedullary brainstem tumors, coma caused by metabolic or structural lesions, and corroboration in suspected brain death. A clinical interpretation of abnormal auditory-evoked potentials is suggested by Spehlmann [1985], and this classification can be adapted to pediatric diseases of unknown cause involving the brainstem, including degenerative disorders. In addition to CNS dysfunction, audiologic studies use auditory-evoked potentials to determine the type and severity of hearing defects in children who cannot be examined with conventional audiometric tests.

Visual-evoked responses

Assessment of visual function constitutes another important aspect of neurologic evaluation of the child. Besides the specific information concerning the integrity of the visual pathway, visual function can help to predict later intellectual performance [Miranda et al., 1977]. The following three techniques can assess visual processing: (1) behavioral testing; (2) pattern-preference testing; and (3) visual-evoked responses. Only the latter is discussed.

Visual-evoked responses can be elicited by a stimulus of light delivered either as a flash from a stroboscope or by a checkerboard. The responses are recorded from the occipital regions of the scalp near the primary visual cortex. The latter stimulus requires maintenance of fixation during testing; therefore flash responses have been applied to infants younger than 3 months of age. The earliest response to flash visual-evoked responses is at 24 weeks' gestational age, and the maturational changes in the visual-evoked responses waveforms have been described [Umezaki and Morrell, 1970; Watanabe et al., 1972b]. The earliest waveform is initially surface-negative, and only after 35 weeks' gestational age is it preceded by a positive wave.

The most stable and readily identifiable component of the neonatal visual-evoked response is a major positive waveform with a latency of approximately 190 msec. The P2 peak latency will rapidly decrease by 2 months after term, followed by slower changes throughout childhood (Figure 6-29). Waking and sleep states may alter the latency of visual-evoked responses, and it is generally recommended that the testing be obtained during non–rapid eye movement (quiet) sleep in newborns. Latencies are expected to be 50 msec shorter during the waking state [Harden, 1982].

Abnormal visual-evoked responses can be encountered in rarely occurring generalized neurodegenerative disorders that may involve the visual system [Harden and Pampiglione, 1977] and in the more commonly encountered generalized brain insults, such as asphyxia. In general, high-risk neonates with severe respiratory disease can demonstrate abnormal visual-evoked re-

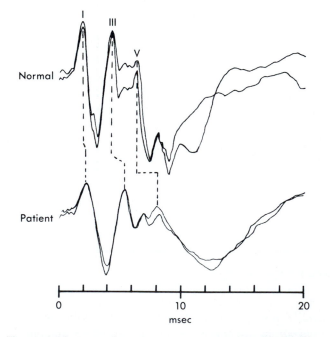

Figure 6-28 An auditory brainstem response to 70 dBnHl click stimuli for a normal 38 weeks' gestation, postconception newborn (*top*) and a newborn with glycine encephalopathy (*bottom*) who was also tested at 38 weeks' gestation, postconception. *Dash lines* denote the difference in component wave latencies of the two infants. (See Figure 6-26 depicting EEG of patient with glycine encephalopathy.) (From Scher MS, et al. Neuropediatrics 1986; 17:137.)

sponses [Graziani et al., 1972]. Specific ischemic cerebrovascular disorders, such as cavitary periventricular leukomalacia, may also result in abnormal visual-evoked responses [DeVries et al., 1986]. Under such clinical circumstances, crude correlations have been suggested between the severity of visual-evoked response disruption and long-term neurodevelopmental outcome. Unfortunately, normal flash visual-evoked response results can be seen in patients with abnormal visual function. It is therefore generally recommended to re-evaluate a patient at risk with pattern visual-evoked response at an older age when visual acuity and attention has matured. Pattern visual-evoked response can be performed reliably as early as 3 months of age.

In conjunction with careful ophthalmologic evaluation, visual-evoked responses can be helpful throughout the childhood years in the investigation of prechiasmal, chiasmal, and postchiasmal lesions [Spehlmann, 1985]. This anatomic distinction may require using pattern-reversal, half-field stimulation in the older child. Monocular full-field stimulation may be preferable for the young child with a decreased level of cooperation. Less specific but helpful information can be obtained by using full-field testing in the evaluation of lesions within the visual pathways, especially demyelination. Although full-field studies can provide sufficient evidence for prechiasmal lesions, if the visual-evoked response abnormality is clearly monocular, lesions of the chiasmal and retrochiasmal portions must be considered with abnormal full-field visual-evoked responses. Further investigation with half-field stimulation is recommended in the cooperative child. For children who cannot sufficiently communicate their responses during these studies because of age or disease, monocular visual-evoked responses can be useful in the evaluation of visual acuity and refraction.

Electroretinogram. The electroretinogram is an electrophysiologic procedure that can assist in the evaluation of retinal disease, in concert with the evaluation of visual pathways by the visual-evoked response. As with the visual-evoked response, the electroretinogram can be obtained by either unstructured flashes of light, or to patterned stimuli. The electroretinogram is an electrical response of the retina that is a consequence of light energy stimulating retinal photoreceptors [Sherman, 1986]. After the stimulus, three major deflections occur in this evoked response (Figure 6-30). An initial negative deflection called the *A wave* corresponds to photoreceptor activity. The second wave is positive deflection termed the *B wave*, which reflects activity presumably from the inner nuclear layer (i.e., Mueller cells). The final C wave is a second positive deflection that apparently has its cellular origins in the retinal pigment epithelium. Given that the flash electroretinogram only represents overall retinal activity, diseases limited to the macular region may not be detected by only a flash electroretinogram procedure. Such flash procedures may be useful, however, with widespread retinal abnormalities, such as retinitis pigmentosa. Patterned stimuli can better detect the 1% of total retinal area comprised by the macula, which may be important to evaluate patients with suspected macular degeneration.

During childhood, the visual system including the retina continues to develop. Rod and cone components, which comprise the electroretinogram signal, are functionally present in the infant, but electrographically are lower in amplitude and longer in latency than the adult electroretinogram [Armington, 1974]. By 1 year of age, pediatric electroretinogram amplitudes are comparable with adult amplitudes. In combination the electroretinogram and visual-evoked potential can be valuable diagnostic tools in the evaluation of a child's visual system. However, the pattern electroretinogram has not yet been aggressively applied to pediatric populations because of the technical difficulties with applying the contact lens electrode in an uncooperative, awake patient. However, certain pathologic conditions that affect mid and far peripheral retinal function (i.e., retinitis pigmentosa) will have a greater effect on the electroretinogram than visual-evoked response. Abnormalities of foveal function, however, such as amblyopia and maculopathy will be manifested in near normal electroretinogram patterns, despite significant visual-

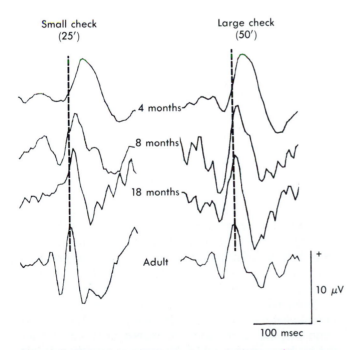

Figure 6-29 Series of visual-evoked responses at increasing ages for both small and large pattern checkerboard images. Decreasing latencies and morphologies of the major positive waveforms are seen. (Courtesy Dr. K. Aso, Nagoya, Japan.)

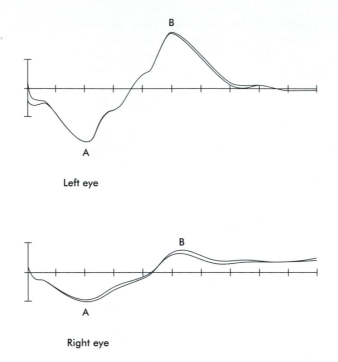

Figure 6-30 An electroretinogram of a 22-month-old male with right eye estropia. Monocular ERG tracings demonstrate diminished amplitude of the A/B wave in the right eye, suggestive of right optic atrophy. The ERG of the left eye is normal. (Courtesy of Dr. R. Sclabassi, Pittsburgh, PA.)

evoked response abnormalities [Sokol, 1986]. The combination of these two studies, therefore, can aid the neurologist in the assessment of the visual system when considering either static or progressive diseases of the nervous system that may involve the visual pathways or retina.

Somatosensory-evoked potentials

Somatosensory-evoked potentials are elicited by percutaneous electrical stimulation of the peripheral nerves. The median nerve is principally used, with cerebral recording over the contralateral-parietal somatosensory cortex. A complex sequence of waveforms results, with significant changes in the early components between groups of different gestational ages, reflecting the postnatal myelination of the sensory fibers of the central somatosensory pathway. Peripheral conduction velocities are largely within the adult range by 3 years of age, whereas spinal cord velocities do not attain adult values until 5 years of age [Cracco et al., 1975]. The somatosensory-evoked potential studies in neonates and infants indicate that the first negative waveform, with a peak latency of 20 msec, is remarkably consistent in its changes over 8 years into the adult pattern. Techniques and results can vary between authors, but short-latency, somatosensory-evoked potentials in infants appear to be easily recorded and well tolerated.

The somatosensory-evoked potential may assist in the localization of brain dysfunction by testing the integrity of the dorsal column mediolemniscal system. Abnormal somatosensory-evoked potentials may suggest impairment, which carries a less favorable prognosis for specific high-risk groups, such as children at risk for hemiplegia [Willis et al., 1984] or preterm neonates surviving periventricular hemorrhage [Laget et al., 1976]. In addition, somatosensory-evoked potential abnormalities associated with lesions in the spinal cord, brain lesions caused by malformation [Duckworth et al., 1976; Dorfman et al., 1980], or neurodegenerative disease [Dorfman et al., 1978] may prove helpful in formulating a prognostic statement.

Somatosensory-evoked potential types consist of either arm or leg electrical stimulation (Figure 6-31). Recording these potentials in children of various ages provides helpful information concerning maturation of the brain and somatosensory-evoked potential abnormalities associated with focal and diffuse neurologic deficits. Different types of spine and scalp somatosensory-evoked potential abnormalities have been found in children with various spinal cord diseases, including those of traumatic, degenerative, and inflammatory etiologies [Cracco and Cracco, 1986]. As with auditory and visual evoked potentials, somatosensory-evoked potential evaluation has a role in the evaluation of patients with diffuse cere-

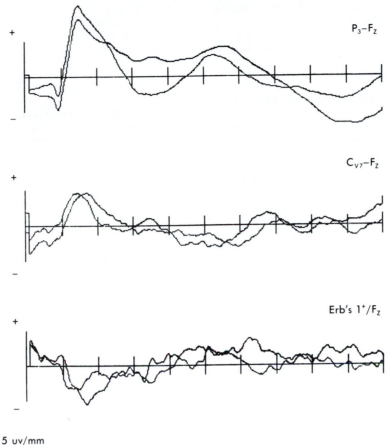

Right median

P₃–Fᵤ

C_{V7}–Fᵤ

Erb's 1⁺/Fᵤ

5 uv/mm
Band width .3   1000 Hᵤ

Figure 6-31 Somatosensory-evoked potential with stimulation of the right medial nerve as recorded at Erb's point, cervical vertebrae, and the somatosensory area of the cortex. (Courtesy Dr. R. Sclabassi, Pittsburgh, Pennsylvania.)

bral disorders with reduced consciousness or altered mental status.

Event-related potentials

Event-related potential refers to both evoked potentials and other types of potentials that are the result of cognitive processes after a stimulus. Such potentials occur substantially later than the standard evoked potential. However, these potentials depend on cognitive processes rather than on the physical characteristics of the stimuli. For instance, the measurement of the most commonly studied event-related potential is the positive peak, which occurs 300 msec after an unexpected stimuli (P300). Attempts have been made to relate abnormalities of the P300 to the condition of altered cognitive functioning in a variety of conditions occurring during childhood, such as learning disabilities [Ollo and Squires, 1986], infantile autism [Novick et al., 1980], and elevated lead levels [Otto et al., 1982]. Although a

number of interesting findings have been reported concerning event-related potentials of children, the data have neither illuminated the nature of the process nor have been diagnostically useful for clinical purposes.

REFERENCES

Aird RB, Gastaut Y. Occipital and posterior electroencephalographic rhythms. Electroencephalogr Clin Neurophysiol 1959; 11:637.

Aird RB, Masland RL, Woodbury DM. The epilepsies. A critical review. New York: Raven Press, 1984.

Ajmone-Marsan C, Zivin LS. Factors related to the occurrence of typical paroxysmal abnormalities in the EEG records of epileptic patients. Epilepsia 1970; 11:361.

American electroencephalographic society guidelines in EEG and evoked potentials. J Clin Neurophysiol 1986; 3:1.

Anders T, Emde R, Parmelee A. A manual of standardized terminology, techniques and criteria for scoring of states of sleep and wakefulness in newborn infants. Los Angeles: NINDS Neurological Information Network, 1971.

Anderson CM, Torres F, Faoro A. The EEG of the early premature. Electroencephalogr Clin Neurophysiol 1985; 60:95.

Aoki Y, Lombroso CT. Prognostic value of electroencephalography in Reye's syndrome. Neurology 1973; 23:333.

Arfel G, Fischgold H. EEG-signs in tumours of the brain. Electroencephalogr Clin Neurophysiol 1961; 19:36.

Arfel G, Leondardon N, Mousali E. Densité et dynamique des encoches pointues frontales dans le sommeil du nouveau-né et du nourisson. Rev EEG Neurophysiol 1977; 7:351-60.

Armington JC. The electroretinogram. New York: Academic Press, 1974.

Ashwal S, Schneider S. Brain death in children. Part II. Pediatr Neurol 1987; 3:69.

Aso K, Scher MS, Barmada M. Nconatal electroencephalography and neuropathy. J Clin Neurophysiol 1989; 6:103-23.

Ayala GF, Dichter M, Gumnit RS, et al. Genesis of epileptic interictal spikes. New knowledge of cortical feedback systems suggests a neurophysiological explanation of brief paroxysms. Brain Res 1973; 52:1.

Beaumanoir A, Ballis T, Varfis G, et al. Benign epilepsy of childhood with rolandic spikes. A clinical, electroencephalographic and telencephalographic study. Epilepsia 1974; 15:301.

Beckwith L, Parmelee AH Jr. EEG patterns of preterm infants, home environment, and later IQ. Child Dev 1986; 57:777-89.

Benda GI, Engel RCH, Zhang Y. Prolonged inactive phases during the discontinuous pattern of prematurity in the electroencephalogram of very low-birthweight infants. Electroencephalogr Clin Neurophysiol 1989; 72:189-97.

Berger H. Uber das elektroencephalogramm des merschen s mittlg. Arch Psychiatr Nervenkr 1932; 98:231.

Blume WT. Clinical and electroencephalographic correlates of the multiple independent spike foci pattern in children. Ann Neurol 1978; 4:541.

Blume WT. Atlas of pediatric electroencephalography. New York: Raven Press, 1982.

Blume WT, David RB, Gomez MR. Generalized sharp and slow wave complexes. Associated clinical features and long-term follow-up. Brain 1973; 96:289.

Brenner RP. Artifacts. Atlanta: American Electroencephalographic Society Annual Course, 1981.

Browne TR, Penry JK, Porter RJ, et al. Responsiveness before, during and after spike-wave paroxysms. Neurology 1974; 24:659.

Celesia CG. Pathophysiology of periodic EEG complexes in subacute sclerosing panencephalitis (SSPE). Electroencephalogr Clin Neurophysiol 1973; 35:293.

Challamel MJ, Isnard H, Brunon AM, et al. Asymétrie EEG transitoire a l'entrée dans le sommeil calme chez le nouveau-né: étude sur 75 observations. Rev Electroencephalogr Neurophysiol Clin 1984; 14:17-23.

Chatrian GE, Shaw C, Leffman H. The significance of periodic lateralized epileptiform discharges in EEG. Electroencephalogr Clin Neurophysiol 1964; 17:177.

Chevrie JJ, Aicardi J. Childhood epileptic encephalopathy with slow spike-wave. A statistical study of 80 cases. Epilepsia 1972; 13:259.

Clancy RR, Fischer RA. Midline sagittal epileptogenic foci in children. Epilepsia 1984; 25:652.

Clancy RR, Legido A. The exact ictal and interictal duration of electroencephalographic neonatal seizures. Epilepsia 1984; 18:537-41.

Clancy RR, Malis S, Laragie D, et al. Focal motor seizures heralding stroke in full-term neonates. Am J Dis Child 1985; 139:601.

Clancy RR, Spitzer AR. Cerebral cortical function in infants at risk for sudden infant death syndrome. Ann Neurol 1985; 18:41.

Clancy RR, Tharp BR. Positive rolandic sharp waves in the electroencephalograms of premature neonates with intraventricular hemorrhage. Electroencephalogr Clin Neurophysiol 1984; 57:395.

Cobb WA, Guiloff RJ, Cart J. Breach rhythm. The EEG related to skull defects. Electroencephalogr Clin Neurophysiol 1979; 47:251.

Coen RW, McCutchen CB, Wermer D, et al. Continuous monitoring of the electroencephalogram following perinatal asphyxia. J Pediatr 1982; 100:628.

Connell JA, Oozeer R, Dubowitz V. Continuous 4-channel EEG monitoring: a guide to interpretation with normal values in preterm infants. Neuropediatrics 1987; 18:138-45.

Cooper R, Osselton JW, Shaw JC. EEG technology. London: Butterworth, 1980.

Cracco RQ, Bodis-Wollner I, eds. Evoked potentials. New York: Alan R. Liss, 1986.

Cracco JB, Cracco RQ. Spinal, brainstem and cerebral somatosensory-evoked potential in the pediatric age group. In: Cracco RQ, Bodis-Wollner I, eds. Evoked potentials. New York: Alan R. Liss, 1986.

Cracco JB, Cracco RQ, Graziani LJ. The spinal evoked response in infants and children. Neurology 1975; 25:31.

Cukier F, Andre M, Monod M, et al. Apport de l'EEG au diagnostic des hemorragies intraventriculaires du prematur. Rev Electroencephalogr Neurophysiol Clin 1972; 2:318.

Currie S, Heathfield K, Henson R, et al. Clinical course and prognosis of temporal lobe epilepsy. Brain 1971; 94:173.

Curzi-Dascalova L, Peirano P, Morel-Kahn Inserm F. Development of sleep states in normal premature and full-term newborns. Dev Psychobiol 1988; 21:431-44.

Dalby MA. Epilepsy and 3 per second spike and wave rhythms. Acta Neurol Scand 1969; 40:1.

Dalla Berbnardina B, Beghini G. Rolandic spikes in children with and without epilepsy (20 subjects polygraphically studied during sleep). Epilepsia 1976; 17:161.

Daly DD. Brain tumors and other space occupying processes. In: Handbook of electroencephalography and clinical neurophysiology, vol 14. Clinical EEG. Amsterdam: Elseview, 1975.

Daly DD, Markand ON. Focal brain lesions. In: Daly DD, Pedley TA, eds. Current practice of clinical electroencephalography, 2nd ed. New York: Raven Press, 1990; 335-700.

Dela Paz D, Brenner RP. Bilateral independent periodic lateralized epileptiform discharges. Arch Neurol 1981; 38:713.

Despland POA. Maturational changes in the auditory system as reflected in human brainstem evoked responses. Dev Neurosci 1985; 7:73.

DeVries LS, Dubowitz LMS, Dubowitz V, et al. Correlation of the pattern of cerebral palsy with the distribution of multicystic brain lesions in preterm infants. Jerusalem: International Child Neurology Congress, 1986.

Dittrichová J, Paul K, Pavliková E. Rapid eye movement in paradoxical sleep in infants. Neuropaediatrie 1972; 3:248-57.

Doose H, Gerken H, Hlen-Volpel KF, et al. Genetics of photosensitive epilepsy. Neuropediatrics 1969; 1:56.

Doose H, Gerken H, Morstmann F, et al. Genetic factors in spike-wave absences. Epilepsia 1973; 14:57.

Dorfman LJ, Pedley TA, Tharp BR, et al. Juvenile neuroaxonal dystrophy. Clinical, electrophysiological and neuropathological features. Ann Neurol 1978; 3:419.

Dorfman LJ, Perkash I, Bosley TM, et al. Use of cerebral evoked potentials to evaluate spinal somatosensory function in patients with traumatic and surgical myelopathies. J Neurosurg 1980; 2:654.

Dreyfus-Brisac C. Neonatal electroencephalography. In: Scarpelli EM, Cosmi EV, eds. Reviews in perinatal medicine, vol 3. New York: Raven Press, 1979.

Dreyfus-Brisac C. Ontogenesis of sleep in human prematures after 32 weeks of conceptional age. Dev Psychobiol 1970; 3:91-121.

Dreyfus-Brisac C. Sleep ontogenesis in early human prematurity from 24 to 27 weeks of conceptional age. Dev Psychobiol 1968; 1:162-9.

Dreyfus-Brisac C, Fischgold H, Samson-Dollfus D, et al. Veille, sommeil, réactivité sensorielle chez le prématuré, le nouveau-ne le nourisson. Electroencephalogr Clin Neurophysiol 1957; 6(suppl):417-40.

Dreyfus-Brisac C, Monod N. Electroclinical studies of status epilepticus and convulsions in the newborn. In: Hrakovy P, Petersen I, eds. Neurological and electroencephalographic correlative studies in infancy. New York: Grune & Stratton, 1964.

Dreyfus-Brisac C, Samson-Dreyfus D, Fischgold H. Activite electrique crebrale du premature et du nouveau-ne. Ann Pediatr 1955; 31:1.

Duckworth T, Yamashita T, Franks CI, et al. Somatosensory evoked cortical responses in children with spina bifida. Dev Med Child Neurol 1976; 18:19-24.

Earle JM, Baldwin M, Penfield W. Incisural sclerosis and temporal lobe seizures produced by hippocampal herniation at birth. Arch Neurol Psychiatr 1953; 69:27.

Eeg-Oloffsson O. The development of the electroencephalogram in normal adolescents from the age of 16 through 21 years. Neuropaediatrie 1971; 3:11.

Elian M. Herpes simplex encephalitis. Prognosis and long-term follow-up. Arch Neurol 1975; 32:39.

Ellingson RJ. Cortical electrical responses to visual stimulation in the human infant. Electroencephalogr Clin Neurophysiol 1960; 12:663-77.

Ellingson RJ. Electroencephalograms of normal fullterm newborns immediately after birth with observations on arousal and visual evoked responses. Electroencephalogr Clin Neurophysiol 1958; 10:31-50.

Ellingson RJ. Studies of the electrical activity of the developing human brain. In: Himwich WA, Himwich EH, eds. The developing brain—progress in brain research, Amsterdam: Elsevier, 1964, 26-53.

Ellingson RJ, Peters JF. Development of EEG and daytime sleep patterns in low risk premature infants during the first year of life. Longitudinal observations. Electroencephalogr Clin Neurophysiol 1980; 50:165.

Engel J, Rapin I, Giblin DR. Electrophysiological studies in two patients with cherry red spot-myoclonus syndrome. Epilepsia 1977; 18:73.

Ersuykova II. Oculomotor activity and autonomic indices of newborn infants during paradoxical sleep. Hum Physiol 1980; 6:57-64.

Eyre JA, Nanei S, Wilkinson AR. Quantification of changes in normal neo-natal EEGs with gestation from continuous five-day recordings. Dev Med Child Neurol 1988; 30:599-607.

Falconer MA. Genetic and related etiological factors in temporal lobe epilepsy. A review. Epilepsia 1971; 12:13.

Falconer MA, Taylor DC. Surgical treatment of drug resistant epilepsy due to mesial temporal sclerosis. Arch Neurol 1968; 19:353.

Frantzen E, Lennox-Buchthal M, Nygard A. Longitudinal EEG and clinical study of children with febrile convulsions. Electroencephalogr Clin Neurophysiol 1968; 24:197.

Fukumoto M, Mochizuki N, Takeishi M, et al. Studies of body movements during night sleep in infancy. Brain Dev 1981; 3:37-43.

Gastaut H. A physiopathogenic study of reflex anoxic cerebral seizures in children (syncopes, sobbing spasms and breath-holding spells). In: Kelloway P, Petersen I, eds. Clinical electroencephalography of children. New York: Grune & Stratton, 1968.

Gastaut H, Roger J, Soulayrol R, et al. Childhood epileptic encephalopathy with diffuse slow spike-waves (otherwise known as "petit mal variant") or Lennox syndrome. Epilepsia 1966; 7:139.

Gibbs FA, Gibbs EL. Atlas of electroencephalography, vol 1. Normal controls. Reading, Massachusetts: Addison-Wesley, 1950.

Gibbs FA, Gibbs EL. Atlas of electroencephalography, vol 3. Reading, Massachusetts: Addison-Wesley, 1964.

Gibbs FA, Rich CL, Gibbs EL. Psychomotor variant type of seizure discharge. Neurology 1963; 13:991.

Gloor R, Kalabay O, Giard N. The electroencephalogram in diffuse encephalopathies. Electroencephalographic correlates of gray and white matter lesions. Brain 1968; 91:779.

Gloor R, Rasmussen T, Altuzzara A: Role of the intracarotid amobarbital-pentylenetetrazol EEG test. The diagnosis and surgical treatment of patients with complex seizure problems. Epilepsia 1976; 17:15.

Goldensohn ES. Use of the EEG for evaluation of focal intracranial lesions. In: Klass DS, Daly DD, eds. Current practice of clinical electroencephalography. New York: Raven Press, 1979a.

Goldensohn ES. Neurophysiologic substrates of EEG activity. In: Klass DS, Daly DD, eds. Current practice of clinical electroencephalography. New York: Raven Press, 1979b.

Goldie L, Svedsen-Rhodes U, Easton J, et al. The development of innate sleep rhythms in short gestation infants. Dev Med Child Neurol 1971; 13:40-50.

Gotman J. The use of computers in analysis and display of EEG and evoked potentials. In: Daly DD, Pedley TA, eds. Current practice of clinical electroencephalography, 2nd ed. New York: Raven Press, 1990; 51-84.

Graziani LJ, Weitzman ED, Peneda G. Visual-evoked responses during neonatal respiratory disorders in low weight infants. Pediatr Res 1972; 6:203.

Harden A. Maturation of the visual-evoked potentials. In: Chiarenza GA, Papakostopoulos D, eds. Clinical application of cerebral-evoked potentials in pediatric medicine. Amsterdam: Excerpta Medica, 1982.

Harden A, Pampiglione G. Visual evoked potentials, electroretinogram, and electroencephalogram studies in progressive neurometabolic "storage" diseases of childhood. In: Desmedt JE, ed. Visual-evoked potentials in man. Oxford: Clarendon Press, 1977.

Harper RM, Leake B, Miyahara L, et al. Development of ultradian periodicity and coalescence at 1 cycle per hour in electroencephalographic activity. Exp Neurol 1981; 73:127-43.

Hayakawa F, Watanabe K, Hakamada S, et al. FZ theta/alpha bursts: a transient EEG pattern in healthy newborns. Electroencephalogr Clin Neurophysiol 1987; 67:27-31.

Harris R, Tizard JPM. The electroencephalogram in neonatal convulsions. J Pediatr 1970; 57:501.

Heijel J, Blom S, Rasmuson M. Benign epilepsy of childhood with centrotemporal EEG foci. A genetic study. Epilepsia 1975; 16:285.

Hellbrugge T. The development of circadian rhythms in infants. Cold Spring Harbor Symp Wuant Biol 1960; 25:311-23.

Hellbrugge T. Ontogenese des rhythmes circadaires chez l'enfant. In: Ajuriaguerra J de, ed. Cycle biologiques et psychiatrie. Geneva: Masson, 1968, 159-83.

Hess R, ed. Brain tumors and other space-occupying processes. In: Handbook of electroencephalography and clinical neurology, vol 14. Clinical EEG. Amsterdam: Elsevier, 1975.

Hildebrandt G. Functional significance of ultradian rhythms and reactive periodicity. J Interdisc Cycle Res 1986; 17:307-19.

Hockaday JM, Whitty CW. Factors determining the electroencephalogram in migraine. A study of 560 patients, according to clinical type of migraine. Brain 1969; 92:769.

Holmes G. Diagnosis and management of seizures in children. Philadelphia: WB Saunders, 1987.

Hrachovy RA, Mizrahi EM, Kellaway P. Electroencephalography of the newborn. In: Daly DD, Pedley TA, eds. Current practice of clinical electroencephalography, 2nd ed. New York: Raven Press, 1990, 201-42.

Hughes JR, Fino J, Gagnon L. Periods of activity and quiescence in the premature EEG. Neuropediatrics 1983; 14:66-72.

Hughes JR, Fino JJ, Hart LA. Premature temporal theta. Electroencephalogr Clin Neurophysiol 1987; 67:7-15.

Hughes JR, Miller JK, Fino JJ, et al. The sharp theta rhythm on the occipital areas of prematures (STOP): a newly described waveform. Clin Electroencephalography 1990; 21:77-87.

Jeavons PM, Bower BD. Infantile spasms. In: Vinken PJ, Bruyn GW, eds. Handbook of clinical neurology, vol 15. The epilepsies. New York: American Elsevier, 1974.

Jeffreys JGR. Basic mechanisms of focal epilepsies. Exp Physiol 1990; 75:127-62.

Jewett DL, Romano MN. Human auditory development potential averaged from the scalp of rat and cat. Brain Res 1972; 36:101.

Joseph JP, Lesevre N, Dreyfus-Brisac C. Spatio-temporal organization of EEG in premature infants and full-term newborns. Electroencephalogr Clin Neurophysiol 1976; 40:153-68.

Karbowski K, Nencka A. Right mid-temporal sharp EEG transients in healthy newborns. Electroencephalogr Clin Neurol 1980; 48:461-9.

Keen J, Lee D. Sequelae of neonatal convulsions. Study of 112 infants. Arch Dis Child 1973; 48:542.

Kellaway P. The development of sleep spindles and of arousal patterns in infants and their characteristics in normal and certain abnormal states. Electroencephalogr Clin Neurophysiol 1952; 4:369.

Kellaway P. An orderly approach to visual analysis parameters of the normal EEG in adults and children. In: Klass DW, Daly DD, eds. Current practice of clinical electroencephalography. New York: Raven Press, 1979.

Kellaway P, Bloxsom A, MacGregor M. Occipital spike foci associated with retrolental fibroplasia and other forms of retinal loss in children. Electroencephalogr Clin Neurophysiol 1955; 7:469.

Kellaway P, Fox BJ. Electroencephalographic diagnosis of cerebral pathology in infants during sleep. I. Rationale, technique, and the characteristics of normal sleep in infants. J Pediatr 1952; 41:262.

Kellaway P, Petersen I. Neurological and electroencephalographic correlative studies in infancy. New York: Grune & Stratton, 1964.

Kellaway P, Crawley JW. A primer of electroencephalography of infants, sections I & II: methodology and criteria of normality. Baylor University College of Medicine, Houston, Texas, 1964.

Kershmann J, Conde A, Gibson WC. Electroencephalography in differential diagnosis of supratentorial tumors. Arch Neurol Psychiatr 1949; 62:255.

Kindt GW, Waldman J, Kohl S, et al. Intracranial pressure in Reye syndrome. Monitoring and control. JAMA 1975; 231:822.

Klass DW, Reiher J. Extracerebral uses for electroencephalography. Med Clin North Am 1965; 52:941.

Kooi KA. Voltage-time characteristics of spikes and other rapid electroencephalographic transients. Semantic and morphological considerations. Neurology 1966; 16:59.

Laget P, Salbreux R, Raimbault J, et al. Relationship between changes in somesthetic-evoked responses and electroencephalographic findings in the child with hemiplegia. Dev Med Child Neurol 1976; 18:620.

Lairy GC, Harrison A. Functional aspects of EEG foci in children—clinical data and longitudinal studies. In: Kellaway P, Peterson I, eds. Clinical electroencephalography of children. New York: Grune & Stratton, 1968.

Landau WM, Kleffner FR. Syndrome of acquired aphasia with convulsive disorder in children. Neurology 1957; 7:523.

Legido A, Clancy RR, Berman PH. Neurologic outcome after electroencephalographically proven neonatal seizures. Pediatrics 1991; 88:583-96.

Lennox WG. The petit mal epilepsies, their treatment with tridione. JAMA 1945; 129;1069.

Levy SR, Abroms IF, Marshall PC, et al. Seizures and cerebral infarction in the full-term newborn. Ann Neurol 1985; 17:366.

Lindsley DB, Cutts KK. Electroencephalograms of "constitutionally inferior" and behavior problem children. Comparison with those of normal children and adults. Arch Neurol Psychiatr 1940; 44:1199.

Lombroso CT. Quantified electrographic scales on 10 pre-term healthy newborns followed up to 40-43 weeks of conceptional age by serial polygraphic recordings. Electroencephalogr Clin Neurophysiol 1979; 46:460.

Lombroso CT. Normal and abnormal EEGs in full-term neonates. In: Henry CE, ed. Current clinical neurophysiology. Update on EEG and evoked potentials. Amsterdam: Elsevier/North Holland, 1980.

Lombroso CT. A prospective clinical electrophysiological study on intracranial hemorrhages in the newborn. In: Fukuyama Y, Arima M, Maekawa K, et al., eds. International Congress Series 010 No. 579. Tokyo: Elsevier, 1981. Child neurology. Proceedings of the IYPD commemorative international symposium on developmental disabilities, 1982.

Lombroso CT. Neonatal electroencephalography. In: Niedermeyer E, Lopez-Desilva F, eds. Electroencephalography, basic principles, clinical applications in related fields. Baltimore: Urban and Schwarzenberg, 1989; 599-637.

Lombroso CT. Neonatal polygraphy in full-term and premature infants. A review of normal and abnormal findings. J Clin Neurophysiol 1985; 2:105.

Lombroso CT, Erba G. Primary and secondary bilateral synchrony in epilepsy. Arch Neurol 1970; 22:321.

Lombroso CT, Schwartz IH, Clark NM, et al. Ctenoids in healthy youths. Neurology 1966; 16:1152.

Lynch JA, Aserinsky E. Developmental changes of oculomotor characteristics in infants when awake and in the active state of sleep. Behav Brain Res 1986; 20:175-83.

Mantovani JF, Landau WM. Acquired aphasia with convulsive disorder: course and prognosis. Neurology 1980; 30:524.

Markand ON. Slow spike-wave activity in EEG and associated clinical features, called "Lennox" and "Lennox-Gastaut" syndrome. Neurology 1977; 27:746.

Martinius J, Matthes A, Lombroso CT. Electroencephalographic features in posterior fossa tumors in children. Electroencephalogr Clin Neurophysiol 1968; 25:128.

Maulsby RL. Some guidelines for assessment of spikes and sharp waves in EEG tracing. Am J EEG Technol 1971; 11:3.

McCutchen CB, Coen R, Iragui VJ. Periodic lateralized epileptiform discharges in asphyxiated neonates. Electroencephalogr Clin Neurophysiol 1985; 61:210.

Ment LR, Freedman RM, Ehrenkranz RA. Neonates with seizures attributable to perinatal complications. Am J Dis Child 1982; 136:548.

Metrakos K, Metrakos JH. Genetics of epilepsy. In: Vinken PJ, Bruyn GW, eds. Handbook of clinical neurology, vol 15. The epilepsies. New York: American Elsevier, 1974.

Miranda SB, Hack M, Fantz F, et al. Neonatal pattern vision. A predictor of future mental performance. J Pediatr 1977; 91:642.

Mises J, Moussalli F, Plovin P: Eture du-trac des premiers jours devie dansles amino-acidopathies. Rev Electroencephalogr Clin Neurophysiol 1977; 7:371.

Mizrahi EM, Dorfman LJ. Sensory-evoked potentials. Clinical application in pediatrics. J Pediatr 1980; 97:1.

Mizrahi EM, Kellaway P. Cerebral concussion in children: assessment of injury by electroencephalography. J Pediatr 1984a; 73:419.

Mizrahi EM, Kellaway P. Characterization of seizures in neonates and young infants by time-synchronized electroencephalography/polygraphic/video monitoring. Ann Neurol 1984b; 16:383.

Mizrahi EM, Tharp BR. A characteristic EEG pattern in neonatal herpes simplex encephalitis. Neurology 1982; 32:1215.

Monod D, Dreyfus-Brisac C, Ducas P, et al. L'EEG du nouveauné à terme. Étude comparative chez le nouveau-né en présentation céphalique et en présentation de siége. Rev Neurol 1960; 102:375-9.

Monod N, Garma L. Auditory responsibility in the human premature. Biol Neonate 1971; 17:292-316.

Monod N, Pajot N, Guidasci S. The neonatal EEG. Statistical studies and prognostic value in fulterm and preterm babies. Electroencephalogr Clin Neurophysiol 1972; 32:529.

Monod N, Tharp B. Activité électroencéphalographique normale du noveau-né et du prématuré au cours des états de veille et de sommeil. Rev EEG Neurophysiol 1977; 7:302-15.

Morrell F, Torres F. Electrophysiological analysis of a case of Tay-Sachs disease. Brain 1960; 83:213.

Nelson KB, Ellenberg JH. Febrile seizures. In: Dreyfuss FE, ed. Pediatric epileptology. Boston: John Wiley & Sons, 1983.

Niedermeyer E, Lopes da Silva F. Electroencephalography. Baltimore: Urban and Schwarzenberg, 1981.

Noriega-Sanchez A, Markand OH. Clinical and electroencephalographic correlation of independent multifocal spike discharges. Neurology 1976; 26:667.

Novick B, Kurtzberg D, Vaughan HG, et al. An electrophysiologic indication of auditory processing defects in autism. Psychiatr Res 1980; 3:107.

Novotny EJ, Tharp BR, Coen RW, et al. The significance of positive sharp waves in the electroencephalogram of premature infants. Neurology 1986; 36(suppl):279.

Novotny, EJ, Tharp BR, Coen RW, et al. Positive rolandic sharp waves in the EEG of the premature infant. Neurology 1987; 37:1481.

Nunez PL. Electric fields of the brain. New York: Oxford University Press, 1981.

Obrien MJ, Lem SYL, Prechtl HR. Transient flattenings in the EEG of newborns—a benign variation. Electroencephalogr Clin Neurophysiol 1987; 67:16-26.

Okamato Y, Kirikae T. Electroencephalographic studies on brain of foetus, of children of premature birth and newborn, together with a note of foetus brain upon drugs. Folia Psychiatr Neurol Jpn 1951; 5:150.

Ollo C, Squires N. Event-related potentials in learning disabilities. In: Cracco RQ, Bodis-Wollner I, eds. Evoked potentials. New York: Alan R. Liss, 1986.

Otto DA, Benignus VA, Muller KE, et al. Effects of age and body lead burden on CNS function in young children. I. Slow cortical potentials. Electroencephalogr Clin Neurophysiol 1982; 52:229.

Ounsted C, Lindsay J, Norman R. Biological factors in temporal lobe epilepsy. In: Clinics in developmental medicine, no. 22. London: William Heinemann Medical Books, 1966.

Pampiglione G, Harden A. Resuscitation after cardiocirculatory arrest. Lancet 1968; 1:1261.

Pampiglione G, Harden A. Neurophysiologic identification of a late infantile form of "neuronal lipidosis." J Neurol Neurosurg Psychiatry 1973; 36:68.

Parmalee AH Jr. Changes in sleep patterns in premature infants as a function of brain maturation. In: Minkowski A, ed. Regional development of the brain in early life. Philadelphia: F.A. Davis, 1967.

Parmalee AH, Akiyama Y, Stern E, et al. A periodic cerebral rhythm in newborn infants. Exp Neurol 1969; 25:575-84.

Parmelee AH, Schulte FJ, Akiyama Y, et al. Maturation of EEG activity during sleep in premature infants. Electroencephalogr Clin Neurophysiol 1968; 24:319-29.

Pedley TA, Traub RD. Physiological basis of the EEG. In: Daly DD, Pedley TA, eds. Current practice of clinical electroencephalography, 2nd ed. New York: Raven Press, 1990; 107-38.

PeBenito R, Cracco JB. Periodic lateralized epileptiform discharges in infants and children. Ann Neurol 1979; 6:47.

Penfield W, Jasper H. Highest level seizures. Res Publ Assoc Nerv Ment Dis 1946; 26:252.

Penry JK, Porter RJ, Dreifuss FE. Simultaneous recording of absence seizures with videotape and electroencephalography. A study of 374 seizures in 48 patients. Brain 1975; 98:427.

Peterson I, Eeg-Olofsson O. The development of the electroencephalogram in normal adolescents from the age of 1 through 15 years—non-paroxysmal activity. Neuropaediatrie 1971; 2:247.

Pope SS, Werner SS, Bickford RG. Atlas of neonatal electroencephalography. New York: Raven Press, 1992.

Prechtl HFR. Continuity of neural functions from prenatal to postnatal life. Spastics International Medical Publications. Oxford: Blackwell Scientific Publications, Philadelphia: JB Lippincott, 1984; 94:1-255.

Prechtl HFR, Fargel JW, Weinmann HM, et al. Postures, motility and respiration of low risk preterm infants. Dev Med Child Neurol 1979; 21:3-27.

Prechtl HRF, Lenard HG. A study of eye movements in sleeping newborn infants. Brain Res 1967; 5:477-93.

Prechtl HFR, Weinmann H, Akiyama Y. Organization of physiological parameters in normal and neurologically abnormal infants. Neuropaediatrie 1969; 1:101.

Prensky AL, Sommer D. Diagnosis and treatment of migraine in children. Neurology 1979; 29:506.

Prince DA. Physiological mechanisms of focal epileptogenesis. Epilepsia 1985; 26:1.

Prince DA. Neurophysiology of epilepsy. Ann Rev Neurosci 1978; 1:395.

Prince DA, Gutnick M. Neuronal activities in epileptogenic foci of immature cortex. Brain Res 1972; 45:455.

Reilley EW, Peters JF. Relationship of some varieties of electroencephalographic photosensitivity to clinical convulsive disorders. Neurology 1973; 23:1040.

Remillard GM, Ethier R, Andermann F. Temporal lobe epilepsy and perinatal occlusion of the posterior cerebral artery. Neurology 1974; 24:1001.

Rhee RS, Goldensohn ES, Kim RC. EEG characteristics of solitary intracranial lesions in relationship to anatomic location. Electroencephalogr Clin Neurophysiol 1975; 38:553.

Richey ET, Norman R. EEG instrumentation and technology. Springfield, Illinois: Charles C. Thomas, 1976.

Robertson SS. Intrinsic temporal patterning in the spontaneous movement of awake neonates. Child Devv 1982; 53:1016-21.

Robertson SS. Human cyclic motility: fetal-newborn continuities and newborn state differences. Dev Psychobiol 1987; 20:425-42.

Rose AL, Lombroso CT. Neonatal seizure states. A study of clinical, pathological and electroencephalographic features in 137 full-term babies with a long-term follow-up. Pediatrics 1970; 45:404.

Rowe RJ, Holmes GL, Hafford J, et al. Prognostic value of electroencephalograms in term and preterm infants following neonatal seizures. Electroencephalogr Clin Neurophysiol 1985; 60:183-96.

Salamy A. Maturation of the auditory brainstem response from birth through early childhood. J Clin Neurophysiol 1984; 1:293.

Samson-Dollfus D. L'électroencéphalogramme du prématuré jusqu'à l'âge de trois mois et du nouveau-né à terme. Thèse Méd (Paris). Foulon éd., 1955.

Scher MS. The clinical significance of spikes and sharp waves in neonatal EEG. Am J EEG Technol 1991; 31:145-72.

Scher MS. Cerebral neurophysiological assessment of the high-risk neonate. In: Guthrie RD, ed. Recent advances in neonatal care. Clinics in critical care medicine. New York: Churchill Livingstone, 1987a.

Scher MS. Midline electrographic abnormalities and cerebral lesions in the newborn brain. J Child Neurol 1988; 3:135-44.

Scher MS. Neonatal electroencephalography: normal features. In: Holmes G, Moshe S, eds. Pediatric clinical neurophysiology. Norwalk, Connecticut: Appleton & Lang, 1993a.

Scher MS. Neonatal electroencephalography: abnormal features. In: Holmes G, Moshe S, eds. Pediatric clinical neurophysiology. Norwalk, Connecticut: Appleton & Lang, 1993b.

Scher MS. Physiologic artifacts in neonatal electroencephalography. Am J EEG Technol 1985; 25:257.

Scher MS, Ahdab-Barmada M. Gestational age by electrographic, clinical and anatomical criteria. Pediatr Neurol 1987b; 3:256.

Scher MS, Ahdab-Barmada M, Fria T. Neurological and anatomical correlations in neonatal nonketotic hyperglycinemia. Neuropediatrics 1986; 17:137.

Scher MS, Aso K, Beggarly ME, et al. Electroclinical seizures in preterm and fullterm neonates: comparisons of diagnostic criteria, associated brain lesions, and risk for neurological sequelae. Pediatrics (in press).

Scher MS, Barmada M. Estimation of gestational age by electrographic, clinical, and anatomical criteria. Pediatr Neurol 1987; 3:256-62.

Scher MS, Beggarly ME. Periodic discharges in neonatal EEG recordings. Epilepsia 1986a; 27:609.

Scher MS, Hamid MY, Steppe DA, et al. Ictal and interictal durations in preterm and term neonates. Epilepsia (in press).

Scher MS, Painter MJ, Bergman I, et al. EEG diagnoses of neonatal seizures: clinical correlations and outcome. Pediatr Neurol 1989; 5:17-24.

Scher MS, Sun M, Hatzilabrou GM, et al. Computer analyses of EEG sleep in the neonate: methodological considerations. J Clin Neurophysiol 1990; 7:417-41.

Scher MS, Tharp B. Significance of focal abnormalities in neonatal EEG-radiologic correlation and outcome. Ann Neurol 1982; 12: 217.

Schulte FJ, Hinze G, Schrempf G. Maternal toxemia, fetal malnutrition and bioelectric brain activity of the newborn. Neuropaediatrie 1971; 2:439.

Schulz H, Labie P. Ultradian rhythms in physiology and behavior. Berlin: Springer-Verlag, 185; 1-340.

Schwartzkroin PA, Prince DA. Changes in excitatory and inhibitory synaptic potentials leading to epileptogenic activity. Brain Res 1978; 147:117.

Seshia SS, Chowq PN, Sankaran K. Coma following cardiorespiratory arrest in childhood. Dev Med Child Neurol 1979; 21:143.

Sherman J. ERG and VEP as supplemental aids in the differential diagnosis of retinal versus optic nerve disease. In: Ciacco R, Bodis-Wollner I, eds. Evoked potentials. Frontiers of clinical neuroscience, vol 3. New York: Liss, 1986.

Shewmon DA. What is a neonatal seizure? Problems in definition and quantification for investigative and clinical purposes. J Clin Neurophysiol 1990; 7(3):315-68.

Shewmon DA, Ervin RJ. Focal spike-induced cerebral dysfunction is related to the after-coming slow wave. Ann Neurol 1988; 23:131-7.

Shoumaker RD, et al. Clinical and EEG manifestations of an unusual asphasic syndrome in children. Neurology 1974; 24:10.

Silverman D. Electroencephalographic study of acute head injury in children. Neurology 1962; 12:273.

Slater GE, Torres F. Frequency-amplitude gradient. A new parameter for interpreting pediatric sleep EEGs. Arch Neurol 1979; 36: 465.

Slatter KH. Some clinical and EEG findings in patients with migraine. Brain 1968; 91:85.

Smith JMB, Kellaway P. Central (rolandic) foci in children. An analysis of 200 cases. Electroencephalogr Clin Neurophysiol 1964; 17:460.

Sokol S. Clinical applications of the ERG and VEP in the pediatric age group. In: Cracco R, Bodis-Wollner I, eds. Evoked potentials. New York: Liss, 1986.

Spehlmann R. Evoked potential primer. Stoneham, Massachusetts: Butterworth, 1985.

Statz A, Dumermuth G, Mieth D, et al. Transient EEG patterns during sleep in healthy newborns. Neuropediatrics 1982; 13:115-22.

Sternberg B, Lerique-Koechin A, Misès J, et al. Morphological studies of so-called periodic abnormalities in children. Electroencephalogr Clin Neurophysiol 1972; 32:574.

Stratton P. Rhythmic functions in the human newborn. In: Stratton P, ed. Psychobiology of the human newborn. New York: John Wiley & Sons, 1982.

Tanguay PE, Ornitz EM, Kaplan A, et al. Evolution sleep spindles in childhood. Electroencephalogr Clin Neurophysiol 1975; 38:175.

Task Force for the Determination of Brain Death in Children. Guidelines for the determination of brain death in children. Neurology 1987; 37:1677.

Tharp BR. The 6-per-second spike and wave complex. Arch Neurol 1966; 15:533.

Tharp BR. Orbital frontal seizures. An unique electroencephalographic and clinical syndrome. Epilepsia 1972; 13:627.

Tharp BR. Neonatal electroencephalography. In: Korobkin R, Guilleminalt C, eds. Progress in perinatal neurology, vol 1. Baltimore: Williams and Wilkins, 1981a.

Tharp BR. Neonatal and pediatric electroencephalography. In: Aminoff MJ, ed. Electrodiagnosis in clinical neurology. New York: Churchill Livingstone, 1986.

Tharp BR, Cukier F, Monod N. The prognostic value of the electroencephalogram in premature infants. Electroencephalogr Clin Neurophysiol 1981b; 51:219.

Tharp BR, Laboyrie PM. The incidence of EEG abnormalities and outcome of infants paralyzed with neuromuscular blocking agents. Crit Care Med 1983; 11:926.

Torres F, Anderson C. The normal EEG of the human newborn. J Clin Neurophysiol 1985; 2:89.

Trauner DA, Stockard JJ, Sweetman L. EEG correlation with biochemical abnormalities in Reye syndrome. Arch Neurol 1977; 34:116.

Trojaborg W. Changes in spike foci in children. In: Hrakovy P, Peterson I, eds. Clinical electroencephalography in children. New York: Grune & Stratton, 1968.

Umezaki H, Morrell F. Developmental study of photic-evoked responses in premature infants. Electroencephalogr Clin Neurophysiol 1970; 28:55.

Vignaendra V, Matthews RL, Chatrian GE. Positive occipital sharp transients of sleep. Relationships to nocturnal sleep cycle in man. Electroencephalogr Clin Neurophysiol 1974; 37:239.

Volpe JJ. Neonatal seizures. In: Neurology of the newborn, vol 22. Major problems in clinical pediatrics. Philadelphia: WB Saunders, 1987.

Watanabe K. Behavioral state cycles, background EEGs and prognosis of newborns with perinatal hypoxia. Electroencephalogr Clin Neurophysiol 1980; 49:618.

Watanabe K, Iwase D. Spinkle-like fast rhythms in the EEGs of low birthweight infants. Dev Med Child Neurol 1972a; 14:373.

Watanabe K, Iwase K, Hara K. Maturation of visual-evoked responses in low-birthweight infants. Dev Med Child Neurol 1972b; 14:425.

Watanabe K, Hara K, Miyazaki S, et al. Electroclinical studies of seizures in the newborn. Folia Psychiatr Neurol Jpn 1977; 31:383.

Watt J, Strongman K. The organization and stability of sleep states in fullterm, pre-term and small-for-gestational age infants: A comparative study. Dev Psychobiol 1985; 18:151-62.

Weiner SP, Painter MJ, Scher MS. Neonatal seizures: electroclinical disassociation. Pediatr Neurol 1991; 7:363-8.

Weitkunat R. Digital biosignal processing in techniques in the behavioral and neural sciences, vol 3. Amsterdam: Elsevier, 1991.

White JC, Langston JW, Pedley T. Benign epileptiform transients of sleep. Clarification of the "small sharp spike" controversy. Neurology 1977; 27:1061.

Willis J, Seales D, Frazier E. Short latency somatosensory-evoked potentials in infants. Electroencephalogr Clin Neurophysiol 1984; 59:366.

Worster-Drought C. An unusual form of acquired aphasia in children. Dev Med Child Neurol 1971; 13:563.

Zivin L, Ajmonel-Marsan C. Incidence and prognostic significance of "epileptiform" activity in the EEG in non-epileptic subjects. Brain 1968; 91:751.

7

Spinal Fluid Examination

Kenneth F. Swaiman

CEREBROSPINAL FLUID FUNCTION

There are a number of postulated functions for cerebrospinal fluid (CSF). Undoubtedly, CSF acts as a buffer of the brain against trauma. More important, however, CSF provides a means by which various brain constituents in the intracellular spaces may be returned to the venous circulation. CSF is an integral part of the mechanism that maintains the proper chemical milieu for the brain and spinal cord in both normal and pathologic situations [Hochwald, 1984]. The extracellular compartment of the brain is in close communication with CSF in the ventricles and the subarachnoid space.

CSF, brain parenchyma, and blood constitute the three fundamental intracranial compartments [Truex and Carpenter, 1971]. Because of the rigidity of the bony cranium, the total volume of these three constituents may vary only within a small range before a change in intracranial pressure ensues.

The measured pressure varies with the site and method of measurement. Normal CSF pressure in adults and older children is 120 to 200 mm water. Normal CSF pressure in a young, relaxed child varies from 60 to 180 mm water [Clark, 1969]. The range of pressure in newborns varies between 90 to 120 mm water [Munroe, 1928; Levinson, 1928].

CSF FORMATION, FLOW, AND ABSORPTION

The choroid plexus of the ventricles, through an energy-consuming active process, secretes most of the CSF volume. The rate of CSF formation in the choroid plexus is highly variable. The rate of secretion is approximately 750 ml/day in adults, less in children, and as little as 25 ml/day in newborns. Total CSF volume ranges from 5 ml in neonates to 150 ml in adults. Administration of acetazolamide decreases CSF formation ostensibly by interference with carbonic anhydrase activity in the chorioid plexus [Welch et al., 1972].

Normal CSF is as clear and colorless as pure water; specific gravity ranges from 1.004 to 1.007.

Although most of the CSF is formed in the choroid plexus, water and other substances gain entrance into the ventricles and subarachnoid space through meningeal blood vessels and the ependyma.

CSF secreted by the choroid plexus in the lateral ventricles traverses the foramina of Monro and flows into the third ventricle, then passes through the third ventricle and subsequently through the relatively narrow aqueduct of Sylvius to reach the fourth ventricle. The fluid passes out of the ventricular system through the paired lateral foramina of Luschka or the unpaired midline foramen of Magendie. The CSF that passes through the foramina of Luschka generally flows around the brainstem into the prepontine cisterns or the cerebellopontine angles. The CSF that leaves the fourth ventricle through the foramen of Magendie exits directly into the cisterna magna. The flow from this area is upward within the subarachnoid space over the cerebellar hemispheres, downward into the spinal subarachnoid space, or into the basal cisterns around the brainstem, including the interpeduncular cistern. Flow within the spinal subarachnoid space is predominantly downward posterior to the spinal cord and upward anterior to the cord, continuing to the basal cisterns. From the basal cisterns, the fluid continues upward over the brain convexity. Most CSF eventually passes through the arachnoid villi and then mingles with venous blood in the sagittal sinus. The villi are concentrated over the convexity of the brain, primarily near the midline in proximity to the sagittal sinus (Figure 7-1).

CSF reabsorption, to a lesser extent, also takes place through intrathecal blood vessels (capillaries and veins). Some absorption occurs through the lymphatic system through perineural pathways [Guyton, 1971].

There is evidence that excess cerebral fluid and its molecular constituents are removed through the custom-

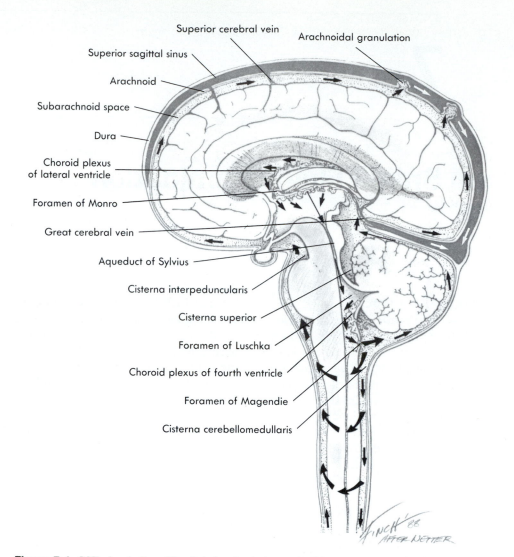

Superior cerebral vein

Arachnoidal granulation

Superior sagittal sinus

Arachnoid

Subarachnoid space

Dura

Choroid plexus
of lateral ventricle

Foramen of Monro

Great cerebral vein

Aqueduct of Sylvius

Cisterna interpeduncularis

Cisterna superior

Foramen of Luschka

Choroid plexus of fourth ventricle

Foramen of Magendie

Cisterna cerebellomedullaris

Figure 7-1 CSF circulation. The lightly stippled area indicates the position of the lateral ventricle.

ary reabsorption channels [Bruce et al., 1979]. Much effort has gone into studying CSF turnover because the understanding of the dynamics of formation, absorption, pressure, and flow is so important to the therapy of hydrocephalus [Welch, 1975].

The epithelium of the choroid plexus secretes sodium ions. Cations, including chloride, are subsequently attracted. The resultant increase in osmotic pressure causes entrance of water and other soluble materials into the CSF through the choroid plexus and other adjacent tissues. The concentration of ions in CSF and their ratios with counterparts in plasma are different than what would be expected if the CSF were merely a dialysate of plasma [Davson, 1967]. Sodium, chloride, and potassium are found in increased concentrations in the CSF when compared with the concentrations in serum. On the other hand, only small amounts of phosphate, calcium, sulfate, and uric acid are present.

Protein is partially restricted from entering CSF because of its molecular size and relative insolubility; therefore CSF protein content is much less than in plasma. It is noteworthy that the bulk of CSF protein originates in plasma [Widdel, 1958; Fishman, 1980].

The site of origin of cellular elements in CSF remains controversial. Neutrophilic, lymphocytic, and monocytic responses occur. Lymphocytic responses are associated with cellular and humoral immune systems; other cellular responses are associated with phagocytosis. The monocyte has nonspecific phagocytic activity, and the neutrophil primarily phagocytizes bacteria. Eosinophiles are rarely found in CSF except in parasitic disease.

LUMBAR PUNCTURE PROCEDURE

At times, lumbar puncture is necessary even when there is increased intracranial pressure, which can be deduced from the presence of papilledema, lack of venous pulsations over the optic disc, effacement of the cortical sulci on CT and MRI scans, and nuchal rigidity resulting from early tonsillar herniation. In young infants the anterior fontanel may be bulging. In children younger than the age of 10, separation of the cranial sutures, particularly with long-standing increased intracranial pressure, may be evident on plain skull radiographs. Securing spinal fluid may be essential in certain conditions, specifically meningitis. In the presence of asymmetric masses or spinal cord tumors with resultant shift of intracranial contents, severe consequences may result from the puncture procedure when unbalanced hydrostatic forces cause compression of blood vessels or nervous tissue.

The site of puncture should not be infected, and an area of dysmorphic skin should not be selected. The presence of a coagulopathy requires cautious puncture by an experienced operator with a small-caliber needle.

It is often necessary for a second person to aid the physician during the puncture. The helper must position and hold the patient. Utmost care, particularly with infants, must be exercised so that the airway is not compromised by the holding procedure. The puncture sites commonly used are the interspaces between L_3 and L_4, L_4 and L_5, or L_5 and S_1. After the skin is prepared, a 20- or 22-gauge needle, 2.5 to 5 cm, is used. The needle is beveled and has a stylet in place. Using a needle without a stylet is not recommended.

Local anesthesia is optional and required infrequently because the pain of injection of the anesthetic agent approaches that of the puncture itself. The needle is inserted in the exact midline and the tip aimed on a plane with the umbilicus. The bevel of the needle is turned so that it passes between the vertically running fibers of the dura. Needle puncture with this orientation is also less likely to injure the spinal nerve rootlets.

The needle is gradually advanced from 2 to 4 cm (depending on the depth of the overlying tissue) until the ligamentum flavum and dura mater are encountered. As the tip of the needle pierces the dura, a slight popping sensation may be felt. At this point the stylet is removed. If no fluid appears, the needle should be rotated a quarter turn so that the bevel of the needle has changed position. If no fluid appears, the needle should be slowly withdrawn. Another interspace should be selected for a second attempt.

The opening pressure should be measured when the child is relaxed and in the lateral decubitus position. There should be no direct pressure on the abdomen and little or no flexion of the legs or hips during the measurement.

If the spinal subarachnoid space and the manometer are properly connected, there may be pulsation of the fluid column in the manometer. The Queckenstedt test should not be performed. CSF pressure should be ascertained again after the fluid has been removed.

The clinician should carefully document the details of the lumbar puncture. The appearance of the fluid should be studied and recorded accurately. The volume of fluid required depends on the analyses planned. In general, studies should include quantitative and qualitative protein examination (1.0 ml), quantitative and qualitative cytologic studies (1.0 ml), glucose content determination (0.5 ml), and routine cultures and smears for bacteria and other organisms when appropriate (0.5 ml). Commonly, no less than 5 ml of fluid is collected. For routine studies the fluid should be collected in three tubes. Approximately 1 ml should be collected in the first tube. This fluid may be contaminated by small clots of blood. If bloody, it should be used for microorganism studies; if not bloody, glucose determination can also be performed on this fluid. The second and third tubes, containing 1 to 2 ml each, should be collected. A fourth tube containing 2 ml may also be collected for determination of xanthochromia after the specimen has been centrifuged. Xanthochromia indicates that blood breakdown products were present before the puncture was performed. For optimal observation, centrifugation for the determination of xanthochromia should take place immediately after the puncture, before the fluid is sent to the laboratory. Additional fluid for the study of enzymes, electron microscopic observation of cellular morphology, and special cultures can be obtained.

Although relatively unusual, complications of lumbar punctures in infants and children do occur. Most complications are transient and usually occur in the form of a postpuncture headache.

Postlumbar puncture headache may be due to lowered CSF pressure after CSF loss with subsequent stretching of pain-sensitive intracranial structures. Intracranial CSF volume, measured noninvasively in adults by an MRI technique, corroborates the loss of fluid, mostly from the areas in the cortical sulci. Losses are evident in most patients 24 hours after puncture. Very large reductions in intracranial CSF volume are frequently associated with postpuncture headache, but some patients develop headache with relatively little alteration in the intracranial CSF volume. There is not a measurable change in position of the intracranial structures after puncture [Grant et al., 1991]. The headache usually occurs within 24 hours of the puncture and lasts up to several days. Using small-diameter needles appears to reduce the incidence of this complication [Tourtellotte et al., 1972].

The more serious complications of lumbar punctures are spinal subarachnoid, subdural, and epidural hematomas [Masdeu et al., 1979]. These hematomas result from breeching the epidural venous plexus vessels or radicular arteries or veins. Usually symptoms are those of meningeal irritation or local pain. Only rarely does sensory dysfunction, paresis of the legs, or sphincter impairment occur; in these cases, surgical evacuation of hematomas may prove necessary [Kirkpatrick and Goodman, 1975].

In special situations, CSF can be obtained by ventricular or cisternal punctures. These procedures are best performed by a neurosurgeon. The basilar cistern may be very small in young infants, rendering cisternal puncture both risky and unproductive.

STUDY OF CSF

Techniques for the handling and study of CSF are recorded in detail elsewhere [Barringer, 1970; Cole, 1969].

Cells

A standard counting chamber technique is used for quantitative evaluation of cells. The fluid should be fresh so that no disintegration of red or white cells occurs. Although difficult, examiners accustomed to the technique can, with some precision, identify erythrocytes and polymorphonuclear cells. However, for precise evaluation, stained smears of the fluid are required. Red cells are uncommonly found in the fluid of older children and adults if a traumatic puncture has not occurred. A mean of 120 red cells/mm^3 in the CSF of term newborns has been reported [Widell, 1958]. CSF from preterm infants may contain as many as 10 white cells/mm^3 [Samson, 1930; Otila, 1948; Gyllensward and Malmstrom, 1962]. In general, newborns have a mean CSF white cell count of 7.5 cells/mm^3 [Widell, 1958], and children up to the age of 1 year may have a white cell count as great as 10 cells/mm^3. Between 1 to 4 years of age, 8 cells/mm^3 has been cited as the upper limit of normal [Clark, 1969]. In a study of normal juveniles and adults, Dyken [1974] found the mean value of 2.6 ± 1.7 leukocytes/mm^3 to be present. In one report, seizures did not appear to change CSF cell count, glucose, or protein [Portnoy and Olson, 1985]. In another report, only slight increases in leukocytes were present (range was 1 to 16/mm^3) and slight changes in spinal fluid protein concentration (range was 18 to 48 mg/dl) [Woody et al., 1988] occurred.

Qualitative studies of cells within CSF require special techniques and staining [Rich, 1972; Dyken and Mulina, 1973; Dyken et al., 1980]. Collection of cells on special membranes or the use of sedimentation enhances the likelihood of identifying abnormal cells in CSF, particularly tumor cells. The presence of neoplastic cells, plasmacytes, stem cells, and eosinophiles is always abnormal. CSF obtained after a traumatic puncture with excessive red blood cells usually has an accompanying increase in neutrophilic and polymorphonuclear cells.

Excessive red cells in CSF may indicate a hemorrhage or a traumatic puncture. Unfortunately, a traumatic (i.e., bloody) puncture may follow a properly performed procedure. Although there have been assurances to the contrary [Bonadio et al., 1990], experience dictates that calculation of leukocyte-to-erythrocyte ratios after traumatic punctures does not safely discount the absence of pleocytosis. Centrifugation with observation of the supernatant fluid should indicate the presence of xanthochromia and previous hemorrhage. Clear supernatant fluid indicates a traumatic lumbar puncture. Increased polymorphonuclear reaction is present in bacterial meningitis but may also occur in early viral and neoplastic meningitides. Chemical meningitides may also cause an early polymorphonuclear cell response.

Microorganisms

The initial fluid obtained should be studied for microorganisms, particularly bacteria; usually 1 to 2 ml of fluid will suffice. Gram smears using 0.5 ml of fluid should be performed. Identification of the shape and Gram-stain characteristics of the bacteria allows for a presumptive, rapid diagnosis. Routine studies for tuberculosis are usually unnecessary, as are routine India ink preparations and cultures for fungal organisms.

In addition to inoculation in broth, several culture media should be inoculated (e.g., blood agar, chocolate agar, thioglycolate). The common bacteria that cause bacterial meningitides are usually successfully cultured in chocolate agar under a carbon dioxide atmosphere at 35° to 37° C.

Additional studies are available that may afford rapid determination of microorganisms. The studies include counterimmunoelectrophoresis, latex agglutination, and limulus lysate assay. These studies are of great aid when Gram's stain studies are not definitive. Counterimmunoelectrophoresis can distinguish among the capsular polysaccharide of *Haemophilus influenzae*, *Neisseria meningitidis*, group B streptococcus, and *Streptococcus pneumoniae*. However, test insensitivity and a high incidence of false-negative findings may prove confounding.

Latex agglutination is more sensitive than counterimmunoelectrophoresis, especially for *H. influenzae* and *N. meningitidis* [Overturf and Hoeprich, 1983] but can also identify *S. pneumoniae* and group B streptococcus. Latex agglutination requires only a small quantity of fluid. Limulus lysate assay of CSF is useful in Gram-negative bacterial meningitis but is nonspecific and does not discriminate among different types of Gram-negative organisms [Martin, 1983]. The C-reactive protein assay is a nonspecific test for bacterial infections and is readily performed [Putto et al., 1986]. The value of CSF lactate determination in bacterial meningitis remains undetermined [Jordan et al., 1983; Rutledge et al., 1981]. Newer tests based on immunologic methods or gene-amplification techniques hold great promise for diagnosis of infections caused by organisms that are difficult to culture or present in small numbers [Greenlee, 1990].

Glucose

Glucose enters CSF through a carrier-mediated transport system that is stereospecific, saturable, competitively inhibitory, and that manifests countertransport capability [Fishman, 1964]. There are several methods of determination of CSF glucose concentration. Most techniques are specific for glucose and do not detect other reducing agents. In general, it is advantageous to compare the simultaneous content of blood and CSF glucose. The CSF glucose concentration is normally two thirds of the blood glucose concentration. Obviously, any cause of hypoglycemia will lead to CSF glucose decrease. This parallel decrease can be detected by studying the simultaneously obtained data.

Independently decreased CSF glucose occurs most commonly in bacterial meningitis, although it may occur in meningitis caused by fungi, spirochetes, protozoa, and yeast. The precise mechanism of glucose decrease is not fully explained [Menkes, 1969]. At times there is decreased CSF glucose concentration in subarachnoid hemorrhage, carcinomatosis, sarcoidosis, and chemical meningitis. Lymphocytic reactions secondary to meningeal inflammation by viruses (e.g., lymphocytic choriomeningitis, herpes simplex, mumps) may also lead to decreased CSF glucose concentration.

Protein

Total protein content of CSF is relatively high at birth, falls to a low at approximately 10 months of age (20 mg/dl), and gradually climbs to adult values thereafter. Most of CSF protein is albumin that is not synthesized in brain but is derived from the plasma. Widell's study of neonates revealed a range of 50 to 120 mg/dl with a mean of 80 mg/dl. The mean protein content between 1 and 2 years was approximately 17 mg/dl with a standard deviation of ± 2.7 (Table 7-1 and Figure 7-2).

Total CSF protein concentration varies with the anatomic area from which the fluid is sampled. Often the ventricular fluid protein content is less than 5 mg/dl. Cisterna magna fluid protein content ranges from 10 to 25 mg/dl. In older children and adults, CSF collected at the lumbar level has a protein content of 15 to 45 mg/dl. Protein concentration also varies with age in younger children [Widell, 1958].

CSF protein content increases below the obstruction when there is a blockage of the spinal canal, ostensibly because of lack of a reabsorption by the arachnoidal villi. Rarely, CSF removed below such an obstruction clots (Froin's syndrome), ostensibly because of the entrance of serum fibrinogen into the CSF compartment. A protein content greater than 500 mg/dl may be caused by a spinal cord tumor and resultant block of CSF flow. The amount of fluid that can be collected during the lumbar puncture is usually limited.

Protein content is also increased in various meningit-

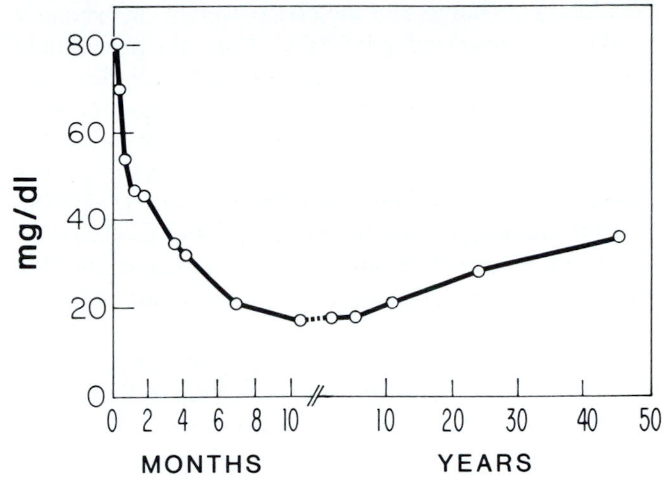

Figure 7-2 Changes in average CSF protein content associated with maturation (see also Table 7-1). (Modified from Widell S. Acta Paediatr 1958; 47[suppl. 155]:1).

Table 7-1 Total protein content (mg/dl) in CSF from healthy children

Age			Age		
0 to 6 days	n*	11	5 to 8 months	n	7
	m	80.9		m	20.4
	s	20.8		s	2.4
7 to 13 days	n	7	9 to 11 months	n	5
	m	70.4		m	16.6
	s	23.6		s	2.6
14 to 27 days	n	13	12 to 23 months	n	8
	m	53.9		m	16.8
	s	17.8		s	2.7
28 to 41 days	n	10	2 to 7 years	n	21
	m	46.5		m	17.7
	s	15.4		s	3.1
42 to 59 days	n	11	8 to 13 years	n	19
	m	45.6		m	20.8
	s	14.2		s	4.1
2 to 4 months	n	9			
	m	34.8			
	s	12.0			

From Widell S. Acta Paediatr 1958; 47(Suppl. 115):1.
*n, Number; m, mean; s, standard deviation.

ides, particularly those caused by bacteria. Minor-to-marked protein elevations usually can be found in viral meningoencephalitides. Increased protein content may also occur in a number of degenerative, demyelinating, and neoplastic diseases. Protein content is increased frequently in peripheral neuropathy.

A number of techniques are available for determination of the components of CSF protein. Studies using electrophoresis permitted delineation of proteins based on electrical charge and molecular weight. Subsequent studies demonstrated that CSF contains one prealbumin fraction, albumin, and globulin. The globulins are further subdivided into alpha, beta, and gamma portions. Beta-globulin content in CSF is usually twice that of gamma globulin, in contradistinction to the prominence of gamma-globulin in the serum. Gamma globulin in CSF originates from the plasma [Cutler et al., 1970]. Normal CSF gamma-globulin content ranges up to 15% of the total protein concentration [Savory and Heintges, 1973].

Subsequent use of immunoelectrophoresis (i.e., electrophoresis for separation of proteins followed by immune precipitation-reaction techniques) further separated the protein bands under each electrophoretic peak [Fishman, 1980]. Normal CSF contains prealbumin, albumin, alpha-1-globulin, alpha-2-globulin, glyco-protein, alpha-1-antitrypsin, haptoglobins, ceruloplasmin, hemopexin, transferrin, beta-1-globulin, and the following immunoglobulins: A (IgA), M (IgM), and G (IgG). The changes in immunoglobulins may be expressed as percentage of total protein, percentage of albumin, or ratios of CSF IgG/serum IgG to CSF albumin/serum albumin. The major proteins found in CSF are listed in Tables 7-2 and 7-3 [Fishman, 1980].

The concentrations of various CSF proteins have been used as measures of blood-brain barrier function in infants, children, and adults [Eeg-Olofsson et al., 1981]. Increased concentration of CSF immunoglobulins has been reported in many inflammatory conditions. Identification of other immunoglobulins in normal CSF notwithstanding, virtually all immunoglobulin in normal CSF is IgG. IgG in the CSF of children is 0.7 to 1.7 mg/dl (3.5% to 8% of total protein).

Table 7-2 Proteins identified in CSF with electrophoresis and immunoelectrophoresis

Electrophoretic fraction	Prealbumin	Albumin	Alpha$_1$ globulin	Alpha$_2$ globulin	Beta globulin	Gamma globulin
Immunoelectrophoretic proteins	Prealbumin	Albumin	Alpha$_1$ antitrypsin	Alpha$_2$ macro-globulin	Beta lipo-protein	IgG
			Alpha$_1$ lipo-protein	Alpha$_2$ lipo-protein	Transferrin	IgA
			Alpha$_1$ glyco-protein (orosomu-coid)	Haptoglobulin	Tau fraction (modified transferrin) Plasminogen	IgM
				Ceruloplasmin	Complement	IgD
				Erythropoietin	Hemopexin	IgF
					Beta-trace	Gamma-trace

Data from Laterre, 1965; Schultze and Heremans, 1966; Dencker, 1969; Link and Olsson, 1972; Lumsden, 1972; Nerenberg et al., 1987; and Williams et al., 1978 as cited by Fishman RA. Cerebrospinal fluid in diseases of the nervous system. 2nd ed. Philadelphia: WB Saunders, 1992.

Table 7-3 Concentrations of proteins in plasma and CSF

Protein	Molecular weight	Hydrodynamic radius (Å)	Plasma concentration (mg/L)	CSF concentration (mg/L)	Plasma/CSF ratio
Prealbumin	61,000	32.5	238	17.3	14
Albumin	69,000	35.8	36,600	155.0	236
Transferrin	81,000	36.7	2040	14.4	142
Ceruloplasmin	152,000	46.8	366	1.0	366
IgG	150,000	53.4	9870	12.3	802
IgA	150,000	56.8	1750	1.3	1346
Alpha$_2$ macroglobulin	798,000	93.5	2220	2.0	1111
Fibrinogen	340,000	108.0	2964	0.6	4940
IgM	800,000	121.0	700	0.6	1167
Beta lipoprotein	2,239,000	124.0	3728	0.6	6213

Data from Felgenhauser, 1974 as cited by Fishman RA. Cerebrospinal fluid in diseases of the nervous system. 2nd ed. Philadelphia: WB Saunders, 1992.

Oligoclonal IgG bands can be detected in unconcentrated CSF using isoelectric focusing and immunolabeling. The bands are found in the cathodal region on electrophoresis. In normal CSF, there is no evidence of discrete banding in this region but only a homogenous grouping of protein. Oligoclonal IgG bands signal the presence of an abnormal humoral immune response in the CSF-CNS compartment that is most often associated with infections but is sometimes associated with tumors, migraine, and seizures [Kostulas et al., 1986; Siemes et al., 1981; Gerbaut and Ponsot, 1984].

Alterations in the qualitative protein profile also occur independent of an increase in total protein. In multiple sclerosis and subacute sclerosing panencephalitis, there is a marked increase in the IgG fraction, but total protein content is unchanged. The IgG level is both absolutely elevated and elevated as a relative percentage of total protein. The IgG molecule contains two heavy (lambda) and two light (kappa) chains. Free light chains of IgG have been reported in increased concentrations in the CSF of multiple sclerosis patients; the specificity of this finding appears to be high [Rudick et al., 1986].

Myelin-basic protein (encephalitogenic protein) can be quantitated in spinal fluid by radioimmunoassay. Although the presence of myelin-basic protein in CSF is not an indicator of specific disease, increased concentrations are found in the acute phases of multiple sclerosis [Warren and Catz, 1987] and other conditions in which acute demyelination occurs [Olsson et al., 1990].

Antimyelin-basic protein (bound and unbound fractions) has also been identified in the CSF of multiple sclerosis patients. Higher titers of free antimyelin-basic protein were associated with acute exacerbations and of bound antimyelin-basic protein with chronic, progressive disease [Warren and Catz, 1986; Warren and Catz, 1987].

Myelin-associated glycoprotein has also been identified in both normal subjects and patients with neurologic disease [Yanagisawa et al., 1985].

There have been occasional reports of qualitative protein alterations in tuberculous meningitis, brain tumors, and meningitis.

Other Substances

Other substances have been studied in CSF in an attempt to gain information concerning brain metabolism. They are discussed in the appropriate portions of this book in association with specific pathologic conditions. Among them are lactate, glycine, pyruvate, creatine kinase, aspartic acid, acetylcholine, phospholipids, lipoproteins, cephalin, and many more. Serologic studies for determining the presence of toxoplasmosis, cytomegalic inclusion virus disease, rubella, rubeola, and herpes simplex are performed when appropriate.

REFERENCES

Barringer R. A simplified procedure for spinal fluid cytology. Arch Neurol 1970; 22:305.

Bonadio WA, Smith DS, Goddard S, et al. Distinguishing cerebrospinal fluid abnormalities in children with bacterial meningitis and traumatic lumbar puncture. J Infect Dis 1990; 162:251.

Bruce DA, Ter Weeme C, Kaiser G, et al. Mechanisms and time course for clearance of vasogenic cerebral edema. In: Popp AJ, et al., eds. Neural trauma. New York: Raven Press, 1979.

Clark D. Lumbar puncture. In: Nelson W, ed. Textbook of pediatrics, 9th ed. Philadelphia: WB Saunders, 1969.

Cole M. Examination of the cerebrospinal fluid. In: Toole J, ed. Special techniques for neurologic diagnosis. Philadelphia: F.A. Davis, 1969.

Cutler RWP, Watters GV, Hammerstad JP. The origin and turnover of cerebrospinal fluid albumin and gamma globulin in man. J Neurol Sci 1970; 10:259.

Davson H. Physiology of the cerebrospinal fluid. London: Churchill Livingstone, 1967.

Dyken PR. Cerebrospinal fluid cytomorphology: n.c. the effect of air and oil instillation within the subarachnoid spaces, and cerebrospinal fluid cellular defense. Ann Arbor: Xerox University Microfilms, 1974.

Dyken PR, Mulina JL. The normal cellular population of the cerebrospinal fluid by sedimentation-flocculation techniques at various ages. Proc Child Neurol Soc 1973; 2:26.

Dyken PR, Shirley S, El Gammal T. Comparison of cytocentrifugation and sedimentation techniques for CSF cytomorphology. Acta Cytol 1980; 24:2.

Eeg-Olofsson O, Link H, Wigertz A. Concentrations of CSF proteins as a measure of blood brain barrier function and synthesis of IgG within the CNS in "normal" subjects from the age of 6 months to 30 years. Acta Paediatr Scand 1981; 70:167.

Fishman RA. Carrier transport of glucose between blood and the cerebrospinal fluid. Am J Physiol 1964; 206:836.

Fishman RA. Cerebrospinal fluid in diseases of the nervous system. 2nd ed. Philadelphia: WB Saunders, 1992.

Gerbaut L, Ponsot G. Semeiology of the gammaglobulinic patterns of cerebrospinal fluid in children. In: Peeters H, ed. Protides of the biological fluids. Oxford: Plenum Press, 1984.

Grant R, Condon B, Hart I, et al. Changes in intracranial CSF volume after lumbar puncture and their relationship to post-LP headache. J Neurol Neurosurg Psychiatry 1991; 54:440.

Greenlee JE. Approach to diagnosis of meningitis: Cerebrospinal fluid evaluation. Infect Dis Clin North Am 1990; 4:583.

Guyton AC. The cerebrospinal fluid system. In: Guyton AC, ed. Textbook of medical physiology, 4th ed. Philadelphia: WB Saunders, 1971.

Gyllensward A, Malmstrom S. The cerebrospinal fluid in immature infants. Acta Paediatr Scand Suppl 1962; 135:54.

Hochwald GM. Cerebrospinal fluid. In: Baker AB, Baker LH, eds. Clinical neurology. New York: Harper & Row, 1984.

Jordan GW, Statland B, Halsted C. CSF lactate in diseases of the CNS. Arch Intern Med 1983; 143:85.

Kirkpatrick D, Goodman SJ. Combined sub-arachnoid and subdural spinal hematoma following spinal puncture. Surg Neurol 1975; 3:109.

Kostulas V, Eeg-Olofsson O, Olsson T, et al. Demonstration in children of oligoclonal IgG bands in unconcentrated CSF using agarose isoelectric focusing and immunolabeling. Pediatr Neurol 1986; 2:286.

Levinson A. Cerebral spinal fluid in infants and children. Am J Dis Child 1928; 36:799.

Martin WJ. Rapid and reliable techniques for the laboratory detection of bacterial meningitis. Am J Med 1983; 75(suppl. 1B):119.

Masdeu JH, Breuer AC, Schoene WC. Spinal subarachnoid hematomas. Clue to a source of bleeding in traumatic lumbar puncture. Neurology 1979; 29:872.

Menkes J. The causes for low spinal fluid sugar in bacterial meningitis. Another look. Pediatrics 1969; 44:1.

Munroe D. Cerebrospinal fluid pressure in the newborns. JAMA 1928; 90:1688.

Olsson T, Bang S, Höjeberg B, et al. Antimyelin basic protein and antimyelin antibody-producing cells in multiple sclerosis. Ann Neurol 1990; 27:132.

Otila E. Studies on the cerebrospinal fluid in premature infants. Acta Paediatr Scand 1948; 35(suppl. 8):72.

Overturf GD, Hoeprich PD. Bacterial meningitis. In: Hoeprich PD, ed. Infectious diseases, Philadelphia: Harper & Row, 1983.

Portnoy JM, Olson LC. Normal cerebrospinal fluid values in children: another look. Pediatrics 1985; 75:484.

Putto A, Ruuskanen O, Meurman O, et al. C-reactive protein in the evaluation of febrile illness. Arch Dis Child 1986;61:24.

Rich JR. A membrane filter technique for cerebrospinal fluid cytology. J Neurosurg 1972; 36:661.

Rudick RA, Pallant A, Bidlack JM, et al. Free kappa light chains in multiple sclerosis spinal fluid. Ann Neurol 1986; 20:63.

Rutledge J, Benjamin MB, Hood L, et al. Is the CSF lactate measurement useful in the management of children with suspected bacterial meningitis? J Pediatr 1981; 98:20.

Samson K. Der normale liquor cerebrospinalis im ersten lebenstrimenon. Z Neurolog Psychiatr 1930; 128:494.

Savory J, Heintges M. Cerebrospinal fluid levels of IgG, IgA, and IgM in neurologic disease. Neurology 1973; 23:953.

Siemes H, Siegert M, Hanefeld F. Occurrence of oligoclonal gamma-globulin in the CSF of children with prolonged and chronic CNS infections. Acta Paediatr Scand 1981; 70:91.

Tourtellotte WW, Henderson WG, Tucker RP, et al. A randomized double-blind clinical trial comparing the 22 versus 26 gauge needle in the production of the post-lumbar puncture syndrome in normal individual animals. Headache 1972; 12:73.

Truex RC, Carpenter MB. Cerebrospinal fluid. In: Truex RC, Carpenter MB, eds. Human neuroanatomy. Baltimore: Williams & Wilkins, 1971.

Warren KG, Catz I. Diagnostic value of cerebrospinal fluid anti-myelin basic protein in patients with multiple sclerosis. Ann Neurol 1986; 20:20.

Warren KG, Catz I. A correlation between cerebrospinal fluid myelin basic protein and anti-myelin basic protein in multiple sclerosis patients. Ann Neurol 1987; 21:183.

Welch K. The principles of physiology of the cerebrospinal fluid in relation to hydrocephalus including normal pressure hydrocephalus. In: Friedlander WJ, ed. Advances in neurology. New York: Raven Press, 1975.

Welch K, Araki H, Arkins T. Electrical potentials of the lamina epithialis choroidea of the fourth ventricle of the cat in vitro: Relationship to the CSF blood potential. Dev Med Child Neurol 1972; 14 (suppl. 27):146.

Widell S. On the cerebrospinal fluid in normal children and in patients with acute abacterial meningoencephalitis. Acta Paediatr Scand 1958; 47(suppl. 115):1.

Woody RC, Yamauchi T, Bolyard K. Cerebrospinal fluid cell counts in childhood idiopathic status epilepticus. Pediatr Infect Dis J 1988; 7:298.

Yanagisawa K, Quarles RH, Johnson D, et al. A derivative of myelin-associated glycoprotein in cerebrospinal fluid of normal subjects and patients with neurological disease. Ann Neurol 1985; 18:464.

Part Three

Disease Characteristics and Categories

Signs and Symptoms Found in Selected Diseases Associated with Mental Retardation

Eye Abnormalities	Seizures

Cataracts
  Cockayne syndrome
  Cretinism
  Down syndrome
  Galactosemia
  Lowe syndrome
  Marinesco-Sjögren syndrome
  Myotonic dystrophy
  Oculocerebral syndrome and keratosis follicularis
  Pseudohypoparathyroidism
  Rubella (gestational)
Cherry-red spot in macular area
  GM_1 gangliosidosis (generalized)
  Mucolipidoses
  Niemann-Pick disease
  Tay-Sachs disease
Chorioretinitis
  Congenital lues
  Cytomegalic inclusion body disease
  Prenatal Rubella (gestational)
Clouding of cornea
  Congenital lues
  Hunter syndrome
  Hurler syndrome
  Lowe syndrome
  Oculocerebral syndrome and keratosis follicularis
Corneal ulcers
  Familial dysautonomia
Dislocated lenses
  Homocystinuria
  Sulfite oxidase deficiency
Glaucoma
  Lowe syndrome
  Oculocerebral syndrome and keratosis follicularis
Nystagmus
  Hyperpipecolatemia
  Hypervalinemia
  Joubert syndrome
Photophobia
  Cockayne syndrome
  Hartnup disease
  Homocystinuria
Retinitis pigmentosa
  Ataxia-telangiectasia
  Cockayne syndrome
  Hallervorden-Spatz syndrome
  Hyperpipecolatemia
  Kearns-Sayre syndrome
  Laurence-Moon-Biedl syndrome
  Mitochondrial encephalomyopathies
  Neuronal ceroid-lipfuscinosis
  Scleral telangiectasia
	Generalized tonic-clonic
	  Argininosuccinic aciduria
	  Neuronal ceroid-lipofuscinosis
	  Citrullinemia
	  Glycogen synthetase deficiency
	  Hyper-beta-alaninemia
	  Hyperammonemia
	  Hyperlysinemia
	  Hyperonithinemia-hyperammonemia and homo-citrullinuria hyperprolinemia I
	  Hypoglycemia, particularly associated with glycogen storage diseases I, III, IV, and VI
	  Idiopathic hypoglycemia of infancy
	  Joseph syndrome
	  Ketotic hypoglycemia
	  Kinky hair disease (Menkes disease)
	  Lactic acidosis
	  Lysine intolerance with periodic ammonia intoxication
	  Maple syrup disease
	  Methionine malabsorption syndrome
	  Mitochondrial encephalomyopathies (e.g., MERRF, MELAS)
	  Neuroaxonal dystrophy
	  Nonketotic hyperglycinemia
	  Phenylketonuria
	  Tay-Sachs disease
	Seizures in neonatal period
	  Argininosuccinic acidura
	  Hyperammonemia I and II
	  Hyperprolinemia I
	  Hypoxic-ischemic encephalopathy
	  Isovaleric acidemia
	  Joseph syndrome
	  Lactic acidosis
	  Maple syrup disease
	  Mitochondrial encephalomyopathy
	  Methylmalonic acidemia
	  Propionic acidemia

Signs and Symptoms Found in Selected Diseases Associated with Mental Retardation—cont'd

Skin Abnormalities

Café-au-lait spots
    Ataxia-telangiectasia
    Bloom syndrome
    Neurofibromatosis
    Tuberous sclerosis
Depigmented nevi
    Tuberous sclerosis
Eczema
    Phenylketonuria
Keratosis follicularis
    Oculocerebral syndrome with keratosis follicularis
        [Adler and Nyhan, 1969], with cerebral atrophy
        [Cantu et al., 1974]
Malar flush
    Homocystinuria
Photosensitivity
    Hartnup disease
    Tryptophanuria
Synophrys
    Cornelia de Lange syndrome
    Cretinism

Hair Abnormalities

Fine hair
    Homocystinuria
    Hypothyroidism
Friable and tufted hair (trichorrhexis nodosa)
    Argininosuccinic aciduria
    Kinky hair disease (Menkes disease)
Loss of scalp hair
    Familial lactic acidosis with necrotizing encephalopathy
Premature gray hair
    Ataxia-telangiectasia
    Progressive cerebral hemisphere atrophy [Gomez and Moore, 1974]
White hair (patches)
    Methionine malabsorption syndrome
    Tuberous sclerosis

Hearing Abnormalities

Conduction deafness
    Hunter syndrome
    Hurler syndrome
Hyperacusis
    GM1 gangliosidosis (generalized)
    Krabbe disease
    Subacute sclerosing pancencephalitis
    Sulfite oxidase deficiency
    Tay-Sachs disease
Sensorineural deafness
    CHARGE syndrome [Menenzes and Coker, 1990]
    Kearns-Sayre syndrome
    MELAS
    MERRF
    Refsum syndrome

Hepatosplenomegaly

Argininosuccinic aciduria
Gaucher disease
GM1 gangliosidosis (generalized)
Glycogen storage disease types I and III
Hydroxykynureninuria
Hyperpipecolatemia
Mucopolysaccharidoses
Neuronal ceroid-lipofuscinosis
Niemann-Pick disease

Vomiting

Hyperammonemia (all types)
Hyperglycinemia
Hyperlysinemia
Hypervalinemia
Increased intracranial pressure
Lactic acidosis
Maple syrup disease
MELAS

Metabolic Acidosis

Ketotic hypoglycemia
Lactic acidosis
Maple syrup disease
Methionine malabsorption syndrome
Methylmalonic acidemia
Mitochondrial encephalomyopathy
5-Oxoprolinuria (pyroglutamic aciduria)
Propionic acidemia

Signs and Symptoms Found in Selected Diseases Associated with Mental Retardation — cont'd

Other Abnormalities

Anterior horn cell disease (includes electrodiagnostic evidence of normal nerve conduction time in the presence of muscular denervation potentials)
    Neuroaxonal dystrophy
Ataxia
    Argininosuccinic aciduria
    Ataxia-telangiectasia
    Cockayne syndrome
    Hartnup disease
    Hyperammonemia from any cause
    Joubert syndrome
    Kearns-Sayre syndrome
    Marinesco-Sjögren syndrome
    MERRF
    Metachromatic leukodystrophy
    5-Oxoprolinuria (pyroglutamic aciduria)
    Pyruvate decarboxylase deficiency
    Tryptophanuria
Broad thumbs and toes
    Rubinstein-Taybi syndrome (Rubinstein and Taybi, 1963)
Choreoathetosis (see Chapters 18 and 57)
    Hallervorden-Spatz syndrome
    Huntington chorea
    Joseph syndrome
    Lesch-Nyhan disease
    Phenylketonuria
Dystonia
    Hallervorden-Spatz syndrome
    Wilson disease
Enlarged head
    Alexander disease
    Canavan disease
    GM2 gangliosidosis (generalized)
    Histiocytosis X
    Hydrocephalus
    Mucopolysaccharidoses
    Sandhoff disease
    Spongy degeneration
    Subdural effusion
    Subdural hematoma
    Tay-Sachs disease

Micromelia
    Cornelia de Lange syndrome
Odors
    Isovaleric acidemia
    Maple syrup disease
    Methionine malabsorption syndrome
    Phenylketonuria
Peripheral neuropathy (includes electrodiagnostic evidence of decreased conduction time)
    Cockayne syndrome
    Krabbe syndrome
    Metachromatic leukodystrophy
    Niemann-Pick disease
Short stature
    Bird-headed dwarf (Seckel type)
    Cockayne syndrome
    Cornelia de Lange syndrome
    Cretinism
    Leprechaunism (Dekaban, 1965)
    Mucolipidoses
    Mucopolysaccharidoses
    Prader-Willi syndrome
    Rubinstein-Taybi syndrome
Tremor
    Citrullinemia
    Hartnup disease
    Hyperpipecolatemia
    Hypersarcosinemia

chromosomal studies. Physical anomalies, particularly when there are several, are also indications for chromosomal studies.

The study of dermatoglyphics has become less important in recent years because of the availability of sophisticated and readily obtainable cytogenetic studies. Nevertheless, abnormal chromosomal patterns often are signaled by abnormal dermatoglyphic patterns [Rodewald et al., 1986].

As stated, although many chromosomal abnormalities are associated with conditions that include mental retardation, it has been recognized in recent years that the fragile X syndrome, an X-linked recessive condition, is responsible for a relatively high percentage of mental retardation, primarily in males [Wisniewsky et al., 1991; Johnson et al., 1991]. In one study, 10% of mildly retarded and 6% of severely retarded males had the chromosomal abnormality [Blomquist et al., 1982]. At

Table 8-2 Ferric chloride screening test for urine

Diseases or conditions	Compound	Color
Alkaptonuria	Homogentisic acid	Green (fades quickly)
Drug ingestion	Phenothiazine derivatives, salicylates	Purple (stable)
Histidenemia	Imidazolepyruvic acid	Green or blue-green
Hyperbilirubinemia	Bilirubin	Blue-green
Hypervalinemia, systemic acidosis	Pyruvic acid, α-Ketosisovaleric acids	Yellow
Malignant melanoma	Melanin	Gray with precipitate, turning black
Maple syrup disease	α-Ketoisocaproic acid, α-Ketoisovaleric acid, α-Ketomethylvaleric acid	Gray with green tinge
Normal metabolite	α-Ketobutyric acid	Purple (fades to red-brown in 1 to 2 minutes)
Phenylketonuria	Phenylpyruvic acid	Green or blue-green
	o-Hydroxyphenylacetic acid	Mauve
Systemic acidosis	ρ-Aminosalicylic acid, acetoacetic acid	Red-brown
Transient tyrosinosis	ρ-Hydroxyphenylpyruvic acid	Green (fades quickly)
Trytophan load	3-Hydroxyanthranilic acid	Immediate deep brown
Tryptophan load, hydroxykynureninuria	Xanthurenic acid	Deep green, turning later to brown
No known clinical relevance	Vanillic acid	Red-brown to green-blue or mauve

Modified from Henry RJ. Clinical chemistry. New York: Harper & Row, 1964.

least two types of fragile X syndromes have been recognized [Sutherland, 1979; Carpenter et al., 1982]. In one type the testes are enlarged, and in the other the testes are normal. Some females with mild mental retardation also appear to have fragile X sites [Blomquist et al., 1982].

Using a 15-item checklist proved to be helpful in the clinical diagnosis of fragile X syndrome [Butler et al., 1991]. When compared with mentally retarded boys without the fragile X syndrome, fragile X syndrome boys had a statistically significant greater incidence (P < 0.01) of hyperactivity; shorter attention span; more tactile defensiveness, hand-flapping, perseverative speech, and hyperextensibility; larger ears and testes; higher frequency of simian creases or Sydney lines and plantar creases; and a higher frequency of positive family histories of mental retardation. An overall correct classification rate of 93% was achieved based on six variables (i.e., plantar crease, simian crease, hyperflexibility, large testes, large ears, and positive family history of mental retardation) [Butler et al., 1991].

There is evidence that these boys become more impaired as they mature [Curfs et al., 1991].

EEG and sensory-evoked potentials. A specific diagnosis rarely rests on interpretation of EEG studies; however, pseudoretardation, which is the result of frequent, brief, generalized seizures and little or no motor component (absence episodes), may be indicated by spike-and-wave or polyspike-and-wave activity.

Visual-evoked potentials have facilitated assessment of the integrity of the visual pathways in children who appear profoundly retarded (see Chapter 6). Some of these children have gross visual impairment, whereas others appear to be unable to process visual information correctly after it has reached the occipital cortex.

Brainstem auditory-evoked potentials indicate the integrity of the audiologic system and are of particular value in retarded individuals (see Chapter 6). These studies can be performed in very young children; thus detection of hearing impairment may be performed early in life.

Other studies. CT and MRI have become the most common means of assessing brain structure. The presence of old blood, subdural hematomas, porencephalic cysts, and intracranial calcifications is easily determined with these studies. Small areas of calcification may be overlooked in routine skull radiographic studies but are readily visualized with CT; calcium deposits may indicate tuberous sclerosis, cytomegalic inclusion body disease, toxoplasmosis, old intracranial hemorrhage, and other diseases. Plain skull radiographs may also reveal bony orbit changes and neurofibromatosis, asymmetry of the skull, old skull fracture, or craniosynostosis [Schey, 1974].

MRI has provided a means of assessing neuronal migratory defects to a degree not previously available. Gross changes of the cortical gray ribbon, such as those associated with lissencephaly, micro/pachygyria, and failure of operculization of the temporal lobe, are readily diagnosed in vivo. Ectopic gray matter can also be readily distinguished with these studies. Unusual stores of lipid, failure of myelination, and irregular patterns of myelination are also detectable. The utility of this technique makes it highly desirable that all infants and children without otherwise explainable intellectual retardation should have cranial MRI scans. Unfortunately, because the process is sometimes of lengthy duration, most young children require sedation and a few require general anesthesia.

The use of positron emission tomography, single photon emission computed tomography, and nuclear magnetic tomography (NMR) may have future impact on the diagnosis of underlying conditions that lead to mental retardation.

Pneumoencephalography is now rarely performed. Occasionally, arterioangiography is necessary to detect and delineate certain types of vascular malformations, vascular arteritis, or dural venous sinus thrombosis. Focal neurologic findings require appropriate neuroimaging study [Naheedy and Schnur, 1979].

Genetics

The biologic origins of mental retardation remain controversial. Birth injury is probably less of a factor than previously believed, although reliable data are difficult to develop [Chaney et al., 1986]. The theory that multiple, additive genes are responsible for mild mental retardation is not well substantiated [Akesson, 1986].

Obviously, the family of children with specifically identifiable diseases can usually be provided with information concerning specific hereditary patterns. For other patients, such a genetic pattern cannot be delineated. In one study of 214 first-degree relatives of 40 patients with profound retardation of unknown causes, 53 (24.8%) were mentally retarded or dull normal. Among the group were 23 parents and 30 siblings. A total of 73 (7.9%) of 928 first-degree, second-degree, and third-degree relatives were retarded; 21% of the siblings were included. Certainly the group was heterogeneous; however, an autosomal-recessive mode of inheritance was the likely pattern in many of the families [Becker et al., 1977].

Rett syndrome, which occurs almost exclusively in girls and includes mental retardation, autistic behavior, seizures, unusual hand movements, and other characteristics, is discussed in Chapter 55.

ASSESSMENT OF FUNCTIONING

Whenever mental retardation appears likely, a suitable evaluation of motor, perceptual, and cognitive abilities should be undertaken. This endeavor is particularly necessary as children reach school age. Fre-

quently, multidisciplinary teams that include a physician, psychologist, speech and language consultant, social worker, and educational consultant can provide the best evaluation and planning for the child. Any neuropsychologic evaluation should provide measures of the child's verbal and nonverbal problem-solving abilities, social adaptation, and motor evaluation. The child who has inadequacies in one or two areas must be distinguished from the child who has global mental retardation.

Normal function in one or more areas should serve to warn the clinician that the child may not be mentally retarded, and the diagnosis of mental retardation should be made only after multiple measures and testing sessions have occurred. The clinician should be particularly leery of assessments of a child younger than 3 and sometimes 4 years of age. The data may be unreliable and may reflect specific areas of developmental delay, such as perceptual and motor skills. Nevertheless, when a child is cooperative, a neuropsychologist experienced in assessing preschool children can be reasonably accurate in estimating ability. Several tests may be used for such evaluation (Table 8-3).

In addition to the assessment of intelligence through measures of verbal and nonverbal problem-solving ability, adaptive behavior scales are used to assess the level of social functioning of the older child. Although a diagnosis cannot be made on the basis of one of these parent interview-based scales, nonacademic skills are assessed rather well with the following two scales:

1. Vineland Adaptive Behavior Scale (VABS) (1984)—a set of scales that measure communication, daily living skills, socialization, motor skills, and maladaptive behavior domains. It has 297 items with a structured interview format. It is well standardized.
2. Woodcock Johnson Scales of Independent Behavior (SIB) (1984)—14 scales organized into four clusters that include motor, social interaction and communication, personal independence, and community independence skills.

For the younger child, the Minnesota Child Development Inventory (1972), a parent questionnaire, yields information about general development, gross motor, fine motor, expressive language, comprehension (conceptual), situation comprehension, self help, and personal social skills.

For the moderately retarded child, the Adaptive Behavior Scale (AAMD), 1974 version, includes scales of functioning level in various activities and maladaptive behaviors with norms for moderately retarded children. The Cain Levine Social Competency Scale (1964) is also geared to this population, with scores on five adaptive scales.

Table 8-3 Measures of intelligence used for the diagnosis of mental retardation and other cognitive defects

Date of publication	Age range for test	Scores yielded from test and administration time	Description of test
Wechsler Intelligence Scale for Children—III			
1991	Ages 6 to 17	Full scale, verbal, performance IQ Mean = 100 Standard deviation = 15 Subtests: information, similarities, arithmetic, vocabulary, comprehension, digit span, picture completion, picture arrangement, block design, object assembly, symbol search, coding, mazes Mean = 10 Standard deviation = 3 Administration time: 1¾ hours	The standard measure of children's intelligence. It yields the most useful information because of the diversity of the tasks. Provides an excellent opportunity to observe approaches to problem solving. Heavily weighted on timed tests, motor skills, and processing tasks. Well standardized. Not appropriate for severely retarded children.
Wechsler Adult Intelligence Scale—revised			
1981	Ages 16 and older	Full scale, verbal, performance IQ Mean = 100 Standard deviation = 15 Subtests: information, digit span, similarities, arithmetic, vocabulary, comprehension, picture completion, digit symbol, picture arrangement, block design, object assembly Mean = 10 Standard deviation = 3 Administration time: 1½ hours	The standard measure of adolescent and adult intelligence. It yields the most useful information because of the diversity of the tasks. Provides an excellent opportunity to observe approaches to problem solving. Heavily weighted on timed tests, motor skills, and processing tasks. Well standardized. Not appropriate for severely retarded adolescents.
Stanford Binet Intelligence Scale—fourth edition			
1985	Ages 2½ to adulthood	Standard Age Scores for composite, verbal reasoning, abstract visual reasoning, quantitative and short-term memory scales Mean = 100 Standard deviation = 16 Subtests vary by age and ability Mean = 50 Standard deviation = 8 Administration time: 1 to 2 hours	This is a restandardized and reorganized verson of the test most frequently used to assess retarded individuals. It is difficult to administer, especially in children with uneven abilities for whom the starting levels may be too high. It is a power test. There are few timed tests, few tasks that involve motor skills. Heavy on learned material. Different subtests at different ages and abilities. Question adequacy of normative data.
Kaufman Assessment Battery for Children			
1983	Ages 2½ to 12½	Mental processing composite, sequential processing score, simultaneous processing score, achievement score Mean = 100 Standard deviation = 15 Subtests vary by age Mean = 10 Standard deviation = 3 for processing scales Mean = 100 Standard deviation = 15 for achievement scales Administration time: 45 minutes	The only test based on a theory of intelligence and processing styles. Good norms for minority children, attractive materials, easy and short to administer. No language or motor tasks. Most of the subtests involve processing tasks. It is questionable if processing scores actually measure sequential and simultaneous processing. Different tasks at different ages. Test not designed for significantly impaired children.

Compiled by Elsa G. Shapiro, Ph.D.

Continued.

Table 8-3 Measures of intelligence used for the diagnosis of mental retardation and other cognitive defects—cont'd

Date of publication	Age range for test	Scores yielded from test and administration time	Description of test
McCarthy Scales of Children's Abilities			
1972	Ages 2½ to 8½	General cognitive index Mean = 100 Standard deviation = 15 Verbal, perceptual performance, quantitative, memory, and motor development scales Mean = 50 Standard deviation = 10 Administration time: 1 to 1½ hours	A purportedly culture-fair test but often misclassifies learning-disabled children as retarded. Rote material, not many problem-solving or processing tasks. Separate memory and motor scales, which are useful separately. Sometimes difficult for the child to interpret instructions. Not a good sample of behaviors for observational purposes.
Wechsler Preschool and Primary Scale of Intelligence—Revised			
1989	Ages 3 to 7	Full scale, verbal, performance IQ Mean = 100 Standard deviation = 15 Subtests: information, similarities, arithmetic, vocabulary, comprehension, sentences, object assembly, picture completion, geometric design, mazes, block design, animal pegs. Mean = 10 Standard deviation = 3 Administration time: 1½ hours	New norms are very good and has excellent materials for observation. Heavily weighted on timed tests, motor skills, and processing tasks. Not appropriate for severely retarded children.
Bayley Scales of Infant Development: Mental and Motor Scales			
1969	Age 2 to 30 months	Mental development index Motor development index Mean = 100 Standard deviation = 15 Mental age and motor age also obtainable Administration time: 45 minutes	Measures sensory motor development in infants, thus it is a poor predictor of later intelligence. It requires little sustained attention. Appropriate for the assessment of older, severely impaired children. Requires much skill and experience to administer.
Merrill Palmer Scales of Mental Development			
1937	Ages 24 months to 5½ years	IQ, mental age Administration time: 45 minutes	A largely nonverbal test with good assessment of perceptual and motor skills. Not predictive of overall intelligence. Many retarded children score well on this test. Appropriate specifically for language-impaired children. Very interesting materials for preschoolers and retarded children. Norms are outdated.
Leiter International Scale—Arthur Adaptation			
1948	Ages 2 to 18	IQ, mental age Administration time: 30 minutes	Completely nonverbal. Appropriate for deaf or non-English speaking–children. A highly structured and repetitive test that yields limited information. Norms are outdated.
Pictorial Test of Intelligence			
1964	Ages 3 to 8	IQ, mental age Subtests: picture vocabulary, form discrimination, information and comprehension, similarities, size and number, immediate recall Administration time: 45 minutes	Appropriate for children with severe motor and speech impairments. A test of auditory and visual processing; only requires pointing as a response. Materials lack interest.

Table 8-3 Measures of intelligence used for the diagnosis of mental retardation and other cognitive defects—cont'd

Date of publication	Age range for test	Scores yielded from test and administration time	Description of test
Hiskey Nebraska Test of Learning Aptitude			
1966	Ages 3 to 16	Deviation IQ, age equivalents Subtests: bead patterns, memory for color, picture identification, picture association, paper folding, visual attention span, block patterns, completion of drawings, memory for digits, puzzle blocks, picture analogies, spatial reasoning Administration time: 1 to 1½ hours	This test is especially good for children who are deaf or have severe language impairments. It is also good for younger children. The materials are interesting and varied and provide good observation material. Norms available for deaf children.
Peabody Picture Vocabulary Test—revised			
1981	Ages 2 to adulthood	Standard score Mean = 100 Standard deviation = 15 Administration time: 15 to 30 minutes	A test of receptive vocabulary that is often used as an estimate of potential. It is a good measure of a single function but should not be used as an estimate of general intelligence.
Raven Progressive Matrices			
1983	Ages 5 to adulthood	Three forms, colored for young children, a general form, and an advanced form Percentile ranks for age Administration time: 15 to 45 minutes	A test of nonverbal problem solving that, like the PPVT, has often been used as a way to estimate intelligence. It has also been described as culture-fair but measures a narrowly defined function.

Evaluation of the patient

Great caution must be exercised in evaluating infants during the first year of life. At best only motor function is reasonably assessed, and long-term prediction for children under 2 or 3 years of age is unwise unless the children are grossly retarded. For those children who are not profoundly involved, it may be difficult to make assessments until 4 to 6 years of age, when a more reliable prediction of academic skills can be made. Preschool testing is best used for planning short-term educational intervention and not for long-term management or prognosis. It must be remembered that most of the standardized measures allow an IQ to be calculated that reflects the child's ability when compared with children of the same age. These few scores are intended to characterize many skills. The characteristics of children who have wide variation in their abilities may not be adequately represented by IQ scores, and caution should be exercised. Table 8-4 summarizes the frequency of occurrence of IQ categories in the population, indicates IQ score ranges, and provides terms frequently used [Kirk, 1972]. Although IQ is relatively consonant with performance in many areas in normal children, children with impaired abilities have greater variability and developmental variation during their early years. IQ

Table 8-4 Classification of intellectual level

IQ range	Interpretation	Frequency (percent) WISC-R
130 and above	Very superior	2.3
120 to 129	Superior	7.4
110 to 199	Above average	16.5
90 to 110	Average	49.4
80 to 89	Below average	16.2
70 to 79	Borderline retarded	6.0
67 and below	Mentally retarded	2.2
52 to 67	Mildly (educably) retarded	
36 to 51	Moderately (trainably) retarded	
20 to 35	Severely retarded	
Less than 20	Profoundly retarded	

Data from material in the manual of the Weschler Intelligence Scale for Children—Revised, and from Heber R. Am J Ment Defic 1961; 65:500.

scores are only meaningful when compared with other psychologic, social, and medical data.

Children who do not babble by 7 to 9 months of age should have a competent audiologic evaluation, including brainstem auditory-evoked potentials (see Chapter 21). Additionally, a speech and language consultant should evaluate the characteristics of delayed development of speech and language.

A social worker may develop a most useful and detailed developmental history and family assessment. The expectations and attitudes of the family members may be most important in the management of the retarded child. The ability of the family to accept the child's disability and to expend the necessary energy in helping the child live with the disability is important. Counseling may be essential for the parents and family to help them accept future educational plans for the child and to help them with decisions regarding in-home or out-of-home placement. Observation, play, interviews, and simple projective testing allow the examiner of the moderately or mildly retarded child to gain some sense of the child's personality. Emotional and behavioral difficulties may be significant, some of which may arise from poor parenting techniques and inadequate school placement. Other innate factors, such as temperament, may be important. The child and family may benefit through changes made by counseling of parents, school consultation, behavior modification techniques, and medications.

MANAGEMENT

The day-to-day management of the physical needs of mentally retarded children embraces all those areas of care required for normal children. Some facets of care are rendered more difficult because of the handicap. Nutrition can often be a problem. Gross motor/self-feeding impairment, oral-motor dysfunction, lack of appetite, and food aversions may interfere with adequate intake. Alternate feeding practices, including prolonged assisted feeding and use of pureed foods, may be necessary. Because of these conditions and requirements nutrition may not be optimal [Thommessen et al., 1991]. Dental care for retarded children is another area of management that is often inadequate, and the problems are unrecognized.

The management of mentally retarded individuals requires a multitude of services and accompanying expenditure of funds. There has been a modest, overall increase in public funding in the United States for services to the retarded during the past decade. The estimated expenditure in the United States for these services in fiscal 1984 was 16.59 billion dollars [Braddock and Hemp, 1986].

Many variables contribute to the optimum management of patients with mental retardation. The trend in the past 2 decades has been away from institutionalization and toward keeping the child in the home; however, certain families are unable to cope with the stresses created by the presence of a retarded child. Foster home

placement has proved to be a viable alternative. The stimulation provided by a home or home-substitute environment provides the opportunity for developing normal socialization and interpersonal relationships.

Most placements outside the home occur before 5 years of age. The lack of adequate school programs is one of the primary reasons cited for outside placement [Koch et al., 1977].

Many individuals live in over 200 institutions in the United States [Nelson and Crocker, 1978]. One study indicates that males outnumber females in residential placement [Richardson et al., 1986]. Unfortunately, large institutions are usually poorly equipped to provide individual planning and implementation of individual programs.

Day activity centers and the increasing involvement of the public school systems in the education of the mentally retarded has brought about more systematic efforts in socialization and education.

There has been a trend toward the use of group homes for adolescent and adult mentally retarded individuals in the United States. These group homes provide supervision but also allow some degree of independence and development of interpersonal relationships. Group-home living coupled with sheltered workshops and similar occupational opportunities allows these individuals to function relatively independently and to develop everyday living skills.

It is unlikely that large institutions for the housing and management of the mentally retarded will disappear completely. Severely retarded children and those who require the special and continuous ministrations of physical therapists, speech therapists, occupational therapists, physicians, and other professional personnel are probably best housed in such large institutions.

The pervasive practice of sterilization of mentally retarded individuals has been a matter of legal controversy in the United States. Most states have legal statutes that allow persons to sue physicians who perform sterilization on minor retarded individuals for malpractice, assault and battery, negligence, or infringement of civil rights. Suits have been brought even after such operations were performed under the direction of a court order [Dowben and Hartwell, 1970]. Thus it is evident that mentally retarded individuals require sex education and other counseling concerning parenthood and methods of contraception. Most retarded persons are capable of understanding the implications of sterilization and require adequate and practical education.

Siblings of handicapped children when compared with control children feel lonely more often and more often have peer problems. They commonly regard handicapped siblings as a burden. Siblings often do not know why their handicapped brother or sister is different from other children. There are also more behavior disturbances in the siblings of retarded children [Bagenholm and Gillberg, 1991].

PROGNOSIS

When mental retardation is associated with a specific underlying condition, prognosis is most accurately predictable. Regrettably, most children with mental retardation do not have easily determined, specific underlying etiologic conditions. Children with mild retardation, good general physical health, and no disease of the cardiorespiratory system are likely to have a relatively normal life expectancy. Conversely, profoundly retarded children with significant general health and nutritional problems may die prematurely. In an older study, 17 of 48 profoundly retarded children were dead by 8 years of age, and 22 of 44 were dead by 17 years of age [Koch et al., 1977].

It is noteworthy that attempts to estimate life expectancy based on various categorizations are fraught with imprecision because of the individual circumstances of each child. Although deficits in cognitive ability combined with immobility, requirement for gastrostomy or nasogastric tube feeding, and incontinence have been designated as life-limiting, the data were collected over a relatively short period of time (3½ years) and statistical extrapolations were made for selected age groups (including those who were 60 years of age and older) without regard to individual quality of care [Eyman et al., 1987; 1990]. These data require confirmation from other studies that survey data collected over a longer time period and monitor quality of medical care and individual living circumstances.

REFERENCES

Akesson HO. The biological origin of mild mental retardation. A critical review. Acta Psychiatr Scand 1986; 74:3.

Bagenholm A, Gillberg C. Psychosocial effects on siblings of children with autism and mental retardation: a population-based study. J Ment Defic Res 1991; 35:291-307.

Becker JM, Kaveggia EG, Pendleton E, et al. A biologic and genetic study of 40 cases of severe pure mental retardation. Eur J Pediatr 1977; 124:231.

Blomquist HK, Gustavson K-H, Holmgren G, et al. Fragile site X chromosomes and X-linked mental retardation in severely retarded boys in a northern Swedish county. A prevalence study. Clin Genet 1982; 21:209.

Bodensteiner JB, Schaefer GB. Wide cavum septum pellucidum: a marker of disturbed brain development. Pediatr Neurol 1990; 6:391.

Braddock D, Hemp R. Governmental spending for mental retardation and developmental disabilities, 1977-1984. Hosp Community Psychiatry 1986; 37:702.

Butler MG, Mangrum T, Gupta R, et al. A 15-item checklist for screening mentally retarded males for the fragile X syndrome. Clin Genet 1991; 39:347.

Carpenter NJ, Leichtman LG, Say B. Fragile X-linked mental retardation. Am J Dis Child 1982; 136:392.

Chaney RH, Givens CA, Watkins GP, et al. Birth injury as the cause of mental retardation. Obstet Gynecol 1986; 67:771.

Curfs LM, Wiegers AM, Fryns JP. Intelligence and the [fra(X)] syndrome: a review. Genet Couns 1991; 2:55.

Dexter LA. Screening and prevention of high-grade mental retardation—to what purpose? Under what circumstances? On what premises? Bull NY Acad Med 1975; 51:169.

Dowben C, Heartwell SF. Legal implications of sterilization of mentally retarded. Am J Dis Child 1979; 133:697.

Eyman RK, Grossman HJ, Chaney RH, et al. The life expectancy of profoundly handicapped people with mental retardation. N Engl J Med 1990; 323:584.

Eyman RK, Grossman HJ, Tarjan G, et al. Life expectancy and mental retardation. A longitudinal study in a state residential facility. Monogr Am Assoc Ment Defic 1987; 1.

Frankenburg WK, Dodds JB. Denver developmental screening test. J Pediatr 1967; 71:181.

Frankenburg WK, Dodds JB, Archer P, et al. The Denver II: a major revision and restandardization of the Denver developmental screening test. Pediatrics 1992; 89:91.

Freytag E, Lindenberg R. Neuropathologic findings in patients of a hospital for the mentally deficient. A survey of 359 cases. Johns Hopkins Med J 1967; 121:379-92.

Ghose S, Chandra Sekhar G. The eye in idiopathic mental retardation. Jpn J Ophthalmol 1986; 30:431.

Hagberg B, Kyllerman M. Epidemiology of mental retardation—a Swedish survey. Brain Dev 1983; 5:441.

Harbord MG, Boyd S, Hall-Craggs MA, et al. Ataxia, developmental delay and an extensive neuronal migration abnormality in 2 siblings. Neuropediatrics 1990; 21:218.

Huttenlocher PR. Dendritic and synaptic pathology in mental retardation. Pediatr Neurol 1991; 7:79.

Johnson VP, Carpenter NJ, Skorey PA. Martin-Bell syndrome segregating in a large kindred with normal transmitting males: clinical, cytogenetic, and linkage study. Am J Med Genet 1991; 38:275.

Joubert M, Eisenring JJ, Anderman F. Familial dysgenesis of the vermis: a syndrome of hyperventilation, abnormal eye movements, and retardation. Neurology 1968; 18:302-3.

Kazee AM, Lapham LW, Torres CF, et al. Generalized cortical dysplasia. Clinical and pathologic aspects. Arch Neurol 1991; 48:850.

Kinsbourne M. Early identification of mental retardation. Reactions and comments. Ann NY Acad Sci 1986; 477:277.

Kirk S. Educating exceptional children. New York: Houghton-Mifflin, 1972.

Koch R, Strickland G, Graliker B. A 17-year longitudinal study of 117 children with mental retardation, starting in infancy: their present status. Clin Pediatr 1977; 16:1015.

Madhavan T, Narayan J. Consanguinity and mental retardation. J Ment Defic Res 1991; 35:133.

McKusick VA. Mendelian inheritance in man, 7th ed. Baltimore: Johns Hopkins University Press, 1986.

Menenzes M, Coker S. CHARGE and Joubert syndromes: are they a single disorder? Pediatr Neurol 1990; 6:428-30.

Naheedy MH, Schnur JA. The value of computerized tomography scanning in syndromes associated with mental retardation: preliminary report. Comput Tomogr 1979; 3:1.

Nelson RP, Crocker AC. The medical care of mentally retarded persons in public residential facilities. N Engl J Med 1978; 299:1039.

Nelson KB, Deutschberger J. Head size at one year as a predictor of four-year I.Q. Dev Med Child Neurol 1970; 12:487.

O'Connell EJ, Feldt RH, Stickler GB. Head circumference, mental retardation, and growth failure. Pediatrics 1965; 36:62.

Opitz JM. Diagnostic/genetic studies in mental retardation. Postgrad Med 1979; 66:205.

Pearson PH. The physician's role in diagnosis and management of the mentally retarded. Pediatr Clin North Am 1968; 15:835.

Richardson SA, Koller H, Katz M. A longitudinal study of numbers of males and females in mental retardation services by age, IQ and placement. J Ment Defic Res 1986; 30:291.

Rodewald A, Froster-Iskenius U, Kab E, et al. Dermatoglyphic peculiarities in families with X-linked mental retardation and fragile site Xq27: collaborative study. Clin Genet 1986; 30:1.

Rossi LN, Candini G, Scarlatti G, et al. Autosomal dominant microcephaly without mental retardation. Am J Dis Child 1987; 141:655.

Schellinger D, Grant EG, Manz HJ, et al. Ventricular shapes, distortions, and deformities: mirrors of past cerebral insults. A study based on early sonographic follow-up studies. Pediatr Neurol 1986; 2:193.

Schey WL. Intracranial calcifications in childhood: frequency of occurrence and significance. Am J Roentgenol 1974; 122:495.

Shapiro BK, Palmer FB, Capute AJ. The early detection of mental retardation. Clin Pediatr 1987; 26:215.

Stein Z, Durkin M, Belmont L. "Serious" mental retardation in developing countries: an epidemiologic approach. Ann NY Acad Sci 1986; 477:8.

Streissguth AP, Aase JM, Clarren SK, et al. Fetal alcohol syndrome in adolescents and adults. JAMA 1991; 265:1961.

Sutherland GR. Heritable fragile sites on human chromosomes. III. Detection of fra (X)(q27) in males with X-linked mental retardation and their female relatives. Hum Genet 1979; 53:23.

Thommessen M, Riis G, Kase BF, et al. Energy and nutrient intakes of disabled children: do feeding problems make a difference? J Am Diet Assoc 1991; 91:1522.

Wellesley D, Hockey A, Stanley F. The aetiology of intellectual disability in Western Australia: a community-based study. Dev Med Child Neurol 1991; 33:963.

Wisniewski KE, Segan SM, Miezejeski CM, et al. The Fra(X) syndrome: neurological, electrophysiological, and neuropathological abnormalities. Am J Med Genet 1991; 38:476.

9

Intellectual and Motor Deterioration

Kenneth F. Swaiman

Many progressive, serious, and usually irreversible diseases of the CNS cause intellectual and motor decline. Intellectual deterioration is characterized by a decrease in the ability to learn, decrease in systematic intellectual processing, loss of previously acquired information, personality instability, and impairment of judgment. Because these complex "higher cortical" functions are mediated by many areas of the brain acting in concert, intellectual loss rarely is the result of focal disruption. Motor deterioration, in a parallel fashion, is the impairment or loss of previously acquired motor skills. Often the patient is unable to acquire new motor skills. The motor strip in the frontal lobe contains the motor neurons from which impulses are generated that must eventually reach effector muscles; however, the frontal, parietal, and temporal lobes are involved in the synthesis of sensory data necessary for directing skilled motor activity.

CORRELATIVE NEUROANATOMY

As intimated, on rare occasions a child's deterioration may occur subsequent to single lobe involvement. Usually a number of lobes are involved. Function of the individual lobes can be characterized generally.

Lobar dysfunction is briefly described in the following section; Table 9-1 summarizes lobar impairment.

The frontal lobes, which are located anterior to the central sulcus and superior to the sylvian fissure [Haymaker, 1969], comprise a number of important functional portions. The anterior poles of the frontal lobes stabilize emotion and personality, implement systematic activities over a time increment, provide smooth transition from one activity to another, instigate proper affect, and store recent memory. Overt intellectual deterioration may result from extreme dysfunction of the frontal lobes.

The motor strip or motor cortex is found in the posterior portion of the frontal lobe. When involvement of this area occurs, the expected signs of upper motor neuron unit dysfunction, including spasticity, result. Functional impairment of the premotor areas causes apraxia, ataxia, and reestablishment of primitive reflexes (e.g., rooting, sucking, grasping). Directly anterior to the portion of the motor strip that controls head and eye movements is an area that subserves synchronized contralateral rotation of the head and eyes. Involvement of this area results in faulty contralateral execution and coordination of head-eye movements. After several years of age, severe involvement of the Broca speech center in the dominant hemisphere results in motor aphasia.

Temporal lobe compromise in the form of irritative foci may result in unusual seizure manifestations (e.g., hallucinations of smell and taste, unusual and terrifying dreams, unexplained episodes of fright). These seizures, which may progress to loss of consciousness, are classified as simple, partial seizures with somatosensory or special-sensory symptoms. Temporal lobe impairment may also result in gross personality changes that may be indistinguishable from those associated with frontal lobe dysfunction. Language function is centered in the temporal lobe of the dominant hemisphere. Deterioration or destruction of this area results in major language compromise of both auditory and visual functions, which are associated with reception, storage, and language construction. Involvement of the superior and middle gyri of the temporal lobe in the dominant hemisphere causes Wernicke aphasia. Varying degrees and combinations of disability involve the ability to write, read, and understand speech. Nondominant temporal lobe function, when disturbed, is manifested by disordered perception of spatial interrelation-

Table 9-1 Symptoms associated with compromise of lobes of the cerebrum

Lobes	Either or both	Dominant hemisphere	Nondominant hemisphere
Frontal	Akinetic mutism Difficulties with chewing and swallowing Distractibility; incapability of performing sequential activities Instability of mood; inappropriate excitement Irritability Lack of initiative or spontaneity Loss of recent memory Loss of voluntary movement of contralateral side Motor, ideational, and ideokinetic apraxia (includes apraxia of gait) Motor inactivity Personality changes (impulsivity, irritability, emotional lability) Reappearance of primitive reflexes Reduction of general intelligence Sphincter incontinence	Broca aphasia	
Temporal	Auditory illusions and hallucinations Gross learning impairment with bilateral ablation of hippocampus Homonymous superior quadranopia Labyrinthine and auditory functional impairment with bilateral dysfunction Psychotic, aggressive behavior Seizures with sensory hallucinations (e.g., taste and smell), abberation of orientation, vertigo, and vegetative and autonomic symptoms and signs	Amusia Dysnomia Difficulty with verbal tests in which material is presented orally Wernicke aphasia	Agnosia for nonlexical qualities of music Difficulty with judgment of spatial relationships Difficulty with tests in which material is presented visually
Parietal	Cortical deafness Failure of recognition of contralateral visual field Growth retardation in contralateral limbs with mild weakness Homonymous hemianopia Impairment of cortical sensory function (sterognosis, two-point discrimination, position sense) Loss of opticokinetic nystagmus Sham rage	Gerstmann syndrome Gross language difficulties Ideomotor apraxia Tactile agnosia	Lack of awareness of contralateral hemiparesis and hemianesthesia Lack of awareness of contralateral side of body
Occipital	Cortical blindness in presence of bilateral regions Homonymous field defect (congruous) Loss of visual recognition		

Modified from Adams RD, Victor M. Syndromes due to focal cerebral lesions. In: Wilson JD, Braunwald E, Isselbacher KJ, Petersdorf RG, Mortin JB, Fauci AS, Root RK, eds. Harrison's principles of internal medicine. 12th ed. New York: McGraw-Hill, 1991.

ships and faulty appreciation of changes in musical pitch.

Parietal lobe dysfunction manifests in the form of sensory impairment. It may involve graphesthesia, two-point discrimination, appreciation of shape, size, and texture of objects, and facility to distinguish between simultaneous, cutaneous stimulation of bilateral homologous body parts. Impairment of the parietal lobe during the first 2 to 3 years of life often results in growth retardation, which causes a decrease in both volume and length—predominantly distal—of the involved extremity.

Language impairment and apraxia are the result of dominant parietal lobe disruption. It is noteworthy that Gerstmann syndrome, which includes acalculia, agraphia, right-left disorientation, and inability to recognize body parts, is also a sequel to dominant parietal lobe dysfunction. Ideomotor apraxia may also accompany this syndrome.

Dysfunction of the nondominant parietal lobe also produces characteristic difficulties. The patient may experience impairment or distortion of perception of superficial and deep sensation, including pain, on the contralateral side. The patient may be unable to recognize contralateral body parts and may have difficulty with visual recognition of objects in the visual field on the contralateral side.

Visual defects are the result of occipital lobe lesions. The dysfunction may lead to actual deficiency but also may result in distorted recognition of visual objects. If both occipital lobes are involved, cortical blindness frequently is manifest. The patient may have gross difficulty in recognizing visual objects. A varying pattern of difficulty emerges depending on the affected area; the patient may experience varying degrees of loss of ability to interpret objects in the visual field. Patients with adequate visual acuity who cannot identify visual objects are said to have visual agnosia; examination reveals the pupillary reflexes to be intact. If one occipital lobe is affected, homonymous field defects in the contralateral field frequently are present.

Because of the large size and widespread location of the brain regions that determine intellectual function, small focal lesions are not likely to impair brain function significantly unless there is associated (1) obstruction or diminution of blood flow of a major artery or vein, (2) obstruction of CSF passages, or (3) action by the lesion as an epileptogenic focus. Therefore the most common conditions that impair intellectual and motor development are chronic, diffuse or scattered, and progressive.

Documentation of progression of neurologic dysfunction in the intellectual or motor spheres requires demonstration of regression or loss of attained skills. The distinction between retardation, intellectual and/or motor, and deterioration, intellectual and/or motor, is crucial because the differential diagnosis for each situation varies. Standardized test instruments, such as those discussed in Chapter 8, are most helpful in evaluating the patient's motor and intellectual abilities, as well as changes in these abilities.

Patient history is as important as formal documentation and frequently is more readily available because parents and other observers can describe previous loss of intellectual and/or motor abilities. The availability of home movies or videotapes, as well as photographs, may convincingly demonstrate motor and intellectual loss.

APRAXIA

Apraxia implies the inability of a patient to perform useful motor acts, previously mastered, in the absence of overt motor deficiency. The emergence of apraxia is one form of intellectual deterioration. The term *apraxia* cannot be defined precisely, but it continues to be a clinical concept of value [Geschwind, 1975; Luria, 1966]. There is no ataxia, paresis, or alteration in muscle tone. Sensation is intact. The original conceptualization of apraxia was based on the hypothesis that voluntary motor acts are the result of the formulation of a mental idea of the motor act and the necessary motor sequence. By following this reasoning, the entire motor act was subdivided into portions.

Motor apraxia is the result of lack of neurologic connections within the brain that are required for origination and execution of motor movements. The patient usually has the mental image of the necessary movements. Often, one hand or arm is involved; motor acts, such as twisting a door knob or closing a simple clasp, may be compromised.

Ideational apraxia results in the inability to plan a sequence of movements. The patient may initiate and implement discrete movements, but the complete sequence of acts cannot be consummated. The patient, for example, may grasp a coin from a surface but then does not deposit it in a purse and close the clasp. Another example is the failure of an older child to strike a match after it has been removed properly from its book.

Ideokinetic apraxia is the dissociation of the motor act and the idea. Although the patient may be able to spontaneously blow, suck, or whistle, the patient is unable to perform these acts on command.

These oversimplified classifications are of some use in clinical neurology. Apraxia usually is the result of frontal lobe dysfunction. Synthesis and integration of information generated in other parts of the brain occur in the precentral and postcentral sulcal areas. This information ultimately is processed to plan and modulate voluntary movements. Although great emphasis is placed on efferent motor impulses that originate in the motor cortex because they have a final role in instigation of the motor act, basic input and preparation are provided by afferent impulses that originate in other brain areas. The formulation of motor movements is complex. The organization of voluntary movements is the result of the synthesis of information concerning spatial relationships of objects and the changing positions of muscles and joints, as well as information generated by brain areas associated with speech and symbol formulation. Therefore these movements are the result of a number of nervous system discharges that commission and inhibit the nervous impulses that control motor function and successively integrate impulses to allow smooth motor activity. Much efferent integration probably occurs in the premotor area.

The processing of sensory information is vital to proper motor function of limbs. There may be no loss of strength or changes in muscle tone, but the patient may find it impossible to control the movement in a meaningful manner or there may be uncontrolled and sometimes simultaneous contractions of agonist and antagonist muscles. Assuredly, many areas of brain are used to originate, formulate, and execute voluntary motor movements. Dysfunction of the frontal lobe (particularly the premotor area), the motor cortex, the parietal sensory cortex, confluent areas of the parietal, occipital, and temporal lobes, and the cerebellum may result in disordered motor function. Difficulties experienced may vary from minor problems with initiating an action to functional limb paresis.

EVALUATION OF THE PATIENT

The child's level of function in several areas should be assessed. General categories include social, behavioral, gross motor, fine motor, and language skills. When compared with history, the likelihood of regression should be evident. The clinician should be knowledge-able about developmental milestones. A list of signs and symptoms that may be associated with diseases that cause progressive brain dysfunction is provided in Chapter 8. Abnormalities of the eyes, skin, liver and spleen, visual pathways, auditory pathways, as well as the presence of seizures, abnormal head circumference, and failure-to-thrive must be studied further. The presence of involuntary movements should be diligently sought. On rare occasions, unusual body odors are present and should be identified (see Chapter 8). The general history and neurologic examinations should provide the clinician with a working differential diagnosis.

DIFFERENTIAL DIAGNOSIS

Intellectual and motor deterioration may be caused by numerous conditions, including many uncommon diseases. Many of these conditions are listed in Tables 9-2, 9-3, and 9-4.

Table 9-2 Selected metabolic causes of childhood intellectual deterioration

Age of onset	Disease	Major symptoms and signs
Below age 2	Adrenoleukodystrophy (neonatal)	Abnormal at birth, developmental delay followed by regression, hypotonia, seizures
	Biotinidase deficiency	Seizures, hyperventilation, ataxia, hearing loss, developmental delay, optic atrophy, dermatitis
	Fructose intolerance	Hypoglycemia after fructose ingestion, failure-to-thrive; generalized aminoaciduria, albuminuria, fructosuria, and jaundice with hepatomegaly after fructose ingestion; moderate mental retardation frequently present
	Fucosidosis	Progressive intellectual motor deterioration, early hypotonia gradually transforming to spastic quadriplegia, decorticate rigidity, anhydrosis, cardiomegaly, failure to thrive, and repeated respiratory infections. Angiokeratoma corporis diffusum may be present
	Galactosemia	Jaundice, hepatosplenomegaly, cataracts, seizures secondary to hypoglycemia
	Gaucher disease (infantile)	Opisthotonus, dysphagia, squint, spasticity, splenomegaly, hepatomegaly
	Glutaric acidemia, Type I	Mental retardation, movement disorder (chorea, dystonia), ataxia, acidosis
	Glycogen storage disease (type I of Cori)	Hepatomegaly, seizures, hypoglycemia
	Glycogen storage disease (type II of Cori: infantile)	Enlarged tongue, hypotonia, muscle induration, cardiomegaly, profound muscle weakness
	Glycogen storage disease (type III of Cori)	Muscle weakness, hepatomegaly, hypoglycemia, seizures
	Glycogen storage disease (type IV of Cori)	Liver atrophy, jaundice, hypoglycemia, failure-to-thrive
	Glycogen synthetase deficiency	Seizures, hypoglycemia
	GM1 gangliosidosis	Intellectual and motor retardation, seizures, dull facies, frontal bossing, depressed nasal bridge, cherry-red spot (50% of patients), hepatosplenomegaly

Table 9-2 **Selected metabolic causes of childhood intellectual deterioration—cont'd**

Age of onset	Disease	Major symptoms and signs
Below age 2—cont'd	Propionic acidemia	Metabolic acidosis in infancy, intermittent lethargy, psychomotor retardation
	Pyridoxine dependency state	Neonatal seizures (frequently myoclonic), failure-to-thrive
	Sandhoff disease	Hyperacusis, seizures, megalencephaly, blindness associated with cherry-red spots, decerebrate rigidity
	Tay-Sachs disease	Blindness, seizures, hyperacusis, hypotonia, muscle weakness, megalencephaly (later stages)
	Wolman disease	Diarrhea, hepatosplenomegaly, adrenal calcification, death in the first year
	Zellweger syndrome	Craniofacial dysmorphism, seizures, profound developmental delay, hepatic cirrhosis, renal microcysts
Between ages 2 to 5	Adrenoleukodystrophy	Increased pigmentation of extremities, adrenal insufficiency, spasticity, blindness, deafness, behavioral disturbances, dementia, increased gamma globulin fraction in CSF
	GM2 gangliosidosis (juvenile GM2 gangliosidosis)	Seizures, ataxia, spasticity, athetosis, late blindness
	Leigh syndrome	Swallowing difficulty, hypotonia, ataxia, peripheral neuropathy, external ophthalmoplegia, impaired hearing and vision, seizures, vomiting
	MELAS syndrome	Mitochondrial myopathy, encephalopathy, lactic acidosis, stroke syndrome
	MERFF syndrome (Fukahara syndrome)	Myoclonus, epilepsy, dementia, ataxia, muscular atrophy, lactic acidosis
	Metachromatic leukodystrophy (sulfatide lipidosis, late infantile form)	Ataxia, weakness, hypotonia, arreflexia; followed by spasticity, amaurosis, macular degeneration with cherry-red spot at times, supranuclear bulbar palsy
	Niemann-Pick disease (late infantile-moderate course group)	Myoclonic seizures, mild hepatosplenomegaly, spasticity, ataxia, amaurosis
	Sanfilippo syndrome	Short stature, slight hepatosplenomegaly, moderate osteoporosis, keel breast, short neck, prominent maxilla
	Wilson disease	Acute hepatic necrosis, hyperbilirubinemia, occasional dystonia, rare choreoathetosis, Kayser-Fleischer rings
	GM2 gangliosidosis (generalized)	Hypotonia, hepatomegaly, blindness, splenomegaly, Hurler facies, short stubby fingers, frontal bossing, peripheral edema
	Hunter syndrome (MPS II)	Boys only; contractures of joints at elbows and knees, flattened nasal bridge, large tongue and thick lips, hirsutism, deafness, umbilical hernia, chronic nasal discharge
	Hurler syndrome (MPS I)	Kyphosis, contractures of joints (particularly of the elbows), hepatomegaly, corneal clouding, large head, broad hands and short fingers, flattened nasal bridge, thickened lips, spurring of the first or second lumbar vertebrae
	Hyperammonemias	Variability in level of consciousness ranging from lethargy to coma, intellectual retardation, vomiting, seizures, aversion to high-protein diet
	Krabbe disease	Tonic seizures, hyperacusis, increased startle response, spasticity
	Mannosidosis	Mental retardation, skeletal changes (kyphosis), hepatosplenomegaly, hearing loss, Hurler-like facies
	Menkes disease (kinky hair disease)	Spasticity, seizures, monilethrix, pili torti; X-linked recessive
	Methylmalonic acidemia	Metabolic acidosis in infancy, intermittent lethargy, psychomotor retardation

Continued.

in hydrocephalus. Other deformities associated with basilar impression (platybasia) or Klippel-Feil malformation may disrupt the passage of spinal fluid with resultant hydrocephalus. The Dandy-Walker malformation, which stems primarily from absence or imperforation of the foramina of Luschka and Magendie, is another malformation that may cause deterioration secondary to increasing intracranial pressure.

Generalized, increased intracranial pressure may result from simultaneous closure of sagittal and coronal cranial sutures. Premature closure of either suture alone does not result in increased intracranial pressure. Coronal suture closure may be accompanied by increased pressure on the orbital contents, including the optic nerve.

Early symptoms and signs of increased intracranial pressure in older children may not appear to be neurologic in origin in the early stages. Complaints include nausea and vomiting in the early morning, and headache and appetite loss may follow. Only later, when pressure has increased considerably, will there be disorientation and impairment of higher cortical function. Tonsillar herniation may be signaled by nuchal rigidity. Papilledema may be clearly evident.

In contrast, increased intracranial pressure in infants may be relatively insidious if the process develops slowly. The anterior fontanel bulges, and the cranial sutures separate. Anorexia, vomiting, and lethargy ensue. Papilledema and nuchal rigidity usually manifest later. Serial measurements of the occipitofrontal circumference reveal rapid increases, reflecting the increased pressure.

Metabolic conditions

Numerous metabolic conditions have resulted in intellectual and motor deterioration. The number of large groupings increases with the passage of time and requires the clinician to remain cognizant of the current metabolic literature. The aminoacidurias, exemplified by phenylketonuria and maple syrup urine disease, are usually not associated with deterioration but rather with delayed development.

Storage conditions represented by the sphingolipidoses usually are characterized by a period of normal development followed by declining function. Conditions such as metachromatic leukodystrophy and Gaucher disease typify these storage conditions. Although leukodystrophies are a mixed group, some of which have been characterized metabolically, there are many that remain descriptive (e.g., Pelizaeus-Merzbacher disease, Alexander disease).

Progressive deterioration may also occur with various mitochondrial encephalopathies, peroxisomal diseases, glycoproteinoses, and neuronal ceroid-lipofuscinoses.

Endocrinologic conditions

For the most part, delayed development or intellectual and motor decline has been associated with hypothyroidism. Hypothyroidism in the newborn period, termed *cretinism*, is the result of failure of development or only partial development of the thyroid gland, thyroid malfunction secondary to maternal autoimmunization, ectopic thyroid gland that is limited in size and/or secretory capability, defect in enzymatic synthesis of thyroxin, or the influence of goitrogenic substances including iodine, propylthiouracil, cobalt, PAS, and goiterin.

Acquired hypothyroidism may result in intellectual deterioration. This diagnosis is made by appropriate laboratory studies and should be suggested by the clinical pattern of hypothyroidism, which includes dry skin, intolerance to cold, growth retardation, hoarse cry, delayed bone and tooth development, and deafness (Pendred syndrome).

Idiopathic panhypopituitarism results in multiple endocrine abnormalities that engender hypoglycemia, difficulties with water balance, and growth failure. In particular, hypothyroidism may result in impaired intellectual and motor function.

Epilepsy

Uncontrolled seizure activity, particularly of the generalized type, may lead to intellectual deterioration. Patients with absence or akinetic seizures may have hundreds of episodes per day. Concomitant EEG abnormalities indicating generalized discharges of spike-and-slow wave patterns are frequently observed. Seizure control may lead to a reversal of intellectual and motor decline. Unfortunately, seizure activity may be a signal of an underlying degenerative disease that is responsible for the intellectual and motor impairment rather than seizures.

Speech disturbance as a result of epileptiform discharges may be transient or take the form of a prolonged acquired aphasia. This syndrome is termed the *Landau-Kleffner syndrome* [Landau and Keffner, 1957].

Toxic conditions

Toxic conditions can be classified as endogenous or exogenous. Endogenous toxins are those that result from failure of normal body systems. Most endogenous toxins result from hepatic or renal failure, although other disease processes may be involved; therefore it is essential that the clinician consider and investigate the possibility of nonnervous system disease as a cause of deterioration of nervous system function. A general examination and laboratory screening tests are indicated.

Exogenous toxins may be inhaled, absorbed through the skin or mucosa, injected, or ingested. Exogenous toxins may be present as a pollutant in the environment, introduced into the body in the form of "recreational drugs," or in the form of drugs intended for therapeutic benefit. Most antiepileptic drugs are capable of causing dementia or interfering with learning and memory. Exogenous toxins are discussed in detail in Chapter 62.

INFANTILE AUTISM

Kanner [1943] described a syndrome characterized by failure to establish communication with others, obsession to continue "sameness," failure of language communication, aloofness, preoccupation with handling small objects, and an inability to anticipate with appropriate body positioning the likelihood of being picked up. Although much has been written, autism continues to be poorly defined in neurologic terms, and it is most likely that infantile autism is associated with varied conditions that affect language, behavior, and usually intellect [Lockman et al., 1979; Rapin and Allen, 1987]. The most common manifestations of the condition are present by the ninth or tenth month of life and are represented by diminution in crying, general motor activity, and feeding. Language development appears delayed, and children do not appropriately respond to noises. Motor milestones are often normal.

Some children will appear normal until 18 to 24 months of age when there appears to be loss of social and language milestones and a relative lack of communication. The children seek repetitive tactile, visual, vestibular, and auditory stimulation. The child may forcefully refuse any tactile interaction with others.

Some authorities have suggested that autism is a combination of maladaptive factors in the environment and a basic genetic defect. The definition and diagnosis of autism remain controversial; the need for precise diagnostic guidelines and the determination of the various subsets subsumed under the autism umbrella are critical. Autism is discussed in Chapter 55 .

Rett syndrome, a disease that afflicts girls after the first year of life with intellectual deterioration, followed by unusual posturing, hyperventilation, bruxism, and myoclonic seizures, has been identified as part of the autism spectrum [Hagberg, 1983]. It is discussed in Chapter 55.

DEPRESSION

Occasionally, children may suffer severe depression and cannot maintain previously acquired levels of intellectual and motor skills. Symptoms include headache, lethargy, insomnia, withdrawal, decreased school performance, and appetite loss. Diagnosis may necessitate detailed assessment of the child's environment, as well as projective psychometric evaluation [Brumback et al., 1977; Katz, 1977].

REFERENCES

Brumback RA, Dietz-Schmidt SG, Weinberg WA. Depression in children referred to an educational diagnostic center: diagnosis and treatment and analysis of criteria and literature review. Dis Nerv Syst 1977; 38:529.

Geschwind N. The apraxias: neural mechanisms of disorders of learned movement. Am Sci 1975; 63:188.

Hagberg B, Aicardi J, Dias K, et al. A progressive syndrome of autism, dementia, ataxia, and loss of purposeful hand use in girls: Rett's syndrome: report of 35 cases. Ann Neurol 1983; 14:471.

Haymaker W. Bing's local diagnosis in neurological disease, 15th ed. St. Louis: Mosby, 1969.

Kanner L. Autistic disturbances of affective contact. Nerv Child 1943; 2:217.

Katz J. Depression in children. Med J Aust 1977; 1:592.

Landau WM, Kleffner FR. Syndrome of acquired aphasia with convulsive disorder in children. Neurol 1957; 7:523.

Lockman LA, Swaiman KF, Drage VS et al., eds. Workshop on the neurobiological basis of autism. Bethesda, Md., 1979, National Institute of Neurological and Communicative Disorders and Stroke, Monograph No. 23.

Luria AR. Higher cortical functions in man. New York: Basic Books, 1966.

Rapin I, Allen DA. Developmental dysphasia and autism in preschool children: characteristics and subtypes. In: Proceedings of the first international symposium on specific speech and language disorders in children. London: Association for All Speech Impaired Children, 1987.

10

Speech and Language Disorders

Carl J. Crosley

The evaluation of a child with a speech or language disturbance demands an understanding of basic definitions and a developmental perspective. The physician must distinguish among disorders of voice, speech, language, and cognition. Language can be defined as a system of learned symbols that contain socially shared meanings and provide categories for classifying experiences [Berry, 1969]. Speech, on the other hand, is the production and perception of oral symbols. Voice consists of the acoustic characteristics of both speech and nonspeech sounds. The interrelation between these functions produces a complex array of possible disorders. Each may be affected individually by a single process, although many disturbances affect more than one function. Similarly, dysfunction in one area may impair development in another.

DEVELOPMENT OF THE VOCAL TRACT

The subglottic component of the vocal tract consists of the tracheobronchial tree and the pulmonary system. Ordinarily exhalation is passive and only half the duration of inspiration. During activity (e.g., exercise, speech, singing) exhalation is actively controlled and may be 20 times as long as inspiration. The normal respiratory rate of the neonate is 40 to 70 breaths per minute, but by adolescence the rate falls to 13 to 18 breaths per minute.

The vocal cords are the essential structures of the glottic portion of the vocal tract. During inhalation the cords abduct. This movement is accentuated during speech. Voice pitch is proportionate to the vocal fold length tension, and air flow. The larynx, which contains the structures necessary to produce these vocal elements, grows and molds along with the growth of the child. The three notable phases of laryngeal growth include the following: from newborn to 3 years, 3 years to puberty, and after puberty [Rood, 1983].

The supraglottic component of the vocal tract in-cludes the hypopharynx, the oropharynx, the nasopharynx, and the oral and nasal cavities. The sound produced by the glottic and subglottic components of the vocal tract is thin and reedy. The resting shape and the varied changes in the shape and length of the supraglottic component produce the complex sounds that make up the elements of speech and nonspeech sounds.

The ability to vary that shape and to regulate the glottic pressure through respiratory control requires a complex adjustment of the muscles of the pharynx, the vocal cords, and the muscles of respiration. This ability appears by the time an infant is able to produce polysyllabic babbling at 7 to 8 months of age [Lenneberg, 1967]. Further maturation of speech sounds is in part effected by the descent of the larynx into the neck and the elongation of the supraglottic pharynx.

DEVELOPMENT OF ARTICULATION

The ability to produce specific speech sounds depends intimately on developmental factors. The physician must recognize that simple mispronunciation of sounds is not synonymous with misarticulation. Younger children normally omit speech sounds, substitute one sound for another, or distort speech sounds. The consonants /m/, /p/, /t/, /k/, and /f/ are pronounceable by 3 years of age, but /l/ and /s/ may not be clear until 8 years of age [Curlee and Shelton, 1983]. By 2 years of age the normal child is intelligible to strangers about half of the time. Total intelligibility is expected by 4 years of age. Articulation errors may be self-correcting to some degree. Although almost 10% of children have significant articulation disorders in the first grade, only 0.5% of twelfth-grade students are similarly affected [Hull et al., 1976].

Control of the muscles of speech is directed by the lower cranial nerves, including the hypoglossal, vagus, facial, and trigeminal nerves. Damage to any of these nerves produces dysfunction of one or several components of the vocal tract, which results in one of several

other disturbances of language or cognitive function. Categorization of dyslexia is fraught with many pitfalls. However, a reasonable paradigm has been outlined by Mattis et al. [1975]. These authors believed most of their patients could be classified into 3 independent syndromes. A language disorder had prominent dysnomia, poor imitative speech, and speech sound discrimination, as well as a selective comprehension deficit. Children with an articulatory and graphomotor dyscoordination syndrome performed poorly on sound blending and graphomotor tests but had normal hearing and receptive language. A visuospatial perceptual disorder was characterized by a verbal IQ much greater than the performance IQ with abnormal scores on the Raven's Coloured Progressive Matrices and the Benton Test of Visual Retention.

EVALUATION OF THE PATIENT

Parents will commonly bring concerns about their child's language to the physician when the child is 18 to 36 months of age. The alert physician should recognize abnormal language development before this juncture. Diagnosis of speech and language disorders requires not only a knowledge of specific disorders and a sense of the normal development of speech and language but anticipation of these disorders by knowledge of the at-risk factors for disruptions of speech and language in children.

In the newborn a history of any insult potentially damaging to the CNS, such as prematurity, asphyxia, and congenital intrauterine infections, should alert the physician. Children who have had a family history of deafness, who have had bacterial meningitis, as well as those with visible defects of the structures of the ear, nose, and throat should be considered suspect. The prevalence of deafness in childhood is at least two or three per thousand at birth and double that when acquired hearing loss is included [Schein and Delk, 1974]. Unfortunately, the consequences of deafness, even when recognized early in life, are significant and may be cumulative. Alternative communications systems are incomplete in their ability to provide full communication for events that are not contemporary or about principles and complex issues. This translates into deficient reading skills and the knowledge that reading provides; therefore deaf children are information deprived [Rapin, 1979].

Recurrent episodes of otitis media or persistent serous otitis media may well be expected to produce a partial hearing loss both in degree and in duration. Even this partial sensory deprivation has been documented to have resulted in significant expressive language delays. Impairment in expressive language has been reported in children as early as 1 year of age when they have had recurrent episodes of otitis media [Wallace et al., 1988].

In a recent review of deafness, profound congenital hearing loss was most commonly not recognized until 24 months of age with lesser degrees not recognized until 48 months of age [Coplan, 1986]. The delay was clearly a failure of the physician to be aware of or to heed the implications of the physical abnormalities or the specific historical risk factors as listed. Moreover, even in the presence of an alert physician, an office examination was not adequate and formal audiometric evaluation was required to make the diagnosis in several instances. Only with early recognition can amplification be provided and the child allowed to optimize the use of his or her residual hearing.

Infants provide additional clues about their hearing abilities in their behavior. Children whose prelinguistic behaviors are abnormal also may have speech and language disorders. Poor visual responsiveness or failure to alert to elementary sounds are signals of potential speech and language abnormality. Concern should be raised if the child were to exhibit poor swallowing or other components of feeding.

Language acquisition depends strongly on hearing others speak; therefore an assessment of the language environment of the child is necessary. The physician must ask whether there is adequate language stimulation for the child and whether there is disordered, confusing, or deficient language stimulation.

Recognition of articulation disorders and delays is also important. By listening to the speech or other sounds a child makes the physician should be able to determine whether the child has a voice disorder. In addition, it must be determined whether the child's difficulty in speaking is compromised by the structure or function of the peripheral speaking mechanism.

By the time a child is 3 years of age the experienced physician should have distinguished mental retardation, hearing loss, and some of the more readily recognizable developmental language disorders including autism. However, there remains a cadre of children whose language development is unfortunately simply described as slow. On occasion the perception of slow is simply just that. A child whose parents' abilities and expectations are superior may be regarded as abnormal by their parents when they are simply below average. Conversely, such a child may be regarded as normal by parents whose own abilities are limited. Although severe environmental deprivation can result in delayed language, the effect of lesser degrees of deprivation is unclear [Bishop, 1987].

In the absence of specific risk factors for hearing or language deficits the examining physician is challenged to distinguish not only the significant and specific language disorders but to predict those children whose language abnormality is of no great long-term significance. In a prospective study of almost 100 preschool language-impaired children, 47% were indistinguishable from a control group within 1 year when their nonverbal abilities were within normal limits at initial examination [Bishop and Edmundson, 1987]. Even without that caveat, 37% were normal at exit from the study. The authors were able to predict good or poor outcome with 90% accuracy by tests performed at 4 years of age. In particular the children's abilities to relate a standardized story appeared to be the most sensitive indicator of outcome. In looking at patterns of deficits the authors concluded that global impairments were more likely to have poor outcomes than isolated impairments and that the initial patterns of language impairment were subject to change with time, which blurred the distinctions between them. Further, they concluded that the vulnerability of language in any area was proportional to the number of areas involved. In children who were least severely involved, only phonology was distorted. As severity of impairment increased, other expressive functions, such as syntax, morphology, and semantics, became abnormal before receptive language was impaired. Although the data were applied to a narrow age range, the patterns should be clinically useful.

There is a variety of instruments that facilitate office recognition of speech and language abnormalities. Many screening scales include elements that specifically evaluate language. One instrument that fully screens language and is amenable to quantification is the Early Language Milestone Scale (ELM Scale) developed by Coplan [1983] (Figure 10-1). This instrument provides detailed assessment of each of the essential components of visual and auditory language from birth to 36 months of age. A history is taken, and the child is examined by observation and direct testing. The test has excellent validity when used both in normal and high-risk populations [Coplan et al., 1982; Coplan and Gleason, 1990; Walker et al., 1989]. After 36 months of age, the complexity of language makes any of the so-called screening tests fraught with error. For instance, the easily administered Peabody Picture Vocabulary Test correlates well with overall intelligence in normal subjects but may miss expressive, vocal, syntactic, and pragmatic disorders.

TREATMENT

The treatment of speech disorders is predicated on a recognition of the interrelated components of voice, speech, language, and cognition in any one child. It may appear that children with craniofacial anomalies would be most responsive to their voice and bulbar motor speech dysfunctions. Yet even in these children, associated hearing and cognitive defects can compound locally caused defects in resonance and phonation. For motor speech disorders (the dysarthrias) the components of respirations, phonation, articulation, resonation, and prosody need to be assessed [Dworkin, 1991]. Ideally these components are first approached in that sequence;

as skill is achieved in one area the next is approached. Coexistent language, cognitive, emotional, social, and other disturbances vary this simplified concept.

Exercises to achieve respiratory control may focus on relaxation, postural support, pressure generation, and rate and rhythm control. Resonation is more difficult to improve and may require the use of prosthetic devices. Phonation therapies face even greater difficulties. However, a logical program of intervention can be devised for most dysarthrias. In spastic speech relaxation, vowel prolongation and yawn and sigh exercises may provide a foundation for intelligible sentence production. A profile of exercises is also available for dyskinetic cerebellar dysarthria. Articulation therapies introduce both more complex imitative exercises and lip, tongue, and jaw-strengthening exercises. Finally, prosody can be reestablished with practiced pitch, loudness, rate, and intonation and stress exercises.

Therapies for aphasia have less clearly established scientific bases and even less well demonstrated evidence of efficacy. The number of variables, the role of spontaneous recovery, the relative worth of various modes of therapy, and the relative effectiveness of any mode of therapy are all problems that have not been clearly assessed by individual studies. However, several facilitative and compensatory approaches have shown promise [LaPointe, 1978].

Applying modes that appear effective in adults to children with developmental language disorders requires an understanding not only of the components of language and cognition but also their place in a child's changing environment. If preschool children use multiple modes of communication naturally to expand their linguistic skills, a parallel to that can logically be part of their therapy. One such system starts with nonverbal intervention [Wilcox, 1986]. This approach is particularly useful in the child who is unable to use communication as an interpersonal tool. The techniques begin with nonconditional exercises to establish attention-getting behavior and then placing conditions on the attention sought. For the child who does communicate but fails to do so conventionally the initial general idea is to establish a core lexicon of a dozen or so words used in varied situations. The subsequent training of the child in semantic relationships and order should fully imprint a solid pragmatism. In school-age children the majority of those with developmental language disorders disappears into the population of the learning disabled [Snyder, 1986]. Although individual vocabulary may appear adequate, their use of syntactic modes and their production of the indirect form and complex pragmatic forms are likely to be inadequate. In adolescents with restricted difficulties in the higher order pragmatic functions, problems occur in topic maintenance, sensitivity, tonal misunderstandings, and group problem solving [Prather, 1986]. In an age at which self confidence

ing and language models provided by the families of these children may be deficient and effectively subject these children to cultural deprivation [Swisher, 1985].

Developmental language disorders

Although mental retardation is the most common developmental language disorder, the astute physician must be aware of those disorders that may masquerade as mental retardation. Disordered expression must be assessed regarding its semantic correctness and its pragmatic appropriateness. For instance, some children with hydrocephalus who are indeed mentally retarded speak in complete sentences but appear to have little comprehension of what they are saying. They have been described as hyperverbal [Swisher and Pinsker, 1971] or as having a cocktail party syndrome [Hadneius et al., 1962]. Several of the primary developmental language disorders are distinguishable on the basis of their particular semantic or articulatory disturbances or lack thereof. Although they are uncommon, these disorders can be disabling because the child may act differently and even have no spoken language.

Autism perhaps represents the most severe such disturbance. It is a pervasive language disorder, involving both auditory and visual language wherein spoken language that persists may appear perverse. The phenomenon of delayed echolalia, for instance, may result in the repetition of apparently learned nursery rhymes and television commercials, yet the autistic child will not be using this speech to communicate. Mental deficiency is not an essential feature of autism. However, many children with autism have variable degrees of associated mental retardation. In a subgroup of autism, called *Asperger syndrome*, verbal skills of these children are actually superior to their performance skills [Cox, 1991].

Acquired language disorders

Closed-head injury is a significant childhood disorder [Craft, 1972]. Cobbs et al. [1985] reported a high frequency of dysgraphia, naming disorders, and decreased verbal output in children who suffered closed-head injuries. Approximately 10% of the children were aphonic. In addition, they noted that specific classical aphasic syndromes were distinctly infrequent; therefore, in caring for any child who has suffered a closed-head injury, an assessment of the likely patterns of language disorder is important.

Hearing loss

The problem of hearing loss cannot be overemphasized. Not only can hearing loss accompany other neurologic insults (e.g., prematurity, meningitis, cerebral palsy) but individuals with recognized hearing loss are at risk for the expression of complementary problems, such as mental retardation, cerebral palsy, and visual difficul-

ties. Hearing loss is certainly more frequent than any of the specific developmental language disorders, and the majority of children with hearing loss have congenital hearing loss [Schein and Delk, 1974]. The import of less than total hearing loss and unilateral hearing loss is also considerable. Sound localization and speech discrimination, especially in a noisy situation, can provide considerable difficulties for children with partial or unilateral hearing loss. School failure in the absence of easily discernible cognitive or speech impairment is likely to result in the referral of these children for a comprehensive neurologic evaluation, whereas a simple audiometric examination would suffice.

Dysarthria

Dysarthrias in children range from almost complete unintelligibility to minor deviations that are indistinguishable from developmental articulation disorders. Classification of dysarthrias in children has been made by specific speech characteristics, by etiology, and by the neurologic localization of the responsible lesion. Many children with dysarthria have abnormal feeding patterns that may simply be the persistence of primitive reflexes, such as the swallow or bite reflexes. There may be limitation of the ability to produce or reproduce voluntary oral nonspeech movements (i.e., of the tongue and lips). Although the correlation between nonspeech and speech difficulties has not been found to be high by some investigators [Irwin, 1955], it is of enough value to be used as an indicator of risk.

Dysarthria of laryngeal origins is usually the consequence of cranial nerve abnormalities. Involvement of the cranial nerve X at the brainstem or anywhere above the superior laryngeal nerve may produce almost total aphonia. The voice will be breathy with decreased volume. In unilateral vagus nerve paralysis the peculiar phenomenon of diplophonia secondary to the presence of a second frequency in the vibration of the vocal folds will occur. In central involvement of the vagus nerve a spastic or strangled characteristic will be heard. Vowels will be prolonged, and crying and wailing will flutter. Subtle degrees of weakness of the vagus nerve can be detected by simply asking the patient to cough. When the abductors are weak, the cough or the glottal attack on a vowel will be noticeably weaker. When there is weakness of the velopharyngeal musculature, distinct hypernasality is heard. On occasion this defect can be better seen than heard. Ask the child to say words like *we*, *cheese*, or *please*, with a mirror near the nares to detect air leakage. Examination of the oral musculature is performed most simply by having the patient perform the tasks of the standard examination of cranial nerves V, VII, and XII.

Psychogenic dysarthrias exist but are less common in children than in adults. Aphonia, breathiness, and hoarseness are all potential functional phenomena.

Characteristic inconsistencies in these abnormalities in functional disorders help to distinguish them from organic neurologic disorders.

The most common origin of dysarthria in children is cerebral palsy. The incidence of cerebral palsy is 6 per 1000, and a considerable portion of these children have significant dysarthrias [Ingram, 1955]. The pseudobulbar palsy that is the origin of dysarthria in children with spastic cerebral palsy produces a persistence of the glottic closing reflex, which results in involuntary opening and closing or overclosure of the glottis. In addition, the respiratory efforts of these children are irregular, which produces deficiencies in voice and resonance [Lencione, 1976]. Voiced consonants, nasals, and lip sounds are more easily produced than nonvoiced consonants and nonnasal, tongue, and palate sounds, respectively. Children with spasticity are unable to execute tongue motions, whereas children with athetoid disorders are able to execute tongue motions but are unable to control extraneous motions of the tongue. Children with cerebral palsy may also have mental retardation, specific developmental language disorders, and hearing loss, all of which may contribute to their speech abnormalities.

One in 750 children are born with a cleft palate [McWilliams, 1983]. At least one fourth of these children will have hypernasal speech; some will actually be hyponasal. Other disturbances include combinations of hypernasality and hyponasality, nasal turbulence, and hoarseness [McWilliams, 1983]. This defect, the most frequent anatomic basis for articulatory disorders, may occur alone or in combination with other anomalies, including those of the CNS. Children with cleft palate are subject to a greater frequency of otitis media than other children. All of these factors compound a situation that already produces many articulatory disorders. Altogether, 40% of children with cleft palate are unintelligible at 3 years of age [Brown, 1985].

Speech characteristics of specific syndromes

Those neurologic syndromes with primary motor unit, bulbar, pseudobulbar, or common visible anatomic defects, such as cleft palate, can be logically expected to produce voice defects consistent with those abnormalities. Most syndromes and anomalous disorders of the CNS produce language deficiencies because of varying degrees of mental retardation or hearing loss. Some disorders have characteristic voice patterns, such as the chromosome 5p-syndrome (cri-du-chat syndrome) in which the infant's mewing cry is readily apparent. This cry has been ascribed to abnormal laryngeal development (Table 10-3). Even these characteristic patterns may be inconsistent within syndromes and may change as the child ages. Language is disturbed in most instances of neurologic disease in a nonspecific pattern. The

Table 10-3 Neurologic Syndromes/Diseases with Unusual/Abnormal Voice*

Syndrome/Disease	Characteristic
5p-syndrome	mewing
Bloom syndrome	high-pitched
Cornelia de Lange syndrome	low-pitched, weak, growling
Dubowitz syndrome	high-pitched, hoarse
Happy puppet syndrome	paroxysms of inappropriate laughter, absent speech
Hypothyroidism	hoarse
Trisomy 17/18	sea gull-like
Weaver syndrome	hoarse, low-pitched
Williams syndrome	hoarse

*Data from Jones KL. Smith's recognizable patterns of human malformation. Philadelphia: WB Saunders, 1988.

association of particular syndromes with specific language disorders is fraught with the problems of evolving and age-dependent patterns, as well as the confounding factors of pervasive cognitive and behavioral abnormalities. In Williams syndrome a prominent semantic pragmatic dysphasia has been noted, and autism is commonly associated with Joubert syndrome [Holroyd et al., 1991]. Although individual children with fetal alcohol syndrome have also been reported to have semantic pragmatic dysfunction [Shaywitz et al., 1981], the majority of children with fetal alcohol syndrome exhibit no such predilection, and their language is disturbed more as a reflection of mental retardation [Iosub et al., 1981].

The effect of sex hormones on language development is now acknowledged. Geschwind and Galaburda [1985] postulated and have received support for a detailed and complex interrelationship of hemispheric dominance, the immune system, and sex hormones. Consistent with their construct, we should expect a clustering of language disorders in children with sex chromosome aberrations. Although not all studies are supportive of this hypothesis, accumulating evidence suggests that XXX girls' language deficiency is merely parallel to their cognitive deficiencies, whereas boys with XXY are characteristically afflicted with selective expressive language deficits with good phonology but disordered semantics and relatively intact pragmatics [Bender et al., 1983; Graham et al., 1988; Linden et al., 1988]. On the other hand, XO girls are less likely to be selectively language deficient. In these children, perceptual organization and fine motor skills are most severely affected [Bender et al., 1984]. Although the degree and character of these language abnormalities are far from pathognomonic, the association is one which should be attended to in anticipating language problems in these children.

In children with specific anatomic syndromes, claims of specific language dysfunctions have been less striking. Perisylvian abnormalities have been reported in specific language-impaired boys [Plante et al., 1989; 1991], but the degree of abnormality is not sufficient to be clinically useful. Similarly, although phonologic processing deficiencies have been demonstrated as isolated abnormalities in several children with agenesis of the corpus callosum [Temple et al., 1990], the association of this defect with more extensive anatomic defects and with significant mental retardation diminishes the clinical utility of the findings. Attempts to delineate characteristic language disturbances in children with selected disorders of intermediate metabolism have produced interesting results but no clear pattern has emerged [Nyhan et al., 1989]. Similar ventures in children with diffuse or multifocal disorders have produced few useful results.

Differentiating these disorders of voice, speech, language, and cognition can be accomplished only when the physician is willing to record a complete and directed history and take the time not only to examine the child but to obtain an adequate language sample. A 10-minute period of observation is not enough. Moreover, norm-referenced test instruments and questionnaires are an essential part of the process. Once the risk factors have been recognized and the elements of speech and language appreciated, a useful diagnosis can be made.

REFERENCES

Allen DV, Bliss LS. Evaluation of procedures for screening preschool children for signs of impaired language development. Bethesda: National Institute of Communicative Disorders and Stroke, 1978; Report of Project No. NO1-NS-6-2355.

Beadle KR. Speech and language disturbances in childhood development. In: Darby JK Jr, ed. Speech evaluation in medicine. New York: Grune and Stratton, 1981.

Bender BG, Fry E, Pennington B, et al. Speech and language development in 41 children with sex chromosome anomalies. Pediatrics 1983; 71:262.

Bender B, Puck M, Salenblatt, et al. Cognitive development of unselected girls with complete and partial X monosomy. Pediatrics 1984; 73:175.

Berry M. Language disorders of children. New York: Appleton-Century-Crofts, 1969.

Biklen D. Communication unbound: autism and praxis. Har Educ Rev 1990; 60:291.

Bishop DVM. The causes of specific developmental language disorder ("developmental dysphasia"). J Child Psychol Psychiatry 1987; 28:1.

Bishop DVM, Edmundson D. Language-impaired 4-year-olds: distinguishing transient from persistent impairment. J Speech Hear Disord 1987; 52:156.

Brown JK. Dysarthria in children-neurologic perspective. In: Darby JK, ed. Speech and language evaluation in neurology: childhood disorders. New York: Grune and Stratton, 1985.

Cobbs LE, Fletcher JM, Landry SH, et al. Language disorders after pediatric head injury. In: Darby JK, ed. Speech and language evaluation in neurology: childhood disorders. New York: Grune and Stratton, 1985.

Coplan J. Deafness: ever heard of it? Delayed recognition of permanent hearing loss. Pediatrics 1987; 79:206.

Coplan J. The early language milestone scale. Tulsa: Modern Education Corporation, 1983.

Coplan J, Gleason JR. Quantifying language development from birth to 3 years using the early language milestone scale. Pediatrics 1990; 86:963.

Coplan J, Gleason JR, Ryan R, et al. Validation of an early language milestone scale in a high risk population. Pediatrics 1982; 5:677.

Cox AD. Is Asperger's syndrome a useful diagnosis? Arch Dis Child 1991; 66:259.

Craft AW. Head injury in children. In: Vinken PD, Bruyn GW, eds. Handbook of clinical neurology, Vol 23. New York: Elsevier, 1972.

Crossley R. Lending a hand: a personal account of the development of facilitated communication training. Am J Speech Lang Pathol 1992; 1:15.

Curlee RF, Shelton RL. Disorders of articulation, voice and fluency. In: Bluestone CD, Stool SE, eds. Pediatric otolaryngology. Philadelphia: WB Saunders, 1983.

Curtiss S. Genie: a psycholinguistic study of a modern day "wild child." New York: Academic Press, 1977.

Dworkin JP. Motor speech disorders, a treatment guide. St. Louis: Mosby, 1991.

Ferry PC, Hall SM, Hicks JL. "Dilapidated" speech: developmental verbal dyspraxia. Dev Med Child Neurol 1975; 17:749.

Geschwind N, Galaburda AM. Cerebral lateralization: biological mechanisms, associations, and pathology. A hypothesis for research. Arch Neurol 1985; 42:428.

Graham JM, Bashir AS, Stark RE, et al. Oral and written abilities of XXY boys: implications for anticipatory guidance. Pediatrics 1988; 81:795.

Hacaen H. Acquired aphasia in children and the ontogenesis of hemispheric functional specialization. Brain Lang 1976; 43:114.

Hadenius A, Hagberg B, Hyttnas-Bensch K, et al. The natural prognosis of infantile hydrocephalus. Acta Pediatr 1962; 51:117.

Holroyd S, Reiss AL, Bryan RN. Autistic features in Joubert syndrome. Biol Psychiatry 1991; 29:287.

Hull FM, Mielke PW, Willefore JA, et al. National speech and hearing survey. Fort Collins: Office of Education, Bureau of Education for the handicapped, U.S. Department of Health, Education, and Welfare, 1976; Final report, Project No. 50978.

Ingalls R. Mental retardation: the changing outlook. New York: John Wiley, 1978.

Ingram T. A study of cerebral palsy in the childhood population of Edinburgh. Arch Dis Child 1955; 30:85.

Iosub S, Fuchs M, Bingol N, et al. Fetal alcohol syndrome revisited. Pediatrics 1981; 68:475.

Irwin OC. Phonetic speech development in cerebral palsied children. Am J Phys Med 1955; 34:325.

Kinsbourne M, Swisher L. Disorders of voice, speech and language in children. Prac Pediatr 1977; 4:1.

Landau WM, Goldstein R, Kleffner FR. Congenital aphasia: a clinicopathologic study. Neurology 1960; 10:915.

LaPointe LL. Aphasia therapy: some principles and strategies for treatment. In: Johns DF, ed. Clinical management of neurogenic communicative disorders. Boston: Little, Brown, 1978;129.

Lencione R. The development of communication skills. In: Cruickshank WM, ed. Cerebral palsy, a developmental disability. Syracuse: Syracuse University Press, 1976.

Lenneberg EH. Biologic foundations of language. New York: John Wiley, 1967.

Linden MG, Bender BG, Harmon RJ, et al. 47,XXX: what is the prognosis? Pediatrics 1988; 82:619.

Mattis S, French JH, Rapin I. Dyslexia in children and young adults: three independent neuropsychological syndromes. Dev Med Child Neurol 1975; 17:150.

McWilliams BJ. Multiple speech disorders (cleft palate and cerebral palsy speech). In: Bluestone CD, Stool SE, eds. Pediatric otolaryngology. Philadelphia: WB Saunders, 1983.

Miller JF, Campbell TF, Chapman RS, et al. Language behavior in acquired childhood aphasia. In: Costello JM, Holland AL, eds. Handbook of speech and language disorders. San Diego: College-Hill Press, 1986; 599.

Nye S, Foster SH, Seaman D. Effectiveness of language intervention with the language/learning disabled. J Speech Hear Disord 1987; 52:348.

Nyhan WL, Wulfeck BB, Tallal P, et al. Metabolic correlates of learning disability. Birth Defects 1989; 25:153.

Plante E, Swisher L, Vance R. Anatomic correlates of normal and impaired language in a set of dizygotic twins. Brain Lang 1989; 37:643.

Plante E, Swisher L, Vance R. MRI findings in boys with specific language impairment. Brain Lang 1991; 41:52.

Prather EM. Developmental language disorders: adolescents. In: Costello JM, Holland AL, eds. Handbook of speech and language disorders. San Diego: College-Hill Press, 1986; 701.

Rapin I. Effects of early blindness and deafness on cognition. In: Katzman R, ed. Congenital and acquired cognitive disorders. New York: Raven Press, 1979.

Rapin I, Allen DA. Developmental language disorders: nosologic considerations. In: Kirk U, ed. Neuropsychology of language, reading, and spelling. New York: Academic Press, 1983.

Rapin I, Allen DA. Syndromes in developmental dysphasia and adult aphasia. In: Plum F, ed. Language, communication, and the brain. New York: Research Publications ARNMD Raven Press, 1988.

Rapin I, Mattis S, Rowan AJ, et al. Verbal auditory agnosia in children. Dev Med Child Neurol 1977; 19:192.

Rood SR. Anatomy and physiology of speech. In: Bluestone CD, Stool SE, eds. Pediatric otolaryngology. Philadelphia: WB Saunders, 1983.

Rutter M, Schopler E. Autism and pervasive developmental disorders: concepts and diagnostic issues. J Autism Dev Disord 1987; 17:159.

Schein JD, Delk MT Jr. The deaf population of the United States. Silver Springs: National Association for the Deaf, 1974.

Schlanger B. Mental retardation. Indianapolis: Bobbs-Merrill, 1973.

Shaywitz SE, Caparulo BK, Hodgson E. Developmental language disability as a consequence of prenatal exposure to ethanol. Pediatrics 1981; 68:850.

Snyder LS. Developmental language disorders: elementary school age. In: Costello JM, Holland AL, eds. Handbook of speech and language disorders. San Diego: College-Hill Press, 1986; 671.

Stevenson J, Richman N. The prevalence of language delay in a population of three-year-old children and its association with general retardation. Dev Med Child Neurol 1976; 18:431.

Swisher L, Pinsker J. The language characteristics of hyperverbal hydrocephalic children. Dev Med Child Neurol 1971; 13:746.

Swisher L. Language disorders in children. In: Darby JK, ed. Speech and language evaluation in neurology: childhood disorders. New York: Grune and Stratton, 1985.

Temple CM, Jeeves MA, Vilarroya OO. Reading in callosal agenesis. Brain Lang 1990; 39:235.

Walker D, Guggenheim S, Downs MP, et al. Early language milestone scale and language screening of young children. Pediatrics 1989; 83:284.

Wallace IF, Gavel JS, McCarton CM, et al. Otitis media and language development at 1 year of age. J of Speech Hear Disord 1988; 53:245.

Wilcox MJ. Developmental language disorders: preschoolers. In: Costello JM, Holland AL, eds. Handbook of speech and language disorders. San Diego: College-Hill Press, 1986; 643.

Wolpaw TM, Nation JE, Aram DM. Developmental language disorders: a follow-up study. In: Burns MS, Andrews JR, eds. Selected papers in language and phonology. Evanston: Institute for Continuing Professional Education, 1977.

Woods B, Carey S. Language deficits after apparent clinical recovery from childhood aphasia. Ann Neurol 1978; 6:405.

11

Sleep Disorders in Children

Stephen A. Smith

Sleep is an active process with cycling of different states. There are changes in awareness and responsiveness with alterations of muscle tone and temperature regulation. As understanding about the nature of sleep at various ages from preterm life on has developed, it has become clear that sleep-related disturbances are problems facing children, parents, and clinicians. The organization of sleep into sleep stages is developmentally determined, and the quality of sleep depends on numerous factors, including environmental influences. A number of specific sleep-related problems have been identified requiring recognition and oftentimes detailed study. In this chapter the term *sleep* will refer to a necessary physiologic process, during which an individual is not readily in contact with his or her environment on a conscious level.

SLEEP PHYSIOLOGY

Sleep can be divided into stages (Figure 11-1) based on the EEG, muscle tone, and eye movements. For example, during light sleep, designated as stage 1 or drowsy sleep, an individual can be easily aroused. In this stage an EEG discloses a loss of waking rhythms, which are replaced by low-voltage 3- to 7-Hz activities. Deeper stage 2 sleep is characterized by the presence of sleep spindles and K complexes at the vertex with mild slowing of background activities. In stage 3 and 4, which is often referred to as *delta sleep*, it is very difficult to arouse an individual; increased slow-wave activity, especially over the posterior head regions, is observed. As the night progresses, there are periods of rapid eye movement (REM) sleep [Aserinsky and Kleitman, 1955], which are referred to as *active sleep*. It is during these periods that most dreaming occurs [Dement and Kleitman, 1957]. REM sleep is distinct from delta sleep (Table 11-1).

The importance of REM sleep is underscored by the fact that it emerges at 29 weeks of gestation. It persists throughout life with the amount of REM sleep in late childhood, adolescence, and adult life remaining approximately 25% of the total sleep time at night. REM sleep is marked by low-amplitude, sawtooth waves on the EEG, REMs, and loss of muscle tone. The remainder of sleep is designated as non-REM (NREM) sleep. NREM sleep emerges as an easily recognized state between 32 and 35 weeks of gestation.

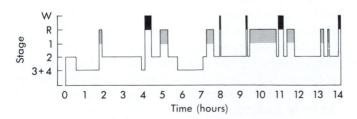

Figure 11-1 Normal sleep in a 3-year-old child. Total sleep time is 531 minutes divided into stage 2 sleep (58%), stage 3 to 4 sleep (20%), and REM sleep (22%). The first REM epoch (*R* and shading) occurs 71 minutes after falling asleep. Note the typical, brief arousals throughout the night (*W* and black coloring). (Courtesy Minnesota Regional Sleep Disorders Center, Hennepin County Medical Center.)

Table 11-1 Sleep stages

Physiologic parameter	Delta (Stages 3 and 4)	REM
Heart rate, respiratory rate, and blood pressure	Slow and stable	Variable
Muscle tone	Lower than awake	Absent
Time of night	First third	Second half
Arousals	Difficult to arouse	Easily awakened
EEG	Synchronized slow waves	Desynchronized
Dreaming	Absent	Typical

There are many physiologic factors that differentiate NREM from REM sleep. During NREM sleep the heart rate, respiratory rate, blood pressure, and muscle tone remain constant and regular. By contrast, REM sleep is denoted by irregular heart and respiratory rates, variable blood pressure, and decreased muscle tone. This decrease in muscle tone is one of the parameters used to monitor the appearance of REM sleep periods. Oxygen consumption increases during REM sleep compared with NREM, but responsiveness to carbon dioxide decreases. During NREM sleep, responsiveness to carbon dioxide is similar to that in the waking state. Responsiveness to hypoxia, however, remains the same during both NREM and REM sleep and is similar to that observed in awake individuals. Temperature control during NREM sleep is maintained, but an individual becomes poikilothermic during REM sleep. Penile tumescence occurs regularly and frequently during REM sleep.

Polysomnograms obtained in sleep laboratories monitor the EEG, eye movements, muscle tone recorded at the chin, oxygen saturation, and respiratory patterns, including air flow, chest movement, and abdominal movement. Leg and arm movements may also be monitored and videotaping conducted. In studies of gastroesophageal reflux, pH may be monitored in the lower esophagus.

DEVELOPMENT OF SLEEP PATTERNS

During the second half of gestation, sleep patterns that are definable in the same terms used in postnatal life and childhood begin to emerge [Booth et al., 1980; Parmelee et al., 1967]. Preterm studies are based on findings in premature infants, and, just as other parameters of premature function develop relatively constantly at various ages, sleep stages emerge at approximately the same time in most infants.

A uniform sleeping pattern manifests electrically between 24 and 27 weeks of gestation. At 28 weeks a tracé discontinue pattern is identified so that up to 3 minutes of suppression of electrical activity can be observed. Chin muscle tone has not yet developed on a regular basis. By 29 weeks, REM sleep can be identified because of an increased respiratory rate and increased eye movements. Temperature is important for respiratory control in the fetus [Dawes, 1968; Gluckman et al., 1983]. Near term, smiling during periods of REM sleep can be observed. REM sleep appears to develop first and is dominant, but after 7 to 8 months of gestation NREM sleep emerges as a separate sleep stage [Sterman and Hoppenbrouwers, 1971]. NREM sleep is characterized by an absence of body and eye movements. Sucking-like movements also may develop, and startle responses have been observed [Nijhuis et al., 1982]. The heart rate and respiratory rate are quite stable at this stage, and the EEG often demonstrates a tracé alternans pattern of 2- to 6-second bursts of activity followed by 4 to 6 seconds of lower voltage or near absence of activity. Both REM and NREM sleep are well established at birth.

As postterm development continues, sleep spindles can be identified by 1 month of age, and K complexes by 5 to 6 months. Newborns sleep more than 16 hours per day. Until 3 months of age, infants go directly into REM sleep from the awake state but between 3 and 5 months a change occurs so that they enter NREM sleep first [Hoppenbrouwers, 1986; Schulz et al., 1983]. Approximately 50% of sleep for a term infant is REM. The percentage decreases to 30% by age 2 and to 20% to 25% in adolescents and adults. The decrease in REM sleep is due to a decrease in the number of REM episodes during the night [Hoppenbrouwers et al., 1988]. At 3 months of age, NREM sleep is more frequent in the early portion of the night as it is after infancy [Coons and Guilleminault, 1982]. In the second half of the first year a maximum of NREM sleep occurs after sleep onset, and NREM and REM sleep alternate throughout the night [Schulz et al., 1989]. Between 1 and 6 years of age, the alternating pattern is replaced, with most NREM sleep occurring in the first part of the night [Hirai et al., 1968; Kohler et al., 1968]. Recent studies suggest that two types of NREM sleep occur in infants, one with and one without slow-wave sleep [Bes et al., 1991].

In the infant, temperature plays a significant role in respiratory control [Johnson, 1985]. Chemoreflexes become important for respiratory control at several months of age [Fleming et al., 1984]. Sleep/wake cycles begin to organize by 1 month of age. At 3 months of age, good organization of sleep/wake cycles is observed, resulting in longer periods of daytime wakefulness and a greater percentage of sleep occurring for longer periods of time at night [Kleitman and Engelmann, 1953; Meier-Koll et al., 1978]. The total amount of sleep time, however, remains approximately the same throughout this time of improved organization. Infants 1 to 3 months of age sleep 15 to 15.5 hours per day, whereas 12- to 18-month-old infants sleep 13.5 hours per day. The average 1-year-old sleeps 11 hours at night and obtains an additional 2½ hours sleep from two naps during the day. By 2 years of age, the average amount of sleep per day is 13 hours, and by age 3, the average is 12 hours per day, usually including one nap. The amount of sleep per day continues to fall so that by school age most children are sleeping approximately 10 hours per night and 8 to 9 hours by adolescence.

DISORDERS OF INITIATING AND MAINTAINING SLEEP
Sleeplessness in infants and preschool children

The inability of infants, toddlers, and preschool children to fall asleep or maintain sleep is a relatively common disorder. A number of reasons may contribute to initiating or continuing insomnia once it develops.

The more common problems are those associated with the parents' inappropriate expectations and improper limit setting [Ferber and Boyle, 1986]. The establishment of a routine of placing infants into their cribs for sleep facilitates the development of an appropriate wake-sleep cycle. The failure to establish a routine schedule often results in the infant's inability to establish a regular sleeping pattern. The circumstances under which a child falls asleep early on become the expected circumstances from the child's point of view under which sleep will occur. Alteration of these circumstances, such as being in a different location, kept awake for irregular periods, or with strangers, may produce sleeplessness. Under such circumstances fears may become magnified, leading to further sleep disruption.

Discussing with parents their routine of placing their infant or toddler into the crib for sleep at nap time during the day and bedtime at night will often uncover problems that prevent establishing a practice that is appropriate for the child. Parental expectations should be age appropriate. Resistance to going to bed is a frequent complaint of parents who have children with insomnia. Bedtime struggles may lead to loss of sleep for many family members.

At this age, medical problems are uncommon causes of sleeplessness, although colic, gastroesophageal reflux, otitis media, and CNS disease may produce altered sleep/wake cycles. The use of various medicines also may disrupt the normal sleep/wake cycle. Sleeplessness is more common in mentally retarded children than it is in children of normal intelligence. Children with upper motor neuron dysfunction or static encephalopathy are often impulsive during the daytime and are poor nappers. They have difficulty getting to sleep until late in the evening and often awaken early in the morning.

More significant disorders of the sleep/wake cycle may occur at an early age. Some children have been taught to go to sleep earlier than expected, and of course, they will awaken earlier in the morning than usual. The child who has been trained to go to bed later will have difficulty falling asleep when asked to go to bed earlier. This child will also be tired in the morning because he or she has become accustomed to sleeping much later. Various techniques have been used to retard or advance the sleep/wake cycle.

Recognizing pavor nocturnus, or night terrors, is important because this normal phenomenon, which develops out of slow-wave sleep, is self-limiting. The child may suddenly awaken from a seemingly sound sleep, sit upright in bed, appear terrified, and then scream quite loudly. In some instances, children will walk or run about the house and may be at some risk of hurting themselves. As a rule, these children are not fully awake during these episodes and have no remembrance of the event the following day. Helping the child cope with the night terror and then resettle to sleep is appropriate.

Sleeplessness in adolescents

Sleeplessness in adolescents is typically a result of a delayed sleep-phase cycle, which causes adolescents to gear themselves to fall asleep much later than is ideal. Adolescents typically have difficulty falling asleep at a normal time and are difficult to arouse in the morning. The need for more sleep in adolescence compared with other ages is common [Strauch and Meier, 1988]. It has been established that as teenagers move from early to late adolescence, they actually require more, rather than less, sleep, compounding the problem [Carskadon et al., 1983]. Unfortunately, social norms dictate staying up late at night, struggling to get to school early in the morning, and then sleeping through the entire morning on weekends to catch up on lost sleep. In severe instances, adolescents cannot fall asleep and stay awake all night. Trying to move their sleep phase back to normal may prove nearly impossible, and the only other course of action is to advance their sleep phase by 2 to 3 hours per night until enough cycles have passed to bring them back into normal compliance with an appropriate bedtime. A wide variety of drugs, including alcohol, may also interfere with normal sleep. Only 3.3% of adolescents report getting sufficient sleep. Adolescents with inadequate sleep have excessive morning tiredness, called the *morning-tiredness syndrome*.

DISORDERS OF EXCESSIVE SLEEPINESS
Narcolepsy

Narcolepsy is a dyssomnia with life-long and often disabling symptoms, specifically the tetrad of sleep attacks, cataplexy, sleep paralysis, and hallucinations [Yoss and Daly, 1957]. The condition affects approximately 0.06% to 0.1% of the population [Dement et al., 1973], and it initially develops during childhood or adolescence. Years may pass before the proper diagnosis is made [Kales et al., 1987]. The presence of sleep attacks plus cataplexy is diagnostic of narcolepsy.

The onset of narcolepsy occurs between the ages of 10 and 20 years. A positive family history increases the likelihood of narcolepsy up to 50% from the less than 1% prevalence in the general population [Kessler et al., 1974]. The genetic basis for the condition remains uncertain. Two modes of inheritance are considered. One is an autosomal-dominant inheritance with low penetrance and variable expressivity [Baraister and Parkes, 1987]. The second possible inheritance pattern involves multiple genes interacting with environmental factors [Kessler et al., 1974; Honda et al., 1983; and Guilleminault et al., 1989].

Excessive daytime sleepiness is present 75% of the time, cataplexy 33%, sleep paralysis 50%, and hypna-

Gastrointestinal system. Certain gastrointestinal events may cause paroxysmal arousals, and at times may be difficult to detect. Gastroesophageal reflux may cause laryngospasm [Guilleminault and Miles, 1980]. Cardiac arrhythmias have been initiated by esophageal spasm [Bortolotti et al., 1982; Fontan et al., 1984]. Gastroesophageal reflux may mimic seizures in infants [Wyllie et al, 1988].

REFERENCES

Abe K, Shimakawa M. Predisposition to sleep walking. Psychiatr Neurol 1966; 2:446.

Armstrong D, Sachis P, Bryan C, et al. Pathological features of persistent infantile sleep apnea with reference to the pathology of sudden infant death syndrome. Ann Neurol 1982; 12:169.

Aserinsky E, Kleitman N. A motility cycle in sleeping infants as manifested by ocular and gross bodily activity. J Appl Physiol 1955; 8:11.

Babson SG, Clarke NG. Relationship between infant death and maternal age: comparison of sudden infant death incidence with other causes of infant mortality. J Pediatr 1983; 103:391.

Baraister M, Parkes JD. Generic study of narcoleptic syndrome. J Med Genet 1987; 15:254.

Barnes PJ. Circadian variation in airway function. Am J Med 1985; 79:5.

Barnes PJ, Greening AP, Neville L, et al. Single-dose slow-release aminophylline at night prevents nocturnal asthma. Lancet 1982; 1:299.

Berger RM, Maizels M, Moran GC, et al. Bladder capacity (ounces) equals age (years) plus 2 predicts normal bladder capacity and aids in diagnosis of abnormal voiding patterns. J Urol 1983; 129:347.

Bergman AB. Sudden infant death syndrome in King County, Washington: epidemiolgical aspects. In: Bergman AB, Beckwith JB, Ray GC, eds. Sudden infant death syndrome: proceedings of the second international conference on causes of sudden death in infants. Seattle: University of Washington Press, 1970;47.

Bes F, Schulz H, Navelet Y, et al. The distribution of slow-wave sleep across the night: a comparison for infants, children, and adults. Sleep 1991; 14:5.

Billiard M. Narcolepsy. Clinical features and aetiology. Ann Clin Res 1985; 17:220.

Billiard M, Seignalet J. Extraordinary association between HLA-DR2(DRW15) and narcolepsy. Lancet 1985; i:226.

Booth CL, Leonard HL, Thoman EB. Sleep states and behavior patterns in preterm and fullterm infants. Neuropediatrics 1980; 11:354.

Bortolotti M, Cirignotta F, Labo G. Atrioventricular block induced by swallowing in a patient with diffuse esophageal spasm. J Am Med Assoc 1982; 248:2297.

Brooks JG. Apnea of infancy and sudden death syndrome. Am J Dis Child 1982; 136:1012.

Brouillette RT, Fernbach SK, Hunt CE. Obstructive sleep apnea in infants and children. J Pediatr 1982; 100:31.

Brown RW, McLeod WR. Sympathetic stimulation with temporal lobe epilepsy. Med J Aust 1973; 2:274.

Bruhn FW, Mokrohisky ST, McIntosh K. Apnea associated with respiratory syncytial virus infection in young infants. J Pediatr 1977; 90:382.

Carskadon MA, Dement WC. Normal human sleep: an overview. In: Kryger MH, Roth T, Dement WC, eds. Principles and practice of sleep medicine. Philadelphia: WB Saunders, 1989; 3.

Carskadon MA, Dement WC, Mitler MM, et al. Guidelines for the multiple sleep latency test (MSLT): a standard measure of sleepiness. Sleep 1986; 9:519.

Carskadon M, Harvey K, Duke P, et al. Evolution of sleep and daytime sleepiness in adolescents. In: Guilleminault C, Lugaresi E, eds. Sleep/wake disorders: natural history, epidemiology and long-term evolution. New York: Raven Press, 1983.

Catterall JR, Douglas NJ, Calverley PMA, et al. Irregular breathing and hypoxaemia during sleep in chronic stable asthma. Lancet 1982; i:301.

Chen WY, Chai H. Airway cooling and nocturnal asthma. Chest 1982; 81:675.

Cirignotta F, Zucconi M, Mondini S, et al. Enuresis, sleep walking and nightmares: an epidemiological survey in the Republic of San Marino. In: Guilleminault C, Lugaresi E, eds. Sleep/wake disorders: natural history, epidemiology and long-term evolution. New York: Raven Press, 1983.

Clancy RR, Spitzer AR. Cerebral cortical function in infants at risk for sudden infant death syndrome. Ann Neurol 1985; 18:41.

Coe CI, Barnes PJ. Reduction of nocturnal asthma by an inhaled anticholinergic drug. Chest 1986; 90:485.

Coons A, Guilleminault C. The development of sleep-wake patterns and non-rapid eye movement sleep stages during the first six months of life in normal infants. Pediatrics 1982; 69:793.

Davidson SL, Keens TG, Chan LS, et al. Sudden infant death syndrome in infants evaluated by apnea programs in California. Pediatrics 1986; 77:451.

Davis RS, Larsen GL, Grunstein MM. Respiratory response to intraesophageal acid infusion in asthmatic children during sleep. J Allergy Clin Immunol 1983; 72:393.

Dawes GS. Fetal and neonatal physiology. Chicago: Year Book Medical, 1968.

Dement WC, Carskadon M, Levy A. The prevalence of narcolepsy. Sleep Res 1973; 11:147.

Dement W, Kleitman N. Cyclic variations in EEG during sleep and their relation to eye movements, body motility, and dreaming. Electroencephalogr Clin Neurophysiol 1957; 9:673.

DeRoeck J, Van Hoof E, Cluydts R. Sleep-related expiratory groaning. A case report. Sleep Res 1983; 12:237.

Dexter JD, Riley TL. Studies in nocturnal migraine. Headache 1975; 15:51.

Dexter JD, Weitzman ED. The relationship of nocturnal headaches to sleep stage patterns. Neurology 1970; 20:513.

Ditta SD, Geoge CFP, Singh SM. HLA-D-region genomic DNA restriction fragments in DRw15(DR2) familial narcolepsy. Sleep 1992; 15:48.

Dunne KP, Matthews TG. Apnea monitors and sudden infant death. Arch Dis Child 1985; 60:688.

Dunne G, Matthews TP. Near-miss sudden infant death syndrome: clinical findings and management. Pediatrics 1987; 79:889.

Elias-Jones AC, Higenbottam LW, Barnes ND, et al. Sustained release theophylline in nocturnal asthma. Arch Dis Child 1984; 59:1159.

Evans J. Rocking at night. J Child Psychol Psychiatry 1961; 2:71.

Ferber R, Boyle MP. Six year experience of a pediatric sleep disorders center. Sleep Res 1986; 15:120.

Fleming PJ, Cade D, Bryan MH, et al. Congenital central hypoventilation and sleep state. Pediatrics 1980; 66:425.

Fleming PJ, Goncalves AL, Levine MR, et al. The development of stability of respiration in human infants: changes in ventilatory responses to spontaneous sighs. J Physiol 1984; 347:1.

Fontan JP, Heldt GP, Heyman MB. Esophageal spasm associated with apnea and bradycardia in an infant. Pediatrics 1984; 73:52.

Foxman B, Burciaga VZR, Brook RH. Childhood enuresis: prevalence, perceived impact and prescribed treatments. Pediatrics 1986; 77:482.

Frank Y, Kravath RE, Pollack CP, et al. Obstructive sleep apnea and its therapy. Clinical and polysomnographic manifestations. Pediatrics 1983; 71:737.

Froggatt P, Lynas MA, Marshall TK. Sudden death in babies: epidemiology. Am J Cardiol 1968; 22:457.

George CFP, Singh SM. Juvenile onset narcolepsy in an individual with Turner syndrome. A case report. Sleep 1991; 14:267.

Gluckman PD, Gunn TR, Johnston BM. The effect of cooling on breathing and shivering in unanaesthetized fetal lambs in utero. J Physiol 1983; 343:495.

Goel KM, Thoman RB, Gibbs EM, et al. Evaluation of nine different types of enuresis alarms. Arch Dis Child 1984; 59:748.

Gould JB, Lee AFS, James O, et al. The sleep state characteristics of apnea during infancy. Pediatrics 1976; 59:182.

Guilleminault C. Disorders of arousal in children: somnambulism and night terrors. In: Guilleminault C, ed. Sleep and its disorders in children. New York: Raven Press, 1982; 243.

Guilleminault C, Eldridge F, Simmons F, et al. Sleep apnea in eight children. Pediatrics 1976; 58:23.

Guilleminault C, Mignot E, Grumet FC. Familial patterns of narcolepsy. Lancet 1989; ii:1376.

Guilleminault C, Miles L. Differential diagnosis of obstructive sleep apnea syndrome: the abnormal exophagela reflux and laryngospasm during sleep. Sleep Res 1980; 9:200.

Guilleminault C, Motta J. Cardiac dysfunction during sleep. Ann Clin Res 1985; 17:190.

Guilleminault C, Nino-Marcia G, Heldt G, et al. Alternative treatment to tracheostomy in obstructive sleep apnea syndrome: nasal continuous positive airway pressure in young children. Pediatrics 1986; 78:797.

Guilleminault C, Pool P, Motta J, et al. Sinus arrest during REM sleep in young adults. N Engl J Med 1984a; 311:1106.

Guilleminault C, Souquet M, Ariagno RL, et al. Five cases of near miss sudden infant death syndrome and development of obstructive sleep apnea syndrome. Pediatrics 1984b; 73:71.

Herman JH, Blaw ME, Steinberg JB. REM behavior disorder in a two year old male with evidence of brainstem pathology. Sleep Res 1989; 18:242.

Herson VC, Schmitt BD, Rumack BH. Magical thinking and imipramine poisoning in two school-aged children. JAMA 1979; 241:1926.

Hirai T, Takano R, Uchinuma Y. An electroencephalographic study on the development of nocturnal sleep. Folia Psychiatr Neurol Jpn 1968; 22:157.

Honda Y, Asaka A, Tanimura M, et al. A genetic study of narcolepsy and excessive daytime sleepiness in 308 families with narcolepsy or hypersomnia proband. In: Guilleminault C, Lugaresi E, eds. Sleep/wake disorders. New York: Raven Press 1983; 187.

Honda Y, Juji T, Matsuki K, et al. HLA-DR2 and Dw2 in narcolepsy and in other disorders of excessive somnolence without cataplexy. Sleep 1986; 9:133.

Hoppenbrouwers T. Ontogenesis of sleep and waking. In: Sterman MB, Hodgman JE, Start CR, et al., eds. Ontogeny of sleep and cardiopulmonary regulation: factors related to risk for the sudden infant death syndrome. Washington, DC: NICHD, 1986.

Hoppenbrouwers T, Hodgman J, Arakawa K, et al. Sleep and waking states in infancy: normative studies. Sleep 1988; 11:387.

Hoppenbrouwers T, Hodgman JE, Harper RM, et al. Polygraphic studies of normal infants during the first six months of life. III. Incidence of apnea and periodic breathing. Pediatrics 1977; 60:418.

Jensen NB, Joensen P, Jensen J. Chronic paroxysmal hemicrania: continued remission of symptoms after discontinuation of indomethacin. Cephalalgia 1982; 2:163.

Johnson P. The development of breathing. In: Jones CT, ed. The physiological development of the fetus and newborn. New York: Academic Press, 1985; 201.

Juji T, Satake M, Honda Y, et al. HLA antigens in Japansese patients with narcolepsy. All patients are DR2(DRW15) positive. Tissue Antigens 1984; 24:316.

Kales A, Vela-Bueno A, Kales JD. Sleep disorders: sleep apnea and narcolepsy. Ann Intern Med 1987; 106:434.

Kales JD, Kales A. Nocturnal psychophysiological correlates of somatic conditions and sleep disorder. Int J Psychiatry Med 1975; 6:43.

Kayed K, Godtlibsen OB, Sjaastad O. Chronic paroxysmal hemicrania. IV. "REM sleep locked" nocturnal headache attacks. Sleep 1978; 1:91.

Kelly DH, Shannon DC. Home monitoring of infants at risk for apnea. Pediatrics 1980; 65:1054.

Kelly DH, Shannon DC. Treatment of apnea and excessive periodic breathing in the full-term infant. Pediatrics 1981; 68:81.

Kessler S, Guilleminault C, Dement WC. A family study of 50 REM narcoleptics. Acta Neurol Scand 1974; 50:503.

Klackenberg G. Somnambulism in childhood: prevalence, course and behavioral correlation. Acta Paediatr Scand 1982; 71:495.

Kleitman N, Engelmann TG. Sleep characteristics in infants. J Appl Physiol 1953; 6:269.

Kohler WC, Dean Coddington R, Agnew HW. Sleep patterns in 2-year-old children. J Pediatr 1968; 72:228.

Krongrad E. Post neonatal risk factors: The NIH Cooperative Epidemiological Study of Sudden Infant Death Syndrome (SIDS) Risk Factors. Proceedings of the American Pediatric Society—Society for Pediatric Research. Washington, DC, May 1982.

Kurth VE, Gohler I, Knaape HH. Utersuchungen uber der pavor nocturnus bei kindern. Psychiatr Neurol Med Psychol 1964; 17:1.

Langdon N, Welsh KI, Van Dam M, et al. Genetic markers in narcolepsy. Lancet 1984; 1178.

Lind MG, Lundell BPW. Tonsillary hyperplasia in children. Arch Otolaryngol 1982; 108:650.

Lipowski ZJ. Delirium (acute confusional state). Am Med Assoc J 1987; 258:1789.

Mahowald MW, Rosen GM. Parasomnias in children. Pediatrician 1990; 17:21.

Mahowald MW, Schenck CH. REM sleep behavior disorder. In: Kryger MH, Roth T, Dement WC, eds. Principles and practice of sleep medicine. Philadelphia: WB Saunders, 1989; 389.

Martin ME, Grunstein MM, Larsen GL. The relationship of gastroesophageal reflux to nocturnal wheezing in children with asthma. Ann Allergy 1982; 49:318.

Martin RJ, Miller MJ, Waldemar AC. Medical progress. Pathogenesis of apnea in preterm infants. J Pediatr 1986; 109:733.

Matsuki K, Juji T, Tokunaga K, et al. Human histocompatibility leukocyte antigen (HLA) haplotype frequencies estimated from the data on HLA class I, II, and III antigens in 111 Japanese narcoleptics. J Clin Invest 1985; 76:2078.

May HJ, Colligan RC, Schwartz MS. Childhood enuresis—important points in assessment, trends in treatment. Postgrad Med 1983; 74:111.

Meier-Koll A, Hall U, Hellwig U, et al. A biological oscillator system and the development of sleep-waking behavior during early infancy. Chronobiologia 1978; 5:425.

Merritt TA, Valdes-Dapena M. SIDS research update. Pediatr Ann 1984; 13:193.

Milner AD. Apnea monitors and sudden infant death. Arch Dis Child 1985; 60:76.

Mitler MM, Gujavarty KS, Browman CP. Maintenance of wakefulness test: a polysomnographic technique for evaluating treatment in patients with excessive somnolence. Electroencephalogr Clin Neurophysiol 1982; 53:658.

Mitler MM, Hajdukovic R. Relative efficacy of drugs for the treatment of sleepiness in narcolepsy. Sleep 1991; 14:218.

Montplaisir J, Walsh J, Malo JL. Nocturnal asthma: features of attacks, sleep and breathing patterns. Am Rev Respir Dis 1982; 125:18.

Morgan AD, Connaughton JJ, Catterall JR, et al. Sodium cromoglycate in nocturnal asthma. Thorax 1986; 41:39.

Morgan AD, Rhind GB, Connaughton JJ, et al. Breathing patterns during sleep in patients with nocturnal asthma. Thorax 1987; 42:600.

Naeye RL, Ladis B, Drage JS. Sudden infant death syndrome: a prospective study. Am J Dis Child 1976; 130:1207.

ance. In 68 patients with hemolytic uremic syndrome, 22 experienced major neurologic symptoms (convulsions and/or coma). In 9 patients who also had dysregulation of breathing, 8 died despite adequate seizure control, replacement of renal function, and assisted ventilation [Bos et al., 1985].

Endocrinologic disorders. In diabetes mellitus, coma can occur as a result of either hyperglycemia or hypoglycemia. Diabetic coma occurs gradually over several hours as a result of osmotic diuresis, with concomitant glycosuria, dehydration, ketoacidosis, and salt depletion. Repeated episodes of diabetic coma can lead to permanent neurologic deficit. Blunt head injury and other CNS disturbances can also be accompanied by hyperglycemia and renal glycosuria; thus further laboratory confirmation is needed before the diagnosis of diabetic origin can be made in a comatose patient. Insulin overdose or failure to consume adequate carbohydrates in relation to a given dose can lead to hypoglycemic coma, which probably poses a greater threat of permanent neurologic injury. Confusion and decreased level of consciousness can occur in Wernicke encephalopathy, usually a condition of alcoholic adults but which also has been reported in children with nutritional problems, such as vomiting, anorexia, inadequate formula, or malabsorption. Recently it has been associated with malignancy and decreased nutrition [Pihko et al., 1989].

When complicating adrenocortical or medullary failure, hypothyroidism, or hyperthyroidism, coma usually occurs after other signs of endocrine abnormality. Coma without specific episode-related metabolic derangement has been noted rarely in Lesch-Nyhan syndrome [Watts RWE et al., 1982; Lynch and Noetzel, 1991].

Seizure and postictal depression. Although usually observed after a tonic-clonic convulsion, postictal depression can also occur after less-severe seizures. Occasionally the seizure is not witnessed, and the diagnosis rests on finding tongue lacerations or incontinence. So-called subclinical status epilepticus unresponsiveness associated with continuous epileptiform discharges on EEG must be specifically considered.

Prognosis

When coma lasts more than a few hours, an estimate of the probable outcome is often desired to plan treatment and to provide the family with some perspective of the severity of the problem. The various coma scales were designed to permit prognostication in patients with trauma. In general the lower the score, the greater the likelihood of neurologic sequelae or even death.

In a study of outcome of nontraumatic, prolonged coma in 16 patients between 6 months and 16 years of age, only 3 diagnoses were represented in the patients: encephalitis (8), anoxia (5), and Reye's syndrome (3).

Prolonged coma was defined as lasting longer than 15 days. None of the patients in coma of anoxic origin did well. Patients who experienced stage 3 coma for more than 2 weeks' duration had some sequelae, as did patients who experienced stage 4 coma for any length of time. Eleven patients who had assisted ventilation, either electively (two patients) or by necessity, had a less satisfactory outcome.

In a stepwise, multivariate, discriminate analysis of outcome in 102 patients with nontraumatic coma, seven clinical variables found on the initial examination (within 2 to 12 hours of the onset of coma) correlated best with outcome: coma severity, extraocular movements, pupils, motor patterns, blood pressure, temperature, and seizure type [Johnston and Seshia, 1984]. Patients could be classified into one of five outcomes. Only eight patients were severely misclassified using these variables. In assessing the 66 patients remaining in coma at 20 to 28 hours after onset, five variables correlated with outcome: age, coma severity, motor patterns, blood pressure, and seizure type. There were two serious classification errors. About 25% of the comas were caused by either intracranial infection, anoxia-ischemia (including cardiorespiratory arrest), or metabolic causes; 17% were caused by epilepsy. The results underscore the value and importance of a directed and accurate neurologic examination at the time of first contact with a comatose patient. Further analysis of these patients [Johnston and Seshia, 1984; Seshia et al., 1983] indicated that of the patients younger than 1 year of age, 44% died and 24% were normal; of the patients 6 to 17 years of age, 24% died and 73% were normal. All patients who died had either absent extraocular movements or nonreactive pupils, or hypothermia or inability to maintain body temperature.

Monitoring brain function in comatose children using electrophysiologic techniques provides diagnostic, therapeutic, and prognostic information [Talwar and Torres, 1988]. The Cerebral Function Monitor provides amplitude data from a single channel of EEG. It provides data about variability and response to stimuli. The compressed spectral array provides frequency spectral information from two channels and thus permits comparison of the hemispheres. A monotonous, slow pattern portends a grave prognosis, as does failure of the pattern to change with external stimuli or medications that usually cause faster EEG rhythms [Bricolo et al, 1978]. Compressed spectral array has been used to predict outcome in patients with prolonged coma; return of theta or alpha frequency range in the first 10 days of coma was found in all patients who made a good recovery. Conversely, if either frequency did not return or was lost again, the survivors usually had neurologic residua.

Prognostic variables were evaluated in 51 nearly drowned, comatose children and included mean cerebral perfusion pressure and mean intracranial pressure. Estimated submersion time and mean intracranial pressure and mean cerebral perfusion pressure determined survival but could not predict the neurologic outcome [Nussbaum, 1985]. In 66 patients admitted to Los Angeles Children's Hospital after a severe near-drowning episode who had required full CPR and who had a score of 3 on the Glasgow Coma Scale, 24% had intact survival. No patient who arrived at the intensive care unit with a Glasgow Coma Scale of less than 3 (flaccid) survived neurologically intact. Of the 37 patients who had a Glasgow Coma Scale score of 3 or less, 26 died and 11 suffered severe brain damage [Allman et al., 1986].

In a study of four self-asphyxiated children, Ashwal et al. [1991] found that poor outcome was associated with initial blood glucose greater than 300 mg/dl; CBF/P_{CO_2} response less than 2.0 ml/min/100 gm/torr P_{CO_2}; and cardiac index less than 2.0 L/min/m^2 for longer than 12 to 24 hours.

Evoked responses may have some usefulness in predicting outcome. Somatosensory-evoked responses repeated after at least a week were more reliable than visual-evoked responses [Taylor and Farrell, 1989]. Brainstem auditory-evoked responses were not helpful [De Meirleir and Taylor, 1986]. On the other hand, normal somatosensory potentials have been reported in children with persistent coma [Tsao and Ellingson, 1989].

Thus, at best, an estimate of the course and outcome of the patient can be derived from attempts at prognosis.

BRAIN DEATH

Brain death was first described clinically in 1959 when Mollaret and Goulon [1959] identified a condition they called *coma depassé,* literally a state beyond coma. All of the classic features of brain death are found in this early report.

Controversy surrounds the means of reliably diagnosing brain death in young children, whereas there is general agreement on brain death criteria for adults; these latter guidelines are based on the criteria established in 1968 by the ad hoc committee of the Harvard Medical School [1968], which were subsequently refined and modified. Some authors have proposed that the adult brain death criteria are applicable to children as well [Rowland et al., 1983; Pitts 1984; Robinson, 1981]; others disagree or at least urge caution in applying adult brain death standards to children. Many types of confirmatory testing have been advocated, but all have been demonstrated to be at least somewhat unreliable, especially in the very young.

Pediatric brain death guidelines must consider the need for criteria that preclude the chance of recovery, while avoiding rigid rules that would unnecessarily prolong life or the dying process. The criteria should be clear and distinct; the tests performed should yield vivid and unambiguous results, and the analysis should include an evaluation of the permanence or the irreversibility of the absent functions.

Historically the brain death literature has not made a clear distinction regarding children. In 1972 the National Institute of Neurologic Disease and Stroke [Task Force on Death and Dying of the Institute of Society, Ethics, and the Life Sciences, 1972] did a collaborative study to determine criteria that would reliably predict irreversible loss of brain function. The purpose was to improve on the Harvard criteria by increasing accuracy and inclusivity. The major differences from the Harvard criteria were the shorter interval required (6 versus 24 hours), a different definition of apnea, the irrelevance of spinal reflexes, and the introduction of a blood flow test as a definitive confirmatory procedure. No mention of specific pediatric criteria or exception was made. Of the 503 patients in the National Institute of Neurologic Disease and Stroke study, 43 were 1 to 9 years of age and 58 were 10 to 19 years of age. Walker and Molinari [1975] concluded that this study cannot be applied to infants and young children. Furthermore, Green and Lauger [1972] suggested that brain death criteria for adults are not valid for children because younger patients may have greater resistance to hypoxic damage.

The President's Commission for the Study of Ethical Problems in Medicine and Biomedical and Behavioral Research [1984] proposed a Uniform Determination of Death Act in 1981 in which they reaffirmed the applicability of clinical criteria alone in the diagnosis of brain death. They viewed ancillary testing, such as EEG and cerebral blood flow to be necessary only when "objective documentation of clinical findings was needed." Younger than 5 years of age was considered a complicating criterion; because children have increased resistance to hypoxic damage, they may recover function even after demonstrating neurologic unresponsiveness for periods longer than those detrimental in adults. The cutoff of 5 years of age appears arbitrary.

An editorial [Robinson, 1981] commented on the insufficiency of attempts to assess the applicability of the brain death criteria to children and argues for delaying the diagnosis of brain death in small children (particularly infants who have suffered extensive cerebral trauma) because the lack of evidence does not allow the diagnosis of brain death in these young patients with complete confidence.

In agreement with reports that the diagnosis of brain death in adults can be made by clinical criteria alone is a series of 15 patients [Rowland et al., 1984], 2 months to 13 years of age, who met the following criteria:

1. The patient is deeply comatose and without verbal or purposeful motor response to external stimuli.
2. The patient has no spontaneous respiration.

3. There are no brainstem reflexes; pupillary, corneal, gag, oculovestibular, or oculocephalic.
4. Drugs, hypothermia, and metabolic causes for coma have been excluded.
5. All appropriate diagnostic and therapeutic tests have been performed, and a period of observation has passed during which the previous findings are consistent (usually 6 to 24 hours).

None of the 15 patients who met these criteria survived, and each of 11 autopsies performed revealed marked liquefactive necrosis of the brain. These criteria, distilled from the literature, represent a core concept of the clinical diagnosis of brain death. The endpoints to test the criteria are either the eventuality of irreversible cardiac standstill and/or severe brain necrosis at postmortem examination. In a related editorial, Crone [1983] agreed that clinical criteria for the diagnosis of brain death could be applied to children with certainty but noted the need for flexibility in each situation and that sensitivity to the psychosocial issues of the family might influence the need for additional confirmatory testing.

A recent review [Drake et al., 1986] of 61 pediatric patients (ranging from newborn to 18 years of age, with a mean of 34 months) with suspected brain death led to proposed brain death criteria. The absence of cerebral blood flow, as demonstrated by radionuclide bolus, provided nearly absolute information in suspected brain death (none of the 27 patients with absence of cerebral blood flow recovered any brain function). Brainstem auditory-evoked potentials (BAEPs) were not recommended. Drake et al. considered the use of ancillary testing to confirm brain death as a medicolegal requirement rather than as providing medical certainty.

Ashwal et al. [1977] studied 15 patients ranging from 32 weeks to 11 years of age. There was complete correlation of clinical examination, absence of cerebral blood flow, and electrical cerebral silence in 79% of patients. They concluded that radioisotope bolus testing for cerebral blood flow in conjunction with the clinical examination and EEG in patients 1 year of age and older represented a reasonable and conclusive approach to the diagnosis of brain death.

Of special concern in children is apnea testing. Results in children may differ from those of adults because metabolic rate, oxygen consumption, and functional reserve capacity (FRC) of the lung are age-dependent and size-dependent [Crone, 1983]. Special guidelines have been published [Outwater and Rockof, 1984; Rowland et al., 1984].

One criterion of absent brainstem function is the failure of spontaneous respiration. The apnea test, performed by removing ventilatory support for a period of time and observing signs of spontaneous respiration is widely used, but uniform standards have not yet been determined. Avoiding hypoxia and achieving a P_{CO_2} of 60 torr is commonly used. However, an intact brainstem may well respond to much more physiologic P_{CO_2} levels [Riviello et al., 1988]. The debate on the best ancillary test to confirm brain death is still unresolved. Since the publication of the Harvard criteria, the use of the EEG has been widely accepted. Two isoelectric EEGs recorded 24 hours apart are a commonly accepted indication of brain death. However, children with electrocerebral silence have recovered brain function [Green and Lauber 1972; Trojaborg and Jorgensen, 1973]. The limits of the EEG in the diagnosis of brain death in children have been emphasized [Ashwal et al., 1977].

Although evoked potentials may be helpful in supporting a diagnosis of brain death [Steinhart and Weiss, 1985; Goldie et al., 1981], the absence of evoked potentials is not conclusive evidence of brain death [Aminoff, 1984; Dear and Godfrey, 1985; Boyd and Harden, 1985]. Brainstem reflexes that are evaluated in brain death determinations are not consistently present in normal infants under 32 weeks' postconceptional age [Ashwal and Schneider, 1979].

Doppler ultrasound studies via the anterior fontanel have been suggested as a noninvasive way of correlating blood flow in the anterior cerebral artery with brain death [McMenamin and Volpe, 1983], but at least one child who had no pulsations survived [Furgiule et al., 1984]. Doppler carotid flow studies are also being investigated as indicators of cerebral flow [Ahman et al., 1985].

Radionuclide imaging appears to be a very useful confirmatory test in brain death determinations [Holzman et al., 1983; Schwartz et al., 1984]. It is rapid, portable, and relatively noninvasive; however, Ashwal et al. [1977] reported that one patient with a bolus study demonstrating no cerebral activity and electrocerebral silence and having a clinical examination consistent with brain death subsequently recovered. Korein [1978] also cautioned about the limitations of the radionuclide bolus technique for confirming brain death in infants and children. This technique also is primarily suited for confirming neocortical death but is poor for diagnosing brainstem death.

Four-vessel cerebral angiography, currently definitive in diagnosing brain death, is invasive and hazardous in critically ill children. Digital subtraction angiography may be a reasonable compromise [Vatne et al., 1985; Lee et al., 1984], although anuria is a contraindication. As reported, small areas of perfusion may exist, along with some EEG activity, even though the patient is clinically brain dead [Fackler and Rogers, 1987]. MRI angiography can demonstrate blood flow but is of little use in these patients because life support requirements make scanning difficult.

Estimation of cerebral blood flow using xenon CT was applied to 21 children, 10 of whom were clinically brain dead [Ashwal et al., 1989]. Flow of less than 5 ml/min/100 g was the equivalent of no flow by radionuclide techniques, and flow below 10 ml/min/100 g was consistent with clinical brain death. Patients with flow of greater than 10 to 15 ml/min/100 g had the potential to survive.

It is clear that there is confusion over what tests reliably document whole brain death.

An ad hoc committee on brain death at Children's Hospital, Boston [1987], addressed the entire issue. Clinical examination was given great emphasis, with laboratory studies only as adjuncts or as a means of confirming irreversibility. Even these guidelines are not without controversy. The requirement for absent sagittal sinus flow on radionuclide angiogram is probably too stringent; the value of auditory brainstem potentials is problematic. Rarely, a patient may recover, at least transiently, after meeting all of the criteria (Kohrman et al., 1990).

Only rarely can the diagnosis of brain death be established using standard criteria in anencephalic newborns [Ashwal et al., 1990]. A Task Force for the Determination of Brain Death in Children, with representatives of all major American pediatric, neurologic, and pediatric neurologic societies, published the following guidelines [1987] that resulted from their deliberations:

History

The critical initial assessment is the clinical history and examination. The most important factor is determination of the proximate cause of coma to ensure absence of remediable or reversible condition. Most difficulties with the determination of death on the basis of neurologic criteria have resulted from overlooking this basic fact. Especially important are detection of toxic and metabolic disorders, sedative-hypnotic drugs, paralytic agents, hypothermia, hypotension, and surgically remediable condition. The physical examination is necessary to determine the failure of brain function.

Physical examination criteria

1. Coma and apnea must coexist. The patient must exhibit complete loss of consciousness, vocalization, and volitional activity.
2. Absence of brainstem function as defined by:
   (a) Midposition or fully dilated pupils that do not respond to light. Drugs may influence and invalidate pupillary assessment.
   (b) Absence of spontaneous eye movements and those induced by oculocephalic and caloric (oculovestibular testing).
   (c) Absence of movement of bulbar musculature, including facial and oropharyngeal muscles. The corneal, gag, cough, sucking, and rooting reflexes are absent.

   (d) Respiratory movements are absent with the patient off the respirator. Apnea testing using standardized methods can be performed but is done after other criteria are met.
3. The patient must not be significantly hypothermic or hypotensive for age.
4. Flaccid tone and absence of spontaneous or induced movements, excluding spinal cord events, such as reflex withdrawal or spinal myoclonus, should exist.
5. The examination should remain consistent with brain death throughout the observation and testing period.

Observation periods according to age

The recommended observation period depends on the age of the patient and the laboratory tests used.

7 days to 2 months. The task force recommends two examinations and EEGs separated by at least 48 hours.

2 months to 1 year. The task force recommends two examinations and EEGs separated by at least 24 hours. A repeat examination and EEG are not necessary if the concomitant radionuclide angiographic (CRAG) study demonstrates no visualization of cerebral arteries.

Over 1 year. When an irreversible cause exists, laboratory testing is not required and the Task Force recommends an observation period of at least 12 hours. There are conditions, particularly hypoxic-ischemic encephalopathy, in which it is difficult to assess the extent and reversibility of brain damage. This is particularly true if the first examination is performed soon after the acute event. Therefore in this situation the Task Force recommends a more prolonged period of at least 24 hours of observation. The observation period may be reduced if the EEG demonstrates electrocerebral silence or the concomitant radionuclide angiographic study does not visualize cerebral arteries.

Laboratory testing

EEG. EEG to document electrocerebral silence should, if performed, be done over a 30-minute period, using standardized techniques for brain death determinations. In small children, it may not be possible to meet the standard requirement for 10-cm electrode separation. The interelectrode distance should be decreased proportional to the patient's head size. Drug concentrations should be insufficient to suppress EEG activity.

Angiography. A cerebral radionuclide angiogram confirms cerebral death by demonstration of the lack of visualization of the cerebral circulation. A technically satisfactory cerebral radionuclide angiogram that demonstrates arrest of carotid circulation at the base of the skull and absence of intracranial arterial circulation can be considered confirmatory of brain death, even though there may be some visualization of the intracranial venous sinuses. The value of this study in infants under 2 months of age is under investigation. Contrast angiography can document lack of effective blood flow to the brain.

Techniques under investigation. The task force recognizes that other tests, including xenon CT, digital subtraction angiography, visualization of cerebral arterial pulsations by real-time cranial ultrasound, Doppler determination of cerebral blood flow velocity, and evoked potential are under investigation.

REFERENCES

Ad Hoc Committee of the Harvard Medical School to Examine the Definition of Brain Death. JAMA 1968; 205:337.

Ad Hoc Committee on Brain Death, The Children's Hospital, Boston. Determination of brain death. J Pediatr 1987; 110:15.

Ahman PA, Carrigan TA, Carlton D, et al. Carotid arterial blood velocity patterns in brain dead children. Ann Neurol 1985; 18:416.

Allman FD, Nelson WB, Pacentine GA, et al. Outcome following cardiopulmonary resuscitation in severe pediatric near-drowning. Am J Dis Child 1986; 140:571.

American Psychiatric Association. Diagnostic and statistical manual of mental disorders, 3rd ed., revised. Washington, DC: The Association, 1987.

Aminoff MJ. The clinical role of somatosensory evoked potential studies: a critical appraisal. Muscle Nerve 1984; 7:345.

Ashwal S, Peabody JL, Schneider S, et al. Anencephaly: clinical determination of brain death and neuropathologic studies. Pediatr Neurol 1990; 6:233-9.

Ashwal S, Perkin RM, Thompson JR, et al. CBF and CBF/Pco_2 reactivity in childhood strangulation. Pediatr Neurol 1991; 7:369-74.

Ashwal S, Schneider S. Failure of electroencephalography to diagnose brain death in comatose children. Ann Neurol 1979; 6:512.

Ashwal S, Schneider S, Thompson J. Xenon computed tomography measuring cerebral blood flow in the determination of brain death in children. Ann Neurol 1989; 25:539-546.

Ashwal S, Smith AJK, Torres F, et al. Radionuclide bolus angiography: a technique for verification of brain death in infants and children. J Pediatr 1977; 91:722.

Bos AP, Donckerwolcke RA, van Vught AJ. The hemolytic-uremic syndrome: prognostic significance of neurological abnormalities. Helv Paediatr Acta 1985; 40:381.

Boyd SG, Harden A. Neonatal auditory brainstem response cannot reliably diagnose brainstem death (letter). Arch Dis Child 1985; 60:396.

Bricolo A, Turazzi S, Faccioli F, et al. Clinical application of compressed spectral array in long-term EEG monitoring of comatose patients. Electroencephalogr Clin Neurophysiol 1978; 45:211-25.

Crone R. Brain death (editorial). Am J Dis Child 1983; 137:545.

De Meirleir LJ, Taylor MJ. Evoked potentials in comatose children: auditory brainstem responses. Pediatr Neurol 1986; 2:31-4.

Dear PRF, Godfrey DJ. Neonatal auditory brainstem response cannot reliably diagnose brainstem death. Arch Dis Child 1985; 60:17-9.

DiMario FJ Jr, Packer RJ. Acute mental status changes in children with systemic cancer. Pediatrics 1990; 85:353-60.

Drake B, Ashwal S, Schneider S. Determination of cerebral death in the pediatric intensive care unit. Pediatrics 1986; 78:107.

Fackler JC, Rogers MC. Is brain death really cessation of all intracranial function? J Pediatr 1987; 110:84.

Furgiule TL, Frank LM, Riegle C, et al. Prediction of cerebral death by cranial sector scan. Crit Care Med 1984; 12:1.

Goldie D, Chiappa KH, Young RR, et al. Brainstem auditory and short-latency somatosensory evoked responses in brain death. Neurology 1981; 31:248.

Green JB, Lauber A. Recovery of activity in young children after ECS. J Neurol Neurosurg Psychiatry 1972; 35:103.

Holzman BH, Curless RG, Sfakianakis GN, et al. Radionuclide cerebral perfusion scintigraphy in determination of brain death in children. Neurology 1983; 33:1027.

Huttenlocher PR. Reye's syndrome: relation of outcome to therapy. J Pediatr 1972; 80:845.

Jennett B, Bond M. Assessment of outcome after severe brain damage: a practical scale. Lancet 1975; 1:480.

Jennett B, Teasdale G. Aspects of coma after severe head injury. Lancet 1977; 1:878.

Jennett B, Teasdale G, Galbraith S, et al. Severe head injuries in 3 countries. J Neurol Neurosurg Psychiatry 1977; 40:291.

Johnston B, Seshia SS. Prediction of outcome in non-traumatic coma in childhood. Acta Neurol Scand 1984; 69:417.

Kohrman MH, Spivack BS. Brain death in infants: sensitivity and specificity of current criteria. Pediatr Neurol 1990; 6:47-50.

Korein J. Brain death: interrelated medical and social issues. Ann NY Acad Sci 1978; 315:1.

Lee BC, Voorhies TM, Ehrlich ME, et al. Digital intravenous cerebral angiography in neonates. Am J Neuroradiol 1984; 5:281.

Lipowski ZJ. Delirium, clouding of consciousness and confusion. J Nerv Ment Dis 1967; 145:227.

Lynch BJ, Noetzel MJ. Recurrent coma and Lesch-Nyhan syndrome. Pediatr Neurol 1991; 7:389-91.

Masters SJ, McClean PM, Arcarese JS, et al. Skull x-ray examinations after head trauma. Recommendations by a multidisciplinary panel and validation study. N Engl J Med 1987; 316:84.

McMenamin J, Volpe J. Doppler ultrasonography in the determination of neonatal brain death. Ann Neurol 1983; 14:302.

Mollaret P, Goulon M. Le coma depasse. Rev Neurol 1959; 101:3.

Nussbaum E. Prognostic variables in nearly drowned, comatose children. Am J Dis Child 1985; 139:1058.

Outwater KM, Rockof MA. Apnea testing to confirm brain death in children. Crit Care Med 1984; 12:357.

Pihko H, Saarinen U, Paetau A. Wernicke encephalopathy: a preventable cause of death: Report of 2 children with malignant disease. Pediatr Neurol 1989; 5:237-42.

Pitts LH. Determination of brain death. West J Med 1984; 140:631.

President's Commission for the Study of Ethical Problems in Medicine and Biomedical and Behavioral Research. Guidelines for the determination of death. JAMA 1984; 246:2184.

Pro JD, Wells CE. The use of the electroencephalogram in the diagnosis of delirium. Dis Nerv Syst 1977; 38:804.

Raimondi AJ, Hirschauer J. Head injury in the infant and toddler. Coma scoring and outcome scale. Childs Brain 1984; 11:12.

Reye RDK, Morgan G, Baral J. Encephalopathy and fatty degeneration of the viscera: a disease entity in childhood. Lancet 1963; 2:474.

Riviello JJ Jr, Sapin JI, Brown LW, et al. Hypoxemia and hemodynamic changes during the hypercarbia stimulation test. Pediatr Neurol 1988; 4:213-8.

Robinson RO. Brain death in children. Arch Dis Child 1981; 56:657.

Rowland TW, Donnelly JH, Jackson AH. Apnea documentation for determination of brain death in children. Pediatrics 1984; 74:505.

Rowland TW, Donnelly JH, Jackson AH, et al. Brain death in the pediatric intensive care unit. Am J Dis Child 1983; 137:547.

Schwartz JA, Baxter J, Brill DR. Diagnosis of brain death in children by radionuclide cerebral imaging. Pediatrics 1984; 73:14.

Seshia SS, Johnston B, Kasian G. Non-traumatic coma in childhood: clinical variables in prediction of outcome. Dev Med Child Neurol 1983; 25:493.

Simpson D, Reilly P. Pediatric coma scale (letter). Lancet 1982; 2:450.

Stanczak DE, White JG III, Gouview WD, et al. Assessment of level of consciousness following severe neurological insult. A comparison of the psychometric qualities of the Glasgow Coma Scale and the Comprehensive Level of Consciousness Scale. J Neurosurg 1984; 60:955.

Steinhart CM, Weiss IP. Use of brainstem auditory evoked potentials in pediatric brain death. Crit Care Med 1985; 13:560.

Takahashi H, Nakazawa S. Specific type of head injury in children. Report of 5 cases. Childs Brain 1980; 7:124.

Talwar D, Torres F. Continuous electrophysiologic monitoring of cerebral function in the pediatric intensive care unit. Pediatr Neurol 1988; 4:137-47.

The Task Force on Death and Dying of the Institute of Society, Ethics, and the Life Sciences. Refinements in criteria for the determination of death: an appraisal. JAMA 1972; 221:48.

Task Force for the Determination of Brain Death in Children. Guidelines for the determination of brain death in children. Pediatr Neurol 1987; 3:242.

Taylor MJ, Farrell EJ. Comparison of the prognostic utility of VEPs and SEPs in comatose children. Pediatr Neurol 1989; 5:145-50.

Trauner DA, James HE. Evaluation of coma. In: James HE, Anas NG, Perkin RM, eds. Brain insults in infants and children. Pathophysiology and management. Orlando, Florida: Grune & Stratton, 1985.

Trojaborg J, Jorgensen EO. Evoked cortical potentials in patients with isoelectric EEG's. Electroencephalogr Clin Neurophysiol 1973; 35:301.

Tsao CY, Ellingson RJ. Normal somatosensory evoked potentials in a child in persistent coma. Pediatr Neurol 1989; 5:257-8.

Vatne K, Nakstad P, Lundar T. Digital subtraction angiography in the evaluation of brain death. A comparison of conventional cerebral angiography with intravenous and intraarterial DSA. Neuroradiology 1985; 27:155.

Walker AE, Molinari GF. Criteria of cerebral death. Trans Am Neurol Assoc 1975; 100:29.

Watts RWE, Spellacy E, Gibbs DA, et al. Clinical, post-mortem, biochemical and therapeutic observations on the Lesch-Nyhan syndrome with particular reference to the neurological manifestations. Q J Med 1982; 201:43-78.

Young HA, Gleave JR, Schmidek HH, et al. Delayed traumatic intracerebral hematoma: report of 15 cases operatively treated. Neurosurgery 1984; 14:22.

Zimmerman RA, Bilaniuk LT, Bruce D, et al. Computed tomography of pediatric head trauma: acute general cerebral swelling. Radiology 1978; 126:403.

Zimmerman RA, Bilaniuk LT. Computed tomography in pediatric head trauma. J Neuroradiol 1981; 8:257.

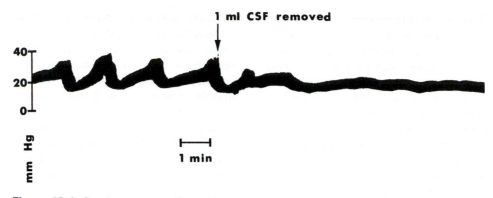

Figure 13-1 Continuous recording of intraventricular pressure in patient with Reye syndrome. Note plateau waves are abolished after CSF removal. (From Trauner DA et al. Ann Neurol 1978; 4:275.)

compliance and lack of accuracy in reflecting true intracranial pressure as a result of signal damping. These drawbacks limit the clinical usefulness of this device.

Surface subarachnoid and subdural monitoring

This technique involves placement of a fluid-filled metal screw or bolt in the subdural or subarachnoid space [James et al., 1975; Dearden et al., 1984]. This bolt is connected to an external transducer similar to the other monitoring devices. Advantages include a low risk of neurologic morbidity because the brain substance is not penetrated; also, the device is secure in the skull and is not likely to be dislodged [Nussbaum and Maggi, 1985]. The method is independent of ventricular size and allows for some assessment of compliance. The disadvantages are the potential risk of meningitis because the dura is penetrated; the tendency for the devices to obstruct; and underreading of pressures, especially at levels of intracranial pressure over 20 torr [Mendelow et al., 1983].

Neonatal intracranial pressure monitoring

Infants with intracranial pathologic conditions present a problem when intracranial pressure monitoring is considered. Because the cranial bones are thin, it is not feasible to insert a heavy metal screw into a surface space. Invasive techniques, such as ventricular catheters, are not popular because of potential risks to the developing brain of a small infant. However, infants do develop increased intracranial pressure as a consequence of hydrocephalus, anoxia, and intracranial hemorrhage despite an open fontanel. Thus there are instances when intracranial pressure monitoring may be needed in the very sick infant. Methods of measuring intracranial pressure in infants include the use of flexible catheters, such as those used for intravenous treatment in older children [Levene and Evans, 1983]. The catheter may be placed within any of the surface spaces by entering through the anterior fontanel, using a conventional subdural puncture procedure. This method offers ease of insertion as an advantage; however, because of the flexibility, it is difficult to prevent movement of the catheter, which may result in air-fluid interfaces or blockage; thus intracranial pressure recordings would be false.

A more popular device, particularly for use in neonates, is the Ladd fiberoptic pressure transducer for measuring fontanel pressure [Vidyasagar and Raju, 1977]. The transducer is placed directly on the anterior fontanel and secured in position with a holding device. If properly fixed, intracranial pressure recordings appear to be reliable. The advantage to this method is its noninvasive nature. The primary drawbacks are those previously described for extradural recordings. Also, a change in position of the sensor may lead to false or inconsistent intracranial pressure recordings. The relationship between fontanel pressure and intracranial pressure is not clearly established [Ivan and Badejo, 1983]. Further refinement of this technique may be necessary before it has widespread clinical use.

Intracranial pressure recordings and plateau waves

A continuous recording of intracranial pressure gives the clinician much more information than the obvious pressure level. Recurrent oscillations are observed in the tracing, reflecting the change in intracranial pressure with each heart beat (Figure 13-2). The wider the oscillations, the lower the brain compliance. The observer may then readily detect changing compliance. A continuous paper tracing is preferred to record intracranial pressure because this affords a permanent record and previous activity can be reviewed to determine whether changes have occurred and whether there has been improvement or deterioration. Minor changes in intracranial pressure are found with respirations as well. Increased intrathoracic pressure increases intracranial pressure. During therapeutic maneuvers, such as chest

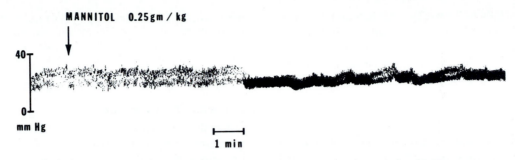

Figure 13-2 Continuous recording of intraventricular pressure in patient with Reye syndrome. Note wide oscillations with heartbeat, indicating poor compliance. Within 5 minutes after intravenous administration of mannitol, intracranial pressure decreases and compliance improves. (From Trauner DA, et al. Ann Neurol 1978; 4:275.)

physiotherapy or suctioning, intracranial pressure can be monitored closely to ensure that a sustained rise is not a result of these treatments.

Plateau waves that occur in association with increased intracranial pressure are rhythmic fluctuations in pressure that arise spontaneously from the baseline intracranial pressure, plateau at a higher pressure, and then return to the previous baseline (see Figure 13-1). Their presence is at times an ominous sign, heralding clinical deterioration [Lundberg, 1960]. The origin of plateau waves is not well-defined, although recent studies suggest that they represent changes in arteriolar tone [Rosner and Becker, 1984].

Lumbar puncture

Measurement of the opening pressure during a lumbar puncture, although of value, may be less accurate in pathologic states in which intracranial pressure is increased. Positioning the patient appropriately for a lumbar puncture can alter the CSF pressure. The technique is unsuitable for prolonged recording and provides only a single measurement over several seconds. In many conditions associated with intracranial pressure elevations the pressure fluctuates between normal values and abnormally high levels; if the lumbar pressure is measured during the trough of these fluctuations, an erroneous impression of normal intracranial pressure may be obtained.

TREATMENT

If increased intracranial pressure is suspected in a comatose child, intracranial pressure control should be approached in a sequential fashion, using only the method or methods necessary to maintain intracranial pressure and cerebral perfusion pressure in safe ranges. An arterial line should be inserted for frequent blood gas evaluations; arterial blood pressure recordings may then be obtained simultaneously with intracranial pressure measurements so that cerebral perfusion pressure may

be readily calculated. The child should have endotracheal intubation so that assisted ventilation may be provided if necessary. Careful chest physiotherapy may be necessary to prevent accumulation of mucous plugs that could increase intrathoracic pressure. The patient's head should be elevated 15 to 30 degrees.

Hyperventilation

Reducing the $Paco_2$ to 25 to 30 torr by controlled hyperventilation is effective in rapidly reducing intracranial pressure. CO_2 response curves indicate that below a $Paco_2$ of about 20 torr, no further decrease in cerebral blood flow occurs [Bruce, 1984]. Thus there is no therapeutic reason for hyperventilating the patient beyond this level. In addition to decreasing cerebral blood flow and cerebral blood volume, hyperventilation helps to reverse tissue and CSF acidosis, a complication common after severe brain injury or metabolic encephalopathy.

Although a theoretic concern exists that vigorous hyperventilation may produce brain ischemia, there is no direct evidence to support this contention; however, hyperventilation is potentially dangerous if performed improperly. If intrathoracic pressure is increased by the use of excessive ventilatory pressures, there may be impairment of venous return with poor cardiac output, a decrease in arterial blood pressure, and an increase in intracranial pressure.

Neuromuscular blockade

Paralysis with a neuromuscular blocking agent, such as pancuronium bromide, has several advantages. The muscle relaxation prevents spontaneous movements, such as thrashing or shivering, which can increase intracranial pressure. It also prevents coughing and spontaneous respiratory efforts by the patient, events that may increase intrathoracic pressure and then intracranial pressure. Respiratory paralysis allows the clinician to more easily administer controlled ventilation. In doses of 0.04 to 0.1 mg/kg, pancuronium bromide is effective as a muscle relaxant for up to 3 hours. The relatively short duration of action allows for frequent determinations of clinical status. If necessary, the effect of this medication can be reversed by administration of physostigmine.

CSF removal

If a ventricular catheter is present, removal of 1 to 2 ml of CSF results in rapid reduction of intracranial pressure and may eliminate plateau waves (see Figure 13-1). The effect is brief, lasting 15 to 60 minutes. It is a useful method when used in combination with mannitol to decrease the amount of diuretic needed.

Diuretic therapy

Diuretic treatment is used extensively in the acute management of intracranial pressure. The aim is to reduce water content in an edematous brain, thus reducing intracranial volume and intracranial pressure.

Osmotic diuretics set up an osmotic gradient across the blood-brain barrier, allowing water to move from brain to intravascular space; the excess water is then excreted in the urine. The most commonly used osmotic diuretic is mannitol. The usual dose is 0.25 to 1.0 g/kg body weight of a 20% solution, administered as a bolus intravenously. This dose reduces intracranial pressure within a few minutes (see Figure 13-2) and can be repeated as often as necessary to control intracranial pressure. The effect typically lasts 2 to 4 hours. Because mannitol works best when there is an osmotic gradient, continuous infusion of this agent is not as likely to be effective. Attention must be given to serum osmolarity because a high osmolarity reduces the response and may lead to impaired renal function (mannitol nephrosis). Serum osmolality should be kept below 310 mOsm when feasible, by altering intravenous fluid rates accordingly. When used in this fashion, mannitol does not lose its effectiveness, even when used frequently for several days. A brisk diuresis accompanies the administration of this agent; electrolyte, and fluid balance must be carefully monitored during its use.

Other hypertonic diuretics have limited usefulness in children. Hypertonic urea is effective in reducing intracranial pressure but rapidly diffuses into tissues, lessening its effect. Glycerol controls intracranial pressure in some situations, but concerns about hemolysis and hematuria have limited its use.

Loop diuretics, especially furosemide, are sometimes used for intracranial pressure control. The intravenous dose is 1 to 5 mg/kg. This agent has been used to reduce cerebral edema and intracranial pressure during subacute and chronic administration [Rose and Millac, 1966]. Its mechanism of action may be related to a reduction of sodium transport into brain, and an inhibition of CSF production [Tornheim et al., 1979]. In acute intracranial hypertension, use has been limited. The association of furosemide and mannitol has been advocated in instances of refractory intracranial pressure problems. Electrolyte and fluid status must be carefully monitored and balance maintained.

Corticosteroid therapy

Corticosteroids have been used in many conditions associated with brain edema and increased intracranial pressure with variable results. Steroids are most effective in patients with mass lesions and less so in patients with head trauma and metabolic encephalopathy. Steroids have multiple effects on neuronal and glial metabolism and may exert a protective effect other than an antiedema role [Hall, 1985]. The typical dose of dexamethasone is 1 mg/kg/dose intravenously. Deleterious side effects include infection and gastric hemorrhage, which are uncommon when this agent is used in an acute situation [James et al., 1979].

Barbiturate therapy

Barbiturates have a number of effects on the brain, including reduction in cerebral blood flow and cerebral metabolic rate for oxygen ($CMRo_2$), that result in reduction of intracranial pressure. Although a cerebral protective effect aside from intracranial pressure control has been suggested for barbiturates, there is no convincing evidence for this phenomenon [Trauner, 1986]. The short-acting barbiturates, pentobarbital and thiopental, are used most often. A typical treatment regimen is to give a loading dose of 10 to 15 mg/kg intravenously over 1 hour, followed by a maintenance schedule of 2 to 3 mg/kg/hour to maintain a serum concentration in the range of 25 to 40 µg/ml. Alternatively, small, intermittent doses may be used when necessary to reduce intracranial pressure.

Continuous barbiturate therapy is associated with significant side effects. The most common are cardiac depression and severe systemic hypotension. Pressor agents may be required to maintain blood pressure in the normal range. Because patients receiving this treatment are in iatrogenic deep coma, intensive supportive care is critical for prolonged periods. It is best to reserve this mode of treatment for severe and intractible intracranial hypertension in only the most seriously ill patients.

PSEUDOTUMOR CEREBRI

Pseudotumor cerebri, sometimes termed *benign intracranial hypertension*, differs from other causes of elevated intracranial pressure because it is characterized by a chronic increase in intracranial pressure with otherwise normal CSF examination, normal radiographic studies, and typically mild symptomatology [Rose and Matson, 1967; Weisberg and Chutorian, 1977]. Pseudotumor cerebri may occur throughout childhood. Symptoms include headache, diplopia, and occasionally tinnitus, vertigo, or decreased visual acuity. Neurologic examination is usually normal with the exception of papilledema and, rarely, cranial nerve VI paresis. Despite sometimes markedly increased intracranial pressure, there is no impairment of consciousness or risk of herniation. The primary potential danger of this condition is permanent visual impairment. Pseudotumor cerebri may be precipitated by a number of problems [Moffat, 1978], including use of antibiotics (e.g., tetracycline, sulfonamides, gentamicin), oral contraceptives, phenothiazines, and vitamin A. Both use of and withdrawal from steroids may cause pseudotumor cerebri. Systemic disorders, such as iron deficiency anemia, histiocytosis X, systemic lupus erythematosus, sinusitis, mastoiditis and otitis media, deficiencies of vitamins D and A, and obesity, as well as intracranial venous sinus thrombosis, have all been associated with development of pseudotumor cerebri.

The pathogenesis of pseudotumor cerebri is controversial. Although intracellular and extracellular edema have been observed in needle-biopsy specimens, these alterations are unlikely to be major factors, given the paucity of symptoms. Other potential factors include an increase in cerebral blood volume [Raichle et al., 1978], impaired CSF absorption [Sklar et al., 1979], and increased CSF production [Donaldson, 1981].

Diagnosis of pseudotumor cerebri is based on the presence of papilledema and absence of other significant neurologic deficits on examination, normal EEG and radiologic studies (except in the presence of cerebral venous sinus thrombosis, which causes the ventricular system to be small on CT scan), elevated CSF pressure (200 mg H_2O or greater) on lumbar puncture, and otherwise normal CSF examination. MRI angiography is particularly useful in documenting dural venous sinus thrombosis.

Pseudotumor cerebri is generally self-limited. The disorder may remit after a single lumbar puncture. If not, the standard treatment consists of repeated lumbar punctures until the intracranial pressure remains normal. Acetazolamide and other diuretics are sometimes effective. Oral corticosteroid administration often controls intracranial pressure, but patients may become dependent on steroids. Lumboperitoneal shunts may be necessary in refractory, long-term cases. The object of treatment is to reduce symptoms, but the most important objective is to prevent permanent visual impairment.

REFERENCES

Bruce DA. Effects of hyperventilation on cerebral blood flow and metabolism. Clin Perinatol 1984; 11:673.

Dearden NM, McDowall DG, Gibson RM. Assessment of Leeds device for monitoring intracranial pressure. J Neurosurg 1984; 60:123.

Donaldson JO. Pathogenesis of pseudotumor cerebri syndromes. Neurology 1981; 31:877.

Duncan CC, Ment LR. Indications and methods of measurement of intracranial pressure. Conn Med 1984; 48:141.

Friden HG, Ekstedt J. Volume/pressure relationship of the cerebrospinal space in humans. Neurosurgery 1983; 13:351.

Hall ED. High-dose glucocorticoid treatment improves neurological recovery in head-injured mice. J Neurosurg 1985; 62:882.

Havill JH. Prolonged hyperventilation and intracranial pressure. Crit Care Med 1984; 12:72.

Ivan LP, Badejo A. Clinical and experimental observations with fontanel pressure measurements. Childs Brain 1983; 10:361.

James HE, Bruno L, Schut L, et al. Intracranial subarachnoid pressure monitoring in children. Surg Neurol 1975; 3:313.

James HE, Madauss WC, Tibbs PA, et al. The effect of high dose dexamethasone therapy in children with severe head injury. Acta Neurochir 1979; 45:225.

Levene MI, Evans DH. Continuous measurement of subarachnoid pressure in the severely asphyxiated newborn. Arch Dis Child 1983; 58:1013.

Lou MC, Lassen NA, Friis-Hansen B. Impaired autoregulation of cerebral blood flow in the distressed newborn infant. J Pediatr 1979; 94:118.

Lundberg N. Continuous recording and control of ventricular fluid pressure in neurosurgical practice. Acta Psychiatr Neurol Scand 1960; 36 (suppl. 149):1.

Mendelow AD, Rowan JO, Murray L, et al. A clinical comparison of subdural screw pressure measurements with ventricular pressure. J Neurosurg 1983; 58:45.

Minns RA. Intracranial pressure monitoring. Arch Dis Child 1984; 59:486.

Moffat FL. Pseudotumor cerebri. J Can Sci Neurol 1978; 5:431.

Nussbaum E, Maggi JC. Intracranial pressure monitoring by subarachnoid bolt in comatose children. Clin Pediatr 1985; 24:329.

Raichle ME, Posner JB, Plum F. Cerebral blood flow during and after hyperventilation. Arch Neurol 1970; 23:394.

Raichle ME, Grubb RL, Phelps ME, et al. Cerebral hemodynamics and metabolism in pseudotumor cerebri. Ann Neurol 1978; 4:104.

Rose A, Matson DD. Benign intracranial hypertension in children. Pediatrics 1967; 39:227.

Rose AL, Millac P. The treatment of benign intracranial hypertension with furosemide. J Neurol Sci 1966; 3:606.

Rosner MJ, Becker DP. ICP monitoring: complications and associated factors. Clin Neurosurg 1976; 23:494.

Rosner MJ, Becker DP. Origin and evolution of plateau waves: experimental observations and a theoretical model. J Neurosurg 1984; 60:312.

Siesjo BK. Cerebral circulation and metabolism. J Neurosurg 1984; 60:883.

Sklar FH, Beyer CW, Ramanathan M, et al. Cerebrospinal fluid dynamics in patients with pseudotumor cerebri. Neurosurgery 1979; 5:208.

Smith RW, Alksne JF. Infections complicating the use of external ventriculostomy. J Neurosurg 1976; 44:567.

Szewczykowski J, Dytko P, Kunick A, et al. A method of estimating intracranial decompensation in man. J Neurosurg 1976; 45:155.

Tornheim PA, McLauren RL, Sawaya R. Effect of furosemide on experimental traumatic cerebral edema. Neurosurgery 1979; 4:48.

Trauner DA, Brown F, Ganz E, et al. Treatment of elevated intracranial pressure in Reye syndrome. Ann Neurol 1978; 4:275.

Trauner DA. Barbiturate therapy for acute brain injury. J Pediatr 1986; 108.

Vidyasagar D, Raju TNK. A simple noninvasive technique of measuring intracranial pressure in the newborn. Pediatrics 1977; 59:957.

Weisberg LA, Chutorian AM. Pseudotumor cerebri of childhood. Am J Dis Child 1977; 131:1243.

14

Microcephaly, Micrencephaly, Megalocephaly, and Megalencephaly

William DeMyer

MECHANISMS AND PATHOPHYSIOLOGY OF CRANIAL AND BRAIN DIMENSIONS

Definitions

Megalocephaly and its antonym, microcephaly, indicate diametrically opposite head sizes (*cephalon* meaning "head"). Megalencephaly and its antonym, micrencephaly, indicate diametrically opposite brain weights (*encephalon* meaning "brain"). These four terms designate the smallness or largeness of the cranium or brain, respectively, without specifying the cause of the abnormal dimension or the integrity of brain function [Friede, 1989]. A small head must contain a small, underweight brain, although the brain may function well. A large head may contain a large cerebrum as occurs in megalencephaly, a small, compressed cerebrum as occurs in chronic subdural hematomas [Cadman et al., 1968], or virtually no cerebrum as occurs in hydranencephaly. In severe hydranencephaly the supratentorial space contains only fluid, which may result in megalocephaly if not absorbed properly. When the pathologic process simultaneously reduces the size of the brain and greatly increases the amount of intracranial fluid, both megalocephaly and micrencephaly coexist [DeMyer, 1993].

Components of cranial dimensions

The OFC is determined by the intracranial volume, the ability of the cranial sutures to expand, and the thickness of the skull bones and scalp. The total intracranial volume is a composite of brain volume, CSF volume in ventricles and subarachnoid spaces as determined by CSF dynamics, blood volume in the intracranial vessels as determined by hemodynamics, and the presence of space-occupying lesions.

Genetic constitution, disease, and age alter all of these factors. Many errors of chromosomal morphology—translocations, trisomies, nondisjunctions, and duplications—cause a small, defective brain. Some genetic disorders such as neurofibromatosis I and achondroplasia regularly cause large brains. Genetic factors determine much of the normal variation in brain size and hence OFC [Weaver and Christian, 1980]. The OFC of males averages 1 to 2 cm more than that of females. In persons older than 1 year of age, the normal range for the OFC equals about 5 cm (two standard deviations above the mean minus two below). The OFC increases linearly with height. The mean circumference of mature tall individuals exceeds that of short individuals by 4 to 5 cm [Bale et al., 1991]. The head size may be proportionate or disproportionate to the somatotype.

Changes in OFC during maturation

At term the average infant's OFC measures about 35 cm, the brain weighs about 350 g, and the infant weighs about 3500 g. The brain weight and body weight roughly double in 6 months and triple by 1 year of age, when the brain reaches 950 of its 1350 g of final weight. At 3.5 years of age the OFC averages about 50 cm. In the immediate postnatal period before normal growth begins the OFC may decrease a centimeter or so, as birth-induced scalp edema, bruising, and head molding resolve. The expansion of the skull by the growing brain normally produces the standard OFC growth curve. During the first year, the OFC increases at an average rate of about 1 cm per month, with growth occurring more rapidly in the first 6 months. In the first few postnatal months the OFC normally increases about 0.4

cm per week. In megalencephaly the OFC increases at a mean rate of approximately 0.6 cm per week [DeMyer, 1972], and in obstructive hydrocephalus, expansion occurs even more rapidly. The circumference of premature or malnourished infants who subsequently receive an adequate diet may increase more rapidly than normal [Sher and Brown, 1975]. When the infant has an abnormally small or large circumference or when successive plots of the circumference cross graph lines upward or downward, abnormal brain growth should be suspected (see Figures 4-1 and 5-12).

Bray et al. [1969] reported that the OFC correlated strongly with the intracranial volume. Gooskens et al. [1988a] advocate multiplying the OFC by the head height as a better measure of volume. New MRI programs allow direct computation of brain volume.

Correlation between brain size and intelligence

In general the brain size as reflected in the OFC correlates with IQ scores; however, with either too large or too small a brain, intellectual function declines. The inverted U curve in Figure 14-1 illustrates the decline in brain function when the brain weighs more or less than the optimum. Although microcephalic individuals can be intellectually normal [Dorman, 1991], the degree of intellectual impairment parallels the smallness of the head. Only 14% of individuals with an OFC two standard deviations below the mean had IQs above 100, whereas 0% of individuals with circumferences three standard deviations below the mean had IQs above 100 [Dolk,

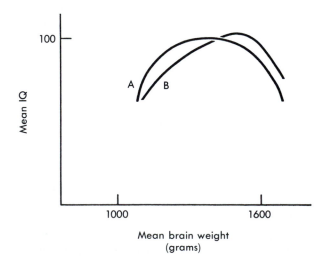

Figure 14-1 Inverted U curve showing a reduction in the dependent variable (Y axis) as the independent variable (X axis) deviates above or below the mean [DeMyer, 1986]. **A,** Theoretical inverted U curve showing IQ as a function of brain weight. **B,** Actual inverted U showing that the zone of optimum brain weight for higher IQ shifts to the right.

1991]. In the Collaborative Perinatal Study of the National Institutes of Health, infants with OFCs slightly greater than the mean also had slightly higher IQ scores at 4 years of age. The IQ scores increased almost linearly from 46 to 47 cm to 52 to 53 cm. Then, however, the IQ scores for three of the four groups decreased with a further increase in the OFC, demonstrating an inverted U curve [Broman et al., 1975]. Correspondingly, male college students with IQs greater than 130 had somewhat larger OFCs than college students who had IQs around 100 [Willerman, 1991]. The literature reports many mentally deficient patients whose brains range from 1600 g upward. The largest human brain on record (2850 g) belonged to a mentally defective individual with epilepsy [van Walsem, 1899].

The strength of association between microcephaly, macrocephaly, and intellectual deficit varies with the population studied [Smith et al., 1984]. In school children consecutively selected solely because of a large OFC, Lorber and Priestly [1981] found retardation in only 7 of 109 with megalencephaly; 9 of the children had epilepsy. In a series of 18 consecutive patients who were highly selected by referral to a specialty hospital, 9 were intellectually deficient [DeMyer, 1972].

Occipitofrontal circumference

Because a deviant circumference warns of an abnormal brain, the OFC of every infant should be measured regularly. Ideally the OFC should be measured monthly during the first year, every 3 months during the second year, every 6 months during years 3 to 5, and once a year thereafter. A tape measure is stretched across the glabella and extended laterally around the head to the occiput to encircle the largest circumference [DeMyer, 1993]. The measurements should be plotted on standard OFC forms (see Figure 14-1). (Figure 5-12 depicts the OFC for premature infants.)

The OFC is customarily plotted in percentiles rather than standard deviations. Expressing the circumference in standard deviations is more useful for comparative purposes. Percentiles and standard deviations of these measurements can be determined from a standard table [Roche et al., 1987]. Statistically an abnormal OFC is one that is more than two standard deviations above or below the mean.

MICROCEPHALY/MICRENCEPHALY

The term *microcephaly* indicates an OFC that falls two or more standard deviations below the mean established for the individual's age and gender. The presence of microcephaly necessitates a small brain (micrencephaly). Microcephaly implies the likelihood of a neurologically impaired individual; however, the OFC of 2.5% of the normal population falls below two standard deviations from the mean.

Pathogenesis

Although hypoplastic, the brain in primary micrencephaly (microcephaly vera) has a fairly normal overall contour and sulcal pattern and has no destructive lesions per se, thus implying a prenatal cause, usually genetic or idiopathic, for the condition. The basal ganglia, brainstem, and cerebellum may appear normal, or in fact enlarged, in comparison with the small cerebrum.

In malformative micrencephaly, more extensive abnormalities are present, such as macrogyria, microgyria, and migratory disturbances [Friede, 1989] or gross deviations of contour as in holoprosencephaly [DeMyer, 1987]; and lissencephaly [Dobyns et al., 1992]. The cause is usually genetic or teratogenic but is sometimes infectious [Hayward et al., 1991].

Secondary or destructive micrencephaly implies a potentially or genetically normal brain that has suffered a prenatal or perinatal insult, usually inflammatory or anoxic or as a result of an exogenous teratogen. Typical lesions consist of single or multifocal porencephaly, thickened meninges, ventriculitis, periventricular calcification, and cortical laminar necrosis. Calcification suggests tuberous sclerosis, cytomegalovirus, toxoplasmosis, Cockayne syndrome, acquired immunodeficiency syndrome, hyperthyroidism, rubella, varicella [Bonnemann et al., 1991; Scheffer et al., 1991], and some forms of familial calcification of the basal ganglia.

Approach

The presence of a small OFC does not predict which developmental abnormalities may ensue in the form of retardation, seizures, and learning or behavioral disabilities [Lewis et al., 1983]. After an appropriate evaluation and follow-up period the clinician ultimately discovers whether the microcephalic patient is neurologically normal or abnormal (asymptomatic or symptomatic). Asymptomatic patients with OFCs that deviate two standard deviations or more below the mean, who have no other syndromic anomalies, and who remain neurologically normal on subsequent examinations finally receive a diagnosis of asymptomatic (benign) microcephaly representing merely an OFC in the lower tail of the normal distribution curve. If the patient has any neurologic deficits or other anomalies, the clinician must consider specific pathologic entities.

The causes for pathologic micrencephaly range from genetic to acquired. The etiologic agent may act at one time as a single teratologic insult, throughout the pregnancy, or only in the perinatal or early postnatal period. Maternal predispositions include the presence or history of viral infections, exposure to ionizing radiation, diabetes, uremia, phenylketonuria, malnutrition, carbon-monoxide intoxication, ingestion of a variety of prescription and street drugs, and alcohol use and smoking. Many drugs taken during pregnancy, especially in the first weeks during the period of organogenesis, may impair brain development. Ironically, the agents that cause microcephaly may also cause hydrocephalus and megalocephaly because of impaired absorption of CSF. The sutures close earlier than normal in microcephaly, but closure usually does not result in palpable ridges. The examiner can easily identify a small head resulting from craniosynostosis because of the abnormal shape, usually oxycephaly, and the readily palpable ridging of the sutures. Plain skull radiographs or scans provide confirmation. Scalp rugae may accompany some microcephaly of prenatal onset that causes collapse of the skull [Russell et al., 1984]. The box on p. 208 lists the most common identifiable causes of microcephaly.

Investigation of micrencephaly requires a systematic consideration of each of the categories listed in the box. Obtain a very careful pedigree, measure the OFC and height of siblings and parents, and ascertain the somatotype of the family. By correcting for normal familial variations in somatotype, mainly in height and OFC [Bale et al., 1991; Weaver and Christian, 1980], the examiner can begin to separate otherwise normal infants whose OFC happens to fall in the lower extreme of the normal distribution curve from those with pathologic microcephaly. When neurologic, facial, or extracephalic abnormalities accompany the microcephaly, the patient generally has a specific, previously described syndrome [Buyse, 1990; Gorlin et al., 1990; Jones, 1988]. (For a more extensive listing of the syndromes and the use of various computerized indices, particularly for genetic syndromes, see McKusick [1988], Opitz and Holt [1990], and Winter and Baraitser [1990].)

The clinician should image the brain by MRI scan in virtually all patients with an abnormal OFC. MRI scans are greatly superior to CT for differentiating gray and white matter and for demonstrating abnormalities of neuronal migration, sulcation, and gyration; the patterns of myelin deposition or demyelination; and the details of basal ganglia, brainstem, and cerebellum.

Screening for prenatal and perinatal infections is routine. Common infections include rubella, herpes simplex, coxsackie virus and cytomegalovirus, acquired immunodeficiency syndrome, syphilis, and toxoplasmosis. In addition to titers for these conditions being performed, the urine and CSF are cultured in a neonate.

The urine or urine and blood are routinely screened for aminoacidurias and organic acidurias. Blood lactic and pyruvic acid levels may suggest the presence of metabolic diseases that restrict energy production. If the developmental course suggests retrogression, a lysosomal enzyme battery, muscle, or skin biopsy should be considered (see Chapter 9).

Common Causes for Microcephaly/ Micrencephaly	

1. Infections
  Cytomegalovirus
  Herpes simplex
  Rubella
  Varicella
  Coxsackie B virus
  Acquired immunode-
    ficiency syndrome
  Toxoplasmosis
  Syphilis
  Postmeningitis
2. Drugs
  Alcohol
  Tobacco
  Marijuana
  Cocaine
  Heroin
  Anticancer
  Antiepileptic
  Prescription
3. Anoxia
  Generalized cerebral
    anoxia
  Poststatus epilepticus
  Porencephaly/
    hydranencephaly
  Carbon monoxide
    poisoning
  Placental insuffici-
    ency
4. Hereditary
  Normal, variation in
    OFC, asymptomatic
  Mendelian pattern,
    symptomatic:
    autosomal domi-
    nant, autosomal re-
    cessive, or X-linked
  Craniosynostosis
  Heredofamilial de-
    generative diseases
  Pelizaeus-
    Merzbacher
    disease
  Neuronal ceroid-
    lipofuscinosis
    (Batten disease)
  Aminoacidurias/
    organic acidurias
	Miscellaneous syn-
	    dromes, frequently
	    with dwarfism
	    (achondroplastic
	    type excluded)
	  Smith-Lemli-Opitz
	    syndrome
	  de Lange syndrome
	  Rubenstein-Taybi
	    syndrome
	  Dubowitz syndrome
	  Proportionate short
	    stature syn-
	    dromes [Buyse,
	    1990; Gorlin
	    et al., 1990]
	5. Chromosomal
	  Down syndrome
	    and other
	    trisomies
	  Ring chromo-
	    somes
	  Deletions
	  Sex chromosome
	    aneuploidy
	6. Malformations
	  Microcephaly vera
	  Atelencephaly
	  Holoprosencephaly
	    [DeMyer, 1987]
	  Lissencephaly
	    [Dobyns, 1992]
	  Encephalocele
	7. Trauma
	  Birth trauma
	  Child abuse
	8. Perinatal metabolic/
	    endocrine imbal-
	    ances
	  Hypoglycemia
	  Hypothyroidism
	  Hypopituitarism
	  Hypoadreno-
	    corticism
	9. Malnutrition
	10. Prenatal Maternal
	    Illness
	  Systemic illness
	  Anemia
	  Malnutrition
	  Toxic exposures

Chromosomal studies are ordered if the history reveals early spontaneous abortions or if the patient is neurologically impaired or dysmorphic.

Asymptomatic (familial) microcephaly. Infants with pathologic micrencephaly must often be separated from those whose OFC falls in the lower ranges of the normal distribution curve but who have normal intelligence and no neurologic defects [Day and Schutt, 1979; DeMyer, 1986; Heney et al., 1992]. Usually these infants have no facial or extracephalic anomalies, but one family has been described with hypotelorism [Evans, 1991]. The diagnosis of asymptomatic familial microcephaly is confirmed by the absence of any risk factors for pathologic microcephaly, small OFCs in family members who are neurologically normal, autosomal dominant transmission, usually a proportionately small body size, and finally and most important, a normal developmental course. If doubts remain about the patient's neurologic status, the clinician should start the workup with an MRI scan and proceed as described.

Symptomatic familial microcephaly. The genetic pattern of familial symptomatic microcephaly may be autosomal-dominant, autosomal-recessive, X-linked, or polygenic [Haslam, 1987; Komai et al., 1955; McKusick, 1988; Opitz and Holt, 1990]. In the less severe autosomal-dominant form the patients may have normal facies and an otherwise normal somatotype. The autosomal-recessive form may be very severe, with a striking discrepancy between the normal size of the face and the small calvarium. Pelizaeus-Merzbacher disease, an X-linked recessive microcephaly, becomes apparent at or shortly after birth by nystagmoid eye movements, ataxia, and profound-to-moderate retardation [Zeman et al., 1964].

Management of symptomatic microcephaly/ micrencephaly

The justification for an exhaustive etiologic search lies in determining the recurrence risk and the possibility for preventing microcephaly in subsequent children. The recurrence risk depends on the risk of the same etiologic agent acting again. The empirical recurrence risk of symptomatic microcephaly without a known etiologic or specific syndromic diagnosis is 6% to 20% [Opitz and Holt, 1990].

The clinician should never declare that a microcephalic infant has a dismal prognosis. The proof must come from the slow developmental course. Delayed visual fixation, head control, smiling, eye-hand use, and vocalizations establish symptomatic microcephaly.

MEGALOCEPHALY

The term *megalocephaly* (macrocephaly) indicates an OFC that exceeds the mean by two or more standard

Most Common Causes for Megalocephaly	

1. Hydrocephalus
   Noncommunicating
      Chiari malformation
      Aqueductal stenosis
      Dandy-Walker
         malformation
         [Pascual-
         Castroviejo et
         al., 1991b]
      Walker-Warburg
         syndrome
         (lissencephaly
         and Dandy-
         Walker)
   Neoplasms, supra-
      tentorial and
      infratentorial
   Arachnoid cyst,
      infratentorial
      [Pascual-
      Castroviejo
      et al., 1991]
   Holoprosencephaly
      with dorsal
      interhemispheric
      sac [DeMyer, 1987]
   Communicating
      External or extra-
         ventricular
         obstructive hydro-
         cephalus
         (dilated subarach-
         noid space) [Al-
         varez et al., 1986;
         Gooskens et al.,
         1988a]
      Arachnoid cyst,
         supratentorial
         [Pascual-
         Castroviejo et al.,
         1991a]
      Meningeal fibrosis/
         obstruction
      Postinflammatory
      Posthemorrhagic
      Neoplastic in-
         filtration
	Vascular
	   Arteriovenous
	      malformation
	   Intracranial
	      hemorrhage
	   Dural sinus
	      thrombosis
	   Galenic vein
	      aneurysm
	   Choroid plexus
	      papilloma
	   Neurocutaneous
	      syndrome
	   Incontinentia
	      pigmenti
	Destructive lesions
	   Hydranencephaly
	   Porencephaly
	Familial, autosomal-
	   dominant, auto-
	   somal-recessive,
	   or X-linked
	   [McKusick, 1988]
	2. Megalencephaly (see
	   box on p. 211)
	   Anatomic
	   Metabolic
	   Hydrodynamic
	   Megalencephaly
	      with hydroceph-
	      alic complica-
	      tion: achondro-
	      plasia and
	      mucopoly-
	      saccharidoses
	3. Subdural fluid
	   Hematoma
	   Hygroma
	   Empyema
	4. Brain edema (toxic-
	   metabolic)
	   Intoxication
	      Lead
	      Vitamin A
	      Tetracycline
	   Endocrine
	      Hypoparathy-
	         roidism
	      Hypo-
	         adreno corticism
	   Galactosemia
	   Spongy degenera-
	      tion of the brain
	   Idiopathic (pseudo-
	      tumor cerebri)

Most Common Causes for Megalocephaly—cont'd	

5. Thick skull
   Familial variation
   Anemia
   Myotonia dystrophica
   Cranioskeletal dysplasia
      Rickets
      Osteopetrosis
      Osteogenesis
         imperfecta
      Orodigitofacial
         dysostosis
      Craniometaphyseal
         dysplasia of Pyle
	Cleidocranial
	   dysostosis
	Hyperphospha-
	   tasemia
	Epiphyseal dysplasia
	Russell dwarf
	Pycnodyostosis
	Leontiasis ossea
	Progressive diaphy-
	   seal dysplasia
	Proteus (elephant
	   man) syndrome

deviations for the age and gender of the patient. The OFC may already exceed two standard deviations by the time of birth, or if the infant has a normal OFC at birth, it may accelerate postnatally. As with microcephaly, megalocephaly constitutes a statistical description, not a diagnosis.

Causes

The five most common causes of megalocephaly are the following [DeMyer, 1993]:

- Hydrocephalus, communicating and noncommunicating
- Megalencephaly
- Subdural fluid collection
- Brain edema (toxic-metabolic)
- Thickened skull (bone dysplasia)

The box provides a more extensive list of the most common causes of megalocephaly.

Approach

History taking and pedigree. Record the infant's birth OFC and determine whether successive OFC measurements parallel the normal curve or accelerate (see Figures 4-1 and 5-12). The clinician should also determine whether the patient is improving developmentally or retrogressing. Retrogression indicates an ongoing, active pathologic process, that is causing deterioration, thus differentiating these patients from those with static causes for megalocephaly. Poor feeding, vomiting, irritability, and a disturbed sleep pattern suggest increased intracranial pressure.

In addition to the routine pedigree, the examiner should specifically inquire about other large-headed babies or individuals in the family. Parents will frequently remember that a grandparent required a very large hat. The examiner should then compare the OFC of the infant with the OFC and somatotype of parents and siblings. If abnormalities are present, investigate the other blood relatives.

Physical examination. Determine the size and contour of the fontanels and palpate the sutures. With the infant relaxed and upright, the normal anterior fontanel has a slightly concave contour. The contour can be best appreciated by palpation and by shining a light tangentially across the fontanel. Increased intracranial pressure causes an enlarged, convex anterior fontanel and palpable separation of the sutures. If hydrocephalus or increased intracranial pressure occurs after 10 to 12 years of age, the sutures will no longer yield and macrocephaly will not result. To complete the neurologic examination, the examiner dilates the pupils and performs ophthalmoscopy. Carefully search for neurocutaneous stigmata, particularly café au lait spots and other pigmentations, hemangiomas, and the ash leaf–contoured, depigmented spots of tuberous sclerosis.

The examiner can recognize some types of megalocephaly from the pedigree or physical examination without an extensive investigation. For achondroplastic dwarfs, patients with Hurler syndrome, or those with craniofacioskeletal dysplasia syndromes with a thickened skull, inspection of the somatotype leads to the correct diagnosis (see the box on p. 209).

The megalocephalic patient who does not display a clinically diagnosable syndrome requires a systematic, carefully planned sequence of ancillary investigations. After radiographic imaging of the brain, preferably MRI, try to assign the patient to one of the five major diagnostic categories listed in the box on p. 209. If the patient is dysmorphic or has a dysplastic body or if an endocrine or metabolic disorder is suspected, consider a radiographic survey of the bones and a metabolic-endocrine evaluation. Urinary screening for abnormal amino acids, increased amino acid excretion, or organic acids is required for infants with unexplained megalocephaly [Hoffman et al., 1991; Leupold et al., 1982; Plochl et al., 1991]. Depending on the history, obtain blood vitamin A and lead levels. Either low or high vitamin A levels may cause macrocephaly [Kasarkis and Bass, 1982].

MEGALENCEPHALY
Mechanisms and pathophysiology

Megalencephaly designates an oversized and overweight brain that exceeds the mean by two or more standard deviations for the age and gender of the patient [DeMyer, 1972]. A more accurate but little used term, *megalobarencephaly*, emphasizes the indispensable requirement of an excessive brain weight. Thus a hydrocephalic brain may have an increased circumference but a reduced weight (excluding ventricular fluid) because of thinning of the cerebral wall. Gooskens et al. [1988b]

define megalencephaly as a brain with a volume exceeding the mean by two standard deviations as calculated from radiographic imaging.

Approach

The approach to megalencephaly is essentially the same as cited for macrocephaly.

Etiology. Two types of megalencephaly occur: anatomic and metabolic [DeMyer, 1972]. Anatomic megalencephaly designates brain enlargement because of an increased number and/or size of cells but with no known metabolic abnormality. Metabolic megalencephaly designates brain enlargement because of the accumulation of a metabolic product, abnormal in type or quantity, without an increased number of cells.

Some authors suggest a third pathogenetic type, hydrodynamic megalencephaly, which is related to increased venous pressure or decreased CSF absorption [Alvarez et al., 1986; Bresnan and Lorenzo, 1975; Gooskens et al., 1985; Gooskens et al., 1988b; Govaert et al., 1991; Portnoy and Croissant, 1978; Talwar et al., 1990]. The box classifies the types of megalencephaly.

The box omits several syndromes with megalocephaly that resist classification because of uncertainty whether true megalencephaly is present or some other cause for megalocephaly exists. These include fragile X syndrome; agenesis of the corpus callosum [Schinzel and Schmid, 1980; Young et al., 1985]; Greig syndrome [Gollop and Fontes, 1985]; Proteus syndrome [Cohen, 1988; Wiedemann et al., 1983]; Weaver-Smith syndrome of excessive growth, dysmorphic facies, mental retardation, and advanced bone age [Amir et al., 1984]; transient macrocephaly with brain edema, hypernatremia, and fluid retention [Marty and Zurbrugg, 1982]; and other rare conditions with macrocephaly [Gorlin et al., 1990]. Although older patients with Duchenne muscular dystrophy commonly have larger than average OFCs [Appleton et al., 1991a], the average brain weight remains controversial. Three of the four patients of Schmidt et al. [1985] with large OFCs showed megalencephaly on CT scans.

Pathology of the anatomic megalencephalies

The most common type of megalencephaly occurs in patients with otherwise normal brains that happen to fall two standard deviations or more above the mean in the upper reaches of the normal distribution curve (see p. 212). Whether such brains contain an increased number and/or increased size of neurons or glia is unknown due to methodologic problems in counting cells and distinguishing glia from small neurons. In symptomatic anatomic megalencephaly, lesions may consist of distorted cells, disturbed cortical lamination, heterotopias that stud the ventricular surface or the white matter, and micropolygyria or pachygyria

Differential Diagnosis of Megalencephaly

1. Anatomic megalencephaly
   Focal megalencephaly
   Oekonomakis malformation [Becker, 1990; Dodgson, 1955]
   Cerebellar, Lehrmitte-Duclos [Gessaga, 1980]
   Other [Choi et al., 1980]
   Unilateral megalencephaly
   Without somatic hemihypertrophy [Dambska et al., 1984]
   With somatic hemihypertrophy and hemangiomatosis/hamartomas [Gorlin et al., 1990]
   Klippel-Trenauny-Weber syndrome [Matsubara et al., 1983]
   Bilateral megalencephaly
   Without extraneural malformations or abnormal stature
   Asymptomatic familial anatomic megalencephaly (neurologically normal individual with excessive brain weight); autosomal dominant heredity [Lorber and Priestly, 1981; Day and Schutt, 1979; DeMyer, 1972; Schrier et al., 1974]
   Symptomatic familial anatomic megalencephaly (neurologically abnormal individual with excessive brain weight who does not match another syndrome, autosomal-dominant or autosomal-recessive transmission [DeMyer, 1986; Lewis et al., 1983])
   Idiopathic (sporadic) symptomatic anatomic megalencephaly (nonfamilial)
   With gigantism
   Sotos syndrome of cerebral gigantism [Winship, 1985]
   Pituitary
   Arachnodactyly
   Adiposogigantism [Wechselberg and Neumann, 1965]
   Weaver-Smith syndrome [Amir et al., 1984]
   With dwarfism/small stature
   Achondroplastic dwarf
   Thanatophoric dwarf
   FG syndrome [Opitz et al., 1982; Thompson et al., 1985]
   Robinow syndrome [Gorlin et al., 1990]
   Multiple endocrinopathy [DeMyer, 1972]

   With neurocutaneous syndrome
   Neurofibromatosis
   Tuberous sclerosis
   Hypomelanosis of Ito [Ross et al., 1982]
   Nevoid basal cell carcinoma [Bale et al., 1991]
   Organoid nevus syndrome [Clancy et al., 1985]
   Ataxia telangiectasia [Scott, 1969]
   With multiple hemangiomatosis, lipomatosis, hamartomas, and tissue overgrowth the Bannayan-Zonana-Ruvacalba-Myhra-Riley-Smith syndromes [DiLiberti et al., 1984; Gorlin et al., 1990; Holden and Alexander, 1970; Miles et al., 1984; Okumura et al., 1986]
   Cowden syndrome of multiple hamartomas and extraneural neoplasia [Civatte et al., 1979; Gorlin et al., 1990]
   With Klinefelter syndrome [Budka, 1978; Choi et al., 1980]
   Miscellaneous
   Dysencephalia splanchoncystica [Hori et al., 1980]
   Endocardial fibroelastosis and microphallus [Jennings et al., 1980]
   Duchenne muscular dystrophy [Appleton et al., 1991a; DeMyer, 1972]
   Beckwith-Wiedemann syndrome
   Collins-Hoshino syndrome [Hoshino, 1981]
   Van Benthem syndrome [Van Benthem, 1970]
   Midfacial deformity and long philtrum [Cole and Hughes, 1991]
2. Metabolic megalencephaly
   Lysosomal diseases
   Tay-Sach disease
   Generalized gangliosidosis
   Mucopolysaccharidoses
   Metachromatic leukodystrophy
   Aminoaciduria/organic aciduria
   Maple syrup urine disease
   Methylglutaryl-CoA lyase-deficiency [Leupold et al., 1982]
   Spongy degeneration of Canavan [Luo and Huang, 1984]
   Alexander disease [Borrett and Becker, 1985; Pietrini et al., 1983]
   Hypoparathyroidism-hypoadrenocorticism
3. Hydrodynamic megalencephaly (decreased venous or CSF outflow) [Alvarez et al., 1986; Bresnan and Lorenzo, 1975; Gooskens et al., 1988b; Portnoy and Croissant, 1978; Talwar et al., 1990]

[Friede, 1989; Lemire et al., 1975; Muller, 1983; Ross et al., 1982].

The brains of some megalencephalic patients display a tendency to hamartomas, neoplasia, or exuberant overgrowth beyond the overall brain enlargement

[Civatte et al., 1979; Gorlin et al., 1990; Halal and Silver, 1989; Ronnett et al., 1990]. Neoplasms of the CNS and peripheral nervous system are common in neurofibromatosis and tuberous sclerosis. In Alexander disease the overweight brain results from an overgrowth of glial

Table 14-1 OFC in megalencephaly in 109 patients

Distance above 98th percentile	No. at presentation	Maximum no.
<2 cm	77	66
2 to 4 cm	23	32
>4 cm	2	11
TOTAL	102*	109

From Lorber J, Priestley BL. Dev Med Child Neurol 1981; 23:494.
*For seven children, initial OFC <98th percentile.

fibers (Rosenthal fibers) [Borrett and Becker, 1985; Pietrini et al., 1983]. It is variously classified as a leukodystrophy, a neoplasm, or a hamartoma. The Bannayan syndrome holds particular interest regarding overgrowth because of the extreme brain size, 2000 g in one case [Okumura et al., 1986], in association with massive extraneural lipomas and extreme macrodactyly [Miles et al., 1984]. In hemimegalencephaly in which the overgrowth is restricted to one hemisphere, the patient may also display hemihypertrophy of the body and extremities and Wilms tumor of the kidney [Dambska et al., 1984; Matsubara et al., 1983]. In an infant with extreme anatomic megalencephaly (1450 g at 16 weeks, born at 34 weeks of gestation), Schoenle et al. [1986] found very high levels of immunoglobulin F II (IGF II), which they postulate is a brain growth factor. Zagon and McLaughlin [1983] produced megalencephaly in rats treated with an opiate antagonist.

Presenting features and occipitofrontal circumference in anatomic megalencephaly. The clinician most commonly encounters megalencephaly during routine OFC measurements of infants or during the examination of an infant or older child displaying psychomotor retardation, delayed speech, seizures, hypotonia, or mild cerebral palsy. Three studies have consistently found overweight brains in victims of sudden infant death syndrome [Kinney et al., 1992], but the association remains unexplained.

The OFC normally increases at a mean rate of approximately 0.4 cm per week in the first 4 months. In megalencephaly the OFC may increase at a mean rate of approximately 0.6 cm per week in the same period. The maximum growth rate is about 1 cm per week [DeMyer, 1972]. The OFC may be normal or enlarged at birth. It may not enlarge rapidly until as late as 1 to 2 years of age, or conversely, it may enlarge too rapidly in the initial months; the rate may then slow and the OFC ultimately may fall within the normal range. The skull may have a normal contour or show asymmetry, dolichocephaly, or frontal bossing. Table 14-1 details the OFC at the time of presentation in anatomic megalencephaly in the large series of Lorber and Priestley [1981].

Asymptomatic (familial) anatomic megalencephaly

Because it follows a bell-shaped distribution curve, the OFC of 2.5% of the normal population will exceed the mean by two standard deviations. In everyday practice the clinician must frequently separate neurologically normal infants who have large OFCs from those with pathologic causes for megalocephaly. In asymptomatic (familial) anatomic megalencephaly the patient displays normal neurologic function, develops normally with no hint of retrogression or progressive hydrocephalus, has no other pathological cause for a large head, and has at least one other neurologically normal family member with a large OFC. After a complete examination of the infant, the clinician should record the OFC and height of all available family members and inspect them for somatic anomalies and neurocutaneous stigmata. Asymptomatic (familial) anatomic megalencephaly generally follows an autosomal dominant pattern, but the condition affects males more than females at a ratio of approximately 4:1 [Day and Schutt, 1979; DeMyer, 1972; Gooskens et al., 1988]. The box on p. 213 lists the diagnostic criteria.

The first six criteria in the box virtually ensure the correct diagnosis. Still the temptation to do a CT or MRI scan is strong, particularly to differentiate some form of familial hydrocephalus from megalencephaly [Alvarez et al., 1986]. If the parents understand the advantages and disadvantages, the clinician can provide frequent follow-up visits instead of performing a scan. If the criteria in the box are not met and frequent follow-up examinations are normal, the need to shuttle every child with megalocephaly through all possible laboratory procedures is obviated.

To designate a medical disorder as asymptomatic or benign requires a retrospective conclusion justified by the benign family history and normal developmental course. Any hint of neurologic deficits, most commonly retardation or seizures, retrogression, or increased intracranial pressure, rules out the diagnosis and necessitates a full-scale investigation that starts with consideration of hydrocephalus and metabolic megalencephaly (Table 14-2).

Symptomatic familial anatomic megalencephaly

Many megalencephalic patients have neurologic deficits ranging from mild learning disabilities to hypothermia [Roubergue et al., 1986] in association with other features that constitute a diagnostic entity (see the box on p. 213). If a megalencephalic patient has neurologic deficits and matches a specific syndrome or diagnosis such as neurofibromatosis, the diagnosis is symptomatic familial anatomic megalencephaly with neurofibromatosis. If the patient does not match another, more specific syndrome, the diagnosis is the same by exclusion

---

Diagnostic Criteria for Asymptomatic (Benign) Familial Anatomic Megalencephaly

1. OFC more than two standard deviations above the mean or above the 98th percentile
2. No clinical evidence of increased intracranial pressure in the form of bulging fontanel, palpably split sutures, or persistent vomiting
3. Normal developmental and neurologic examination
4. Absence of any neurocutaneous signs or craniofacial or somatic anomalies that might indicate a specific syndrome
5. One or more of the parents or siblings having a large OFC but neurologically normal or a family history of an increased OFC in several generations
6. Follow-up visits establishing the normality of the patient's developmental course and the leveling of the OFC curve to a high curve beginning to parallel the normal
7. Radiographic demonstration of normal or only slightly enlarged ventricles in one of the family members with an enlarged OFC, establishing that the condition is megalencephaly and not arrested hydrocephalus or some other lesion
8. Negative chemical screening tests for metabolic disorders or lysosomal enzyme deficits in those patients lacking some of the other criteria

From DeMyer W. Pediatr Neurol 1986; 2:321.

---

and without further qualification. Some megalencephalic individuals in the family may be normal and others, not [Cole and Hughes, 1991]. Refined genetic, biochemical, and dynamic studies of CSF and blood flow should ultimately yield further subgroupings of symptomatic familial anatomic megalencephaly.

Genetic considerations in anatomic megalencephaly. Although Pettit [1980] reported autosomal-recessive inheritance, most anatomic megalencephalies, whether asymptomatic or syndromic, follow an autosomal-dominant pattern, and the incidence in males versus females is 4:1 [Baraitser, 1990; DeMyer, 1972; Gooskens et al., 1988b]. Some autosomal-dominant disorders with megalencephaly have a high mutation rate, including neurofibromatosis, achondroplasia, and tuberous sclerosis. Other autosomal-dominant syndromes include some instances of Sotos cerebral gigantism [Winship, 1985], Bannayan and other overgrowth syndromes with hamartomas [Gorlin et al., 1990; Miles et al., 1984], the midfacial defect reported by Cole and Hughes [1991], and asymptomatic and symptomatic familial anatomic megalencephalies. In contrast, the

Table 14-2 Differential clinical features of hydrocephalus, A-FAM, and metabolic megalencephaly

	Genetic pattern	Birth weight	Head circumference: At birth	Head circumference: Rate of increase	Neurologic regression	Bulging fontanel	Setting-sun irises	High pressure	Skull	Ventricular size	Routine CSF examination
Hydrocephalus	Most often sporadic	Normal	Normal or increased	Often rapid acceleration	Consonant with cause and degree of hydrocephalus	+++	Frequent	+++	Thin*; sutures split widely	Huge	Variable, usually normal
Asymptomatic anatomic megalencephaly	Autosomal dominant	High in some	Large in some	May be rapid in early months	None		None	None	Usually normal; may be thick	Normal or slightly enlarged	Normal
Metabolic megalencephaly	Autosomal or sex-linked recessive	Normal	Normal	Slow acceleration	Severe in relation to OFC increase	+	Rare	++	Varies; + sutures may split	Normal or small except in gargoyles	Frequently abnormal

*Skull is thin unless the hydrocephalus is a complication of cranioskeletal dysplasia such as mucopolysaccharidoses, osteoporosis, or achondroplasia. Skull may be thick in some metabolic megalencephalies such as mucopolysaccharidoses.

metabolic megalencephalies are typically autosomal-recessive.

Conventional karyotypes have generally been normal in these megalencephalies, but the loci controlling brain size remain to be discovered. In rare cases a patient diagnosed as having Klinefelter syndrome has had generalized [Budka, 1978] or focal [Choi et al., 1980] megalencephaly.

Radiographic features of the anatomic megalencephalies

Plain skull radiographs have little value in the diagnosis of asymptomatic familial anatomic megalencephaly but may disclose one of the macrocephaly syndromes with thickened skulls (see the box on p. 209). Some megalencephalics have slight suture diastasis [Day and Schutt, 1979]. MRI scan is by far the most informative procedure, but CT scans differentiate some disorders, such as tuberous sclerosis and frank hydrocephalus. Major points of interest in the scans are the size of the ventricles, the width of the subarachnoid spaces, the presence of migratory disorders or abnormal sulcation or gyration, and the presence of some treatable cause for head enlargement such as increased subdural fluid. An "eyeball" examination usually suffices in evaluating the ventricles in megalencephaly. In asymptomatic familial anatomic megalencephaly the ventricles are usually normal; if slightly enlarged, they generally correspond to the brain size [Day and Shutt, 1979]. Slight ventricular enlargement does not warrant shunting if the OFC curve levels, the fontanel closes, and the child shows no signs of increased intracranial pressure.

Hydrocephalus

MRI or CT scans differentiate noncommunicating from communicating hydrocephalus. In noncommunicating hydrocephalus the ventricles contain the excessive CSF because of obstruction to outflow into the subarachnoid space. In external or communicating hydrocephalus the subarachnoid space contains excessive fluid, and the ventricles are variably enlarged. The obstruction results from lack of absorption of fluid into the venous sinuses or overproduction of fluid. Distinguishing among communicating hydrocephalus, diffuse cerebral atrophy with hydrocephalus ex vacuo, and hypodense subarachnoid fluid (also known as *extraventricular obstructive hydrocephalus* [Gooskens et al., 1985] and *idiopathic external hydrocephalus* [Alvarez et al., 1986; Govaert et al., 1991; Hamza et al., 1987] is difficult. (Table 14-2 aids in differentiating the megalocephaly of hydrocephalus from megalencephaly.) Many patients have external hydrocephalus and true megalencephaly, often familial, and require no treatment [Alvarez et al., 1986]. In normal, full-term infants the subarachnoid space between the cerebral gyri contains little subarachnoid fluid. By 1 year of age the subarachnoid spaces of infants normally enlarge, but by 2 years of age the normal infant again shows no subarachnoid space between the gyri on MRI or CT scans. The examiner has to evaluate the clinical course and the volume of intracerebral and extracerebral fluid in relation to brain size over successive MRI scans to determine whether a given megalencephalic patient also has a progressive hydrocephalus that requires shunting or subdural fluid that requires taps.

On the basis of the location of the intracerebral fluid on CT scans, Gooskens et al, [1985] divided their 14 megalocephalic patients into three groups: group I with normal-sized ventricles and subarachnoid space diagnosed as megalencephaly; group II with enlarged subarachnoid space diagnosed as external obstructive hydrocephalus; and group III with enlarged ventricles and subarachnoid spaces diagnosed as communicating hydrocephalus. To determine ventricular enlargement, the authors used the Evans ratio: maximum ventricular width of the frontal horns divided by the maximum width of the inner table. They considered the ventricles enlarged if the Evans ratio exceeded 0.35 in children to 3 years of age or 0.30 in older children. They considered the subarachnoid space widened if it exceeded 7.5 mm in children younger than 1 year of age and 4 mm in children between 1 and 2 years of age; if any subarachnoid space was evident in children over 2 years of age, it was also considered widened. Evaluation of the width of the subarachnoid space presents many difficulties because of the lack of normal control data. A second problem is determining whether any excessive fluid occupies the subarachnoid or subdural space, which is a difficult task.

In some achondroplastic dwarfs with true megalencephaly the size of the ventricles may progressively increase because of obstructive hydrocephalus, possibly related to a disturbance in venous pressure or outlet obstruction in the posterior fossa [Dennis et al., 1961; Mueller, 1980a]. Doppler studies show a reversal of blood flow in the ophthalmic vein away from the orbit [Mueller, 1980b]. Achondroplastic dwarfs also have megalomyelia but a small foramen magnum and vertebral canal. The patient may suffer cervicomedullary compression with apnea or quadriplegia [Fremion et al., 1984]. Because the brain and spinal cord enlargement are genetic and prenatal in origin, the changes in intracranial fluid dynamics, both vascular and CSF, may represent effect rather than cause. Dynamic factors may also explain the pathogenesis of the excessive subarachnoid fluid. Prospective studies integrating CSF infusion rates, radioactive CSF absorption rates, Doppler flow studies, serial radiographic imaging, and angiography are needed to clarify fully the pathogenesis and nosology of these disorders and their relation to macrocephaly and megalencephaly.

Sotos syndrome of cerebral gigantism

Infants with cerebral gigantism, most commonly males, have a large OFC and body weight at birth. They are mildly to severely retarded and often have slightly large ventricles, but have no clinical signs of increased intracranial pressure. Facial features include a high forehead, downward angulation of the palpebral fissures, and dolichocephaly. Their growth, skeletal maturation, and bone age accelerate, but they do not have sexual precocity. Urinary 17-ketosteroid levels are high, compatible with the advanced bone age. Fasting plasma growth hormone levels are normal and show the normal decrease after glucose ingestion. Cerebral giants have large hands and feet, but pituitary giants have more characteristic acromegalic features and increased levels of growth hormone. Although sometimes an autosomal-dominant disorder [Winship, 1985], Sotos syndrome usually occurs sporadically. Cole and Hughes [1991] describe patients who have some features of Sotos syndrome but who differ by regularly having autosomal-dominant inheritance, infantile hypotonia, midfacial concavity, a long philtrum, and normal rather than accelerated bone age.

Hemimegalencephaly and focal megalencephaly

Some patients have only hemimegalencephaly with no cutaneous or extracephalic abnormalitites, whereas others have neurocutaneous syndromes, such as Klippel-Trenaunay-Weber syndrome or linear sebaceous nevus of Jadassohn (organoid nevus or epidermal nevus syndrome) [Gorlin et al., 1990; Hager et al., 1991; Pavone et al., 1991]. Many have hemihypertrophy of the face or body. The hemihypertrophy of one side of the body may be ipsilateral or contralateral to the enlarged hemisphere [Matsubara et al., 1983; Trounce et al., 1991]. Intractable seizures are also common [Konkol et al., 1990] and may respond to early hemispherectomy [Appleton et al., 1991b; Takashima et al., 1991]. Pathologic changes in the enlarged hemisphere include continued proliferation of immature neurons [Ronnett et al., 1990], pachygryia, subcortical and leptomeningeal glioneuronal heterotopias, and giant cells, which may have an increased deoxyribonucleic acid content indicating heteroploidy [Dambska et al., 1984; Hager et al., 1991; Takashima et al., 1991]. The presence of giant neurons in the ipsilateral brainstem and ipsilateral somatic hypertrophy may indicate a very early increase in growth factors on one side of the embryo.

Another form of focal megalencephaly, the Oekonomakis malformation [Dodgson, 1955], consists of micropolygria with thickening of the insular cortex, frequently bilaterally. Clinically it manifests by a developmental Foix-Chavany-Marie syndrome of facio-oropharyngoglossomasticatory diplegia (pseudobulbar palsy), mental retardation, and seizures [Ambrosetto and Tassimari, 1990; Becker, 1990; Fusco and Vigevano, 1991].

Metabolic megalencephaly

In the metabolic megalencephalies an accumulation of metabolic substances distends the cells. Examples are the gangliosidoses, mucopolysaccharidoses, and metachromatic leukodystrophy. (Appropriate studies for these conditions can be found elsewhere in this text.) Aminoacidurias and organic acidurias that may cause megalocephaly or metabolic megalencephaly are diagnosed by urinary genetic screening tests [Hoffman et al., 1991; Leupold et al., 1982; Plochl et al., 1991].

In some metabolic megalencephalies the brain may be normal in size at birth, enlarge as the metabolic substance accumulates, and then ultimately undergo atrophy and weigh less than normal. In other metabolic megalencephalies such as endocrinopathies the brain may be edematous for a prolonged time [Marty and Zurbrugg, 1982].

In contrast to the anatomic megalencephalies, patients with metabolic megalencephalies typically manifest developmental retrogression rather than a steady, slow progression and often display at least a transient increase in intracranial pressure. In some instances, physical clues, such as retinal degeneration as found in Tay-Sachs disease or an abnormal somatotype as in patients with Hurler syndrome suggest the diagnosis. These patients have a detectable metabolic error by standard urinary screening tests or lysosomal enzyme batteries, and a recessive hereditary pattern is usually present.

When the evaluation discloses an edematous brain but no metabolic disorder and no increased levels of vitamin A or lead in the blood, the possibility of pseudotumor cerebri should be considered (see Chapter 13).

REFERENCES

Alvarez LA, Maytal J, Shinnar S. Idiopathic external hydrocephalus: natural history and relationship to benign familial macrocephaly. Pediatrics 1986; 77:901, 1986.

Ambrosetto G, Tassimari CA. Sleep-related focal motor seizures in bilateral central macrogyria. Ann Neurol 1990; 28:840.

Amir N, Gross-Kieselstein E, Hirsch HJ, et al. Weaver-Smith syndrome. Am J Dis Child 1984; 138:1113.

Appleton R, Bushby K, Gardner-Medwin D, et al. Head circumference and intellectual performance of patients with Duchenne muscular dystrophy. Dev Med Child Neurol 1991a; 33:884.

Appleton R, Gardner-Medwin D, Mendelow D. Hemispherectomy for intractable seizures. Dev Med Child Neurol 1991b; 33:273.

Bale SJ, Amos CI, Parry DM, et al. Relationship between head circumference and height in normal adults and in the nevoid basal cell carcinoma syndrome and neurofibromatosis type I. Am J Med Genet 1991; 40:206.

Baraitser M. The genetics of neurological disorders. No. 18, Oxford Monographs on Medical Genetics. 2nd ed. New York: Oxford Medical, 1990.

Becker PS. Developmental Foix-Chavany-Marie syndrome: polymicrogyria or macrogyria? Ann Neurol 1990; 27:693.

Bonnemann CG, Meinecke P, Reigh H. Encephalopathy with intracerebral calcification, white matter lesions, growth hormone deficiency, microcephaly, and retinal degeneration: two sibs confirming a probably distinct entity. J Med Genet 1991; 28:708.

Borrett D, Becker LE. Alexander's disease: a disease of astrocytes. Brain 1985; 108:367.

Bray PF, Shields WD, Wolcott GJ, et al.: Occipitofrontal head circumference—an accurate measure of intracranial volume. J Pediatr 1969; 75:303.

Bresnan MJ, Lorenzo AV. Cerebrospinal fluid dynamics in megalencephaly. Dev Med Child Neuro Suppl. 1975; 17:51.

Broman SH, Nichols PL, Kennedy WA. Preschool IQ: prenatal and early developmental correlates. New York: John Wiley & Sons, 1975.

Budka H. Megalencephaly and chromosomal anomaly. Acta Neuropathol 1978; 43:263.

Buyse ML, ed. Birth defects encyclopedia. Cambridge Mass.: Blackwell Scientific, 1990.

Cadman TE, Young BL, Tucker SH. Microcephaly associated with massive chronic subdural effusions. J Pediatr 1968; 73:246.

Choi H, Ho KC, Luprecht GL. Chromatin-negative Klinefelter's syndrome with focal megalencephaly. Acta Neurol Scandinav 1980; 62:357.

Civatte J, Belaich S, Delort J, et al. Maladie de Cowden. Syndrome des Hamartomes Multiples. Rev Stomatol Chir Maxillo Fac 1979; 80:257.

Clancy RR, Kurtz MB, Bakker D, et al. Neurologic manifestations of the organoid nevus syndrome. Arch Neurol 1985; 42:236.

Cohen MM Jr. Understanding Proteus syndrome, unmasking the Elephant Man and stemming elephant fever. Neurofibromatosis 1988; 1:260.

Cole TR, Hughes HE. Autosomal dominant macrocephaly: benign familial macrocephaly or a new syndrome? Am J Med Genet 1991; 41:115.

Dambska M, Wisniewski K, Sher JH. An autopsy case of hemimegalencephaly, Brain Dev 1984; 6:60.

Day RE, Schutt WH. Normal children with large heads: benign familial megalencephaly. Arch Dis Child 1979; 54:512.

DeMyer W. Megalencephaly in children: Clinical syndromes, genetic patterns, and differential diagnosis from other causes of megalocephaly, Neurology 1972; 22:634.

DeMyer W. Megalencephaly: types, clinical syndromes, and management. Pediatr Neurol 1986; 2:321.

DeMyer W. Technique of the neurologic examination: a programmed text. 4th ed. New York: McGraw-Hill, 1993.

DeMyer W. Holoprosencephaly (cyclopia-arhinencephaly). In: Vinken PJ, Bruyn GW, Klawans HL, eds. Handbook of clinical neurology. vol 6: malformations. Amsterdam: Elsevier Science, 1987.

Dennis JP, Rosenberg HS, Alvord EC. Megalencephaly, internal hydrocephalus, and other neurological aspects of achondroplasia. Brain 1961; 84:427.

DiLiberti JH, D'Agostino AN, Ruvalcaba RHA, et al. A new lipid storage myopathy observed in individuals with the Ruvalcaba-Myhre-Smith syndrome. Am J Med Genet 1984; 18:163.

Dobyns WB, Elias ER, Newlin AC, et al. Causal heterogeneity in isolated lissencephaly. Neurology 1992; 42:1375.

Dodgson MCH. A congenital malformation of insular cortex in man, involving the claustrum and certain subcorotical centres. J Comp Neurol 1955; 102:341.

Dolk H. The predictive value of microcephaly during the first year of life for mental retardation at seven years. Dev Med Child Neurol 1991; 33:974.

Dorman C. Microcephaly and intelligence. Dev Med Child Neurol 1991; 33:267.

Evans DG. Dominantly inherited microcephaly, hypotelorism and normal intelligence. Clin Genet 1991; 39:178.

Fremion AS, Garg BP, Kalsbeck J. Apnea as the sole manifestation of cord compression in achondroplasia. J Pediatr 1984; 104:398.

Friede RL. Developmental neuropathology. 2nd ed. New York: Springer-Verlag, 1989.

Fusco L, Vigevano F. Reversible operculum syndrome caused by progressive epilepsia partialis continua in a child with left hemimegalencephaly. J Neurol Neurosurg Psychiat 1991; 54:556.

Gessaga EC. Lehrmitte-Duclos disease of the cerebellum. Neurosurg Rev 1980; 3:151.

Gollop TR, Fontes LR. The Greig cephalopolysyndactyly syndrome: report of a family and review of the literature. Am J Med Genet 1985; 22:59.

Gooskens RH, Willemse J, Gielen CC. Cerebrospinal fluid dynamics and cerebrospinal fluid infusion in children. Part II: Clinical application of lumbar cerebrospinal fluid infusion in children with macrocephaly and normal growth rate of the head circumference. Neuropediatr 1985; 16:121.

Gooskens RH, Gielen CC, Hanlo PW, et al. Intracranial spaces in childhood macrocephaly: comparison of length measurements and volume calculations. Dev Med Child Neurol 1988a; 30:509.

Gooskens RH, Willemse J, Bijlsma JB, et al. Megalencephaly: definition and classification. Brain Devel 1988b; 10:1.

Gorlin RJ, Cohen Jr MM, Levin LS, eds. Syndromes of the head and neck. 3rd ed. New York: Oxford University Press, 1990.

Govaert P, Oostra A, Matthys D, et al. How idiopathic is idiopathic external hydrocephalus? Dev Med Child Neurol 1991; 33:274.

Hager BC, Dyme IZ, Guertin SR, et al. Linear nevus sebaceous syndrome: megalencephaly and heterotopic gray matter. Pediatr Neurol 1991; 7:45.

Halal G, Silver K. Slowly progressive macrocephaly with hamartomas: a new syndrome. Am J Med Genet 1989; 33:l82.

Hamza M, Bodensteiner JB, Noorani PA, et al. Benign extracerebral fluid collections: a cause of macrocrania in infancy. Pediatr Neurol 1987; 3:208.

Haslam RHA. Microcephaly. In: Vinken PJ, Bruyn GW, Klawans HL, eds. Handbook of clinical neurology. Amsterdam: Elsevier, 1987; 267-284.

Hayward JC, Titelbaum DS, Clancy RR. Lissencephaly-pachygyria associated with congenital cytomegalovirus infection. J Child Neurol 1991; 6:109.

Heney D, Mueller R, Turner G, et al. Familial microcephaly with normal intelligence in a patient with acute lymphoblastic leukemia. Cancer 1992; 69:962.

Hoffman GF, Trefz FK, Barth PG, et al. Macrocephaly: an important indication for organic acid analysis. J Inherit Metab Dis 1991; 14:329.

Holden K, Alexander F. Diffuse neonatal hemangiomatosis. Pediatrics 1970; 46:411.

Hori A, Orthner H, Kohlschutter L, et al. CNS dysplasia in dysencephalia splanchnocystica (Gruber's syndrome). Acta Neuropathol (Berl) 1980; 51:93.

Hoshino A. Megalencephaly: a report of 4 children including a previously undescribed congenital syndrome and review of the literature (in Japanese) No To Shinkei (Tokyo) 1981; 33:377.

Jennings MT, Hall JG, Kukolich M. Endocardial fibroelastosis, neurologic dysfunction and unusual facial appearance in two brothers, coincidentally associated with dominantly inherited macrocephaly, Am J Med Genet 1980; 5:271.

Jones KL. Smith's recognizable patterns of human malformation. 4th ed. Philadelphia: WB Saunders, 1988.

Kasarskis AJ, Bass NH. Benign intracranial hypertension induced by deficiency of vitamin A during infancy. Neurology 1982; 32:1292.

Kinney HC, Filiano JJ, Harper R. The neuropathology of the sudden infant death syndrome. J Neuropath Exp Neurol 1992; 51:1l5.

Komai T, Kiskimoto K, Ozaki Y. Genetic study of microcephaly based on Japanese material. Am J Human Genet 1955; 7:51.

Konkol RJ, Maister BH, Wells RG, et al. Hemimegalencephaly: clinical EEG, neuroimaging, and IMP-SPECT correlation. Pediatr Neurol 1990; 6:414.

Lemire RJ, Loeser JD, Leech RW, et al. Normal and abnormal development of the human nervous system. New York: Harper & Row, 1975.

Leupold D, Bojasch M, Jakobs C. 3-Hydroxy-3-methylglutaryl-CoA lyase deficiency in an infant with macrocephaly and mild metabolic acidosis, Eur J Pediatr 1982; 138:73.

Lewis BA, Aram DM, Horwitz SJ. Language and motor findings in benign megalencephaly. Ann Neurol 1983; 14:364.

Lorber J, Priestley BL. Children with large heads: a practical approach to diagnosis in 557 children, with special reference to 109 children with megalencephaly. Dev Med Child Neurol 1981; 23:494.

Luo Y, and Huang K. Spongy degeneration of the CNS in infancy. Arch Neurol 1984; 41:164.

Marty H, Zurbrugg RP. Passagere neonatale makrozephalie: Zur differentialdiagnose des abnorm raschen Schadelwachstums beim Neugeborenen. Helv paediat Acta 1982; 37:273.

Matsubara O, Tanaka M, Takashi I, et al. Hemimegalencephaly with hemihypertrophy (Klippel-Trenaunay-Weber syndrome). Virchows Arch [Pathol Anat] 1983; 400:155.

McKusick VA. Mendelian inheritance in man: catalogs of autosomal-dominant, autosomal-recessive, and X-linked phenotypes. 8th ed. Baltimore: Johns Hopkins University, 1988.

Miles JH, Zonana J, McFarlane J, et al. Macrocephaly with hamartomas: Bannayan-Zonana syndrome, Am J Med Genet 1984; 19:225.

Mueller S: Enlarged cerebral ventricular system in infant achondroplastic dwarf. Neurology 1980a; 30:767.

Mueller S, Reinertson JE: Reversal of emissary vein blood flow in achondroplastic dwarfs. Neurology 1980b; 30:769.

Muller J. Congenital malformations of the brain. In: Rosenberg RN, ed. The clinical neurosciences. vol. III. Neuropathology. New York: Churchill-Livingston, 1983.

Okumura K, Sasaki Y, Ohyama M, et al. Bannayan syndrome-generalized lipomatosis associated with megalencephaly and macrodactyly. Acta Pathol Jpn 1986; 36:269.

Opitz JM, Holt MC. Microcephaly: general considerations and aids to nosology. J Craniofac Biol Dev Biol 1990; 10:175.

Opitz JM, Kaveggia EG, Adkins WN, et al. Studies of malformation syndromes of humans XXXIIIC: the FG syndrome—further studies on three affected individuals from the FG family. Am J Med Genet 1982; 12:147.

Pascual-Castroviejo I, Roche MC, Bermejo AM, et al. Primary intracranial arachnoidal cysts: a study of 67 cases. Child Nerv Syst 1991a; 7:257.

Pascual-Castroviejo I, Velez A, Pascual-Pascual SI, et al. Dandy-Walker malformation: analysis of 38 cases. Child Nerv Syst 1991b; 7:88.

Pavone L, Curatolo P, Rizzo R, et al. Epidermal nevus syndrome: a neurologic variant with hemimegalencephaly, gyral malformation, mental retardation, seizures, and facial hemihypertrophy. Neurology 1991; 41:266.

Pettit RE. Macrocephaly with head growth parallel to normal growth pattern. Arch Neurol 1980; 37:518.

Pietrini V, Tagliavini F, Tedeschi F, et al. Megalencephaly with formation of Rosenthal fibers in symmetric subependymal gliomatous proliferations: clinicopathologic report. Clin Neuropath 1983; 2:16.

Plochl E, Christensen E, Colombo JP et al. Macrocephaly and dystonic cerebral palsy in a child with type I glutaric aciduria. Pediatr Pathol 1991; 26:97.

Portnoy HD, Croissant PD. Megalencephaly in infants and children: the possible role of increased dural sinus pressure. Arch Neurol 1978; 35:306.

Roche AF, Mukherjee D, Guo S, et al. Head circumference reference data: birth to 18 years. Pediatrics 1987; 79:706.

Ronnett GV, Hester LD, Nye JS, et al. Human cortical neuronal cell line: establishment from a patient with unilateral megalencephaly. Science 1990; 248:603.

Ross DL, Boleslaw HL, Chun RWM, et al. Hypomelanosis of Ito (incontinentia pigmenti achromians)—a clinicopathologic study: macrocephaly and gray matter heterotopias. Neurology 1982; 32:1013.

Roubergue A, Beauvais P, Richardet JM. Hypothermie spontanee recidivante et megalencephalie: une observation. Revue de la litterature. Ann Pediatr (Paris) 1986; 33:125.

Russell LJ, Weaver DD, Bull MJ, et al. In utero brain destruction resulting in collapse of the fetal skull, microcephaly, scalp rugae, and neurologic impairment: the fetal brain disruption sequence. Am J Med Genet 1984; 17:509.

Scheffer IE, Baraitser M, Brett EM. Severe microcephaly associated with congenital varicella infection. Dev Med Child Neurol 1991; 33:916.

Schinzel A, Schmid W. Hallux duplication, postaxial polydactyly, absence of the corpus callosum, severe mental retardation, and additional anomalies in two unrelated patients: a new syndrome. Am J Med Genet 1980; 6:241.

Schmidt B, Watters GV, Rosenblatt B, et al.: Increased head circumference in patients with Duchenne muscular dystrophy. Ann Neurol 1985; 17:620.

Schoenle EJ, Haselbacher GK, Briner J, et al. Elevated concentration of IGF II in brain tissue from an infant with macrencephaly. J Pediatr 1986; 108:737.

Schreier H, Rapin I, Davis J. Familial megalencephaly or hydrocephalus? Neurology 1974; 24:232.

Scott RD. Ataxia-telangiectasia. Arch Path 1969; 88:78.

Sher, PK, Brown SB. A longitudinal study of head growth in pre-term infants. II. Differentiation between 'catch-up' head growth and early infantile hydrocephalus. Dev Med Child Neurol 1975; 17:711.

Smith RD, Ashley J, Hardesty RA, et al. Macrocephaly and minor congenital anomalies in children with learning problems. Develop Behav Peds 1984; 5:231.

Takashima S, Chan F, Becker LE, et al. Aberrant neuronal development in hemimegalencephaly: immunohistochemical and Golgi studies. Pediatr Neurol 1991; 7:275.

Talwar D, Schwartzman MJ, McGeachie RE. Megalencephaly secondary to occlusion and stenosis of sigmoid sinuses. 1990; 6:51.

Thompson EM et al. FG syndrome: 7 new cases. Clin Genet 1985; 27:582.

Trounce JQ, Rutter N, Mellor DH: Hemimegalencephaly: diagnosis and treatment. Dev Med Child Neurol 1991; 33:261.

Van Benthem LH. Cryptorchidism, chest deformities and other congenital anomalies in three brothers. Arch Dis Child 1970; 45:590.

Van Walsem G. Ueber das Gewicht des schwersten bis jezt beschriebenen Gehirns. Neurol Centralbl 1899; 18:578.

Weaver DD, Christian JC. Familial variation of head size and adjustment for parental head circumference. J Pediatr 1980; 96:990.

Wechselberg K, Neumann D. Zur Ubergrosse des hirn- und gesichtsschaedels bei adiposogiganten. Z Kinderheilk 1965; 92:169.

Wiedemann HR, Burgio GR, Aldenhoff P, et al. The Proteus syndrome: partial gigantism of the hands and/or feet, nevi, hemihypertrophy, subcutaneous tumors, macrocephaly or other skull anomalies and possible accelerated growth and visceral affections. Eur J Pediatr 1983; 140:5.

Willerman L. Science 1991; 254:1584.

Winship IM. Sotos' syndrome—autosomal-dominant inheritance substantiated. Clin Genet 1985; 23:243.

Winter RM, Baraitser M. London dysmorphology data base. London: Oxford University, 1990.

Young ID, Trounce JQ, Levene MI, et al. Agenesis of the corpus callosum and macrocephaly in siblings. Clin Genet 1985; 28:225.

Zagon IS, McLaughlin PJ. Increased brain size and cellular content in infant rats treated with an opiate antagonist. Science 1983; 221:1179.

Zeman W, DeMyer W, Falls H. Pelizeaus-Merzbacher disease: a study in nosology. J Neuropath Exp Neurol 1964; 23:334.

15

Headache

A. David Rothner

Each year at least 80% of the general population will suffer from headache. Headache is also a frequently encountered symptom in children and adolescents. As many as 75% of children will have experienced significant headache by 15 years of age [Bille, 1962]. This symptom represents a dilemma for the practicing pediatrician who must decide if the patient has an underlying CNS disorder or if it is safe to simply reassure the parents and observe the child. In addition, the pediatrician considers whether the symptoms should be treated symptomatically or whether an intensive evaluation should take place. Headache may accompany childhood infectious diseases with or without fever, be part of systemic disorders, be a component of an acute or chronic CNS disorder or, in the case of migraine, be a disease unto itself [Rothner, 1983].

In a population of 9000 Scandinavian school children, Bille reported that by 7 years of age 1.4% of patients had experienced true migraine, 2.5% had frequent nonmigrainous headaches, and 35% had frequent headaches of other varieties [1962]. By 15 years of age, 5.3% had experienced migraine, 15.7% had frequent nonmigrainous headaches, and 54% had infrequent nonmigrainous headaches. In a prepaid health plan, 80% of all enrolled children were examined for headache during a 6-year period [Starfield et al., 1984]. In a recent epidemiologic study, it was noted that many individuals with migraine do not seek a physician's intervention [Stewart et al., 1992].

Despite its common occurrence, medical discussions concerning headache in children remained nonexistent until 1873 when William Henry Day, a British pediatrician, devoted a chapter in *Essays on Diseases in Children* to the subject [Day, 1873]. Literary milestones concerning headache in children include the books *Headaches in Children* edited by Friedman and Harms [1967], *Headaches and Migraine in Childhood* by Barlow [1984] and *Migraine in Childhood* by Hockaday [1988]. Several reviews of headaches in children have been published [Rothner, 1983; Shinnar and D'Souza, 1982]. This chapter discusses the pathophysiology of head pain and the approach to the patient with headache, including the differential diagnosis and treatment. Discussions concerning headache as a component of seizure disorders, trauma, increased intracranial pressure, congenital anomalies, CNS infections, toxins, tumors, vascular disorders, metabolic disorders, systemic medical disorders, and migraine are presented elsewhere in the text.

PATHOPHYSIOLOGY

Both extracranial and intracranial structures may be sensitive to pain. Extracranial structures sensitive to pain include the skin, subcutaneous tissues, muscles, mucous membranes, teeth, and some of the larger vessels. Intracranial tissues that are pain-sensitive include the vascular sinuses, the larger veins, the dura surrounding these larger veins, the dural arteries, and the arteries at the base of the brain. Pain from extracranial and intracranial structures in and about the face and from the front half of the skull is mediated by cranial nerve V. Smaller areas are innervated by branches from cranial nerves VII, IX, and X. Pain from the occipital half of the skull is mediated via the upper cervical nerves. The brain, the cranium, most of the dura, the ependyma, and the choroid plexus are insensitive to pain. Inflammation, irritation, displacement, traction, dilatation, or invasion of any of these pain-sensitive structures will cause pain [Ray and Wolff, 1940]. These stimuli activate nociceptive primary afferents that connect to vascular structures and secondarily affect blood flow. The role of chemical mediators released in response to tissue damage is recognized to further aggravate the pain.

Prostaglandins, once released, contribute to the activation of the primary afferent nociceptors. Acetylsalicylic acid or other nonsteroidal antiinflammatory agents prevent pain by inhibiting the metabolism of arachidonic acid to prostaglandins. The activation of the primary afferents leads to action potentials in their axons that propagate to vascular structures and to the spinal cord. In the spinal cord the sensory axons enter the gray matter of the superficial dorsal horn to synapse on nerve cells, contributing to pain transmission pathways, such as the spinothalamic tract. There are also other neurons located within the superficial dorsal horns that relay information from other primary afferents and another system that inhibits the relay of information to the projection cells. The latter alters the pain messages entering the CNS. The sensation of pain is a complex sum of activity of nociceptive and nonnociceptive afferents [Fields and Levine, 1984].

CLASSIFICATION

The classifications of headaches that currently exist are based on the presumed location of the abnormality, its origin, its pathophysiology, or the symptom complex with which the patient presents. Prior to 1991 the major classification used was one provided by the American Medical Association [1962] (Table 15-1) [AMA ad hoc committee, 1962]. In 1988 the International Headache Society published its lengthy classification [Olesen, 1988]. Its primary use is in research studies.

Clinically, it is also helpful to classify headaches using the temporal pattern of the headache [Rothner, 1978]. By plotting the severity of the headache over time, one of the following five patterns is identified: acute, acute-recurrent, chronic-progressive, chronic-nonprogressive, and mixed (Figure 15-1).

An acute headache is defined as a single event with no history of previous similar events. If this acute event is associated with a clinically ill child with neurologic symptoms or signs, the diagnosis should be made quickly because intervention may be lifesaving. The differential diagnosis involves a wide variety of disorders, including CNS infections, subarachnoid hemorrhage, systemic illness, and hypertension.

Acute recurrent headaches are periodic events that are separated by pain-free intervals. When associated with nausea and vomiting, these headaches are usually migrainous in nature. A nonmigrainous form of recurrent headache is cluster headache (discussed below). The migraine syndrome is discussed in Chapter 48.

Chronic, progressive headache worsens in frequency and severity over time. If these headaches are accompanied by symptoms of increased intracranial pressure, such as vomiting, lethargy, personality change, and/or abnormal neurologic signs, an organic process, such as brain tumor or hydrocephalus, should be suspected.

Chronic, nonprogressive headache occurs constantly, daily, or frequently, and is mild-to-moderate in severity. It is not associated with symptoms of increased intracranial pressure or abnormal neurologic signs. Headache is frequently related to overt or covert stress.

The mixed headache syndrome, the fifth category, is a combination of acute, recurrent headache, superimposed on a pattern of daily chronic, nonprogressive headache. The superimposed headache is episodic in nature, with nausea and vomiting, and the daily headache is similar to that described in chronic, nonprogres-

Table 15-1 Classification of headache

Vascular headache	Muscle contraction headache	Traction and inflammatory headache
Migraine		
Classic—with aura	Depressive equivalents	Mass lesions (i.e., tumors, hematomas, cerebral hemorrhage)
Common—without aura	Conversion reactions	
	Anxiety reactions	Hydrocephalus, abscess
Complicated migraine		
Hemiplegic	Adjustment reactions	Diseases of the eye, ear, nose, throat, teeth
Ophthalmoplegic		Arteritis and cranial neuralgias
Basilar artery		Occlusive vascular disease
Confusional		Atypical facial pain
		Temporomandibular joint disease
Variant		
Cyclic vomiting		
Paroxysmal vertigo		
Paroxysmal torticollis		
Periodic syndrome		
Epilepsy equivalent syndrome		

Modified from AMA Ad Hoc Committee on Classification of Headache. JAMA 1962; 179:717.

sive headache. The patient is easily able to differentiate the two types of headache when prompted. Symptoms of increased intracranial pressure are absent, and the neurologic examination is normal. This added dimension of severity and time may suggest a specific diagnosis, as well as an evaluation and treatment plan (Table 15-2).

EVALUATION OF THE PATIENT

A properly obtained history is the key to correct diagnosis. Questions must be directed at both the patient and parents. A private interview with adolescents is often useful. Children and adolescents respond to pain in a widely variable manner. Younger children commonly react to pain by crying, rocking, and hiding. If the pain becomes chronic, developmental regression, depression, anxiety, or behavioral difficulty may occur. Chronic pain may also affect eating, sleeping, and

playing. A more mature child can better perceive, localize, and remember pain. Emotional and personality considerations assume greater importance in the older child. Chronic pain may present as a developmental disorder of eating, sleeping, playing, as well as school function. Absenteeism and problems in interaction with peers, family, and authority are common. Depression and anxiety also commonly result. The younger the child, the less specific the information obtained. The interaction between the child and parents during the interview should be noted because it may reflect problems not directly discussed including depression, family conflict, hostility, or anxiety [Schechter, 1984].

Specific questions may provide a data base on which to formulate a diagnosis (see box on p. 222). Additional questions relating to increased intracranial pressure or progressive disease relate to specific neurologic symptoms, such as ataxia, lethargy, seizures, visual disturbance, focal weakness, personality change, and loss of abilities. The standard pediatric history regarding pregnancy, labor, delivery, growth and development, academic function, behavior, previous encephalopathic events, medications, drugs, and systems review completes the search for any details that may be pertinent to the headache evaluation. Problems, such as hypertension, chronic sinus disease, recurrent abdominal pain, previous emotional disorders and trauma, may be pertinent to better understanding the headache problem.

Important clues regarding potentially ominous headaches include the severity of the headache, headache that occurs in the absence of previous headache, changes in a chronic headache pattern, consistently localized pain, pain that awakens the patient, pain that occurs early in the morning, or pain that is associated with straining or neurologic symptoms or signs.

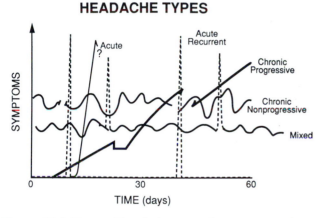

Figure 15-1 Types of headaches according to temporal patterns.

Table 15-2 Examples of syndromes that cause headaches

Acute generalized	Acute localized	Acute recurrent	Chronic progressive	Chronic nonprogressive
Systemic infection	Sinusitis	Migraine	Tumor	Muscle contraction
CNS infection	Otitis	Complex migraine	Pseudotumor	Conversion
Toxins: lead, CO_2	Ocular abnormality	Migraine variants	Brain abscess	Malingering
Postseizure	Dental disease	Cluster	Subdural hematoma	Postconcussion
Electrolyte imbalance	Trauma	Periodic syndrome	Hydrocephalus	Depression
Hypertension	Occipital neuralgia	Paroxysmal hemi-		Anxiety
Hypoglycemia	Temporomandibular	crania		Adjustment reaction
Postlumbar puncture	joint dysfunction	Postseizure		
Trauma				
Embolic				
Vascular thrombosis				
Hemorrhage				
Collagen disease				
Exertional				

Questions for Use in Evaluating Patients

- Do you have only one kind of headache, or are there two distinct types?
- When did you first begin to have headaches?
- How frequently do they recur?
- Are the headaches becoming more severe or occurring more frequently?
- How do the headaches usually begin?
- Do the headaches occur at any special time or under any special circumstances?
- Can you tell when a headache is about to begin?
- Where does it hurt?
- What does the pain feel like?
- When you are having a headache, do you feel nauseous or dizzy?
- Do you have to stop what you are doing?
- Does anything make it worse?
- Does anything make it go away?
- How long does the headache typically last?
- Does anyone else in your family have bad headaches?
- Do you have any other medical problems?
- Are you taking any medicines regularly?
- Has anything particularly good or bad happened to you recently?
- What do *you* think is causing your headaches?

The physical examination should disclose any abnormalities that could cause or be associated with headaches [Paine and Oppe, 1966]. A well child with a history of migraine headache or muscle contraction headache usually has a normal examination. The presence of fever may indicate an infectious process. Blood pressure must be measured because hypertension can cause headaches. The skin must be examined closely because café-au-lait spots, petechiae, or striae may indicate a disorder associated with headache. The sinuses and the occipital area should be palpated to determine whether focal tenderness is present, and the mouth and jaws should be examined in the open and closed position to determine temporomandibular joint function.

The neurologic examination begins with the head and neck. Signs of trauma and nuchal rigidity should be sought. Head circumference should be measured; if it is enlarged, hydrocephalus may be present. Auscultation of the cranium, seeking an asymmetric machinery-like bruit, may indicate an underlying vascular malformation. Cranial nerve examination with close examination of the optic fundus and eye movements follow. Patient strength, muscle bulk, tone, and reflexes should be observed carefully. Normal patients should have symmetric findings, and any abnormality must be further evaluated because it may indicate nonlocalizing increased intracra-

nial pressure or a specific pathologic process. Once again, the patient's orientation to time, place, and person, their language, affect, and level of consciousness should be monitored throughout the history and physical examination. When the pain is described as severe and the patient looks rather unconcerned, the diagnosis of conversion reaction should be suspected.

DIFFERENTIAL DIAGNOSIS AND CLINICAL LABORATORY TESTS

At this point, the differential diagnosis of the patient's headache must be considered (see Figure 15-1 and Table 15-2). Laboratory tests should be ordered based on the history, the character and temporal pattern of the headache, and the physical and neurologic examinations. Skull radiographs are only rarely used in the evaluation of headache patients. In most patients, radiographs are normal, but when an abnormality is found, the finding is nondiagnostic. EEG is of limited value in the routine evaluation of headache unless the patient is suspected of having an epileptiform disorder. If the headache is part of an ictal event where alteration or loss of consciousness has occurred, then EEG is mandatory. Epileptiform abnormalities occur to a slightly greater degree in migraine patients than in the general population, but their clinical significance and relevance to therapy are rarely important [Kinast et al., 1982]. CT is an accurate method of evaluating intracranial contents. It is useful in a variety of disorders, including malformations, infections, neoplasms, and vascular disorders. It initially replaced skull roentgenograms, angiograms, pneumoencephalograms, and isotope scans as the single most valuable test in evaluating a patient suspected of having an organic disorder.

MRI is a diagnostic modality that has surpassed CT in the evaluation of patients suspected of having intracranial abnormalities [Johnson et al., 1983]. It is more accurate than CT in delineating abnormalities in the vicinity of the sella turcica, posterior fossa, and temporal lobe, as well as the cervical-medullary junction. It demonstrates vascular problems, neoplasms, white matter abnormalities, and congenital anomalies not visible on CT. When magnetic resonance angiography and/or magnetic resonance venography is added to the basic MRI scan, detailed information concerning large arteries and large veins can also be obtained. When a patient has a focal symptom, a progressive disorder, symptoms of increased intracranial pressure or a neurologic examination that is abnormal, MRI is necessary. MRI scan routinely visualizes the paranasal sinuses.

Lumbar puncture is useful in determining whether an infectious process or increased pressure exists. If an intracranial lesion is suspected, lumbar puncture may be contraindicated and should be preceded by neuroimaging. In pseudotumor cerebri it is a useful diagnostic and therapeutic procedure. Projective psychologic tests may be useful in individuals with chronic, nonprogressive headaches that are believed to be functional. A psychologic interview is even more helpful. In children with school-related issues, psychoeducational testing can also be useful [Harrison, 1975].

SPECIFIC HEADACHE SYNDROMES

For purposes of discussion of specific syndromes, headache is separated into acute generalized headache, acute localized headache, acute and recurrent headache, chronic-progressive headache, chronic-nonprogressive headache, and mixed headache syndromes.

Acute generalized headache

An isolated, acute, generalized headache presents a difficult diagnostic problem. When the headache is associated with neurologic symptoms or signs, an organic disorder must be suspected. If the patient is clinically ill, the diagnosis should be arrived at in a rapid fashion. Approximately 2% to 6% of all emergency visits by adults and adolescents are due to headache. Specific data regarding emergency room visits for headache in the pediatric population are meager. In one study, 25% of all patients examined in the emergency room with headache were younger than 17 years of age. Of the entire group of patients, 39% had noncentral nervous system infections, 19% had tension headaches, 9% had headaches related to trauma, 5% had vascular headaches, and 5% had headaches related to high blood pressure [Dhopesh et al., 1979]. In the presence of elevated temperature, elevated blood pressure, nuchal rigidity, papilledema, retinal hemorrhages, focal neurologic signs, altered affect, or impaired consciousness, rapid intervention is needed. In 1987, Kandt and Levine studied 37 children with acute headaches seen in a walk-in clinic. Disorders included infections, head injuries, and a variety of other etiologies. Further studies of this nature are needed.

An unusual form of acute, generalized headache is related to exertion. Adolescents may experience acute headaches during running, playing football, or lifting weights. These headaches may be severe, throbbing and generalized, and may last from a few minutes to a few hours. Unless recurrent, they require only symptomatic treatment. When recurrent they may respond dramatically to indomethacin [Diamond, 1982]. A similar severe, generalized headache is frequently observed after a seizure or lumbar puncture. The latter is believed to be caused by CSF leak and is aggravated by the upright position. It may be treated by a blood patch.

Acute localized headache

Acute localized headache may be caused by paranasal sinusitis, otitis, ocular processes, dental problems, temporomandibular joint dysfunction, and head trauma. Some of these processes can also cause chronic, nonprogressive headache.

In sinusitis, pain may be the only symptom or it may be associated with rhinorrhea, cough, allergy, and fever. Pain may be localized to the face or forehead or referred to the occipital area or vertex. In chronic sinusitis the patient is usually afebrile and respiratory symptoms are less prominent. This clinical syndrome may mimic chronic tension headache. Plain sinus radiographs are, in my experience, less valuable than CT or MRI of the sinuses. Total opacification, mucosal thickening, and air-fluid levels are commonly seen in this disorder. The maxillary sinuses are most frequently affected, and treatment includes prolonged use of antibiotics, short-term use of decongestants and, rarely, surgical drainage [Faleck et al., 1988].

Otitis media is a common cause of pain. Infants and children are at highest risk, and severe pain is usually localized to the ear. Pain in very young children is not well localized and is manifested by irritability. Examination reveals a hyperemic, opaque bulging tympanic membrane with poor mobility. Therapy includes the use of antibiotics.

Ocular abnormalities are frequently believed to cause headaches in children but, in my experience, are only rarely causal. Astigmatism, refractory areas, and squinting occasionally cause headaches localized to the eyes and may be precipitated by prolonged reading or watching television. Ophthalmologic examination or refraction is indicated if this type of headache is present. Rarer ocular causes of headache include glaucoma, orbital cellulitis, and retrobulbar neuritis [Behrens, 1978].

Caries, dental abscesses, and malocclusion, as well as temporomandibular junction dysfunction, usually cause pain in the ear, jaw, or mouth, unilaterally or bilaterally. The localized nature of the pain and its relation to chewing suggest the correct diagnosis. The diagnostic criteria for temporomandibular joint dysfunction are not clear, but jaw locking and inability to open the mouth completely are frequently present. Patients who chew gum excessively, grind their teeth, bite their lips, or are anxious are at increased risk for this disorder [Belfer and Kaban, 1982].

Localized or generalized headache may be associated with head trauma immediately and/or several days after injury. The pain usually resolves over a period of days to weeks. When altered consciousness, vomiting, or focal abnormalities occur, neuroimaging is necessary. When prolonged headache is present, re-examination is indicated. Neuroma formation or the development of a leptomeningeal cyst are rare complications of mild head trauma. The second form of protracted generalized headache related to trauma is the postconcussion or posttraumatic syndrome. When patients have chronic headaches for longer than 12 weeks after trauma in the absence of symptoms of increased intracranial pressure and with normal neurologic examinations and laboratory studies, they should be evaluated for a stress-related disorder.

Occipital neuralgia is pain in the occipital and upper cervical region and may be related to sports or automobile injury or to malformation, such as platybasia, Klippel-Feil syndrome, or Chiari malformation. Patients with occipital neuralgia have tenderness and pain in the suboccipital region in the distribution of the second and third cervical dermatomes. The pain may occur in the retroauricular area or in the distribution of the lesser occipital nerve [Dugan et al., 1962]. Sensory changes may be present. Reflex spasm of the neck muscles produces pain. MRI scanning of the cervico-medullary region is necessary to eliminate dislocation or malformation. Improvement is often achieved with the use of a soft cervical collar, range-of-motion and cervical isometric exercises, muscle relaxants, and analgesics.

Acute recurrent headache

The migraine syndrome in pediatric and adolescent patients is the classic example of an acute recurrent headache. This disorder is characterized by episodic, periodic, and paroxysmal attacks of pain separated by pain-free intervals associated with vasoconstriction and vasodilatation and leading to nausea, vomiting, phonophobia, photophobia, and a desire to sleep (see Chapter 48) [Rothner, 1986].

Cluster headaches rarely occur in children but may begin in later adolescence [Curless, 1982]. There are two forms, the typical cluster headache and the chronic cluster headache without remission. Cluster consists of unilateral, periorbital pain, which does not alternate sides. Tearing, unilateral rhinorrhea, nasal stuffiness, and facial flushing coexist. The pain is brief, lasting 20 to 60 minutes, and severe and may occur once or twice daily at the same time for days or weeks and then disappear for months or years. It will frequently awaken the patient 1 to 2 hours after falling asleep on a regular basis. Chronic cluster headaches do not remit. Treatment is difficult and involves the use of steroids, oxygen, lithium carbonate, nonsteroidal antiinflammatory drugs, and methylsergide maleate.

Chronic paroxysmal hemicrania was described by Sjaastad in 1980 [Sjaastad and Spierings, 1984]. This is a syndrome with strictly unilateral headaches unaccompanied by nausea and vomiting. Episodes occur several to many times per day. The pain is severe and causes the child to cry or be excessively irritable. The pain is dramatically relieved by indomethacin therapy. The response to indomethacin is the sine qua non of paroxysmal hemicrania. The treatment must be continued indefinitely.

Chronic progressive headache

Chronic progressive headache implies a pathologic process within the cranial vault. Increased intracranial pressure is usually present. The symptoms and signs by definition are progressive. Prominent in this group of disorders are hydrocephalus, brain tumor, pseudotumor cerebri, brain abscess, and chronic subdural hematoma. When the disorder is rapidly progressive, rapid intervention with regard to diagnosis and treatment is mandatory. If increased intracranial pressure is present, associated symptoms may include nausea, vomiting, focal weakness, ataxia, personality change, lethargy, visual disturbances, intellectual deterioration, and seizures. In some patients the examination may be normal or may demonstrate papilledema cranial nerve VI palsy. When neurologic signs are present, they may be localized, leading to a specific diagnosis. MRI should be used when a CNS abnormality is suspected. Lumbar puncture should only be considered as an initial diagnostic test when an acute infection or hemorrhage is suspected and a mass lesion has been excluded.

Hydrocephalus is a condition in which increased ventricular volume with or without increased pressure is secondary to obstruction or decreased absorption of CSF. It may be secondary to a congenital anomaly such as aqueductal stenosis, or it may be a sequela of subarachnoid hemorrhage or bacterial meningitis. Symptoms and signs are those of nonlocalized, increased intracranial pressure. If the disorder is chronic, macrocephaly may be present. MRI is diagnostic, and a shunting procedure is the treatment of choice.

Brain tumors are the second most frequent type of neoplasm in children and adolescents. The headaches are invariably progressive in frequency and severity, although temporary plateaus in the patient's course may occur. The pain is secondary to traction on pain-sensitive structures or obstruction of CSF flow with resultant hydrocephalus. The location of the headache is not always helpful. Supratentorial tumors may cause frontal headache, and a posterior fossa tumor may cause occipital headache. A hemispheric tumor may cause unilateral pain. Changing positions, defecating, coughing, or exertion may exacerbate the pain. The quality of pain is not diagnostic. It may be more severe in the morning and may be associated with and relieved by vomiting. Approximately 70% of children with brain tumors have headache as the presenting symptom. It is diffuse in the majority of patients, awakens them at night in 65% of patients, and can usually be diagnosed by MRI. Surgical treatment, radiation therapy, and chemotherapy may be used singly or in combination to treat this disorder (see Chapter 50).

Pseudotumor cerebri is increased intracranial pressure without evidence of infection, mass lesion, or hydrocephalus [Corbett et al., 1982]. Patients usually have headache and papilledema, as well as an associated cranial nerve VI palsy. Diplopia may be present. Visual field testing reveals an enlarged blind spot, and MRI reveals normal-to-small ventricles. Lumbar puncture demonstrates normal chemistries, but the pressure is elevated. The disorder has been associated with a variety of conditions including obesity, menstrual irregularity, chronic otitis, and steroid therapy. Treatment consists of careful observation, repeated lumbar puncture with removal of sufficient CSF to return the pressure to normal each time, and diuretics or steroids. If vision is threatened, surgical decompression of the optic nerve is indicated (see Chapter 13) [Corbett et al., 1982].

Brain abscess is rare but can occur in patients with cyanotic congenital heart disease, chronic infections, or immunosuppression secondary to chemotherapy or HIV infection. There may be single or multiple abscesses. The symptoms include fever, headache, and focal weakness; signs include papilledema and focal neurologic abnormalities. MRI is diagnostic and antibiotics and surgical drainage are the treatment of choice.

A chronic subdural hematoma may be secondary to head trauma from accident, abuse, or blood dyscrasia. Symptoms include headache, vomiting, lethargy, and focal neurologic symptoms. The neurologic examination may reveal macrocephaly, papilledema, and focal neurologic abnormality. MRI will usually demonstrate the abnormality. Therapy includes surgical drainage or a shunting procedure.

Chronic nonprogressive headache

Headaches believed to be precipitated by or associated with emotional causes with no organic substrate are called *tension* or *muscle contraction headaches*. This category includes stress-related headaches, headaches caused by conversion reaction, headaches that are depressive equivalents, and headaches related to malingering. This group does not include migraine headaches that are precipitated by stress. Chronic, nonprogressive headaches are less common in children under 10 years of age but become more frequent in adolescents. In my experience, females are more frequently affected. The frequent nonmigrainous headaches described by Bille are muscle contraction headaches and occur in 16% of adolescents by 15 years of age [1962]. Details concerning the clinical features of muscle contraction headaches in adolescents have not been well-studied, but in my experience, the symptoms are similar to those seen in adults [Friedman et al., 1954]. The patients have no aura.

The pain is less severe than migraine, is bitemporal or bifrontal, and is rarely associated with nausea or vomiting. The patients have daily headaches or headaches several times per week. The headaches usually have been present from months to years. Some of these individuals have prolonged absences from school despite being honor students. The patients describe the headaches in a nonspecific manner and may have associated symptoms, such as blurred vision, fatigue, and dizziness. In obtaining the history, details concerning school absence, headaches in other family members, alcoholism, divorce, parental absence from the home, a sibling leaving home, and recent death of a close relative are important. Some of these patients have previous histories of abdominal or limb pain for which no cause was found. Others have histories of chronic behavioral difficulties. The physical and neurologic examinations in these patients are normal. Laboratory testing generally is not needed, although parents will frequently press for them to be performed. A psychosocial evaluation is mandatory. An interview with a psychologist and projective testing are used. Only rarely is a more severe psychopathologic process noted, such as major depression and/or schizophrenia.

Moderate depression may be a concomitant of chronic, nonprogressive headaches. Manifestations of depression in childhood and adolescence include withdrawal, poor school performance, sleep disturbance, aggressive behavior, self-deprecation, lack of energy, somatic complaints, mood changes, weight loss, and school phobia [Ling et al., 1970].

Posttraumatic headaches usually diminish over time. However, when a patient with concussion or head injury is examined months to years later for chronic nonprogressive headache, a coexisting psychologic problem should be suspected. The severity of the headache does not correlate with the severity of the injury. A thorough physical examination and laboratory tests are needed to eliminate organic disorders, such as leptomeningeal cyst or subdural hematoma.

If chronic headache has been present continuously for more than 8 weeks in the absence of neurologic signs and symptoms and the physical and neurologic examinations are negative, the headache is usually stress-related. This finding is especially true when headache is coupled with a prolonged absence from school. When this diagnosis is suspected, it should be discussed openly at the first visit with both the parents and child. Investigations regarding the psychologic aspects of the family should be undertaken promptly. Although data concerning the various treatment modalities for this disorder are not available, family counseling, individual counseling, and biofeedback alone or in combination with medication are reported to be successful [Burke and Andrasik, 1989]. In my experience, amitriptyline is a useful adjunct even in patients without obvious depression [Couch and Hassanein, 1979]. At subsequent examinations, measurement of blood levels and the performance of an EKG are useful guides to measure both compliance and safety. Treatment based solely on medication is not in the best interest of the patient. To design a comprehensive treatment program, the patient's age, the family's responsiveness to the concept of psychologic illness, and the availability of services in the community must be taken into account. Conversion reaction, major depression, and malingering are more complex problems and require psychiatric evaluation and treatment. No definitive data regarding the ultimate outcome of children and adolescents with stress-related headaches are available.

Mixed headaches

The combination of daily nonprogressive headache without neurologic symptoms or signs and superimposed acute recurrent migrainous headache is not uncommon in adolescents. Stress commonly precipitates both forms of headache in the predisposed patient. The history is negative for symptoms of increased intracranial pressure and the neurologic examination is normal. Imaging studies are needed to eliminate an intracranial abnormality and sinusitis and to reassure the patient and parents. A thorough psychologic evaluation is indicated. A combination of individual counseling or family counseling, biofeedback, and amitriptylene therapy is often useful.

REFERENCES

AMA Ad Hoc Committee on Classification of Headache. Classification of headaches. JAMA 1962; 179:717.

Barlow CF. Headaches and migraine in childhood. Philadelphia: Oxford Blackwell Scientific Publishers, 1984.

Behrens MM. Headaches associated with disorders of the eye. Med Clin North Am 1978; 62:507.

Belfer ML, Kaban LB. Temporomandibular joint dysfunction. Pediatrics 1982; 69:564.

Bille BS. Migraine in school children. Acta Paediatr Scand 1962; 52(suppl 136):1.

Burke EJ, Andrasik F. Home- vs. clinic-based biofeedback treatment for pediatric migraine: results of treatment through one-year follow-up. Headache 1989; 29:434-40.

Corbett JJ, Savino PJ, Thompson HS, et al. Visual loss in pseudotumor cerebri. Arch Neurol 1982; 39:461.

Couch JR, Hassanein RS. Amitriptyline in migraine prophylaxis. Arch Neurol 1979; 36:695.

Curless RG. Cluster headaches in childhood. J Pediatr 1982; 101:393.

Day WH. Essays on diseases of children. London: J & A Churchill 1873.

Dhopesh V, Anwar R, Herring C. A retrospective assessment of emergency department patients with complaint of headache. Headache 1979; 19:37.

Diamond S. Prolonged benign exertional headache: its clinical characteristics and response to indomethacin. Headache 1982; 22:96.

Dugan MC, Locke S, Gallagher JR. Occipital neuralgia in adolescents and young adults. N Engl J Med 1962; 267:1166.

Faleck H, Rothner AD, Erenberg G, et al. Headache and subacute sinusitis in children and adolescents. Headache 1988; 28:96-8.

Fields HL, Levine JD. Pain: mechanisms and management. West J Med 1984; 141:347.

Friedman AP, Von Stortch TJS, Merritt HH. Migraine and tension headaches: a clinical study of two thousand cases. Neurology 1954; 4:773.

Friedman AP, Harms E. Headaches in children. Springfield, Illinois: Charles C. Thomas, 1967.

Harrison RH. Psychological testing in headaches: a review. Headache 1975; 14:177.

Hockaday JM. Migraine in childhood and other nonepileptic paroxysmal disorders. Butterworth, 1988.

Honig PJ, Charney EG. Children with brain tumor headaches. Am J Dis Child 1982; 136:99.

Johnson MA, Pennock JM, Bydder GM, et al. Clinical NMR imaging of the brain in children: normal and neurologic disease. AJRN 1983; 4:1013-26.

Kandt RS, Levine RM. Headache and acute illness in children. J Child Neurol 1987; 2:22-7.

Kinast M, Lüeders H, Rothner AD, et al. Benign focal epileptiform discharges in childhood migraine (BFEDC). Neurology 1982; 32:1309.

Ling W, Oftedal G, Weinberg W. Depressive illness in childhood presenting as severe headache. Am J Dis Child 1970; 120:122.

Olesen J. Classification and diagnostic criteria of headache disorders, cranial neuralgias, and facial pain. Cephalagia 1988; 8:1-96.

Paine RS, Oppe TE. Neurologic examination of children. Clin Dev Med 20/21, 1966, pp. 1-279.

Ray BS, Wolff HG. Experimental studies on headache. Pain-sensitive structures of the head and their significance in headache. Arch Surg 1940; 41:813.

Rothner AD. Diagnosis and management of headache in children and adolescents. Neurol Clin 1983; 1:511.

Rothner AD. Headaches in children: a review. Headache 1978; 18: 169.

Rothner AD. The migraine syndrome in children and adolescents. Pediatr Neurol 1986; 2:121.

Schechter NL. Recurrent pains in children: an overview and approach. Pediatr Clin North Am 1984; 31:949.

Shinnar S, D'Souza BJ. Migraine in children and adolescents. Pediatr Rev 1982; 3:527.

Sjaastad O, Spierings EL. Hemicrania continua: another headache absolutely responsive to indomethacin. Cephalagia 1984; 4:65.

Starfield B, Katz H, Gabriel A, et al. Morbidity in childhood: a longitudinal view. N Engl J Med 1984; 310:824.

Stewart WF, Lipton RB, Celentano DD, et al. Prevalence of migraine headache in the United States. JAMA 1992; 267:64.

16

Muscular Tone

Kenneth F. Swaiman

Tone can be conventionally separated into phasic and postural types. Phasic tone is the result of rapid stretching of a tendon, attached muscle, and most important, the muscle spindle. The response is rapid and short-lived. Postural tone is the result of a steady, restrained stretch on tendons and attached muscles, with resultant protracted contraction of the involved muscle. Gravity is the most common stimulus for this response. It is postural tone that is primarily discussed in this chapter and referred to simply as *tone*.

Tone is functionally defined as resistance to passive movement (i.e., the resistance experienced by the examiner while the patient's relaxed limbs are moved about the joints). Hypotonia is a decreased resistance to passive movement. Hyperextensibility is an abnormally increased range-of-joint movement. Hyperextensibility of the elbows, wrists, knees, and ankles usually accompanies hypotonia but is not pathognomonic. The combination of hypotonia and hyperextensibility allows an infant to adopt unusual and awkward-appearing postures.

The term *floppy* is frequently used to describe hypotonic children. This term is useful only if the clinician does not believe that the "classification" constitutes a diagnosis rather than a shorthand description of clinical manifestations.

It is essential that hypotonia be separated from hyporeflexia or muscle weakness. For example, patients with Down syndrome commonly have normal deep tendon reflexes and normal strength and yet are usually hypotonic. Conversely, patients with anterior horn cell disease are weak and manifest hypotonia, as well as hyporeflexia.

There have been a number of reviews of this subject, and the reader is advised to refer to them for further information.*

---

* References Brooke et al., 1979; Dubowitz, 1980; Dubowitz, 1985; Smith and Swaiman, 1983; Swaiman and Wright, 1979.

PATHOLOGY

Both the central and peripheral nervous systems modify tone, but intrinsic physical characteristics of the tendons, joints, and muscles and the anatomic interrelationships of these structures also contribute significantly to tone.

In childhood CNS dysfunction, upper motor neuron (unit) disease may cause either increased or decreased muscle tone [Teddy, 1984]. Disease involving the lower motor neuron (unit) results in hypotonia and weakness.

The final common pathway of upper or lower motor unit modification of tone is through the gamma loop (fusimotor) system [Granit, 1975; Gordon and Ghez, 1991]. Intimately involved with monitoring and effecting tone are the two stretch-sensitive muscle receptors—the muscle spindles and the Golgi tendon organs (Figure 16-1).

Stationed in all areas of the skeletal muscle is the fusiform-shaped receptor structure, the muscle spindle (Figure 16-2). The spindle is composed of contractile fibers at each end and a capsule covering a central fluid-filled dilatation. Sensory endings wrap around the central sections of the intrafusal fibers and monitor the stretch of these fibers; they communicate through the afferent axons that are described later. Through efferent axons, gamma neurons within the anterior horn of the spinal cord innervate the contractile muscle portions on each end of the intrafusal fiber and enhance the sensitivity of the sensory endings to stretch [Gordon and Ghez, 1991]. Gamma motor neurons that innervate muscle spindles comprise the fusimotor system.

A further division of labor occurs; the intrafusal muscle fibers are divided into three types—nuclear chain fibers, dynamic nuclear bag fibers, and static nuclear bag fibers. These fibers derive their names from the configuration of their nuclei in the fiber center. Chain fibers have nuclei arranged in a single column, whereas bag fibers have nuclei aligned in rows of two or three. A solitary Ia afferent fiber provides primary sensory

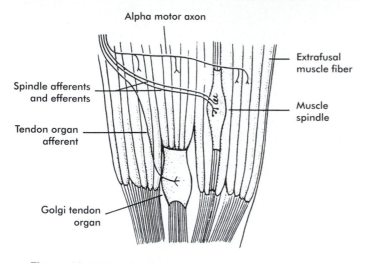

Figure 16-1 Muscle spindles and Golgi tendon organs are encapsulated structures found in skeletal muscle. The main skeletal muscle fibers, or extrafusal fibers, are innervated by large-diameter alpha motor axons. The muscle spindle has a fusiform shape and is arranged in parallel with extrafusal fibers. It is innervated by both afferent and efferent fibers. The Golgi tendon organ is found at the junction between a group of extrafusal fibers and the tendon; it is therefore in series with extrafusal fibers. Each tendon organ is innervated by a single afferent axon. (Adapted from Houck JC, Crago PE, Rymer WZ. Functional properties of the Golgi tendon organs. In: Desmedt JE, ed. Spinal and supraspinal mechanisms of voluntary motor control and locomotion, vol 8, Progress in clinical neurophysiology. Basel: Karger, 1980:33.)

innervation for all three types of intrafusal fibers. A Group II afferent fiber innervates chain and static bag fibers providing secondary sensory endings. The various sensory endings on the different types of intrafusal fibers have different characteristics of sensitivity in regard to rate of change of length. Dynamic gamma motor axons innervate the contractile portions of dynamic nuclear bag fibers, and static gamma motor axons innervate the contractile portions of the static bag fibers [Gordon and Ghez, 1991].

This intricate system of muscle spindle innervation allows the muscle stretch receptors to monitor muscle tension, length, and velocity of stretch and thus provide input for maintenance of tone [Carew, 1985].

It is through their effect on the gamma motor neuron that portions of the CNS (e.g., motor cortex, thalamus, basal ganglia, vestibular nuclei, reticular formation, and cerebellum) modify tone, with ensuing hypotonia or hypertonia (spasticity) [Alexander and Delong, 1985; Brooks and Stoney, 1971; Ghez, 1985; Carew, 1985].

The Golgi tendon organs, unlike the muscle spindles, are found in series with the skeletal muscle fibers (Figure 16-3) and are attached at one end to the muscle and at

the other to the tendon. A number of individual skeletal muscle fibers enter a Golgi tendon organ through a constricted collar. The muscle fibers are attached to collagen fibers within the Golgi tendon organ. A single Ib axon enters each capsule and forms branches that are interlaced among the collagen fibers. The afferent axon branches are compressed when muscle contraction occurs and impulses are transmitted. Tendon organs are much more sensitive to muscle contraction than muscle spindles. Furthermore, tendon organs appear to be less sensitive to stretch than muscle spindles. Each of these sensitivities has different value during the performance of varying motor tasks [Gordon and Ghez, 1991].

EVALUATION OF THE PATIENT
History

Because several conditions characterized by hypotonia are hereditary, a careful genetic history must be sought. Questioning of grandparents and parents, when possible, may prove most valuable.

The age at which hypotonia is first evident may be all-important diagnostically. The presence of hypotonia at birth or shortly thereafter serves to differentiate among a number of conditions. Weak fetal movements or the change from apparently normal fetal movements to those of decreased amplitude and vigor should be determined.

The association of hypotonia and polyhydramnios signals prenatal interference with the swallowing mechanism.

Examination

Observation and manipulation of fixed contractures of the limbs in the neonatal period may demonstrate that the hypotonia is associated with an antenatal insult. Premature infants are normally hypotonic even when not ill; therefore their corrected ages should be considered when assessing premature infants during the first few months of life.

The tendency of the infant to assume unusual positions, including the "frog's legs" configuration in which the supine infant assumes a position with the lower limbs externally rotated and abducted, may indicate the presence of hypotonia.

The hypotonic infant may have difficulties evident at birth. Weakness is often associated with hypotonia, with resultant poor suck, cry, and respiratory effort. There may be a paucity of spontaneous limb movements. Weakness should be suspected if the infant does not briskly withdraw a limb in response to painful stimuli. The infant may be unable to raise a limb or sustain the position of a raised limb.

Passive pronation, supination, flexion, and extension of the limbs, gently shaking the hands and feet while

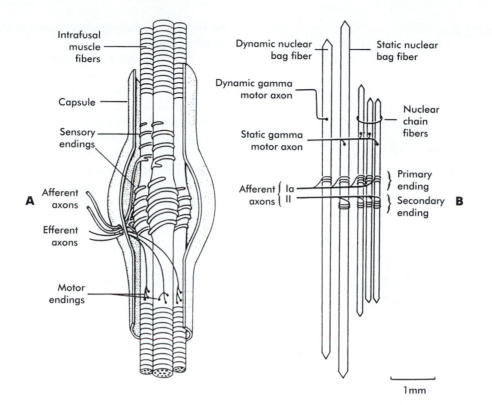

Figure 16-2 The main components of the muscle spindle are intrafusal fibers, sensory endings, and motor axons. **A,** The intrafusal fibers are specialized fibers; their central regions are not contractile. The sensory endings spiral around the central regions of the intrafusal fibers and are responsive to stretch of these fibers. Gamma motor neurons innervate the contractile polar regions of the intrafusal fibers. Contraction of the intrafusal fibers pulls on the central regions from both ends and increases the sensitivity of the sensory endings to stretch. **B,** The muscle spindle contains three types of intrafusal fibers: dynamic nuclear bag, static nuclear bag, and nuclear chain fibers. A single group Ia afferent fiber innervates all three types of intrafusal fiber, forming a primary ending. A group II afferent fiber innervates chain and static bag fibers, forming a secondary ending. Two types of efferent axons innervate different intrafusal fibers. Dynamic gamma motor axons innervate only dynamic bag fibers; static gamma motor axons innervate various combinations of chain and static bag fibers. (**A,** adapted from Hullinger M. Rev Physiol Biochem Pharmacol 1984; 101:1; **B,** adapted from Boyd IA. Trends Neurosci 1980; 3:258.)

grasping the wrists or ankles are common means of assessing tone. The hands move over a large amplitude when the arms are shaken at the wrists. Often the elbows can be extended beyond their normal range. The Scarf sign assessment involves wrapping the infant's arm across the chest and is positive when the elbow can be readily moved beyond the midline. One of the best means of evaluating tone is use of the traction maneuver, during which observation of head control, flexion of elbows during infant participation, and general body and back posture are performed (see Figure 3-6). The hypotonic infant's foot may be brought to the opposite ear, and extreme passive foot dorsiflexion may be possible when hypotonia is profound.

The hypotonic infant will slip through the hands of the examiner when held by the axillae (vertical suspension maneuver). If the hypotonic infant is supported by the trunk in an outstretched prone position (horizontal suspension maneuver), gravity will cause flexion, or

droop of the head and extremities. The normal infant will hold the head erect and flex the limbs against gravity while holding the back straight.

Facial weakness, weak suck, weakness of muscles of deglutition, and paresis of the elevators of the eyelid and the extraocular muscles are often associated with unusual myopathies. The tongue should be carefully examined for atrophy and fibrillations. Evaluation of muscle weakness can be facilitated with the traction maneuver and by ascertaining the withdrawal response to appropriate stimuli and the ability to resist gravity. Paucity of movement signals the likely presence of concomitant weakness. If limb weakness is present, localization of the weakness to the proximal or distal extremities should be attempted. Older children will manifest talipes planus, pronation at the ankles, and genu recurvatum.

The pectus excavatum deformity and a bell-shaped chest may indicate predominate strength of the dia-

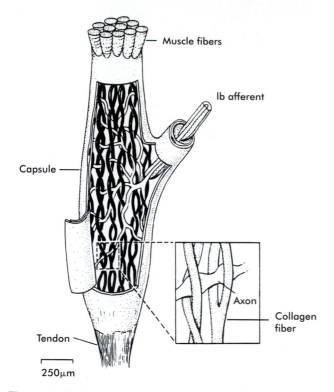

Muscle fibers

Ib afferent

Capsule

Axon

Collagen fiber

Tendon

250μm

Figure 16-3 Golgi tendon organs are specialized structures found at the junctions between muscle and tendon. Collagen fibers in the tendon organ attach to the muscle fibers. A single Ib afferent axon enters the capsule and branches into many unmyelinated endings that wrap around and between the collagen fibers. When the tendon organ is stretched (usually because of contraction of the muscle), the afferent axon is compressed by the collagen fibers (see insert at lower right) and increases its rate of firing. (Adapted from Schmidt RF. Motor systems. In: Schmidt RF, Thews G, eds. Human physiology, Biederman-Thorson MA, trans, Berlin: Springer, 1983:81; inset adapted from Swett JE, Schoultz TW. Arch Ital Biol 1975; 11:328.)

phragm over the intercostal muscles during respiratory efforts. Skeletal deformities and fixed contractures are often present in congenital myotonic dystrophy and some congenital myopathies.

Fixed contractures of the limbs may signal the presence of arthrogryposis multiplex congenita, which results from dysfunction at a number of lower motor neuron unit sites [Lebenthal et al., 1970; Yuill and Lynch, 1974].

Fasciculations of limb muscles cannot be observed in infants because of the overlying, abundant, subcutaneous tissue; however, the experienced examiner can palpate the muscle beneath the fat and estimate the adequacy of muscle bulk.

The deep tendon reflexes in the premature and term newborn should always be elicited. These reflexes may be difficult to elicit in the triceps, variably obtainable at

the biceps, and almost always present at the patellar and Achilles tendons.

In the early infantile period, development of weakness and hypotonia that is progressive and profound suggests the possibility of infantile botulism [Kao et al., 1976; Pickett et al., 1976; Thompson et al., 1980].

In addition to most of the above-mentioned characteristics, hypotonia in the ambulatory child may manifest with a waddling gait, genu recurvatum, and talipes planus. There may be pronation of the feet at the ankles. The presence of scoliosis suggests associated weakness and neuromuscular disease.

In the older child, more formal and discrete muscle testing is possible as described in Chapter 2. Observation of gait may indicate weakness (Chapter 17). Furthermore, elicitation of the deep tendon reflexes, toe signs, and myotonic response to percussion, as well as scrutiny of muscles for evidence of fasciculations, is relatively easily accomplished in older children.

When the lower motor unit is involved, the deep tendon reflexes are usually hypoactive and at times are absent. The reflexes are absent in infantile spinal muscular atrophy [Bundey and Lovelace, 1975; Smith and Swaiman, 1983]. When the upper motor unit is involved, the reflexes tend to be normal or increased.

Further neurologic examination is necessary and should include the search for fasciculations, ptosis, squint, myotonia, and extensor toe signs. The presence of squint and/or ptosis should suggest the possibility of congenital myopathies [Clancy et al., 1980; Fukuhara et al., 1978; Fukuyama et al., 1960; Kamoshita et al., 1976; McComb et al., 1979], myotonic dystrophy, myasthenia gravis [Holmes et al., 1980; Namba et al., 1970], or mitochondrial myopathies (see Chapters 23 and 69).

Specific laboratory studies may be essential in establishing the diagnosis. When lower motor unit diseases are considered, serum enzyme determinations, nerve conduction velocities, electromyography, and nerve or muscle biopsies may be of importance. When upper motor unit diseases are involved, careful history-taking, EEG and evoked-response testing, brain scanning, specific endocrine evaluations, and specific enzyme determinations may be required.

DIAGNOSIS

For didactic purposes and simplification, the motor pathway from the motor neuron in the motor strip to the skeletal muscle fiber can be divided into upper and lower motor neuron units. The upper motor neuron (unit) includes the motor neuron in the motor strip and the myelinated nerve fiber, which traverses the corticospinal tract and eventually terminates in the internuncial pool in the spinal cord adjacent to the anterior horn cell. The lower motor neuron (unit) consists of the anterior horn cell, peripheral nerve, neuromuscular junction, and

---

Conditions associated with hypotonia

Combined Central and Peripheral Nervous System Disease

Adrenoleukodystrophy (neonatal)
Cerebellothalamospinal degeneration
Fukuyama muscular dystrophy and encephalopathy
Infantile neuroaxonal dystrophy
Krabbe disease (globoid cell leukodystrophy)
Metachromatic leukodystrophy
Prader-Willi syndrome
Zellweger syndrome

Upper Motor Unit Disease (CNS Diseases)

Acute cerebral insult
Cerebrovascular accident (e.g., hemorrhage, thrombosis, embolism)
Hypoxic-ischemic encephalopathy
Infection (e.g., viral, bacterial, fungal, parasitic)
Chromosomal abnormality
　Down syndrome
　Prader-Willi syndrome
Congenital motor disease (cerebral palsy)
　Ataxia
　Atonic diplegia or paraplegia (periventricular leukomalacia)
Incontinentia pigmenti
Metabolic diseases
　Carnitine deficiency
　Cytochrome c oxidase deficiency
　Fucosidosis
　Gangliosidosis (GM1)
　Hyperammonemia
　Hypercalcemia
　Hyperglycinemia
　Hyperlysinemia
　Hypocalcemia
　Niemann-Pick disease
　Mannosidosis
　Oculocerebrorenal syndrome (Lowe syndrome)
　Organic acidemias
　Renal tubular acidosis
　Tay-Sachs disease (and other GM2 gangliosidoses)
Toxicity
　Bilirubin
　Magnesium
　Phenobarbital
　Phenytoin
　Sedative drugs
Trauma
　Brain
　Cord

Conditions associated with hypotonia, cont'd.

Lower Motor Unit System Diseases

Arthrogryposis multiplex congenita
Carnitine deficiency
Connective tissue disease, such as Ehlers-Danlos syndrome
Anterior horn cell
　Infantile spinal muscular atrophy
　Kugelberg-Welander disease
　Poliomyelitis
Peripheral nerve
　Familial dysautonomia
　Guillain-Barré syndrome
　Hereditary motor-sensory neuropathies
　Polyneuropathy
Neuromuscular junction
　Botulism
　Myasthenia gravis
　Myasthenic syndrome
　Neonatal myasthenia gravis (immune- and nonimmune-mediated)
　Neonatal transient myasthenia gravis
Muscle
　Congenital myopathies (central core disease, congenital fiber type disproportion, myotubular myopathy, nemaline myopathy)
　Glycogen storage disease (acid maltase deficiency, phosphofructokinase deficiency, phosphorylase deficiency)
　Hypothyroidism
　Polymyositis

---

muscle. Disorders affecting muscular tone are divided into upper and lower motor unit disorders. Combined disorders also occur. It cannot be stressed too emphatically, in contradistinction to the usual residua in older children and adults, that upper motor unit disease may result in either increased or diminished muscle tone in infants and young children.

Functional impairment of the lower motor unit causes both hypotonia and weakness. In addition, hyporeflexia, fasciculations, and muscle atrophy result.

Certain conditions (e.g., Krabbe disease) cause combined upper and lower motor unit impairment and produce hypotonia.

The most common cause of hypotonia is inadequate brain control of the motor pathways, or central hypotonia. The presence of normoactive or brisk deep tendon reflexes suggests that the child is probably not suffering from lower motor unit impairment. The examiner should be alert for other signs of brain dysfunction, such as lethargy, unresponsiveness to the environment (visual and auditory stimuli), lack of development of social skills in the early months of life, and, in older children, delayed development of language and reasoning skills.

Diseases of the upper motor unit may be classified according to pathophysiologic cause (i.e., toxic, metabolic, degenerative, traumatic, congenital, or infectious). A similar classification may be used for lower motor unit diseases; additionally, such diseases may be categorized by the anatomic site of involvement.

A number of specific diseases will be suggested by historic and physical findings. Marked arching of the back and irritability suggests Krabbe disease. Obesity with small male genitalia suggests Prader-Willi syndrome; chromosomal studies are indicated.

Down syndrome is often evident on clinical grounds alone, although confirmatory chromosomal studies are necessary. Visceromegaly, particularly hepatomegaly, is found with some diseases associated with hypotonia, including Niemann-Pick disease and cerebrohepatorenal syndrome. Blindness, seizure activity, and hyperacusis suggest Tay-Sachs disease. Muscle wasting and flexion contractures are characteristic of arthrogryposis multiplex congenita.

The presence of hypothyroidism is suggested by decreased height and weight, a large tongue, and developmental delay. The conditions associated with hypotonia are listed in the box on p. 231 and are discussed in detail elsewhere in this book.

CLINICAL LABORATORY STUDIES

Usual laboratory studies such as hemogram, erythrocyte sedimentation rate, urinalysis, and serum electrolyte determinations are usually of no help in assessing hypotonia. Hypothyroidism can be diagnosed from conventional thyroid studies. Some conditions linked to hypotonia require special tests to yield a precise diagnosis. Pertinent portions of this text should be consulted to determine special laboratory testing requirements.

Neuroimaging techniques using X-ray techniques or MRI may be helpful in the diagnosis of CNS abnormalities. MRI is of particular value in the diagnosis of white matter diseases, including leukodystrophies.

Spinal fluid studies may demonstrate pleocytosis or increased and/or abnormal proteins suggesting demyelinating conditions or peripheral neuropathy.

Testing for leukocyte enzyme activities associated with certain lipid storage diseases may provide definitive diagnoses for conditions that affect the brain alone, the brain and anterior horn cells, or the brain and peripheral nerves. Obviously some of these conditions affect other nonneural organs.

Determination of activities of serum muscle enzymes (i.e., those enzymes that have escaped the muscle cells and are detectable in serum) infrequently aids the diagnosis of hypotonia; however, activities are sometimes elevated in certain congenital muscular dystrophies and mitochondrial myopathies. The ease of obtaining serum creatine kinase and aldolase activities thus makes such determinations worthwhile.

Some neuromuscular diseases are associated with cardiomyopathies, and electrocardiography or echocardiography may be of aid in establishing a diagnosis.

Electromyography differentiates neurogenic from myopathic conditions and should inspire more intense considerations of some diagnostic categories. Studies in infants and young children require patience and experience for optimal studies and interpretation. The conventional assessment of insertion potentials and potentials at rest and during movement are as essential in infants as they are in older children and adults.

The diagnosis of peripheral neuropathy, particularly in those conditions that involve both the central and peripheral nervous system, may be readily overlooked without the determination of nerve conduction velocities. Norms are available for all age groups [Gamstorp, 1963].

The value of muscle biopsy is well established in the diagnosis of neuromuscular conditions and is discussed elsewhere in this book. It is virtually obligatory that biopsies, preparation of the muscle specimens, and light and microscopic studies be performed by individuals specially trained and experienced in these endeavors.

REFERENCES

Alexander G, Delong M. Organization of supraspinal motor systems. In: McKhann A, McDonald W, eds. Diseases of the nervous system: clinical neurology. Philadelphia: WB Saunders, 1985.

Boyd IA. The isolated mammalian muscle spindle. Trends Neurosci 1980; 3:258.

Brooke MH, Carroll JE, Ringel SP. Congenital hypotonia revisited (review). Muscle Nerve 1979; 2:84.

Brooks VB, Stoney SD. Motor mechanisms: the role of the pyramidal system in motor control. Ann Rev Physiol 1971; 33:337.

Bundey S, Lovelace RE. A clinical and genetic study of chronic proximal spinal muscular atrophy. Brain 1975; 98:455.

Carew T. Posture and locomotion. In: Kandel E, Schwartz J, eds. Principles of neural science, 2nd ed. New York: Elsevier Science Publishing, 1985.

Clancy RR, Kelts KA, Oehlert JW. Clinical variability in congenital fiber type disproportion. J Neurosci 1980; 46:257.

Dubowitz V. The floppy infant, 2nd ed. Philadelphia: J.B. Lippincott, 1980.

Dubowitz V. Evaluation and differential diagnosis of the hypotonic infant. Pediatr Rev 1985; 6:237.

Fukuhara N, Yuasa T, Tsubaki T, et al. Nemaline myopathy: histological, histochemical and ultrastructural studies. Acta Neuropathol 1978; 42:33.

Fukuyama Y, Haruna H, Kawazura M. A peculiar form of congenital progressive muscular dystrophy. Paediatr Univ Tokyo 1960; 4:5.

Gamstorp I. Normal conduction velocity of ulnar, median and peroneal nerves in infancy, childhood and adolescence. Acta Paediatr Scand (Suppl.) 1963; 146:68.

Ghez C. Introduction to the motor systems. In: Kandel E, Schwartz J, eds. Principles of neural science, 2nd ed. New York: Elsevier Science Publishing, 1985.

Gordon J, Ghez C. Muscle receptors and spinal reflexes: the stretch reflex. In: Kandel E, Schwartz J, Jessell T, eds. Principles of neural science, 3rd ed. New York: Elsevier Science Publishing, 1991.

Granit R. The basis of motor control. New York: Academic Press, 1970.

Granit R. The functional role of the muscle spindles—facts and hypotheses. Brain 1975; 98:531.

Holmes LB, Driscoll SG, Bradley WG. Contractures in a newborn infant of a mother with myasthenia gravis. J Pediatr 1980; 6:1067.

Houk JC, Crago PE, Rymer WZ. Functional properties of the Golgi tendon organs. In: Desmedt JE, ed. Spinal and supraspinal mechanisms of voluntary motor control and locomotion, vol 8, Progress in Clinical Neurophysiology. Basel: Karger, 1980:33.

Hullinger M. The mammalian muscle spindle and its central control. Rev Physiol Biochem Pharmacol 1984; 101:1.

Kamoshita S, Konishi Y, Segawa M, et al. Congenital muscular dystrophy as a disease of the central nervous system. Arch Neurol 1976; 33:513.

Kao I, Drachman DB, Price DL. Botulinum toxin. Mechanism presynaptic blockade. Science 1976; 193:1256.

Lebenthal E, Ben-Bassat M, Reisner SH, et al. Arthrogryposis multiplex congenita—myopathic type. Isr J Med Sci 1973; 9:463.

Lebenthal E, Shochet SB, Adam A, et al. Arthrogryposis multiplex congenita: twenty-three cases in an Arab kindred. Pediatrics 1970; 46:891.

McComb RD, Markesbery WR, O'Connor WN. Fatal neonatal nemaline myopathy with multiple congenital anomalies. J Pediatr 1979; 94:47.

Namba T, Brown SB, Grob D. Neonatal myasthenia gravis: report on two cases and review of the literature. Pediatrics 1970; 45:488.

Pickett J, Berg B, Chaplin E. Syndrome of botulism in infancy: clinical and electrophysiologic study. N Engl J Med 1976; 295:770.

Schmidt RF. Motor systems. In: Schmidt RF, Thews G, eds. Human physiology, Biederman-Thorson MA, trans. Berlin: Springer, 1983:81.

Smith S, Swaiman K. Hypotonic infant. In: Moss A, ed. Pediatrics update. New York: Elsevier Biomedical, 1983.

Swaiman KF, Wright FS. Pediatric neuromuscular diseases. St. Louis: Mosby, 1979.

Swett JE, Schoultz TW. Mechanical transduction in the Golgi tendon organ: a hypothesis. Arch Ital Biol 1975; 113:374.

Teddy PJ, Silver JR, Baker JH, et al. Traumatic cerebral flaccid paraplegia. Paraplegia 1984; 22:320.

Thompson JA, Glasgow LA, Warpinski JR, et al. Infant botulism: clinical spectrum and epidemiology. Pediatrics 1980; 66:936.

Yuill GM, Lynch PG. Congenital non-progressive peripheral neuropathy with arthrogryposis multiplex. J Neurol Neurosurg Psychiatry 1974; 37:316.

17

Gait Impairment

Kenneth F. Swaiman

Gait disturbances are a common manifestation of neurologic disease in children. Gait is a demanding, complicated skill that requires integration of many functional components of the nervous system and is the result of a repetitive sequence of limb movements. Optimal gait requires the least expenditure of energy possible. Mechanical energy must be generated and then dissipated in a controlled fashion during each cycle [Gage et al., 1984; Õunpuu et al., 1991]. During the gait cycle, posture and balance must be maintained, and the feet must clear the ground without scraping.

Obviously gait must be assessed when the patient's chief complaint focuses on walking or running; however, assessment of gait allows the clinician rapid appraisal of a number of significant nervous system units when patient complaints are other than those relating to gait.

PHYSIOLOGIC CONSIDERATIONS

Skills required for standing must be synthesized into the walking procedure. The walking sequence requires that the non–weight-bearing leg moves forward while weight is shifted smoothly from leg to leg. The definitive components of support and forward movement require separate consideration; the rhythm and duration of each phase require monitoring [Gage and Õunpuu, 1989; Paine and Oppe, 1966]. Conventionally, the period of time from one heel-ground contact to the next heel-ground contact of one foot is one gait cycle; walking can be divided into "stance" and "swing" phases. The instant from which heel-ground contact occurs until the instant when contact terminates is the stance phase. The stance phase can be divided into the following four parts: initial contact, loading response, midstance, and terminal stance (Figures 17-1 and 17-2). The period beginning immediately after the toe leaves the ground until the heel contacts the ground is the swing phase (Figures 17-1 and 17-2) [Burnett and Johnson, 1971a; 1971b; Norlin et al., 1981]. The swing phase can also be divided into the following four parts: preswing, initial swing, midswing, and terminal swing. The stance phase occupies 60% of the duration of the cycle, and the swing phase occupies 40%. Elaborate methods for the assessment of phases of gait have been devised [Burnett and Johnson, 1971a; Õunpuu et al., 1991]. The center of gravity is

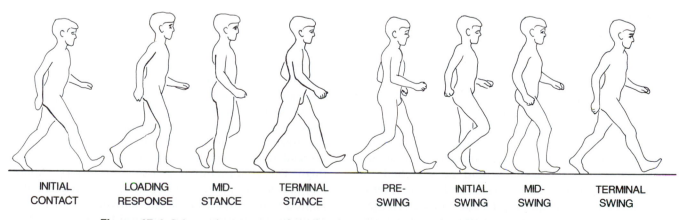

| INITIAL CONTACT | LOADING RESPONSE | MID-STANCE | TERMINAL STANCE | PRE-SWING | INITIAL SWING | MID-SWING | TERMINAL SWING |

Figure 17-1 Schematic representation of various phases of a child walking. (Adapted from Õunpuu S, et al. J Pediatri Orthop 1991;11:341.)

facial muscles, choreiform movements of the trunk and limbs, and irregular breathing patterns and sounds.

Steppage gait

Weakness of dorsiflexion of the feet and toes and fixed contracture in plantar flexion result in a steppage gait. The contracture most often accompanies weakness of the peroneal and anterior tibial muscles. To avoid stumbling, the child lifts the foot disproportionately high at the start of each stride. Flexion at the hip and knee is exaggerated, followed by a forward flinging of the foot. The toe precedes the heel or ball of the foot in hitting the ground, thus emitting the first portion of a split sound. This pattern of ground contact wears away the tips of shoes. The steps are similar to one another and rhythmic. This unusual gait may be isolated to one leg but is more often bilateral.

This condition is most often associated with anterior horn cell and peripheral neuropathy involvement in disease processes such as progressive muscular atrophy, poliomyelitis, Charcot-Marie-Tooth disease, Guillian-Barré syndrome, and distal myopathy.

Hip weakness gait

Severe weakness of the abductors and extensors of the hip lead to a pathologic gait. The child walks with a marked lordosis of the thoracolumbar spine, and the gait is "waddling." The pelvis is unstable and the gait broad-based. The pelvis markedly pivots and rotates sharply from side to side as weight shifts. The movement pattern allows balance to be maintained despite hip muscle weakness.

Stability may be further compromised by accompanying equinovarus deformities. These deformities are frequently present in various muscular dystrophies, myositides, and spinal muscular atrophies, including Kugelberg-Welander disease.

Gait apraxia

Occasionally, severe frontal lobe problems result in gait disturbances. These patients have no direct motor or sensory impairment. Although the child may successfully complete certain simple and automatic movements with the legs, he or she is unable to implement more complex activities, such as tracing a circle with the feet, kicking an object, or attempting to walk in a prescribed pattern. The gait is deliberate. The patient may have difficulty initiating the walking process when already standing and have further problems with execution of the serial acts of rising, standing, or walking. Other characteristics, such as perseveration of leg movements and rigidity, are often present. A curious phenomenon in which a leg becomes rigid when the limbs are passively manipulated occurs during fluctuating resistance (gegenhalten). Other frontal lobe manifestations, such as dementia and reappear-

ance of primitive grasp reflexes, rooting, and palmomental reflexes, may be present.

ANTALGIC GAIT (PAINFUL GAIT)

Pain can arise from any leg and foot structures, including nails, skin, joints, bone, and muscles. The associated limp is caused by a decreased weight support on the painful leg and increased weight support on the unaffected leg [Chung, 1974]. The examiner may require prolonged observation to determine the precise nature of the limp. The exact limp pattern is determined by the location of the pain [Hensinger, 1977].

CONVERSION REACTION GAIT

Conversion reaction may result in patterns that simulate hemiplegia, monoplegia, and paraplegia. Children between 10 and 16 years of age are most commonly affected. The gait pattern may vary from one moment to the next; this phenomenon should alert the examiner to the possible diagnosis of conversion reaction. The clinician will find no abnormalities of coordination, tone, or strength when the patient is sitting or lying down.

The gaits may be outrageously intricate and may vary from time to time in the same child. Short periods of normal walking activity may occur. Tremulousness of the fingers and hands during standing or walking may be associated. It is noteworthy that patients with conversion reaction resembling hemiplegia or monoplegia usually drag the foot along the floor or push it ahead in contradistinction to patients with corticospinal tract difficulty who elevate and circumduct the leg during each step. When both legs are involved, the patient may be bedridden or use crutches. On rare occasions the child will lurch out of control but not fall, demonstrating remarkable coordination and strength. During Romberg testing the swaying is often at the hips or higher trunk. Patients with conversion reactions occasionally do not separate their feet, whereas children with neurologic problems often separate their feet to maintain their balance because they tend to sway from the ankles. They may have associated rapid random movements of the head, hands, and hips. If the patient were to fall, there may be a dramatic aspect to the mishap. The patient may be able to run or walk backward without difficulty. However, as noted, patients with dystonia musculorum deformans may walk backward smoothly, although they have problems with forward ambulation.

Patients with conversion reaction gait difficulties require skillful intervention that is supportive and empathetic. Patients and parents must receive experienced and measured professional therapy and counseling.

REFERENCES

Brown JR. Diseases of the cerebellum. In: Baker AB, Baker LH, eds. Clinical neurology. 4th ed. Baltimore: Harper & Row, 1980.

Burnett CN, Johnson EW. Development of gait in childhood, I. Dev Med Child Neurol 1971a; 13:196.

Burnett CN, Johnson EW. Development of gait in childhood, II. Dev Med Child Neurol 1971b; 13:207.

Chung SM. Identifying the cause of acute limp in childhood: some informal comments and observations. Clin Pediatr 1974; 13:769.

Cotton DG. Acute cerebellar ataxia. Arch Dis Child 1957; 32:181.

Gage JR. Gait analysis in cerebral palsy. London: MacKeith Press, 1991.

Gage JR, Fabian D, Hicks R, et al. Pre and postoperative gait analysis in patients with spastic diplegia: a preliminary report. J Pediatr Orthop 1984; 4:715-725.

Gage JR, Õunpuu S. Gait analysis in clinical practice. Semin Orthop 1989; 4:72-87.

Hensinger RN. Limp. Pediatr Clin North Am 1977; 24:723.

King G, Schwarz GA, Slade HW. Acute cerebellar ataxia of childhood. Pediatrics 1958; 21:731.

Mendez-Cashion D, Sanchez-Longo LP, Valcarcel M, et al. Acute cerebellar ataxia in children associated with infection by polio virus I. Pediatrics 1962; 29:808.

Norlin R, Odenrick P, Sandlund B. Development of gait in normal children. J Pediatr Orthop 1981; 1:261.

Õunpuu S, Gage JR, Davis RB. Three-dimensional lower extremity joint kinetics in normal pediatric gait. J Pediatr Orthop 1991; 11:341.

Paine R, Oppe T. Posture and gait. In: Paine R, Oppe T, eds. Neurological examination of children. London: William Heinemann (Medical Books), 1966.

Saunders JB de CM, Inmann VT, Eberhart HD. The major determinants in normal and pathological gait. J Bone Joint Surg 1953; 35A:543.

Weiss S, Carter S. Course and prognosis of acute cerebellar ataxia in children. Neurology 1959; 9:711.

Winter DA. The biomechanics and motor control of human gait. 2nd ed. Toronto: John Wiley and Sons, 1990.

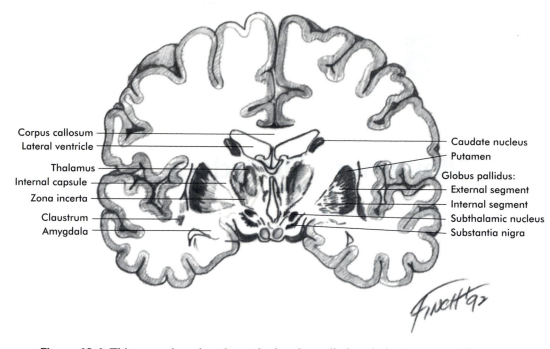

Figure 18-1 This coronal section shows the basal ganglia in relation to surrounding structures. (Adapted from Nieuwenhuys et al., The human central nervous system: a synopsis and atlas, 2nd ed. Berlin: Springer, 1981.)

The corticostriate connections comprise the basic input into the basal ganglia, although some input to the putamen is derived from the centromedian nucleus of the thalamus. Cortical neurons project axons through and around the internal capsule, which is composed primarily of the corticobulbar and corticospinal tracts. The projected fibers release glutamate, an excitatory neurotransmitter.

Internuclear connections in the basal ganglia originate in neurons that form and release gamma-aminobutyric acid, acetylcholine, and various neuropeptides, including vasoactive intestinal polypeptide and somatostatin (Table 18-1). Intrastriatal connections are subserved by the neurotransmitters acetylcholine, somatostatin, and neuropeptide Y. Other connecting fibers include those emanating from the striatum, which terminate in the globus pallidus (external and internal segments) and the pars reticulata of the substantia nigra. The striatal neurons that issue axons that connect with the globus pallidus release substance P, gamma-aminobutyric acid, and enkephalin (Figure 18-2). The striatal fibers that terminate in the pars reticulata of the substantia nigra are known to transmit gamma-aminobutyric acid, dysnorphin, and substance P. Other fibers originate in the external segment of the globus pallidus and terminate in the subthalamic nucleus, and in return, fibers originate in the subthalamic nucleus and terminate in the external segment of the globus pallidus. Fibers connect neurons in the pars compacta of the substantia nigra with the striatum (Figure 18-2); the

neurons in the substantia nigra (pars compacta) that are associated with striatal connections synthesize and release dopamine, an inhibitory transmitter.

The globus pallidus, predominantly the internal segment, projects many fibers to the thalamus; these fibers constitute a major basal ganglia output pathway. Many of these efferent fibers traverse the internal capsule, whereas others skirt the area (Figure 18-3) and eventually terminate in the ventral lateral and ventral anterior thalamus, where they link with the major cerebellar ascending outflow (dentatorubrothalamic tracts). Projections are sent to the motor cerebral cortex and its adjacent areas. The intralaminar thalamic nuclei, including the centromedian nucleus, also receive fibers from the internal segment of the globus pallidus; the centromedian nucleus in turn projects fibers to the striatum [Growdon and Young, 1987].

The pars reticulata of the substantia nigra maintains connections with the superior colliculus and the thalamic nuclei.

The result of this complex axonal and neurochemical network is an intricate system of subcortical loops that modulate motor function by combining input from many sources, including impulses from sophisticated feedback circuits, and issuing excitatory and inhibitory impulses to the motor cortex and associated areas.

Neurotransmitters

As indicated, basal ganglia contain a number of confirmed and putative neurotransmitters that are

Table 18-1 Major neurotransmitters in the basal ganglia

Origin	Termination	Transmitters
Afferent pathways		
Cortex	C + P, STh	Glutamate
Locus ceruleus	C + P, SN	Norepinephrine
Raphe nuclei	C + P, SN	Serotonin
Thalamus (intralaminar nuclei)	C + P	Acetylcholine
Efferent pathways		
GPm, SNr	Thalamus	GABA
Intrinsic connections		
SNc	C + P	Dopamine, CCK
C + P	C + P (interneurons)	Acetylcholine, somatostatin, neuropeptide Y
C + P	SNr	GABA, dynorphin, substance P
C + P	GPl	GABA, enkephalin
C + P	GPm	GABA, substance P
GPl	STh	?GABA
STh	GPm, GPl	?glutamate

Note: C + P, caudate nucleus and putamen (striatum); GP, globus pallidus (l = lateral, m = medial); SN, substantia nigra (c = compacta, r = reticulata); STh, subthalamic nucleus; CCK, cholecystokinin; GABA, gamma-aminobutyric acid.
Modified from Riley DE, Lance AE. Movement disorders. In: Bradley WG et al., eds. Neurology in clinical practice. Stoneham, MA: Butterworth-Heinemann, 1991, p. 1565.

synthesized, stored, released, and inactivated among these nuclear masses. Many transmitters are found in relatively high concentrations in specific areas but are often found in lower concentrations elsewhere in the nervous system, including the spinal cord and the peripheral nerves. This varying distribution sometimes renders interpretation of neurotransmitter functions difficult. Neurotransmitters are synthesized in presynaptic neurons and are often stored in vesicles. The propagation of an electric impulse along an axon will cause release of the neurotransmitter into the synaptic cleft; after reaching the area of the postsynaptic membrane, the neurotransmitter becomes attached (binds) to highly specific receptor sites with resultant development of postsynaptic potentials that may lead to propagation of an electrical impulse. The neurotransmitters that are associated with basal ganglia functions include acetylcholine, gamma-aminobutyric acid, dopamine, and glutamate. Other substances, neuromodulators (e.g., substance P), appear to exert critical influence on

neurotransmitter effects. A thorough understanding of the mechanisms of action of some of these substances and the pharmacologic modification of their effects have been helpful in the therapy of several conditions [Campanella et al., 1987]. A brief summary of pharmacologic agents currently used in the therapy of extrapyramidal disease is found in Table 18-2.

Acetylcholine is active in both the central and peripheral nervous systems. It is formed in the brain from choline that has been transported either free or as a phospholipid, and from acetyl-CoA; the latter compound is ubiquitous because of its pivotal role in energy metabolism at the intersection of the Embden-Meyerhof pathway and the tricarboxylic acid cycle. The rate-limiting synthesizing enzyme, choline acetyltransferase (ChAT), shares control of the rate of acetylcholine formation with the mechanisms that provide choline. Choline-acetyltransferase activity is greatest in the caudate nucleus. Acetylcholine is inactivated by a unique mechanism: cholinesterase hydrolyzes the molecule with resultant formation of choline, which may be once again used for synthesis by the presynaptic neuron. The effect of acetylcholine is blocked by atropine at receptor sites.

Although acetylcholine influence is widespread throughout the brain, it appears particularly important as a neurotransmitter in the striatum, hippocampus, and ascending reticular activating system. Compromise of its actions appears to be a major factor in Alzheimer disease. Acetylcholine is also used as a neurotransmitter by the cochlear nucleus, brainstem, cortical pyramidal cells, posteromedial portions of the thalamus, supraoptic nucleus, lateral geniculate body, caudate nucleus, and ventral thalamus. Afferent axons of the visual and auditory pathways use acetylcholine as a neurotransmitter. Atropine and related drugs reduce the concentration of brain acetylcholine.

Gamma-aminobutyric acid is synthesized from glutamic acid (Figure 18-4) by the rate-limiting enzyme glutamic acid decarboxylase (GAD). Pyridoxal phosphate is a cofactor for both glutamic acid decarboxylase and gamma-aminobutyric acid transaminase (GABA-T) activities. Gamma-aminobutyric acid is rendered inactive by gamma-aminobutyric acid transaminase through the formation of succinic semialdehyde. Gamma-aminobutyric acid is concentrated in the globus pallidus, substantia nigra, hypothalamus, and, to a lesser degree, in the caudate and putamen. The neurotransmitter has a pivotal role in the interneurons of the striatum, the descending pallidonigral pathways, and the striatonigral pathways.

Dopamine is formed in the brain from tyrosine under the auspices of tyrosine hydroxylase and then dopadecarboxylase (Figure 18-5). Pyridoxine is a cofactor for the reaction. Because it is a highly polar molecule, dopamine does not cross the blood-brain barrier.

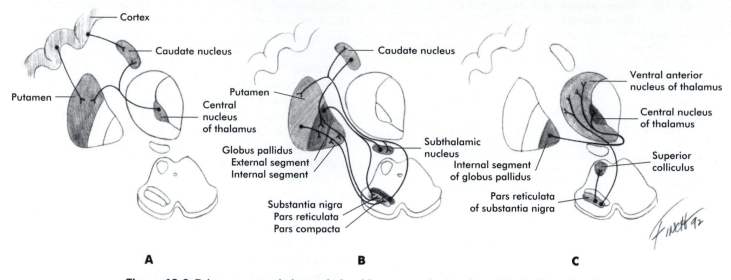

A **B** **C**

Figure 18-2 Primary anatomic interrelationships among the basal ganglia. **A,** Virtually all afferent input to the basal ganglia is directed to the caudate nucleus and putamen. **B,** Internuclear connections constitute topographically organized pathways among all the nuclei of the basal ganglia. **C,** The thalamus is the primary recipient of efferent connections from the basal ganglia. (Redrawn and modified from Côté L, Crutcher MD. The basal ganglia. In: Kandel ER, Schwartz JH, Jessell TM. eds. Principles of neural science, 3rd edition. New York: Elsevier, 1991.)

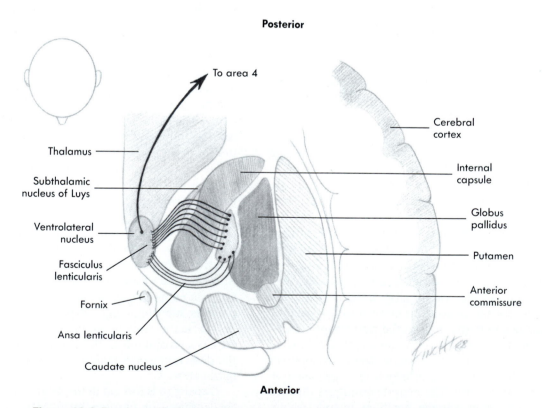

Figure 18-3 Basal ganglia in the horizontal plane, illustrating the main efferent projections from the medial segment of the pallidum to the ventral nuclei of the thalamus. (Adapted from Adams RD, Victor M. Principles of neurology, 3rd ed. New York: McGraw-Hill, 1985.)

Table 18-2 Pharmacologic agents associated with movement disorders

Agent	Actions	Clinical use
D-amphetamine	Displaces endogenous norepinephrine	Attention deficit disorders
L-amphetamine	Displaces endogenous norepinephrine and dopamine	
	Stimulates dopamine receptors	Emetic, test of dopamine responsiveness
Belladonna alkaloids	Decrease brain acetylcholine content; block acetylcholine receptors	Parasympathetic blockers
Benztropine	Anticholinergic	Parkinson disease
Bromocriptine	Dopaminergic agonist	Amenorrhea/galactorrhea
Butyrophenones	Block dopamine receptors	Tranquilizers, chorea, and Tourette syndrome
Clonidine	Dopaminergic agonist	Antihypertensive
Disulfiram	Inhibits dopamine-beta-hydroxylase	Alcoholism
L-5-hydroxytryptophan	Serotonin precursor	
Imipramine, other tricyclic antidepressants	Inhibit serotonin and catecholamine reuptake	Antidepressants
Levodopa (L-dopa)	Stimulates dopamine receptors	Rigidity and akinesia in Parkinson disease, and Huntington chorea
Lithium	Reduces catecholamine receptor sensitivity	Manic-depressive illness
Methysergide	Blocks serotonin receptors	Migraine prophylaxis
Alpha-Methyldopa	Inhibits dopamine-beta-hydroxylase (peripheral)	Hypertension
Monoamine-oxidase inhibitors	Inhibit monoamine oxidase	Antidepressants, antimigraine, hypertension, and angina
Phenothiazines	Block dopamine receptors	Tranquilizers and antiemetics
Physostigmine	Inhibits acetylcholinesterase	Cholinesterase inhibitors
Propranolol	Blocks beta-adrenergic receptors	Cardiac arrhythmias and essential tremor
Reserpine	Inhibits reuptake of dopamine, norepinephrine, and serotonin	Hypertension and Huntington chorea
Tetrabenazine	Inhibits reuptake of dopamine, norepinephrine, and serotonin	Similar to reserpine but less potent

Modified from Lockman LA. Movement disorders. In: Swaiman KF, Wright FS, eds. The practice of pediatric neurology. St. Louis: Mosby, 1982.

Dopamine is highly concentrated in the substantia nigra and is released at the postsynaptic area in the striatum from axons originating in the substantia nigra. Striatal dopamine concentration is markedly decreased if the nigrostriatal pathway is disrupted, such as occurs after administration of 6-hydroxydopa. After release of dopamine from storage sites in the striatum, it combines with a receptor on the postsynaptic membrane; it is inactivated by reuptake in the presynaptic terminal. A feedback mechanism appears to regulate the rate of release of dopamine into the synaptic cleft. Autoreceptors, receptor sites on the presynaptic terminal, may bind with specific neurotransmitters. Such autoreceptors are involved in dopamine action; their stimulation results in decreased synthesis and release of dopamine.

It has been possible with refined pharmacologic techniques to subclassify postsynaptic dopamine receptors. Stimulation of D-1 receptors activates adenylate cyclase, but stimulation of D-2 receptors has no effect on adenylate cyclase activity. Various medications used in the therapy of basal ganglia diseases can be classified by their affinity to these receptors.

In addition to reuptake the neurotransmitter is degraded by two separate pathways, one of which involves catechol-O-methyltransferase and the other by monoamine oxidase (Figure 18-6). Homovanillic acid (HVA) is the end-product of dopamine catabolism. In the presence of decreased dopamine synthesis, spinal fluid and urine concentrations of homovanillic acid are reduced.

Reserpine and tetrabenazine cause depletion of the presynaptic vesicles of dopamine and also inhibit presynaptic dopamine reuptake. Some active pharmacologic agents (e.g., pimozide, haloperidol, and related butyrophenones) block dopamine binding to the specific postsynaptic receptor. Because deficient dopamine production and binding are usually associated with brady-

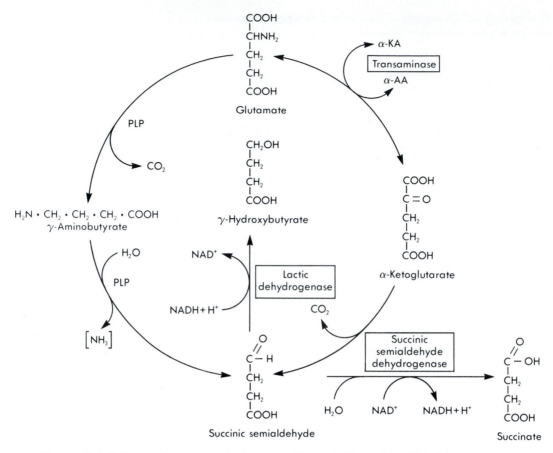

Figure 18-4 Pathway of gamma-aminobutyric acid metabolism. *alpha-KA*, alpha-keto acids; *alpha-AA*, alpha-amino acids; *PLP*, pyridoxal phosphate.

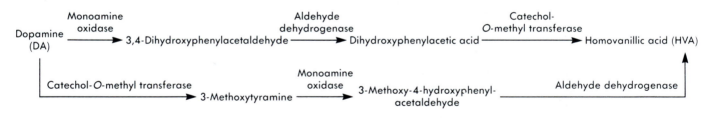

Figure 18-5 Outline of dopamine catabolism.

kinesia, as in Parkinson disease, the movement is alleviated by levodopa therapy [Duvoisin, 1987].

Some movement disorders, including chorea, have been associated with levodopa therapy in patients with Parkinson disease, most likely as a result of denervation sensitivity of dopaminergic neurons. Drugs that facilitate levodopa activity, as well as levodopa itself, have been associated with the onset of Tourette syndrome. Accordingly, drugs such as haloperidol that inhibit dopamine activity are effective in the treatment of Tourette syndrome.

As seen in Figure 18-5, in the process of catabolism,

dopamine is converted to norepinephrine by the enzyme dopamine-beta-oxidase. This relationship of norepinephrine and dopamine is the likely reason that reserpine and phenothiazine reduce both norepinephrine and dopamine brain content. Some drugs, such as tricyclic antidepressants and cocaine, impair norepinephrine uptake but have no effect on dopamine uptake. Other drugs, such as pimozide and haloperidol, affect only dopamine receptor activity and do not modify norepinephrine binding or reuptake.

Serotonin (5-hydroxytryptamine) is formed from 5-hydroxytryptophan (5-HTP); 5-hydroxytryptophan is

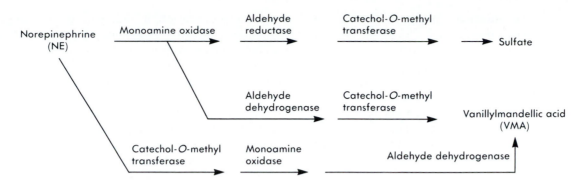

Figure 18-6 Outline of norepinephrine catabolism.

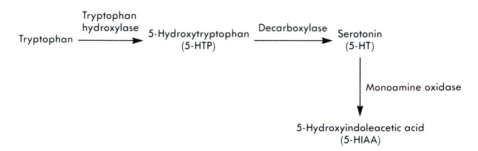

Figure 18-7 Outline of serotonin metabolism.

synthesized from tryptophan under the aegis of the rate-limiting enzyme, tryptophan hydroxylase, and then the decarboxylase transforms 5-hydroxytryptophan to serotonin (Figure 18-7). Serotonin is degraded by monoamine oxidase to 5-hydroxyindoleacetic acid (5-HIAA); however, the primary means of inactivation is through reuptake into the presynaptic terminals.

Serotonin, an inhibitory neurotransmitter, is synthesized in the median raphe nuclei of the brainstem (pons and midbrain). These neurons project axons rostrally to the diencephalon, telencephalon, limbic system, and striatum. Apparent connections also exist between the raphe nuclei and both the substantia nigra and the globus pallidus.

Glutamic acid is an excitatory neurotransmitter that is primarily involved in the pathway leading from the cerebral cortex to the striatum. During electrophysiologic studies the application of glutamate to the cerebral motor cortex causes a marked excitatory effect.

Other molecules, not classified as neurotransmitters but rather as neuromodulators (e.g., substance P, somatostatin, enkephalin), serve to modify, positively or negatively, the actions of neurotransmitters.

EVALUATION OF THE PATIENT

It is essential that the clinician observe the patient's movements at rest and if possible under stress. Unfor-

tunately, there is no substitute for observational skills and experience. Video tapes and films, particularly if recording periods are prolonged over several hours, may be helpful for the assessment of movement disorders, the results of therapy, and documenting the natural course of the condition.

CHOREA

Choreiform movements are quick, random jerks of skeletal muscle involving virtually all body parts. The complaints may involve difficulties with eating and the attendant motor components, impairment of gait, general clumsiness, or fidgetiness.

The trunk and face, as well as the limbs, may be involved; the limbs may be primarily involved proximally, distally, or both. Most commonly the movements are bilateral, although hemichorea occurs. The movements may be evident and literally jump from one body part to the next. The clinician may wish to hold the patient's hands and arms to provide some indication of more subtle choreiform movements. The child may be asked to sit on the examining table, to extend the arms and legs, to place the tongue between the lips, and to attempt to remain as still as possible. This awkward position tends to enhance the most subtle forms of chorea. The classic "milkmaid" sign is the result of the patient's choreiform movements interfering with the constancy of the patient's grip on the clinician's fingers with resultant intermittent squeezing movements. The patient is incapable of maintaining a concerted effort.

The pronator sign consists of hyperpronation of the hands to cause the palms to face outward when the arms are held over the head; this sign has received more notoriety than it deserves. Deep tendon reflexes are usually present, although hypotonia may coexist. The responsiveness of the deep tendon reflexes may vary from moment to moment because of the coincidence of choreiform movements with the elicited tendon stretch. Another classic sign, "spooning," occurs when the arms and hands are extended, the wrists flex slightly, and the metacarpophalangeal joints hyperextend.

Differential diagnosis

Choreiform movements are evident during the examination of many children, particularly those younger than 8 years of age, who do not have persistent movement disorders after maturation. However, these movements are usually inconstant and of small amplitude and do not interfere with motor activities. Sydenham (rheumatic) chorea, which is associated with streptococcal infection, was once common but is now a less common form of chorea because of widespread use of throat culture techniques and effective antibiotic therapy. Rheumatic heart disease is found in one third of patients [Aron et al., 1965]. The chorea may appear weeks to months after the streptococcal pharyngitis, and there may be little or no evidence, clinical or laboratory, of the streptococcal infection at the time when chorea is at its height. Recurrences of Sydenham chorea do not necessarily indicate a recurrence of active rheumatic fever [Berrios et al., 1985]. Sydenham chorea is often accompanied by some emotional lability and hypotonia. Therapy with haloperidol, diazepam, or valproic acid is often beneficial [Alvarez and Novak, 1985].

Tardive dyskinesia usually results from long-term therapy with neuroleptic drugs, including dopamine-receptor antagonists. Other drugs such as anticholinergics, antihistamines, and dopamine agonists have also been associated with the condition or at least movement disorders that are very similar. Tardive dyskinesia is relatively uncommon in childhood. Children with schizophrenia who undergo termination of neuroleptic therapy will often develop a dyskinesia that is generalized and choreiform in nature, resolves in weeks to months, and is sometimes termed the *withdrawal-emergent syndrome*. Although the movements have a choreiform quality, there are some distinguishing characteristics from other forms of chorea. The movements are stereotypic, rapid, and often are in the form of a lingual-facial-buccal dyskinesia. Frequently there is lip smacking, quick protrusion and retraction of the tongue, and movements of the tongue in the oral cavity. Volitional movements of the tongue are often unimpaired and impede the pathologic tongue movements. Patients may walk or march in place and have body rocking. Withdrawal of the offending agent may not lead to dissipation of symptomatology for months or years, and sometimes movements appear to be permanent. Patients should be followed closely for manifestations of the condition and drug therapy terminated promptly if they occur. The mechanism of causation remains unknown although speculation has been plentiful.

Huntington chorea is a genetically determined (autosomal-dominant) disease in which the proximal muscles are primarily more involved. Both dementia and emotional lability are often evident; the disease is progressive and eventually leads to death [Menkes, 1988; Young et al., 1986]. Children are prone to seizures and rigidity, a marked difference from the situation in adult patients who rarely manifest these symptoms. The disease is transmitted as an autosomal-dominant trait. The form that afflicts children and causes marked rigidity is known as the *Westphal variant*.

The differential diagnosis beyond the choreiform conditions already discussed is lengthy and varied. The clinician is advised to consider carefully the history, the presence of infection [Burstein and Breningstall, 1986], exposure to medications [Driesen and Wolters, 1987; Filloux and Thompson, 1987], familial incidence, age of onset, and pattern at time of onset (Table 18-3).

ATHETOSIS

Athetosis is a distinctive, irregular, often continuous, writhing movement of the extremities, primarily the distal portions. The arm movements consist of alternating supination and pronation in combination with various degrees of flexion and extension. The gross movements center about the long axis of the limb. Often there is accompanying hyperextension and then flexion of the fingers. Stress intensifies the frequency and range of these movements.

The causes of athetosis associated with hypoxic-ischemic encephalopathy of the neonate include destructive lesions of the putamen, caudate nucleus, and globus pallidus. The cortex, internal capsule, and thalamus may also be involved. The so-called athetotic form of cerebral palsy is associated with irregularly placed, abnormally myelinated fibers in the globus pallidus and putamen; this marbled pattern is termed *status marmoratus*.

Differential diagnosis

The differential diagnosis of athetosis is similar to that of chorea because of the common association of chorea in the combined movement disorder, choreoathetosis. The causes of athetosis (usually with accompanying chorea) range from infectious processes (e.g., viral

Table 18-3 Differential diagnosis of chorea

Congenital	Degenerative (of unknown cause)	Genetic	Infectious
Cerebral palsy	Canavan spongy degeneration	Ataxia-telangiectasia Bassen-Kornzweig disease Benign familial chorea of early onset Dystonia musculorum deformans Fabry disease Familial microcephaly with curvilinear bodies Familial microcephaly, retardation, and chorea Familial paroxysmal choreoathetosis Friedrich ataxia Glutaric aciduria Huntington chorea Incontinentia pigmenti Lesch-Nyhan syndrome Phenylketonuria Porphyria Sturge-Weber syndrome Tardive dyskinesia Wilson disease	Diphtheria Encephalitis (St. Louis, inclusion body, epidemic, rubeola, mumps, varicella) Neurosyphilis (congenital, meningovascular) Pertussis Poststreptococcal (Sydenham) Typhoid fever

Metabolic-endocrinologic	Neoplastic	Toxic	Traumatic	Unknown and miscellaneous	Vascular
Addison disease Beriberi Cerebral lipidoses Hypocalcemia Hypoglycemia Hypomagnesemia Hypernatremia Hypoparathyroidism Kernicterus Phenylketonuria Polycythemia Porphyria Pregnancy Thyrotoxicosis Vitamin B_{12} deficiency in infants Wilson disease	Brain tumors	Carbon monoxide Isoniazide Lithium Mercury Oral contraceptives Phenothiazine Reserpine Scopolamine	Burns in children	Hyperkinetic syndrome Intranuclear hyaline inclusion disease Nevus unius lateralis Parietal chorea	Anaphylactoid purpura (Henoch-Schönlein purpura) Cerebral infarction Lupus erythematosus Posthemiplegic chorea

Modified from Barbeau A. Birth defects 1971; 7:156; from Greenhouse AH. Arch Intern Med 1966; 117:389.

encephalitis) to inborn errors of metabolism, including phenylketonuria and Wilson disease. The clinician should consider the conditions listed in Table 18-3, in particular those conditions that are appropriate for the child's age, family history, and pattern of onset.

DYSTONIA

Dystonia is characterized by sustained simultaneous contraction of agonist and antagonist muscles, resulting in unusual postures that are transiently maintained. Both appendicular and axial muscles may be involved together or separately. If the contraction of the agonist and antagonist muscles is balanced, there may be little initial movement, only tightening of the muscles. As imbalance ensues, there is a slow, continuous movement of the body part. After full excursion the extreme posture may remain fixed for a minute or more. Occasionally the movements may be of short duration and confound the diagnosis. There may be an associated tremor, particularly when the patient attempts to volitionally impede the dystonic movements.

Frequent manifestations of dystonia include twisting (spasmodic torticollis) or extension of the neck (spasmodic retrocollis); spasms of the trunk that may result in grotesque positioning and interfere with standing, ambulation, sitting, or lying; and variable or intermittent inversion of the leg with accompanying equinovarus posturing. Involvement of the skeletal muscles in the oral cavity, including the tongue, often leads to major distortion of speech. Athetosis, unlike dystonia, does not result in the prolonged maintenance of unusual postures and is almost always distal in location; the delineation between dystonia and athetosis may be difficult at times.

Focal dystonias differ from the previously described pattern because they are confined to specific anatomic muscle groups [Scherokman et al., 1986]. Among the focal dystonias are writer's cramp, spasmodic dysphonia, and blepharospasm. Fluctuation of symptomatology in focal dystonias often occurs [Deonna and Ferreira, 1985].

Differential diagnosis

The predominant causes of dystonia are listed in Table 18-4. The sometimes bizarre nature of the movements, spontaneous remissions and exacerbations, and the accentuation of difficulty in the presence of stress often lead to the erroneous supposition that the patient is suffering from a conversion reaction. Many patients with dystonia have inherited their condition in the form of dystonia musculorum deformans (idiopathic torsion dystonia), Wilson disease, Hallervorden-Spatz syndrome [Swaiman et al., 1983], and neuronal ceroid-lipofuscinosis [Zeman and Whitlock, 1968]. Diurnal fluctuation characterizes one form of hereditary dystonia [Segawa et al., 1987]. Dystonia may be transient when caused by the administration of certain drugs, particularly phenothiazines and butyrophenones.

Dystonia musculorum deformans (torsion dystonia) may be inherited in an autosomal-recessive, autosomal-dominant, or X-linked recessive fashion. Torsion dystonia is discussed in detail in Chapter 57.

Certain abnormal movements may be apparent in carriers of the autosomal-dominant inherited dystonias and may be the forerunners of more severe symptoms in affected patients. These movement disorders include dystonic movements and postures during voluntary activity; so-called passive dystonia, and irregular change in tone, both increasing and decreasing, on passive movement; and focal dystonic disturbances (e.g., writer's cramp, sustained muscle spasms in restricted areas) [Zeman and Dyken, 1967; Deonna and Ferreira, 1985]. At times tremor may be evident in carriers. Examination

Table 18-4 Differential diagnosis of dystonia

Congenital and development	Benign dystonia of infancy [Willemse, 1986]
	Cerebral palsy (dystonic form)
	Dyspeptic dystonia with hiatus hernia
	Paroxysmal torticollis in infancy
Degenerative disorders of unknown cause	Ataxia-telangiectasia
	Dystonia musculorum deformans
	Focal dystonias
	Hallervorden-Spatz syndrome
	Hemidystonia
	Idiopathic torsion dystonia
	Leber disease (variant) [Novotny et al., 1986]
	Myoclonic dystonia (paroxysmal) [Fahn, 1987]
	Segawa dystonia with diurnal fluctuation
	Subacute necrotizing encephalomyelopathy [Campistol et al, 1986]
	Dystonia-Parkinsonian syndrome
Infectious diseases	Viral encephalitis
Metabolic conditions	GM1 gangliosidosis (adult)
	GM2 gangliosidosis
	Phenylketonuria
	Triosephosphate isomerase deficiency
	Wilson disease
Medication reaction	Bethanechol
	Butyrophenones
	Carbamazepine
	Phenothiazine
	Reserpine
	Tetrabenazine
Psychogenic	Münchausen syndrome simulating dystonia
Sleep abnormalities	Paroxysmal sleep dystonia [Lugaresi et al., 1986]

of possible and obligate carriers is important to determine whether an autosomal recessive or dominant inheritance is operative.

Abnormalities of central catecholamine metabolism may be important in the pathophysiology of dystonia because certain obligate carriers and some presymptomatic patients display marked sensitivity to phenothiazine drugs (see Chapter 57) [Eldridge, 1970].

Hexosaminidase A and B deficiency has been associated with a severe, progressive dystonic disease that appears by 10 years of age, manifested by dysarthria, hyperreflexia, and severe dystonic posturing of all extremities. Prominent incoordination is also evident [Goldie et al., 1977; Oates et al., 1986].

Carbamazepine, when administered in antiepileptic doses that result in therapeutic blood concentrations, has engendered dystonia in neurologically impaired children [Crosley and Swender, 1979]. Other drugs that have engendered dystonia are bethanechol and phenothiazine.

A hereditary dystonia with juvenile onset progresses into a combination of lower limb and axial dystonia, as well as juvenile parkinsonism [Nygaard and Duvoisin, 1986]. Leber disease has also been associated with dystonia in a single kindred [Novotny et al., 1986]. Dystonia appearing during infancy that spontaneously resolves has been described in four infants [Willemse, 1986]. Subacute necrotizing encephalomyelopathy has also been associated with dystonia in infancy [Campistol et al., 1986]. Dystonia may be associated with basal ganglia calcification [Di Rocco, 1986]. Curiously, segmental dystonia has been associated with peripheral trauma and pain in adults [Schott, 1985].

Hallervorden-Spatz syndrome, a subacute or chronic condition, often appears in the first decade of life and is characterized by spasticity, dystonia, optic atrophy, and frequently dementia. Rigidity and other characteristics of parkinson-like disease may be prominent. At times choreoathetosis occurs. Intellectual impairment is not uniformly present but frequently manifests during the second decade. Extreme rigidity tends to obscure the dystonic posturing after a number of years in the more chronic forms [Swaiman, 1991].

Infantile paroxysmal torticollis (benign paroxysmal vertigo) is an unusual condition of infants in which repetitive episodes occurring at weekly or biweekly intervals and lasting for approximately 2 to 3 days (range: 10 minutes to 14 days) has been reported [Snyder, 1969]. No patients have been reported who continue to have the episodes beyond 5 years of age.

Hiatus hernia accompanied by dystonia of the head and neck (Sandifer syndrome) has been reported [Kinsbourne, 1964]. Many of the children have abnormal feeding patterns during infancy that improve with age. The children frequently extend and flex the head intermittently, sometimes spontaneously but more often associated with feeding. The condition is uniformly associated with the presence of hiatus hernia. The symptoms decrease rapidly after surgical intervention. The age of diagnosis is 4 to 14 years of age.

Hyperthyroidism has been associated with a number of movement disorders including dystonia. At least one case of dystonia appeared after overvigorous treatment with levothyroxine. The symptoms abated when the medication was withdrawn [Remillard et al., 1974].

Reflex sympathetic dystrophy may mimic the posturing of dystonia and often seemingly occurs secondary to minor trauma [Ashwal et al., 1988]. The associated changes in skin color and pain serve to distinguish this entity from dystonia.

TREMOR

Tremor is a prolonged or continuous, rhythmic movement of a body part (e.g., head, jaw, tongue, hands, or feet). There are many types of tremor. Tremor results from alternating contractions of antagonist muscles. Unfortunately, they are not classified uniformly in authoritative writings. Classification according to frequency, amplitude, presence during rest, and distribution is generally stressed, although other etiologic or presumed etiologic types have been reported.

Classification into resting tremor, postural tremor, and intention tremor appears to be a useful approach [Weiner and Lang, 1989].

Resting tremor is present when there is no voluntary movement. Postural tremor is present when the tremor accompanies attempts to maintain a fixed position, such as extending the arms. Intention tremor is manifest when a body part is moved between fixed objects. Other terms generally are used to describe combinations of the three types cited [Weiner and Lang, 1989].

Resting tremor is uncommon in childhood but occurs in juvenile Parkinson disease and Wilson disease. The frequency ranges from 4 to 8 Hz. Volitional movement suppresses the tremor. It commonly involves the hands but may involve the tongue. Rigidity may accompany this condition. The typical characteristics of Parkinson disease, including festinating gait, bradykinesia, and handwriting that becomes progressively smaller and illegible may be present. Other causes are phenothiazine and butyrophenone toxicity or idiosynchratic reaction and mercury poisoning.

Postural tremor (also often termed *physiologic tremor*) occurs when the patient extends the arms forward. The tremor or its frequency is unrelated to cardiac impulse or function [Marsden et al., 1969]. The tremor appears to be related to norepinephrine and can be suppressed by beta-adenergic blockers (e.g., propranolol) [Marsden et al., 1969]. Stress enhances the tremor and the tremor may become obvious during eating, while carrying an object, or writing. Essential-familial tremor is a postural tremor usually inherited as an autosomal-dominant trait. Occasionally essential tremor may occur without apparent familial basis. Although commonly evident in the second or third decade, the tremor may be manifest in the first decade and confound the diagnostician. The tremor is greatly ameliorated by beta-adrenergic blockers (e.g., propranolol) and alcohol.

Intention tremor is usually the result of cerebellar impairment, drugs, and toxins.

Unusual tremors are associated with the bobble-head

doll syndrome, and spasmus nutans; these conditions are discussed elsewhere in this text.

BALLISMUS

Ballismus, the least common of the generally recognized movement disorders, consists of rapid movements usually involving the shoulders and sometimes the hips. The movements are violent, with flinging, hurling, and throwing of the arms and circumduction or kicking of the legs. The movements are irregular. Hemiballismus (unilateral ballismus) is most common. Ballismus and hemiballismus are usually absent during sleep but are almost continuously present during the waking state. There appears to be only minimal diminution in the tone and strength of the affected limbs. Precision of coordinated movements is decreased. Distinguishing ballismus from chorea may be virtually impossible at times; it is probable that ballismus and chorea are a single entity and represent a range of abnormal activity.

The underlying anatomic basis for ballismus or hemiballismus appears to be involvement of the subthalamic nucleus, which in turn impairs the modulatory effect on the globus pallidus. Adults who suffer from hemiballismus frequently have a vascular lesion in the contralateral subthalamic nucleus; however, any lesion in this region can lead to ballismus. Ballismus in children is most often a markedly exaggerated form of chorea, usually Sydenham chorea. Nevertheless, the movements may be the result of other etiologic conditions that involve the basal ganglia, particularly those of infectious, vascular, neoplastic, or toxic (e.g., drug-induced— phenytoin, dopaminergic agents) origin.

Blocking dopaminergic receptors with appropriate medication is often beneficial. Surgery has been occasionally successful. Stereotactic lesions have been introduced in the ventrolateral thalamus, globus pallidus, and thalamic fasciculus.

MYOCLONUS

Myoclonus is characterized by involuntary, extremely rapid, often repetitive contractions of a muscle or groups of muscles in any body part. Active muscle contraction is termed *positive myoclonus*. Negative myoclonus indicates episodes when ongoing muscle activity is acutely but transiently disrupted by inhibition.

The patterns of myoclonic movement are varied and complicate diagnosis. Myoclonus may be symmetric or asymmetric, as well as rhythmic or arrhythmic. Myoclonus is usually arrhythmic although repetitive. Myoclonus is often facilitated by visual or tactile stimuli or purposeful motor activity (intention myoclonus) [Aigner and Mulder, 1960; Van Woert, 1983].

Myoclonus can be classified electrophysiologically as nonepileptic or epileptic. Myoclonus can also be classified according to any accompanying change in consciousness; those movements accompanied by change in consciousness are presumed to be epileptic. This discussion refers to nonepileptic myoclonus. Epileptic myoclonus is discussed in Chapter 30.

The broad description of myoclonus reflects the large group of involuntary movements that are the result of disruption of diverse neuroanatomic units and involvement by many pathophysiologic conditions [Van Woert and Hwang, 1979].

Etiologic classification is also possible because myoclonus occurs in various physiologic and pathologic conditions. Myoclonus may be a manifestation of a benign or normal physiologic condition. These myoclonic movements include sleep jerks (hypnagogic jerks), exercise myoclonus, or stress myoclonus.

Pathologic myoclonus occurs in conditions that are accompanied by hyperexcitability of the gray matter of many parts of the CNS including the cerebral cortex, basal ganglia, brainstem, and spinal cord. Pathologic myoclonus is facilitated by fatigue and emotional stress; it is often most active just after awakening in the morning.

Myoclonus has been classified using assumed areas of origin. In one scheme, myoclonus has been divided on the basis of whether it originates subcortically, in the brainstem, or in the spinal cord; further categorization depends on whether myoclonus is generalized or whether it is segmental and thus relatively localized [Swanson et al., 1962]. Table 18-5 outlines this system of classification.

Another approach was suggested by Van Woert and Hwang [1979]. They distinguished between arrhythmic and rhythmic myoclonus. Arrhythmic myoclonus is due to compromise of functioning of one or more supraspinal systems that control motor activity. Rhythmic myoclonus is the result of brainstem or spinal cord dysfunction. The differences between these two categories are summarized in Table 18-6.

Arrhythmic myoclonus originates in various brain regions and results from different pathologic mechanisms. It is synchronous or asynchronous, symmetric or asymmetric, unilateral or bilateral, and generalized or focal. Arrhythmic myoclonus may be facilitated by visual, tactile, and auditory stimuli; voluntary movements; changes in posture; fatigue; and psychologic stresses. It is facilitated in the premenstrual period.

Arrhythmic myoclonus may be due to the interruption of supraspinal (cerebral, cerebellar, and brainstem) inhibitory actions that normally influence responses of the reticular formation to broad sensory input [Denny-Brown, 1968; Paolozzi and Guizzaro, 1982]. The myoclonic response to stimuli—internal or external—may be the result of a compromised inhibitory spinobulbospinal reflex [Paolozzi and Guizzaro, 1982]. Ascending sensory impulses reach nuclei in the medial medullary reticular

Table 18-5 Classification of myoclonus

I. Segmental
  A. Type
    1. Brainstem
      a. Eye
      b. Palate
      c. Jaw
      d. Face
      e. Neck and tongue
    2. Spinal cord
      a. Limb
      b. Trunk
      c. Diaphragm
  B. Etiology
    1. Vascular
    2. Infectious
    3. Demyelinating
    4. Neoplastic
    5. Traumatic
    6. Unknown
II. Generalized myoclonus (subcortical, brainstem, or spinal-cord involvement)
  A. Acute and subacute
    1. Encephalomyelitic (including poliomyelitis)
    2. Toxic
      a. Other infections
        (1) Tetanus
        (2) Nonspecific
      b. Strychnine
      c. Other (including drugs)
    3. Anoxic
    4. Metabolic (uremia, hepatic insufficiency, other)
    5. Degenerative (including inclusion body encephalitis)
  B. Chronic
    1. Progressive myoclonus epilepsy (Lafora-bodies, lipidoses, system degeneration; Ramsay Hunt syndrome)
    2. Nonprogressive intermittent myoclonus with epilepsy
    3. Essential myoclonus (paramyoclonus multiplex)
    4. Nocturnal myoclonus

Modified from Swanson PO, Luttrell CM, Magladery JW. Medicine 1962; 41:339; from Swaiman KF. Neurol Clin 1985; 3:197.

formation and generate descending impulses that are transmitted along the reticulospinal tract to various spinal segments [Halliday, 1975]. Studies suggest that the cortical loop reflex [Denny-Brown, 1968] also has a profound effect on the spinobulbospinal reflex.

The conceptualization of these two interdependent modulating systems takes into account the various sites of dysfunction involved in arrhythmic myoclonus. Because different neurotransmitters are included in these various nervous system areas, different therapeutic pharmacologic approaches are indicated. This brief analysis encapsulates the background of theory, mostly based on experimental work, that has led to the separation of two groups of arrhythmic myoclonus: reticular loop reflex myoclonus and cortical loop reflex myoclonus. Table 18-7 summarizes the differences between these two reflex systems.

Negative myoclonus is often characterized by rapid loss of tone, particularly in axial and leg muscles, with subsequent bobbing or actually falling. Asterixis, the flapping movements found when the arms and hands are outstretched in some patients with hepatic disease and other metabolic conditions, is thought to be a form of negative myoclonus.

Rhythmic myoclonus is synonymous with segmental myoclonus categorization in other classifications (see Table 18-5). It is localized to various levels of the brainstem or spinal cord segments. Rhythmic contractions, which remain unmodified by the stimuli that alter arrhythmic myoclonus and that continue during sleep, characterize this group. The prototypic example is palatal myoclonus. Therapy of rhythmic myoclonus is often unsatisfactory, although on rare occasions, antiepileptic drugs (e.g., phenytoin) have been of value.

Myoclonus can be classified on the basis of whether it is static or progressive. Progression usually indicates the presence of a metabolic, hereditary, or infectious process.

Differential diagnosis

Numerous conditions are associated with myoclonus and several strategies may be used to group these

Table 18-6 Characteristics of myoclonus (arrhythmic vs rhythmic)

Classification	Body part involved	Rhythm	Stress response	Sleep response	Sensory stimuli response	Motor activity response
Arrhythmic	Varies (often fluctuates)	Irregular and variable	Enhanced	Movements absent	Enhanced	Enhanced
Rhythmic	Segmental	Regular	Movements unchanged	Movements present	Movements unchanged	Movements unchanged

From Swaiman KF. Neurol Clin 1985; 3:197.

Table 18-7 Arrythmic myoclonus

Reticular reflex myoclonus	Cortical reflex myoclonus
Primarily affects proximal muscles	Primarily affect distal muscles
Generalized myoclonic response to sensory stimuli	Sensory stimuli evoke myoclonus that is limited to distal muscles
Specific EEG abnormalities, related but not synchronous with movements	EEG abnormalities usually synchronous with the myoclonic jerks
Sensory-evoked potentials of normal voltage	Sensory-evoked potentials of high voltage
Brainstem activation caudorostral	Brainstem activation is rostrocaudal

Modified from Hallett M, et al. J Neurol Neurosurg 1977; 40:253; and from Paolozzi C, Guizzaro A. Neurologica (Napoli) 1982; 37:135; from Swaiman KF. Neurol Clin 1985; 3:197.

conditions. Myoclonus may be grouped by the following general categories [Van Woert, 1983]:

1. Genetic: essential myoclonus, progressive myoclonus epilepsy (e.g., Lafora disease), and storage conditions (e.g., lipidosis)
2. Seizure disorders: idiopathic epilepsy and infantile spasms
3. Brain injury: anoxia, toxins and metabolic disorders
4. Viral infections
5. Miscellaneous: opsoclonus, nocturnal myoclonus and palatal myoclonus

Any approach to the problems of a child with myoclonus must be the result of a systematic appraisal for known associated conditions (Table 18-8).

Historic data, including any familial incidence of movement disorders, are essential. Exposure to anoxia, toxins, or trauma should be ascertained. The examination should determine whether myoclonus is focal,

Table 18-8 Selected causes of myoclonus

Congenital

Aicardi syndrome
Cerebral agenesis
Holoprosencephaly
Porencephaly
Syringomyelia

Toxic

Antihistamines
Lead intoxication
Minamata disease
Pentylenetetrazol
Tranquilizers

Trauma

Anoxia
Intracerebral hemorrhage
Subdural hematoma

Vascular

Thrombosis: cortex, cerebellum, brainstem, and spinal cord

Metabolic and endocrinologic

Aminoacidopathies
 Hyperglycinemia
 Hyperornithinemia
 Maple syrup disease
 Phenylketonuria
Hallervorden-Spatz syndrome
Hepatic failure
Hypoglycemia
Hypoxia
Kwashiorkor
Menkes disease

Metabolic and endocrinologic — cont'd

Neuronal ceroid-lipofuscinosis
Pyridoxine dependency
Tay-Sachs disease
Uremia
Wilson disease

Unknown

Myoclonic encephalopathy of infancy (with or without neuroblastoma)

Degenerative

Familial progressive myoclonic epilepsy
Infantile myoclonic spasms
Incontinentia pigmenti
Lafora body disease
Multiple sclerosis
Progressive degeneration of gray matter (Alpers disease)
Ramsay Hunt syndrome
Sturge-Weber syndrome
Sudanophilic leukodystrophy
Tuberous sclerosis
Unverricht-Lundborg disease

Infectious

Acute and chronic encephalitis
Herpes zoster meningoencephalitis
Malaria
Polio
Postencephalitic syndrome
Postimmunization syndrome
Smallpox
Subacute sclerosing panencephalitis
Tuberculous meningitis

rhythmic, or associated with or enhanced by stimuli. When possible, review of video tapes may be helpful when the myoclonus is variably present. The differentiation from tics may be difficult.

Laboratory studies may prove crucial in the diagnostic process. Both EMG and EEG studies may be necessary to classify properly the myoclonic movements. Clearly, incidents related to toxins, trauma, and anoxia should be appropriately evaluated. A number of metabolic diseases can be delineated by the use of proper laboratory studies. The clinician must be cognizant of the usual caveats associated with these studies. For example, study of qualitative or quantitative amino acids in urine or serum are of dubious value unless the patient has had an ongoing adequate protein diet. A severely ill, malnourished child with little intake of protein may have an amino acidopathy that will be undetected by routine laboratory studies. Family histories of lipidoses may be absent except for involvement of siblings because most of the sphingolipidoses are transmitted as autosomal-recessive traits. Therefore it is necessary to obtain the specific white cell or fibroblast enzyme studies needed to diagnose the various sphingolipidoses associated with myoclonus.

TICS

Tics may be motor or vocal or both. They may persist during sleep, which sets them aside from most other movement disorders. Tics may be curtailed by volitional control, but the necessary concentration is disconcerting and not effective over significant time intervals. Emotional stress and excitement enhance the frequency of tics. Tics may be evident from 2 years of age through the geriatric age group; they are particularly prevalent in the last half of the first decade of life. Tics may be transient or life-long. Etiologic classification of tics is unsatisfactory because most underlying causes are not understood. Table 18-9 lists some of the more common categories. The diagnosis of tics is confounded because of the prevalence of frequent movements in hyperactivity states, personal mannerisms, compulsive behavior, and excessive startle responses.

Motor tics are stereotyped, rapid movements of the muscles, usually of the face, neck, and shoulders. The tics are usually jerky in nature although rarely they may be more prolonged. The movements persist for less than a second, are irregular, and may be clustered over a few minutes. Motor tics may persist during sleep. They may be divided into simple and complex types. Simple motor tics are exemplified by eye blinking, grimacing, tongue protrusion, head jerking, shoulder shrugging, arm or leg jerks, and toe curling. Complex motor tics include rubbing, bruxism, wrist shaking, jumping, skipping, squatting, smelling of objects or body parts, copropraxia, and echopraxia [Weiner and Lang, 1989].

Table 18-9 Etiologic classification of childhood tics

Idiopathic
  Acute simple transient tic (< 1 year)
  Persistent simple or multiple tic of childhood (remits before adulthood)
  Chronic simple or multiple motor tics (persists throughout life)
  Gilles de la Tourette syndrome

Secondary tics
Postencephalitic
  Sydenham chorea
  Head trauma
  Carbon monoxide poisoning
  Poststroke
  Acanthocytosis
  Drugs—stimulants, levodopa, neuroleptics (tardive Tourette syndrome), carbamazepine, phenytoin, phenobarbital
  Mental retardation syndromes, including chromosomal abnormalities
  Others

Modified from Lockman LA. Movement disorders. In: Swaiman KF, Wright FS, eds. The practice of pediatric neurology. St. Louis: Mosby, 1982.

The movements usually remain focal or stereotyped and usually disappear without therapy. They may wax and wane over long time intervals. Because of this natural occurrence, there is a general supposition that some tics are the manifestations of psychogenic difficulties. The fact that tics are made worse during emotional stress and are usually quiescent during sleep does not indicate that the condition is psychogenic; these attributes are common to virtually all movement disorders. Some tic disorders may persist and become progressive, such as Tourette syndrome [Shapiro et al., 1978]. It is unusual for tics to be confused with other movement disorders.

Vocal tics are stereotyped, brief, and irregular, but may be clustered. Vocal tics may also be characterized as simple or complex. Simple vocal tics include grunting, throat clearing, sniffing, barking, yelping, snorting, growling, and coughing. Complex vocal tics are exemplified by coprolalia, neologisms, formed but incomprehensible sounds, whistling, echolalia, stuttering, and panting. Common examples include throat clearing, sniffing, pulling on facial parts, and generating guttural noises.

Tourette syndrome (maladie des tics)

This disorder was first comprehensively described in 1885 by Gilles de la Tourette; component symptoms had been described before. The symptoms usually begin in childhood with an age range of 2 to 13 years [Bruun and

Shapiro, 1972]. The disease often manifests with simple involuntary tic-like movements involving the facial muscles, including twitching of the eye muscles [Shapiro and Shapiro, 1986]. Associated vocalizations (e.g., grunts, snorts, barks, or clucks) may become evident; in about one half of the patients the vocalizations become words. Coprolalia and echolalia are unusual. The tics frequently move from area to area. Dementia does not occur, although behavioral abnormalities are common [Bruun and Shapiro, 1972; Golden, 1986].

Tourette syndrome appears to be inherited as an autosomal dominant trait [Pauls and Leckman, 1986]. There is also evidence of a disorder of central neurotransmitters. Development of Tourette syndrome has been associated with methylphenidate and antiepileptic drug treatment [Denckla et al., 1976; Burd et al., 1986].

The use of dopamine antagonist drugs (e.g., haloperidol) has greatly improved the outlook for patients with Tourette syndrome [Sweet et al., 1975]. Other drugs such as pimozide, clonidine, and tetrabenazine have been reported to have merit [Golden, 1986].

RIGIDITY, HYPOKINESIA, AND BRADYKINESIA

Rigidity is marked by persistent increased tone. There is continuous muscle contraction and resultant resistance to passive movement in all fields of muscle action (lead pipe phenomenon). This continuous resistance occurs in contradistinction to the increased resistance (spasticity) that accompanies corticospinal tract impairment. The classic "clasp knife" phenomenon typifies spasticity. A small degree of range of motion during passive movement is normal until the muscles have been slightly stretched; further stretching causes marked resistance through a greater arc of motion followed by a sudden release of tone with yet further muscle stretch. Increased tone and resistance are usually present in the flexor muscles of the upper extremities and the extensor muscles of the lower extremities.

Rigidity is typical of some basal ganglia diseases (e.g., Parkinson disease).

Bradykinesia is decreased velocity of movement. Hypokinesia refers to a paucity of movements, particularly of normal automatic movements, such as crossing the legs, moving the head with lateral gaze, and attendant small movements that accompany the act of rising from the sitting position. These phenomena are most typical of Parkinson disease but may be seen in conditions such as Hallervorden-Spatz syndrome and other conditions in which there are Parkinson-like symptoms.

REFERENCES

Aigner BR, Mulder DW. Myoclonus. Arch Neurol 1960; 2:600.

Alvarez LA, Novak G. Valproic acid in the treatment of Sydenham chorea. Pediatr Neurol 1985; 1:317.

Aron et al. The natural history of Sydenham's chorea. Am J Med 1965; 38:83.

Ashwal S, Tomasi L, Neumann M, et al. Reflex sympathetic dystrophy syndrome in children. Pediatr Neurol 1988; 4:38.

Bruun RD, Shapiro AK. Differential diagnosis of Gilles de la Tourette's syndrome. J Nerv Ment Dis 1972; 155:955.

Burd L, et al. Anticonvulsant medications: an iatrogenic cause of tic disorders. Can J Psychiatry 1986; 31:419.

Campistol J, et al. Dystonia as a presenting sign of subacute necrotising encephalomyelopathy in infancy. Eur J Pediatr 1986; 144:589.

Crosley CJ, Swender PT. Dystonia associated with carbamazepine administration: experience in brain-damaged children. Pediatrics 1979; 63:512.

DeLong MR, Georgopoulos AP. Motor functions of the basal ganglia. In: Brooks VB, ed. Handbook of physiology, section I, the nervous system, vol. 2, motor control, part 2. Bethesda, Maryland: American Physiological Society, 1981.

Denckla MB, Bemporad JR, MacKay MC. Tics following methylphenidate administration: a report of 20 cases. JAMA 1976; 235:1349.

Denny-Brown D. Quelques aspects physiollgiques des myoclonies. In: Bonduelle M, Gastaut H, eds. Les myoclonies. Paris: Masson et Cie, 1968; l121.

Di Rocco M. Dystonia and calcification of the basal ganglia: another case (letter). Neurology 1986; 36:306.

Eldridge R: The torsion dystonias: literature review and genetic and clinical studies. Neurology 1970; 20:1.

Fahn S. Paroxysmal myoclonic dystonia with vocalisations. J Neurol Neurosurg Psychiatry 1987; 50:117.

Golden GS. Tourette syndrome: recent advances. Pediatr Neurol 1986; 2:189.

Goldie WD, Holtzman D, Suzuki K. Chronic hexosaminidase A and B deficiency. Ann Neurol 1977; 2:156.

Halliday AM. The neurophysiology of myoclonic jerking. A reappraisal. Excerpta Medica Int Congress 1975; 307:1.

Kinsbourne M. Hiatus hernia with contortions of the neck. Lancet 1964; 1:1058.

Lugaresi E, Cirignotta F, Montagna P. Nocturnal paroxysmal dystonia. J Neurol Neurosurg Psychiatry 1986; 49:375.

Marsden CD, et al. The role of the ballistocardiac impulse in the genesis of physiological tremor. Brain 1969; 92:647.

Nieuwenhuys R, Voogol J, van Huijzen C. The human central nervous system: a synopsis and atlas, 2nd ed. Berlin: Springer, 1981.

Novotny EJ Jr, et al. Leber's disease and dystonia: a mitochondrial disease. Neurology 1986; 36:1053.

Nygaard TG, Duvoisin RC. Hereditary dystonia-parkinsonism syndrome of juvenile onset. Neurology 1986; 36:1424.

Oates CE, Bosch EP, Hart MN. Movement disorders associated with chronic GM2 gangliosidosis: case report and review of the literature. Eur Neurol 1986; 25:154.

Paolozzi C, Guizzaro A. Physiopathology of myoclonus: a review. Neurologica (Napoli) 1982; 37:135.

Pauls DL, Leckman JF. The inheritance of Gilles de la Tourette's syndrome and associated behaviors: evidence for autosomal dominant transmission. N Engl J Med 1986; 315:993.

Remillard GM, Colle E, Andermann F. On the relation of dystonic movements to serum thyroxine levels. Can Med Assoc J 1974; 110:59.

Schott GD. The relationship of peripheral trauma and pain to dystonia. J Neurol Neurosurg Psychiatry 1985; 48:698.

Segawa M, Nomura Y, Kase M. Hereditary progressive dystonia with marked diurnal fluctuation: clinicopathophysiological identification in reference to juvenile Parkinson's disease. Adv Neurol 1987; 45:227.

Shapiro E, Shapiro AK. Semiology, nosology, and criteria for tic disorders. Rev Neurol 1986; 142:824.

Shapiro AK, et al. Gilles de la Tourette syndrome. New York: Raven Press, 1978.

Snyder CH. Paroxysmal torticollis in infancy. Am J Dis Child 1969; 117:458.

Swaiman KF, Smith SA, Trock GL, Siddigui AR. Sea-blue histiocytes, lymphocytic cytosomes, and ^{59}Fe-studies in Hallervorden-Spatz syndrome. Neurology 1983; 33:301.

Swaiman KF. Hallervorden-Spatz syndrome and brain iron metabolism. Arch Neurol 1991; 48:1285.

Swanson PO, Luttrell CM, Magladery JW. Myoclonus—a report of 67 cases and review of the literature. Medicine 1962; 41:339.

Sweet RD, et al. Presynaptic catecholamine antagonists as treatment for Tourette syndrome. Arch Gen Psychiatry 1975; 31:857.

Van Woert MH, Hwang CE. Myoclonus. In: Vinken PJ, Bruyn GW, eds. Handbook of clinical neurology. Amsterdam: North Holland Publishing, 1979.

Van Woert MH. Myoclonus and L-5-hydroxytryptophan (L-5HTP). Orphan drugs and orphan diseases: clinical realities and public policy. New York: Alan R. Liss, 1983.

Weiner WJ, Lang AE. Movement disorders: a comprehensive survey. Mount Kisco, New York: Futura; 1989.

Willemse J. Benign idiopathic dystonia with onset in the first year of life. Dev Med Child Neurol 1986; 28:355.

Zeman W, Dyken P. Dystonia musculorum deformans: clinical genetic and pathoanatomical studies. Psychiatr Neurol Neurochir 1967; 70:77.

Zeman W, Whitlock CC. Symptomatic dystonias. In: Vinken PJ, Bruyn GW, eds. Handbook of clinical neurology, vol 6. Amsterdam: North Holland Publishing, 1968.

SUGGESTED READINGS

Asconape J, Penry JK. Some clinical and EEG aspects of benign juvenile myoclonic epilepsy. Epilepsia 1984; 25:108.

Bateman DN, Rawlins MD, Simpson JM. Extrapyramidal reactions to prochlorperazine and haloperidol in the United Kingdom. Q J Med 1986; 59:549.

Berrios X, Quesney F, Morales A, Blazquez J, Bisno AL. Are all recurrences of "pure" Sydenham chorea true recurrences of acute rheumatic fever? J Pediatr 1985; 107:867.

Blitzer A, et al. Electromyographic findings in focal laryngeal dystonia (spastic dysphonia). Ann Otol Rhinol Laryngol 1985; 94:591.

Burstein L, Breningstall GN. Movement disorders in bacterial meningitis. J Pediatr 1986; 109:260.

Campanella G, Roy M, Barbeau A. Drugs affecting movement disorders. Annu Rev Pharmacol Toxicol 1987; 27:113.

Comings DE, Comings BG. Tourette syndrome: clinical and psychological aspects of 250 cases. Am J Hum Genet 1985; 37:435.

Delgado-Escueta AV, Enrile-Bacsal F. Juvenile myoclonic epilepsy of Janz. Neurology 1984; 34:285.

Deonna T. DOPA-sensitive progressive dystonia of childhood with fluctuations of symptoms--Segawa's syndrome and possible variants. Results of a collaborative study of the European Federation of Child Neurology Societies (EFCNS). Neuropediatrics 1986; 17:81.

Deonna T, Ferreira A. Idiopathic fluctuating dystonia: a case of foot dystonia and writer's cramp responsive to L-dopa. Dev Med Child Neurol 1985; 27:819.

Driesen JJ, Wolters EC. Oral contraceptive induced paraballism. Clin Neurol Neurosurg 1987; 89:49.

Duvoisin RC. To treat early or to treat late? Ann Neurol 22:2.

Erenberg G, Cruse RP, Rothner AD. Gilles de la Tourette's syndrome: effects of stimulant drugs. Neurology 1985; 35:1346.

Filloux F, Thompson JA. Transient chorea induced by phenytoin. J Pediatr 1987; 110:639.

Growdon JH, Young RR. Paralysis and other disorders of movement. In: Braunwald E, et al., eds. Harrison's principles of internal medicine, 11th ed. New York: McGraw-Hill, 1987.

Hammann KP, et al. Hemichorea associated with varicella-zoster reinfection and endocarditis. A case report. Eur Arch Psychiatry Neurol Sci 1985; 234:404.

Hrachovy RA, et al. Double-blind study of ACTH vs prednisone therapy in infantile spasms. J Pediatr 1983; 103:641.

Hughes M, McLellan DL. Increased co-activation of the upper limb muscles in writer's cramp. J Neurol Neurosurg Psychiatry 1985; 48:782.

Jankovic J, Svendse CN, Bird ED. Brain neurotransmitters in dystonia (letter). N Engl J Med 1987; 316:278.

Klawans HL, Barr A. Recurrence of childhood multiple tic in late adult life. Arch Neurol 1985; 42:1079.

Klawans HL, Paleologos N. Dystonia-Parkinson syndrome: differential effects of levodopa and dopamine agonists. Clin Neuropharmacol 1986; 9:298.

Larsen TA, et al. Dystonia and calcification of the basal ganglia. Neurology 1985; 35:533.

Marsden CD, et al. Familial dystonia and visual failure with striatal CT lucencies. J Neurol Neurosurg Psychiatry 1986; 49:500.

Martinelli P, et al. Different clinical features of essential tremor: a 200-patient study. Acta Neurol Scand 1987; 75:106.

Menkes, JH. Huntington's disease: finding the gene and after. Pediatr Neurol 1988; 4:73.

Mitchell IJ, et al. Common neural mechanisms in experimental chorea and hemiballismus in the monkey. Evidence from 2-deoxyglucose autoradiography. Brain Res 1985; 339:346.

Newman RP, et al. Dystonia: treatment with bromocriptine. Clin Neuropharmacol 1985; 8:328.

Price RA, et al. Gilles de la Tourette's syndrome: tics and central nervous system stimulants in twins and nontwins. Neurology 1986; 36:232.

Reynolds EH, Trimble MR. Adverse neuropsychiatric effects of anticonvulsant drugs. Drugs 1985; 29:570.

Riikonen R. Infantile spasms. Modern practical aspects. Acta Paediatr Scand 1984; 73:1.

Robinson RO, Thornett CE. Benign hereditary chorea–response to steroids. Dev Med Child Neurol 1985; 27:814.

Scherokman B, et al. Peripheral dystonia. Arch Neurol 1986; 43:830.

Schwartz A, Hennerici M, Wegener OH. Delayed choreoathetosis following acute carbon monoxide poisoning. Neurology 1985; 35:98.

Shafrir Y, et al. Acute dystonic reaction to bethanechol–a direct acetylcholine receptor agonist. Dev Med Child Neurol 1986; 28:646.

Spitz MC, Jankovic J, Killian JM. Familial tic disorder, parkinsonism, motor neuron disease, and acanthocytosis: a new syndrome. Neurology 1985; 35:366.

Thal LJ, et al. Ventricular fluid somatostatin concentration decreases in childhood-onset dystonia. Neurology 1985; 35:1742.

Thompson PD, et al. Focal dystonia of the jaw and the differential diagnosis of unilateral jaw and masticatory spasm. J Neurol Neurosurg Psychiatry 1986; 49:651.

Treves T, Korczyn AD. Progressive dystonia and paraparesis in cerebral palsy. Eur Neurol 1986; 25:148.

Van Woert MH, Hwang CE. Myoclonus. In: Vinken PJ, Bruyn GW, eds. Handbook of clinical neurology. Amsterdam: Elsevier—North Holland, 1979.

Walevski A, Radwan M. Choreoathetosis as toxic effect of lithium treatment. Eur Neurol 1986; 25:412.

Wang BJ, Chang YC. Therapeutic blood levels of phenytoin in treatment of paroxysmal choreoathetosis. Ther Drug Monit 1985; 7:81.

Willemse J. Benign idiopathic dystonia with onset in the first year of life. Dev Med Child Neurol 1986; 28:355.

Young AB, et al. Huntington's disease in Venezuela: neurologic features and functional decline. Neurology 1986; 36:244.

19

Cerebellar Dysfunction and Ataxia in Childhood

Kenneth F. Swaiman

BASIC CEREBELLAR MECHANISMS AND FUNCTION

The underlying cause of ataxia is virtually always primary or secondary dysfunction of the cerebellum. Secondary impairment results from failure of necessary information to be relayed to the cerebellum or failure of integrity of the cerebellar efferent pathways.

The cerebellum is fundamentally involved in error detection and correction. Although the cerebellum seems readily comprehensible due to its relatively simple organization, the precise functional interaction within it is still fairly obscure despite intensive investigative efforts. Because the cerebellum has a servomechanistic function, any disruption of component input systems (e.g., cerebral cortex, brainstem, posterior columns of the spinal cord, peripheral nerves) may have a profoundly detrimental effect. In the simplest terms the hemispheres modulate limb movement of the ipsilateral side, and the midline vermis is primarily involved in station and gait.

The input of the cerebellum (afferent systems) consists of two major circuits. Virtually all cerebellar activity is inhibitory and mediated through pathways effectuated by γ-aminobutyric acid.

In the mossy fiber system the fibers form synaptic contacts with the granule cell layer (Figure 19-1). The mossy fibers originate primarily in the cord and brainstem centers. They excite granule cells, and impulses are transmitted through them. The mossy fibers parallel the molecular layer and subsequently impinge on and excite Purkinje cells. Numerous granule cells are associated with one Purkinje cell. In addition, interneurons provide inhibitory feedback to Purkinje and granule cells (e.g., Golgi, stellate, and basket cells).

The other primary afferent circuit is composed of climbing fibers that literally climb on the Purkinje cell dendritic system (see Figure 19-1). Climbing fibers originate from the contralateral inferior olive. There is one climbing fiber for each Purkinje cell.

Unlike the motor cortex, each cerebellar folia appears to have virtually all parts of the body represented—resulting in so-called fractured somatopy (Figure 19-2).

The general functional plan of the cerebellum appears to be delineated by sagittal zones (Figure 19-3): the lateral, which is associated with limb movements and gamma loop function through its thalamic and cortical projections; the intermediate, which is associated with tremor and cerebellorubroolivary circuitry; and the medial, which is associated with locomotion and vestibular function (e.g., posture, gait).

The dorsal spinocerebellar tract emanates from cells of the dorsal horn, particularly in the region of the nucleus dorsalis (Clarke column). The ventral spinocerebellar tract originates in a small number of special cells in the ventral horn. Both of these tracts terminate in the cortex of the cerebellum, primarily in the region of the vermis of the anterior lobe [Rasmussen, 1951].

The inferior olive receives fibers that ascend in the spinal cord and some fibers from higher brain centers. The fibers of the latter generally pass through the thalamoolivary fasciculus of the central tegmental tract. A large feedback loop exists in which the cerebellar nuclei are eventually connected with the inferior olive through the red nucleus. The inferior olive then sends fibers across the midline to the cortex of the opposite cerebellar hemisphere; the accessory olive is connected similarly with the cortex of the vermis.

Other cerebellar connections emanate from the nucleus gracilis and nucleus cuneatus via the dorsal or direct external arcuate fibers through the inferior cerebellar peduncle (the restiform body) of the same side. The nucleus cuneatus and gracilis receive ascending fibers from their corresponding tracts except for a

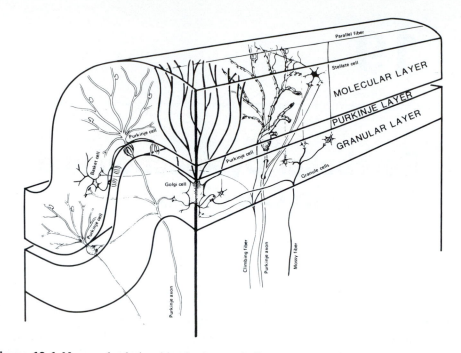

Figure 19-1 Neuronal relationships in the cerebellar cortex. This diagram contains a synthesis of the predominant interconnections in the monkey and cat and is simplified for clarity. (From Gilman S, Bloedel JR, Lechtenberg R. Disorders of the cerebellum. Philadelphia: FA Davis, 1981.)

few fibers that continue through the restiform body directly to the cerebellar cortex.

The outflow of the cerebellar hemispheral cortex is primarily through the dentate nucleus and then the brachium conjunctivum (superior cerebellar peduncle); fibers eventually terminate in the red nucleus and lateral and ventral portions of the contralateral thalamus. The midline vermal structures project to the fastigial and vestibular nuclei, allowing their participation in postural and locomotion functions. The rubrospinal tract originates from the large cells of the red nucleus. The tract crosses immediately and descends to all levels of the spinal cord. Many of the fibers traversing the superior cerebellar peduncle cross the midline before entering the red nucleus, bifurcate, and extend a descending branch in the ventral medial portion of the reticular formation as far as the inferior olive.

EVALUATION OF THE PATIENT
History

The history may provide much information about the underlying process. An explosive onset often indicates an infectious, traumatic, or toxic etiology. The clinician should search carefully for a history of antecedent trauma in the presence of acute ataxia and ascertain the use of prescribed medications, over-the-counter drugs, and illegal drugs. The clinician should also determine

unusual circumstances regarding the environment to exclude the inhalation of or other exposure to toxins. Metabolic conditions may occasionally cause acute ataxia, although slow onset is more common. A slow, insidious course occurs relatively often in the presence of brainstem and cerebellar tumors. Personality and behavioral changes or headaches may signal the presence of increased intracranial pressure.

Congenital abnormalities usually cause signs and symptoms that remain relatively unchanged during maturation. However, examiners may not readily recognize the coordination difficulties until maturational motor milestones are delayed or gross incoordination of hand manipulation and gait occurs.

Hereditary ataxia can often be established from the history. Clinicians need to consult parents and records to exclude the possibility of an inherited ataxia because many inherited causes cannot be confirmed by laboratory studies and frequently do not precisely meet the criteria of conventionally designated hereditary ataxias. The presence of visual or auditory disabilities enhances the likelihood of inherited ataxia.

Clinical examination

The primary clinical manifestations of cerebellar dysfunction reflect asynergia of muscular activity [Haymaker, 1969], but many other manifestations are com-

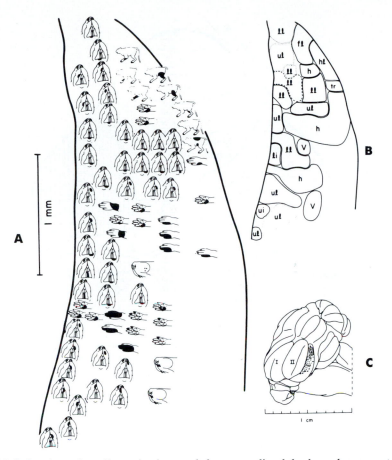

Figure 19-2 Patches of tactile projections to left paramedian lobe homologue portrayed by both figurine (**A**) and patch-mosaic (**B**) methods. (From King JS, ed. Neurology and neurobiology. vol. 22. New York: AR Liss, 1987.) Black patches on body figurines depict receptive fields, which optimally activate multiple units in granular cell layer at sites shown by black dots in (**C**). Contralateral receptive fields are shown on figurines of the right side of the body. In **B** a line surrounds those adjacent figurines having similar peripheral receptive fields. Boundaries between adjacent columnar patches appear discrete. *fl*, Forelimb; *h*, hand; *hl*, hindlimb; *li*, lower incisor; *ll*, lower lip; *ui*, upper incisor; *ul*, upper lip; *V*, mystacial vibrissae.

mon [Gilman et al., 1981]. Cerebellar deficit is often notable in disturbances of voluntary movement, equilibrium, and posture.

Beginning sometime between the ages of 4 and 6 years, most children of normal intelligence participate in a screening motor examination. Components of a neurologic examination directed at the problem of ataxia are listed in the box. The child stands in front of the examiner, and the examiner demonstrates the desired motor acts. The child is asked to hop on each foot in place (first one and then the other), tandem walk forward and backward, toe walk, and heel walk. The child is then asked to arise from a squatting position. Next the child is asked to stand with the feet close together, eyes closed, and arms and hands outstretched. With this maneuver, the examiner can simultaneously assess Romberg sign and the presence of adventitious

movements, particularly of the face, arms, and hands.

The child is then asked to perform finger-to-nose movements while the eyes are closed. The patient often manifests an action or intention tremor when attempting to place the finger on the nose during this part of the examination. Error in estimation of the amplitude of movement is termed *dysmetria*. Dysmetria and action tremor often occur during the same movement. Finger(patient's)-to-finger(examiner's)-to-nose movements may also be performed for further evaluation.

Cerebellar disease frequently decreases muscle tone and may decrease tendon reflexes because of changes in gamma-loop responsiveness. Enhancement of tendon reflex response when reflexes are seemingly absent can be facilitated by having the child squeeze an object such as a block or ball or perform the more traditional Jendrassik maneuver (hooking the flexed fingers of each

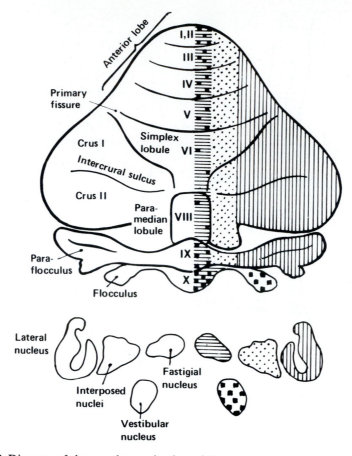

Figure 19-3 Diagram of the zonal organization of the cerebellum. In the upper part of the figure, the cerebellum is separated into three sagittal zones, each of which connects with the deep cerebellar or vestibular nucleus depicted in the lower part of the figure. This pattern of organization was obtained from studies of the projections of Purkinje cells onto the cerebellar nuclei in cats. (From Gilman S, Bloedel JR, Lechtenberg R. Disorders of the cerebellum. Philadelphia: FA Davis, 1981.)

hand together and then attempting to pull them apart).

Head tilt may be associated with tumors of the cerebellum. The tilt is usually ipsilateral to the involved cerebellar hemisphere, but exceptions commonly occur. Other causes include herniation of cerebellar tonsils through the foramen magnum secondary to increased intracranial pressure and neoplasms other than those of the cerebellum that induce increased intracranial pressure.

An adequate sensory examination must be performed. The examiner should assess light touch and pinprick and carefully evaluate both position sense and vibration sense, particularly in the lower extremities. Moderate to profound sensory impairment may result in ataxia because of inadequate input into cerebellar circuits.

Cranial titubation, a bobbing of the head usually in a predominant anteroposterior direction, may also be a conspicuous feature in these children.

Nystagmus arising from cerebellar dysfunction is usually horizontal, although vertical and rotary nystagmus may occur in the presence of cerebellar impairment. In affected patients, lateral gaze fixation in any horizontal direction most often results in nystagmus; the rapid movement is toward the side of gaze, and the slow movement is toward the position of rest. In cerebellar hemispheral lesions the nystagmus is coarser and slower when gaze is directed toward the same side as the affected cerebellar hemisphere. Cerebellar-induced nystagmus may be transient or intermittent.

Cerebellar function is assessed in a number of ways. Impaired ability to perform rapid alternating movements is termed *dysdiadochokinesia*. Hand patting (alternating pronation and supination of the hand on the thigh while the other hand remains stationary on the other thigh) is a good method for assessing dysdiadochokinesis. The maneuver is repeated with each hand independently to assess the presence of mirror movements (synkinesis).

Neurologic Examination

Classic findings of cerebellar dysfunction

Hypotonia
Nystagmus
Staggering gait
Titubation

Other symptoms and signs in cerebellar dysfunction

Action tremor
Asthenia
Ataxia
Decompensation of movements
Dysdiadochokinesis
Dysmetria
Dyssynergia
Hypotonia
Impaired rebound
Nystagmus
Pendular deep tendon reflexes

Examination of arms and hands

Finger-to-nose
Finger-to-finger-to-nose
Rapid alternating movements (hands, fingers, tongue)
Rebound
Tone evaluation

Examination of gait

Foot tapping
Heel-to-shin maneuver
Heel and toe-walking
Hopping in place (one foot)
Romberg or modified Romberg maneuver
Routine walking and running
Tandem walk (forward and backward)
Walking in circle

Tests that monitor cerebellar integrity include repetitive finger tapping (thumb to forefinger), foot tapping, and finger-to-nose, finger-to-finger (examiner's)-to-nose, and heel-to-knee-to-shin stroking. These rapid alternating movements are an index of cerebellar function when limb strength and sensation are intact. Breaks in rhythm and nonfluidity of movement are evident during this phase of the examination.

Changes in muscle tone are also a manifestation, although not exclusively, of cerebellar dysfunction. The abnormality results from the failure of cerebellar impulses to impinge properly on the rubroreticular tract, the cerebral cortex, or both. The limbs may be placed in abnormal positions. Hypotonia may be demonstrable by decreased resistance to passive movement imposed by the examiner. Another means of demonstrating the abnormality is to have the patient's outstretched arms rest on a bar or stick held by the examiner. The patient is asked to relax. After a brief period with the arms resting on the bar, the examiner suddenly removes the bar and the patient's affected arm or arms fall farther and more readily than expected. In the case of asymmetry the abnormal arm will fall farther than the other. During the elicitation of deep tendon reflexes the activated limb may swing unusually freely and may spontaneously repeat the movement arc—this phenomenon is most likely the result of hypotonia and is a pendular reflex.

An abnormal "rebound" phenomenon may be present. This form of difficulty may be demonstrated by the examiner resisting the flexion of the patient's arm, pulling on the patient's forearm, and then suddenly releasing the forearm. The patient's hand will fly up with considerable force and may even strike the patient in the face. Little of this rebound response occurs normally.

Cerebellar gait is characterized by staggering, irregularity, unsteadiness, wide-based lurching movement in any direction, and in the case of hemispheric lesions a tendency to veer in one lateral direction. When walking clockwise around a chair (as viewed from above), a child with a right cerebellar hemispheric lesion will stumble into the chair after a few circles. At times the gait is indistinguishable from the gait of an individual intoxicated with alcohol or drugs. Lesions in the vermis and midline structures result primarily in ataxic gait. When disturbed, important connections in the brainstem may lead to manifestation of cerebellar difficulties; however, the presence of associated corticospinal tract difficulties, Horner's syndrome, and cranial nerve palsies indicates that the brainstem is the site of difficulty.

Certain clinical maneuvers may be used to demonstrate that the brainstem is the affected site. Unsteadiness may be evident when the child is asked to rise from a chair and walk and then suddenly asked to stop and quickly turn 180 degrees. In the presence of significant cerebellar difficulty the patient will have difficulty standing with the feet together with eyes either open or closed. If Romberg sign is positive in this assessment, the patient sways with the feet together and eyes closed but not with the eyes open. This response indicates posterior column dysfunction and not primary cerebellar dysfunction. Less severe forms of ataxia become evident when the patient walks heel-to-toe along a straight line.

Cerebellar gait may not be associated with intention or action tremor of the arms or legs and difficulties with fine coordination. These signs depend on involvement of cerebellar hemispheres as opposed to the anterior lobe of the cerebellum or other midline cerebellar structures. Involvement of the cerebellar hemispheres results in compromise of actions of the ipsilateral limbs.

There may be changes in the voice, including slowing

Selected Causes of Ataxia in Childhood

Congenital

Agenesis of vermis of the cerebellum
Aplasia or dysplasia of the cerebellum
Chiari malformation, type 1
Cerebellar dysplasia with microgyria, macrogyria, or agyria
Cervical spinal bifida with herniation of the cerebellum (Chiari malformation, type 3)
Dandy-Walker syndrome
Encephalocele
Hydrocephalus (progressive)
Hypoplasia of the cerebellum (Chiari malformation, type 4)
Basilar impression

Degenerative

Acute disseminated encephalomyelitis
Acute intermittent cerebellar ataxia [Hill and Sherman*]
Ataxia, retinitis pigmentosa, deafness, vestibular abnormality, and intellectual deterioration [Francois and Descampas*]
Ataxia-telangiectasia
Biemond posterior column ataxia
Cerebellar ataxia with deafness, anosmia, absent caloric responses, nonreactive pupils, and hyporeflexia [Brown, 1959]
Cockayne syndrome
Dentate cerebellar ataxia (dyssynergia cerebellaris progressiva)
Familial ataxia with macular degeneration [Foster and Ingram*]
Friedreich ataxia

---

*Cited in Brown, 1962.

Hereditary cerebellar ataxia, intellectual retardation, choreoathetosis, and eunuchoidism [Altchule and Kotowski*]
Hereditary cerebellar ataxia with myotonia and cataracts [Brown, 1959]
Hypertrophic interstitial neuritis
Marie ataxia
Marinesco-Sjögren syndrome
Olivopontocerebellar ataxia (Dejerine syndrome)
Olivopontocerebellar atrophy with retinal degeneration—dominant inheritance [Weiner et al.*]
Pelizaeus-Merzbacher disease
Periodic attacks of vertigo, diplopia, and ataxia—autosomal dominant inheritance [Farmer and Mustian*]
Posterior and lateral column difficulties, nystagmus, and muscle atrophy [Burge and Wuthrich*]
Progressive cerebellar ataxia and epilepsy [von Bogaert and Colle*]
Ramsay Hunt disease (myoclonic seizures and ataxia)
Roussy-Lévy disease

Endocrinologic

Acquired hypothyroidism
Cretinism

Infectious or postinfectious

Acute cerebellar ataxia
Cerebellar abscess
Coxsackievirus
Diphtheria
Echovirus
Fisher syndrome
Infectious mononucleosis (EBV infection)
Infectious polyneuropathy
Japanese B encephalitis

---

of speech, jerkiness, uneven articulation, and phonation. Speech is often "scanning" or "staccato." This slowing of speech and other changes are believed to be manifestations of dysadiadochokinesia.

Laboratory examination

A toxicologic screen should be performed in any child with unexplained acute ataxia. The metabolic causes of ataxia as indicated in the box on p. 267 should be excluded by proper study. Quantitative amino acid determinations on blood and urine, lactate-pyruvate concentration, urinary organic acid screen, and blood ammonia studies should be performed. In the presence of suggestive historic and examination findings, investigation of lysosomal enzymes, inclusions in circulating lympho-

cytes, and enzymes in the electron transport chain may be indicated.

Imaging studies of the brain, particularly the posterior fossa, may be most important in the diagnosis of trauma, demyelination, or mass lesions. MRI is superior to CT for detection of brainstem and posterior fossa lesions.

SENSORY ATAXIA

Sensory ataxia is the result of disruption of input to the cerebellum from peripheral nerves, posterior roots, posterior columns of the spinal cord, or the pathway from posterior columns to the parietal lobes by way of the medial lemnisci.

No discrete muscle weakness occurs, but standing or

Selected Causes of Ataxia in Childhood—cont'd	
Mumps encephalitis Mycoplasma pneumoniae Pertussis Polio Postbacterial meningitis Rubeola Typhoid Varicella **Metabolic** Abetalipoproteinemia Argininosuccinic aciduria GM2 gangliosidosis (late) Hartnup disease Hyperalaninemia Hyperammonemia I and II Hypoglycemia Kearns-Sayre syndrome Leigh disease Maple syrup urine disease (intermittent) MERRF Metachromatic leukodystrophy Mitochondrial complex defects (I, III, IV) Multiple carboxylase deficiency (biotinidase deficiency) NARP Neuronal ceroid-lipofuscinosis Niemann-Pick disease (late infantile) 5-Oxoprolinuria Pyruvate decarboxylase deficiency Refsum disease Sialidosis Triose-phosphate isomerase deficiency Tryptophanuria Wernicke encephalopathy	**Neoplastic** Frontal lobe tumors Hemispheric cerebellar tumors Midline cerebellar tumors Neuroblastoma Pontine tumors (primarily gliomas) Spinal cord tumors **Primary psychogenic** Conversion reaction **Toxic** *Endogenous* Neuroblastoma *Exogenous* Alcohol Carbamazepine Clonazepam Lead encephalopathy Phenobarbital Phenytoin Primidone Tic paralysis poisoning **Traumatic** Acute cerebellar edema Acute frontal lobe edema **Vascular** Angioblastoma of cerebellum Basilar migraine Cerebellar embolism Cerebellar hemorrhage Cerebellar thrombosis Posterior cerebellar artery disease von Hippel-Lindau disease

walking is extremely difficult, and the child has a wide-based gait. The child has little perception of the relationship of the feet to the ground and consequently lifts the feet high and stamps them down vigorously with each step. The heel contacts the ground first. The toe then strikes the ground, causing a split sound. The child attempts to compensate by watching the ground. Steps frequently change in length, and the body is flexed slightly forward.

Examination reveals a positive Romberg sign, loss of position sense of the toes, and loss of vibration sense in the feet and legs. Pain, light touch, and temperature are not affected unless a severe peripheral neuropathy is the basis of the patient's difficulty. Patients with posterior column degeneration secondary to Friedreich ataxia [Friedreich, 1863], subacute combined degeneration, meningomyelitis, polyneuritis, and demyelinating diseases may be affected. Tabes dorsalis is the classic adult disease of the posterior columns.

HEREDITARY ATAXIAS

The classification of hereditary ataxia (hereditary spinocerebellar conditions) defies reasonable ordering because of the large number of case reports and pedigrees that deviate from attempts at precise categorization [Brown, 1959]. Attempts to classify ataxia according to the site of most prominent pathology (e.g., spinal, cerebellar) provide an imperfect framework in which order can supposedly be superimposed [Greenfield, 1954]. Under this scheme, spinal hereditary atax-

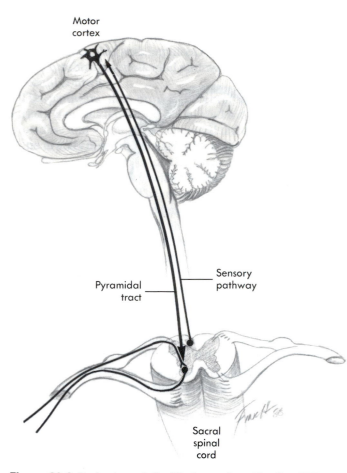

Figure 20-3 Paths 4a and 4b. (Redrawn from Bradley WE. Physiology of the urinary bladder. In: Walsh PC, Gittes BF, Perlmutter AD, et al., eds. Campbell's urology. Philadelphia: WB Saunders, 1986.)

ganglia, anterior hypothalamus, and anterior midbrain inhibit the reflex detrusor contraction that is induced by bladder filling. Although connections between the cerebellum and urinary bladder have been established and possible cerebellar influence on micturition hypothesized [Bradley, 1986], little specific information is available concerning this relationship.

The brainstem detrusor motor nucleus is located in the caudal portion of the dorsal tegmental area of the pons rostral to the nucleus locus coeruleus [Tohyama et al., 1978]. The following two projections emanate from this nucleus: one to the lateral hypothalamic area and one to the sacral spinal cord [Satoh et al., 1978a].

Detrusor muscle and the urethral sphincter striated muscles act in a complex reciprocal manner during bladder filling and voiding. Concurrent relaxation of the striated muscles of the internal and external urethral sphincters and contraction of detrusor muscle results in voiding. Reverse interaction results in bladder filling.

The stretch receptors [Bradley, 1986; Bradley et al., 1974] in the detrusor muscle are activated by bladder filling and initiate the micturition reflex. Some of these stretch receptor-initiated impulses travel in the pelvic nerve afferents, which synapse with the pudendal neurons in the sacral cord (path 3; see Figure 20-2). Impulses inhibit the pudendal neurons, with resultant relaxation of the striated muscles of the internal and external urethral sphincters. Other afferents are directed over a long pathway to the brainstem pudendal nucleus; from there they travel down the reticulospinal tract to terminate on the sacral detrusor neurons, with resultant muscle contraction (path 2).

The voluntary control of the urethral sphincter is mediated through path 4a, which originates in the neurons of the corticospinal tract (pyramidal tract) in the medial anterior frontal cortex. The axons of the pyramidal tract terminate on the pudendal neurons in the sacral cord and by effecting activity in path 4b exert voluntary control over the sphincter muscle (cerebrospinopudendal pathway) [Nakagawa, 1980]. Tonic activity in the pudendal nerves innervating the urethral sphincter maintains closure of the sphincter during both waking and sleeping states. The muscle stretch receptors in the sphincter striated muscle modulate and maintain this tonic activity. Commanding the patient to contract the sphincter provides a test for evaluating these neural connections. Because the innervation of the urethral and anal sphincter is the same for purposes of analysis, anal sphincter monitoring is useful for assessing urethral sphincter function as well. An anourethral reflex has also been described [Shafik, 1992]. Urethral sphincter function may also be assessed electromyographically by examination of the pelvic floor muscles.

The frontal lobes exert some voluntary control over the detrusor muscle. The integrity of this pathway can be readily demonstrated by the ability of the patient to suppress the detrusor reflex contraction on command during micturition and cystometric examination. Pathologic compromise of this pathway results in detrusor hyperreflexia, which is characterized during the cystometric examination by the reaction of a detrusor reflex at a low-volume threshold; the reflex cannot be interdicted volitionally by the patient. The impairment may be so subtle that the clinical manifestations may be evident only on postural change or during walking.

Bilateral pathologic involvement of the pyramidal tract, usually in the spinal cord, results in impaired volitional control of the urethral sphincter; therefore the urethral sphincter may undergo inappropriate relaxation, or increased sphincter activity may occur during detrusor contraction. This imbalance is termed *detrusor-urethral sphincter dyssynergia* [Hinman, 1980].

Anatomic and functional classifications of the disorders of micturition are provided in the boxes on p. 277.

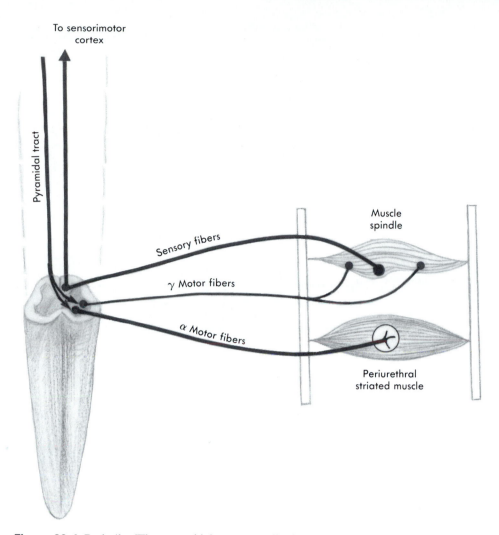

Figure 20-4 Path 4b. (The pyramidal tract actually de-scends on the same side as the ascending tract to the sensorimotor cortex.) (Redrawn from Bradley WE. Physiology of the urinary bladder. In: Walsh PC, Gittes BF, Perlmutter AD, et al., eds. Campbell's urology. Philadelphia: WB Saunders, 1986.)

Evaluation of the patient

History. A detailed history is essential in eliciting clues regarding onset and the site of pathologic involvement in disorders of micturition. The presence or absence of incontinence or change in urinary habits must be ascertained. Frequency, urgency, force of the urinary stream, urinary volume, pattern of incontinence, and associated discomfort are crucial aspects of the history. Interrogating a child concerning these symptoms requires patience and imagination. Allowing the child to describe the urinary dysfunction, with particular emphasis on the sensations associated with urination and the procedures and sensations associated with initiating and terminating micturition, may be crucial to ascertaining the correct diagnosis.

Intact afferent and efferent connections to the detrusor muscle are prerequisites for instigation of the desire to void. Lesions in the afferent pathways from the bladder result in an absence of the desire to void. Sensations of imminent micturition and of ongoing micturition indicate that the requisite sensory pathways are intact. Lesions of the efferent pathways to the bladder lead to a dysfunction of micturition in the presence of a normal desire to void. In this situation, structural obstruction to the flow of urine must be excluded.

In spinal cord lesions the level of injury determines the symptom complex. In lesions of the spinal cord at or below T_{10} the sensation of suprapubic fullness is generally preserved. If the lesion is rostral to T_6, autonomic overactivity may be present and manifested by bradycardia, chills and diaphoresis, piloerection, paroxysmal hypertension, headache, and suffusion of the head and neck. This overactive autonomic response is

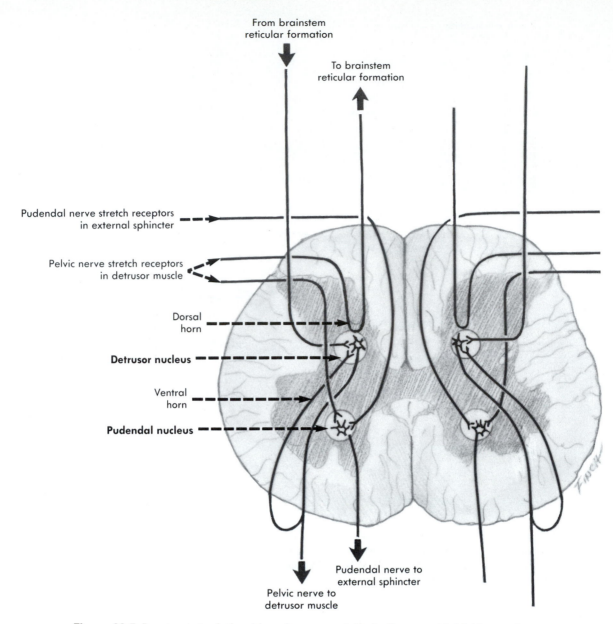

Figure 20-5 Input-outut relationships of conus medullaris. Recurrent inhibition pathways are observed in the pelvic motor nerves. (Redrawn from Bradley WE. Physiology of the urinary bladder. In: Walsh PC, Gittes BF, Perlmutter AD, et al., eds. Campbell's urology. Philadelphia: WB Saunders, 1986.)

the result of exaggerated reflex sympathetic activity in the isolated spinal cord. Plasma catecholamine concentrations are elevated, and peripheral sympathetic activity is increased [Frankel and Mathias, 1976].

Circumstances surrounding the initiation and termination of urination provide further evidence of the type of neural lesion involved. The abrupt urge to void, with resultant sudden micturition, signifies an incomplete suprasegmental lesion. When the lesion is complete, the patient has no warning and no sensation associated with reflex micturition. In peripheral motor lesions involving injury of S_2 to S_4 segments (conus medullaris lesions), bladder pressure must be increased with the use of the abdominal muscles and/or the bladder must be manually compressed to effect voiding. In this instance, micturition may cease when the patient discontinues straining or applying pressure to the abdominal wall. In suprasegmental lesions a momentary, involuntary interruption of the urinary stream may occur. If the patient can volitionally interrupt and resume urination, the efferent pathway may be presumed to be intact.

Micturition Disorders: Sites of Dysfunction
Upper motor neuron unit lesions
Frontal and parietal lobes
Limbic system and hypothalamus
Basal ganglia
Brainstem
Cerebellum
Spinal cord
Lower motor neuron unit lesions
Afferent (sensory) pathways
Efferent (motor) pathways
Preganglionic
Postganglionic
Muscle fibers
Detrusor vesicle outlet—structural alterations

Functional Classification of Urinary Incontinence
A. Impaired urine storage
1. Detrusor dysfunction
a. Hyperreflexia
b. Increased tone
c. Decreased elasticity
2. Altered outflow resistance
a. Incompetent sphincter
b. Structural abnormalities
B. Impaired bladder emptying
1. Detrusor dysfunction
a. Hypotonicity
b. Areflexia
2. Increased outflow resistance
a. Sphincter dyssynergia
b. Structural abnormalities

Nocturnal enuresis is defined as persistent night time bedwetting beyond 5 years of age because 85% of children are urinary bladder continent by this age. In a child who never achieved complete bladder control the enuresis is said to be primary. Secondary enuresis is bedwetting after a dry period indicating successful urinary bladder control. Diurnal or nocturnal enuresis occurring beyond the expected age of urinary control requires systematic evaluation. Associated impairment of sensory or motor function, particularly of the legs and perianal areas, should be carefully delineated because of the possibility of cord involvement.

When present, incontinence should be categorized. Overflow incontinence, relatively rare in childhood, may accompany involvement of central or peripheral motor mechanisms. Loss of urine when lifting objects, coughing, or walking indicates stress incontinence, which may result from a peripheral motor lesion compromising either the detrusor muscle or the muscles of the pelvic floor. Abrupt, uncontrolled voiding is associated with lesions, such as those involving the cerebral hemispheres or the suprasegmental areas of the spinal cord.

Neurologic examination. The classic neurologic conceptualization of disease resulting from either upper or lower motor neuron unit involvement is inadequate for evaluating problems of micturition. Effects of CNS lesions vary widely because these lesions, depending on location, have significant inhibitory or facilitatory influences on micturition. Other confounding factors associated with these lesions are chronic infection and bladder distention, which lead to alterations in detrusor muscle contractility and neuronal excitability; these changes must be differentiated from primary neurologic conditions.

Uninhibited neurogenic bladder may occur with bilateral involvement of the medial frontal lobe areas (e.g., superior sagittal sinus thrombosis). Frequency and urgency of urination are increased; bladder sensation is preserved. As the bladder fills, the detrusor contracts and increases intravesical pressure. The bladder may become so contracted that a minute quantity of urine induces micturition. Ultimately, automatic micturition develops [Haymaker, 1969]. Suprasegmental lesions of the spinal cord above the lumbar segments are accompanied by urgency, incontinence, increased frequency, and nocturia.

The neurologic examination should be directed at excluding focal or progressive spinal cord lesions. The cutaneous area over the spine should be scrutinized for midline abnormalities that may indicate underlying congenital malformations. The spine should be evaluated for tenderness and scoliosis. Skeletal muscle spasticity, hyperreflexia, clonus, and extensor toe signs accompany suprasegmental lesions. Muscle atrophy, muscle weakness, and decreased or absent deep-tendon reflexes accompany lower motor neuron unit lesions originating in the lumbosacral cord; associated sensory changes are often evident. Syndromes of the cauda equina, conus medullaris, and epiconus are distinguishable by clinical findings [Haymaker, 1969; Wright, 1982] (Table 20-1).

When the epiconus (L_4, L_5, S_1, and S_2) is involved, profound motor involvement of the lower legs and feet occurs [Haymaker, 1969]. External rotation and dorsiflexion of the thigh are most affected. Abduction at the hip, flexion at the knee, and flexion and extension at the ankle are also involved. The Achilles tendon reflex is absent.

When the conus medullaris (S_3 to Coc_1) is involved (conus syndrome), paralytic bladder incontinence and,

Table 20-1 Differentiating features of lower spinal cord lesions

	Epiconus L_4-S_2	Conus medullaris S_3-Coc$_1$	Cauda equina L_3-Coc$_1$ roots
Onset	Variable	Usually sudden and bilateral	Usually gradual and unilateral
Motor	Considerable motor dysfunction in the lower extremities (see text for details)	Usually mild, symmetric motor dysfunction; fasciculations may be present	Asymmetric, marked motor dysfunction; fasciculations uncommon
Sensory	Disturbances in L_4-S_2 segments	Bilateral, symmetric saddle distribution; dissociation of sensory loss may be present	Asymmetric, saddle distribution; may be unilateral; no dissociation of sensation
Reflexes	Achilles tendon reflex absent	Achilles tendon reflex may be diminished	Patellar and Achilles tendon reflexes may be absent
Bladder and rectal symptoms	Small, contracted "spastic" bladder, loss of voluntary control with incontinence	Paralytic, distended bladder and patulous anus, incontinence	Paralytic, distended bladder and patulous anus, incontinence; involvement late and less severe
Pain	Variable	Absent or symmetric bilateral mild pain in perineum or thighs	Radicular pain; asymmetric, unilateral pain that may be severe and prominent

usually, bladder distention occur [Haymaker, 1969]. Bowel incontinence is also present. There is loss of perianal sensation consonant with impairment of the lower sacral (S_3 and S_4) and coccygeal cord segments. Rectal sphincter reflex (anal wink) is absent, and denervation of the voluntary anal sphincter causes loss of anal sphincter tone. No motor abnormalities of the legs and feet occur. The Achilles tendon reflex is uninvolved. In a study of traumatic conus lesions the prognosis was somewhat better than has been widely appreciated [Taylor and Coolican, 1988]. In the cauda equina syndrome, there is involvement of nerve roots from spinal segments L_3 to Coc$_1$. It may be difficult to distinguish cauda equina from conus lesions. All forms of sensibility are involved. Spontaneous pain, especially in the perineum over the sacrum and bladder, may dominate the clinical pattern [Haymaker, 1969]. Peroneal weakness, including foot drop, may occur. Fibrillary twitching in affected muscles is common. When preferential interruption of motor innervation occurs, detrusor contraction is greatly compromised, although bladder sensation is preserved (motor paralytic bladder).

Clinical laboratory tests. Studies are chosen to clarify the nature of the bladder dysfunction. Urinalysis and urine culture, blood urea nitrogen, and serum creatinine are necessary studies. Results of these tests may indicate primary renal or other nonneurologic conditions. Ultrasonography of the kidneys and bladder have been of great value in rapidly assessing structural changes. In one series of children studied with ultrasonography, 32% of 74 children with voiding problems had one or more of the following: thickened detrusor; large bladder capacity with or without residual urine; fecal impaction; suspected bladder neck obstruction, which later required internal urethrotomy; and small

bladder capacity [Maizels et al., 1987]. Wide bladder neck anomaly has been recognized as a common cause of incontinence in children [Murray et al., 1987]. Abnormal cystic masses, bladder diverticula, and other structural abnormalities may be recognized; however, interpretation may occasionally be difficult and lead to erroneous diagnoses [Vick et al., 1983].

Urodynamic study of the free-flow curve provides valuable data without invasive instrumentation or an extensive urodynamic study. If the free-flow curve is normal and there is no residual urine, then significant voiding abnormality, whether of functional or anatomic origin, is unlikely [Griffiths and Scholtmeijer, 1984]. Study methods particularly adapted to children and norms for children have been developed [Di Scipio et al., 1986; Pompino and Hoffmann, 1983]. Video urodynamic study of children with grossly intact neurologic function often reveals detrusor dysfunction and abnormal sphincter activity [Webster et al., 1984]. Computer-monitored voiding studies can provide useful information concerning detrusor muscle function and allow categorization of the dysfunction [van Mastrigt and Griffiths, 1986]. Urodynamic evaluation and follow-up care is important in diagnosis and optimal management of many children with micturition problems [Churchill et al., 1987].

Plain radiographs of the lumbosacral area, intravenous pyelography, and a voiding cystourethrogram all provide further information. Bladder prolapse, with the bladder neck situated below the upper margin of the pubic symphysis, has been described as a urographic radiologic sign of urethral sphincter denervation in children with myelodysplasia [Zerin et al., 1990]. Conventional invasive urologic examinations, now less commonly required because of modern imaging techniques, should be performed when other examinations

Table 20-2 Drugs used in neurogenic bladder dysfunction

Bladder dysfunction	Drug	Action	Usual minimum dose per day	Usual maximum dose per day
Impaired urine storage				
Decreased bladder capacity	Propantheline	Anticholinergic	1.0 mg/kg	2.0 mg/kg
	Oxybutynin	Anticholinergic	0.4 mg/kg	0.8 mg/kg
	Flavoxate	Direct muscle action	6.0 mg/kg	9.0 mg/kg
	Dicyclomine	Anticholinergic	1.0 mg/kg	2.0 mg/kg
	Terodiline	Calcium antagonist	12.5 mg/day	25 mg/day
Decreased outflow resistance	Phenylpropranolol	Sympathomimetic	5.0 mg/kg	7.5 mg/kg
	Ephedrine	Sympathomimetic	1.0 mg/kg	3.0 mg/kg
	Imipramine	Complex	1.4 mg/kg	2.4 mg/kg
Impaired bladder emptying				
Increased bladder capacity	Bethanecol	Cholinergic	2.0 mg/kg	3.0 mg/kg
Increased outflow resistance	Phenoxybenzamine	Sympatholytic	0.6 mg/kg	1.5 mg/kg
	Dantrolene	Direct muscle action	1.0 mg/kg	8 to 10 mg/kg

Modified from Bauer SB. Urodynamic evaluation and neuromuscular dysfunction. In: Kelalis PP, King LR, Belman AB, eds. Clinical pediatric urology. 2nd ed. Philadelphia: WB Saunders, 1985.

have not provided sufficient data [Walther and Kaplan, 1979].

Detrusor muscle function can be evaluated by cystometry if other methods are insufficient. A slow-fill cystometrogram triggers bladder contraction after dilatation with instilled fluid. Detrusor tone, reflex threshold, sensation, and volitional ability to inhibit detrusor contraction can be assessed. Reflex abnormality of the detrusor (i.e., hyperreflexia, hyporeflexia, or areflexia) may be documented [Bradley and Andersen, 1977]. Voiding cystourethrography and other radiologic techniques provide useful additional information [Bisset et al., 1987; Lebowitz, 1985].

Although infrequently performed, peripheral reflex pathways can be monitored by percutaneous stimulation of the sacral roots in conjunction with transducer placement in the bladder [Markland et al., 1967]. Intact preganglionic pathways to the bladder are necessary for optimal detrusor response after percutaneous stimulation [Markland et al., 1965].

Testing of the postganglionic pathways is more complex. The effect of percutaneous stimulation is assessed, as well as the detrusor contraction in response to direct electrical stimulation applied through a cystoscope and the intravesical pressure response to bethanechol chloride [Lapides et al., 1962]. Muted or absent response to percutaneous and direct electrical stimulation and denervation hypersensitivity to bethanechol suggest impaired postganglionic pathways. Lack of contractile response to direct stimulation and lack of denervation hypersensitivity may indicate myopathic detrusor changes, which result from bladder overdistention or infection. Bladder muscle biopsy may demonstrate col-

lagen accumulation [Bradley et al., 1965]. An increase in creatine kinase activity occurs after experimental bladder muscle injury [Swaiman and Bradley, 1969].

Differential diagnosis

Nocturnal enuresis is the most common disorder of micturition in childhood. Neurologic disease must be excluded in any child who either does not develop or subsequently loses urinary continence. The box on p. 280 presents a list of differential diagnoses in disorders of micturition.

Management

Precise diagnosis is required for a systematic and effective therapeutic approach. Neurogenic bladder dysfunction must be countermanded so that urinary control and normal renal function are allowed to continue. Optimal therapy prevents infections (Table 20-2).

Hyperreflexic bladder, the result of impairment of suprasegmental governance of the detrusor muscle, is associated with increased resting bladder tone, uncontrollable bladder contraction with incontinence, frequency and urgency of urination, and diminished bladder volume. Therapeutic measures are directed at these cardinal features.

Administration of anticholinergic drugs decreases contractility. Therapy with propantheline bromide is often effective. Oxybutynin may be used in some children. Trials with new anticholinergic agents demonstrate promise [Otto-Unger, 1985; Hehir and Fitzpatrick, 1985]. Unfortunately, anticholinergic therapy may be associated with urinary retention and an increase in residual urine; therefore residual urine volume should

followed by an increase in abdominal pressure and simultaneous relaxation of rectal sphincters, causing defecation.

Interaction of tone and reflex activity is essential in the physiology of continence. Reflex and voluntary contractions of the puborectalis muscle and internal and external sphincters are important components of continence during sleep and waking [Scharli and Kiesewetter, 1970]. Because of the intricate relationship of the sphincters, determining their contribution to maintenance of resting pressure is difficult; however, the resting pressure appears primarily to be the result of contraction of the internal sphincter [Ito et al., 1977; Varma and Stephens, 1972; Verder et al., 1974; Pemberton and Kelly, 1986].

Incontinence results when the pressure induced by the peristaltic movement in the distal rectum overcomes the anorectal pressure. There are three types of incontinence: true incontinence, partial incontinence, and overflow incontinence [Wright, 1982]. Deficient anorectal muscles (e.g., imperforate anus) or impaired neuromuscular function results in true incontinence. There may be insufficient anorectal pressure or impaired sensation of peristaltic movement and bowel distention. Fecal soiling is the result of partial incontinence, because the final stage of defecation is inadequate and is followed by continuing passage of small amounts of stool. Overflow incontinence, not a true form of incontinence, results from chronic fecal impaction and leakage of liquid feces through the dilated anorectal ring.

Evaluation of the patient

History. Fecal incontinence is the usual complaint of patients seeking help. It is essential to determine whether bowel control was lost after it had been achieved or whether bowel control was never present. The age at onset, frequency, related circumstances (e.g., time of day, association with sleep, behavioral aspects), and alterations in bowel habits, stool mass, stool color, and stool consistency should be established. Overall integrity of afferent and efferent pathways may be evaluated by further questioning. Inquiries should be designed to ascertain whether rectal sensation, including pressure of fecal volume and need to defecate, as well as the ability to differentiate between passage of flatus and feces, is present. Similarly, efferent function can be evaluated by questions related to volitional inhibition of defecation.

Neurologic examination. Because the neural pathways are similar, neurologic evaluation of bowel incontinence parallels that described for disorders of micturition.

In lesions above the sacral cord (suprasegmental lesions), voluntary control over the sphincter ani is lost. Sphincter tone is increased, and fecal retention occurs,

leading to chronic fecal impaction and consequent soiling. During rectal examination the patient should be able to contract and relax the sphincter on request. Sphincter tone is often increased and contracted with suprasegmental lesions [Wright, 1982]. Paralysis of the sphincter ani accompanies sacral cord disturbance. The anus is patulous, the anal sphincter reflex is lacking, and the patient is unable to contract the sphincter on command. In contrast to bladder the extent of preservation or return of anal and rectal sensation in conus medullaris lesions is important in achieving bowel control. The involuntary passage of flatus is a distressing symptom in such patients if they cannot distinguish it from feces for which sensory input is essential [Taylor and Coolican, 1988]. Further information on lower cord and cauda equina lesions can be found in the section on urinary incontinence.

Clinical laboratory tests. Proctoscopy and fiberoptic studies of the lower bowel are efficient methods of excluding the presence of structural abnormalities. Barium enema studies are sometimes necessary.

Special studies include anal sphincter electromyography [Waylonis and Powers, 1972; Shafik, 1992]. Denervation potentials indicate a recent lower motor neuron process. A manometric study may also be useful [Varma and Stephens, 1972]. However, the correlation between the clinical findings and the manometric assessment of sphincters in response to rectal distention is often poor. CT allows imaging of the puborectal muscle and external sphincters and identification of associated anomalies [Ikawa et al., 1985; Kohda et al., 1985].

Differential diagnosis

Bowel dysfunction is produced by the conditions listed in the box on p. 280. Lumbosacral defects may be associated with reduced or absent external sphincter function, which is demonstrated by sphincter electromyography. Denervation potentials or reduced, large-amplitude potentials may be observed. In Hirschsprung disease, manometric studies demonstrate an absence of rectoanal inhibitory reflex; that is, the internal sphincter fails to relax in response to a transient rectal distention. The relaxation wave is absent.

The most common cause of bowel incontinence is encopresis, which is not associated with neurologic dysfunction. Encopresis is fecal incontinence without organic cause. Males outnumber females 3.5 to 1 [Bellman, 1966]. The cardinal feature of encopresis is withholding of stools, and the condition is often not recognized by the parents. Neurogenic and other organic conditions causing bowel dysfunction must be excluded.

Management

Assessment of contributing factors, including psychosocial milieu, anorectal examination, and appropriate neurologic evaluation, is necessary for adequate management. Therapeutic approaches include behavioral, pharmacologic, and surgical methods [Wald, 1986].

Dietary measures to harden stools may be attempted for some patients. The stools can then be evacuated by manual pressure over the abdomen and by straining of the abdominal muscles. Some children may perceive the urge to defecate when the stools are bulkier, which can be achieved by using stool-bulking agents (e.g., Metamucil). Rectal suppositories (bisacodyl) or a saline enema may empty the rectum before it fills and cause reflex relaxation of the internal sphincter. This approach may prevent soiling in some children. Excessive flatus and soiling may also be controlled by avoiding certain foods, such as legumes, and by giving attention to strict dietary and bowel habits.

Biofeedback training [Owen-Smith and Chesterfield, 1986], behavior modification [Whitehead et al., 1986], muscle training, and medications are often of benefit [Scharli, 1987]. New devices to control both fecal and urinary incontinence have shown promise [Numanoglu, 1987]. Surgical intervention may be considered if conservative treatment fails [Kottmeier et al., 1986; Chen and Zhang, 1987; Bass and Yazbeck, 1987].

REFERENCES

Ambrosini PJ. A pharmacological paradigm for urinary incontinence and enuresis. J Clin Psycopharmacol 1984; 4:247.

Baskin LS, Kogan BA, Benard F. Treatment of infants with neurogenic bladder dysfunction using anticholinergic drugs and intermittent catheterization. Br J Urol 1990; 66:532.

Bass J, Yazbeck S. Reoperation by anterior perineal approach for missed puborectalis. J Pediatr Surg 1987; 22:761.

Bellman M. Studies in encoparesis. Acta Paediatr Scand [suppl] 1966; 170:1.

Bisset GS III, Strife JL, Dunbar JS. Urography and voiding cystourethrography. Findings in girls with urinary tract infection. Am J Roentgenol 1987; 148:479.

Bradley WE. Physiology of the urinary bladder. In: Walsh PC, Gittes BF, Perlmutter AD, et al., eds. Campbell's urology. Philadelphia: WB Saunders, 1986; 129-185.

Bradley WE, Andersen JT. Techniques for analysis of micturition reflex disturbances in childhood. Pediatrics 1977; 59:546.

Bradley WE, Rockswold GL, Timm GW, et al. Neurology of micturition. J Urol 1976; 115:481.

Bradley WE, Swaiman KF, Markland C, et al. Biochemical assay techniques for estimation of bladder fibrosis. Invest Urol 1965; 3:59.

Bradley WE, Timm GW, Scott FB. Innervation of the detrusor muscle and urethera. Urol Clin North Am 1974; 1:3.

Cass AS, Luxenberg M, Gleich P, et al. Clean intermittent catheterization in the management of the neurogenic bladder in children. J Urol 1984; 132:526.

Chen YL, Zhang XH. Reconstruction of rectal sphincter by transposition of gluteus muscle for fecal incontinence. J Pediatr Surg 1987; 22:62.

Churchill BM, Gilmour RF, Williot P. Urodynamics. Pediatr Clin North Am 1987; 34:1133.

Davies J. Human developmental anatomy. New York: Ronald Press, 1963; 177-198.

Di Scipio WJ, Smey P, Kogan SJ, et al. Impromptu micturitional flow parameters in normal boys. J Urol 1986; 136:1049.

Duthie HL. Progress report: anal continence. Gut 1971; 12:844.

Fidas A, Elton RA, McInnes A, et al. Neurophysiological measurement of the voiding reflex arcs in patients with functional disorders of the lower urinary tract. Br J Urol 1987; 60:205.

Frankel HL, Mathias CJ. The cardiovascular system in tetraplegia and paraplegia. In: Vinken PJ, Bruyn GW, eds. Handbook of clinical neurology: injuries of the spine and spinal cord, vol 26. Part II. Amsterdam: North Holland Publishing, 1976; 313-333.

Frost F, Nanninga J, Penn R, et al. Intrathecal Baclofen infusion effect on bladder management programs in patients with myelopathy. Am J Phys Med Rehabil 1989; 68:112.

Greenfield SP, Fera M. The use of intravesical oxybutynin chloride in children with neurogenic bladder. J Urol 1991; 146:532.

Griffiths DJ, Scholtmeijer RJ. Place of the free flow curve in the urodynamic investigation of children. Br J Urol 1984; 56:474.

Hakelius L, Gierup J, Grotte G. Urinary incontinence in children. Treatment with free autogenous muscle transplantation. Prog Pediatr Surg 1984; 17:155.

Haldeman S, Bradley WE, Bhatia NN, Johnson BK. Pudendal somatosensory evoked potentials. Arch Neurol 1982a; 39:280.

Haldeman S, Bradley WE, Bhatia NN, Johnson BK. Evoked responses from pudendal nerve. J Urol 1982b; 128:974.

Haymaker W. Bing's local diagnosis in neurological diseases. 15th ed. St. Louis: Mosby, 1969; 105-113.

Hehir M, Fitzpatrick JM. Oxybutinin and the prevention of urinary incontinence in spina bifida. Eur Urol 1985; 11:254.

Hellström AL, Hjälmäs K, Jodal U. Rehabilitation of the dysfunctional bladder in children: method and 3-year followup. J Urol 1987; 138:847.

Hensle TW, Burbige KA. Bladder replacement in children and young adults. J Urol 1985; 133:1004.

Himsel KK, Hurwitz RS. Pediatric urinary incontinence. Urol Clin North Am 1991; 18:283.

Hinman F. Syndromes of vesical incoordination. Urol Clin North Am 1980; 7:311.

Ikawa H, Yokoyama J, Sanbonmatsu T, et al. The use of computerized tomography to evaluate anorectal anomalies. J Pediatr Surg 1985; 20:640.

Ito Y, Donahoe PK, Hendren WH. Maturation of the rectoanal response in premature and perinatal infants. J Pediatr Surg 1977; 12:477.

Jerkins GR, Noe HN, Vaughn WR, et al. Biofeedback training for children with bladder sphincter incoordination. J Urol 1987; 138:1113.

Joseph DB, Bauer SB, Colodny AH, et al. Clean, intermittent catheterization of infants with neurogenic bladder. Pediatrics 1989; 84:78.

Kato K, Kondo A, Saito M, et al. In vitro intravesical instillation of anticholinergic, antispasmodic and calcium blocking agents to decrease bladder contractility. Urol Int 1991; 47(suppl 1):36.

Keating MA, Rink RC, Bauer SB, et al. Neurological implications of the changing approach in management of occult spinal lesions. J Urol 1988; 140:1299.

Khoury AE, Churchill BM. The artificial urinary sphincter. Pediatr Clin North Am 1987; 34:1175.

King LR, Webster GD, Bertram RA. Experiences with bladder reconstruction in children. J Urol 1987; 138:1002.

Kohda E, Fujioka M, Ikawa H, et al. Congenital anorectal anomaly. CT evaluation. Radiology 1985; 157:349.

Kottmeier PK, Velcek FT, Klotz DH, et al. Results of levatorplasty for anal incontinence. J Pediatr Surg 1986; 21:647.

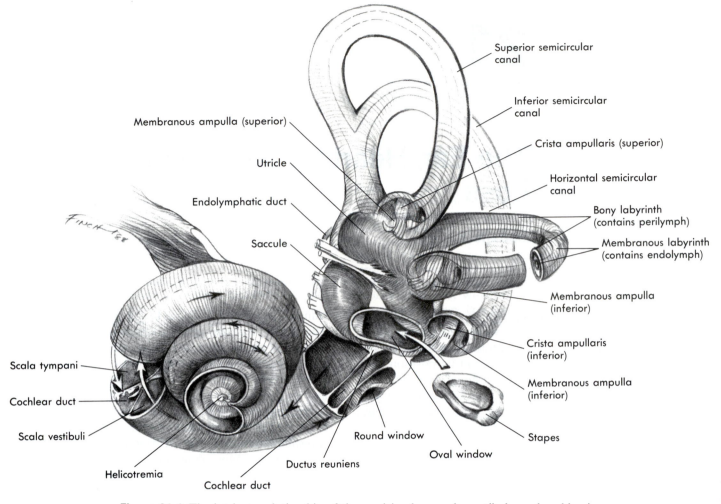

Superior semicircular canal

Inferior semicircular canal

Crista ampullaris (superior)

Horizontal semicircular canal

Bony labyrinth (contains perilymph)

Membranous labyrinth (contains endolymph)

Membranous ampulla (inferior)

Crista ampullaris (inferior)

Membranous ampulla (inferior)

Stapes

Oval window

Round window

Ductus reuniens

Cochlear duct

Helicotremia

Scala vestibuli

Cochlear duct

Scala tympani

Saccule

Endolymphatic duct

Utricle

Membranous ampulla (superior)

Figure 21-1 The intricate relationship of the semicircular canals, vestibule, and cochlea is depicted. The membranous labyrinth is separated from the bony labyrinth by perilymph and contains endolymph. The ampullae at the terminus of each semicircular canal open into the vestibule. A crista is contained within each ampulla. The superior portion of the vestibule is the utricle. The inferior portion is the saccule. The stapes footplate fits in the oval window. Direction of flow of perilymph is indicated by the arrows. (Courtesy Division of Pediatric Neurology, University of Minnesota Medical School.)

neonates but barely detected, if at all, in adults. Patency of the cochlear aqueduct in early life may be a factor responsible for the much higher prevalence in young children than in adults of profound bilateral deafness with vestibular impairment after bacterial meningitis. The pathology of postmeningitic hearing loss is a purulent endolabyrinthitis, which suggests continuity between the subarachnoid space and the perilymph. The endolymphatic duct leads from the utriculosaccular duct of the vestibule to the endolymphatic sac located within the dura on the posterior surface of the petrous bone, close to the internal acoustic meatus. Menière syndrome, which is uncommon but may occur in children, is characterized by episodes of vertigo and tinnitus, and a fluctuating, later progressive sensorineural hearing loss.

Its pathology is hydrops of the endolymphatic spaces, including the endolymphatic sac. One approach to its treatment is drainage of endolabyrinthic fluid by creation of a fistula in the endolabyrinthic sac or the scala vestibuli [Thomsen, 1988].

The first-order neurons of the auditory system reside in the spiral ganglion of Corti, located in the modiolus or axis of the cochlea. The first-order neurons of the vestibular system form Scarpa ganglion, which is located at the base of the internal auditory meatus. The meatus contains the cochlear and vestibular divisions of cranial nerve VIII, including the descending fibers of the inhibitory olivocochlear tract, as well as the facial nerve, chorda tympani, and internal auditory artery and vein.

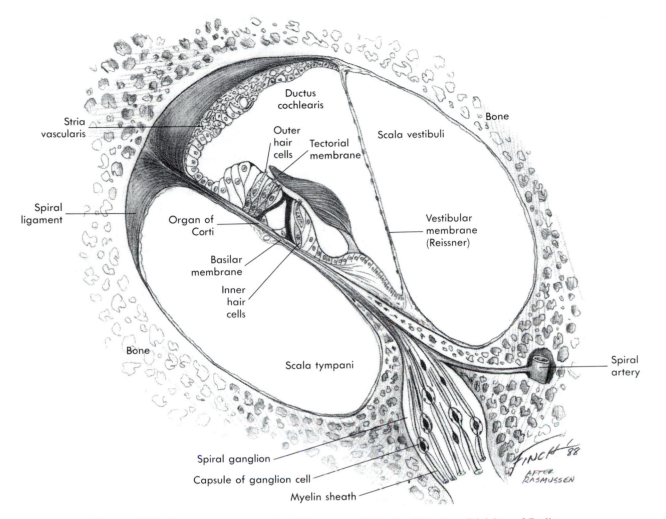

Figure 21-2 Structural components of the organ of Corti.   (Courtesy Division of Pediatric Neurology, University of Minnesota Medical School.)

The scala media contains the organ of Corti. In cross-section the scala media has the shape of a right-angle triangle whose apex is directed medially toward the modiolus and whose vertical side, the stria vascularis, is apposed to the osseous outer wall of the cochlea (Figure 21-2). The floor of the scala media is formed by the basilar membrane and osseous spiral lamina, which separate the scala media from the scala tympani. The roof of the scala media is formed by Reissner membrane, separating it from the scala vestibuli.

The scala media is filled with endolymph. The organ of Corti rests on the basilar membrane, a coiled, truncated triangular membrane whose stiffer, narrower end is located at the base of the cochlea and whose wider, more pliable end is located at the apex. The organ of Corti includes the auditory receptor cells, consisting of a single row of inner hair cells that are the main auditory receptors and three rows of outer hair cells that modulate acoustic reception. The hair cells are surrounded by specialized supporting cells, including the pillar cells that form the tunnel of Corti filled by the high-sodium cortilymph. Hair cells have many stereocilia on the upper surface; some of the longer cilia of the outer hair cells are embedded in the tectorial membrane, a gelatinous membrane attached to the medial limbus, as well as to supporting cells of the organ of Corti. There are about 3500 inner hair cells in each cochlea; each is innervated by about 20 spiral ganglion neurons, whereas each neuron innervates about 20 of the 25,000 outer hair cells [Allen, 1988]. The inhibitory efferent olivocochlear bundle innervates the outer hair cells directly, whereas it terminates indirectly on the dendrites of spiral ganglion cells that innervate the inner hair cells.

Axons of the spiral ganglion neurons project to the cochlear nuclei of the medulla. Axons from the base of the cochlea, which carry high-frequency sounds, project to the ventral cochlear nucleus and ventral portion of the

Averaging techniques enable the recording from the scalp of the negative compound action potential of the auditory nerve. It is called wave I of the brainstem auditory evoked response and occurs with a latency of some 1.5 msec at high intensity to 5.5 msec near threshold. The five waves of the brainstem auditory evoked response are attributed to activation of the auditory nerve, cochlear nucleus, superior olive, nucleus of the lateral lemniscus, and inferior colliculus or structures in their vicinity. Their latency ranges from 1.8 msec for wave I to 5.9 msec for wave V in adults in response to high-intensity clicks. Latency is longer at low-intensity levels and in infants [Picton et al., 1986; Stapells, 1989]. Wave V is the largest. Increased latency (>4 msec) between waves I and V suggests a pathologic process in the brainstem, whereas absence of wave I signifies peripheral hearing loss. Absence of wave I with persistence of the cochlear microphonic indicates that the hearing loss results from damage in the spiral ganglion or auditory nerve with preservation of the hair cells.

Physiologic activation of higher relays of the central auditory pathway also can be recorded. The somewhat inconstant waves VI and VII of the brainstem response are believed to reflect activity in the vicinity of the medial geniculate body and auditory radiations. So-called middle potentials [Mendel, 1985], which have a latency of about 15 to 80 msec, may correspond to the initial activation of the auditory cortex. Later obligatory potentials clearly originate in the primary and secondary auditory cortex; they are recorded with maximum amplitude at the vertex of the scalp because of the geometry of the auditory cortex, which lies horizontally in the sylvian fissure. Later waves, with a complex topography, correspond to later perceptual and discriminative auditory and language operations [Karrer et al., 1984; Steinschneider et al., 1992].

PATHOLOGY OF HEARING LOSS

Conductive hearing loss may result from atresia of the external canal, which usually is associated with gross malformation of the pinna; malformation, dislocation, or destruction of the ossicular chain; fluid or a mass in the tympanic cavity; fixation of the stapes footplate; tympanosclerosis (i.e., calcium deposits and stiffening of the tympanic membrane); destruction of the tympanic membrane; or a combination of these pathologic conditions. In children the most common of these conditions is middle ear effusion resulting from eustachian tube dysfunction. As stated earlier, complete destruction of the middle ear produces a hearing loss of at most 60 dB because the skull transmits sound above this level directly to the inner ear.

Sensorineural hearing loss usually results from hair cell loss, with or without associated damage to the cells of the spiral ganglion [Dublin, 1976; Michaels, 1988]. Infections, including bacterial meningitis, congenital rubella, trauma, and vascular disease, are unselective and regularly damage all elements of the cochlea and vestibule. Some viral infections are surprisingly selective, producing only a high-tone loss rather than total destruction of the cochlea [Nadol et al., 1989]. Genetic disease, toxins (e.g., ototoxic drugs) [Ryback and Matz, 1988; Shulman, 1979], and sound trauma [Alberti, 1979] may affect one cell type selectively. The cells of the organ of Corti and spiral ganglion are end-state cells that are incapable of cell division [Ruben, 1967], which explains the irreversibility of most sensorineural hearing losses. Loss of spiral ganglion cells leads to wallerian degeneration in the acoustic nerve and to transneuronal degeneration in the central auditory pathway [Ruben and Rapin, 1980]. True nerve deafness — that is, deafness resulting from selective damage to the axons of cranial nerve VIII — is rare except in the context of an acoustic neurinoma or of infiltration of the leptomeninges by an infectious or neoplastic process.

Some genetic deafness syndromes appear to be entirely selective for the cochlea, whereas others, such as Waardenburg syndrome [Hageman and Delleman, 1977], may affect the vestibule, the cochlea, both, or neither. Some syndromes, such as Usher syndrome, regularly affect both [Konigsmark and Gorlin, 1976]. It is crucial to diagnose Usher syndrome in childhood because it causes retinitis pigmentosa and, ultimately, blindness in adulthood [Karp and Santore, 1983]. Therefore all children with congenital deafness of unknown origin who have absent vestibular function must be referred to an ophthalmologist who is aware that the diagnosis of Usher syndrome is being considered. Electroretinography should be considered because this test is more sensitive than ophthalmoscopy in the early stages of retinitis pigmentosa.

Because of inaccessibility of the middle and inner ears, remarkably little is known about the cellular pathology of deafness, compared with what is known about pathologic processes in all other organ systems. Examination of the ear requires sawing into the petrous bone, lengthy decalcification of the specimen, and serial sectioning. Because of the long interval between diagnosis of hearing loss and the patient's death, physicians are unlikely to remember that the patient was hearing impaired; thus the ear is rarely removed at autopsy. There are few laboratories equipped to study the ear. Temporal bone banks have been established in some teaching institutions and at the Armed Forces Institute of Pathology. These laboratories often are willing to study specimens, provided they are accompanied by adequate information regarding the patient's hearing and clinical status. The pathology and biology of hearing loss are areas that require further study.

EVALUATION OF THE PATIENT

Tests of hearing

There are two broad categories of hearing tests: those that assess a patient's subjective hearing experience and those that measure the activation of the auditory system. The former require the subject to provide a behavioral response, which can be verbal or nonverbal, to indicate that an auditory stimulus was perceived. Averaged auditory evoked responses provide a physiologic measure of auditory sensitivity, whereas tympanometry assesses the mechanical properties of the middle ear. There are clear and important distinctions between screening and quantitative tests of hearing. In an office setting the clinician can only screen for hearing loss and perform tympanometry [Feldman and Wilber, 1976]. At best, screening tests are confirmatory of normal function in children in whom there is no suspicion of auditory impairment or a flag signaling the need for referral for quantitative testing. Quantitative audiometry requires a soundproof room and an audiologist skilled in working with young children [Northern and Downs, 1978; Jerger, 1984; Katz, 1985; Gravel, 1989].

Failure to detect a hearing loss in infancy has such detrimental consequences for the child that clinicians must proceed immediately to a definitive hearing test whenever a parent or other caretaker suspects hearing loss, whenever the response to auditory screening is dubious, whenever language is delayed, and whenever the results place the infant on the high-risk registry for deafness (see box below) [Joint Committee, 1982; Gottlieb and Krasnegor, 1985]. Definitive tests are noninvasive and widely available, and the cost is rela-

tively modest, considering the consequences of overlooking childhood hearing impairment.

Behavioral hearing tests

Screening tests. Perhaps the most convincing auditory screen is to speak softly to the child and observe whether the response is appropriate. There are many pitfalls in this approach, such as giving the child nonverbal tactile and/or visual cues, speaking more loudly than intended, or interpreting lack of response as unwillingness to cooperate rather than as lack of comprehension. Producing a loud sound out of an infant's or toddler's field of vision is often done; this technique is not recommended because hand claps and dropped metal basins are likely to provide somatosensory cues, as well as auditory cues, that may falsely reassure both physician and parents that the child hears. Crumpling paper or ringing a small bell out of the child's sight and observing whether the child turns the head and eyes promptly in the direction of the sound is more appropriate, keeping in mind that a reliable head turn in the horizontal plane may not occur before 6 months of age and in the vertical plane until almost 1 year of age. There also are screening instruments available, such as a 3000-Hz warbler of variable and calibrated intensity. As with all biologic measurements, a single observation does not suffice; a reproducible one is required, with the caveat that habituation occurs after a few presentations, as soon as the stimulus has lost its novelty and alerting properties.

It is dangerous to rely on such responses as eye widening and cessation of activity because they are subject to observer bias. Lack of behavioral response to sound does not necessarily indicate a peripheral hearing loss in autistic and severely retarded children, but the presence of another handicap must raise, rather than lower, suspicion and mandates definitive testing that includes a physiologic test.

None of these tests is more than a screening method. Any doubt by the child's parent, caretaker, or physician concerning the child's responsiveness to sound or speech development is sufficient to mandate referral for a definitive, quantitative test of hearing without wasting time on repeated and unreliable behavioral tests. This statement also is true of any child who has a hearing-impaired member in the immediate family; who has a malformation of the external ear, face, or palate; who has Down syndrome or another syndromic condition known to be associated with hearing loss; or who manifests any other condition on the High-Risk Registry for Deafness Joint Committee, 1982 (see box at the left), such as prematurity, neonatal jaundice, exchange transfusion, or meningitis. Formal hearing testing is mandatory in all children with delayed acquisition of language, regardless of any other probable cause, such as mental deficiency or autism, because a child can be mentally deficient or autistic and also hearing impaired [Jure et al., 1991].

High-Risk Registry for Deafness

1. Parental suspicion that the child does not hear
2. Family history positive for childhood deafness
3. Congenital perinatal infection (e.g., toxoplasmosis, rubella, cytomegalovirus)
4. Malformation of the pinna, face, palate (cleft or submucous cleft, bifid uvula), Down syndrome, other syndromic or nonsyndromic dysmorphology
5. Low birth weight (<1500 g)
6. Hyperbilirubinemia at a level indicating need for an exchange transfusion
7. Bacterial meningitis
8. Severe neonatal asphyxia with Apgar scores of 0 to 3; need for a ventilator
9. Use of ototoxic drugs

Adapted from Joint Committee on Infant Hearing: Position statement 1982. Pediatrics 1982; 70:496.

22

Vertigo

Lydia Eviatar

Vertigo and dizziness are often used interchangeably in the medical literature, although each word indicates a different set of symptoms. In 1901, Gowers introduced the classic definition of vertigo that is commonly accepted today. He defined vertigo as "any movement or sense of movement, either in the individual himself or in external objects, that involves a defect, real or seeming, in the equilibrium of the body." This definition is broader and less restrictive than the etymologic one that implies only a whirling or turning motion, and as such, covers the broader range of equilibrium disturbances. The maintenance of equilibrium depends on proper sensory afferent input from the vestibular, visual, and proprioceptive systems that provide the information necessary to initiate appropriate postural reactions in response to changes in the center of gravity, controlled by the pyramidal, extrapyramidal, and cerebellar systems.

ANATOMY AND PHYSIOLOGY OF THE VESTIBULAR SYSTEM

The vestibular organ, specifically the membranous labyrinth, is fully developed in a 30-mm embryo [Dekaban, 1970]. Oculovestibular reflexes are first detected around the twelfth week of gestation and fully established by the twenty-fourth week [Gesell and Amatruda, 1945]. The vestibular nerve appears to be fully myelinated by the sixteenth week of gestation, and the vestibular receptors of the inner ear are fully activated by the thirty-second week. A Moro reflex can thus be elicited by 32 weeks' gestation and, at times, even earlier [Hamilton and Mossman, 1972]. The paired organs of equilibrium—the labyrinths—consist of three semicircular canals, the utricle, and saccule. The labyrinths monitor any changes of position of the head and body in space. The cristae in the ampules of the semicircular canals are primarily stimulated by angular acceleration of the head and body, whereas the macules of the utricle and saccule act as transducers that collect information from gravitational forces and from vertical acceleration. The information that is received simultaneously by both labyrinths is conveyed via the vestibular nerve to the vestibular nuclei, impulses ascend in the medial longitudinal fasciculus to cranial nerves III, IV, and VI and contribute to the oculovestibular responses. In addition, impulses from the vestibular nuclei descend in the medial and lateral vestibulospinal tracts and provide excitatory stimuli to the extensor muscles of the head, trunk, and extremities that counteract gravity and maintain the upright posture. The cerebellum receives afferent impulses from the vestibular nuclei and serves as a major center for integration of oculovestibular and postural responses. Efferent impulses from the flocculonodular lobe of the cerebellum are transmitted directly to the peripheral vestibular organ and to the vestibular nuclei and modulate their responses. Widespread diffuse connections throughout the brain are known to exist and modulate vestibular responses. The connections extend to the reticular activating system of the midbrain, thalamus, and subthalamic nuclei. The cortical representation is at the level of the posterior temporal gyrus adjacent and posterior to the Heschl gyrus. Penfield's experiments documented that direct stimulation of this cortical area produces a definite vertiginous sensation [Carpenter, 1974].

The oculovestibular reflex (which permits ocular fixation on stationary objects while the head and body are in motion) and the intensity of nystagmus induced in response to perrotatory and caloric stimulation of the labyrinths can be used as parameters of vestibular function. During clockwise rotation, performed with the head inclined 30 degrees forward for maximum stimulation of the horizontal canal, the endolymphatic fluid in the semicircular canal and the cupula of the horizontal canal shift in the counterclockwise direction. As a result, labyrinthine impulses reach the homolateral abducens and the contralateral oculomotor nuclei and induce a slow eye deviation in the direction of flow of the endolymphatic fluid, namely counterclockwise in this instance. Once maximal eye deviation is achieved, a quick conjugate ocular realignment back to the midposition takes place. This slow deviation of the eyes in the direction of motion of the endolymphatic current, followed by a brisk realignment, is termed *nystagmus*. By definition the direction of nystagmus is designated in accordance with the direction of the fast component. However, it is the slow component of nystagmus that represents the oculo- vestibular response, and calculating the velocity of the slow component gives an estimate of the response to vestibular stimulation. The fast component of nystagmus or ocular realignment is controlled by paramedian pontine centers. In the early stages of rotation and during acceleration the nystagmus and sensation of motion are in the direction of rotation, whereas during deceleration it is opposite the direction of rotation.

Another specific neurophysiologic response used during vestibular testing is the ability to induce endolymphatic flow by caloric stimulation of the ear canal. Irrigation of the external auditory canal with water or air that is cooler or warmer than body temperature transfers a temperature gradient from the external auditory canal to the internal ear by convection. The horizontal semicircular canal develops the largest temperature gradient because it is closest to the source of temperature change. This response is best achieved with the patient in the supine position, head tilted 30 degrees up,

thus placing the horizontal canals in the vertical plane. The endolymph circulates because of the difference in specific gravity on the two sides of the canal when the semicircular canal being investigated is either in or near the vertical plane. When a warm caloric stimulus (44° C) is applied, the column of endolymph nearest the middle ear rises because of its decreased density. As a result the cupula deviates toward the utricle (ampullopetal flow) and produces horizontal nystagmus, with the fast component directed toward the stimulated ear. A cold stimulus (33° C) produces the opposite effect on the endolymphatic column, causing ampullofugal endolymphatic flow and a nystagmus directed away from the stimulated ear. A useful mnemonic for this is COWS: Cold-Opposite, Warm-Same. This specific response to caloric stimulation is the most widely used clinical test of vestibular function, testing each labyrinth separately.

THE NEUROVESTIBULAR EXAMINATION

The neurovestibular examination consists of three parts:
1. History; detailed prenatal and perinatal history and a detailed description of the presenting complaint.
2. General neurologic examination with special emphasis on cranial nerves, proprioception, pyramidal tract function, and cerebellar function.
3. Specific neurovestibular testing adapted to the patient's age, emphasizing:
   a) Postural reactions
   b) Electronystagmography

History

The examiner should inquire about the presence of perinatal asphyxia, hyperbilirubinemia, prenatal or perinatal exposure to infections, such as *tox*oplasmosis, *r*ubella, *c*ytomegalovirus, *h*erpes (TORCH), bacterial meningitis or viral meningitis, acquired immune deficiency syndrome (AIDS) or AIDS-related complex. In addition, exposure to ototoxic drugs, for example, aminoglycosides, ethacrynic acid, furosemide (Lasix), isoniazid, quinine, or acetylsalicylic acid in large amounts, should be determined.

Symptomatology

Vertigo, described as a hallucination of motion of the individual or the environment, is the most common manifestation of vestibular dysfunction. Conversely, dizziness is a nonspecific symptom that suggests cardiovascular dysfunction, hyperventilation, or psychoneurosis. Vertigo may begin acutely as a sudden impairment of equilibrium, most frequently accompanied by autonomic symptoms, such as nausea, vomiting, and diaphoresis. Nystagmus is often present. This symptomatology is suggestive of a peripheral vestibular dysfunction (see box on the left). The presence of hearing loss, tinnitus, or a

---

Symptoms and Signs of Peripheral Vestibular Disease

Sudden onset of vertigo, no loss of consciousness
Disequilibrium, swaying, and falling toward affected side
Nausea, vomiting, autonomic dysfunction
Nystagmus ±
  Toward unaffected side
  Induced by changing head position (Bruins sign)
  Maximal with affected ear down
  Latency of onset—3 to 10 seconds
  Duration ≤60 seconds
  Fatigue with repeated positioning
  Inhibited by visual fixation
Preferred supine position—affected ear up
Sensation of tilt or body motion
Head tilt
Paroxysmal torticollis or tortipelvis in infants

±, present or absent.

sensation of fullness in the ear further localizes the condition to the inner ear because the cochlea and labyrinth are in close proximity and may both be affected by the same inflammatory, metabolic, toxic, or vascular process.

Chronic, unremitting vertigo is more likely to occur in the presence of central vestibular dysfunction.

Neurologic examination

Examination of cranial nerves, visual fields, and the observation of spontaneous or induced nystagmus are very important. Hearing responses can be tested with tuning forks, and the Weber and Rinne tests are helpful in differentiating between conductive and sensorineural hearing loss. Deep tendon reflexes, postural reflexes, and equilibrium reactions are assessed because postural instability may result from the inability of the body to respond to afferent vestibular input with appropriate postural reactions, thus causing dysequilibrium and falling. Cerebellar testing is most important because the cerebellum participates in the modulation and integration of vestibular responses.

Tests of nystagmus

Physiologic nystagmus (end-point nystagmus) is observed in normal individuals, primarily at a 40-degree lateral deviation of the eyes. Pathologic nystagmus implies an underlying abnormality of peripheral or central oculovestibular controls. It is well documented that visual fixation may inhibit mild vestibular nystagmus, and using Frenzel glasses (+10 diopters) or recording the nystagmus in the dark with electronystagmography is helpful to prevent this inhibitory effect. Nystagmus of central origin is often found in conjunction with other brainstem signs and is not effectively inhibited by fixation. Positional nystagmus frequently occurs after traumatic lesions of the labyrinth, lesion of the otoliths, or when the specific gravity of the cupula is changed by structural or metabolic factors (alcohol or drug intoxication).

The Hallpike-Dix positioning maneuver can be used during the neurologic examination to elicit paroxysmal positional nystagmus. The test is performed with the patient sitting on the examining table and then rapidly moved from a sitting to a head-hanging position, with the head extended 45 degrees below horizontal. The patient is then returned to the sitting position for a few minutes until the sensation of vertigo subsides. The head is then turned 45 degrees laterally, and the patient is moved to the supine position, with the head below the horizontal position. This is performed both with the head once to the right and once to the left, to induce paroxysmal positional nystagmus, vertigo, or both. Frenzel glasses can be used and allow better observation of the nystagmus. The most common variety of paroxysmal positional nystagmus is benign paroxysmal positional

nystagmus of Dix and Hallpike and often results as a sequela of acute labyrinthitis, stapedectomy, perilymphatic fistula, or traumatic labyrinthine injury that has displaced one of the otoliths. It usually has a 3- to 10-second latency before onset and generally lasts less than 60 seconds. The paroxysmal positional nystagmus is most prominent in one head-hanging position and has a rotatory component directed toward the unaffected ear; it subsides with subsequent maneuvers. The initially severe vertigo subsides and becomes less intense with repeated positioning. When, in addition to paroxysmal positional nystagmus, unilateral labyrinthine hypoexcitability is observed, the most likely diagnosis is vestibular end-organ disease, such as seen after head injury, viral labyrinthitis, or occlusion of the vasculature to the inner ear. Positional nystagmus that is associated with brainstem or cerebeller disease is a nonfatiguing nystagmus that does not decrease in amplitude or duration with repeated positioning of the head. Usually no obvious latency occurs before its appearance, and it frequently lasts longer than 60 seconds, sometimes for as long as the head position is maintained [Baloh and Honrubia, 1979] (see box below).

Clinical Testing

Hallpike Barany: Positioning Maneuver

Nystagmus and vertigo with affected ear down
Nystagmus latency around 10 seconds duration
  ≤ 60 seconds
Nystagmus fatigues with repeated procedures

Stepping Test

45-degree deviation toward affected side
50 cm forward displacement in peripheral disease

Part Pointing

Toward affected side

Extended Romberg

Fall toward affected side

Tandem Gait (Blindfolded)

Sway toward affected side

Sharp Turns

Fall toward affected side

Righting Responses (6 to 24 months)/Equilibrium Reaction (>24 months)

Doll's-eye responses
Vertical acceleration   } Infants
Faulty toward affected side

Central Vestibular Dysfunction

Clinical Symptoms

Unremitting dizziness or vertigo
Nystagmus ±
  Not inhibited by fixation
  No change with head position
  No latency and no fatiguing
Cranial nerve deficits likely (nerves V, VI, VII, and
  cochlear nerve)
Cerebellar and pyramidal signs frequent

Clinical Testing

Hallpike-Dix maneuver
Nystagmus in all positions
No change in intensity or direction
All clinical tests may be positive with eyes opened or
  closed

Specific neurovestibular testing: postural and equilibrium reactions (see box above)

In infants the most primitive form of labyrinthine reactions, namely tonic neck reflexes, is observed. These reflexes depend on input from the labyrinth, proprioceptive input from the cervical vertebrae, and appropriate tonic reaction of the extremities that depend on the integrity of the pyramidal tract system. A more specific vestibular test described by Eviatar and Eviatar [1978] is called the *vertical acceleration test*. The infant is held in the supine position at arm's length with the head properly aligned with the body. Vertical acceleration is provided while the examiner abruptly descends to a semicrouched position. The normal response in all infants is abduction and extension of the upper extremities followed by an embrace. This maneuver tests the utricular response to gravitational and vertical acceleration.

The doll's-eye response checks responses to angular acceleration. The infant is maintained at arm's length with the head flexed at 30 degrees and rotated around the examiner for 360 degrees several times. In newborns the eyes deviate in the opposite direction of rotation. By 2 to 3 weeks of age, nystagmus is superimposed in the direction of rotation.

By 6 months of age, righting responses appear and persist throughout life, although modified or inhibited voluntarily after the age of 2 years. A righting response is the ability of the child to right the head (align the horizontal semicircular canals parallel to the ground) and extend the upper extremities in a propping reaction in the direction of tilt. Because optical and vestibular righting reactions are identical, labyrinthine tests should be performed with the infant blindfolded to eliminate

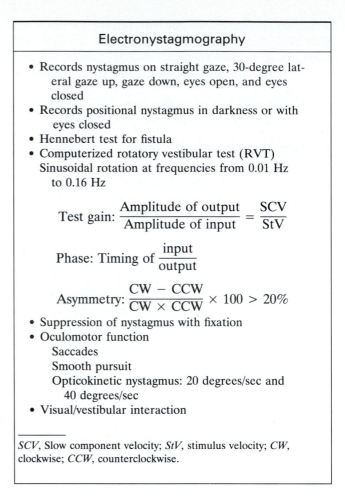

Electronystagmography

- Records nystagmus on straight gaze, 30-degree lateral gaze up, gaze down, eyes open, and eyes closed
- Records positional nystagmus in darkness or with eyes closed
- Hennebert test for fistula
- Computerized rotatory vestibular test (RVT)
  Sinusoidal rotation at frequencies from 0.01 Hz to 0.16 Hz

$$\text{Test gain:} \frac{\text{Amplitude of output}}{\text{Amplitude of input}} = \frac{\text{SCV}}{\text{StV}}$$

$$\text{Phase: Timing of } \frac{\text{input}}{\text{output}}$$

$$\text{Asymmetry: } \frac{\text{CW} - \text{CCW}}{\text{CW} \times \text{CCW}} \times 100 > 20\%$$

- Suppression of nystagmus with fixation
- Oculomotor function
  Saccades
  Smooth pursuit
  Opticokinetic nystagmus: 20 degrees/sec and 40 degrees/sec
- Visual/vestibular interaction

SCV, Slow component velocity; *StV*, stimulus velocity; *CW*, clockwise; *CCW*, counterclockwise.

---

the optical righting responses. By the age of 4 years, equilibrium reactions can be tested with the help of a tilting board in the prone, supine, sitting, or kneeling position. After an acute labyrinthine injury the child will be unable to right his or her head or prop the upper extremities in the direction of tilt. Moreover, the patient is likely to fall in the direction of tilt. In time, compensatory mechanisms develop and help substitute for the loss of labyrinthine function. Visual and proprioceptive cues are essential in this condition.

After the age of 4 years, additional tests, such as tandem gait blindfolded, Romberg, and tandem Romberg, can be performed with a cooperative child. In the presence of unilateral labyrinthine involvement the patient sways toward the side of the lesion while walking with closed eyes and falls toward it during the Romberg test. During tandem Romberg testing the patient is asked to stand in a tandem position with one foot in front of the other, the arms folded, and eyes closed. Normal children are able to maintain this position for about 30 seconds. However, in the presence of a unilateral labyrinthine disease the patient falls toward the affected side.

Computerized Rotary Vestibular Test

Unilateral Peripheral Lesions

Acute

Asymmetric response to rotational stimuli because:
1. Direct current bias resulting from spontaneous nystagmus
2. Difference in response to clockwise and counter-clockwise stimulation of the intact labyrinth

Chronic

Direction changing bias gradually disappears
1. Gain asymmetry between clockwise and counter-clockwise decreases; remains most pronounced at high frequencies: 0.16 Hz and 0.32 Hz
2. Decreased gain and increased phase lead at low frequencies of sinusoidal stimulation: 0.01 and 0.02 Hz

Bilateral Peripheral Lesions

1. Decreased but recordable responses to high-frequency stimulation
2. Decreased gain and increased phase lead at low frequencies
3. Early damage detected at low frequencies less than 0.05 Hz

---

Bithermal Caloric Testing

Labyrinthine Preponderance

$$\frac{(RW + RC) - (LW + LC)}{RW + RC + LW + RC} \times 100 > 14\%$$

Directional Preponderance

$$\frac{(RW + LC) - (LW + RC)}{RW + LC + LW + RC} \times 100 > 18\%$$

- Ice-cold calorics: prone, supine, prone
  Infants to 36 months
  Non-responsive labyrinth
- Binaural or bithermal

RC, Right cold; *RW*, Right warm; *LC*, Left cold; *LW*, left warm.

The stepping test is a modification of Fukuda's original stepping test. The child is asked to take 60 steps with eyes closed at the 90-degree intersection of two straight lines. The examiner reports the angle of lateral displacement, as well as the extent of forward or backward displacement. The test is performed with arms extended parallel to the ground and eyes closed. There is a general tendency to rotate at an angle greater than 45 degrees toward the affected side in a unilateral lesion. In bilateral lesions, forward displacement or backward displacement that is generally greater than 20 inches from the starting position may occur.

Past pointing. The patient is asked to sit in front of the examiner with eyes closed to eliminate visual cues. The arms are extended forward while the patient places an extended index finger on that of the examiner, closes the eyes, raises the extended arm and index finger to a vertical position, and attempts to return the index finger to the examiner's. A consistent deviation to one side is called *past pointing* and suggests vestibular dysfunction on the ipsilateral side.

Electronystagmography (see boxes on pp. 300-301). Electronystagmography permits the recording of eye movements during positional testing, visual pursuit, and in response to vestibular stimulation by rotation or caloric irrigation. Each eyeball acts as an electric dipole oriented in the direction of the long axis of the eyes, with the cornea being electropositive and the retina electronegative. The changes in the magnetic field created around the orbit during ocular displacement can be recorded by placing two electrodes bitemporally and a reference ground electrode on the nasion (binocular recording). The difference in potential between the electrodes is amplified and used to control the displacement of a pen recorder that provides a permanent record of eye movements. The advantage of this technique is the availability of a permanent recording for measurement of eye movements that can be used as future reference. The recommended test battery is described in the box on p. 300. Electronystagmography detects abnormalities of oculovestibular control during visual pursuit, abnormalities of opticokinetic nystagmus, and abnormal saccades in which the motion of the target and resulting eye movement can be simultaneously displayed. The perrotatory nystagmus at frequencies of chair rotation ranging from 0.01 to 0.32 Hz can also be recorded simultaneously with the recording of the chair motion. The maximum slow component velocity of nystagmus elicited by sinusoidal stimulation increases linearly with the log of stimulus intensity. Unfortunately there is a variability in the oculovestibular reflex function measured in normal subjects that depends on stress, fatigue, level of mental alertness, and habituation. The intrasubject variability is much less than intersubject variability. To compare the response to clockwise (CW) versus counterclockwise (CCW) stimulation, the following formula is used: (CW − CCW)/CW + CCW × 100. The mean value for the normalized difference between clockwise and counterclockwise responses is approximately 0 at each stimulus. A difference greater than 20% indicates a directional preponderance of nystagmus, the significance of which is similar to the directional preponderance in bithermal caloric testing. In addition the "gain," which is the ratio of the total amplitude of the eye movement excursion to the total chair rotation excursion, can be measured. It does not take into account timing of their movements. Gain can also be defined as the peak slow-phase eye velocity divided by the peak stimulus velocity. Phase describes the temporal (timing) relationship between the input and output. If there is proper timing of compensatory eye movements to the chair rotation in a sinusoidal rotation test, the eye movement will be 180 degrees out of phase with head movement or by convention will be said to have zero phase level.

Perrotatory stimulation and ice-cold caloric (see boxes on p. 301) stimulation are performed on patients younger than 3 years of age to determine the presence of peripheral versus central vestibular dysfunction. The perrotatory test induces bilateral labyrinthine stimulation, whereas the ice-cold caloric test stimulates each labyrinth individually. Normative data for torsion swing and ice-cold caloric stimulation are available for all age groups [Eviatar and Eviatar, 1979]. Normative data for the computerized rotary chair–induced nystagmus in children are available from Staller et al. [1986] and Cyr et al. [1985].

After 36 months of age, bithermal caloric irrigation can be performed instead of ice-cold caloric stimulation (see box on p. 301). Directional preponderance on bithermal caloric irrigation usually suggests a central vestibular dysfunction. Labyrinthine preponderance is indicative of a peripheral labyrinthine disorder or a hypoactive labyrinth.

Neurotologic examination. A neurotologic examination is important in the evaluation of the child with vertigo, and it is usually best performed by the otologist. However, neurologists and pediatricians can learn to use a pneumatic otoscope. In addition to visualizing the eardrums and determining that no infection or cholesteatoma is present, it is important to test for a fistula sign or Hennebert sign by inducing negative pressure in the ear with the help of the pneumatic otoscope. The positive sign consists of an ocular deviation toward or away from the affected ear followed by a few beats of nystagmus. The patient usually experiences severe vertigo when the test is positive. A positive Hennebert sign may occur with a perforated tympanic membrane or an erosion of the bony labyrinth secondary to chronic infection, trauma, or surgery. In the presence of an intact tympanic membrane, conditions such as congenital syphilis, Meniere syndrome, and perilymphatic fistula should be considered.

DIFFERENTIAL DIAGNOSIS AND MANAGEMENT

Guided by a detailed account of the history and symptomatology, as well as the results of the neurovestibular examination, the physician can consider the differential diagnosis in a rational manner. The diagnostic algorithm (Fig. 22-1) and the flow sheet presented in the box on p. 304 should help to single out the most common disease accounting for the specific symptomatology [Baloh and Honrubia, 1979].

Acute paroxysmal vertigo with hearing loss

Labyrinthitis. A history of infection before the onset of vertigo and the presence of hearing impairment suggest the diagnosis of labyrinthitis. The autonomic symptoms in this condition are marked, as are the instability of gait and the personal discomfort. A spontaneous nystagmus with the fast component directed toward the normal ear is often found on examination. The patient's most comfortable position is lying on the unaffected side; any attempt to move causes severe vertigo, nausea, and vomiting. After a few days the episodes generally subside. Recurrences are possible and can result from recurrent infections or an underlying anomalous labyrinth.

Electronystagmography performed shortly after the acute episode generally demonstrates a poorly reactive labyrinth and the presence of positional nystagmus. Although the hypoactivity of the labyrinth may subside, the positional nystagmus is likely to remain for a long time.

Treatment of this condition is primarily directed toward control of the underlying disease, namely, antibiotics in bacterial infections and symptomatic treatment of vertigo in viral or toxic conditions. Dimenhydrinate administered intramuscularly is likely to alleviate the symptoms during the acute stage; the use of diazepam is also helpful. When vomiting is a prominent symptom, administration of meclizine and/or Compazine alleviate the symptoms.

Meniere syndrome. Meniere syndrome is not very common in children and consists of the famous tetrad of vertigo, fluctuating hearing loss, pressure in the ear, and tinnitus. Meniere syndrome is usually the result of a cochlear hydrops that can be of toxic, allergic, or metabolic origin. Recurrent episodes are common, with progressive hearing loss found after each one. The treatment is similar to that described for labyrinthitis.

Perilymphatic fistula. Head trauma or abrupt change in barometric pressure (decompression syndrome) can cause the sudden onset of hearing loss and vertigo resulting from a ruptured round or oval window into the vestibule, creating a perilymphatic fistula. In children the condition is far more frequent than initially suspected and is often caused by minor trauma that may be forgotten by both parents and patients. A positive fistula sign is diagnostic, and a high index of suspicion should be maintained. Such patients should be referred immediately to neurotologists because surgery may restore some hearing and cause cessation of vertigo (Supance and Bluestone, 1983).

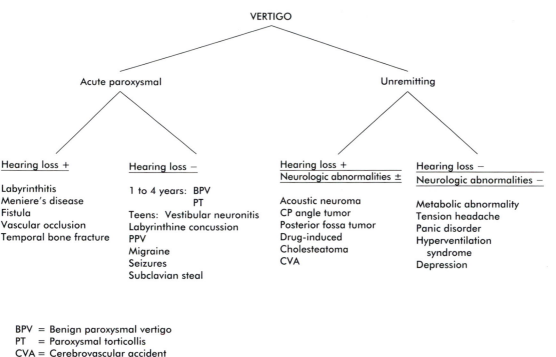

VERTIGO

Acute paroxysmal | Unremitting

Hearing loss +

Labyrinthitis
Meniere's disease
Fistula
Vascular occlusion
Temporal bone fracture

Hearing loss −

1 to 4 years: BPV
                PT
Teens: Vestibular neuronitis
Labyrinthine concussion
PPV
Migraine
Seizures
Subclavian steal

Hearing loss +
Neurologic abnormalities ±

Acoustic neuroma
CP angle tumor
Posterior fossa tumor
Drug-induced
Cholesteatoma
CVA

Hearing loss −
Neurologic abnormalities −

Metabolic abnormality
Tension headache
Panic disorder
Hyperventilation
   syndrome
Depression

BPV = Benign paroxysmal vertigo
PT = Paroxysmal torticollis
CVA = Cerebrovascular accident
PPV = Paroxysmal positional vertigo
+   = Present
−   = Absent
±   = Present or absent

Figure 22-1 Diagnosis of vertigo (flow diagram).

Paroxysmal vertigo without hearing loss

Vestibular neuronitis primarily occurs in adolescents after a history of respiratory infection. Onset is acute with vertigo, nausea, vomiting, and postural instability being the hallmark of the disease. There is no hearing loss in this condition, and the episodes are self-limited but tend to recur periodically with lesser intensity with each recurrence. The neurologic, neurotologic and hearing evaluations are normal between attacks; the only positive findings may be electronystagmography that demonstrates positional nystagmus, a hypoactive labyrinth on bithermal caloric stimulation, and an asymmetric response to sinusoidal rotation. Use of dimenhydrinate, meclizine, and antihistamines may be helpful [Lindsay 1967; Eviatar and Eviatar, 1977].

Benign paroxysmal vertigo. First described by Basser (1969) and subsequently by Koenigsberger et al. (1970), this benign condition of early childhood first appears at about 16 months to 2 years of age and occurs at intervals of weeks or months, subsiding spontaneously by the age of 4 to 4½ years. There is no hearing impairment, and the neurologic examination between episodes is normal. During an episode the child is extremely unsteady and sometimes unable to maintain the upright position. There is often arrest of motor activity and search for immediate support by crouching,

kneeling, or holding onto the parent; nystagmus is frequently present during the attacks. However, vomiting and diaphoresis are uncommon. Although fearful and anxious during the episode, the child remains mentally lucid and fully cognitive of the environment, which helps differentiate this condition from partial complex seizures of childhood. An EEG is essential because it eliminates the possibility of a seizure disorder (partial complex seizures), and electronystagmography is sometimes helpful because it may reveal the presence of a hypoactive labyrinth. Long-term follow-up of patients with benign paroxysmal vertigo indicates that migraines develop later in life in a significant proportion of these children. A strong family history of migraine should alert the physician to a possible vascular cause for this condition [Holguin and Fenichel, 1967].

Paroxysmal torticollis, retrocollis, and tortipelvis. There are clearly several etiologies conducive to paroxysmal torticollis in infants and children. Before 1 year of age the condition is often accompanied by vomiting and gastroesophageal reflux and is known as the *Sandifer syndrome.* Vestibular studies performed in our laboratory on 20 infants with paroxysmal torticollis disclosed a vestibular imbalance in the majority of children. Gastroesophageal reflux was also documented in many of these infants. Snyder [1969] described 12 infants with

Diagnostic Workup	
All patients	Neurologic examination
	Neurotologic examination to rule out infection, malformation, cholesteatoma, fistula
	Hearing test
	Brainstem auditory evoked response in infants
	Electronystagmography
Vertigo plus loss of consciousness	Electroencephalogram
Nonspecific or unremitting vertigo	Metabolic workup: CBC with sickle cell preparation, glucose tolerance test, electrolytes, Ca, P, Mg, T_3, T_4, TSH
Vertigo plus sensorineural hearing loss, ± neurologic findings	CT scan of brain with thin cuts through temporal bones.
	MRI plus gadolinium when tumor is suspected; magnetic resonance angiography when vascular malformation is suspected.

+ present, − absent, ±, present or absent.

the reticular activating system of the brainstem and become secondarily generalized through the thalamo-cortical pathways. Cantor [1971] was the first to describe vestibulogenic seizures in a patient with missile wounds affecting the temporal bone. Testing by simultaneous caloric irrigation of the ear canals and EEG recording from the temporoparietal cortex elicits paroxysmal discharges during ice-cold caloric stimulation.

Both vertiginous and vestibulogenic seizures respond to antiepileptic medication, such as phenytoin, carbamazepine, or primidone.

Unremitting vertigo or dizziness with neurologic signs

Complaints of unremitting, protracted vertigo or dizziness accompanied by cranial nerve deficits, pyramidal tract signs, or cerebellar abnormalities are suggestive of space-occupying lesions at the level of the cerebellopontine angle or in the posterior fossa. Cranial CT with contrast is likely to detect the presence of a structural abnormality within the cerebellum, brainstem, or cerebellopontine angle. In the latter, however, if the lesion is intracanalicular, there is advantage in performing cranial MRI with special cuts through the temporal bone. MRI is particularly helpful in detecting in a patient with a demyelinating disease with vertigo. Additional laboratory tests that help in the diagnosis of demyelinating diseases, such as multiple sclerosis or CNS lyme disease, are lumbar puncture demonstrating elevation of the protein immunoglobulin fraction and oligoclonal bands or the detection of a high lyme virus titer in CNS lyme disease. Abnormal visual-evoked responses and brainstem auditory evoked responses are often present in multiple sclerosis. The recording of abnormal calorics on electronystagmography in multiple sclerosis is suggestive of a demyelinating vestibulopathy.

Unremitting vertigo accompanied by progressive intellectual deterioration and neurologic findings is suggestive of a degenerative brain disease. A combination of peripheral neuropathies, angiokeratoma corposis diffusion, ataxia, and retinitis pigmentosa is characteristic of Refsum disease and can be diagnosed by an increased level of phytanic acid in the blood. Dizziness related to vestibular dysfunction is often present in Friedreich ataxia. Abnormalities of visual pursuit, abnormal saccades, and poor visual inhibition of perrotatory nystagmus are also recorded.

Unremitting vertigo without neurologic abnormalities

Metabolic disorders, such as diabetes or latent diabetes, endocrine abnormalities, blood dyscrasias, and dysgammaglobulinemias, as well as sickle cell disease, may cause dizziness and at times, vertigo. Labile hypertension and cardiovascular conditions causing intermittent vertebrobasilar insufficiency may also contribute to dizziness or vertigo. The subclavian steal syndrome should also be excluded. Ototoxic drugs, particularly aminoglycosides, phenytoin quinine, and ethacrynic acid, may cause a progressive peripheral vestibular neuropathy that also accounts for unremitting dizziness and, rarely, true vertigo. Hearing loss is often present after ingestion of these drugs. The absence of metabolic disorders, the lack of hematologic or cardiovascular abnormalities, and normal laboratory test results suggest the diagnosis of a psychosomatic disorder. Indeed, the complaint of nonspecific dizziness is frequently the first symptom of a depressive reaction in adolescence, of an anxiety syndrome, or of panic attacks. The patient who continues to complain despite a normal neurologic examination and negative laboratory test results often benefits from psychologic counseling or antidepressive medication.

SUMMARY

The differential diagnosis of vertigo in children and adolescents is complex and requires a systematic review of systems and careful evaluation of the patient's complaint. Because of the many possible causes, assessment of the patient's complaint, age, and clinical and laboratory findings may allow the clinician to reach an accurate diagnosis (see box on p. 304). The success of treatment ultimately depends on the clinician's ability to establish the cause of the condition.

REFERENCES

Alpers BJ. Vertiginous epilepsy. Laryngoscope 1960; 70:631.

Baloh RW, Honrubia V. Clinical neurophysiology of the vestibular system. Philadelphia: RA Davis, 1979; 101.

Basser LS. Benign paroxysmal vertigo and vestibular neuronitis. Brain 1969; 87:141.

Behrman S, Wyke, BD. Vestibulogenic seizures. Brain 1958; 81:529.

Bickerstaff ER. Basilar artery migraine. Lancet 1961; 1:15.

Cantor FK. Vestibular-temporal lobe connections demonstrated by induced seizures. Neurology 1971; 21:507.

Carpenter MB. Core text of neuroanatomy. Baltimore: Williams & Wilkins, 1974; 347.

Chutorian AM. Benign paroxysmal torticollis, tortipelvis, retropelvis and retrocollis of infancy. Neurology 1974; 24:366.

Cyr GD, Brookhouser PE, Valente M, et al. Vestibular evaluation of infants and preschool children. Otolaryngol Head Neck Surg 1985; 93:463.

Dekaban A. Neurology of early childhood. Baltimore: Williams & Wilkins, 1970; 270.

Deonna T, Martin D. Benign paroxysmal torticollis in infancy. Arch Dis Child 1981; 56:956.

Eviatar L, Eviatar A. Neurovestibular examination of infants and children. Adv Otorhinolaryngol 1978; 23:169.

Eviatar L, Eviatar A. The normal nystagmic response of infants to caloric and perrotatory stimulation. Laryngoscope 1989; 89:1036.

Eviatar L. Eviatar A. Vertigo in children, differential diagnosis and treatment. Pediatrics 1977; 59:833.

Eviatar L. Vestibular testing in basilar artery migraine. Ann Neurol 1981; 9:126.

Eviatar L, Bergtraum M, Malat Randel R. Post-traumatic vertigo in children: a diagnostic approach. Pediatr Neurol 1986; 2:61.

Gesell A, Amatruda CS. The embryology of behavior: the beginning of the human mind. New York: Harper & Row, 1945; 210.

Gowers WR. Epilepsy and other chronic convulsive disorders: their causes, symptoms and treatment, 2nd ed. London: J & A Churchill, 1901; 189.

Hamilton WJ, Mossman HW. Human embryology: prenatal development of form and function, 4th ed. Cambridge, Mass.: Hoffer, 1972.

Holguin J, Fenichel G. Migraine. J Pediatr 1967; 70:290.

Koenigsberger MR, Chutorian AM, Gold AP, et al. Paroxysmal vertigo of childhood. Neurology 1970;20:1108.

Lapkin ML, French JH, Golden GS, et al. The EEG in childhood basilar artery migraine. Neurology 1977; 27:583.

Lindsay JR. Paroxysmal postural vertigo and vestibular neuronitis. Arch Otolaryngol 1967; 85:544.

McCabe BF, Ryn JH, Sekitani T. Further experiments on vestibular compensation. Laryngoscope 1972; 82:381.

Snyder CH. Paroxysmal torticollis in infancy. Am J Dis Child 1969; 117:458.

Staller SJ, Goin DW, Hildebrandt M. Pediatric vestibular evaluation with harmonic acceleration. Otolaryngol Head Neck Surg 1986; 95:471.

Supance JS, Bluestone CD. Perilymphatic fistulas in infants and children. Otolaryngol Head Neck Surg 1983; 91:663.

23

Oxidative Metabolism Disorders

Galen N. Breningstall

For most cell types, provided the oxygen supply is adequate, the bulk of energy requirements is generated in mitochondria by oxidation of pyruvate, fatty acids, or ketone bodies. These substances enter as acetyl-CoA into the citric acid cycle and the respiratory chain. Impairment of oxidative metabolism may occur as the result of disorders of substrate transport, substrate utilization, citric acid cycle function, or respiratory chain (see the box on p. 310). Tissues most reliant on oxidative metabolism, including brain, skeletal muscle, and cardiac muscle, are most jeopardized by disorders of oxidative metabolism, producing a variety of symptoms related to their dysfunction (Table 23-1). Metabolic acidosis and lactic acidemia, with or without acidosis, are frequent biochemical markers for disorders of oxidative metabolism, as are hypoglycemia and hyperammonemia.

OVERVIEW OF OXIDATIVE METABOLISM

The two primary substrates for mitochondrial energy production are carbohydrates and fats (Figure 23-1). The glycolytic pathway, which is localized in the cytosol, produces pyruvate. Pyruvate diffuses through the outer mitochondrial membrane. It then is processed through the impermeable mitochondrial inner membrane by enzyme pyruvate dehydrogenase [Wallace, 1986]. Pyruvate dehydrogenase produces an energized two-carbon molecule, acetyl-CoA, as well as $NADH + H$. Acetyl-CoA then enters the citric acid cycle. In the process, three additional reduced nicotinamide-adenine dinucleotide (NADH) carriers are converted to $NADH + H$. A lower energy carrier (flavin adenine dinucleotide [FAD]) in the enzyme succinate dehydrogenase also is reduced to $FADH_2$. Free fatty acids are converted to fatty acyl-CoA derivatives at the outer mitochondrial membrane. The fatty acids are transferred through the inner mitochondrial membrane, using carnitine as a transport protein. Carnitine palmitoyl transferase 1 (CPT1) converts carnitine to acylcarnitine, and CPT2 reverses this process after a translocase moves the acylcarnitine to the inner border of the inner mitochondrial membrane. Once inside the mitochondria, fatty acids are oxidized by the beta oxidation cycle. Each turn of this cycle reduces the length of the fatty acid chain by two carbons and generates one $NADH + H$, one $FADH_2$ carried on the electron transfer flavoprotein (ETF), and one acetyl-CoA. Acetyl-CoA then enters the citric acid cycle. Extra $NADH + H$ molecules generated in the cytoplasm can also be oxidized by the mitochondria which enter the mitochondria by two shuttles: glycerol-3-phosphate dehydrogenase and malate-aspartate. The mitochondrial respiratory chain, which comprises alternating hydrogen and electron carriers, transfers reducing equivalents from $NADH + H$ and $FADH_2$ to molecular oxygen in a series of oxidation-reduction steps [Wallace, 1986]. Hydrogen from $NADH + H$ is delivered to the first enzyme of the chain, NADH dehydrogenase (complex 1). Hydrogen from succinate enters through succinate dehydrogenase (complex 2). Hydrogen from fats carried on ETF is delivered through ETF dehydrogenase. These three flavin enzymes pass their electrons through iron-sulfur carriers to the common lipid-soluble carrier coenzyme Q (CoQ) or ubiquinone. Reduced coenzyme Q (QH_2), in turn, donates electrons to complex 3. Complex 3 transfers the electrons through an iron-sulfur protein and cytochromes b and c_1, delivering them to cytochrome c. Cytochrome c is located on the outside of the inner mitochondrial membrane. Cytochrome c donates electrons to cytochrome c oxidase (COX). In COX the electrons pass through cytochrome a and a_3 and their associated copper carriers, finally combining with an oxygen atom and two hydrogen ions to produce water. Energy released during mitochondrial oxidation is utilized by complexes 1, 3, and 4 to pump hydrogen ions through the mitochondrial inner membrane, producing a transmembrane proton electrochemical gradient. Adenosine

tinue to elude specific diagnosis. In one series of 28 patients with congenital lactic acidosis whose fibroblasts were assayed for disorders of pyruvate metabolism and of the respiratory chain, 20 had no specific enzymatic defect assigned [Miyabayashi et al., 1985].

TREATMENT

Management is directed toward buffering life-threatening acidosis, correcting other injurious metabolic abnormalities, removing the accumulation of toxic metabolites, replacing or supplementing cofactors or vitamins, and preventing recurrent crises through dietary manipulation [Evans, 1989]. Therapy for lactic acidosis begins by correcting any cardiac, pulmonary, or circulatory disorder. Administration of bicarbonate is indicated when pH is less than 7.10. Cardiac contractility is impaired below this level. Sodium bicarbonate replacement is determined by calculating the base deficit from arterial blood gases. The base deficit of the extracellular fluid most accurately reflects the metabolic component of acidosis. The amount of bicarbonate needed for correction is calculated by multiplying the base deficit by the volume of distribution (about 0.4 L/kg) and the weight (kg). Half or less of the calculated replacement is given, and then the calculation is repeated for further adjustment. Overzealous correction of acidosis with bicarbonate can result in paradoxical acidosis of the central nervous system, impaired tissue oxygenation, salt and water overload, and further metabolic disturbances, such as hypokalemia, hypercapnia, and overshoot alkalosis [Evans, 1989].

Dietary therapy can remove the offending metabolite and, in many cases, prevent or ameliorate further metabolic crises. Infants with acute metabolic acidosis and children with episodic acidosis should immediately cease protein intake because protein is the usual source of the amino acids that cause most of the organic acidemias. Restriction of protein to less than 0.5 g/kg/day should be instituted until a presumptive diagnosis is determined. Glucose should be administered for caloric intake. Insulin inhibits protein degradation. Administering insulin at 0.05 U/kg/hr with simultaneous glucose infusion to maintain a blood glucose concentration of 150 mg/dl may reduce the endogenous production of toxic metabolites during periods of acute acidosis. However, in patients with pyruvate dysmetabolism, zealous glucose administration may be harmful. Careful monitoring of the patient during the early phase of therapy and circumspection regarding any therapy instituted is critical. High-calorie, protein-restricted diets of about 1.5 g/kg/day of dietary protein can prevent some of the complications of organic acidemias when compliance is maintained. Special diets deficient in specific amino acids are also beneficial in certain instances. In patients with disorders of pyruvate metab-

olism a ketogenic diet may be used, decreasing reliance on glycolysis for energy production. Conversely, in patients with disorders of fatty acid oxidation, a low-fat, relatively high-carbohydrate diet may be used to decrease reliance on fatty acid oxidation for energy production. Patients with disorders of oxidative metabolism are at particular risk when oral intake is decreased because of intercurrent illness or lethargy. Intercurrent illness and catabolism may provoke metabolic crises in these patients, requiring administration of intravenous nutrition.

Carnitine supplementation may reverse the cardiomyopathy of carnitine transport deficiency and prevent episodes of acute encephalopathy in these patients [Stanley et al., 1991]. Carnitine may be depleted as a result of excessive acylcarnitine excretion in the organic acidemias and in disorders of beta oxidation; carnitine supplementation buffers toxic acyl-CoA compounds in these disorders and promotes their excretion. Glycine supplementation promotes excretion of toxic metabolites, such as isovalerylglycine in isovaleric acidemia; it may serve a similar function in other disorders of organic acid metabolism or beta oxidation. Vitamin supplementation with thiamine, biotin, or B_{12} may be helpful in some disorders of amino or organic acid metabolism. Attempts have been made to treat pyruvate dysmetabolism with thiamine, lipoic acid, biotin, and dichloroacetate. In disorders of the respiratory chain, coenzyme Q and riboflavin may be administered, as may menadione and ascorbate.

REFERENCES

Aicardi J, Gordon N, Hagberg B. Holes in the brain. Dev Med Child Neurol 1985; 27:249.

Breningstall GN. Carnitine deficiency syndromes. Pediatr Neurol 1990; 6:75-81.

Breningstall GN, Lockman LA. Massive focal brain swelling as a feature of MELAS, Pediatr Neurol 1988; 4:366.

Campistol J, Fernandez Alvarez E, Cusi V. CT scan appearance in subacute necrotising encephalomyelopathy. Dev Med Child Neurol 1984; 26:519.

Diamantopoulos N, Painter MJ, Wolf B, et al. Biotinidase deficiency: accumulation of lactate in the brain and response to physiologic doses of biotin. Neurology 1986; 36:1107.

DiMauro S, Bonilla E, Lombes A, et al. Mitochondrial encephalomyopathies. Neurol Clin 1990; 8:483.

Evans OB. Lactic acidosis in childhood. Part 1. Pediatr Neurol 1985; 1:325.

Evans OB. Lactic acidosis in childhood. Part 2. Pediatr Neurol 1986; 2:5.

Evans OB. Metabolic acidosis. In: Swaiman KF, ed.: Pediatric neurology. Principles and practice. St. Louis: CV Mosby, 1989; 975.

Fishman RA. Cerebrospinal fluid in diseases of the nervous system. Philadelphia: WB Saunders, 1980; 223.

Grodd W, Krageloh-Mann I, Klose V, et al. Metabolic and destructive brain disorders in children: findings with localized proton MR spectroscopy. Radiology 1991; 181:173.

Hermansen L, Maehlum S, Pruett EDR, et al. Lactate removal at rest and during exercise. In: Howald H, Portman JR, eds.: Metabolic adaptation to prolonged physical exercise. Basel: Birkhauser Verlag, 1975; 101.

Hug G, Bove KE, Soukup S. Lethal neonatal multiorgan deficiency of carnitine palmitoyltransferase II. N Engl J Med 1991; 325:1862.

Kollee LAA, Willems JL, DeKort AFM, et al. Blood sampling techniques for lactate and pyruvate estimation in children. Ann Clin Biochem 1977; 14:285.

Leigh D. Subacute necrotizing encephalomyelopathy in an infant. J Neurol Neurosurg Psychiatry 1951; 14:216-21.

Lloyd MH, Iles, RA, Simpson BR, et al. The effect of simulated metabolic acidosis on intracellular pH and lactate metabolism in the isolated perfused rat liver. Clin Sci Mol Med 1973; 45:543.

Matthews PM, Allaire C, Shoubridge EA, et al. In vivo muscle magnetic resonance spectroscopy in the clinical investigation of mitochondrial disease. Neurology 1991; 41:114.

Medina L, Chi TL, DeVivo CD, et al. MR findings in patients with subacute necrotizing encephalomyelopathy (Leigh syndrome): correlation with biochemical defect. AJNR 1990; 11:379.

Millington DS, Roe CR, Maltby DA. Application of high resolution fast atom bombardment and constant B/E ratio linked scanning to the identification and analysis of acylcarnitine in metabolic disease. Biomed Mass Spectrom 1984; 11:236.

Miyabayashi S, Ito T, Narisawa K, et al. Biochemical study in 28 children with lactic acidosis, in relation to Leigh's encephalomyelopathy. Eur J Pediatr 1985; 143:278.

Munnich A, Rustin P, Rotig A, et al. Clinical aspects of mitochondrial disorders. Int Pediatr 1992; 7:28.

Pappenheimer JR. The ionic composition of cerebral extracellular fluid and its relation to control of breathing. In: The Harvey Lectures 1965-1966. New York: Academic Press, 1967; 71.

Posner JB, Plum F. Independence of blood and cerebrospinal fluid lactate. Arch Neurol 1967a; 16:492.

Posner JB, Plum F. Spinal fluid pH and neurological symptoms in systemic acidosis. N Engl J Med 1976b; 277:605.

Relman AS. Metabolic consequences of acid-base disorders. Kidney Int 1972; 1:347.

Rinaldo P, O'Shea JJ, Coates PM, et al. Medium chain acyl-CoA dehydrogenase deficiency. Diagnosis by stable-isotope dilution measurement of urinary N-hexanoylglycine and 3-phenylpropionylglycine. N Engl J Med 1988; 319:1308.

Roe CR, Millington DS, Maltby DA, et al. Diagnostic and therapeutic implications of medium chain-acylcarnitines in the medium chain acyl-CoA dehydrogenase deficiency. Pediatr Res 1985; 19:459.

Robinson BH. Lactic acidemia. In: Scriver CR, Beaudet AL, Sly WL, et al., eds.: The metabolic basis of inherited disease, 6th ed. New York: McGraw Hill, 1989; 869.

Robinson BH, Taylor J, Sherwood WG. The genetic heterogeneity of lactic acidosis: occurrence of recognizable inborn errors of metabolism in a pediatric population with lactic acidosis. Pediatr Res 1980; 14:956.

Siesjo BK. The regulation of cerebrospinal fluid pH. Kidney Int 1972; 1:360.

Stanley CA, DeLeeuw S, Coates PM, et al. Chronic cardiomyopathy and weakness or acute coma in children with a defect in carnitine uptake. Ann Neurol 1991; 30:709.

Swaiman KF, Lockman LA. Metabolic acidosis. In: Swaiman KF, Wright FS, eds.: The practice of pediatric neurology. St. Louis: CV Mosby, 1982; 309.

Van Coster R, Lombes A, DeVivo DC, et al. Cytochrome c oxidase-associated Leigh syndrome: phenotypic features and pathogenetic speculations. J Neurol Sci 1991; 104:97.

Wallace DC. Mitochondrial genes and disease. Hosp Pract 1986; 21:77.

24

Principles of Genetics

William B. Dobyns

In the broadest sense, genes are simply units of hereditary information, and genetics is the study of genes and their disorders. The modern field of genetics began with the concept of single gene inheritance, which was formulated in 1865 by Gregor Johann Mendel based on his classic experiments with garden peas. From his careful observations, Mendel discovered that individual traits sorted independently in meiosis and proposed what is now known as his law of segregation. From these simple observations the field of genetics has grown to encompass the fundamental basis of life itself. An important part of genetics during this time has been the study of the human genome, which contains about 50,000 to 100,000 genes that control all aspects of growth, development, and metabolism, as well as many other functions. Fully one third of all these genes are expressed in the nervous system.

Rapid progress in the technology of molecular genetics during the past 10 years has led to the discovery of the chromosomal location and DNA sequence of many of these genes. Important examples include Duchenne and Becker muscular dystrophies, myotonic dystrophy, fragile X syndrome, neurofibromatosis 1, and many inborn errors of metabolism. Many more genes have been localized to a specific chromosome region, although the DNA sequence has not yet been discovered. The scientific basis of genes and genetic disorders has become critical to all fields of medicine, and to pediatric neurology in particular. This chapter reviews many of the basic principles of genetics that underlie these recent advances. More detailed information on genetics is available in many excellent texts, such as *Genetics in Medicine* by Thompson et al. [1991].

CHROMOSOMAL BASIS OF HEREDITY

Years after Mendel described independent sorting of genetic traits, occasional exceptions to his law of segregation were discovered. Certain traits were found that were typically inherited as a group. These observations were later explained by the discovery of chromosomes. The nuclear material of a cell, which is known as *chromatin,* appears relatively homogeneous during most of the cell cycle, but condenses into a number of rod-shaped organelles during cell division. These tiny structures were called chromosomes because they stain darkly with various biologic dyes.

Chromosomes

Each human somatic cell contains 46 chromosomes that consist of 22 matched pairs known as *autosomes* and two sex chromosomes: XX in females and XY in males. In contrast, human germ cells contain only 23 chromosomes consisting of one of each kind of autosome and a single sex chromosome. The former is known as the *diploid* or 2n number, and the latter is known as the *haploid* or 1n number. The autosomes are numbered according to length, with chromosome 1 being the longest and chromosome 21 the shortest. Although chromosome 21 is slightly shorter than chromosome 22, the numbers were retained for historic reasons. The two members of each pair of autosomes and the two X chromosomes in females carry the same genes and are known as *homologous chromosomes* or *homologs.* Although they appear similar under the microscope, homologs are not strictly identical. They contain essentially the same genes, but the nucleotide sequence differs at thousands of positions.

Chromosome identification

Individual chromosomes may be seen only when contracted during cell division as described below. Each chromosome consists of two chromatids, which are joined at the primary constriction or centromere. In standard cytogenetic nomenclature the centromere is used to divide the chromosome into two arms, designated the p or short arm, and the q or long arm. The tip

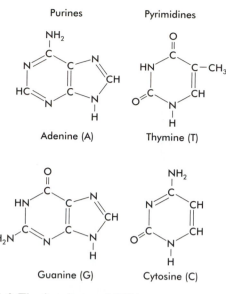

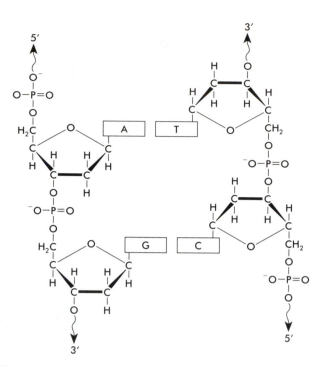

Figure 24-4 The four bases of DNA.

Figure 24-5 The chemical structure of DNA depicts the sugar-phosphate backbone and 3'-5' phosphodiester bonds.

normally exists as a single- rather than double-stranded molecule.

Structure of human chromosomes

Nuclear chromosomes. Human chromosomes consist of a single, uninterrupted strand of DNA that contains 50 to 250 million base pairs (bp), and a group of associated proteins that form the scaffolding. The latter includes five basic proteins called histones, and several acidic proteins. Two copies of each of four histones (H2A, H2B, H3, and H4) join to form an octamer. The DNA double helix wraps almost twice around the octamer, which involves about 140 bp. Adjacent octamers are separated by a short spacer segment of 20 to 60 bp that is associated with histone H1. The complex of DNA and core histones is known as a *nucleosome* (Figure 24-6, *B*).

The strings of nucleosomes are further compacted into a secondary helical structure known as a *solenoid,* which has a diameter of about 30 nm (Figure 24-6, *C*). Each turn of the solenoid contains six nucleosomes. The solenoids are then packed into large loops of 10 to 100 kb (1000 bp = 1 kb), which attach to a non-histone protein scaffolding. These loops pack together loosely to form interphase chromosomes (Figure 24-6, *D*). During early prophase, they pack together more closely to form knoblike thickenings called *chromomeres,* which coalesce further to form the bands observed in metaphase chromosomes. The differences between the light- and dark-staining bands are only partly understood. The dark-staining G bands observed with the G banding technique are AT rich, replicate late in the S phase, and contain relatively few genes. The light-staining R bands (which stain darkly with the R-banding technique) are GC rich, replicate early, and contain many genes.

Mitochondrial chromosome. Each mitochondrion contains multiple copies of a small circular DNA molecule that codes for 13 structural protein genes and some structural RNA genes. The protein packaging is less complex than for nuclear chromosomes.

Organization of the genome

The organization of DNA in the human genome is complex [Thompson et al., 1991]. About 75% represents unique or single copy DNA, of which only 10% actually codes for genes. The function of the remaining 65% is unknown. Most of this is found in short stretches of several kilobases or less, interspersed with several classes of repetitive DNA. The latter consists of DNA whose nucleotide sequence is repeated, either exactly or with some minor variation, hundreds to millions of times in the genome.

Several classes of repetitive DNA have been described, some clustered and others dispersed throughout the genome. Clustered, repeat sequences comprise 10% to 15% of the genome and are collectively called *satellite DNA* because of their separation from other DNA on density centrifugation. These satellite DNA consist of tandemly arrayed (head-to-tail) repeat sequences that can extend for several thousand kilobases. For example the heterochromatic regions of distal Yq and the pericentromeric regions of chromosomes 1, 9, and 16

STRUCTURE AND FUNCTION OF CHROMOSOMES AND GENES

A. DOUBLE HELIX **B.** NUCLEOSOME FIBER ("beads-on-a-string") **C.** SOLENOID **D.** INTERPHASE NUCLEUS

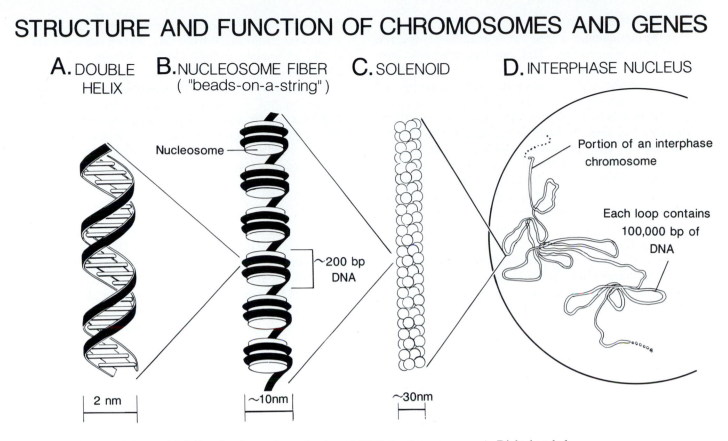

Nucleosome

~200 bp DNA

Portion of an interphase chromosome

Each loop contains 100,000 bp of DNA

2 nm   ~10nm   ~30nm

Figure 24-6 Levels of protein packaging of DNA in chromosomes. **A,** Right-handed double helix proposed by Watson and Crick. **B,** A DNA molecule wrapped around the histone core to form nucleosomes. **C,** Nucleosomes packed into a solenoid structure. **D,** The loops of solenoids that comprise an interphase chromosome. (Modified from Thompson MW, McInnes RR, Willard HF, et al. Genetics in medicine, 5th ed., Philadelphia: WB Saunders, 1991, p.35.)

consist of very long arrays of repeats as short as 5 bp. The centromeric regions contain extensive repeats of an approximately 171-bp unit called *alpha-satellite DNA,* which differs slightly between each chromosome.

Dispersed, repeat sequences comprise 6% to 10% of the genome and belong to several different classes. Minisatellite or variable number of tandem repeat (VNTR) sequences are dispersed, intermediate-length (15 to 65 bp) repeats that usually span only several kilobases. The Alu family of DNA repeats includes about 500,000 related sequences that are each about 300 bp in length, and together comprise about 3% of the genome. The L1 family of repeats includes about 10,000 related sequences that extend up to 6 kb in length and comprise another 3% of the genome. The CA repeat family includes 50-100,000 sequences consisting of short tandem repeats of the cytosine-adenine dinucleotide (or guanine-thymine on complementary strand). Although their origin is not known, all of these families have

proved useful as DNA markers. They may also be "hot spots" for mutation. Based on available data, it appears that a large proportion of genomic DNA has no identified function. It has been proposed that much of this DNA has no function, but simply exploits cellular processes to propagate itself.

Central dogma: DNA-RNA-protein

Genetic information is stored in DNA by means of a genetic code in which the specific base sequence determines the amino acid sequence of the polypeptide. The two major steps in this process are known as *transcription* and *translation.* Transcription is the process by which messenger RNA is synthesized from the DNA template and transported to the cytoplasm. Translation is the process by which the messenger RNA sequence is decoded to allow synthesis of the protein. The flow of information from DNA to RNA to protein is called the *central dogma* of molecular biology.

Gene structure

In the introduction a gene was defined simply as a unit of genetic information. This concept gradually progressed to a more useful definition, which states that a gene is a sequence of chromosomal DNA that is required for production of a functional product, whether the product is RNA or protein [Thompson et al., 1991]. Many studies over the past decade have shown that the structure of a gene is complex and includes much more than the coding sequence of the protein [Schon, 1989b].

Genetic information, whether encoded in DNA or RNA, is always read in the 5' to 3' direction, which is also known as the *upstream to downstream direction*. The nomenclature regarding the 5' and 3' positions of the sugar backbone can be confusing. This convention means that the 5' carbon of the first nucleotide of a sequence will be either unused or joined to a nucleotide not involved in the sequence, whereas its 3' carbon has a phosphodiester bond joining it to the 5' carbon of the second nucleotide and so on. The last nucleotide of the sequence has an open 3' carbon or joins another uninvolved nucleotide.

A model of a typical human gene is shown in Figure 24-7. Various promoter sequences that are important for initiation of RNA transcription and regulation of the gene are present at the 5' end of the gene. Examples include the CAT and TATA boxes whose sequences are conserved among many different genes. Downstream from the promoter region is a start sequence, which signals the start of transcription of DNA to RNA. Further downstream is an initiator codon, which signals the start of the actual coding sequence for the polypeptide product. The region between the transcription and translation start sites is known as the *5' untranslated region*. The coding sequences of genes are called *exons*. Most are not continuous, but rather are interrupted by one or more noncoding regions called *introns*. In most genes the cumulative length of introns is much greater

than that of exons. Special sequences mark the boundaries of the exons and introns. The coding sequence ends at the terminator codon, which is followed by the 3' untranslated region. The latter contains a signal to add a long sequence of adenosine nucleotides, which is called the *poly-A tail*. It is not known whether transcription ends at a specific site within the 3' untranslated region. The length of a gene may vary from less than 1 kb to several hundred kilobases. The longest gene known, which codes for dystrophin, spans more than 2000 kb.

Transcription

Synthesis of messenger RNA begins at the transcription start site and continues in a 5' to 3' direction with regard to the RNA product. The DNA strand that corresponds to the RNA sequence is known as the *coding* or *"sense" strand*. However, the opposite DNA strand, known as the *noncoding* or *"antisense" strand*, actually serves as the template for the messenger RNA and is read in the 3' to 5' direction [Schon, 1989b].

The primary messenger RNA transcript is processed within the nucleus by the addition of a CAP structure to the 5' end, cleavage of the 3' end at a specific point downstream from the end of the coding sequence, and addition of the poly-A tail at a site specified in part by the sequence AAUAAA, which is located in the 3' untranslated region. The poly-A tail appears to increase the stability of the messenger RNA. The fully processed messenger RNA is transported to the cytoplasm where translation occurs.

Translation

The genetic code. The mechanism by which the base sequence of messenger RNA specifies the amino acid sequence of a polypeptide chain is known as the *genetic code*. In this nearly universal code, each set of three adjacent bases in the messenger RNA molecule constitutes a codon, and the different combinations of bases

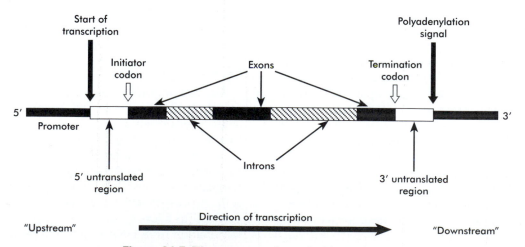

Figure 24-7 The structure of a typical human gene.

within the codon specify the individual amino acids (Table 24-1). The molecular links between messenger RNA codons and amino acids are the small *transfer RNA* molecules. One segment of each transfer RNA molecule contains a three-base anticodon that is complementary to a specific codon on the messenger RNA, whereas another segment contains a binding site for one of the 20 amino acids.

Because there are only 20 amino acids and 64 possible codons, most amino acids are specified by more than one codon. For some of the different amino acids the base in the third position in the triplet may be either of the purines, either of the pyrimidines, or sometimes any of the four bases. Arginine and leucine are each specified by six codons, whereas only methionine and tryptophan are specified by a single codon. Three of the codons are called *stop codons*, which signal termination of translation.

Translation process. The complex process of translation or protein synthesis takes place in the cytoplasm

Table 24-1 The genetic code

First Base		Second Base								Third Base
		U		C		A		G		
U		UUU	phe	UCU	ser	UAU	tyr	UGU	cys	U
		UUC	phe	UCC	ser	UAC	tyr	UGC	cys	C
		UUA	leu	UCA	ser	UAA	stop	UGA	stop	A
		UUG	leu	UCG	ser	UAG	stop	UGG	trp	G
C		CUU	leu	CCU	pro	CAU	his	CGU	arg	U
		CUC	leu	CCC	pro	CAC	his	CGC	arg	C
		CUA	leu	CCA	pro	CAA	gln	CGA	arg	A
		CUG	leu	CCG	pro	CAG	gln	CGG	arg	G
A		AUU	ile	ACU	thr	AAU	asn	AGU	ser	U
		AUC	ile	ACC	thr	AAC	asn	AGC	ser	C
		AUA	ile	ACA	thr	AAA	lys	AGA	arg	A
		AUG	met	ACG	thr	AAG	lys	AGG	arg	G
G		GUU	val	GCU	ala	GAU	asp	GGU	gly	U
		GUC	val	GCC	ala	GAC	asp	GGC	gly	C
		GUA	val	GCA	ala	GAA	glu	GGA	gly	A
		GUG	val	GCG	ala	GAG	glu	GGG	gly	G

Abbreviations

ala (A)	alanine	leu (L)	leucine
arg (R)	arginine	lys (K)	lysine
asn (N)	asparagine	met (M)	methionine
asp (D)	aspartic acid	phe (F)	phenylalanine
cys (C)	cysteine	pro (P)	proline
gln (Q)	glutamine	ser (S)	serine
gluc (E)	glutamic acid	thr (T)	threonine
gly (G)	glycine	trp (W)	tryptophan
his (H)	histidine	tyr (Y)	tyrosine
ile (I)	isoleucine	val (V)	valine
stop	termination codon		

Codons are shown in terms of messenger RNA, which are complementary to the corresponding DNA codons.
From Thompson MW, McInnes RR, Willard HF. Genetics in medicine, 5th ed. Philadelphia: WB Saunders, 1991.

on small structures known as *ribosomes,* which are macromolecules composed of ribosomal RNA and several associated proteins. Ribosomal RNA comprises 18S and 28S subunits that are encoded by genes on the short arms of the acrocentric chromosomes.

Translation begins with binding of the 5′ end of processed messenger RNA to the ribosome, which then moves along the messenger RNA molecule in a 5′ to 3′ direction until encountering the base triplet AUG. In addition to specifying methionine, this codon serves as the start signal for synthesis of the polypeptide chain and establishes the reading frame of the messenger RNA. The ribosome then slides along the messenger RNA exactly three bases, allowing recognition of the next codon. Bonding between the messenger RNA codon and transfer RNA anticodon brings the appropriate amino acid into position on the ribosome for attachment to the carboxyl end of the growing polypeptide chain by formation of a peptide bond. This process continues until one of the stop codons is reached. Thus proteins are synthesized from the amino to the carboxy terminus, which corresponds to translation from the 5′ to 3′ end of messenger RNA, and methionine is always the first amino acid of each polypeptide chain, although it is usually removed before protein synthesis is completed.

TECHNOLOGY OF MOLECULAR GENETICS

Molecular genetics is that branch of genetics concerned with the structure and function of genes at the DNA molecule level. The rapid gains in this field during the past decade have resulted from discovery of several new techniques that have made detailed analysis of both normal and abnormal genes possible. These discoveries have in turn led to better understanding of many important biologic processes, as well as the basis for many genetic diseases. Several of these methods have proved to be of particular importance and are used in many current research studies. Some familiarity with these procedures is helpful in understanding the nature and significance of new discoveries in this area. This section serves as an introduction to some of the more important procedures.

Restriction enzymes

Restriction endonucleases are bacterial enzymes that recognize short, double-stranded DNA sequences and cut the DNA molecule at or near the recognition site [Ray, 1989]. When a mutation occurs that changes as little as one of the base pairs in the sequence, it is no longer recognized and cut by the enzyme. Several hundred restriction endonucleases have been isolated. Most of the recognition sites are palindromes, which means that they read the same in the 5′ to 3′ direction on both strands, and most of the enzymes leave short overhangs of single-stranded DNA, the so-called sticky ends. For example, the enzyme *Bam*HI recognizes the sequence GGATCC and cuts it between the two guanine bases, leaving a four-base overhang:

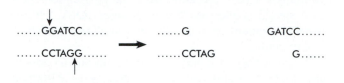

Restriction endonucleases have several important uses in molecular biology. First, they cut or "digest" large DNA molecules into a reproducible collection of as many as a million smaller and more manageable DNA fragments that can be identified based on their size. Second, a mutation at any of the recognition sites that changes the sequence or a mutation elsewhere that creates a new recognition site can potentially be detected. Finally, all DNA molecules cut with the same restriction endonuclease have the same sticky ends and may be joined by using the enzyme DNA ligase. This condition allows specific DNA sequences of interest to be inserted into the DNA of living cells, known as *vectors,* such as the bacterium *Escherichia coli* or the yeast *Saccharomyces cerevisiae* (common bakers' yeast), which then can be propagated to produce large amounts of the sequence of interest. DNA sequences inserted into a vector are known as *recombinant DNA.*

Vectors

A vector is a DNA molecule that can replicate itself without outside control in a host cell, such as bacteria or yeast. Cloning of human or other DNA fragments of interest by using restriction endonucleases and DNA ligase results in propagation of the DNA fragment along with the vector, thus producing large quantities of the fragment of interest, which then can be isolated along with the vector. Four major types of vectors are used in molecular biology.

Plasmids. Plasmids are small circular molecules of double-stranded DNA found in bacteria and less often in yeast, which often contain genes that confer resistance to antibiotics. The plasmids commonly used for cloning are only several kilobases in size and contain an origin of replication sequence, one or more antibiotic resistance genes for use as selectable markers, and one or more restriction endonuclease recognition sites for use in cloning small DNA fragments of interest.

Phage. Bacteriophage lambda is a bacterial virus that contains a single 45 kb double-stranded DNA molecule. The virus replicates rapidly in *E. coli* to produce enormous numbers of progeny, from which DNA molecules can be isolated. Almost one third of the genome can be replaced with other DNA segments, permitting cloning of fragments as large as 20 kb.

Cosmids. Cosmids are man-made DNA molecules constructed from the ends of lambda phage and the middle of a large plasmid. They may contain DNA fragments as large as 35 to 45 kb. Like lambda phage itself, they may be infected into bacterial cells by a technique known as *in vitro packaging*. The recombinant cosmids are mixed with separate protein building blocks of the phage. Under the correct conditions in vitro the phage self-assembles and becomes an infectious particle. After infection of a bacterial cell, cosmids recircularize and replicate as a large plasmid.

Yeast artificial chromosomes. Yeast artificial chromosomes are even larger man-made DNA molecules constructed by combining yeast centromeres and telomeres with large fragments of DNA. They may contain up to 1000 kb of DNA and will replicate and segregate in yeast cells just like the normal yeast chromosomes.

Clones and libraries

A clone is a small molecule of recombinant DNA in a vector that may have come from any of several different sources. The methods used to generate them are known as *cloning*. Many clones are chosen at random from clone libraries, which are large collections of clones originating from a specific source, such as the total DNA (called *genomic DNA*) of a human or other organism [Sylvester and Schmickel, 1989]. Libraries also have been constructed from DNA enriched for a specific chromosome, such as a flow-sorted chromosome 17 library, and from complementary DNA, which consists of synthetic molecules copied from messenger RNA by the enzyme reverse transcriptase. Complementary DNAs have often proved useful because they contain only the coding sequence of a gene. Other clones have been obtained from several classes of dispersed, repetitive DNA elements, including the variable number of tandem repeats, Alu, and L_1 families. Clones may also be synthesized directly when the desired nucleotide sequence is known. Choosing which clones to use in any given project, such as a gene mapping project, is one of the most critical steps.

Probes and southern blots

Probes are either clones or synthetic DNA molecules that have been labeled with a tracer to allow their detection during Southern blot or other experiments. They are used to detect DNA or RNA fragments with a complementary base sequence from a patient or research subject. The most commonly used tracers are radioisotopes such as ^{32}P. Although probes are used in several different laboratory procedures, the most widely used and best known is a technique developed by Dr.

E.M. Southern and known as *Southern blotting* [Ray, 1989].

To perform a Southern blot, DNA must first be isolated from some accessible source, such as genomic DNA from lymphocytes or fibroblasts, and then cut by one or more restriction endonucleases into as many as a million fragments. The fragments are separated by size through electrophoresis on an agarose gel, with smaller fragments moving more rapidly and farther than larger fragments. They are then denatured with a strong base to separate the two strands, transferred to a nitrocellulose or nylon filter membrane by blotting and capillary movement, and finally fixed to the filter by baking.

Because both the DNA fragment of interest and the probe are now single-stranded DNA, they will hybridize or bond to form a new double-stranded DNA fragment under appropriate laboratory conditions when the base sequences are complementary. This is usually done by sealing the filter and probe in a plastic bag and submerging it in a water bath. The filter is then washed to remove unbound probe and exposed to x-ray film to reveal where the probe has bound. The x-ray film shows a characteristic and reproducible pattern of bands that indicate the relative sizes of the marked DNA fragments (Figure 24-8).

Pulsed-field gel electrophoresis

The standard method for agarose gel electrophoresis can separate DNA molecules up to about 20 kb in size. Pulsed-field gel electrophoresis is a technique that allows separation and analysis of much larger fragments of DNA. The DNA source is first cut with special "rare cutting" restriction endonucleases with longer recognition sequences that therefore occur less frequently in the genome. The resulting fragments are consequently larger than those used for standard electrophoresis. The DNA fragments are placed in an agarose gel and subjected to an electric field as for standard electrophoresis, but the potential difference is pulsed to alternatively invert the electric field, which results in separation of molecules up to about 2000 kb in size.

Restriction fragment length polymorphisms

Restriction fragment length polymorphisms are differences in the size of DNA fragments derived from corresponding regions of homologous chromosomes in diploid cells [Ray, 1989]. They are generally detected by restriction endonuclease digestion of a DNA source followed by Southern blotting (Figure 24-8) but may also be identified by other methods, such as pulsed-field gel electrophoresis and allele-specific oligonucleotides (described below). Restriction fragment length polymorphisms are a measure of naturally occurring variations or polymorphisms of normal DNA and are inherited according to mendelian principles. The level of human

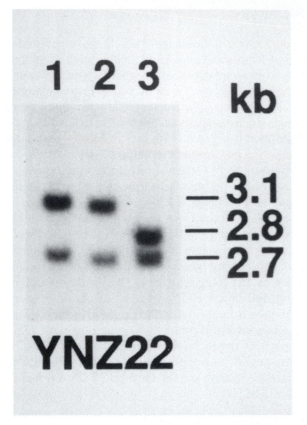

Figure 24-8 Southern blot using the variable number of tandem repeats probe YNZ22 from the short arm of chromosome 17 shows the inheritance of different fragments or alleles in a child *(lane 2)*. He inherited the 3.1-kb fragment from his mother *(lane 1)* and the 2.7-kb fragment from his father *(lane 3)*.

DNA polymorphism is high because one base in 250 to 500 differs in any pair of chromosomes chosen at random. When restriction fragment length polymorphisms are located within or physically close to a cloned gene or other DNA sequence of interest, they may be used for prenatal or presymptomatic diagnosis and gene mapping.

The physical basis for restriction fragment length polymorphisms is the difference in DNA sequence in homologous chromosomes. It may be as small as a single base pair change that alters a restriction endonuclease recognition site, or as large as a chromosome rearrangement that is visible under the microscope. These DNA changes do not always affect the restriction site directly. A restriction fragment length polymorphism will be produced by any change that alters the size of the DNA fragment on which the restriction site is located. Thus several different types of restriction fragment length polymorphisms have been discovered. The first consists of a point mutation or other small DNA alteration that destroys or creates a new restriction endonuclease

recognition sequence. Second, larger DNA changes, such as deletions and duplications, may increase or decrease fragment size without altering any restriction sites. In the last type the polymorphisms consist of variable numbers of tandemly repeated DNA sequences (see below). The size of the fragment is altered by the number of repeat segments so they will be separated on the agarose gel.

Variable number of tandem repeats (VNTR) and CA repeats

Several of the most useful types of restriction fragment length polymorphisms involve repetitive DNA elements, especially minisatellite or VNTR sequences and CA repeats. Variable numbers of tandem repeat sequences are intermediate length (15 to 65 bp) DNA sequences that are repeated one to several dozen times in tandem, and usually span several kilobases in total length. Each copy number may be detected as a separate allele, making them highly polymorphic.

CA repeats (also called *GT repeats*) are an abundant class of repetitive DNA that consists of short tandem repeats of the dinucleotide CA on one strand and GT on the complementary strand, thus taking the form $(CA)_n*(GT)_n$ with n in the range of 6 to 30 [Weber and May, 1989]. The number of repeats within a $(CA)_n$ block varies greatly among different members of a species, producing a set of alleles that always differs in size by multiples of two bases. About 70% of the human population is heterozygous at any given $(CA)_n$ repeat locus, making them highly polymorphic. The human genome contains about 50,000 to 100,000 interspersed $(CA)_n$ blocks, which is enough to place one block every 30 to 60 kb if evenly spaced. For both variable number of tandem repeats and CA repeat sequences, the combination of a high frequency in the genome and a high rate of polymorphism has made them extremely useful for gene mapping.

Polymerase chain reaction

The polymerase chain reaction is a simple but elegant method to amplify a small amount of DNA over a millionfold within a matter of hours [Thompson et al., 1991]. It allows the detection of specific base sequences in DNA samples without the use of cloning or Southern blots. First, a small region of DNA for which the base sequence is known, such as part of a gene, is selected for amplification. A short sequence of about 10 to 15 bp just upstream (on the 5′ side) of the target sequence on one strand is chosen as a starting site, and an oligonucleotide that is complementary to this short upstream sequence is synthesized for use as a primer. Another short sequence upstream of the target sequence on the opposite strand is also chosen, and a second complementary oligonucleotide is synthesized. The two primers thus flank the region of interest on opposite strands.

The DNA and primers are denatured to separate the strands, after which the primers are hybridized to the complementary sequences. The short oligonucleotides then serve as primers for synthesis of a complete complementary strand by the enzyme DNA polymerase. Because both strands are copied, one round of amplification results in a complete second copy of the original target sequence. Repeated cycles of heat denaturation, hybridization of the primers, and DNA synthesis result in the exponential amplification of the target sequence. Within a few hours, more than a million copies of the sequence may be made.

DNA sequence analysis

The most widely used method to determine the nucleotide sequence of a segment of DNA uses synthetic nucleotide analogs (2′, 3′-dideoxynucleoside triphosphates) that inhibit chain lengthening because they lack the 3′-hydroxyl group required for addition of the next base. The target DNA is placed in special plasmid or phage vectors that contain many of the common restriction enzyme recognition sites to allow easy insertion. Synthetic oligonucleotides that are complementary to a short sequence of the plasmid DNA flanking the insert are used as primers for synthesis by the enzyme DNA polymerase I. The enzyme proceeds along the DNA template, incorporating either ^{32}P- or ^{35}S-radiolabeled nucleotides into the newly synthesized sequence.

The sequence is determined by adding the appropriate inhibitory analog into each of four separate sequencing reactions, one for each of the four nucleotide bases. When a guanine analog is added, DNA synthesis of a proportion of the newly synthesized DNA strands stops at each guanine residue that the enzyme encounters. Depending on the relative amount of guanine base and guanine analog in the reaction, some newly synthesized strands are inhibited and stop at the first guanine, some at the second guanine, some at the third, etc. The synthesized DNA molecules are separated by electrophoresis on a polyacrylamide gel and exposed to x-ray film. A series of radioactive bands is observed at lengths corresponding to the locations of each guanine residue. Similar reactions for the other three bases provide corresponding information. The set of four reactions then can be read as a directional sequencing ladder [Thompson et al., 1991].

Allele-specific oligonucleotide probes

Specific mutations causing a disease phenotype, especially point mutations, can sometimes be detected by their hybridization or lack of hybridization with short synthetic DNA molecules known as *allele-specific oligonucleotide* probes [Thompson et al., 1991]. This tech-

nique is only possible when the base sequence and precise point mutation responsible for the abnormal phenotype in at least some individuals are known.

For this method, separate allele-specific oligonucleotide probes complementary to either the normal or the mutant allele are synthesized. The probes consist of the point mutation or its normal counterpart and up to about 9 bp flanking it on either side, for a total length of up to 19 bp. The probes are then hybridized to the DNA source under relatively stringent conditions. Because the probes are short, they are highly sensitive to sequence changes at even a single nucleotide. A probe complementary to the normal allele will hybridize to the normal allele but not to the mutant allele and vice versa. Thus DNA from an individual homozygous for the normal gene will hybridize to the allele-specific oligonucleotide probe complementary to the normal DNA sequence but not to the probe complementary to the point mutation. DNA from persons homozygous for the mutation will hybridize to the allele-specific oligonucleotide probe complementary to the mutation but not to the normal probe. Only DNA from heterozygotes will hybridize to both probes. It is important to remember that DNA from individuals who are homozygous or heterozygous for different mutations in the same gene will also hybridize to the normal probe.

Somatic cell hybrids

Somatic cell hybrids are cells created from the fusion of two separate somatic cells, usually from different species [Bruns, 1989]. In most cases the cells of origin include a human cell line and either a mouse or Chinese hamster cell line. To construct a hybrid the two cell lines are mixed in the presence of either polyethylene glycol or inactivated Sendai virus, which promotes fusion of cell membranes. The mixture is then cultured in special media containing hypoxanthine, aminopterin, and thymidine that helps select for growth of hybrid cells. Two separate nuclei are maintained in each cell at first, but after mitosis and cell division are mixed in a single hybrid nucleus. The human chromosomes are preferentially lost from the hybrid nucleus with even short-term culture, leaving only 2 to 15 in all. After prolonged culture the number is further reduced to one to three chromosomes per clone. This parasexual system allows the study of individual human chromosomes in the laboratory and has made somatic cell hybrids invaluable for mapping genes to specific chromosomes.

When the residual human chromosomes present in a panel of independent somatic cell hybrids are compared with regard to the presence or absence of a particular human gene in the same hybrid panel, the human gene will correlate with the presence or absence of a single chromosome. In a typical hybrid panel, each of the 10 or 20 hybrids contains a different group of human chromosomes. As an example, one such panel was tested for the presence or absence of human hexosaminidase A, mutations that cause Tay-Sachs disease. All hybrids that contained a human chromosome 15 expressed the human hexosaminidase A gene, whereas those that lacked chromosome 15 did not. This perfect concordance was observed only for chromosome 15, and not for any other human chromosome, thus proving that the human hexosaminidase A gene is located on chromosome 15. It is also possible to map genes to specific segments of chromosomes by using hybrids with fragmented human chromosomes or by constructing a hybrid from a human cell line containing a structural chromosome rearrangement.

In situ hybridization

In situ hybridization is a technique that allows direct visualization of the chromosomal location of a DNA or RNA probe by hybridizing the probe to metaphase chromosome spreads on a slide. The chromosomes are first gently denatured, then a labeled probe is added under conditions that permit hybridization. When this technique was first developed, the probes were radiolabeled, which required long exposure under photographic emulsion, analysis of many metaphase spreads to distinguish true signals from background radioactivity, and finally, chromosome banding to identify the specific chromosome involved.

This technically demanding method has been largely replaced by use of probes labeled with fluorescent compounds that can be seen with a fluorescent microscope. With this method, which requires only 1 or 2 days, the position of the gene can be visualized in a single metaphase. When combined with banding techniques, fluorescence in situ hybridization can be used to map genes or other DNA sequences to within a specific band, or about 1 to 2 million bp.

MUTATION AND NORMAL VARIATION

A mutation is a permanent change in the DNA of an individual, specifically a change in the nucleotide sequence anywhere in the genome [Thompson et al., 1991]. Genetic diseases are caused by mutations that adversely affect function of one or more genes. The same is true for many types of cancer. But most mutations have little or no effect on gene function and therefore do not change the survival or reproductive fitness of an individual. Some of these mutations persist in the population as morphologic variants known as *polymorphisms*. By convention a genetic polymorphism is defined as the occurrence of two or more variants or alleles in a region of DNA where at least two alleles appear with frequencies greater than 1%. Alleles with frequencies of less than 1%, which include most mutations causing genetic diseases, are known as *rare variants*. The accumulation

over time of mutations at many different loci is the basis for both normal variation in the population and genetic diseases. Several of the methods used in modern molecular biology, such as restriction fragment length polymorphisms, take advantage of the normal variation between individuals.

Mutations have been subdivided into three main types including genome, chromosome, and gene mutations. They may occur in either somatic or germ cells, although only germ cell mutations can be transmitted to offspring. All three occur often enough to be observed in clinical medicine.

Genome and chromosome mutations

Genome mutations are caused by abnormal segregation of chromosomes during mitosis or meiosis that results in abnormal numbers of chromosomes in the daughter cells or offspring. Examples include trisomy 21, which is the most frequent cause of Down syndrome, and monosomy X, which causes Turner syndrome. The estimated rate of abnormal segregation in germ cells is one per 25 to 50 meiotic cell divisions. Chromosome mutations consist of several different types of rearrangements, including large deletions, duplications, insertions, inversions, and translocations. The frequency is about one per 1700 cell divisions. Both genome and chromosome mutations are rarely perpetuated because most are lethal during early pregnancy and result in spontaneous abortions. Thus the frequencies cited are probably underestimates.

Gene mutations

Gene mutations differ from genome and chromosome mutations because the segment of DNA involved is much smaller and the mechanisms are different. The most common types are base pair substitutions and small deletions or insertions that can be caused by an error during DNA replication or by base changes induced by an extrinsic agent referred to as a *mutagen*. Because genome and chromosome mutations are usually lethal, most significant heritable mutations are gene mutations.

Replication errors. DNA replication is normally a very accurate process. DNA polymerase, the enzyme responsible for DNA replication, inserts an incorrect base only once in every 10 million bp. A series of DNA repair enzymes exist that are able to recognize and replace noncomplementary bases, correcting more than 99.9% of errors. Thus the overall mutation rate is only 10^{-10} per base pair per cell division. The human genome consists of about 6×10^9 bp, so this mutation rate results in less than one base pair mutation per cell division. However, an estimated 10^{15} cell divisions occur during the lifetime of an adult human. Thus thousands of new mutations occur at virtually every position in the genome. Not surprisingly, inherited defects in DNA replication and repair enzymes lead to a striking increase in the frequencies of all types of mutations.

Most of the mutations occur in somatic cells, where they may cause cancer or a genetic disease affecting only part of the body, such as segmental neurofibromatosis. Fewer mutations occur in germ cells. Oogenesis consists of about 22 mitoses during fetal life and one meiosis that begins in fetal life and is then frozen until shortly before ovulation. Spermatogenesis consists of about 30 mitoses from conception until puberty, then about 20 to 25 per year thereafter. Thus the opportunity for mutations in sperm is expected to be greater than for ova. This finding has been observed in several genetic disorders, including some chromosome abnormalities, neurofibromatosis 1, achondroplasia, and hemophilia A. It has been estimated that as many as one in 10 sperm may carry a new deleterious mutation. Most are recessive or lethal and therefore are not apparent in liveborn children.

Mutation rate. The mutation rate for any given gene or other DNA segment depends on both its size and location. The location may be important because certain areas of the genome are known to be "hot spots" for recombination. The average mutation rate is about 1×10^{-6} mutations per locus per generation, but the rate varies over a thousandfold for different genes. For example, the number of new mutations per 10^6 gametes is 40 to 100 for Duchenne muscular dystrophy and neurofibromatosis 1, but only two to five for aniridia and hemophilia B. These statistics include only mutations causing genetic diseases. The rate of change of protein polymorphisms suggests a rate as high as 6×10^{-6} per locus per generation (a locus is defined as the position of a gene on a chromosome).

Molecular basis of mutations

The development and widespread use of modern molecular techniques has led to the discovery of specific mutations at many different loci. From among these, many different types of mutations have been recognized, all of which have the potential for causing genetic diseases. They may be divided by size into single and multiple base changes. The latter may involve only one or a few bases, or may involve millions of base pairs. In any specific gene, mutations are almost always heterogenous, although some types may be more common than others. Thus the specific mutations in unrelated individuals with the same genetic disease are often different.

Nucleotide substitutions

Point mutations or single-base substitutions represent one of the most common types of mutation. Most are related to an error in DNA synthesis by the enzyme DNA polymerase that was not corrected by DNA repair enzymes. However, more than 30% of point mutations discovered in some genetic diseases are the result of cytosine to thymine transitions, which are caused by

methylation of cytosine residues to 5-methylcytosine, especially cytosine residues occurring as the first base in a 5'-CG-3' dinucleotide pair. The latter then undergoes spontaneous deamination to thymidine. Thus the 5'-CG-3' doublet represents a "hot spot" for mutation in the human genome.

Deletions, duplications, and insertions

The remainder of mutations consists of loss or gain of nucleotide bases somewhere in the genome. A deletion consists of any loss of DNA sequence. A duplication consists of a second copy of a DNA sequence that is usually located immediately adjacent to the first copy. An insertion consists of a DNA sequence that has been removed or copied from one location and moved to a nonhomologous region elsewhere on the same chromosome or on a different chromosome. Deletions, duplications, and insertions that involve one or a few base pairs can only be detected by nucleotide sequencing. Large abnormalities may be detected by sequencing, restriction fragment length polymorphisms, fluorescence in situ hybridization, and several other methods.

Mechanisms. Several mechanisms resulting in deletions and duplications have been proposed, including recombination-, replication-, and repair-based models [Krawczak and Cooper, 1991]. The most frequent cause is probably nonhomologous pairing and unequal crossing over during meiosis 1. Many genes exist that are members of large multigene families that share substantial homology in their DNA sequences. The origin of these families is presumed to be ancient duplication events, followed by accumulation of different mutations in the two daughter genes. The alpha- and beta-globin gene families are good examples. Similarly, several of the repetitive DNA elements, especially the minisatellite, Alu, and L_1 families, consist of many short DNA segments, with similar or identical DNA sequences scattered throughout the genome. When the members of multigene or repetitive DNA families are located in tandem (head to tail) in the same chromosomal region, they may misalign and pair incorrectly during meiosis 1. A recombination event between the mispaired homologs results in a duplication or deletion, as shown in Figure 24-9.

Insertions occur much less frequently than either deletions or duplications, and the mechanisms are not well understood. The best example involves the L_1 family of interspersed repetitive sequences, which are capable of moving to different sites in the genome through an RNA-mediated process. In two unrelated patients with hemophilia A, L_1 sequences several kilobases long were inserted into an exon in the factor VIII gene, interrupting the coding sequence and inactivating the gene.

Effects of mutations on gene function

The effect of mutations on gene function depends as much or more on the specific location of the mutation as

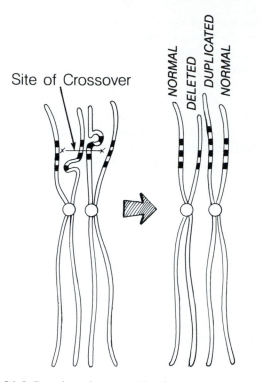

Site of Crossover

NORMAL
DELETED
DUPLICATED
NORMAL

Figure 24-9 Drawing of a recombination event between mispaired homologs during meiosis 1. On the left side of the drawing, the far right and far left chromatids have paired correctly, whereas the middle two chromatids have paired incorrectly. A crossover within the mispaired region results in one daughter chromosome with a duplication and another with a deletion, shown on the right side of the drawing. The *dark squares* represent a repetitive sequence.

on the size. Mutations that occur in DNA outside functioning genes usually have no consequences. Mutations within the boundaries of a gene may inactivate it, or have little or no effect, depending on the nature of the change.

Missense mutations. A point mutation within the coding region of a gene can alter the genetic code by changing the nucleotide triplet and cause the replacement of one amino acid by another in the gene product. Function of the gene product may be altered. Such mutations are called *missense mutations,* and do not change the reading frame of the DNA sequence. The best known example is the adenine to thymine substitution in the sixth codon of the beta-globin gene, which causes sickle cell anemia, by substituting valine for glutamic acid in the beta-globin chain; however, not all mutations within the coding region result in a missense mutation. All but two of the 20 amino acids are specified by more than one codon, most often differing in the third position of the triplet. The gene product will be identical if the new triplet codes for the same amino acid.

Transcriptional control mutations. Mutations involving the 5′ promoter region or 3′ untranslated regions of a gene may result in a significant decrease in the amount of mature, processed messenger RNA produced. Both base substitutions and nucleotide loss or gain mutations may result in transcriptional control mutations.

Chain termination (nonsense) mutations. Mutations that generate one of the three stop codons result in premature termination of translation, whereas those that alter a stop codon allow translation to continue until the next stop codon is reached. Those mutations that result in a premature stop codon are called *nonsense mutations.* In general, these mutations have no effect on transcription (DNA-RNA), but the shortened polypeptide may be so unstable that it is rapidly degraded in the cell. Both base substitutions and nucleotide loss/gain mutations may result in nonsense mutations. A typical example is a mutation in exon 3 of the human phenylalanine hydroxylase gene that changes the codon from CGA (arginine) to TGA (stop). This mutation results in premature chain termination and the classic phenylketonuria phenotype [Eisensmith and Woo, 1992].

RNA splicing mutations. Mutations that occur adjacent to an exon/intron boundary may alter RNA splicing and prevent normal messenger RNA processing. The splicing reactions are guided by specific DNA sequences at both the 5′ and 3′ ends of introns. The upstream or 5′ sequence, called the *donor site,* consists of nine bases, of which two (a GT dinucleotide located on the downstream side of the splice site at the start of the intron) are invariant. The downstream or 3′ sequence, called the acceptor site, consists of about 12 bases of which two (an AG dinucleotide located just upstream of the splice site) are obligatory for normal splicing.

Splicing mutations may either inactivate existing splice sites or create new ones. In the first type the mutation alters either the splice donor or the acceptor site, and the intron at that site will not be spliced out. This mutation effectively results in a large insertion in the processed messenger RNA. A stop codon often occurs as the intron is translated. In the second type, mutations within the intron create alternative donor or acceptor sites that compete with the normal splice sites during RNA processing. A proportion of the mature messenger RNA may contain incorrectly spliced intron sequences. Both base substitutions and nucleotide loss/gain mutations may result in splicing mutations. One example of the first type is a guanine to cytosine transition in the first position of the intron at the donor splice site in the hexosaminidase A gene found in a proportion of Ashkenazi Jewish patients with Tay-Sachs disease [Thompson et al., 1991]. In this example the bases in the exon are underlined, whereas those in the intron are not.

Normal hexosaminidase A allele
5′ . . . CCAGGCTCTGGTAAGGGT . . . 3′
Tay-Sachs allele
5′ . . . CCAGGCTCTGCTAAGGGT . . . 3′

Frameshift mutations. Small nucleotide loss or gain mutations may alter the reading frame of the messenger RNA product from the point of the mutation on, which results in a completely different amino acid sequence at the carboxyl end of the protein product or premature chain termination if a stop codon is encountered in the new reading frame. Any loss or gain mutation that involves a multiple of three bases maintains the reading frame, whereas a mutation that does not involve a multiple of three changes the reading frame. Larger deletions that include one or more introns may also cause a frameshift mutation because exon/intron splice sites may occur at any point in the reading frame, thus splitting codons. If the exon just downstream from the deletion normally begins at a different position in the triplet than the deleted intron, the reading frame will be changed. In contrast, base substitutions do not cause frameshift mutations. Deletions and insertions cause dysfunction of the gene more often than point mutations because of the possibility of a frameshift. One of the best known examples is a single base deletion in the ABO blood group locus that results in the nonfunctional O allele. The deletion alters the reading frame at codon 86 until a premature stop codon is reached 30 codons later. The stop codon is normally out of frame and therefore not read.

Large deletions and insertions. If the DNA segment involved in a deletion, duplication, or insertion is 3 to 5 million bp or more, an abnormality may be visible by high-resolution chromosome analysis or by routine chromosome analysis if the segment is larger. DNA segments of this size may contain 50 to 100 or more genes. Several clinical syndromes caused by deletions or duplications of a small number of genes have been described, which have been variably termed microdeletion, contiguous gene, or segmental aneusomy syndromes. Examples include the WAGR (Wilms tumor, aniridia, genital hypoplasia, retardation) syndrome in chromosome band 11p13, retinoblastoma mental retardation syndrome on 13q14, Prader-Willi and Angelman syndromes in 15q11-13, and Miller-Dieker syndrome in 17p13 [Ledbetter and Cavenee, 1989].

CLINICAL CYTOGENETICS

Chromosome abnormalities may involve either the number or structure of chromosomes. The former are considered genome mutations and the latter chromosome mutations. The mechanisms involved in the two major types of mutations are quite different, but both may result in loss or gain of DNA in the nucleus. Both types may involve all the cells of an organism or only a proportion; in such cases the abnormality is termed *mosaic*.

Abnormalities of chromosome number

For germ and somatic cells the normal chromosome complement consists of the haploid and diploid number, respectively. Any deviation from these numbers is associated with significant abnormalities.

Triploidy and tetraploidy. Occasionally, fetuses with three or four times the normal haploid number have been observed. These abnormal chromosome complements are called *triploidy* (3n) and *tetraploidy* (4n). The few who are liveborn survive only briefly after birth. Triploidy results from failure of a maturational division in either egg or sperm. Tetraploidy results from failure of completion of an early division of the zygote.

Aneuploidy. Aneuploidy is defined as any chromosome complement other than a multiple of the haploid number. In the majority of cases, it consists of either monosomy, which is defined as loss of an entire chromosome, or trisomy, which refers to gain of an entire chromosome. Aneuploidy is the most common and clinically significant type of chromosome disorder, occurring in 3% to 4% of all recognized pregnancies.

Both monosomy and trisomy of autosomes are lethal during early pregnancy in a large majority of affected fetuses. Autosomal monosomy is uniformly lethal except for a few reports of liveborn children with monosomy 21. Monosomy X is prenatally lethal in most affected fetuses, but many survive and will have the phenotype of Turner syndrome. The effects of trisomy vary depending on the chromosome involved. Trisomy 16 is the most frequent autosomal trisomy at conception but is uniformly lethal before birth. The most common type of trisomy in liveborn infants is trisomy 21, which is the chromosome abnormality observed in 95% of children with Down syndrome. The only other autosomal trisomies observed at appreciable frequencies are trisomy 13 and trisomy 18, although trisomy 8 may be observed in mosaic form.

The most common mechanism is nondisjunction, which is the failure of a pair of chromosomes to separate correctly during one of the two stages of meiosis, usually meiosis 1. The consequences of nondisjunction during meiosis 1 and 2 are somewhat different. If the error occurs during meiosis 1, the unbalanced gamete with 24 chromosomes contains both the maternal and the paternal members of the pair. If the error occurs during meiosis 2, the unbalanced gamete will contain either the maternally—or paternally—derived chromosome, but not both.

Abnormalities of chromosome structure

Structural rearrangements consist of loss, gain, or abnormal location in the genome of chromosome segments rather than whole chromosomes. The most common types include deleted or duplicated segments and translocation, in which two chromosomal segments exchange positions. All occur less frequently than aneuploidy. The mechanisms causing rearrangements are not well understood. In many instances, chromosomes may simply break or break and rejoin a different segment from the same or another chromosome that happens to be nearby at the time, producing an abnormal configuration. Another mechanism is unequal crossing over, which is probably the cause of most intrachromosomal deletions and duplications (see Fig. 24-9).

Structural rearrangements are termed *balanced* if the chromosome set has the normal amount of genetic information, regardless of its location. They are termed *unbalanced* if there has been either loss or gain of DNA sequence. The phenotypic effects are usually severe. The chromosomes involved in the reconfiguration are known as *derivative chromosomes.* Many different types of rearrangements have been reported, and the following sections describe them. When the centromere and both telomeres are present and functioning, the derivative chromosome is stable and capable of being transmitted unaltered to daughter cells during mitosis or meiosis. Other types may be unstable during cell division.

Balanced rearrangements

Balanced chromosome rearrangements do not usually have phenotypic effects because the normal amount of genetic information is present; however, exceptions do occur. One of the breakpoints may disrupt a gene, or the

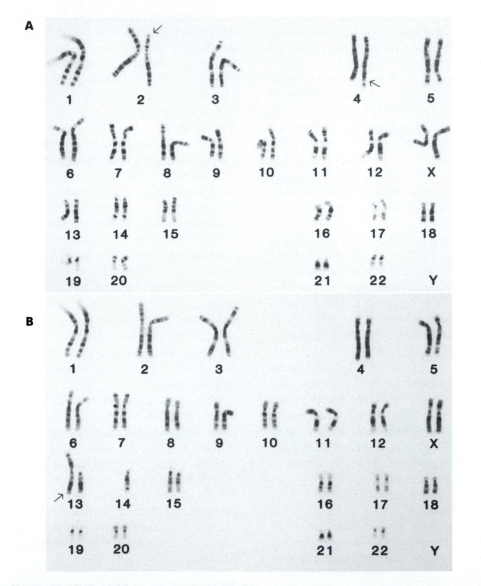

Figure 24-10 Partial karyotypes of several different types of structural rearrangements. **A,** reciprocal translocation; 46,XX,t(2;4)(p22.2;q35.2). **B,** Robertsonian translocation: 45,XX,t(13q14q).   *(Figure continues.)*

rearrangement may appear to be balanced when actually a significant amount of genetic material, but too little to be detected under the microscope, has been lost. Rearrangements pose a much greater risk to the next generation because of the high frequency of unbalanced gametes produced.

Reciprocal translocations. Reciprocal translocations consist of breaks in nonhomologous chromosomes, with reciprocal exchange of the broken segments (Figure 24-10, *A*). Usually only two chromosomes are involved, but rarely complex translocations involving three or more chromosomes have been described. Population studies have detected either reciprocal or Robertsonian translocations in about 1 in 500 newborns.

Reciprocal translocations often result in the production of unbalanced gametes. During meiosis 1 the derivative chromosomes and their normal homologs form a quadriradial shape that may separate into pairs in one of three ways, known as *alternate, adjacent 1,* and *adjacent 2 segregation.* Alternate segregation produces balanced gametes that have either normal chromosomes or both derivatives, which are therefore balanced. Adjacent 1 segregation produces unbalanced gametes in which homologous centromeres separate into different daughter cells. It results in duplication of the distal segment of one derivative chromosome and deletion of the distal tip of the other. The types of balanced and unbalanced offspring conceived by a reciprocal translo-

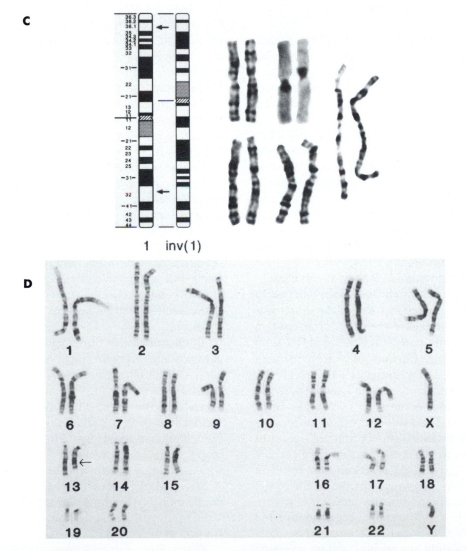

Figure 24-10 cont'd   C, pericentric inversion: 46,XX,inv(1)(p36.1q32). The upper right pair are C-banded chromosomes; the others are G-banded. D, interstitial deletion: 46,XY,del(13)(q21.3q31). (**Karyotypes in A, B,** and **D** courtesy of B. Hirsch, Department of Laboratory Medicine and Pathology, University of Minnesota Hospital and Clinic. C from Johnson DD, Dobyns WB, Gordon H, et al. Hum Genet 1988; 79:315.   *(Figure continues.)*

E

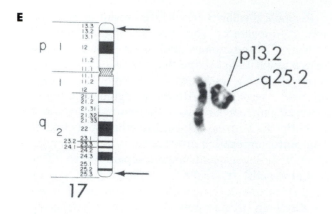

Figure 24-10 cont'd **E,** ring: 46,XY,r(17)(p13.3q25.3). (**E** from Dobyns WB, Stratton RF, Parke JT et al. J Pediatr 1983; 102:552.)

cation carrier and his normal mate are shown in Figure 24-11. Adjacent 2 segregation, which is rare, also produces unbalanced gametes, but homologous centromeres pass to the same daughter cell. Although rare, nondisjunction resulting in 3:1 and even 4:0 segregation may occur.

Reciprocal translocations are often detected in phenotypically normal adults evaluated because of repeated fetal loss or after birth of a child with multiple congenital anomalies related to transmission of the translocation in unbalanced form. Apparently balanced reciprocal translocations are sometimes observed in children with birth defects or abnormal development, in whom the abnormal phenotype may be the result of submicroscopic loss, a disrupted gene, or unrelated factors.

Robertsonian translocations. Robertsonian translocations involve two acrocentric chromosomes that fuse in or near the centromere region with loss of the short arms (see Figure 24-10, *B*). Because the short arms contain repetitive DNA elements, especially ribosomal RNA, no phenotypic effect occurs. Carriers of a Robertsonian translocation involving chromosome 21 have a high risk of producing a child with translocation Down syndrome.

Inversions. Inversions occur when two breaks occur in a single chromosome and the intervening segment is inverted. In paracentric inversions, both breaks occur in the same arm; in pericentric inversions, one break occurs in each arm (see Figure 24-10, *C*). Both may result in production of unbalanced gametes as the result of the effects of recombination within the inverted segment. During meiosis 1 a loop is formed between the inverted chromosome and its homolog. Recombination is somewhat but not completely suppressed within inversion loops, so crossovers are common in larger loops.

Crossovers within a paracentric inversion loop result in acentric or dicentric chromosomes. The genetic imbalance in offspring is so great that almost all are

spontaneously aborted. Recombination within a pericentric inversion loop produces derivative chromosomes in which segments distal to the breaks are duplicated or deleted (Figure 24-12). The phenotypic effects are inversely proportional to the size of the inversion. For small pericentric inversions the distal segments are often large, and most unbalanced offspring are spontaneously aborted. Liveborn children with birth defects are more likely with larger inversions because the distal segments are relatively small.

Insertions. Insertions occur when a small segment of a chromosome is removed and inserted into a different region on the same or another chromosome. If the segment is inserted with the same orientation with respect to the centromere, it is known as a *direct insertion.* The reverse orientation is called an *inverted insertion.* Insertions are rare because three separate chromosomal breaks are required. Segregation during meiosis can produce abnormal offspring with duplication or deletion of the inserted segment in addition to normal offspring and balanced carriers.

Unbalanced rearrangements

Deletions. A deletion consists of loss of a chromosome segment. It may be either interstitial or terminal, the latter including the telomere in the deletion (see Figure 24-10, *D*). Most interstitial deletions are believed to be the result of unequal crossing over (see Figure 24-9); terminal deletions are more likely to result from simple breakage. Alternatively, many or even all terminal deletions may actually be interstitial deletions in which one breakpoint happens to be close to the telomere. Any carrier of a deletion is hemizygous for the information on the corresponding segment of the normal homolog. Thus small but cytogenetically visible deletions involving critical genes occasionally produce mendelian phenotypes, such as retinoblastoma or Duchenne muscular dystrophy.

Duplications. A duplication consists of gain of a chromosomal segment, most often by unequal crossing over. Thus duplicated segments are usually adjacent. In general the phenotypic effects of duplications are less severe than the effects of deletion of a similar segment. Rather unexpectedly, small duplications can also result in mendelian phenotypes. After discovery of submicroscopic duplications of band 17p11.2 in many patients with hereditary motor and sensory neuropathy type I (Charcot-Marie-Tooth disease), a patient with visible duplication of the short arm of 17 proved to have the same neuropathic changes on nerve conduction studies [Lupski et al., 1992].

Rings. Ring chromosomes are formed when a chromosome undergoes two breaks and the broken ends are rejoined (see Figure 24-10, *E*). The segments distal to the breaks are lost, resulting in deletion of both tips of the chromosome. Rings may not segregate properly

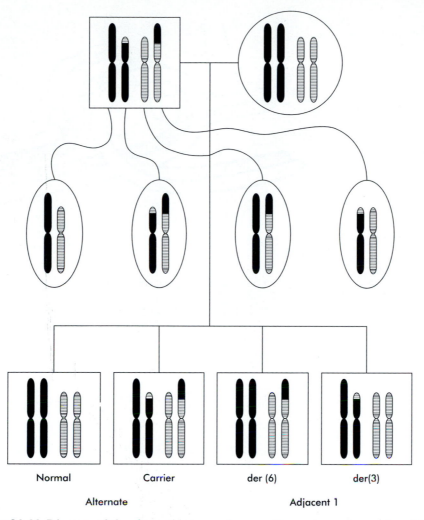

Normal   **Carrier**   **der (6)**   **der(3)**

Alternate   Adjacent 1

Figure 24-11 Diagram of the alternative types of segregation and gametes produced in the carrier of a reciprocal translocation between the short arms of chromosomes 3 *(solid black)* and 6 *(hatched)*. The top line represents the parental chromosome pairs, the middle line represents the four types of gametes produced by the father, and the bottom line represents four possible chromosome combinations that may be observed in offspring. Alternate segregation *(shown on the left)* produces offspring with either normal chromosomes or the balanced translocation. Adjacent 1 segregation *(shown on the right)* produces offspring with unbalanced karyotypes. Children with the derivative *(6)* karyotype have deletion of the distal segment of 6p and duplication of the distal segment of 3p. Children with the derivative *(3)* karyotype have deletion of 3p and duplication of 6p. In both alternate and adjacent 1 segregation, homologous centromeres pass to different daughter cells. In adjacent-2 segregation (not shown), homologous centromeres pass to the same daughter cells, leading to even greater chromosomal imbalance.

during mitosis and meiosis, especially if a crossover occurs. This often results in breakage followed by fusion, which may produce larger or smaller rings.

Isochromosomes and dicentrics. Isochromosomes are chromosomes in which one arm is missing and the other is duplicated as the result of misdivision of the centromere during meiosis 2 or translocation of one arm to its homolog with a breakpoint adjacent to the centromere. The most commonly observed isochromosome involves Xq. Dicentrics are rare chromosomes in

which two segments, each containing a centromere, fuse end to end. They tend to break during mitosis because of the double centromeres.

Nomenclature

Extensive rules regarding nomenclature of chromosomes and chromosome abnormalities have been published [ISCN, 1985]. Examples of each of the major types of abnormalities using the standard nomenclature are listed in Table 24-2. Note that breakpoints on the same

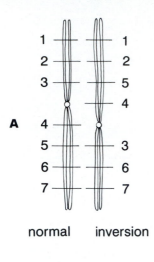

Figure 24-12 The effect of recombination within the loop of a pericentric inversion. **A,** A normal chromosome is shown on the right with loci 1 to 7 in order and the centromere located between loci 3 and 4. A pericentric inversion is shown on the left with the segment containing loci 3 to 5 and the centromere inverted. **B,** Pairing of the normal and inverted chromosomes during meiosis 1, with a crossover occurring within the inversion loop in the middle two chromatids. **C,** The four types of gametes produced after completion of meiosis include a normal chromosome, a derivative chromosome with duplication of the distal short arm and deletion of the distal long arm *(dup p)*, the reverse derivative chromosome with duplication of the distal long arm and deletion of the distal short arm *(dup q)*, and a balanced pericentric inversion.

chromosome are not separated by any punctuation, whereas breakpoints on different chromosomes are always separated by a semicolon.

PATTERNS OF INHERITANCE
Single gene inheritance

Any discussion of single gene inheritance requires familiarity with a special vocabulary. A gene was previously defined as a sequence of DNA that is required for production of a functional product. The position of a gene on a chromosome is known as its *locus.* The alternative forms of a gene that may occupy a given locus are known as *alleles.* When both alleles at a given locus are identical, the individual is said to be homozygous for that trait. When the alleles are different, the individual is heterozygous. When only one allele is present, the individual is hemizygous. The best example of the latter concerns X-linked traits in males, who have only one X chromosome.

The genetic constitution of an individual is the genotype. At any given locus the genotype consists of either a single allele (for genes on the X chromosome in males) or a pair of alleles. The observable expression of the genotype is the phenotype. Penetrance is the percentage of individuals with a particular genotype who are actually affected. It is an all-or-none phenomenon. Expressivity is the extent to which a genetic trait or disease is expressed and may vary greatly between affected individuals. The proband is the family member through whom a family was identified. A pedigree is a diagram of the family history that lists the family members, their relationships to the proband, and their status with regard to the hereditary condition. The standard symbols used for pedigrees in medical genetics are illustrated in Figure 24-13.

The specific pattern of single gene or mendelian inheritance depends on the chromosomal location of the gene and on the genotype required for expression. The trait is autosomal when the gene is located on human chromosomes 1 to 22 and X-linked when located on the X chromosome. A trait is considered dominant when it is expressed in both heterozygotes and homozygotes and recessive when expressed only in homozygotes; therefore the four major patterns of inheritance are autosomal-dominant, autosomal-recessive, X-linked dominant, and X-linked recessive. However, several nonclassic patterns of inheritance have been recognized.

Autosomal-dominant inheritance. The most important attributes of autosomal-dominant inheritance are expression of the trait in heterozygotes and male-to-male transmission. This pattern may be recognized because (1) the trait or disease appears in every generation except that it may arise by new mutation in the first affected family member, (2) any child of an affected person has a 50% risk of inheriting the trait, (3) the offspring of unaffected family members are also unaffected, and (4) the trait may be transmitted by a parent of either sex to a child of either sex, and specifically may be transmitted from father to son, which distinguishes it from X-linked inheritance. A typical pedigree is illustrated in Figure 24-14, *A*.

Autosomal-dominant inheritance is readily identified in most families but may be difficult to discern in others. If the disease is the result of a new mutation, no relatives are affected. Reduced penetrance, low expressivity, and late age of onset may result in failure to recognize other affected family members. Among the best examples for each of these mechanisms are myotonic dystrophy and Huntington disease. Finally, incorrect information on family relationships, such as false paternity, may complicate interpretation of the pedigree.

Most patients with autosomal-dominant disorders are heterozygotes, but occasionally a homozygous individual

Table 24-2 Examples of chromosome abnormalities using standard nomenclature (short system)

Reciprocal translocation	
Balanced	46,XY,t(7;17) (p22.3;p13.3)
Unbalanced	46,XX,-17, + der(17),t(7;17) (p22.3;p13.3)pat
Robertsonian translocation	
Balanced	46,XX,rob(13;21)
Unbalanced	46,XY,-13, + der(13),rob(13;21)mat
Paracentric inversion	46,XX,inv(1) (p32p36.1)
Pericentric inversion	
Balanced	46,XX,inv(1) (p36.1q32)
Unbalanced	46,XY,dup(q),inv(1) (p36.1q32)mat
Deletion	
Terminal	46,XY,del(8) (p21.1)
Interstitial	46,XX,del(17) (p11.2p11.2)
Duplication	46,XY,dir dup (2) (p14p23)
Ring	46,XY,r(17) (p13.3q22.3)

del, deletion; *der*, derivative; *dir*, direct; *dup*, duplication; *inv*, inversion; *mat*, maternal; *pat*, paternal; *r*, ring; *rob*, Robertsonian translocation; *t*, translocation.

is encountered. Generally, the phenotype in homozygous individuals is more severe than in heterozygous persons. For example, one child born to parents who each had hereditary motor and sensory neuropathy type I had a severe phenotype consistent with Dejerine-Sottas disease or hereditary motor and sensory neuropathy type III [Killian and Kloepfer, 1979]. The only known exception to this rule is Huntington disease.

Autosomal-recessive inheritance. The most important attributes of autosomal recessive inheritance are expression in homozygotes and equal sex distribution. This pattern may be recognized because (1) the trait or disease appears in only one generation and in a sibship rather than in parents, children, or other relatives of the affected person, (2) each full sibling of an affected person has a 25% chance of inheriting the trait, (3) the parents are more likely than usual to be related, and (4) with rare exceptions, males and females are equally likely to be affected. A typical pedigree is shown in Figure 24-14, *B*.

In our culture, many and probably most children appear as isolated cases, with no affected relatives because of small family size and the tendency of parents to stop bearing children after the birth of an abnormal child. This finding does not hold true in many other cultures, especially in inbred populations. When the

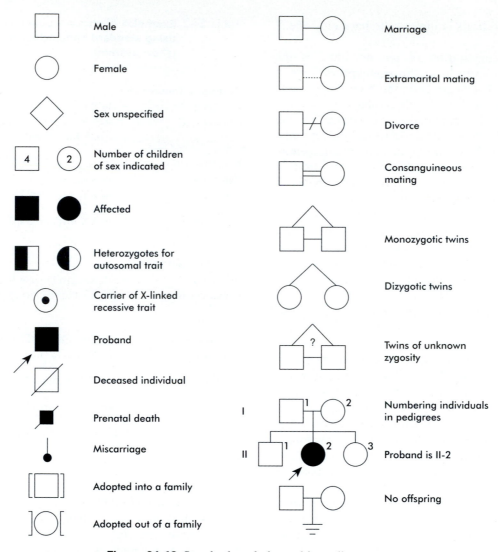

Figure 24-13 Standard symbols used in pedigrees.

frequency of a rare recessive allele is relatively high within a family or population, the disease may appear in more than one generation. This is known as *pseudodominant* inheritance.

Consanguinity. Most of the alleles for autosomal recessive diseases in a population are present in carriers rather than in homozygous affected individuals (refer to the Hardy-Weinberg law in a following section). They can be passed from parent to child for many generations without ever appearing in homozygous form. It is believed that every individual carries several genes (perhaps 10 to 20) that would be disabling or lethal if homozygous. The presence of such hidden recessive genes is not revealed unless the carrier happens to mate with someone who carries the same mutation or a different mutation at the same locus and both disease alleles are inherited by a child.

The chance that a child will inherit two disease alleles is greatly increased if the parents are consanguineous or related by descent. More formally, the probability that

a homozygote has received both alleles of a pair from an identical ancestral source is known as the coefficient of inbreeding. It is also the proportion of loci at which a person is homozygous by descent. For example, any child born to first cousins is homozygous at $\frac{1}{16}$ of all loci. Although the relative risk of abnormal offspring is higher for related than unrelated parents, it is still relatively low, about 5%.

X-linked recessive inheritance. The most important characteristic of X-linked recessive inheritance is expression primarily in hemizygous males. This pattern may be recognized because (1) the incidence of the trait is much higher in males than in females, (2) the gene is never transmitted from father to son but is transmitted from a father to all daughters who are then heterozygous, (3) the trait may be transmitted through a series of carriers or heterozygous females, so that all affected males in a family are related through females, and (4) heterozygous females are, with rare exceptions, unaffected. A typical pedigree is illustrated in Figure 24-14,

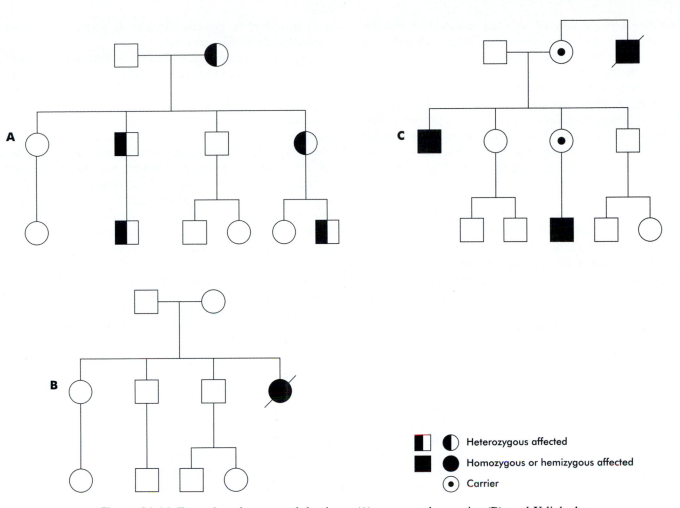

Figure 24-14 Examples of autosomal-dominant **(A)**, autosomal recessive **(B)**, and X-linked recessive pedigrees **(C).**

▮ ◖	Heterozygous affected
◼ ●	Homozygous or hemizygous affected
⊙	Carrier

C. Examples relevant to pediatric neurology include adrenoleukodystrophy, Duchenne and Becker muscular dystrophy, and Menkes disease.

X-linked recessive inheritance may not be apparent in some families for several reasons. First, a large proportion of cases may represent new mutations. For genetically lethal conditions (disorders in which affected persons do not reproduce), such as Duchenne muscular dystrophy, one third of all cases are caused by new mutations. This occurrence was first determined theoretically by Haldane but has since been confirmed by observation. Second, the number of males born in a family may be small.

There are several mechanisms by which females may be affected. The first is lyonization, or the process of X inactivation. In each cell of a female mammal, only one X chromosome is active, and the other is inactive. The process by which one X chromosome becomes inactive is usually random; therefore most females have an even proportion of cells, with one or the other X chromosome inactivated. By chance, some females have a high proportion (such as 90%) of one X chromosome inactivated. If this happens to be the X carrying a disease gene, she will be normal. If this happens to be the X carrying the normal gene, she will manifest signs of the disease. There are several less common reasons why females may have an X-linked recessive disease. Women with Turner syndrome have only one X chromosome and may be hemizygous. Finally, common diseases, such as X-linked color blindness, can occur when a carrier mother mates with an affected father. Half of the daughters from such a mating will be homozygous and affected.

X-linked-dominant inheritance. The most important characteristics of X-linked-dominant inheritance are expression in both heterozygous females and hemizygous males and lack of male-to-male transmission. This pattern may be recognized because (1) affected males with normal mates have no affected sons, but all their daughters are affected, (2) both male and female offspring of affected females have a 50% risk for inheriting the condition, (3) the incidence of affected females is twice that of affected males, and (4) the phenotype in affected males is often more severe than in affected females. One example is ornithine transcarbamylase deficiency.

In addition to the known X-linked dominant diseases, a small group of diseases is observed exclusively or almost exclusively in females. It has been proposed that these are all X-linked dominant diseases that are lethal before birth in hemizygous males. Several of these diseases are relevant to pediatric neurology, including Aicardi, Goltz, and Rett syndromes, and orofaciodigital syndrome type I.

Nonclassic patterns of inheritance

Mitochondrial inheritance. Mitochondria are cellular organelles that are primarily responsible for cellular respiration and production of adenosine triphosphate. Each mitochondrion contains multiple copies of a small 16.5 kb circular chromosome that codes for 13 proteins. These proteins are components of the respiratory chain, as well as many ribosomal RNA and transfer RNA genes that differ from the nuclear ribosomal RNA and transfer RNA genes. The remainder of the respiratory pathway enzymes are coded by nuclear genes.

Mitochondria are derived almost exclusively from the mother through the mitochondria of the ovum. Each ova contains hundreds of mitochondria, with a variable proportion being mutant and normal. Thus diseases caused by mutations in mitochondrial DNA must exhibit strict maternal inheritance and should exhibit phenotypic variation within a family because the proportion of mutant and normal mitochondria may vary from individual to individual [Zeviani et al., 1989]. Maternal inheritance may be recognized because (1) the incidence of the disease is equal in males and females, (2) the disease is transmitted from mother to offspring of both sexes, but never from father to offspring, and (3) variable expression is common. These criteria have been met for several diseases, most of which affect the nervous system and muscle. Examples include Kearns-Sayre syndrome, Leber hereditary optic neuropathy, MELAS (*mitochondrial encephalomyopathy, lactic acidosis and strokelike episodes*) syndrome, and MERRF (*myoclonus epilepsy with ragged-red fibers*). Specific mutations of mitochondrial DNA have been discovered in each of the four.

Somatic mosaicism. A mosaic is an individual or tissue that contains two or more cell lines that differ in DNA sequence, although they are derived from a single zygote. Differently stated, all organisms begin with a specific DNA sequence in the cell of origin or zygote. As cell multiplication occurs, some mutations occur that produce small differences among different cell lines. Mosaicism is clinically important in many chromosome disorders and probably explains many other disorders in which only part of the body appears to be affected with a birth defect or genetic disease. A good example is segmental neurofibromatosis.

Germline mosaicism. Autosomal-dominant diseases caused by new mutations usually do not recur in any of the siblings of the patient. However, there are several explanations for the rare occasions when this has been observed. The simplest are reduced penetrance and variable expressivity. Another potentially important cause is germline mosaicism. During early development of the parent a somatic mutation may occur in the germline or its precursors, which may persist in the clonal descendants of that cell, including a proportion of the ova or sperm. When the mutation exists only in the germline, the parent has no signs of the disease but may conceive more than one affected child. If the mutation exists in several different cell lines, the parent may have mild expression of the disease. This occurrence has been documented most often in Duchenne muscular dystrophy and in the autosomal-dominant form of osteogenesis imperfecta, which is caused by mutation in the COL1A2 gene.

Genomic imprinting. With classic mendelian inheritance the expression of a trait or disease is expected to be the same regardless of whether the gene was inherited from the mother or father. However, significant differences in expression based on the sex of the transmitting parent have been observed in several disorders. This phenomenon is known as *imprinting* and is believed to be related to differences in the state of the maternal and paternal contributions to the genome. The mechanism of imprinting is not known. It has been associated with differences in DNA methylation patterns, but these are likely secondary [Hall, 1990].

For example, the severe congenital form of myotonic dystrophy occurs only in affected children born to affected mothers. The age of onset of Huntington disease is usually earlier if the gene was inherited from the father instead of the mother. The expression of neurofibromatosis 1 is, on average, more severe when the disease allele is inherited from the mother. The most striking examples of imprinting are Prader-Willi and Angelman syndromes. Small deletions of chromosome band 15q11-13 result in Prader-Willi syndrome if the deleted chromosome was inherited from the father and in Angelman syndrome if inherited from the mother [Ledbetter and Cavenee, 1989].

Uniparental disomy. Uniparental disomy is defined as the presence of a diploid cell line containing two chromosome homologs inherited from the same parent. When the two homologs are identical, it is called *uniparental isodisomy*. When different, it is known as *uniparental heterodisomy*. This unusual condition is believed to result from nondisjunction, which results in trisomy for a particular chromosome, followed by loss of one of the three homologs, reducing the chromosome number back to normal. It can result in disease by at least two different mechanisms. The first is by identifying recessive diseases that occur only with uniparental isodisomy. Because the two chromosomes are identical, they are homologous at all loci. When any recessive disease loci exist on the chromosome, the individual will be homozygous and thus affected. The second is related to genetic imprinting and may occur with either type of uniparental disomy. Some patients with Prader-Willi syndrome have no deletion of chromosome 15 but do have uniparental disomy, in which both copies of chromosome 15 are inherited from the mother. At first, this finding appears to be contradictory to the paternal origin of deletions, but both mechanisms result in the lack of a paternally derived chromosome 15. Similarly, Angelman syndrome is sometimes associated with uniparental disomy, in which both chromosome 15 homologs are inherited from the father.

Multifactorial inheritance. Among genetic diseases, both single gene and chromosome disorders occur much less frequently than common disorders that appear to run in some families but do not follow any of the known patterns of inheritance. Most of these are believed to have multifactorial inheritance, which is defined as inheritance by a combination of genetic factors and sometimes extrinsic factors, each with a relatively small effect. For most the genetic component is believed to consist of one or a few "major" genes and a larger number of "minor" genes that contribute to the phenotype.

Multifactorial disorders have a number of characteristics that differ from single gene disorders. For example, there is no clear pattern of inheritance within a single family, although more than one relative may be affected. The risk to first-degree relatives is approximately the square root of the population risk. As a consequence, the lower the population risk, the relatively greater the risk for first-degree relatives. The risk is much lower for second-degree than for first-degree relatives, but it declines less rapidly for more remote relatives. Finally, the recurrence risk is higher when more than one family member is affected. There are many examples of diseases with multifactorial inheritance, including neural tube defects, congenital heart defects, and cleft lip and palate.

HUMAN GENE MAP

In the years after rediscovery of Mendel's work, occasional exceptions to his law of segregation were discovered in which the expected segregation ratios were distorted. These observations were eventually explained by proposing that traits that did not sort independently were located on the same chromosome; however, it was not possible to determine which genes were located on which chromosomes. These early efforts gradually evolved into the field of linkage analysis and gene mapping, which now encompasses one of the most ambitious scientific projects ever undertaken, the Human Genome Project.

There are two separate but complementary approaches useful for constructing maps of genes and chromosomes. Genetic mapping is based on family studies of the tendency of certain genes to segregate together. Physical mapping makes use of many of the methods of molecular biology to assign genes to particular locations along a chromosome.

Linkage and genetic mapping

Genetic mapping depends on the behavior of chromosomes during meiosis 1, specifically the occurrence of recombination or crossing over during late prophase [Conneally, 1989; Thompson et al., 1991]. On average, most chromosomes have one to three chiasmata or crossovers per meiotic division, which provides ample opportunity for segregation of genes that are syntenic (i.e., located on same chromosome).

Given this complex process, there are four possible ways for pairs of alleles to segregate during meiosis. Alleles on different chromosomes always sort independently. Alleles located very far apart on the same chromosome also sort independently because the likelihood of one or more recombination events between them is very high. In contrast, alleles located very close together on the same chromosome almost always are transmitted together. Finally, alleles located on the same chromosome but separated by intermediate distances are transmitted together most of the time but are occasionally separated by recombination events, resulting in a distorted segregation ratio in offspring.

Linkage analysis. With this background, genetic linkage may be defined as the tendency for alleles close together on the same chromosome to be transmitted together as a unit during meiosis. The strength of linkage can be used as a unit of measurement to determine the relative distance separating the two loci. The unit of measurement used for linkage, which is called a *morgan,* is the length of a chromosomal segment over which, on average, one recombination event is observed per meiosis. Thus a centimorgan (cM) is the genetic length over which recombination is observed 1% of the time. It translates to approximately one million base pairs of DNA. However, the frequency of recombination is not constant along the length of a chromosome; therefore the genetic distance measured in centimorgans may vary significantly in physical size in different parts of the genome.

The principal value of genetic linkage analysis is to aid in identifying and mapping the genes responsible for inherited diseases. Then a combination of genetic linkage and physical mapping techniques may lead to identification of the gene, even when the nature of the disorder is not understood, as has been accomplished for cystic fibrosis, Duchenne and Becker muscular dystrophies, neurofibromatosis 1, and several other genes. There are two major requirements for successful linkage analysis. First, genetic polymorphisms in the family must be informative; that is, the different alleles present at each loci must be known or be able to be determined. Second, the particular alignment or phase should be known; that is, which alleles at the two (or more) loci are on the same chromosome and which are on the other chromosome of a homologous pair.

To demonstrate the process, assume that two genetic loci, A and B, are to be tested in a series of families to establish linkage. The manner in which the loci are identified does not matter so long as two or more variations or alleles may be recognized. For example, the loci may be a genetic disease identified by phenotype, a biochemical polymorphism, such as a blood group or electrophoretic variant of an enzyme, a restriction fragment length polymorphism, or even a cloned gene. Among informative matings, assume that 90% of offspring have the same combination of alleles as the parents, whereas 10% have a new combination. The recombination frequency is therefore 10%, and the two loci are estimated to lay approximately 10 cM apart. This result is significant only if the number of offspring is large enough to determine that the 90:10 ratio is significantly different from the 50:50 ratio expected for independent assortment. This is determined by evaluating the relative likelihood or odds of obtaining the observed data when the two loci are linked compared to when they are not.

Lod scores. In linkage analysis the likelihood ratios are calculated at various possible recombination frequencies ranging from 0 (or no recombination) to 0.5, which indicates random segregation. The likelihood Z at any given recombination frequency theta (θ) is determined by the following equation:

$$Z = \frac{\text{Likelihood of data if loci linked at } \theta}{\text{Likelihood of data if loci unlinked}}$$

The computed likelihoods are usually expressed as the $\log_{10}$ of this ratio, and are called *lod scores* (for "logarithm of the odds.") Use of the lod score allows data from different families to simply be added together. By convention a combined lod score of $+3$ or greater, which is equivalent to odds of 1000:1 or greater, is considered proof that two loci are linked, whereas a combined lod score of -2 or less is considered proof that two loci are not linked. The value of θ at which Z is greatest is considered the best estimate of the recombination fraction.

Physical mapping

Several physical or laboratory methods for mapping human genes to specific chromosomes and chromosome regions have been developed, including somatic cell hybrids and in situ hybridization, which were described in a previous section, and other methods used for high-resolution mapping. The latter consists of several different strategies to map and clone small regions of DNA from a few base pairs up to about 1000 kb. Long-range restriction mapping makes use of restriction endonucleases with longer recognition sequences, which consequently occur less frequently in the genome than the more common short sequences. These rare-cutting enzymes cleave DNA into larger fragments, usually hundreds to thousands of kilobases, which must be separated by pulsed-field rather than routine electrophoresis.

DNA fragments of up to 1000 kb can be cloned into yeast artificial chromosomes. The large size of the clones allows more rapid screening of an entire chromosome region and consequently fewer steps in moving along a chromosome toward a gene. Finally, smaller DNA fragments must be cloned in cosmids, phage, or plasmids and analyzed by methods such as chromosome walking and jumping, DNA sequencing, and restriction fragment length polymorphisms together with linkage studies.

Status of human gene map

As of 1992, more than 2000 genes and 6000 anonymous DNA segments had been mapped in the human genome. Mutations of many of these genes are known to cause diseases affecting the nervous system and muscle in children and therefore are particularly relevant to the field of pediatric neurology. Some of these mutations and their map locations are listed in Table 24-3.

POPULATION GENETICS

Population genetics is the study of the distribution of genes in populations and of how the frequencies of genes and genotypes are maintained or changed [Thompson et al., 1991]. It is most often used in clinical genetics to calculate carrier (heterozygote) frequencies.

Hardy-Weinberg law

The basic tenet of population genetics is the Hardy-Weinberg law, which states that if two or more alleles occur in a population, their relative proportions will remain the same from generation to generation provided that the population is in equilibrium; that is, there must be random mating, and immigration must be balanced by emigration. At a locus with two alleles A and a, with frequencies of p and q respectively, the frequencies of the genotypes AA, Aa, and aa will be p^2, 2pq and q^2, respectively.

Table 24-3 Selected neurogenetic diseases mapped in the human genome

Disorder	Inheritance	Map location
Kallmann syndrome	XR	Xp22.3
Aicardi syndrome	XD/ml	Xp22
Mental retardation, XMR1	XR	Xp22
Duchenne/Becker muscular dystrophy	XR	Xp21.2
Hereditary motor and sensory neuropathy, XL	XR	Xq13
X-linked dystonia-Parkinsonism	XR	Xq12-21.1
Menkes syndrome	XR	Xq12-13.3
Mental retardation, XMR2	XR	Xq11-12
Kennedy spinal muscular atrophy	XR	Xq21.3-22
Pelizaeus-Merzbacher disease	XR	Xq22
Spastic paraplegia, XL uncomplicated	XR	Xq21-22
Lowe syndrome	XR	Xq25
Fragile X syndrome	XR	Xq27.3
Adrenoleukodystrophy	XR	Xq28
Aqueductal stenosis with adducted thumbs	XR	Xq28
Emory-Dreifuss muscular dystrophy	XR	Xq28
Myotubular myopathy, X-linked	XR	Xq28
Spastic paraplegia, XL complicated	XR	Xq28
Neuronal ceroid lipofuscinosis (infantile)	AR	1p32
Nemaline myopathy (AD form)	AD	1q21-23
Hereditary motor and sensory neuropathy 1B	AD	1q21.2-q23
Holoprosencephaly	del	7q36
von Hippel-Lindau disease	AD	3p25
Postanesthetic apnea (succinylcholine sensitivity)	AD	3q21-26
Huntington disease	AD	4p16.3
Facioscapulohumeral muscular dystrophy	AD	4q35
Spinal muscular atrophy, types 1-3	AR	5q12-14
Limb-girdle muscular dystrophy (AD form)	AD	5q22.3-31.3
Spinocerebellar ataxia (SCA1)	AD	6p23
Narcolepsy	AD	6p21.3
Craniosynostosis	del	7p21
Zellweger syndrome	AR	7q11
Holoprosencephaly	del	7q36
Thomsen disease (AD myotonia congenita)	AD	7q35
Tuberous sclerosis (TSC1)	AD	9q32-34
Friedreich ataxia	AR	9q12-21.1
Familial torsion dystonia	AD	9q34
Beckwith-Wiedemann syndrome	dup	11p15
WAGR syndrome (Wilms tumor, aniridia, genital hypoplasia, retardation)	del	11p13
Cerebellar ataxia with mental retardation	AR	11q14-21
Ataxia telangiectasia	AR	11q23
Retinoblastoma/mental retardation	del	13q14.1
Wilson disease	AR	13q14
Angelman syndrome	del	15q11-13
Prader-Willi syndrome	del	15q11-13
Limb-girdle muscular dystrophy (AR form)	AR	15q15-22
Tuberous sclerosis (TSC2)	AD	16p13
Neuronal ceroid-lipofuscinosis (juvenile)	AR	16p12
Isolated lissencephaly sequence	del	17p13.3
Miller-Dieker syndrome	del	17p13.3
Hereditary motor and sensory neuropathy 1A	AD	17p12
Neurofibromatosis 1	AD	17q11.2
Malignant hyperthermia susceptibility	AD	17q11.2-24
Hyperkalemic periodid paralysis	AD	17q23.1-25.3
Paramyotonia congenita	AD	17q23.1-25.3
Tourette syndrome (unconfirmed)	AD	18q22.1-?

Table 24-4 Recurrence risks in siblings for selected neurologic disorders of childhood

Disorder	Empiric risk (%)	Reference
Brain malformations		
Agenesis corpus callosum	Low*	[Baraitser, 1990]
Dandy-Walker malformation	1-5	[Murray et al., 1985]
Holoprosencephaly	4-6	[Roach et al., 1975]
Hydrocephalus	1-4	[Baraitser, 1990]
Male sibling of male patient	12	[Burton, 1979]
Lissencephaly	5-7	[Dobyns et al., 1992]
Neural tube defects	2-3	[Koch and Fuhrmann, 1985]
Developmental abnormalities		
Autism	4-5	[Jorde et al., 1991]
Cerebral palsy (spastic)		
Symmetric	10	[Baraitser, 1990]
Asymmetric	1-2	[Baraitser, 1990]
Mental retardation	4-5	[Herbst and Baird, 1982]
Male sibling of male patient	6-12	[Herbst and Baird, 1982]
Microcephaly	12	[Baraitser, 1990]
Microcephaly with multiple congenital anomalies	6	[Baraitser, 1990]
Seizure disorders		
Primary generalized epilepsy	4-13	[Metrakos and Metrakos, 1961]
Partial epilepsy	5	[Andermann, 1982]
Benign rolandic epilepsy	15	[Heijbel et al., 1975]
Febrile seizures	8-24	[Hauser et al., 1985]
		[Tsuboi, 1987]
Other neurologic disorders		
Migraine	12-27	[Baraitser, 1990]

*Only an estimate based on personal experience.

unaffected relatives, or the results of some laboratory tests. This is most easily done by using Bayes theorem, which is a method of assessing the relative probability of two alternative possibilities. In genetics the possibilities most often considered are whether an individual carries a particular allele. Although complex, this material is presented because of its importance for counseling for X-linked diseases, especially Duchenne and Becker muscular dystrophies.

The use of Bayesian analysis in Duchenne and Becker muscular dystrophies may be demonstrated by considering several typical pedigrees (Figure 24-15). In family A the consultand is at risk for being a carrier of Duchenne muscular dystrophy because her brother was affected. Their mother is a mandatory carrier because she had an affected brother and an affected son. The risk that the consultand inherited the Duchenne muscular dystrophy allele from her mother is ½. But the consultand has two healthy sons whose tests for muscle disease were normal. Intuitively, this makes it less likely that she actually is a carrier. Bayesian analysis takes this information into account in modifying her risk.

The two alternative possibilities being considered are whether the consultand is or is not a carrier. Four steps are required for this calculation. Before considering the additional data regarding her sons, the consultand's risk for being a carrier is ½; her risk for not being a carrier is also ½. This is the prior probability. Next consider the probability of both of her sons inheriting or not inheriting the normal allele, which is the conditional probability. If she is a carrier, the chance that any son is unaffected is ½, and the chance that two sons are unaffected is ½ × ½ = ¼. If she is not a carrier, then the chance that any son is unaffected is 1 (actually $1 - \mu \approx 1$). The product of the posterior and conditional probabilities is known as the *joint probability*. The joint probability that she is a carrier is ½ × ¼ = ⅛. The joint probability that she is not a carrier is ½ × 1 = ½. The resulting risk figure or posterior probability is merely the ratio of the two values, that is: ⅛:½ or 1:4.

The posterior probability for either condition (carrier or noncarrier) is calculated as a fraction or percentage risk by using the joint probability of the chosen condition as the numerator and the sum of both joint probabilities

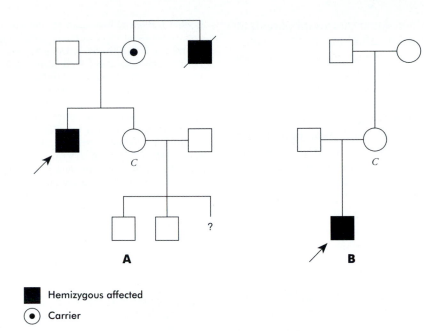

■ Hemizygous affected

⊙ Carrier

Figure 24-15 Examples of Bayesian analysis in two families segregating the gene for Duchenne muscular dystrophy. **A** and **B** designate family pedigrees. In family **B**, the consultand has a normal level of serum creatine kinase. *C*, Consultand.

as the denominator. For the carrier condition, this is $\frac{1}{5}$ or 20%, as shown in the following:

$$(\tfrac{1}{8})/(\tfrac{1}{8} + \tfrac{1}{2}) = (1)/(1 + 4) = \tfrac{1}{5}$$

The computations for this family are summarized below:

	Carrier	Not carrier
Prior probability	$\frac{1}{2}$	$\frac{1}{2}$
Conditional probability	$\frac{1}{4}$	1
Joint probability	$\frac{1}{2} \times \frac{1}{4} = \frac{1}{8}$	$\frac{1}{2} \times 1 = \frac{1}{2}$
Posterior probability	$\frac{1}{5}$	$\frac{4}{5}$

The same process may be used to determine the significance of certain tests if their discriminating value is known. The best example involves serum creatine kinase levels in females at risk for being carriers of Duchenne or Becker muscular dystrophies. Several studies have shown that serum creatine kinase levels are elevated in about 70% of carriers and normal in the remaining 30%. Only 5% or less of normal females have elevated creatine kinase levels. In family B the consultand is the mother of the affected boy. As explained in the section on population genetics, her prior risk for being a carrier is ⅔ or 0.67, and her risk for not being a carrier is therefore 0.33. Serial creatine kinase levels on the consultand were normal. If she is a carrier, the chance of having a normal creatine kinase level is 0.3. If she is not a carrier, the chance of having a normal creatine kinase level is 0.95 or greater. The risk that she is a carrier is 0.4 or 40% as summarized below:

	Carrier	Not carrier
Prior probability	0.67	0.33
Conditional probability	0.3	0.95
Joint probability	0.2	0.3
Posterior probability	0.4	0.6

Although this may appear to be a complicated process, it does allow the genetic counselor to quantify some factors that appear to be intuitively likely. In both of these hypothetical examples the recurrence risk estimate could be substantially lowered by use of Bayesian analysis. In some families the risk becomes so low that carrier evaluation by DNA analysis appears to be superfluous. For example, the chance that a woman with one son with Duchenne muscular dystrophy and eight normal sons is a carrier is less than 1%.

Prenatal diagnosis

Prenatal diagnosis is now possible for hundreds of genetic disorders, including many of those discussed in this chapter. The major methods used include chromosome analysis, enzyme assays and other biochemical tests, molecular genetic tests (including restriction fragment length polymorphisms and direct analysis of the gene), and direct examination of the fetus by ultrasonography. The latter is a far more rigorous procedure than routine prenatal ultrasonography and is usually referred to as high-resolution, level 2, or genetic ultrasonography. The purposes of prenatal diagnosis are to provide (1) a range of informed choices for parents at risk for having a child with an abnormality, (2) reassurance to reduce anxiety, especially among parents at high risk, and (3) an opportunity for parents to conceive and bear healthy children, who otherwise would choose not to have children.

The results of prenatal tests are normal in more than 98% of pregnancies evaluated, and their parents are reassured that the infant will be unaffected by the condition in question. Of course, the infant remains at risk for other disorders just as children born to any parents. In a small number of cases the fetus is indeed found to have a serious defect. Because effective prenatal therapy is not possible for most disorders, the parents may then choose to terminate the pregnancy.

SUMMARY

Genetics has become one of the most rapidly expanding fields in all of biology, and it is likely that this trend will continue. The next few years will see the discovery and isolation of genes and mutations responsible for many more of the disorders seen in pediatric neurology clinics. This new knowledge will eventually include knowledge regarding the genetic components of common disorders such as seizures, learning disabilities, and even migraine.

REFERENCES

Andermann NE. Multifactorial inheritance of generalized and focal epilepsy. In: Anderson VE, Hauser WA, Penry VK, et al., eds. Genetic basis of the epilepsies. New York: Raven Press, 1982; 355.

Baraitser M. The genetics of neurological disorders. Oxford: Oxford University Press, 1990.

Bruns GAP. Assigning genes to chromosomes: family studies, somatic cell hybridization, chromosome sorting, in situ hybridization, translocations. In: Rowland LP, Wood DS, Schon EA, et al., eds. Molecular genetics in diseases of brain, nerve, and muscle. New York: Oxford University Press, 1989; 156.

Burton BK. Recurrence risks for congenital hydrocephalus. Clin Genet 1979; 16:47.

Conneally PM. Assigning genes: linkage, crossing over, lod scores. In: Rowland LP, Wood DS, Schon EA, et al., eds. Molecular genetics in diseases of brain, nerve, and muscle. New York: Oxford University Press, 1989; 184.

Dobyns WB, Stratton RF, Parke JT, et al. Miller-Dieker syndrome: lissencephaly and monosomy 17p. J Pediatr 1983; 102:552.

Dobyns WB, Elias ER, Newlin AC, et al. Causal heterogeneity in isolated lissencephaly. Neurology 1992; 42:1375.

Eisensmith RC, Woo SLC. Molecular basis of phenylketonuria and related hyperphenylalaninemias: mutations and polymorphisms in the human phenylalanine hydroxylase gene. Hum Mutation 1992; 1:13.

Haldane. p. 1103.

Hall JG. Genomic imprinting: review and relevance to human diseases. Am J Hum Genet 1990; 46:857.

Hauser WA, Annegers JF, Anderson VE, et al. The risk of seizure disorders among relatives of children with febrile convulsions. Neurology 1985; 35:1268.

Heijbel J, Blom S, Rasmuson M. Benign epilepsy of childhood with centro-temporal EEG foci: a genetic study. Epilepsia 1975; 16:285.

Herbst DS, Baird PA. Sib risks for nonspecific mental retardation in British Columbia. Am J Med Genet 1982; 13:197.

ISCN (1985). An international system for human cytogenetic nomenclature. In: Harnden DG, Klinger HP, eds. Basel: Karger, 1985.

Johnson DD, Dobyns WB, Gordon H, et al. Familial pericentric and paracentric inversions of chromosome 1. Hum Genet 1988; 79:315.

Jorde LB, Hasstedt SJ, Ritvo ER. Complex segregation analysis of autism. Am J Hum Genet 1991; 49:932.

Killian JM, Kloepfer HW. Homozygous expression of a dominant gene for Charcot-Marie-Tooth neuropathy. Ann Neurol 1979; 5:515.

Koch M, Fuhrmann W. Sibs of probands with neural tube defects—a study in the Federal Republic of Germany. Hum Genet 1985; 70:74.

Krawczak M, Cooper DN. Gene deletions causing human genetic disease: mechanisms of mutagenesis and the role of the local DNA sequence environment. Hum Genet 1991; 86:425.

Ledbetter DH, Cavenee WK. Molecular cytogenetics: interface of cytogenetics and monogenic disorders. In: Scriver CR, et al., eds. The metabolic basis of inherited disease, 6th ed. New York: McGraw-Hill, 1989.

Lupski JR, Wise CA, Kuwano A, et al. Gene dosage is a mechanism for Charcot-Marie-Tooth disease type 1A. Nature Genet 1992; 1:29-33.

Metrakos K, Metrakos JD. Genetics of convulsive disorders, II. Genetic and electroencephalographic studies in centrencephalic epilepsy. Neurology 1961; 11:474.

Murray JC, Johnson JA, Bird TD. Dandy-Walker malformation: etiologic heterogeneity and empiric recurrence risks. Clin Genet 1985; 28:272.

Ray PN. The tools of molecular biology: restriction enzymes, blots, and RFLPs. In: Rowland LP, Wood DS, Schon EA, et al., eds. Molecular genetics in diseases of brain, nerve, and muscle. New York: Oxford University Press, 1989; 123.

Roach E, DeMeyer W, Conneally PM, et al. Holoprosencephaly: birth data, genetic and demographic analyses of 30 families. Birth Defects 1975; 11:294.

Schon EA. Prokaryotic and eukaryotic genomes. In: Rowland LP, Wood DS, Schon EA, et al., eds. Molecular genetics in diseases of brain, nerve, and muscle. New York: Oxford University Press, 1989a; 39.

Schon EA. Transcription and regulatory elements. In: Rowland LP, Wood DS, Schon EA, et al., eds. Molecular genetics in diseases of brain, nerve, and muscle. New York: Oxford University Press, 1989b; 62.

Sylvester J, Schmickel R. Making libraries: using vectors with genomic DNA or cDNA. In: Rowland LP, Wood DS, Schon EA, et al., eds. Molecular genetics in diseases of brain, nerve, and muscle. New York: Oxford University Press, 1989; 132.

Thompson MW, McInnes RR, Willard HF. Genetics in medicine, 5th ed. Philadelphia: WB Saunders, 1991.

Tsuboi T. Genetic analysis of febrile convulsions: twin and family studies. Hum Genet 1987; 75:7.

Watson JD, Crick FHC. A structure for deoxyribose nucleic acid. Nature 1953; 171:737.

Weber JL, May PE. Abundant class of human DNA polymorphisms which can be typed using the polymerase chain reaction. Am J Hum Genet 1989; 44:388.

Zeviani M, Bonilla E, DeVivo DC, et al. Mitochondrial diseases. Neurol Clin 1989; 7:123.

25

Chromosome-Linked Disorders

Bernard G. Lemieux

Each human being begins as a single cell, the fertilized egg (zygote). From this cell, through a process of cellular proliferation (mitosis), trillions of cells (about 3×10^{12}) form approximately 200 different tissues before the mature organism emerges. Cell multiplication continues throughout adult life. Every 24 hours, almost 1% of cells die and are replaced. Different tissues are renewed at different rates. The only cells that are not renewed are the nucleus of adult nerve cells and the macroneurones, which develop predominantly during the first half of gestation [Dobbing, 1970]. Cell division of neuroblasts does not occur in the human nervous system after 6 to 12 months of life; therefore nuclei of adult nerve cells are in a resting or interphase state. In morphologic terms, this resting state indicates that the chromosomes are not visible by photomicroscopy as they are during the mitosis that occurs in other dividing cells.

Embryogenesis is modulated by genes composed of exceedingly small units of deoxyribonucleic acid (DNA); these DNA units provide the guidelines for heredity, controlling the development of each cell and its daughter cells. Chromosomes, threadlike structures composed of genes, are the vehicles of inheritance.

Genes and chromosomes have two primary purposes: (1) maintenance and transmission of hereditary material in germinal cells, and (2) synthesis of agents that modulate cell metabolism so that inherited traits manifest in somatic cells. The final manifestation of an inherited trait depends on two genes, one from each parent. Approximately 50,000 to 100,000 structural genes reside on the 23 homolog pairs of chromosomes of each normal human somatic cell. In contradistinction, only 23 chromosomes are contained in each germinal cell (sperm and ovum). Somatic cells contain the diploid or 2n chromosome complement (diploos, double), whereas germinal cells contain the haploid or n chromosome complement (haploos, single).

The term *genome* refers to the full DNA complement.

An individual's phenotype (morphologic, biochemical, or physiologic characteristics) is the primary result of interaction between the genetic constitution (gene stock) that each individual inherits and its environment. Mutations are the result of an abrupt alteration of the genotype (i.e., a permanent change in the nucleotide sequence or arrangement of DNA in the genome). The change can occur either in the nuclear DNA or in the mitochondrial (cytoplasmic) DNA. Pathologic genotypic states may be produced either by chromosome abnormalities in number (genome mutation) and in structure (chromosome mutation) or by gene abnormalities (gene mutation) in either somatic or germ cells [Vogel and Motulsky, 1986]. Classification of genetic diseases regarding the nuclear DNA mutations is based on these concepts (see the box on page 358).

Moreover, nuclear DNA mutations may be acquired (many forms of cancer) or may be inherited and follow, as a general rule, the principles of mendelian inheritance. In contrast, mitochondrial DNA mutations ("the 25th chromosome") follow a unique pattern of maternal inheritance. Other nonclassical patterns of mendelian inheritance relevant to cytogenetics and neurology include mosaicism, genomic imprinting, and uniparental disomy. The reader should consult Chapter 24 and the references for further insight into this important, newly recognized concept [Austin and Hall, 1992; Thompson et al., 1991].

Several details of the fine structure of chromosome and gene organization are described [Park, 1991]. Virtually all DNA in the nucleus is associated with specific proteins (histones). These proteins keep DNA in a compact and well-ordered structure (chromatin). The fundamental subunit of the chromatin is the nucleosome, the structural quantum of chromosomes. Each nucleosome includes a central core, or chromatosome. Two turns of the double helix of DNA, each containing approximately 83 base pairs, are coiled in the chroma-

---

Classification of Genetic Disease

Germinal Cell Genetic Disease (conventional forms)

Chromosomal (trisomy 21)
Monogenic (locus): classical mendelian mutation
(phenylketonuria)
Multifactorial: multiple genes (loci) and environment
(spina bifida)

Somatic Cell Genetic Disease (neoplasia, some
autoimmune disease, aging, some malformations)

Chromosomal (rearrangements in malignancy)
Genic (point mutation in neurooncogene)
Multifactorial: multigenic and chromosomal combina-
tion with environment

Interplay Between Germinal and Somatic Cell Mutation
(familial retinoblastoma, possibly neurofibromatosis,
tuberous sclerosis ?, etc.)

Modified from McKusick VA. Medicine 1986; 65, Part 1.

---

tosome as a super helix around an octomer (eight molecules) of histones. The adjacent chromatosomes are held tightly together with a DNA segment called a *linker* [Felsenfeld, 1985; Kornberg and Klug, 1981]. Figure 25-1, *A* is a conceptual schematic representation of the structure and condensation of a chromosome in metaphase (original magnification × 10,000). In essence, each chromosome is a long DNA string of letters (A [adenine], T [thymine], G [guanine], C [cytosine] . . .) that continues until the string contains an estimated 3 billion letters.

Modern molecular biology provides a perspective that is useful for understanding the enormous difference in scale between the gene and the chromosome. Known genes vary in size from about 1000 base pairs (bp, nucleotide base of DNA) or 1 kilobase (kb) in length, such as those for insulin or for alpha- and beta-globin, to more than 2300 kb for Duchenne muscular dystrophy [Kunkel, 1986; Monaco et al., 1986]. For simplification, however, a typical gene occupies about 40 kb of space.* The haploid genome of each human cell consists of approximately 3 million kb (or 3×10^9 bp, or 6×10^9 bp for diploid genome), which corresponds to at least 2 meters of DNA in each cell (0.34 nanometer [nm] = 1 bp). Moreover, the length of DNA varies from 249 to 48

bp $\times 10^6$, with an average chromosome approximately 100,000 kb [Southern, 1982].

A small, distinguishable part of a chromosome (band) seen by high-resolution banding is about 100,000 kb, divided by 40, or 2500 kb long, and contains approximately 60 genes. Therefore many genes are involved in even the smallest deletion or duplication. Any visible rearrangements involve at least 2% to 5% of a chromosome. Figure 25-1, *B* is a schematic representation of chromosome 11 that shows the relative size of a chromosome band, the beta-like globin cluster and the beta-globin gene, based on recent mapping [Sparkes, 1985].

At the DNA level, mendelian disorders are coded. A point mutation, deletion, duplication, or inversion, usually involving one gene, has occurred within a single strand of DNA; the end product is an abnormal protein. This change takes place at the molecular level. Chromosome number and gross structure are normal.

At the chromosome level, conventional chromosomal aberrations occur in which a segment of chromosome or a whole chromosome may be missing, present in excess, or even misplaced. These alterations are visible with light microscopy. The changes are mainly quantitative; that is, they involve the omission or repetition of certain parts of DNA chains of normal composition, thus changing the hereditary message.

Between these two levels of DNA and chromosome a group of recognizable syndromes has recently been identified as a result of advances in microcytogenetics and molecular cytogenetics. This group concerns the involvement of adjacent (contiguous) genes on a chromosome and can be considered as disorders of chromosomal organization of genes (see later discussion).

CYTOGENETIC FUNDAMENTALS FOR THE NEUROLOGIST

Chromosomal aberrations may be manifested by changes in the structure or number of chromosomes or both. These changes result from accidents that may arise during meiosis in germinal cell division or in mitosis during somatic cell division. Such accidents may disturb the gene balance and cause aneuploidy, a deviation from a multiple of haploid number. Trisomy or monosomy results when a single chromosome is added to or deleted from a diploid set. When part of a chromosome or supernumerary fragment is added in excess or is deleted, the condition usually is called *duplication* or *deletion* (deficiency). Readers should consult the excellent textbooks of human cytogenetics or chapters of medical genetic books to gain more insight into the pathogenesis of chromosomal aberrations.*

---

*Physical distance (kb pairs) is different from genetic distance expressed in recombination frequency (centimorgan: cM). Total length of the haploid human genome is about 30 morgan. It is generally accepted that 1 cM (1% of recombination) is equivalent to 1000 kb, although the equation is not precise.

*References Epstein, 1986; Priest, 1977; Therman, 1988; Thompson et al., 1991; Yunis and Chandler, 1977.

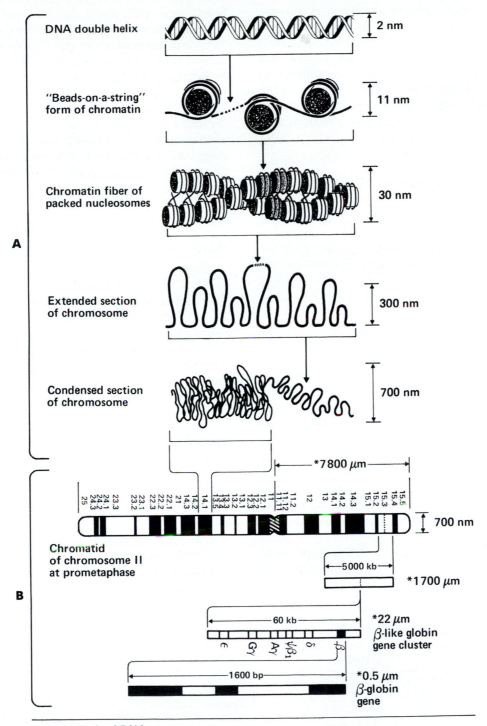

*Total length of DNA

Figure 25-1 Schematic representation of DNA and chromosome organization. **A,** Orders of chromatin packing at metaphase. Width expressed in nanometers (nm). **B,** Relative size of chromosome band, the beta-globin cluster of genes, and the beta-globin gene, expressed in length of DNA (μm) and in the number of base pairs (bp) (1000 bp = 1 kilobase [kb]). (Modified from Albert B, Bray D, Lewis J, et al. Molecular biology of the cell. New York: Garland Publishing, 1983; Schmickel RD. J Pediatr 1986a; 103:235; and Schmickel RD. J Pediatr 1986b; 108:244.)

Cause of chromosomal aberrations

Although the pathogenesis of aberration of chromosome number and structure is better understood, little is known about the cause of meiotic and mitotic accidents [Stene and Mikkelsen, 1984]. Different genetic and environmental factors have been incriminated, both in humans and in animals. Such factors include ionizing radiation, autoimmunity, viral infection, drugs, mutant genes, "nondisjunction gene," rare recessive traits with high frequency of chromosomal breakage, and especially, late maternal and paternal age.

Clinical procedures in chromosomal aberration

The procedures outlined in the following section are not all necessary in each case; they are included for completeness.

Buccal smear analysis (X and Y count). With the increasing availability of cytogenetic laboratories, sex chromatin analysis and Barr body studies are used less frequently, mainly only for screening sex chromosomal aberrations.

Dermatoglyphics. Dermatoglyphics refers to the systematic classification and study of the epidermal ridge pattern on the fingers, palms, and soles. The formation of dermatoglyphic patterns is under genetic influence, but the mode of inheritance is unknown, and the genetic mechanisms involved are obscure. The patterns remain unaltered once they are fully developed. Dermatoglyphics is useful for the study of chromosomal aberrations and some other neurologic disorders. Horizontal palm creases (simian lines) are seen in many persons with chromosomal and nonchromosomal disorders, as well as in the normal population. A single flexion crease on the fifth finger suggests very high probability of a chromosomal aberration.

Readers are referred to more detailed descriptions of dermatoglyphics in chromosomal aberrations [Lemieux, 1982; Loesch, 1983]. Dermatoglyphics is described only briefly here in the major chromosomal syndromes.

Chromosome analysis. Chromosome analysis detects both qualitative and quantitative variations in the normal chromosome complement. For routine analysis, peripheral lymphocytes are the most readily accessible somatic cells. For more specific purposes, other tissues, such as bone marrow, are used for rapid diagnosis [Francke et al., 1979a]; skin fibroblasts are used for identification of mosaicism, and chorionic villus sampling and amniotic fluid cells are used for cytogenetic prenatal diagnosis. Details of the methodology and applications in human chromosome analysis are available [Barch, 1991; Larson, 1983; Rooney and Czepulkowski, 1992].

History of human cytogenetics

Human cytogenetic study has a relatively short history (Table 25-1). The initial step was the establishment of the number of human chromosomes at 46 by Tjio and Levan in 1956. In 1959 Lejeune et al. recognized the first chromosomal abnormality in humans: trisomy 21.

Except for the improvement of tissue cultures, chromosome preparation, and the introduction of autoradiography with tritiated thymine, little new knowledge appeared until 1970. In that year a revolution occurred with the introduction of differential staining techniques, performed first by Caspersson et al. [1970] (Table 25-2). These techniques permit unambiguous identification of each chromosome within the human karyotype.

In an extension of banding techniques available in 1970, several scientists, most notably Yunis [1981], developed high-resolution procedures that permit even more detailed analysis of a chromosome with light microscopy. Basically, high-resolution procedures produce more synchronized cell growth, and a chromosome can be analyzed in the prophase or prometaphase [Yunis

Table 25-1 **History of human cytogenetics**

Phase*	Date	Name	Limit
Classic cytogenetics	1956	Tjio and Levan	Group and number
Modern cytogenetics	1970	Casperson et al.	Midmetaphase banding 350 bands/genome Medium band: 1000 kb†
Microcytogenetics	1976	Yunis	Prophase and prometaphase 850-1200 bands/genome "Super" band: 3 kb†
Molecular cytogenetics	1981	Harper and Gerhard	In situ hybridation (ISH) "Micro" band: 0.5 kb† Chromosome sorting

*Terms used to identify phases are descriptive designations only.
†Arbitrary estimated scale: variable with each chromosome condensation.

and Lewandowski, 1983]. Such techniques produce a more extended or uncoiled chromosome and more than double the observable bands (up to 1250) in the genome compared with standard banding techniques (350 bands). Figure 25-2 shows the schematic anatomy of chromosome 1, including an idiogram at different stages of condensation. Table 25-3 provides a partial list of the nomenclature useful for interpretation of a karyotype.

The application of molecular biologic tools to cytogenetics opened a new vista, molecular cytogenetics, and has returned cytogenetics to its rightful position in the forefront of human genetics [Ferguson-Smith, 1991]. Recent methods emanating from research laboratories are now used as an adjunct to classical banding techniques. They include the techniques discussed in the following sections.

Chromosomal in situ hybridization or hybridocytochemistry. This method is based on the annealing of a single-copy DNA or RNA sequence (probe) to complementary sequences (or targets) of DNA, which are usually fixed to a microscope slide in metaphase or interphase conformation. Single or multiple hybridized probes can be visualized by autoradiographic, colorimetric, and fluorescent in situ hybridization (FISH) detection systems [Dyer and Meyne, 1991]. Nonisotopic chromosome in situ suppression hybridization using flow-sorted chromosome libraries, so-called chromosome painting, may become an important diagnostic tool in clinical cytogenetics [Hulten et al., 1991b]. In addition to its primary use for refined gene mapping, in situ hybridization is a powerful and complementary tool for identifying small chromosome abnormalities; detecting inframicroscopic deletion, duplication, or translocation not revealed by routine karyotype analysis; and defining breakpoints in chromosome rearrangements. In situ hybridization is also essential for studying the various processes of oncogene activation in the development of cancer and for analyzing complex mechanisms implicated in species evolution [Mattei and Mattei, 1986; Taviaux et al., 1989].

Cell sorter flow cytometry. Also known as laser or fluorescent chromosome sorting, cell sorter flow cytometry has been developed and applied to chromosomal analysis [Carrano et al., 1979]. This methodology has contributed to optimizing human chromosome separation for the production of chromosome-specific DNA libraries and has allowed the determination of DNA content of the human chromosome. Moreover, chromosome sorting is a potential tool for objective analysis of chromosomal abnormalities [Harris et al., 1986]. Other new tools of molecular genetics, such as pulsed-field gel electrophoresis, yeast artificial chromosomes, and polymerase chain reaction, fill the gap between the resolution provided by microcytogenetics and molecular genetics. The advances of molecular biology now allow diagnosis of more minute submicroscopic aberrations, representing a few dozen genes, in syndromes previously considered sporadic or familial and of unknown cause (see Table 25-13). Moreover, with these new cytogenetic tools, it is now easier to reveal accurately the meiotic stage and parental origin of numerical or structural chromosomal anomalies and to derive greater insight into the new concepts of mosaicism [Hall, 1988], uniparental disomy [Engel et al., 1991; Schinzel, 1991], and genomic imprinting (differential parental gene expression) [Editorials, Lancet, 1991; Flint, 1992; Hall, 1990, 1991, 1992; Hodgson, 1991; Sapienza, 1990].

Many chromosomal aberrations have been analyzed using a variety of cloned probes or specific or restriction fragment length polymorphisms, which are available in increasing numbers. This trend provides cytogenetics with a new and broadened outlook. DNA probes will prove useful as a complementary tool for analysis of constitutional (germinal) or acquired (somatic) cytogenetic disorders [Jean Pierre and Junien, 1984].

CURRENT MEDICAL INDICATIONS FOR CHROMOSOME ANALYSIS

Chromosome analyses are being used more widely. Their medical applications are summarized as follows:
- Clinical diagnosis of constitutional chromosome aberrations
- Prenatal diagnosis
- Chromosomal polymorphisms (variants or markers)
- Chromosomes and neoplasia
- Human gene mapping
- Specific genetic (mendelian) diseases with cytogenetic landmarks, including chromosomal instability syndrome, atypical monogenic disorder, and fragile X syndrome (X-linked mental retardation).

Clinical diagnosis of constitutional chromosome-linked disorders

Constitutional chromosome aberrations are the major indications summarized in the box on p. 364, based on

---

Table 25-2 Types of chromosome banding techniques

Band	Staining techniques
C	Centric heterochromatin method
Q	Quinacrine fluorescent dye banding
G	Giemsa banding with or without proteolytic enzymes
R	Reverse Giemsa stain
BrdU	Incorporation of 5-bromodeoxyuridine followed by staining with Giemsa stain or acridine orange
SNOR	Silver nucleolar organizing regions

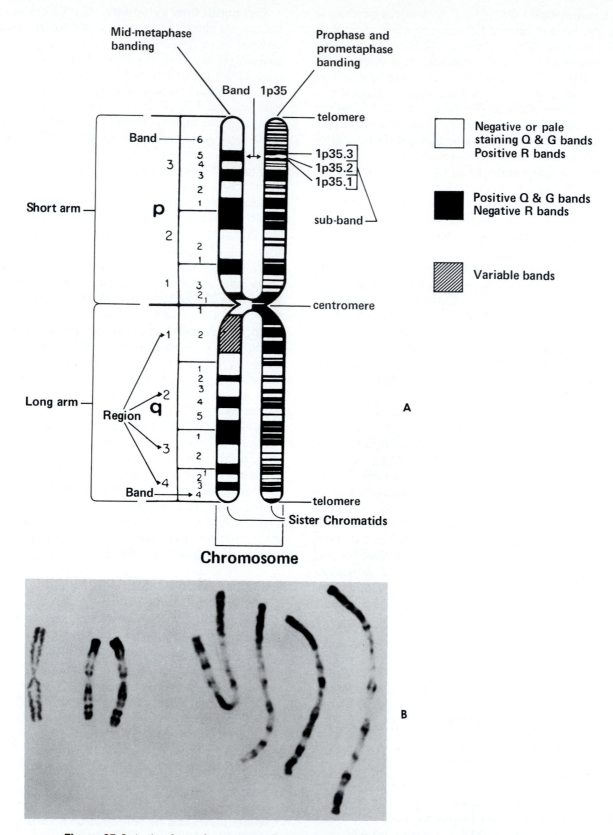

Figure 25-2 A, A schematic anatomy of chromosome 1. **B,** An idiogram at different stages of condensation: R banding. (Courtesy M.G. Mattei, Marseilles, France.)

Table 25-3 Nomenclature symbols (partial list)

Symbol	Explanation
1-22	The autosome numbers
X,Y	The sex chromosomes
/	Separates cell lines in describing mosaicisms (mixoploidy)
ace	Acentric fragment (see also f)
arrow (→)	From-to
asterisk (*)	Used like a multiplication sign
b	Break
cen	Centromere
colon, single (:)	Break
colon, double (::)	Break and reunion
del	Deletion
der	Derivative chromosome
dic	Dicentric
dis	Distal
dmin	Double minute
dup	Duplication
end	Endoreduplication
fra	Fragile site
h	Secondary constriction
i	Isochromosome
ins	Insertion
inv	Inversion
mar	Marker chromosome
mat	Maternal origin
mos	Mosaic
p	Short arm of chromosome
parenthese ()	Used to surround structurally altered chromosome(s)
pat	Paternal origin
prx	Proximal
q	Long arm of chromsome
question mark (?)	Indicates questionable identification of chromsome or chromosome structure
r	Ring chromosome
rcp	Reciprocal
rec	Recombinant chromosome
rob	Robertsonian translocation
s	Satellite
t	Translocation
tan	Tandem translocation
ter	Terminal (end of chromosome)
+ or −	Placed *before* the chromosome number, these symbols indicate addition (+) or loss (−) of a whole chromosome (e.g., +21 indicates an extra chromosome 21, as in Down syndrome); placed *after* the chromosome number, these symbols indicate increase or decrease in the length of a chromosome part (e.g., 5p− indicates loss of the short arm of chromosome 5, as in cri du chat syndrome.)

For further details, see Harndess PG, Klingfer HP, eds. An international system for human cytogenetic nomenclature. Basel: S Karger AG, 1985.

the clinical aspects of chromosome-linked disorders as a whole. These disorders also are discussed in the sections on clinical aspects of chromosome-linked disorders and contiguous gene syndrome.

Prenatal cytogenetic diagnosis

The scope of prenatal diagnosis has greatly increased and has become an accepted part of medical care for mother and child. Noninvasive and invasive sampling techniques provide remarkably increased capability associated with the new molecular tools for prenatal cytogenetic analysis. These techniques include the following:

- Noninvasive techniques as follows:
1. Fetal ultrasonography (transabdominal or recently, transvaginal): used for assessment of mul-

---

Clinical Diagnosis of Constitutional Aberrations

Offspring

Major

- Severe or moderate retardation with or without dysmorphism, particularly males
- Syndrome with multiple congenital anomalies
- Confirmation of suspected classic chromosomal syndrome
- All children of individuals with balanced rearrangement or structural anomalies
- Abnormalities of growth or of primary or secondary sexual development, with or without abnormal bucal smears (X or Y body count)

Minor

- Abnormal dermatoglyphics
- Developmental abnormalities
- Failure to thrive in infancy
- Peculiar-looking infants, children, or adults with or without mental retardation
- Unexplained death in infancy

Parents

- Family history of malformation
- Couple with reproductive problems, including infertility
- Mother with multiple abortions and stillbirths
- Severely malformed offspring
- Young mother with trisomic child
- Offspring with chromosomal rearrangements

Families With Presumed X-linked Recessive or Autosomal Dominant Patterns of Mental Retardation

---

tiple malformations, need for fetal karyotyping in almost 30% [Eydoux et al., 1989].

2. Maternal serum triple test screening: The combined measurement of the maternal serum alpha-fetoprotein level (low), unconjugated estriol level (low), and human chorionic gonadotropin level (high) seems to be more effective in screening for fetal Down syndrome. These markers are evaluated at many centers for detection efficiency of trisomy 21, and possibly for trisomy 18 [Haddow et al., 1992; Robertson, 1991; Staples et al., 1991; Wald et al., 1988; D'Alton et al., 1993].

3. In the foreseeable future, rare fetal trophoblast cells will be harvested from the maternal circulation, allowing prenatal genetic testing without risking harm to the fetus [Mueller, 1990].

- Invasive ultrasound-guided techniques include the following:
1. Chorionic villus sampling, transcervical or transabdominal, performed around 9 to 10 weeks' of gestation; total loss rate of 0.06% to 0.8% [Jackson et al., 1992].
2. Amniocentesis: early—before 15 weeks—or, usually, midtrimester—between 15 and 17 weeks' gestation—with an early amniocentesis total loss rate of about 2% and a midtrimester amniocentesis loss rate of <0.5%.
3. Percutaneous umbilical blood sampling (cordocentesis) for rapid prenatal karyotyping of particular conditions, with a total loss rate of <1.1%.

Problems in prenatal chromosome analysis such as mosaicism, culture failure, and unsuspected adverse findings are beyond the scope of this chapter [Thompson et al., 1991; Johnson, 1991].

The physician should determine the indications for prenatal cytogenetic analysis and should recommend it for the woman whose risk of having a child with chromosomal aberration is greater than 1%. However, a positive, nonrestrictive attitude is recommended. The physician should consider the following facts:

1. Approximately 1 in 175 to 200 children have some chromosomal abnormalities that "nature" overlooked.
2. "Nature" recognizes and disposes of most chromosomal errors by early spontaneous abortion.
3. Population testing for chromosomal aberration currently is not feasible.
4. Determination of the chromosomal constitution of all fetuses is neither feasible nor sensible.

The following are the most commonly accepted indications for prenatal cytogenetic analysis:

- Late maternal age (greater than 35 years)
- Parent with a potentially transmissible chromosome rearrangement
- Previous offspring with chromosomal aberration
- X-linked mental retardation (fragile X syndrome)

Important details about these four situations are described in the following section.

1. Late maternal age and the risk of trisomic chromosomal aberration. All sex chromosomal and autosomal aneuploidies resulting from a nondisjunction occur with increasing frequency with advancing maternal and possibly paternal age [Hook, 1981; Stene et al., 1984]. Data indicate that a woman who becomes pregnant between the ages of 35 and 39 years has a 1% to 2.2% probability of producing a child with a chromosomal abnormality. The risk for a 40-year-old woman is approximately 3.5% to 4.5%, rising to about 8% to 10% by 45 years of age [Milunsky, 1977].

2. Parental carrier of a potentially transmissible

chromosomal rearrangement (either a translocation or an inversion). It is believed that approximately 1 in 1000 persons carries transmissible chromosomal rearrangements. The risk of an unbalanced fetal karyotype is about 5% to 25%, depending on the specific arrangements and their origin (maternal or paternal). Family cytogenetic studies and genetic counseling should be undertaken as early as possible while the parents and close relatives are planning their families.

3. Chromosomal aberrations in previous offspring, including a trisomic child. Regardless of maternal and possibly paternal age the previous birth of a trisomic child yields a risk of roughly 1% to 2% for birth of another trisomic infant. Other chromosomal aberrations in previous offspring result in a risk of less than 1%.

4. Other. Many other generally accepted indications for prenatal cytogenetic analysis vary from center to center. Such indications include familial history of trisomy or mental retardation, previous congenital malformations, spontaneous abortions, acquired and inherited chromosomal breakage conditions, parental sex chromosomal or autosomal mixoploidy and aneuploidy, and X-linked disorders without an available biochemical technique for diagnosis. In normal pregnancies psychologic reasons may include parental anxiety and excessive fear. Finally, chromosomal analysis should be performed on cells from any specimen of amniotic fluid obtained for any reason. A complete karyotype analysis rather than only evaluation of Y or X chromosome fetal cells should be performed for an adequate assessment of sex chromosomes.

Chromosome polymorphic markers (variants)

Modern cytogenetic studies of large populations have revealed minor variations of length and staining properties of certain chromosomal segments. These variations, also called *heteromorphism*, appear frequently, do not usually result in abnormal phenotypic manifestations, and are stable variants inherited as mendelian codominant traits. Variable segments include (1) the fluorescent centrometic regions of chromosomes 3 and 4; (2) the centromeres, short arm, and satellites of all acrocentric chromosomes (13 to 15, 21, 22) where they are detectable by Q banding; (3) the secondary constriction of chromosomes 1, 9, 16, and Y; and (4) variations in C-band heterochromatin such as those of chromosome 18.

Chromosomal variants are distributed widely among cells of humans and are found in 2% or more of the general population [Jacobs, 1977]. Such variations serve as markers within a family and are useful for identifi-

cation purposes and epidemiologic studies of human chromosomal aberrations. Recognition of these markers has allowed insight into the pathogenesis of well-known syndromes, such as trisomies 21 and 13, as well as information regarding the origin of additional chromosomes: paternal or maternal source, first meiotic division, second meiotic division, or zygotic meiotic division [Chamberlin and Magenis, 1980]. These determinations require a precise banding technique and the expertise of an experienced cytogeneticist.

Another group of chromosomal variants are the fragile sites. As defined by Sutherland [1979a, 1979b], fragile sites are morphologic features of chromosomes having specific points or loci in which there is a nonstaining gap of variable width, usually involving both chromatids. The abnormalities are observed at the same locus in patients or relatives and are inherited in a mendelian co-dominant fashion. These sites exhibit fragility by producing, for example, deleted chromosomes, acentric fragments, and multiradial figures. Because of these features the fragile sites are potentially useful for genetic linkage analysis. The number of identified sites has increased over the years; at the Human Gene Mapping Conference 11 [1991], 114 sites were identified. Fragile sites can be classified by mode of induction (the tissue culture conditions required for their cytologic expression) [Sutherland and Hecht, 1985]. Three main types are recognized: primarily folate-sensitive, distamycin A–inducible, and 5-bromodeoxyuridine-requiring.

These sites can also be categorized as heritable (rare) fragile sites and as constitutive (common) fragile sites. The ramifications of the fragile site phenomenon with regard to constitutional chromosomal rearrangements, cancer, and evolution are beyond the scope of this chapter [Daniel, 1986; Petit et al., 1986; Sutherland, 1985b].

Several autosomes have been identified with fragile sites, but only one fragile site on the X chromosome has clearly been associated with phenotypic abnormalities, including mental retardation. (See the section on X-linked mental retardation for a discussion of specific genetic mendelian disorders with cytogenetic effects.)

Chromosomal variants have also been used for genetic linkage studies in families. These variants form a category of genetic cellular probes (markers) (Table 25-4) and should be differentiated from the phenotypic polymorphic markers, such as erythrocyte antigens, human leukocyte antigens, isoenzymes, and serum proteins, which are end products or expressed proteins. This historic category has been superseded by a rapidly growing and highly important category: the genetic variations between DNA sequences of homologous chromosomes. They include the following:

• Restriction fragment length polymorphism, usually

Table 25-4 Genetic cellular probes (markers)

Categories	Description	Numbers
Phenotype	Expressed proteins: blood group, human leukocyte antigen, isoenzme serum proteins	>150
Chromosome	Variants (polymorphisms) including fragile sites (114)	>125
Genotype (DNA)	Restricted fragment length polymorphisms Variable number of tandem repeats (minisatellites) Microsatellites Alumorphs	Clone DNA segments: >7000

*From Human Gene Mapping 11.

related to a base pair substitution and usually biallelic

• Variable number of tandem repeats, usually the result of insertion-deletion polymorphism, usually multiallelic and referred to as minisatellites

• Microsatellites consisting of dinucleotide (GT)n and (CA)n simple sequence repeats, which are extremely polymorphic with each locus having numerous alleles (six to 12) [Weber and May, 1989]

• Alumorphs, with highly repetitive sequences

For further discussion, readers should consult literature on molecular genetics [Cooper and Schmidtke, 1991].

Chromosomes and neoplasia

Theodore Baverin's hypothesis in 1914 that the malignant transformation of cells was secondary to somatic mutations, visible and identifiable in human chromosomes, was not confirmed for almost 70 years. The advances of microcytogenetics and molecular cytogenetics have produced evidence of clonal, nonrandom chromosomal defects (numeric, structural, or both) in neoplasia [Berger and Larsen, 1986; Croce and Klein, 1985; Mitelman, 1991; Nowell, 1992; Solomon et al., 1991]. In certain types of malignancies, this evidence suggests an important link between specific chromosome patterns and the origin and maintenance of neoplastic cells in humans [Yunis, 1983].

Numerous, diverse, nonrandom chromosomal changes, updated in Human Gene Mapping 11 and involving all chromosomes except the X chromosome, have been described in both solid tumors and hemopathies. These are becoming an important part of the management of patients with neoplasia and also have prognostic value in human cerebral astrocytoma [Chung et al., 1992; Kim-

mel et al., 1992]. Cancer is now recognized primarily as a genetic disorder.

The basic mechanism of neoplasia or cancer involves a mutation, either in the germline or, much more frequently, in somatic cells. Neoplasia may be defined as a progressive accumulation of multiple genetic events that occur in a single clone of cells because of an alteration in a limited number of specific genes: the oncogenes and tumor suppressor genes (antioncogenes) [Bishop, 1991; Marshall, 1991; Shapiro, 1986]. Qualitative or quantitative changes appear in these specific genes.

The hypothesis of two "hits" or mutational events, first proposed by Knudson in 1971, is particularly applicable to some neuroectodermal tumors. This hypothesis implies that a primary mutation is recessive to the normal allele at the cellular level. The growth of the tumor ensues only after secondary change, such as chromosome nondisjunction or mitotic recombination, eliminates the normal allele, thereby unmasking the altered allele [Cavenee et al., 1985, 1986; Friend et al., 1986; Koufos et al., 1985]. In this model, patients who have the heritable condition inherit the first of these events as a germline mutation. The second event occurs somatically in the cell that eventually becomes the tumor, which is often bilateral. This situation contrasts with nonheritable (sporadic) cases in which solitary tumors result from the infrequent occurrence of two rare events within the same cell [Murphree and Benedict, 1984; Phillips and Gallie, 1984].

In 1983, Gilbert proposed a classification of chromosome abnormalities in cancer, which included the following:

Class I includes equivalent exchange of chromosome segments between chromosomes (reciprocal translocation) with no significant loss of structural material from the karyotype, as exemplified by the translocation between chromosomes 9 and 22 in chronic myelogenic leukemia. In essence this translocation could serve to place an oncogene next to an activator DNA sequence.

Class II includes deletion or rearrangement resulting in the loss of structural material, such as the 13q− in retinoblastoma or 11p− in Wilms tumors. In essence a deletion could eliminate an antioncogene.

Class III constitutes additional whole chromosomes or chromosome segments, as with trisomy 8 in acute leukemia and an extra 1q in neuroblastoma. In essence a trisomy could be associated with extra gene dosage. In this class, two novel types of acquired cytogenetic changes have been associated with the multiplication of a single gene in cells (gene amplification): double minutes, that is, very small accessory chromosomes, and homogeneously staining regions [Harndess and Klingfer, 1985]. A minute is an acentric fragment smaller than the width of a single chromatid. It may be single or double. In the special situation found in tumor cells, where multiple double minutes are present, the abbreviation dmin may be used. Both double minutes and hemogeneously stained regions are unique cancer cells and alternate manifestations of the same biologic phenomenon (i.e., the breakdown of a homogenously stained region causes double minutes).

Table 25-5 contains a selection of neuroectodermal tumors and lists chromosomes with breakpoints and/or oncogenes involved. A discussion concerning the large group of hemopathies and other solid tumors is beyond the scope of this chapter.

Increased expression or activation of a number of oncogenes has been described in tumors of the nervous system [Breakefield, 1986]. These neurooncogenes include N-myc, erb B, Neu, and Sis among more than 40 known oncogenes. N-myc and erb B are more specific for neural tumors.

The genetic mechanisms of activation include gene amplification, gene loss, alterations in gene structures that affect the gene product, and change in the regulation of gene expression, including the role of antioncogenes [Knudson, 1985; Junien, 1986]. Moreover, fragile sites, familial or constitutional, may also play a role in tumorigenesis [Berger et al., 1985].

In summary, chromosome rearrangements may play a central role in human neoplasia and may exert their effects through related genomic mechanisms.

Table 25-5 Neuroectodermal tumors

Groups	Chromosome with breakpoints	Oncogenes
Tumors of CNS		
Medulloblastoma		
Meningioma*	del 22q	
Glioblastoma		Neu
		Sis
		erb B
Retinoblastoma*	del 13q$_{14}$	N-myc
Acoustic neuroma*†	del 22q	
Tumors of PNS		
Neuroblastoma*	del 1p$_{32-36}$	Nmyc
		Nras
		Neu
Tumors of pigment cells		
Melanoma	del 6q	

*Related to neurofibromatosis.
†Two "hit kinetics" (Knudson): As few as two genes are sufficient for tumorigenesis, i.e. first can be inherited or can occur in somatic target cells, second occurs in somatic cells. This applies also to familial forms of Wilms tumor (del 11p$_{13}$), the third childhood malignancy.

Gene mapping

Human gene mapping has been one of the most active areas in human genetics as indicated by serial Human Gene Mapping Workshops since 1973. This subject is well reviewed by Thompson et al. [1991]. Just as multiple maps exist to represent the earth, the human genome can be represented by three types of maps: cytogenetic (chromosomal bandings), genetic (linkage), and physical (including restriction, contiguous, and sequence-tagged site maps) [Bernheim, 1991; Green and Waterson, 1991]. The following are some current methods used for gene mapping:

- Linkage analysis with genetic cellular probes (markers)
- Intraspecific somatic cell hybridization with DNA and phenotypic markers
- Gene dosage analysis
- In situ DNA or RNA hybridization to chromosomes
- Laser or fluorescent chromosome sorting
- Comparative mapping (linkage homology between species)

Other methods are also used; readers should refer to the rapidly growing literature resources on human gene mapping [Donis-Keller, 1991].

Knowing the precise position of a gene on the human chromosome "map" is considered to be so important for medicine and science that there is a large international project under way to map all 50,000 or more human genes, with the objective of completing this mammoth task by the year 2005. This epochal project has had and will have a profound impact on clinical medicine [Friedmann, 1990]. "A neurologic gene map" can be constructed for many chromosomes where the location of some important serious hereditary neurologic disorders is now known [Harding and Rosenberg, 1993; Brice and Mallet, 1991; Landrieu, 1992; Kapland and Fontaine, 1991; McKusick, 1986, 1990, 1992]. Already there is an avalanche of disease genes mapped (>2000), together with a growing number actually cloned [McKusick, 1992]. Indeed, the majority of serious human genetic diseases are now mapped with sufficient accuracy to allow prediction within families, whereas for some, such as Duchenne muscular dystrophy, neurofibromatosis, and fragile X syndrome, a detailed exploration of molecular pathology is becoming possible [Conneally, 1992].

Specific genetic mendelian disease with cytogenetic landmarks

1. Chromosomal instability and cancer-prone hereditary diseases with DNA processing anomalies. With the advances of cytogenetic analysis and its increased availability, chromosomes of individuals with rare hereditary syndromes have been investigated. An interrelationship has been discovered

among cytogenetic aberrations, an inability to repair diverse genetic damage, an immune deficiency, and an early development of malignancies in adolescence and adulthood. Table 25-6 summarizes the most important diseases; others, such as Itai-Itai disease, Werner syndrome, and Robert syndrome, are rare [Shiraishi, 1975; Schroeder, 1982; Maraschio et al., 1986]. Although nonspecific, the discovery of these rare hereditary genomic normal instabilities may be of diagnostic value. Their importance in relation to cancer is more than academic.

2. Atypical monogenic disorders. A chromosomal analysis usually is not indicated for inborn errors of metabolism or for any known single-gene mutation transmitted as a mendelian trait because they do not manifest any visible chromosome defects. However, recent "experiments of nature" recognized by astute clinicians can be of benefit for localizing and subsequently mapping a disease on a specific chromosome. This approach has been useful for sex-linked diseases and particularly for the location and isolation of the gene for Duchenne muscular dystrophy, either rare female patients with Duchenne muscular dystrophy phenotype and X-autosomal translocation, or minor Xp21 chromosome deletion in a patient with multiple mendelian disorders [Bartley et al., 1986; Dunger et al., 1986; Francke et al., 1985; Jacobs et al., 1981].

Unusual findings in frequent autosomal-recessive or dominant neurologic disorders occasionally associated with visible cytogenetic abnormalities, such as translocation or deletion. These rare circumstances may provide the crucial first step for positional cloning, and identifying the physical location of a gene [Edwards, 1982; Ledbetter and Canavee, 1989].

Microcytogenetic and molecular cytogenetic techniques for discovery of new chromosomal submicroscopic rearrangements or deletions. Such findings represent an excellent opportunity to explore unexplained genetic defects, particularly single-gene abnormalities and the contiguous gene syndrome (i.e., complex phenotypes of many multisystem diseases related to the involvement of genes related to each other by their physical proximity on a chromosome rather than by their function) [Schmickel, 1986b; Schinzel, 1988].

3. The fragile X syndrome. This syndrome is discussed in detail in the following section.

X-LINKED MENTAL RETARDATION (FRAGILE X SYNDROME)

History. Mental retardation occurs in approximately 3% of the general population. About 20% to 25% of mental retardation may be the result of major oligogenes located on the X chromosome. At most, the oligogenes represent 6% of the haploid genome and contain thus far 240 or more known gene mutations, 25% of which are associated with mental retardation.

The concept of X-linked mental retardation has been developed during the past 50 years through excellent and exhaustive studies [Herbst and Miller, 1980; Lehrke, 1984; Penrose, 1938; 1963; Reed and Reed, 1965]. X-linked mental retardation appears to be a very heterogenous group; precise classification is not yet possible and awaits clinical delineation and gene localization [Glass, 1991; Howard-Peebles, 1982]. A cytologic marker has been identified for approximatively 40% of X-linked mental retardation: a fragile site (see previous discussion on cellular probes), which is a constriction near the distal end of q (Xq27.3) [Harrison, 1983]. The combination of a single mutant gene and a specific cytogenetic abnormality is unique in medical genetics. The association was first described by Lubs in 1969, and a reproducible cytogenetic test was proposed by Sutherland in 1977. The discovery in 1991 of the molecular genetic basis of the fragile X syndrome promises to elucidate the cause and treatment of this disorder and perhaps other forms of mental retardation [Oberlé et al., 1991; Yu et al., 1991; Pieretti et al., 1991; Verkerk et al., 1991]. The clinical characteristics, including macroorchidism and the characteristic facial appearance, were reported by Martin and Bell in 1943 and corroborated by Richards et al. in 1981.

The general term *fragile X syndrome/Martin-Bell syndrome* has become accepted for identifying individuals exhibiting the complete clinical pattern. The syndrome should be differentiated from the many various other syndromes, some described years ago and others described more recently [Wilson et al., 1991]. Moreover, a computerized approach to X-linked mental retardation syndrome with a review of 33 syndromes is available [Arena and Lubs, 1991a; 1991b].

Incidence. The frequency of fragile X syndrome remains to be determined. There are problems in gathering and interpreting data. Based on one estimate (1:1250 affected males and 1:5000 nonpenetrant males or normal transmitting males leading to an overall prevalence of about 1:1,000 among male births), the inherited fragile X syndrome rivals the sporadic Down syndrome as a specific cause of mental retardation [Herbst and Miller, 1980]. The possibility exists that fragile X syndrome may exceed Down syndrome in frequency. Fragile X syndrome has been described in all racial groups and is a major public health problem. The population prevalence of affected females is approximately 1:2000 [Webb et al., 1986]. Overall, prevalence of female carriers is estimated to be about 1:700. On the basis of these estimates the gene is present overall in approximatively 1 in 850 people. Because retarded

Table 25-6 Chromosome instability and cancer-prone hereditary disorders with DNA processing abnormalities

Syndrome	Clinical features	Cellular events	Risk of neoplasia	Types	Reference
Ataxia-telangiectasia Louis-Bar syndrome	Cerebellar ataxia Oculocutaneous telangiectaneous parent by 6 years of age Neurologic deterioration Recurrent sinopulmonary infections Increased susceptibility to x-irradiation Small or absent thymus or lymph nodes Occurrence 2:100,000 to 3:100,000 Immunodeficiency: low to absent IgA	Hypersensitivity and hypomutation to ionizing radiations and certain alkylating agents High frequency of chromosome aberrations: random breaks, gaps, and rearrangements Most frequently affected chromosome 14 + 7, 2+/or 22 Complementation groups A, C, and D (97%) Located to 11q 22-23	+++ 20% to 30%	Lymphomas Chronic and acute lymphocytic leukemia Hodgkin disease Lymphosarcoma Reticular cell carcinoma	Kidson and Dambergs, 1982 Aurias, 1986 Shiloh et al., 1986 Gatti et al., 1991 Swift et al., 1991
Fanconi anemia	Prenatal and postnatal growth retardation Pancytopenia Anatomic defect: hypoplasia or plasia of thumb Hyperpigmentation of skin Mental retardation (+)	Hypersensitivity to some cross-linking compounds High frequency of spontaneous chromosome aberrations (triradials) Breakage usually chromatid in type	+	Leukemia Hepatic adenoma Squamous cell carcinoma of the mucocutaneous junctions	Auerback et al., 1981 Moustacchi and Diatloff-Zito, 1985 Pavlakis et al.,
Bloom	Sunlight hypersensitivity Skin abnormalities: vitiligo, café-au-lait spots, facial telangiectatic erythema in a butterfly-like pattern Prenatal and postnatal growth retardation Microcephaly Skeletal deformities Infections	High frequency of spontaneous sister chromatid exchanges and spontaneous chromosome aberrations (quadriradials) No evidence of DNA repair deficiency	15% +++	Acute leukemia (nonlymphocytic) Gastrointestinal malignancies	Shabtai and Halbrecht, 1980 Emerit and Cerutti, 1981
Xeroderma pigmentosum (classic XP): De Sanctis-Cacchione syndrome	Sunlight hypersensitivity Photophobia: ocular defects Often neurologic abnormalities including mental retardation and seizures, microcephaly, spasticity, incoordination Skin abnormalities: freckles, progeric changes Death by 20 years	Hypersensitivity to hypermutable by ultraviolet and chemical carcinogens Defective complementation groups (9) Defective DNA repair No spontaneous chromosome breakage or rearrangement	+++	Angioma Basal and squamous cells carcinoma Malignant melanoma	Hanawalt and Sarasin, 1986 Mimaki et al., 1986
(XP variants) Incontinentia pigmenti syndrome	Same as above, but no neurologic problems Bullous skin lesions at birth or neonatal onset/linear distribution	Increased chromosome breakage	++ +	Acute myelogenous leukemia and pheochromocytoma	Carney, 1976
Cockayne syndrome	Cachetic dwarfism Mental retardation (microcephaly) Premature aging Sunlight hypersensitivity Intracranial calcification Unsteady tremulous gait	Hypersensitive to ultraviolet and chemical carcinogens No chromosomal instability	+		Nance and Berry, 1992

Continued.

Table 25-6 Chromosome instability and cancer-prone hereditary disorders with DNA processing abnormalities—cont'd

Syndrome	Clinical features	Cellular events	Risk of neoplasia	Types	Reference
Basal cell nevus syndrome	Mild to moderate mental deficiency Frontal and biparietal bossing Jaws cysts and basal cell nevi first appear during childhood and increase during adolescence over neck, upper arms, trunk and face; hypertelorism, dyskeratotic pits of palms and soles	Increased breakage	+++ 15%→ 1-5%→	Basal cell carcinoma Others: medulloblastoma, astrocytoma, ovarian carcinoma	Gorlin and Sedano, 1972
Nijmegen breakage syndrome	Microcephaly Stunted growth Mental retardation Skin abnormalities Immunodeficiency	Rearrangement of chromosomes 14	?	?	Weemaes et al., 1981
Werner syndrome	Multiple progeric features: juvenile cataract, retinal degeneration, gray sparse hair, soft tissue calcification, common lyarngeal abnormalities, peripheral osteoporosis, calcific atherosclerosis, muscle hypoplasia/patchy areas of fibrosis, no mental retardation, CNS normal, short stature. Proteoglycan: hyaluronic aciduria Onset: late childhood	Variegated translocation mosaicism in fibroblast (short life) Mild chromosome breakage under right conditions	++	Mesenchymal tumors: sarcoma (10%), meningioma	Salk, 1982

All of the human hereditary disorders listed exhibit autosomal recessive inheritance, except incontinentia pigmenti, which is X-linked dominant, and basal cell nevus syndrome, which is autosomal dominant with new mutation having a paternal age effect.

persons with fragile X syndrome usually do not reproduce, an extraordinarily high new mutation rate, highest of any human gene ($\approx 1 \times 10^3$ in sperm only), must exist to balance the loss of their genes from the gene pool [Webb, 1989]. The incidence in entire populations (including males and females) varies with different studies and is approximately 1:2000 to 2500 live births [Froster-Iskenius et al., 1983; Sherman et al., 1984; Turner and Jacobs, 1983]. The only study of randomly selected neonates (3450 patients, 1810 males) revealed no patients with fragile X syndrome [Sutherland and Hecht, 1985]. The overall prevalence in institutionalized retarded males varies from 1.6% to greater than 6%. Among children at special schools for the retarded the incidence is probably 3% to 5% [Turner et al., 1992] and even higher in autistic children [Blomquist et al., 1985]. With direct diagnosis by DNA analysis of the fragile X

syndrome, more precise data will be available soon from population screening for male and female carrier status.

Clinical features

Males. The triad of moderate mental retardation, typical dysmorphic facies, and macroorchidism can be found in more than 50% of males with fragile X syndrome [Fryns, 1984]. However, many other manifestations are now recognized [Butler et al., 1992]. Table 25-7 summarizes features of males with fragile X syndrome, taking into account that not all affected males have all or many of these characteristics. Although most patients appear to be the same, a wide variation in phenotypic expression is evident (see Figure 25-15). Scoring systems based on easily quantifiable characteristics are available to assist in screening adults and young children at risk for fragile X syndrome [Hagerman et al., 1991; Laing et al., 1991; Butler et al., 1991; Simko et al.,

Table 25-7 Male phenotype with fragile X-linked mental retardation

Parameter	Features
Birth weight	Normal but usually greater than sibs, mean at about 70 percentile
Height	Infancy and childhood: between 50th and 90th percentile Adult: below 50th percentile
Head circumference	Above the 50th percentile
Extermities	Plantar crease, simian crease, abnormal dermatoglyphics
Dysmorpic facies	Long, narrow face with:
Forehead	Prominent, especially in older children and adults
Jaws	Prognathism, especially in adults
Ears	Large (lap), long, mildly dysmorphic: "Dumbo-like"
Nose	Broad-based, large nose
Eyes	Pale irides
Genitalia	Macroorchidism usually seen in adults, occasionally in children. Volume >30 ml in 80%. Penis usually normal length. Scrotal skin sometimes thickened. Possibly increased incidience of hypospadias, cryptorchidism, and other genitourinary problems. Normal semen.
Endocrine	Hypogonadal appearance of some adults: sparse body hair with a female pubic hair distribution and gynecomastia. Striae on the buttocks, abdomen, and axillae. Endocrinologic investigation usually normal, but not extensive.
Connective tissue	Hyperextensibility of joints, particularly fingers. Fine, velvety skin with striae. High-arched or cleft palate. Mitral valve prolapse and dilatation of ascending aorta. Torticollis and kyphoscoliosis. Flat feet. Inguinal hernia.
Neurologic	Seizure, incoordination. Blepharospasm. Stooped posture and gait. Hyperreflexia of lower limbs with bilateral extension plantar response but without abnormal spasticity.
Behavior	Usually before adolescence. Stereotyped with odd mannerisms such as hand flapping and rubbing. Excessive shyness and hypersensitivity. Tactile defensiveness, poor eye contact. Mild self-mutilation, such as hand and wrist biting. Autism. Better visual than auditory learner. Hyperkinetism, attention deficit disorders
Speech	Litany speech, perseveration, echolalia, better language form content.
Cognitive defects	Better verbal than spatial abilities, deficit in verbal abstractions, deficit in digit span, no specific verbal versus performance difference, possible specific left-hemisphere defect. No dementia or progressive intellectual deterioration.

Modified from TIG 1985a; 1:108; Sutherland GR. Ann Hum Genet 1985b; 49:153; Sutherland GR, Hecht F. Fragile sites on human chromosomes. New York: Oxford University Press, 1985. Sutherland GR and Hagerman, RJ. Physical and behavioral phenotype. In Hagerman RJ, Cronister-Silverman A, eds. Fragile X syndrome: diagnosis, treatment, and research, Baltimore, Johns Hopkins Univeristy Press, 1991.

1989]. Dermatoglyphic abnormalities have been described and may be useful as a simple prescreening test [Langenbeck et al., 1988]. No correlation exists between the mental status, phenotype, and the mar (X) expression (% of fragility). Cognitive dysfunction seen in the fragile X male includes deficits in visual short-term memory, visual/spatial abilities, and processing of sequential information [Kemper et al., 1988; Freund and Reiss, 1991]. The physiopathology of mental retardation (cognitive dysfunction) is still unknown. Recently, cyclic adenosine monophosphate metabolism in platelets of a subgroup of patients with fragile X syndrome was demonstrated to be abnormal [Berry-Kravis and Huttenlocher, 1992]. Behavioral problems are the primary feature of the condition and cause parents more coping difficulties than the intellectual deficiency. The problems usually consist of hyperkinesis, emotional instability, and hypersensitivity; however, some children have been labeled as autistic before the diagnosis, whereas others have manifested psychotic features [Brown et al., 1986; Einfeld et al., 1989; Hagerman et al., 1986a; McGillivray et al., 1986; Borghgraef et al., 1987; Reiss and Freund, 1991b]. In general, these behavioral problems appear to improve with age.

Excessive prenatal and postnatal overgrowth in length, weight, and skull and bone age along with macrocephaly, minor craniofacial abnormalities, and language deficit are reminiscent of cerebral gigantism (Sotos syndrome). These disorders have been described with fragile X syndrome [Beemer et al., 1986], stressing the need for appropriate studies in all cases of Sotos syndrome. In the newborn period a relative macrocephaly with mild facial edema is more striking than the long face typical of the adult. Recently, Robin sequence, which is known to be associated with numerous genetic conditions, was reported with fragile X syndrome [Hagerman, 1987; Lachiewicz et al., 1991]. Serial photography during long-term evaluation documents extreme changes in the individual phenotype. Recurrent otitis media in fragile X syndrome has been observed by Hagerman et al. [1987] and could be related to the associated connective tissue dysplasia, hypotonia, or other unknown factors. Differential diagnosis of the fragile X phenotype is vast and complex, but the newly available direct DNA analysis of the gene will greatly facilitate the diagnosis [Arena and Lubs, 1991a; 1991b].

Neurologic impairment, including neurodevelopmental disabilities, recently has been emphasized as a component of the triad. Usually neurologic examination reveals no focal or hard neurologic findings, but most often soft neurologic signs, such as mirror (overflow) movement (synkinesia), clumsiness, hyperreflexia, positive palmomental reflex, and generalized mild hypotonia [Vieregge and Froster-Iskenius, 1989; Wisniewski et al., 1985b; 1989; Finelli, 1985; Veenema et al., 1987]. The presence of neurologic abnormalities does not exclude the diagnosis of fragile X syndrome. Seizures, either generalized tonic-clonic or partial complex, occur with a prevalence ranging from 9.1% to 45% in males with fragile X syndrome [Pueschel, 1985; Hecht, 1991; Musumeci et al., 1991]. Nevertheless, major neurologic aberrations are only occasionally evident on routine diagnostic studies such as neuroimaging and evoked potential monitoring [Arinami et al., 1988; Hagerman and Cronister-Sylverman, 1991; Wisniewski et al., 1991]. Mild, generalized atrophy and ventricular dilatation in affected males and heterozygous females have been reported. MRI did not identify white matter abnormalities that were demonstrated in a few patients postmortem. However, a recent study of neuroanatomy in fragile X in both males and females discloses a significant reduction in the size of the posterior vermal region of the cerebellum with an increase in the volume of the fourth ventricle compared to controls [Reiss et al., 1991a; 1991b]. EEG examination is usually normal except when the condition is associated with seizures. A novel EEG pattern originating from the temporal lobe during sleep has recently been described in fragile X syndrome [Sanfilippo et al., 1986] and subsequently reported by Musumeci et al. [1988a, 1988b] as a paroxysmal focal activity reminiscent of benign rolandic epilepsy in childhood.

Females. Approximately one third or more of female heterozygotes exhibit varying degrees of mental retardation similar in quality but less in severity than those in hemizygous males [Borghgraef et al., 1990]. However, a few severely retarded females with fragile X syndrome have been reported [Sherman et al., 1984].

Although most affected females are reported as phenotypically normal, some have many features of affected males that correlate with the severity of intellectual impairment. Moreover, in demonstrated fragile X syndrome families, most of the affected females express the fragile X site in the 5% to 50% range, not much less frequently than their affected brothers [Pembrey et al., 1986]. Furthermore, a relationship exists between the frequency of fragile X expression and age: a higher frequency of mar (X) expression occurs in the young female carrier. Usually, the percentage of fragility seems to correlate more with physical than with cognitive findings [Hagerman et al., 1992].

Neuropathology. Neuropathologic findings are limited because few postmortem studies have been reported. Rudelli et al. [1985; 1988] confirmed the preferential involvement of cerebral and testicular structure in an adult with fragile X syndrome. Brain weight was normal for age, and no gross abnormalities in either cerebrum or cerebellum were observed. Deep white matter pallor caused by myelin loss and diffuse, spongy edema were also observed. Dendritic spine abnormalities, similar to the type observed in trisomy 21, were associated with synaptic immaturity [Hinton et al., 1991].

A specific hypothalamic lesion responsible for some of the clinical manifestations has been suggested [Fryns et al., 1986] based on the evidence of acquired central nervous system lesions in three patients with a triad suggestive of fragile X syndrome. Dilatation of the ventricular system in affected males as well as in a heterozygous female has been reported [Tajara and Varella-Garcia, 1985; Reiss et al., 1991a]. The occurrence of macroorchidism in affected males and true precocious puberty in a girl with fragile X syndrome also point to an underlying disturbance of hypothalamic-pituitary-gonadal function in patients with fragile X syndrome [Moore et al., 1990]. Further neuropathologic studies are needed and may provide expected correlation with the growing number of recognized phenotypes.

Genetics. Fragile X syndrome is considered an X-linked disorder [McKusick, 1992]. However, the genetic aspects of this syndrome are peculiar and behave as a model for a new class of genetic mutations (see molecular genetics). The condition does not represent a conventional chromosomal aberration or a single-gene defect inherited in a classic X-linked mendelian fashion, either recessive or dominant. The fragile X syndrome is unique among X-linked disorders in that approximately 20% of the males who inherit the gene are unaffected carriers, often referred to as normal transmitting males [Brown, 1990; Sherman et al., 1984; 1985; Sherman, 1991]. There are several large pedigrees in which unaffected males have transmitted the condition to all of their normal daughters who, in turn, are at high risk of having affected sons, thereby proving their carrier status. Moreover, the carrier mothers of normal transmitting males have less chance of having mentally retarded offspring than do the unaffected carrier daughters of these normal transmitting males (Sherman paradox). Several other aspects that are uncharacteristic of a conventional X-linked disorder also have been recognized, including the following: (1) about 50% of heterozygous females have the disorder to some extent, (2) as many as 30% are mentally retarded, (3) mothers of all affected children are considered to be obligate carriers, and (4) no affected offspring arise as a direct result of a new mutation. Different hypotheses have been advanced to explain the inheritance and genetic mechanism [Friedman and Howard-Peebles, 1986; Laird, 1991; Pembrey et al., 1986].

Cytogenetics. The fragile site is induced in vitro by growing the lymphocyte in a special culture that contains reduced concentrations of folic acid and thymidine and uses different systems of induction [De Arce et al., 1986; Jacky, 1991; Sutherland, 1983]. The folate-sensitive fragile phenomenon on the X chromosome in culture is not always observed in affected individuals or in most normal male transmitters; it is not always associated with the obligate carrier of the fragile X syndrome and is observed in only 1% to 80% of cells analyzed and usually in less than 50% of cells. Moreover, a dissociation appears to exist between fragile X q27.3 and clinical expression because males expressing the fragile site but without evidence of intellectual handicap have been described [Romain and Chapman, 1992; Voelckel et al., 1989]. Indeed, until now, the cytogenetic test was considered the definitive means of identifying fragile X syndrome. However, because it is labor intensive and not entirely reliable for prenatal diagnosis or for the detection of the clinically normal carrier (male or female), it is not the ideal method for genetic counseling.

Molecular genetics. The cloning of the fragile X locus in 1991 and the identification of DNA mutations [Oberlé et al., 1991; Yu et al., 1991] and the gene (FMR-1) [Pieretti et al., 1991; Verkerk et al., 1991] involved have significantly changed the diagnostic approach to the fragile X syndrome. The mutations associated with the syndrome affect a small target region and are of a completely new type: DNA expansion of a trinucleotide repeat [(CGG)n] associated with abnormal methylation of the surrounding DNA (which is known to inhibit gene expression) and DNA instability (meiotic and mitotic). A brief summary of these unstable and methylatable mutations causing the fragile X syndrome is found in Table 25-8.

Studies of known fragile X families with direct DNA analysis at the fragile X locus [Fu et al., 1991; Pergolizzi et al., 1992; Rousseau et al., 1991; Yu et al., 1992] have revealed that most (more than 99%) of the fragile X mutations are of this type and are detectable by Southern blot analysis using the appropriate probe. Two types of fragile X mutations exist. "Premutations" are found in nonexpressing carriers (male or female) and correspond to small expansions (of less than 600 bp) not associated with abnormal methylation. The theoretic prevalence of fragile X premutations is about 1:500 women. Premutations are accompanied by a normal phenotype and are transmitted almost unchanged by the normal transmitting males to each of their daughters. When transmitted by a female a premutation has a high risk of converting to a "full mutation" associated with the clinical phenotype (e.g., mental retardation) in 100% of males and about 50% to 75% of females who inherit such a full mutation. "Full mutations" are characterized by large expansions (more than 600 bp) of the target region that are associated with abnormal methylation of the surrounding DNA region on the active X chromosome, which is believed to cause the clinical phenotype by inhibiting expression of the FMR-1 gene.

The fragile X syndrome appears to be the first member of a new family of dynamic mutations where insert-

serious psychologic problems that cannot be explained by environment. However, some specific behaviors have been described in some chromosomal aberrations. For example, in duplication 15p syndrome, psychotic behavior with anxiety, hyperactivity, autoaggressiveness, tremor, low frustration tolerance, and autistic features have been described in addition to seizures.

Autosomal ring chromosome syndromes are associated with few physical abnormalities and moderate mental retardation. Similar features have been reported, however, including aggressiveness, temporal lobe seizures, schizophrenia, and certain characteristics reminiscent of a neurodegenerative disorder as seen in r(18) [Schinzel, 1981a], r(20) [Stewart et al., 1979], and r(22) [Reeve, 1985]. In trisomy 8 M, a schizophrenic-like behavior has been described [Sperber, 1975].

Patterns of dysmorphism

Dysmorphism relates to normal variations in the shape and size of any part of the body, particularly the face, genitalia, and distal limbs. Some stigmata occur singly in normal neonates or infants (Table 25-10). Dysmorphic features usually do not affect function of an organ, but esthetic qualities are diminished. The face is important to evaluate. It is sometimes said that "the face predicts the brain," such as in holoprosencephaly or agenesis of the corpus callosum [Dyken and Miller, 1980]. Dysmorphic features include abnormal size, shape, and position of the ear (Figure 25-3); nonhorizontal eye axes; aberrant palpebral fissures; unusual size and form of the nose, philtrum, and mandible; unusual palatal configuration; neck webbing (pterygium coli); and redundant skin [Aase, 1990; Cohen, 1979; Jones and Higginbottom, 1978].

Interpupillary distance (Figure 25-4) should be mea-

sured to exclude hypotelorism or hypertelorism. Both of these common facial features are defined, respectively, as an absolute decrease or increase in the distance between the inner canthi, pupils, or outer edge of the long orbits [DeMyer, 1977]. Such distances are best used to refer to the position of the bony orbits in relation to each other. Although best ascertained with radiographs, the measurement of interpupillary distance has been standardized and is an objective reliable bedside measurement [Pryor, 1969].

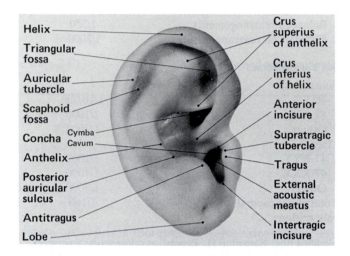

Figure 25-3 Normal descriptive anatomy of the ear.

Table 25-10 Incidence of stigmata in 74 normal children

Anomaly	Percentage
High palate	16.7
Head circumference >1 standard deviation outside normal range	15.3
Adherent ear lobes	14.0
Gap between first and second toe	11.7
Stubbed fifth finger	8.1
Curved fifth finger	7.7
Hypertelorism	6.8
Low-set ears	4.5
Epicanthal folds	3.2
Syndactyly of toes	2.7

From Walker HA. Incidence of minor physical anomalies in autistic patients. In Coleman M, ed. Autistic syndrome. New York: Elsevier-North Holland, 1976.

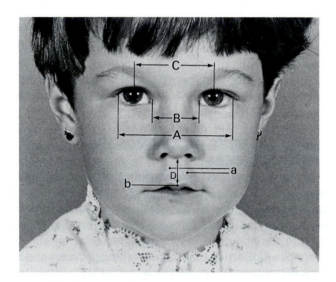

Figure 25-4 Interpupillary distance. **A,** Outer canthal distance; **B,** inner canthal distance; **C,** interpupillary distance; **D,** nasolabial distance; **a,** pillars of philtrum; **b,** cupid's arc. Distances **A** and **B** allow rapid assessment of distance between the eyes. Normally,

$$A = 3 \times B, \text{ and } \frac{A - B}{2} + B = C.$$

(From Pryor HB. Pediatrics 1969; 44:973.)

In autosomal deletion or duplication, hypertelorism is often incorrectly diagnosed because of the associated microcephaly that falsely suggests that the eyes are too widely set [Miller, 1973]. Physiognomic changes occur with age. Adults often do not exhibit the dysmorphic features that are highly evident when they are children. It is important to look at old photographs, if available, to differentiate the constitutional traits from the phenotypic features of a particular chromosome syndrome. In essence a pattern of dysmorphic features that is more characteristic of an autosomal aberration than a single dysmorphic sign should be distinguished. The absence of one or two features of the pattern does not affect the overall clinical impression.

Patterns of multiple organ system distribution of congenital anomalies

When errors of morphogenesis are considered, it is important to understand general concepts and terms [Aase, 1992; Spranger et al., 1982]. Correctly defining the individual alteration of form and structure is essential. The following definitions are used with regard to morphogenesis:

Deformation Abnormal form, shape, or position of a part of the body caused by mechanical forces.

Disruption Morphologic defect of an organ, part of an organ, or a larger region of the body resulting from an extrinsic breakdown of, or an interference with, an originally normal developmental process.

Dysplasia Abnormal organization of cells into tissue along with the morphologic results. In other words, dysplasia is a process (and the consequence) of dyshistogenesis.

Malformation Morphogenic defect of an organ, part of an organ, or a larger region of the body resulting from an intrinsically abnormal developmental process.

Most chromosomal aberrations result in malformation and sometimes in dysplasia.

The patterns of morphologic defects should also be well defined and include the following:

Association Nonrandom occurrence in two individuals of multiple anomalies not known to be a polytopic field defect, sequence, or syndrome (e.g., Vater or anidria-Wilms tumor).

Polytopic field defect Pattern of anomalies derived from the disturbance of a single developmental field, as seen in holoprosencephaly.

Sequence Pattern of multiple anomalies derived from a single known or presumed prior anomaly or mechanical factor (e.g., myelomeningocele, arthrogryposis, Potter malformation, and fetal akinesia/hypokinesia sequence [Moessinger, 1983]).

Syndrome Pattern of multiple anomalies believed to be pathogenetically related and not known to represent a single sequence or a polytopic field defect (e.g., Cornelia de Lange, Prader-Willi, Rubinstein-Taybi syndromes).

In chromosomal aberrations, malformations are multiple and vary in intensity, that is, they are gross or subtle. Gross malformations are life threatening, and subtle ones are detectable only on postmortem examination. In cases of dysmorphism, more reliance should be placed on the total pattern of the abnormalities than on the single malformation [Holmes, 1976]. Visceral malformations should be sought, particularly of the urinary tract and heart, with imaging techniques such as ultrasonography [Egli and Stalder, 1973; Naganuma, 1978]. The boxes on this page and p. 378 list common and uncommon malformations in autosomal chromosomal aberrations.

Dysmorphism and malformations result from multifactorial interaction. In addition to the chromosomal abnormalities that cause approximately 0.6% of the cases, other causes should be considered. Such causes

---

Malformation Outside the CNS Common in Autosomal Chromosome Aberrations

Eyes

Microphthalmia
Ocular coloboma

Gastrointestinal and Abdomen

Cleft palate, cleft lip, or both
Esophageal and duodenal atresia
Tracheoesophageal fistula, anal atresia with fistula
Omphalocele
Common mesentery
Malrotation of the gut

Heart and Great Vessels

Kidney and Urinary Tracts

Extremities

Absence or hypoplasia of radius and thumb
Radial-ulnar synostosis
Postaxial hexadactyly
Edema

Modified from Schinzel A. Catalogue of unbalanced chromosome aberration in man. Berlin: Walter de Gruyter, 1984.

Malformation Uncommon in Autosomal Aberrations
Anencephalus, exencephalus, iniencephalus, otocephalus
Gastroschisis
Situs inversus totalis
Atresia of the jejunum or ileum
Exstrophy of the bladder or cloaca
Sirenomelia, peromelia, amelia, phocomelia
Ulnar or fibular ray defects
Congenital arthrogryposis
Teratoma

Modified from Schinzel A. A catalogue of unbalanced chromosome aberrations in man. Berlin: Walter de Gruyter, 1984.

include environmental-teratogenic factors (e.g., drugs, infections, radiation), maternal factors (e.g., diabetes, phenylketonuria), and mendelian traits (including inborn errors of metabolism; e.g., glutaric acidemia type II, peroxisomal disorders). More fundamental biologic factors appear to be of prime importance. These factors include DNA repair defects; gene dysfunction controlling cellular growth, development, and differentiation; anomalies of both spatial and temporal control of gene expression; anomalies of cell recognition, adhesion, and communication; and finally, anomalies of the extracellular matrix or the cytoskeleton. Investigation of these fundamental biologic factors eventually will explain now-recognized syndromes of unknown cause that manifest as sporadic events and frequently have an impact on CNS development.

Intrauterine and postnatal growth disturbances

Growth may be reduced, normal, or accelerated in autosomal aberrations. Intrauterine growth and postnatal growth retardation are characteristics of many well-known chromosomal aberrations, although genetic background apparently contributes to the degree of retardation.

Severe dwarfism usually does not accompany autosomal chromosome aberration; however, growth hormone deficiency has been associated with cat's eye syndrome and 18p−. Normal growth is common in 18p+, 13q+, trisomy 8 M, and 1q+ or 1q− syndromes. Advanced growth may occur characteristically in patients with trisomy 8 but is otherwise the exception in autosomal chromosome aberrations. Bone age is usually retarded, along with delayed and diminished puberty. Growth may continue until age 22 to 25 years. Height and weight curves, although indicating patients' deviation from values obtained from the normal population, do not reflect the expected values for patients with individual chromosomal aberrations.

Endocrine abnormalities (puberty and fertility)

Most autosomal chromosome abnormalities are associated with delayed or diminished puberty. Male fertility is present in patients with autosomal ring syndromes and cat's eye syndrome. Fertility and normal puberty occur no more often in the female with autosomal aberrations than in the male. Gonadal dysgenesis or ovarian hypoplasia has been reported in some aberrations, including trisomies 13 and 18. Pregnancy has been reported in patients with trisomy 21, various autosomal ring syndromes, deletion 18q, trisomy 8 M, and cat's eye syndrome.

In newborns, the identification of major or minor anomalies is an important facet of the clinical assessment leading to the diagnosis of clinical chromosomal disorders. The examiner should scrutinize the head, face, ears, eyes, mouth, neck, chest, abdomen, genitalia, limbs, and skin. The dermatoglyphic patterns should also be studied. No substitute exists for a serial photographic record obtained at various ages. Serial photography in long-term follow-up can document severe changes in the individual phenotype (see discussion of trisomy 8).

During childhood, puberty, or adulthood the patient with chromosomal anomalies will be referred for evaluation of learning disorders, neurobehavioral problems, cerebral palsy, multiple handicaps, abnormal physical growth, and most often mental retardation. As a part of the neurologic examination, patterns of minor malformation and dysmorphism, often age-dependent and unrecognized at birth, should be excluded. Neurologic signs and symptoms are not always evident. Most patients display abnormal head shape, abnormal tone and movements (tics), seizures, sensory impairment, midline fusion defects, and significant structural anomalies of the skull, brain, and spinal cord and associated vertebrae (Table 25-11). Most of these anomalies are not specific for chromosomal imbalance. For example, holoprosencephaly can result from multiple causes, including monogenic, environmental, and chromosomal causes [Leech and Shuman, 1986]. Others, such as fetal choroid plexus cysts, are being evaluated [McHugo et al., 1991]. Similar to other developmental processes that affect a particular phenotype, most CNS malformations are the product of interaction between the genetic stock and the environment.

Skeletal abnormalities in autosomal chromosome aberrations are also common [Finidori et al., 1983]. Some aberrations are nonspecific, such as abnormal shape and number of vertebrae or ribs, abnormal shape of the pelvis, delayed bone maturation, pseudoepiphysis,

Table 25-11 Malformations of skull and brain, spinal cord and column

Skull

Microcrania	1q−;3p+;4p−;4p+;5p−;5p+;r(6);7q−;9p+;9q+;+9;10q+;11q+;12p−;+13; 13q−;13q+;r(13);15q+;16p+;17q+;+18;18p−;18q−;r(18);19q+;+21;21q−; r(22);triploidy
Macrocrania	12q+
Brachycephaly	1q+;1q−;3p+;6q+;7q+;9p+;10q+;+21
Dolichocephaly	4p+;7p+;9q+;+9;10p+;15q+;+18;18q+;r(21)
Trigonocephaly	**6q+**;7p−;**9p−;11q−;13q+**;14p+;18p−
Turricephaly (oxycephaly)	12p+
Craniostenoses	1q−;3q+;5p+;6q+;**7p−**;7p+;9p−;11q−;12p−;**+13**;3q−;**18p−**;r(21); triploidy
Fontanel and/or suture anomalies	1q+;4p−;7q+;7p+;+8;9p+;9p−;+13;1q−;+18;19q+;+21
Scalp defect	13p+;16p+;4p−
Kleeblattschädel (triphyllocephaly)	13p+;15q+

Brain

Anencephaly	r(13);+18;+21
Holoprosencephaly	**1q+**;3p+;3q+;4p−;6p+;r(16);7q−;9p+;10p−;**11q+;+13**;13q−;13q+;14p+;r(15); 16q+;17q;17p+;+18;**18p−**;r(18);+21;22p−;22q+;**triploidy**
Hydrocephaly	1q+;3q+;4p−;5p+;+8M;9p+;+9 M;+13;+18 triploidy
Cerebellar hypoplasia or dysplasia	**1q+**;2p+;3p+;3q+;4p−;6q+;9p−;9p+;9q+;13q+
Chiari malformation	1q+;3q+;4p−;5p+;+8M;9p+;+9 M;+13;+18 triploidy
Dandy-Walker malformation	3q+;5p+;6p−;8p+;8q+;9p+;17q+;triploidy
Occipital or frontal encephalocele	2q+;6q+;7p+;8q+;+18
Agenesis of corpus callosum	2q−;3q+;4p−;4p+;6q+;r(6);7p−;**+8 M;8p+**;9p−;9p+;+9 M;10q−;10p+;**11q+**; 13q−;r(13);14p+;14q−;17p+;**+18**;18q−;+19 M; **triploidy**
Fusion of thalami	3q+
Fusion of basal ganglia	+13
Migration defect of many aberrations	2p+;3p+;3q+;4p−;6p+;**+13;17p−;+18**;+21
Choroid plexus cysts	+18

Spinal cord and column

Meningomyelocele	2p+;3q+;+9 M;+13;+14;11q+;+18;13q−;13p+;**triploidy**
Vertebrae anomalies	5p−;+8 M;**13q−; r(13)**;+18;21q−;+21
Scoliosis	5p−;7q+;+18;18p−;+20;45X;XYYY;XXXXY
Kyphosis	7q+;18p−;+20

Most frequently seen malformations appear in boldface type.

cone-shaped epiphysis, and minor abnormalities of metacarpals, metatarsals, and phalanges. Other skeletal abnormalities are more specific, such as in trisomy 21, trisomy 8 M, duplication 9p, and deletion 1q, as described in later sections.

In addition to cytogenetic studies, other techniques are useful for the delineation of chromosomal disorders, particularly in the evaluation of a specific organ system. The availability and use of neuroimaging techniques such as CT, MRI, and ultrasonography have become routine.

Neurophysiologic techniques, including EEG with sleep polygraphic studies, evoked potentials, and brain electrical activity mapping, have been of definite but limited use in the delineation of syndromes.

The many syndromes described during the past several years are each associated with different chromosomes. No clustering of abnormalities has occurred on a single chromosome or among a small group of chromosomes. The syndromes often involve different closed breakpoints on the same arm of a chromosome and appear most frequently in families with balanced translocation.

Precise localization is difficult because many phenotypic features depend on both position and extent of deletion or duplication within a chromosome. Because few patients are reported by the same authors, karyotype-phenotype correlations are often imprecise; more correlated reports of karyotype-phenotype manifestations associated with the same breakpoints are necessary. Furthermore, all chromosomes have been involved in a partial duplication-deletion syndrome with the same or, more often, with other segments of autosomal chromosomes and even of sex chromosomes.

Both duplication and deletion contribute to the phenotype, and although karyotypes may appear to be similar, appreciable differences are likely to exist in the amount of duplicated or deleted material [Rudd and Lamarche, 1971]. In duplication the severity of the clinical syndrome appears to be clearly related to the added quantity of material rather than to the specific chromosome or chromosome part duplicated. The effects of deletion are more pronounced than those of duplication for the same segment [de Grouchy, 1983; Lazjuk et al., 1985]. Ring chromosomes, although often unstable, tend to cause phenotypes corresponding to the deletion of the long arm rather than the short arm [Kistenmacher and Punnett, 1970].

This area of investigation is rapidly changing. The use of new techniques in microcytogenetics and molecular cytogenetics will continue to better refine and delineate phenotype-karyotypes. Current journals should be consulted regularly. A prototype is presented in tabular form (Table 25-12) to stress the extent of this growing field and the potential for clarification of more than 1000 unexplained syndromes [Steele and Golden 1984]. *The Handbook of Clinical Neurology* should be consulted for more details.* Further information should be sought in books devoted to cataloging recognized syndromes.† Other atlases, such as those by Goodman and Gorlin [1983], Graham [1988], Gorlin et al. [1989], Holmes et al. [1973], Jones [1988], Nyhan and Sakati [1987], and Salmon [1978], are useful references. In 1980 Kunze presented an overview of neurologic manifestations of major chromosome disorders. For genetic counseling and chromosome anomalies, readers should consult Gardner and Sutherland [1989].

CONTIGUOUS GENE SYNDROMES

Contiguous gene syndromes are recognizable and comprise microdeletion and microduplication syndromes [Schinzel, 1988; Schimckel, 1986b; Emanuel, 1988, Ledbetter and Canavee, 1989].

The application of molecular genetics to microcytogenetics ("new cytogenetics") is instrumental in demonstrating DNA rearrangements involving contiguous genes, also called *segmental aneusomies*. Many develop-

mental disorders suggest a chromosomal aberration because they usually occur sporadically, although occasional familial (recessive or dominant) incidence is observed. An accompanying broad spectrum of distinct dysmorphic features of variable severity, with severe growth and mental retardation, also can be delineated. Many disorders can be grouped together because precise chromosomal alterations have been related to previously established dysmorphic syndromes by dysmorphologists and syndromologists [Jones 1988; Gorlin et al., 1989]. Many were considered to be of probable monogenic inheritance [Schmickel, 1986a].

The contiguous gene syndromes are the experiments of nature that tell us about the organization of genes on a chromosome and where they are. These syndromes tell us where important developmental genes are located, and molecular biology provides the means to explore these areas with genetic probes. If we know where a gene is, we can find out what is defective and ultimately how it should work.

A recent review of this subject was presented by Punnet and Zakai [1990], who added some possible new syndromes: Alagille (del 20p), Pallister-Killian (i 12p), and alpha-thalassemia and mental retardation (del 16p13.3) with a preferential paternal origin. Table 25-13 summarizes the best known syndromes (with established 1 to 8 with preferential origin of parents: maternal, paternal, or random; provisional 9 to 15). In addition, other syndromes associated with a terminal deletion of an autosomal chromosome, such as Wolf-Hirschhorn syndrome (del 4p16) and cri-du-chat syndrome (del 5p16), likely represent phenotypes associated with DNA rearrangement involving contiguous genes.

Two regions of the X chromosome are known to have microdeletions of contiguous genes leading to multiple X-linked disorders in the same male patient. At the X p21 region, various combinations of Duchenne muscular dystrophy, chronic granulomatous disease, glycerol kinase deficiency, retinitis pigmentosa, McCleod phenotype, congenital adrenal hypoplasia, ornithine transcarbamoylase deficiency, and various degrees of mental retardation have been described [Francke et al. 1987]. Similarly, at the X p22 region, combinations of steroid sulfatase deficiency, Kallmann syndrome, chondrodysplasia punctata, and mental retardation have been demonstrated to have been caused by deletions of contiguous genes [Nishimura et al., 1991]. Molecular studies are revealing subsets of genes involved in many other neurodevelopmental disorders and will probably explain the variability found in each of the contiguous gene syndromes.

The increased availability of DNA probes now permits definition of the size of mutations, chromosome changes, and, above all, the parental origin, which may have a profound effect on the function of chromosomes

---

*References Cox and Ray, 1977; Zellweger and Simpson, 1977; Zellweger et al., 1977; Réthoré, 1977; Warkany et al., 1981; Warkany 1985; Zellweger and Patil, 1987a, 1987b; Réthoré and Pinet, 1987.
†References Bergsma, 1979; Emery and Rimoin, 1990; Vinken and Bruyn, 1982; Borgaonkar, 1991; Schinzel, 1984; de Grouchy and Turleau, 1984.

Table 25-12 Autosomal chromosome aberrations

Chromosome	Syndrome	Core findings (including mental retardation for all)	Reference
1	1q−	Round face/prominent "cupid's bow," downturned corners of the mouth, thin vermilion borders of lips, long upper lip/smooth philtrum, short and broad nose, micrognathia. Microcephaly, generalized hypotonia, seizures, abnormal hands and feet (specific x-ray findings), cardiac and genital anomalies.	Johnson et al., 1985 Murayama et al., 1991
	1p+	Phenotype nonspecific, variable, relative macrocephaly/prominent forehead, large fontanel and widely separated sutures, flat nasal bridge, micrognathia, holoprosencephaly.	Michels et al., 1984
2	2p+	Variable phenotype, multiple congenital malformations, growth retardation.	Fineman et al., 1983
	2q+	Specific phenotype more pronounced toward adolescence, psychomotor retardation, hypertelorism, midface hypoplasia, cardiac, urogenital, retinal and optic disc, anomalies, kyphosis/scoliosis, hypotonia	Kyllerman et al, 1984
3	.3p−	Facial changes, congenital heart defects, hypoplasia of male genitalia, holoprosencephaly, limb malformation and gastrointestinal anomalies	Martin and Steinberg, 1983 Reifen et al., 1986
	3p+	Variable phenotype, severe postnatal growth retardation, ptosis, temporal indentation, frontal bossing, hypertelorism, congenital heart anomalies.	Tolmie et al., 1986 Reiss et al., 1986
	3q+	Synophrys; long eyelashes, hypertrichosis, square-shaped face, malformation of auricles, anteverted nares, retracted lower lip, abnormal head shape, microcephaly, seizures, brain anomalies, clinodactyly, heart and renal malformations; similar to de Lange-like: see contiguous gene syndrome.	Wilson et al., 1985b
4	.4p−	See text.	
	4q−	Faunlike ears, snub nose, cleft palate, retrognathia, micrognathia, hypertelorism	Townes et al., 1979
	4p+	Variable phenotype. Aplasia of the nasal bones (boxer nose) in adult, microcephaly, growth retardation, prominent glabella, low-set malformed ears.	Reynolds et al., 1983
	4q+	"Cul de poule" or pursed mouth, no nasal bridge, short and prominent philtrum, abnormal auricles, hypotonia, microcephaly, urinary tract malformations.	Stoll and Roth, 1980
5	.5p−	See text	
	5p+	Hypotelorism, large mandible, dolichocephaly/flat forehead, hypotonia, seizures, ear anomalies.	Leschot and Kim, 1979
6	6q−	Microcephaly, strabismus, low-set malformed ears, broad nasal bridge, micrognathia, short neck, congenital heart defect, hand abnormalities.	Young et al., 1985
	6p+	Large fontanels, blepharophimosis, bulbous nose, small mouth, low-set and malformed ears, congenital heart malformation.	Bernheim et al., 1979
	6q+	Microcephaly/abnormally shaped head, hypertelorism, bow-shaped mouth, flat face profile, micrognathia, short neck/unusual webbing, club feet.	Pivnick et al., 1990
7	.7p−	Psychomotor retardation, craniostenosis, antimongoloid slant of palpebral fissures, hypotelorism, short nose, proptosis, limb and genital abnormalities.	Motegi et al., 1985 Aughton et al., 1991
	7q−	Microcephaly, flat occiput, bulbous nose, palpebral fissures slanted up and downward, redundant subcutaneous tissue.	Young et al., 1984
	7p+	Mild dysmorphism: elongated skull, skeletal and heart anomalies.	Moore et al., 1982
	7q+	Discrete facial dysmorphism: low birth weight, fuzzy hair, small palpebral fissure, micrognathia, abnormal low-set ears, abnormal muscle tone, skeletal abnormalities.	Bartsch et al., 1990

Continued.

Table 25-12 **Autosomal chromosome aberrations—cont'd**

Chromosome	Syndrome	Core findings (including mental retardation for all)	Reference
	18q−	Frontal bossing, deeply set eyes and eye anomalies, depressed midface, carp-shaped mouth and prominent chin, strongly folded ears, hypertelorism, high frequency of whorls, hypoplasia of first metacarpals.	Ehrlich et al., 1983 Miller et al., 1990
	r(18)	Predominance of the features of 18q−, microcephaly, midfacial depression, carplike mouth.	Rethoré, 1977
	18p+	Chubby face, flat nasal bridge, macrognathia.	Gardner et al., 1978
	18q+	Minor clinical features, features of trisomy 18, ambiguous external genitalia.	Razavi-Encha et al., 1985
19	19q+	Craniofacial dysmorphism: failure to thrive, psychomotor retardation.	Zonana et al., 1982
20	r(20)	Seizure/behavior disorders, variable degree of physical anomalies, no severe malformations, severe cardiac and renal anomalies, neurodegenerative-like course.	Burnell et al., 1985
	20p+	Mild to moderate psychomotor retardation, craniofacial anomalies: round face/full cheeks, short chin, oblique palpebral fissures, brachycephaly, major cardiac and renal malformations, hypotonia, poor coordination.	Francke, 1982
21	+21	See text.	
	r(21)	Hypertonia, protuberant nasal bridge, palpebral fissures slanted down; and outward protuberant occiput, large ears, segment distal to the sod-1 locus (i.e., 21q 22.2 → qter) has been lost during ring formation.	Wisniewski et al., 1983
	21q−	Discrete dysmorphism: aplastic nasal bridge, high forehead, wide mandible, stiffness of joints, vertebral anomalies.	Ferrante et al., 1983
22	.+22	Severe growth retardation, micrognathia, asymmetrical cranium, long and deep philtrum, large ears, preauricular skin tag or sinus, palate anomaly, heart and genital anomalies; see trisomy by T (11;22): most frequent translocation.	Wertelecki et al., 1985 Schinzel et al., 1981b Anneren and Gustavson, 1981
	Cat's eye syndrome	Ocular vertical coloboma (6 o'clock), low-set ears, hypertelorism, microphthalmia, epicanthus, microcephaly, heart, urogenital, and intestinal defects (atresia and stenosis).	Duncan et al., 1986 Rosenfeld et al., 1984 Guanti, 1981
	22q−	Microcephaly, ptosis, hypertelorism, large and low-set ears, flat nasal bridge, syndactyly, cardiac anomalies, variable phenotype: behavioral problems See Di George: contiguous gene syndrome.	Watt et al., 1985
	r(22)	Mild craniofacial anomalies: doe eyes, low-set eyebrows, dental malocculsion, neurologic environment of CNS, peripheral nerves and muscles; meningioma and acoustic neuroma.	Reeve et al., 1985
Y	47,XXY Klinefeller syndrome	See text	
	XXXY	Severe mental retardation, microcephaly, minor dysmorphism.	Zollinger, 1969 Ferrier et al., 1974
	XXXXY	Mental retardation, hypotonia, mimics Down syndrome.	Lomelino and Reiss, 1991
	47,XYY	Incidence: 1/1000 male newborns. Unusually tall stature, dull normal IQ, delayed speech and cognitive disorders, minor neurologic findings, behavioral manifestations.	Daly, 1969 Noël et al., 1969
	48,XXYY	Incidence: 1/50,000 newborns. Severe mental retardation hypogonadism and may be increased in height and aggressive behavior	Sorensen et al., 1978 Schlegel et al., 1965
	48,XYYY	Mild retardation, severe behavioral disorders, tallness of stature, genital hypoplasia.	Townes et al., 1965 Ridler et al., 1973

Table 25-12 Autosomal chromosome aberrations—cont'd

Chromosome	Syndrome	Core findings (including mental retardation for all)	Reference
X	45, X Turner syndrome	See text.	
	47,XXX	Incidence: 1/1000 or 2/1000 female newborns. Normal phenotype: usually normal puberty and fertility, secondary amennorhea may be present; 30% mental retardation and seizures.	Pennington et al., 1980 Sills et al., 1978
	48,XXXX	Facies suggestive of Down syndrome. Mild facial hypoplasia, epicanthal folds, micrognathia, mental retardation, variable amenorrhea, speech and behavioral problems.	Tumba et al., 1975
	49,XXXXX	Moderate to severe mental retardation, low nasal bridge, hypertelorism, upslanting palpebral fissures, ptosis, patent ductus arteriosus, mimics Down syndrome, uncoordinated eye movements.	Kassai et al., 1991
Triploidy	69, XXX: 1/3. 69, XXY: 2/3.	Large placenta, many hydatidiform changes, prenatal growth deficiency, microphthalmia, dysplastic ears, coloboma of the iris and choroid, congenital heart defect, large posterior fontanel, hypospadias and cryptorchidism, usually stillborn or early neonatal death, survivors are mosaic.	Uchida and Freeman, 1985 Wertelecki et al., 1976

and genes. Genomic imprinting (origin of parents) is considered to be a possible explanation for the observation that children may have similar chromosomal deletions, but the particular phenotype depends on which parental set of genes is lost. This new "look" (nonclassical mendelian inheritance) seems to apply to many definite or provisional contiguous gene syndromes. Uniparental disomy (two homologous chromosomes from one parent) with or without imprinting effect would be another possible explanation. Both mechanisms could also be applied to other clinically well-defined disorders of unknown cause, which generally occur de novo, and in which undergrowth or overgrowth is an important component, such as in Russell-Silver dwarfism, Sotos syndrome, and Williams syndrome [Bellugi et al., 1990; Greenberg et al., 1990]. This new twist on nonclassical mendelian heritability will be a frequent consideration in the near future.

The paradigm of contiguous syndromes is two rare disorders: Prader-Willi syndrome, first described by Prader, Labhart, and Willi in 1956, and the "happy puppet" Angelman syndrome, first described by Angelman in 1965. Both syndromes reveal a common, indistinguishable molecular chromosome 15 rearrangement, but differ in their complex, distinct, clinical phenotypes, although both are characterized by mental retardation, unusual behavior and growth disturbance, and most importantly, parental origin (see box on p. 388).

Incidence

Prader-Willi syndrome has an incidence between 1 in 5000 and 1 in 30,000 live births and accounts for about 1% of the causes of mental handicap [Bray et al, 1983;

Cassidy, 1984; Holm and Sulzbacher, 1987; Zellweger and Soper, 1979]. Based on published cases, Angleman syndrome appears to occur ten times less frequently, but the precise frequency has not yet been determined.

Prader-Willi syndrome phenotype

Two distinctive clinical stages characterize the course and natural history of Prader-Willi syndrome. Prospective clinical observation of the first stage has recently been expanded because of the possibility of an early cytogenetic diagnosis and follow-up [Aughton, 1990; Stephenson, 1992; Whorton and Bresnan, 1989]. After an uneventful prenatal period, except for possible diminished fetal movement, the neonate is usually floppy with a weak cry, low birth weight, and small stature. Considerable feeding difficulties include poor sucking and swallowing, with failure to thrive. Cardinal manifestations are subtle but distinctive facial dysmorphism, genital hypoplasia, and particularly severe, axial more than rhizomelic, hypotonia of cerebral type, persisting throughout infancy. Serum muscle enzyme tests, electromyography, and muscle biopsy results are usually normal except for some nonspecific changes seen with electron microscopy [Brooke, 1986]. In the past the diagnosis was often delayed until 2 years of age (second stage), when progressive, striking hyperphagia and obesity develop, making Prader-Willi syndrome the most common syndromal cause of marked human obesity (Figure 25-5). In addition to the nervous system manifestations, these symptoms suggest hypothalamic dysfunction, although neuroendocrine investigation has not revealed a consistent abnormality [Theodoridis et al., 1971]. Other findings include hypothalamic hypogo-

Table 25-13 Contiguous gene syndromes

Conditions	Characteristics	Chromosome	Frequency	Reference
Prader-Willi/Angelman syndrome	See text.	del 15q12	+ + + >60%	
Miller-Dieker syndrome p.o: p	Intrauterine and postnatal growth retardation, microcephaly, hydrocephaly, abnormal neuronal migration, lissencephaly, severe mental retardation, high, narrow forehead/bitemporal hallows, downward and narrow slanting palpebral fissures, broad midface/upturned nares. Circulimbal clouding of corneas, micrognathia, short neck, scoliosis, widely spaced nipples, sacral dimple, short fingers, polydactyly and syndactyly, hypotonia followed by hypertonia, seizures (infantile spasms) and EEG disturbances. Renal, cardiac, and genital anomalies.	del 17 p. 13.3	+ + +	Dobyns et al., 1991 Stratton et al., 1984 Dobyns et al., 1985 Alvarey et al., 1986 Greenberg et al., 1986 Kuwano et al., 1991
Langer-Giedion syndrome p.o: m	Physical and mental retardation, microcephaly, sparse hair, bushy eye brows, prominent ears, pear-shaped nose, tented alae, micrognathia, long, broad philtrum, thin upper lip, dental anomalies. Bradydactyly, preaxial polydactyly, muscular hypotonia, skin laxity, multiple exostoses, cone-shaped epiphyses.	del 8q24.1	+ + + >50%	Buhler et al., 1984 Murachi et al., 1984 Langer et al., 1984
DiGeorge syndrome p.o: m	Hypoplasia to aplasia of thymus and parathyroid, hypocalcemia and seizures in early infancy, cellular immunodeficiency, pixie face, short philtrum, downward slanting of palpebral fissures, mental retardation, cardiac defects, diaphragmatic hernia, hydronephrosis, severe brain defects. Most infants die during first month of life. Field defect (or sequence): involves foregut in the region of the third and fourth pharyngeal pouch and the fourth brachial arch.	del 22q11	+ +	Carey, 1980 Greenberg et al., 1984
Beckwith-Wiedemann syndrome p.o: p	Macrosomia, muscular hypertrophy, macroglossia, hypoglycemia, ear creases, hyperplastic visceromegaly, omphalocele, immunodeficiency, high alpha-fetoprotein levels, embryonal cancer-prone: hepatoblastoma Wilms tumor, rhabodmyosarcoma. Biologic markers: INS, RAS, IGF, HBB, TH.	dup 11q15.4	+ +	Waziri et al., 1983 Turleau et al., 1985 Journell et al., 1985 Koufos et al., 1985
Aniridia Wilms tumors association p.o: p	Wilms tumor, aniridia, genitourinary tract defects, mental retardation (WAGR); gonadoblastoma, sexual ambiguity, hemihypertrophy. Markers: Catalase, follicle-stimulating hormone	del 11p13	+ + +	Turleau and de Grouchy, 1985 Narahara et al., 1984 Huff, 1990
Retinoblastoma p.o: p	Microcephaly, prominent nasal bridge, short-webbed neck, small or absent thumbs. Most are severely retarded. Esterase D gene-linked.	del 13q14	+ + +	Sparkes, 1983
Smith-Magenis syndrome p.o: r	Mental retardation, behavioral problems, facial dysmorphism brachycephaly: with broad, flat midface. Short and broad hands. Speech delay, hoarse, deep voice. Clinical sign of peripheral neuropathy, abnormal sleep function.	del 17p11.2	+ + +	Greenberg et al., 1986 Moncla et al., 1991

Table 25-13 Contiguous gene syndromes—cont'd

Conditions	Characteristics	Chromosome	Frequency	Reference
Similar to Cornelia de Lange (de Lange) syndrome	Antenatal and postnatal marked growth retardation, mental retardation, initial hypertonicity, hirsutism, low-pitched cry, malformation of hands and feet. Facies: bushy eyebrows and synophrys, long and curly lashes, small anteverted nose, thin lips, small midline beak of upper lip, downward curving angle of the mouth.	dup 3q dup 13q	+ +	Padfield et al., 1968 Schinzel, 1984
Similar to Rubinstein-Taybi syndrome	Short stature, downward slanting palpebral fissures, hypoplastic maxilla, narrow palate, strabismus, low-set malformed ears, broad thumbs and toes, cryptorchidism, anomalies of bone, eye, heart and kidney.	dup 20p dup 2q	+ +	Beck and Mikkelsen, 1981 Schinzel, 1984 Rubinstein, 1990
Similar to Smith-Lemli-Opitz syndrome	Prenatal and postnatal growth retardation, mental retardation, microcephaly, narrow frontal area, anteverted nostrils, ptosis of eyelids; low-set rotated ears, simian crease, syndactyly of second and third toes, ambiguity of external genitalia, hypospadias and cryptorchidism.	dup 3q dup 2p	+ + +	Steinbach et al., 1981 Yunis et al., 1979
Similar to Seckel syndrome	Prenatal and post-natal growth retardation, mental retardation, microcephaly, premature synostosis, facial hypoplasia, prominent nose, low-set ears, lack of lobules, 11 ribs and cryptorchidism.	del 13q del 2q	+ + +	Schinzel, 1984 Majewski and Goecke, 1982
Aase syndrome	Mild growth deficiency, hypoplastic anemia, triphalangeal thumbs, narrow shoulders, late closure of fontanel, cardiac defects, rarely cleft lip and palate, hip dislocation, malformed ears, hydrocephaly, Dandy-Walker malformation.	?	+	Aase and Smith, 1969
Thrombocytopenia-absent radius (TAR syndrome)	Thrombocytopenia, absence or hypoplasia of megakaryocytes, anemia, bilateral absence of hypoplasia or the radius. Defects of hands, legs, and feet; 40% of patients die as a result of hemorrhage during infancy.	?	+	Hall, 1987
Similar to Hallermann-Streiff syndrome	Malar hypoplasia, micrognathia, microphthalmia, congenital cataracts, small pinched nose, hypoplasia of teeth, atrophy of skin, hypertrichosis, bradycephaly. Eye abnormalities such as blue sclerae, nystagmus, coloboma and chorioretinal pigment alteration.	?	+	Steele and Bass, 1970 Judge and Chalcanovskis, 1971

/ = with; frequency:frequent: + + + greater than 10% to 60%. p.o. preferential origin: maternal (m); paternal (p); random (r).

nadotrophic hypogonadism causing micropenis or microlabia, cryptorchidism, and pubertal insufficiency.

Clinical characteristics of CNS function and behavior include moderate to severe mental retardation, hyperactivity, sleepiness, personality change with maturation, and the habit of picking sores; occasionally seizures are present [Cassidy and Ledbetter, 1989]. Visual problems such as strabismus, nystagmus, and hypopigmentation are encountered in more than 50% of patients with Prader-Willi syndrome. These problems have been attributed to a brain abnormality characterized by misrouting of retinal ganglion fibers at the optic chiasma, a finding previously reported in forms of albinism [Butler, 1989; Creel et al., 1986]. Mild facial dysmorphism, including almond-shaped palpebral fissures, narrow bifrontal diameter, a fishlike mouth, and dental

Comparison of Principal Features in Prader-Willi and Angelman Syndromes

Clinical

Prader-Willi Syndrome	Angelman Syndrome
Mild or moderate mental retardation	Severe mental retardation
Feeding problems	Ataxia
Neonatal and infantile hypotonia	Hyperactivity
Hyperphagia	Convulsions
Obesity	Paroxysms of laughter
Behavioral problems	Clumsy, jerky movements
Genital hypoplasia	Almost-absent speech
Characteristics	Characteristic facies
Dolichocephaly	Microcephaly
Narrow bifrontal diameter	Widely spaced teeth
Almond-shaped eyes	Prognathism (progeria)
Small-appearing mouth	Macrostomia (large mouth)
Downturned corners of the mouth	Tongue protrusion
Short stature	Ocular hypopigmentation
Small hands and feet	Abnormal EEG
Hypopigmentation	

Cytogenetics

Deletion

Micro deletion: 15q11-q13	Micro deletion: 15q11-13
Frequency: 50% to 60%	Frequency: 50% to 60%
Origin: Paternal	Origin: Maternal

Nondeletion

Uniparental maternal disomy	Uniparental paternal disomy
Frequency: 20% to 30%	Frequency: 4% to 5%

Consequence

Absence of paternal Contribution	Absence of maternal Contribution

Modified from Smeets DFCM, Hamel BCJ, Nelen MR, et al. N Engl J Med 1992; 326:807.

anomalies, is often evident. Acromicria (small hands and feet) and scoliosis develop at a later age [Holm and Lauren, 1981; Chitayat et al., 1989]. Most of these findings are present in any one patient, but the syndrome is clinically variable and age related [Berry et al., 1981; Butler, 1990; Butler et al., 1981; Holm et al., 1981; Robinson et al., 1991; Stephenson, 1980].

Expanded forms of Prader-Willi syndrome have been reported with findings that include ventricular septal defects, hypoplastic right side of the heart, renal abnormalities, and bifid uvula [Pauli et al., 1983]. There appears to be some correlation between the severity of the symptoms and the extent of chromosomal alterations [Mattei et al., 1984b; Niikawa and Ishikiriyama, 1985].

Differential diagnosis is extensive and should include Cohen syndrome (which is manifested in hypotonia, obesity, and mental retardation); this is genotypically different from the Prader-Willi syndrome locus [Dunn et al., 1961; Kondo et al., 1990].

Angelman syndrome phenotype

First described in 1965, Angelman syndrome is being diagnosed more frequently. Prominent clinical features are summarized in the box to the left for comparison with Prader-Willi syndrome and have been expanded recently [Shapiro-Fryburg et al., 1991; Robb et al., 1989; Zori et al., 1992]. They include delayed developmental milestones from early infancy, with postnatal onset of microcephaly with flat occiput, frequent hyperkinesia of trunk and limbs, a puppetlike, jerky gait, hypotonia with brisk deep tendon reflex, a happy demeanor—often with episodes of unprovoked or inappropriate outbursts of laughter—and characteristic facial features that evolve over time. The diagnosis is usually made after 2 years of age when the characteristic manifestations become more obvious. Seizures are common, and the syndrome is associated with an unusual EEG, which is now recognized as a key diagnostic feature [Boyd et al., 1988; Gandi and Duncan, 1989]. The recent localization of the gene encoding the GABA receptor beta$_3$ subunit to the Angelman syndrome and Prader-Willi syndrome region suggests a possible role of the inhibitory neurotransmitter GABA in the pathogenesis of one or both of these syndromes [Wagstaff et al., 1991] (Figure 25-6).

Cytogenetic findings

The proximal region on chromosome 15 is of particular interest by virtue of its heterogeneous structural rearrangement involving deletion, duplication, or translocation, all of which can be reflected in abnormal clinical phenotypes [Nicholls et al., 1989]. The "new" cytogenetics data unravel fascinating information, summarized in the box above left. Prader-Willi syndrome and Angelman syndrome have the same apparent cytogenetic and molecular lesion and yet exhibit distinct clinical phenotypes. Most occur sporadically, but some familial patients have been reported in both syndromes.

The focus of molecular DNA rearrangement is in the 15q11-q13 region, mostly subband q11.2, which is about 1 to 3 megabases, sufficient to include 10 to 30 average-size genes of 100 kb each.

De novo interstitial microdeletion is observed in about 60% of affected patients with both syndromes. Deletion occurs at the molecular level in up to 75% [Donlon, 1988; Hamabe et al., 1991; Ledbetter et al., 1981; Pembrey et al., 1989].

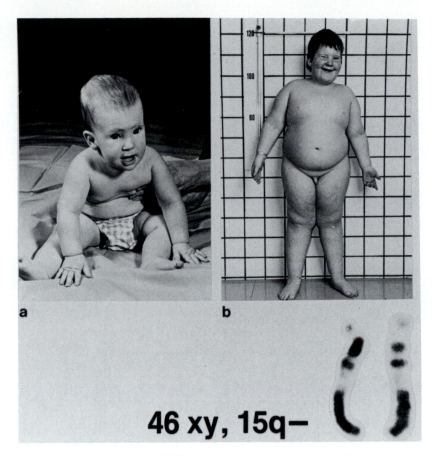

Figure 25-5 Patient with Prader-Willi syndrome at **A,** 7 months, and **B,** 6 years of age. (Karyotype courtesy M.G. Mattei, Marseilles, France.)

To date, cytogenetic and molecular genetic studies have failed to distinguish between the deletion in Prader-Willi syndrome and Angelman syndrome, except with respect to parental origin: paternal in Prader-Willi syndrome and maternal in Angelman syndrome [Knoll et al., 1989; Williams et al., 1990]. Substantial clinical overlap is usually absent between deletion-positive Prader-Willi syndrome and Angelman syndrome patients, except in a few recently reported patients [Kirkilionis et al., 1991].

In the deletion-negative patients, findings indicate that 20% to 30% of cases of Prader-Willi syndrome result from the inheritance of both copies of chromosome 15 from the mother (uniparental disomy; either isodisomy or heterodisomy) with the consequent absence of a paternal chromosome [Nicholls et al., 1989; Trent et al., 1991; Mascari et al., 1992a]. Conversely, Angelman syndrome results from the inheritance of both copies of chromosome 15 from the father as recently described [Smith et al., 1992; Malcolm, 1991], with the consequent absence of a maternal chromosome. Moreover, both syndromes have recently been demonstrated to occur in the same family through different mechanisms [Smeets, 1992]. Normal human development requires genetic input from both parents; however, the absence of a paternal contribution to the region 15q11-q13, whether by paternal deletion or maternal uniparental disomy, appears to result in Prader-Willi syndrome. Conversely, the absence of maternal contribution to the same region, whether by maternal deletion or paternal uniparental disomy, results in Angelman syndrome.

These findings have led to the hypothesis that this region of the genome is "imprinted," "labeled," or "modified" in some epigenetic process (possibly by methylation) so that maternal and paternal copies are not equivalent in development [Magenis et al., 1990; Hulten et al., 1991a; Mascari et al., 1992b]. Some of the most compelling evidence for human genomic imprinting is emerging from the study of both Prader-Willi and Angelman syndromes [Hall, 1992].

Neuropathology

No consistent neuroanatomic lesions have been identified either at autopsy or by neuroimaging (e.g., CT, MRI, or positron emission tomography) for either

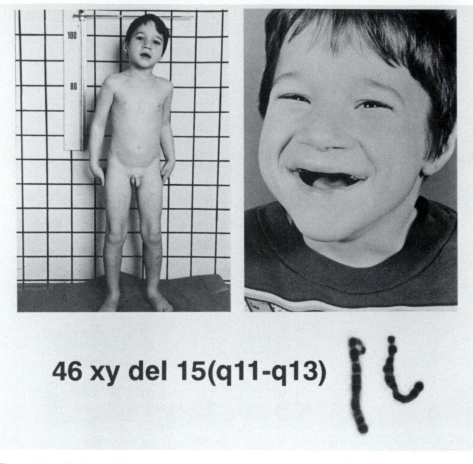

Figure 25-6 Patient with Angelman syndrome at 6 years of age. (Karyotype courtesy of M. Rochon, Sherbrooke, Quebec, Canada.)

Prader-Willi syndrome or Angelman syndrome [Jay et al., 1991; Levin et al., 1989; Kyriakides, 1992].

Management

No specific treatment exists for Prader-Willi syndrome. The profound hypotonia and feeding difficulties eventually improve over the years. The obesity responds poorly to dietary management [Holm and Pipes, 1976; Crnic et al., 1980]. Patients can usually maintain normal weight with 60% of normal caloric intake. Approaches to prenatal diagnosis have been recommended [Schinzel, 1986]. No specific treatment exists except supportive measures for Angelman syndrome.

MAJOR CHROMOSOMAL ABERRATIONS

This section describes autosomal and sex chromosomal aberrations. Autosomal aberrations include numeric (trisomy 21, 18, 13 +8) and structural (4p− and 5p−). Details concerning other syndromes may be found in references provided for each (see Table 25-12) and in the numerous reviews mentioned previously.

Trisomy 21 (Down syndrome)

History. Trisomy 21 was probably described initially by Séguin in 1846 under the name of "furfuraceous" idiocy and was first classified as a nosologic entity [Down, 1866] under the name of "mongolian idiocy." This best-known chromosome syndrome is now the focus of biologic research in premature aging, particularly in relation to Alzheimer disease [Epstein, 1986b, 1989; Pueschel and Rynders, 1982; Sinex and Merril, 1982; Smith and Warren, 1985]. Extensive literature on Down syndrome was reviewed by Zellweger [1977; Zellweger and Patil, 1987a], Breg [1977] and Stewart et al. [1988]. A comprehensive clinical review update has recently been published [Cooley and Graham, 1991].

Incidence. Down syndrome is the most frequent chromosomal aberration, with a rather consistent incidence in different ethnic and socioeconomic groups of approximately 1:700 live births. Most recent calculations suggest that the incidence is closer to 1:1000 or even 1:1100 births, primarily because of increasing use of various approaches for the prevention of pregnancy in

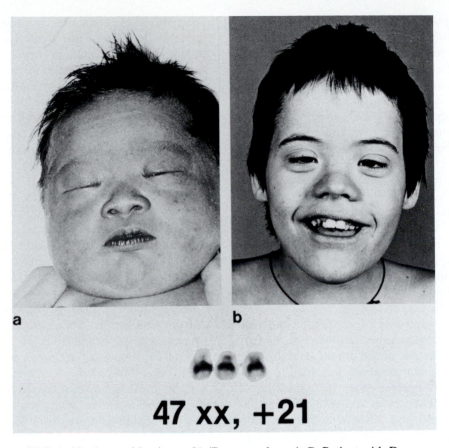

47 xx, +21

Figure 25-7 A, Newborn with trisomy 21 (Down syndrome). **B,** Patient with Down syndrome at 12 years of age. (Karyotype courtesy M. Rochon, Sherbrooke, Quebec, Canada.)

older women, as well as amniotic fluid examination. Approximately one quarter of spontaneous abortions are a result of Down syndrome, and about 20% of the fetuses with this diagnosis are stillborn.

Phenotype. The phenotype of Down syndrome is complex [Smith and Berg, 1976] and comprises a cluster of signs and symptoms accompanying abnormal physical and neurologic maturation (Figure 25-7). Prominent features of diagnostic value that vary with age are of aid to the clinician [Hall, 1970; Jackson et al., 1976]. Although individual characteristics occasionally occur in normal individuals (see Table 25-10), most clinical stigmata are so characteristic that karyotype examination is not required for diagnosis but only to ascertain whether nondisjunction or translocation is the underlying mechanism of chromosomal abnormality.

The phenotype consists of multiple congenital abnormalities with developmental defects of nervous, cutaneous, osseous, ligamentous, cardiac, gastrointestinal, and hematopoietic tissue. Stature and weight are below average, and the adult male with Down syndrome is significantly shorter than other adult males [Cronk et al., 1988; Cowie, 1972]. Recent head circumference standardized curves for males and females with Down

syndrome have been published, providing valuable information in the medical, physical, and developmental management of children with Down syndrome [Palmer et al., 1992].

The infant with trisomy 21 manifests the following: a small brachycephalic head with a large anterior fontanel and widely separated sutures; a flat facial profile with depressed nasal bridge; upward slanted palpebral fissures; epicanthi; narrow palate; loose skin folds on the posterior portion of a short neck; and low-set, small, and misshapen ears with a narrow auditory canal [Aase et al., 1973]. Incurvation of the fifth finger (bradyclinodactyly), which is usually short because of hypoplasia of the middle phalange; broad, short hands; solitary transverse palmar crease (simian line); and a wide gap between the first and the second toe are typically evident but are not of diagnostic value.

The two most prevalent major somatic abnormalities affect the heart in 40% and the gastrointestinal tract in approximately 20% of patients. Cutaneous manifestations are variable and nonspecific [Colomb et al., 1977]. Hyperkeratotic lesions, alopecia areata, adenomas of the sweat glands (syringomas), and alteration of vasomotor control are often present, particularly in older patients.

Cheilitis and blepharitis sometimes are disturbing features; psoriasis, although rare, may be present.

Ophthalmologic features are composed of Brushfield spots (circumferential speckling of the iris resulting from a diminished amount of stroma), squint, and lens opacities. Refractive error and senile cataracts may appear later. In approximately 5% of patients, amaurosis subsequently develops. Neonatal ocular findings include an increased number of retinal vessels arranged in a spokelike configuration. Other neuroophthalmologic manifestations include nystagmus and slowly reactive pupils [Caputo et al., 1989].

Auditory abnormalities include congenital malformation of the bones of the middle ear, permanent fixation of the stapes, and shortening of the cochlear spiral. These findings explain the increased frequency of sensorineural hearing loss and middle ear disease in Down syndrome [Balkany et al., 1979a, 1979b; Brook et al., 1972].

In addition to the decrease of acetabular and iliac angles, radiographs demonstrate narrowing of the cervical canal and subluxation of the atlantoaxial process. Accentuation of these abnormalities may lead to paraplegia or tetraplegia [Finerman et al., 1976; Pueschel et al., 1987; Pueschel, 1990; Roy et al., 1990]. Fortunately, although between 10% and 20% of individuals with Down syndrome are affected, only a small percentage require treatment, such as a posterior bony fusion [Rosenbaum, 1986; William et al., 1987]. A radiograph is recommended at age 5 years or earlier, particularly for children with Down syndrome who wish to participate in sports.

Abnormally slow growth of the cranium occurs [Roche, 1966]. Neuroimaging studies may reveal underdevelopment of the temporal lobes and calcium deposits within the basal ganglia and cerebellar folia [Takashima and Becker, 1985; Pelz et al., 1986].

The neurology of Down syndrome has been reviewed in detail by Lott [1986]. Mental retardation is an outstanding feature in the older child with nonmosaic trisomy 21, varying from the educable retarded state to a noncommunicative bedridden condition. Current reports based on individuals growing up with families in the community setting reveal IQs averaging in the mild to moderate range of mental retardation, with better visual processing than auditory processing [Pueschel et al., 1987]. Functions typically associated with the left cerebral hemisphere appear to be more impaired than those associated with the right hemisphere [Elliott et al., 1987]. No correlation exists between the number or extent of characteristic physical features and the degree of intellectual retardation. Evaluation of the motor, adaptive, and social behavior of trisomic children suggests developmental regression preceding the first birthday [Dicks-Mireaux, 1972]. Denver Developmental Scale studies demonstrate that trisomic infants approximately 6 months of age typically experience a steady progressive deceleration of development that foretells the mental retardation readily evident by 4 years of age. Most patients have poor articulation and an extremely limited vocabulary. Less than 5% are able to read, and even fewer can write. Although most patients have a pleasant, docile, and happy personality, some have pronounced behavorial difficulties consisting of hyperactivity and outbursts of anger with increased frequency during adolescent and adult years [Hartley, 1986; Johnson and Olley, 1971; Lund, 1988].

The language and communication skills of children with Down syndrome are obviously delayed. The majority appear to have expressive language disabilities disproportionate to their general cognitive limitation [Miller, 1988].

Neurologic examination of the newborn often documents apathy with feeding difficulties. Prolonged physiologic jaundice is often present. Profound diffuse hypotonia, hyperextensibility of joints, and slowed response of neonatal reflexes are evident [Loesch-Mdzewska, 1968]. Some characteristics are exaggerated with maturation; however, hypotonia lessens. Generally, children with Down syndrome are maladroit, move slowly, and have an unsteady, wide-based gait [Paulson et al., 1969]. A coincidental association with Tourette syndrome has recently been reported [Barabas et al., 1986; Collacott and Ismail, 1988]. Superficial sensation is normal.

Seizures, including infantile spasms, occur in approximately 2% to 9% of patients [Zellweger, 1977; Romano et al., 1990; Stafstrom et al., 1991]. Infantile spasms, with or without hypsarrhythmia, appear spontaneously or after treatment with 5-hydroxytryptophan [Pollack et al., 1978]. Focal seizures with abrupt onset in a patient with cyanotic heart disease and right-to-left shunt may result from embolism or thrombosis of small cerebral blood vessels. Moyamoya disease has been described as a rare cause of stroke in patients with Down syndrome [Fukushima et al., 1986; Pearson et al., 1985]. A 20% to 25% higher incidence of EEG abnormalities occurs in patients with Down syndrome than in control subjects; abnormalities are more often present in younger patients [Ellingson et al., 1973]. EEG studies of older patients manifesting dementia often demonstrate progressive, although nonspecific, disorganization [Crapper et al., 1975].

Maturational neurophysiologic evaluation of trisomic 21 infants with sleep EEGs and sensory-evoked potentials reveals the absence of a normal response decrement with repetitive stimulation characteristic of both increasing maturation and normal development of the CNS [Ellingson, 1973; Monod and Guidasci, 1976]. Sleep studies document a disproportionate amount of rapid eye movement sleep, suggesting immature cortical function. Electrodiagnostic studies in patients with Down syndrome have been reviewed extensively [Galbraith, 1986].

Neuropathology. No gross malformations occur in Down syndrome in contrast to other trisomies. Pronounced and distinctive deceleration of nervous system development manifests [Benda, 1972]. Mild reduction of brain size and weight occurs; the frontal lobe, brainstem, and particularly the cerebellum are affected. The most constant abnormalities are those of the cerebellum, which may explain the almost uniform presence of profound hypotonia. The gross cortical convolutional patterns are embryonic. A narrow superior temporal gyrus, an exposed insula resulting from lack of development of the third frontal gyrus, and a short frontooccipital diameter with steep inclination of both occipital lobes are the most significant changes. Hippocampal dysgenesis discernible prenatally has been described [Sylvester, 1983; Wisniewski, 1990].

The gross external appearance of the brain affected by Down syndrome is more diagnostic than the minor light microscopic findings described in the past, which are considered nonspecific and secondary to the immediate cause of death, such as congenital heart failure or sepsis; however, cytoarchitectural studies have revealed some consistent findings, such as a reduction in the number of spines along the apical dendrites of pyramidal neurons [Becker et al., 1986; Marin-Padilla, 1976; Suetsugu and Mehraein, 1980; Takashima et al., 1981]. A lack of granular cells is also observed, with a specific decrease in the population of a specific cell type, most likely the aspinous stellate granular cell [Ross et al., 1984; Wisniewski et al., 1986].

The relationship between Down syndrome and Alzheimer disease is a focus of investigation. There is speculation that Alzheimer disease is a part of the pathologic process of Down syndrome. In addition to the documented clinical evidence of dementia in Down syndrome [Wisniewski et al., 1985a; Evenhuis, 1990], an outstanding histologic feature of brains from virtually all young adults older than 30 to 40 years of age with Down syndrome is the early appearance of neurofibrillary tangles, senile plaques, or both, as well as the strandlike cluster of filamentous protein in the perikaryon. These findings are similar to those found in Alzheimer disease.* Other similarities include a high frequency of hematologic cancer, a decrease in cholinergic enzymes (choline acetyltransferase) in the cortex, a decrease in neurotransmitters (dopamine, serotonin, or norepinephrine), and a selective loss of cells in the nucleus basalis of Meynert [Casanova et al., 1985]. Furthermore, iden-

tical dermatoglyphics, late maternal age at the time of delivery, and an increased prevalence of chromosomal aberrations support a postulated pathophysiologic connection between Down syndrome and Alzheimer disease [Wisniewski et al., 1985a]. However, differences in the composition of senile plaques in some neurochemical studies (dolichols) [Wolfe et al., 1985] and immunologic studies are unexplained.

Myelination is incomplete or delayed in some cerebrocortical regions, such as the frontotemporal lobe and especially in the U fibers and the cerebellocortex [Wisniewski et al., 1986]. However, no abnormalities exist in the composition of myelin and synaptosomal lipids [Johnson et al., 1977].

Other neurochemical studies of Down syndrome, particularly in relation to the pathogenesis, have been summarized [Balazs and Brooksband, 1985, 1986].

Biologic studies. There is much information detailing the biologic changes in Down syndrome [de Grouchy and Turleau, 1984; Smith and Warren, 1985; Zellweger and Simpson, 1977, 1987]. In general, studies suggest an overall decrease in the efficiency of cellular metabolism [Hsia et al., 1971; Stern, 1971]. Evidence of immune system derangement in Down syndrome includes increased incidence of lymphatic leukemia, infection, and known carrier status for Australian antigen. Significant quantitative deviations from normal of lymphocyte surface markers, serum immunoglobulin, and nitrogen responsiveness, as well as deficiency of T cells, have been reported [Gershwin et al., 1977; Levin et al., 1979; Ugazio et al., 1990]. The localization of the interferon receptor to the 21q22 region has stimulated new conjecture regarding immunologic impairment in Down syndrome [Epstein et al., 1980].

Thyroid dysfunction, as evidenced in some patients by increased thyroid-stimulating hormone levels and Hashimoto thyroiditis, has been demonstrated in patients with Down syndrome and patients with Alzheimer disease. The underlying pathologic mechanism in both conditions is likely related to immunologic abnormalities [Vladutiu et al., 1984; Pueschel, 1990; Cutler et al., 1986].

Studies of leukocytes, erythrocytes, and platelet enzymes and/or trace elements to clarify the pathogenesis of Down syndrome have been relatively unrewarding. In a recent review of the epidemiology of Down syndrome, no dysmorphic, parental, or environmental factors except maternal age have been proved convincingly [Bell, 1991].

Molecular characterization of Down syndrome is steadily increasing, although the pathogenesis of mental retardation is still poorly understood [Lejeune, 1990]. Recent publications of rare patients with only a part of the long arm of chromosome 21 present in triplicate (partial trisomy q21) and rare patients with no cytoge-

---

*References Ball et al., 1986; Ellis et al., 1974; Ohara, 1972; Prince et al., 1982; Schochet et al., 1973.

netically visible chromosome abnormalities have been useful in defining the region responsible for several phenotypic features of Down syndrome to the distal band 21q 22.2-22.3, called the *"critical region."* This region is expected to contain at least 50 to 100 genes [Stewart et al., 1988; Pattersen and Epstein, 1990].

Identification of specific genes causing features of Down syndrome is being performed by a combination of techniques using molecular analysis, in situ hybridization, fluorescence, and high-resolution chromosome analysis. The results indicate that small regions of chromosome 21 are likely to contain the gene for congenital heart disease of the endocardial cushion type (a region of about 3 megabases), for duodenal stenosis (a region of about 15 megabases), and for severe to mild mental retardation and classic facial appearance. Moreover, this "critical region" appears to exclude the gene superoxide dismutase and amyloid precursor protein [Korenberg et al., 1990].

Dermatoglyphics. Dermatoglyphic patterns have been closely examined in patients with Down syndrome; various nomograms, dermatograms, and other diagnostic indexes have been described [Preus, 1977]. Among the abnormalities are displacement of the palmar triradius distally to the center of the palm (ATD angle, formed between lines drawn from the triradii at the bases of the index and little fingers to the axial triradius, greater than 45 degrees), a tibial arch on the hallucal areas of the sole, and unusual fingerprint patterns, including ulnar loops on all 10 digits [Rignell, 1985].

Cytogenetics. The Down syndrome karyotype may be of three types. It is essential to distinguish among them to ensure adequate genetic counseling.

Most patients (92% to 94%) manifest "free" trisomy 21, that is, an extra copy of chromosome 21 is present in the genome. It has long been known that increasing maternal age is associated with increased risk for trisomy 21, with a sharp rise after age 40 [Jagiello et al., 1987; Lane and Stratford, 1985]. It is now well known that trisomy 21 primarily follows a nondisjunctional event that occurs in about 95% of maternal meiosis and in about 5% of paternal meiosis, both predominantly in meiosis I [Antonarakis et al., 1991].

Translocation is responsible for Down syndrome in 4% to 5% of patients [Lejeune, 1970]. The translocation pattern is usually of the robertsonian type; that is, the long arm of chromosome 21 is relocated to the long arm of one of the other acrocentric chromosomes (usually 14 or 22). (Another rare type is 21q21q translocation.) This condition is not related to maternal age. The normal number (46) of chromosomes is present, but the total chromosomal mass is identical to that in trisomy 21. The translocation may be sporadic or transmitted from one parent who is a "balanced carrier," having her chromosome set with a normal complement of genetic information; 45 chromosomes are present, but a normal total chromosomal mass allows manifestation of a normal clinical phenotype. Translocation 21 trisomy occurs in 1:18,000 live-born infants [Peterson et al., 1991].

A mosaic pattern (46/47, +21) is responsible for 2% to 3% of patients with Down syndrome; at least one cell line is trisomic for chromosome 21. There is a varying percentage of trisomic cells (11% to 70%). In rare instances a child with the complete syndrome results from the pregnancy of a woman who has a mosaic pattern. The clinical features of these progeny are highly variable; patient manifestations range from virtually normal physical and intellectual characteristics to patients with the typical Down syndrome phenotype [Fishler et al., 1976].

Prognosis. Approximately one third of infants with Down syndrome do not survive infancy, and one half die during the first 5 years of life. Death usually results from cardiac complications and respiratory infections. Patients with Down syndrome experience an incidence of acute leukemia 10 to 20 times greater than that in the general population. Although the average life span is diminished, some patients live 50 to 60 years [Thase et al., 1984].

Management. No specific treatment exists for Down syndrome. Medical intervention should be directed toward the prevention and/or treatment of infection, hearing defects, and significant malformations of the heart, gastrointestinal tract, and upper cervical spine [Rubin and Crocker, 1990; Zellweger and Patil, 1987]. Although controversy continues about specific therapies for children with Down syndrome [Golden, 1984; Pruess, 1989], all reasonable efforts should be made to improve the environment.

Family counseling is essential. The likelihood of recurrence, which can be predicted from available data, should be determined and explained to the parents [Ludman et al., 1984]. Several publications are available for family members [Cooley and Graham, 1991; Reisz, 1977; Smith and Wilson, 1973; Wilks and Wilks, 1974]. Table 25-14 summarizes the risk of recurrence with each of the three karyotypes [Lurie, 1979]. This assessment is particularly important because prenatal diagnosis should be recommended only for those women in whom the risk of a child with Down syndrome outweighs the risk of amniocentesis or chorionic villus sampling. The risk varies with the woman's age, the karyotype of the parents, and the reproductive history of the mother and her relatives with respect to Down syndrome and other trisomies.

Trisomy 18 (Edwards syndrome)

Trisomy 18 was reported initially by Edwards et al. [1960]. The syndrome occurs in 1:3500 to 1:9000 live

Table 25-14 Risk for Trisomy 21

"Regular" 47,XY, +21 at different maternal ages

Maternal age groups (years)	In population	In families after one trisomy 21 child
15-19	1/2,400	1/800
20-24	1/1,500	1/500
25-29	1/1,200	1/400
30-34	1/900	1/300
35-39	1/300	1/100
40-44	1/100	1/30
45-49	1/40	1/10

Translocation carriers

Type of translocation	Parental carrier	
	Father	Mother
t (14q 21q)	1/10	1/20
t (21q 22q)	1/6	1/12
t (21q 21q)	100%	100%

Mosaic parent

Based on meiotic studies in the germinal tissues: if the mosaic parents have 50% abnormal cells, about 25% of the children will be affected.

births. There is a 3:1 preponderance of females, which may be explained by the gestational and perinatal death of affected males [Jones, 1988].

Phenotype. Phenotypic characteristics of trisomy 18 are typical (Figure 25-8), although many somatic defects (more than 120) have been described [Hodes et al., 1978]. Greatly decreased fetal activity, abnormal gestational duration, and hydramnios may be present. Low birth weight and subsequent failure to thrive are common. Other neonatal difficulties include apnea, jitteriness, and poor feeding.

Physical features include an elongated, narrow head with a prominent occiput. Microcephaly is uncommon. The ears are low set and the auricles deformed. Blue scleras, corneal opacities, and strabismus may be present [Calderon et al., 1983]. The abnormally shaped mouth, small and triangular, is often associated with micrognathia and a narrow palatal arch. The upper lip is elongated and the philtrum flattened. Other accompanying abnormalities consist of flexed fingers with typical hand clenching, "trigger thumb," short sternum, small nipples, talipes calcaneovalgus, hallux malleus with "rocker bottom feet," and small pelvis with limited hip abduction [Ray et al., 1985b]. Inguinal and umbilical hernias are also found. Most patients have cardiac, renal, and genital malformations, including cryptorchidism in males.

In those patients who survive the first year of life, the neurologic findings include severe motor and intellectual retardation and increased muscle tone. A few patients

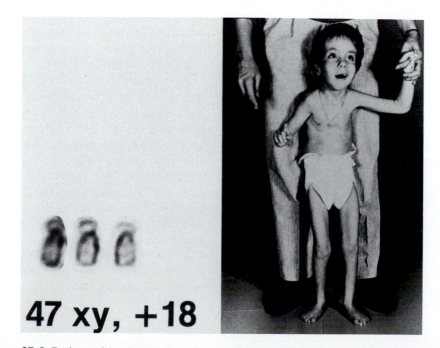

47 xy, +18

Figure 25-8 Patient with trisomy 18 at 7 years of age. (Karyotype courtesy M. Rochon, Sherbrooke, Quebec, Canada.)

have unilateral facial palsy and hearing compromise. Seizures have also been reported [Taylor, 1968].

Neuropathology. Gross anomalies are found in approximately 50% of patients with trisomy 18. Defective rhombencephalic development may occur with ensuing Chiari malformation, with or without neural tube defect [Case et al., 1977]. Various malformations include cleavage defects that result in abnormalities of the prolabium and premaxilla or cyclopia [Lang et al., 1976], cebocephaly [Hunter et al., 1977], and anencephaly [Menashi et al., 1977; Merrild, 1978]. Other anomalies include hydrocephalus and porencephaly. Agenesis of the corpus callosum, occipital lobes, and olfactory nerves and bulbs may be evident.

Widespread heterotopias of both the cerebrum and the cerebellum are present in about 80% of the brains of affected individuals.* Several abnormalities of the inner ears have been reported [Wright et al., 1985].

Cytogenetics. A monoclonal trisomy is present in approximately 80% of the patients with trisomy 18 as a result of meiotic nondisjunction in maternal oogenesis. Parental mosaicism (10%) and acquired or spontaneous structural rearrangements (translocation, inversion, isochromosome: 10%) are underlying explanations. Thus a deletion or incomplete trisomic phenotype occurs with resultant increased life expectancy. No correlation with parental age exists [Bass et al., 1979; Rocci et al., 1979].

Double aneuploidies with another autosome (13 or 21) or a sex chromosome (48,XXY) are sometimes present. A few infants with a trisomy 18 phenotype but a normal karyotype have been reported. Their condition is best understood by invoking a different hypothesis (see discussion of complete trisomy 13).

Dermatoglyphics. An increased incidence of arch patterns of most or all digits is often present in patients with trisomy 18. The pattern is not specific but is characteristic.

Prognosis. The median life expectancy is approximately 48 days [Carter et al., 1985]. Fewer than 10% of patients with trisomy 18 survive the first year of life and fewer than 1% survive the first decade. A greater life span is possible for individuals with mosaicism or for patients with partial trisomy [Crippa et al., 1978; Mehta et al., 1986; Smith et al., 1978]. The survivors are profoundly retarded in both motor and intellectual development. Thin long bones have been documented in long-term survivors [Bensen, 1985].

Management. Patients with trisomy 18 require extensive nursing care. Parental counseling should be provided. In primary trisomy the recurrent risk for subsequent pregnancies is approximately 1:100.

Trisomy 13 (Patau syndrome)

History. Trisomy 13 was described by Patau et al. [1960]. Estimates of the incidence of the condition average from about 1:5000 to 1:8000 live births. Female patients outnumber males.

Phenotype. The midface, central nervous system, hands, and internal organs are primarily affected in trisomy 13 (Figure 25-9). Prenatal and postnatal growth retardation are pronounced. Those patients who survive past 1 year of age experience profound motor and intellectual retardation. Apneic spells, jitteriness, and feeding difficulties complicate early infancy. Atypical petit mal seizures occur in approximately 66% of patients. Hearing impairment results from developmental errors. Variable alterations of tone are observed in patients who have prolonged survival. Cardinal dysmorphic features include microcephaly, areas of cutis aplasia of the scalp, sloping forehead, agenesis of the external olfactory apparatus, and cleft lip and palate or both. Ophthalmic abnormalities consist of anophthalmia, cataracts, coloboma, microphthalmia, and retinal dysplasia [Allen et al., 1977]. Large capillary hemangiomas of the brow and occiput, micrognathia, and low-set, malformed, and rotated pinnas are observed frequently.

Polydactyly, usually postaxial (ulnar and fibular) hexadactyly, occurs in 60% to 80% of patients. Syndactyly and narrow convex fingernails are typically present. "Trigger thumb" and "rocker bottom" feet occur less frequently than in trisomy 18. Assorted cardiovascular defects affect approximately 90% of patients, and urogenital defects affect about 80% of patients. An accessory spleen is often present. Hematologic abnormalities include persistence of fetal hemoglobin and an increased number of projections on the nuclei of neutrophils, reflecting an abnormal intracellular structural pattern [Taylor, 1968].

Neuropathology. Neuropathologic changes are nonspecific but of great magnitude. Varying degrees of holoprosencephaly occur in approximately 80% of infants with trisomy 13.* Fusion of the frontal lobes with an accompanying single ventricle is common. Absence of olfactory nerves or bulbs also occurs. Cerebellar changes are evident in 28%, defects of the corpus callosum in 22%, and hydrocephalus in 15% of patients. Agyria, extensive heterotopias in the subcortical white matter and cerebellum, and absence of the corticospinal tract have been reported [Norman, 1966]. Many neuropathologic anomalies affect the cranial nerves, intracerebral vessels, and leptomeninges [Gilbert et al., 1977]. Defects of the musculoskeletal system are numerous [Pettersen et al., 1979].

---

*References Gullota et al., 1981; Kakulas et al., 1968; Passarge et al., 1966; Sumi, 1970; Terplan et al., 1970; Warkany et al., 1966.

*References Agbata et al., 1979; Escobar et al., 1979; Gullota et al., 1981; Lorch et al., 1978; Warkany et al., 1966.

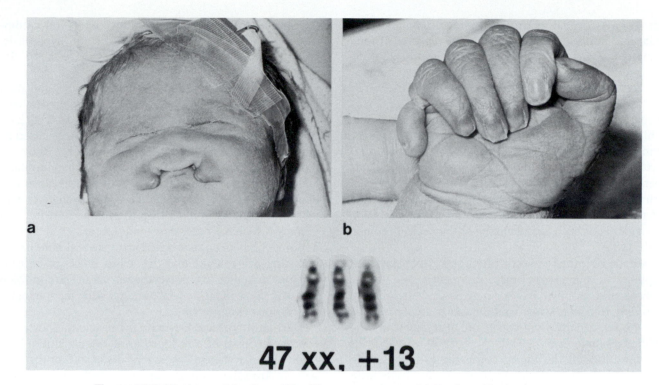

47 xx, +13

Figure 25-9 Newborn with trisomy 13. (Karyotype courtesy M. Rochon, Sherbrooke, Quebec, Canada.)

Unusual temporal bone findings, including a type of anomaly classified as Mondini or Mondini-Alexander, have been described [Tomoda et al., 1983].

Cytogenetics. The most frequent karyotype associated with trisomy 13 contains 47 chromosomes, with an extra chromosome 13 in about 80% of patients. Parents manifest no chromosomal abnormalities. Similar to other primary trisomies, advanced maternal age predisposes to the condition. Approximately 20% of infants have the normal complement of 46 chromosomes but also have a translocation. The translocation may develop de novo or may be inherited from a balanced parental carrier; it is usually of the robertsonian type, affecting chromosome 13 or 14 [Perez-Castillo and Abrisqueta, 1978]. Double aneuploidies, seldom occurring parental mosaicism, and complex rearrangements such as pericentric inversion have been described. A few infants have some characteristics of the trisomic syndrome but have a normal karyotype. Some of these patients may have a mosaic pattern involving trisomy 13, others have Meckel syndrome, and some may have an undescribed contiguous syndrome.

Dermatoglyphics. An increase in arch patterns on the fingertips and distal axial triradii occur with trisomy 13.

Prognosis. One half of patients with trisomy 13 die in the first 2 months of life. By 3 months of age 70% are dead, and by 3 years 95% are dead. A few patients have survived for prolonged periods [Cowen et al., 1979].

Management. No definitive treatment is possible for trisomy 13. Grave management difficulties are associated with the facial anomalies, including feeding problems. Apneic spells, atypical absence seizures, and profound mental deficiencies complicate management.

Trisomy 8 (Warkany syndrome)

History. Trisomy 8 was the first syndrome described in humans with a trisomy affecting a large autosome [de Grouchy et al., 1971] and the first complete trisomy to be corroborated by banding techniques.

Incidence. Trisomy 8 has a relatively high frequency, approximately 1:25,000 live births [Gagliardi et al., 1978; Pfeiffer, 1977; Réthoré et al., 1977; Riccardi, 1977]. Increased parental age may also be a predisposing factor; the greater risk is more often associated with greater male parental age (3:1).

Phenotype. Phenotypic variation is relatively great in trisomy 8. No significant correlation exists between the extent of mosaicism and the severity of clinical abnormalities.

Patients are usually thin and of normal height. Mild to moderate motor and intellectual retardation as well as delayed language skills and poorly articulated speech are common, although not uniformly present [Chandley et al., 1980; Tkeilgaard et al. 1977]. Schizophrenia accompanied by normal intelligence has been reported [Sperber, 1975]. Corneal opacities, nystagmus, and other visual and auditory defects have been reported [Frangoulis and Taylor, 1983]. Agenesis of the corpus callosum is the most frequent anomaly, but aqueductal stenosis and hydrocephalus are often major findings. Seizures and associated abnormal EEGs have been reported. Increased tone with restricted movement of joints and diffuse stiffness become prominent with advancing age. Craniofacial characteristics typically include a long, narrow face with deep-set eyes and prominent forehead, dysmorphic cranium, low-set and/or dysplastic auricles with thickened helixes, broad bulbous nose with anteverted nostrils, thick everted lower lip, micrognathia or retrognathia or both, and webbing of the neck [Breemer et al., 1984].

Skeletal deformities occur often and affect clavicles, scapulas, sternum, vertebrae, ribs, pelvis, and limbs. Scoliosis and spondylolisthesis may be evident. Acutely ascending thin iliac wings and aplasia or hypoplasia of the patellas, usually asymmetric, are also typical abnormalities [Silengo et al., 1979].

Deformities of the digits, consisting of clinodactyly and camptodactyly of the fifth finger, are frequently present. The fingers and toes are elongated and thin; sometimes contractures are exaggerated. A characteristic age-dependent feature is the occurrence of deep, cutaneous furrows on the palms and soles in neonates (pli capitonné) (Figure 25-10).

Visceral changes include various congenital cardiovascular and renal anomalies. Testicular hypoplasia, cryptorchidism, and delayed puberty have been described in males.

Neuropathology. Agenesis of the corpus callosum has been associated with trisomy 8. Few neuropathologic studies have been performed [Gullotta et al., 1981].

Cytogenetics. Many cases of trisomy 8 are caused by mosaicism (trisomy 8 M); approximately 10% are monoclonal in origin. Early studies of skin fibroblasts and circulating lymphocytes are required because evidence suggests that the extent of mosaicism changes with maturation [Berry et al., 1978]. Monozygotic twins with trisomy 8 M have been described [Reyes et al., 1978]. Trisomy 8 has been associated with several conditions, including acute leukemia, the acute phase of chronic myeloid leukemia, and polycythemia vera. The condition also has been identified in patients with meningiomas and various carcinomas.

Dermatoglyphics. Dermatoglyphic characteristics of trisomy 8 consist of a reduced total ridge count, a high frequency of arches in the fingers, distal shift of the axial palmar triradius, simian creases, high palmar and plantar pattern intensity, and increased incidence of whorls in the interdigital regions [Rodewald et al., 1977].

Prognosis. Trisomy 8 is benign when compared with other autosomal trisomies, although exceptions have been described. Affected patients have a relatively

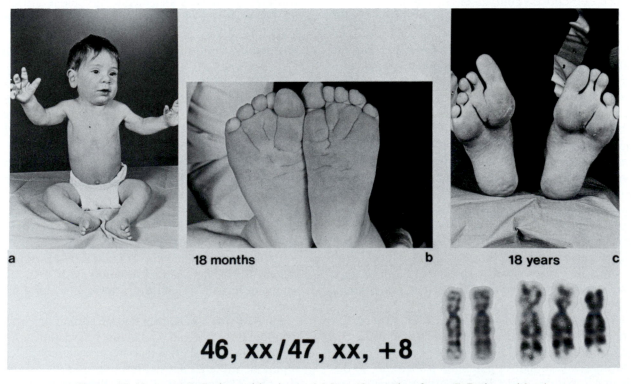

a   **18 months**   b   **18 years**   c

46, xx/47, xx, +8

Figure 25-10 A and **B,** Patient with trisomy 8 M, at 18 months of age. **C,** Patient with trisomy 8 M at 18 years of age. (Karyotype courtesy M. Rochon, Sherbrooke, Quebec, Canada.)

normal life pattern until the second or third decade. A normal adult male is infertile [Chandley, 1980].

Management. No specific therapy is available for trisomy 8 except supportive measures.

Deletion 4p (Midline fusion defect syndrome, Wolf-Hirschhorn syndrome)

History. Deletion 4p syndrome has been well characterized with the techniques of modern cytogenetics and microcytogenetics. The condition was first delineated by Wolf et al. [1965] and by Hirschhorn [1973]. Deletion 4p has been the focus of studies related to the identification of more DNA markers for Huntington disease [Froster-Iskenius et al., 1986b; Gusella et al., 1986; 1985].

Incidence. The precise incidence of 4p deletion is unknown, but it is less than the incidence of 5p deletion, which is estimated to be 1:20,000 live births.

Phenotype. All neonates have low birth weight and manifest failure to thrive. Severe intellectual retardation and a social "insensitivity" occur (Figure 25-11). The phenotype includes a cluster of midline fusion defects. Prominent among these abnormalities are asymmetric microcephaly, scalp defects, arched eyebrows, hyperte-

lorism, ptosis, coloboma of the iris, prominent glabella, cleft lip or palate, flat beaked nose with rectilinear and parallel edges reminiscent of a "Greek warrior" helmet and short philtrum and micrognathia with carp-shaped mouth [Wilcox et al., 1978].

More than 50% of patients have a periauricular dimple and low-set, lobeless ears that contain little cartilage [Delozier-Blanchet et al., 1985; Gutherie et al., 1971]. Males frequently have hypospadias and cryptorchidism. Seizures (occurring in 80% of patients), severe squint, hypotonia, and indifference to pain are often present. Sacral pilonidal dimple or sinus and internal hydrocephalus have been reported. Careful analysis of the phenotype allows for the identification of patients who most likely have a deletion requiring intensive cytogenetic analysis [Preus et al., 1985].

Dermatoglyphics. The dermatoglyphic pattern, often normal, may contain a disproportionately high frequency of arches, hypoplastic dermal ridges, bilateral simian creases, distal axial triradiis, and low ridge count.

Cytogenetics. The length of the deleted segment of the short arm varies from 20% to 80%, with some correlation between the percentage of deletion and

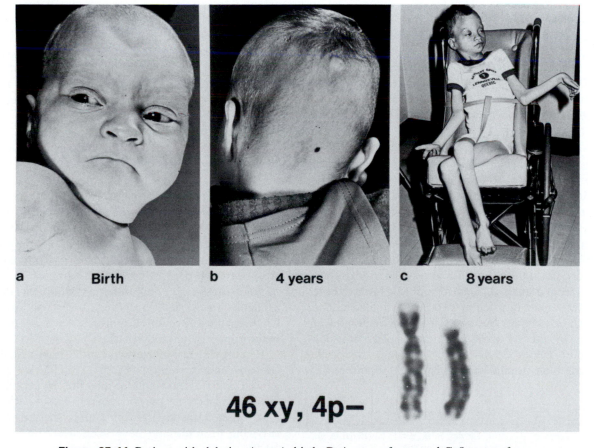

| a | Birth | b | 4 years | c | 8 years |

46 xy, 4p—

Figure 25-11 Patient with deletion 4p at **A,** birth; **B,** 4 years of age; and **C,** 8 years of age. (Karyotype courtesy M. Rochon, Sherbrooke, Quebec, Canada.)

degree of abnormal manifestations. Deficiency in the chromosome 4 mass may result from a de novo deletion or from inheritance of an unbalanced translocation. Most patients lack the terminal 4p16 band.

Origin of the de novo deletion has been demonstrated to be paternal in all patients, suggesting a possible genomic imprinting for the distal part of chromosome 4p. This was postulated to explain the phenomenon that patients with the severe juvenile form of Huntington disease inherit the disease from their fathers [Reik, 1988]. However, imprinting as a mechanism to explain the paternal origin of the 4p deletion cannot yet be proved [Quarrell et al., 1991; Tupler, 1992].

A different and less severe clinical syndrome with interstitial deletion of the proximal portion of 4p has been described [Francke et al., 1977]. Phenotypic "hybrids" with traits of 4p− and other autosomal segment trisomies occur [Stengel-Rutkowski, 1984].

Neuropathology. Few neuropathologic data are available for 4p deletion.* Microalterations occur, such as nerve cell heterotopias or microdysplasia within the cerebellum or cerebrum.

Prognosis. Patient longevity is poorly documented, but death follows congestive heart failure and associated pneumonia during the first year of life in more than one third of the patients with 4p deletion. Some patients may live past the first decade of life.

Management. No specific therapy exists for 4p deletion, and only supportive and psychologic care is indicated.

Deletion 5p (Cat's cry syndrome)

History. Cat's cry syndrome, or cri-du-chat syndrome, is one of the best known syndromes and was described initially by Lejeune et al. [1963].

Incidence. The incidence of cri-du-chat syndrome is approximately 1:20,000 live births. Deletion 5p may be a relatively common cause of profound intellectual retardation. In one report, 1% of patients with IQs less than 35 were demonstrated to have this syndrome [Breg et al., 1970]. A slight female preponderance exists.

Phenotype. The cardinal characteristics of infants who survive are severe mental retardation and a weak mewing cry, not unlike that of a kitten. The bizarre cry emanates from a small, narrow, hypoplastic larynx; there may be accompanying stridor and laryngomalacia. The cry is not evident after the first few weeks or months of life. The voice quality of older patients is often unusual, with higher values of frequency (by spectrographic evaluation) than in unaffected people [Romano et al., 1991].

Craniofacial dysmorphism (Figure 25-12) is characteristic and consists of antimongoloid slant of the palpebral fissures, micrognathia, a round, moonlike face that later becomes thin and asymmetric, and microcephaly [Neu et al., 1982]. Although patients appear to have wide-set eyes (or a broadened nasal bridge), true hypertelorism is rare [Niebuhr, 1978]. Ptosis, strabismus, and astigmatism have been reported [Mansour et al., 1984]. Hypotonia or hypertonia has been described in affected infants, as well as severely delayed developmental milestones. Older patients manifest features of upper motor unit disease, waddling gait, pes planus, scoliosis, and poor muscular development [Platt and Holmes, 1971; Wilkins et al., 1980]. Seizures typically occur.

Many infants with cri du chat syndrome are small for gestational age and fail to thrive; however, a few patients exhibit normal weight and length. Onset and progression of puberty are normal in both sexes.

Malformations are nonspecific and have only occasionally been described; they involve the nervous system, heart, and gastrointestinal tract.

Dermatoglyphics. Abnormalities of the palmar creases are observed, including bilateral simian creases and/or a single crease on digit 5.

Cytogenetics. The deletion associated with the cri-du-chat syndrome consists of the 5p15 band. The extent of the 5p deletion leading to the phenotype varies from almost the entire short arm to a very small deletion composed of 4% to 8% of the short arm. The midportion of the 5p15 segment must be deleted to cause development of the typical clinical pattern of cri-du-chat syndrome [Niebuhr, 1978]. Advanced maternal age is not a predisposing factor. A molecular approach to analyzing the deletion has been rewarding [Carlock and Wasmuth, 1985; Overhauser et al., 1986]. Paternal inheritance of the deleted chromosome 5 in patients with cri-du-chat syndrome has recently been demonstrated [Overhauser et al., 1986].

Ring chromosome formation, interstitial and terminal deletions, unbalanced familial or de novo translocation, and crossing over within a pericentric inversion loop are the most common causes of chromosomal material loss. Deletion 5p mosaicism rarely occurs [Romano, 1991]. Approximately 85% of cases are sporadic.

Neuropathology. Few neuropathologic data are available for 5p deletion [Breg, 1975; Solitaire, 1967]. Changes include microalterations, such as nerve cell heterotopias or microdysplasia.

Prognosis. The mortality of patients with 5p deletion remains undocumented. Feeding difficulties and congenital heart disease may reduce life expectancy; however, life expectancy may be greater than in patients who have other autosomal trisomic abnormalities. Patients surviving to adulthood have been described [Niebuhr, 1979].

---

*References Arias et al., 1970; Citoler et al., 1971; Gottfried et al., 1981; Laziuk et al., 1979; Mikelsaar et al., 1973.

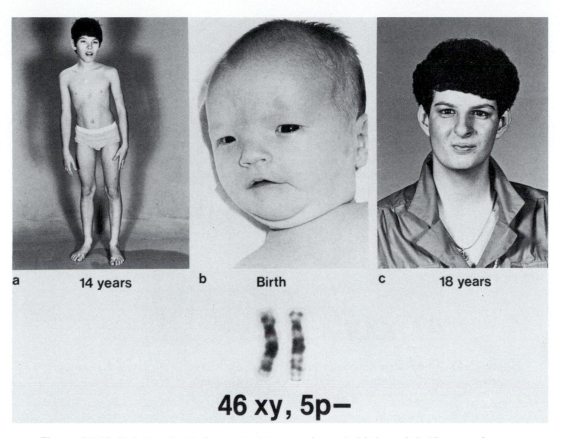

46 xy, 5p−

Figure 25-12 Deletion 5p. Patient at **A,** 14 years of age; **B,** birth; and **C,** 18 years of age. (Karyotype courtesy of M. Rochon, Sherbrooke, Quebec, Canada.)

Management. No definitive therapy exists for 5p deletion, but supportive care should be offered.

SEX CHROMOSOME SYNDROMES

Conditions associated with sex chromosomal aberrations are relatively frequent and occur in 1:1100 live-born females and 1:380 males [Gerald, 1976] (see Table 25-9). Most sex chromosome (X and Y) abnormalities are associated with numeric rather than structural changes.

Five broad categories of clinical features are encountered [de la Chapelle, 1990] as follows:
1. Higher cerebral dysfunction, including mental retardation and learning disorders, is generally less common than in autosomal aberrations. Mental retardation is not a feature in most sex chromosome aberrations in the absence of a Y chromosome; rarely a feature in 45,X; only mild in 47,XXX, 47,XXY, and 47,XYY; but moderate to severe in polysomies of the X and Y chromosomes. Learning disorders are often reported in children with sex chromosome aberrations [Bender et al., 1983; Hier et al., 1980].
2. Dysmorphic patterns are rare and nonspecific, except for the 45,X syndrome.
3. Major malformations are much less common than in autosomal aberrations. A few are rather specific, such as coarctation of the aorta in 45X (Turner syndrome) or radioulnar synostosis in X tetrasomies and X pentasomies.
4. Growth retardation is not a feature in many aberrations containing a Y chromosome and is absent in some structural aberrations of the X chromosome with female phenotype except with gonadal dysgenesis in 45,X. Increased height, highly unusual for autosomal aberrations, is characteristic for 47,XXX and 47,XYY.
5. Endocrine anomalies are more important. In the female, infertility is almost constant in 45,X but occurs less in patients with mosaic patterns and structural X chromosomal aberrations, particularly deletion of smaller Xp segments. Male nonmosaic Klinefelter syndrome and many structural aberrations of X and Y are associated with infertility, whereas fertility is only reduced in individuals with a 47,XYY karyotype. Moreover, karyotype-phenotype correlations are less well delineated and more variable because of the appreciable frequency of mosaicism (e.g., 20% of patients with Klinefelter syndrome and 40% of

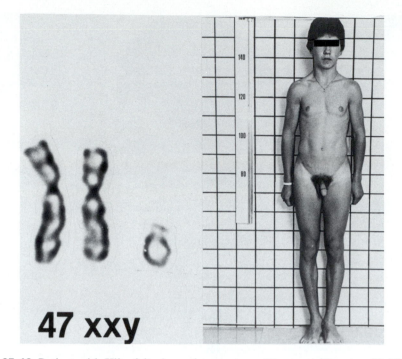

Figure 25-13 Patient with Klinefelter's syndrome at age 13 years. (Courtesy K. Khoury; karyotype courtesy M. Rochon, Sherbrooke, Quebec, Canada.)

individuals with Turner syndrome). In such patients the proportion of mosaic cells varies among affected individuals and also tends to decrease with time (selection). Although considerable geographic variations appear to exist for sex chromosome anomalies, Klinefelter syndrome in males and Turner syndrome in females are described in detail in the following sections. The other most common anomalies, XYY in phenotypic males and XX syndrome in females, are briefly summarized in tabular form (see Table 25-12).

Klinefelter (47,XXY) syndrome

History. Klinefelter syndrome was first described by Klinefelter et al. [1942]. Jacobs and Strong [1959] initially reported the karyotype XXY.

Incidence. The frequency of occurrence of Klinefelter syndrome varies between 1:500 and 1:1000 in male newborns. The frequency is increased by approximately 1% in male inmates in mental institutions, 1% in males with mental illness, and 3% in infertile males [Ferguson-Smith, 1966].

Phenotype. Klinefelter syndrome (XXY) is accompanied by few clinical characteristics. The phenotypic expression is often evident at puberty or later and includes testicular dysgenesis and hypogonadism with resultant azoospermia and sterility.

During puberty, gynecomastia may be manifest (50% of patients). Eunuchoid features may become prominent, including tall stature with large skeleton, large pelvic girdle, muscular hypotrophy, sparse facial and body hair, and lack of libido and potency (Figure 25-13).

Hormonal dysfunction is evident in the thyroid, hypothalamus, pituitary, and pancreas, in addition to the manifestations of gonadal insufficiency [Hsueh et al., 1978].

The phenotypic features are subtle and may be overlooked before puberty. Routine buccal smear studies suggest the diagnosis [Petremand-Hyvarinen, 1978]. The possibility of the condition should be considered when young males have genital anomalies (i.e., cryptorchidism or hypospadias with small penis), or intellectual retardation and somatic defects, particularly in patients with Klinefelter variants [Ferrier et al., 1974; Levy et al., 1978; Schmidt et al., 1978]. Significant abnormalities consist of microcephaly, ocular defects (i.e., astigmatism; severe myopia; bilateral coloboma of the iris, choroid, and uvea; complete bilateral aniridia), and skeletal anomalies (i.e., limitation of range of motion of the elbow; clinodactyly with brachymesophalangia of the fifth finger; coxa valga; deformed toes) [Caldwell and Smith, 1972].

Some patients with Klinefelter XXY (25% to 30%) are mentally retarded or have cognitive disorders that are often less severe than those associated with patients who have the XYY aberration. WISC or WAIS studies demonstrate that verbal IQ is decreased to a greater extent than performance IQ. During early childhood and adolescence, learning disabilities, speech and language defects, stuttering, and antisocial acts including aggressiveness may be present [Garvey and Mutton, 1973; Kessler and Moos, 1973]. It is noteworthy that pro-

spective evaluations suggest fewer accompanying difficulties.*

The reported abnormally increased incidence of neurologic findings, including essential tremor, may be spurious [Boltshauser et al., 1978].

Many variants of Klinefelter syndrome exist. The superfluous Xs typically are associated with more profound dysmorphism, more severe abnormalities of sexual development, and more severe intellectual retardation.

Cytogenetics. Various described karyotypes are listed in Table 25-15; the most frequent type is 47,XXY. Approximately 20% of patients with Klinefelter syndrome exhibit mixoploidy. Advanced maternal age is often a factor. The buccal smear result is positive, as evidenced by the presence of one chromatin mass less than the number of X bodies and one fluorescent Y body.

Table 25-15 Male sex chromosomal aberrations

Karyotypes	Chromatin	Cases (%)
Klinefelter syndrome		
47,XXY	+ (1 X body)	82
48,XXXY	+ (2 X bodies)	3
49, XXXXY	+ (3 X bodies)	<1
Mosaics		8
Other variants	+	6
Polysomies Y		
47,XYY	–	>98
48,XXYY	–	Rare
48,XYYY	–	Rare

*References Harkulich et al., 1979; Puck et al., 1975; Ratcliffe, 1975; Ratcliffe et al., 1982; Walzer et al., 1978.

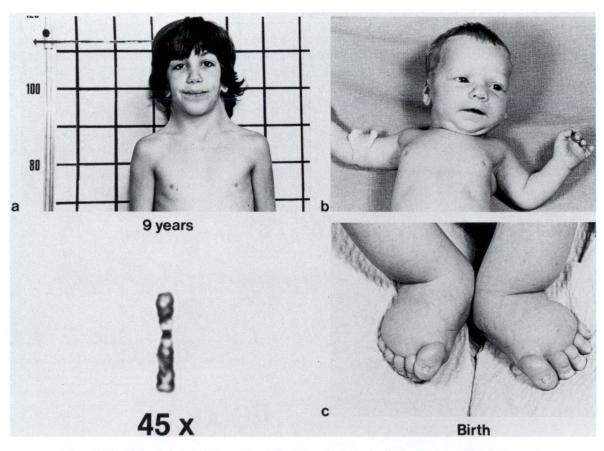

Figure 25-14 Patient with Turner's syndrome at **A,** 9 years of age; **B,** 1 month of age; and **C,** birth. (Courtesy K. Khoury; karyotype courtesy M. Rochon, Sherbrooke, Quebec, Canada.)

Management. Patients with Klinefelter syndrome respond to endocrine therapy. Treatment should begin shortly before or at puberty. The treatment may also improve psychologic status.

Turner syndrome (Gonadal dysgenesis, 45,X)

History. The phenotype of the 45,X syndrome has been well documented since initial reports [Ferguson-Smith, 1973; Turner, 1938] and the first characterization of the cytogenetic abnormalities [Ford et al., 1959].

Incidence. Turner syndrome occurs in approximately 1:2000 to 1:5000 female infants [Rosenfeld, 1990]. Among early spontaneous abortuses, 3.5% have a 45,X karyotype; 95% of these fetuses die in utero.

Phenotype. The phenotype of 45,X syndrome is composed of many anomalies, including somatic features (polymalformations and dysmorphism) and ovarian dysgenesis. Mental retardation is usually absent. Neonatal or infantile somatic characteristics consist of short stature, lymphedema over the dorsum of the feet (Figure 25-14), and facial structural anomalies (epicanthi, high palate, wide mouth, flattened nose, micrognathia). These facial structural abnormalities associated with oral-motor dysfunction and possible pharyngeal and gastrointestinal disorders contribute to the feeding difficulties seen from early age [Mathisen et al., 1992]. Other accompanying features include low-set "Gothic ears," surplus skin over the nape of the neck (cutis laxa), short fourth metacarpals (Archibald sign), nail hypoplasia, and a shieldlike chest with widely spaced hypoplastic nipples. Gonadal and endocrine changes such as clitoral hyperplasia may occur. Congenital heart disease—frequently coarctation of the aorta—is exhibited by 25%

of patients. Malformations of the urinary tract have also been described. Anomalies of the ribs and clavicles are demonstrated by radiography. Intestinal hemorrhage resulting from congenital hemangiomas, venous ectasia, and telangiectasia is experienced by approximately 7% of patients and may occur at any age [Burge et al., 1981].

Prepubertal females are of short stature with or without associated mild somatic features such as webbed neck (pterygium colli) with a lower posterior hairline, cubitus valgus, medial tibial exostosis, and pigmented nevi.

Pubertal and postpubertal females may manifest a lack of sexual development and accompanying primary amenorrhea. Ovarian dysgenesis is indicated by gonadal infantilism and further documented by gonadal streaks observed during surgery. Significant neurologic abnormalities may occur. Approximately 18% of patients are mentally retarded [Nielson, 1990]. The mean overall IQ is near normal, but there is a tendency for diminished nonverbal IQ [Garron and Vander Stoep, 1969].

Most patients have some degree of directional sense dysgnosia, space-form dysgnosia, and a mild numeric disability that may result from developmental parietal lobe impairment [Money, 1973; 1975]. The defect in perceptional organization, which was termed *space-form blindness* by Bender et al. [1984], may explain the learning disabilities. Neuropsychologic aspects of Turner syndrome have been reviewed [Chen et al., 1981; Leviton, 1984; Pidcock, 1984; Waber, 1979].

Table 25-16 Female sex chromosomal aberrations

Karyotypes	Chromatin	Cases (%)
Turner syndrome		
45,X	−	57
46,X,i(Xq) with mosaics	−	17
46,X,del(Xq) with mosaics	−	1
Mosaics 45,X/ 46,XX,45,X/47,XXX	−	12
Mosaics 45,X/46,XY		4
Others (del [Xp], [iX], mosaics)		9
Polysomies X		
47,XXX	+ (2X bodies)	98
48,XXXX	+ (3X bodies)	Rare
49,XXXXX	+ (3X bodies)	Rare
Mosaics		Rare

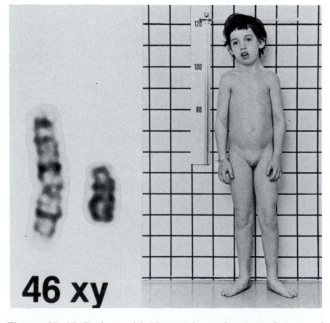

Figure 25-15 Patient with Noonan's syndrome at 8 years of age. (Karyotype courtesy M. Rochon, Sherbrooke, Quebec, Canada.)

Table 25-17 Differential diagnosis between Turner syndrome and Noonan syndrome

Manifestations/features	Turner syndrome	Noonan syndrome
External genitalia	Female	Male or female
Short stature	Constant	Frequent, less Turner syndrome
Amenorrhea	Usually present	Exceptional
Fertility:		
Females	Exceptional	Often present
Males		
Agonadism		In some cases
Cryptorchidism		frequent
Phenotype	Less variable	More variable: association with malignant hyperthermia Neurofibromatosis Multiple lentigines
Dysmorphic stigmata	Present	Present
Neuropsychologic findings	Mild	Prominent
Digital ridge count	High	Normal or low
Dental malocclusion	Rare	Common
Cardiovascular malformations	Mainly aortic coarctation Aortic stenosis	Mainly pulmonary stenosis Septal defects
Electrovectocardiogram (frontal axis)	Inferior	Superior
Sternum deformity	Rare	Frequent
Karyotype	Abnormal 45,X and mixoploidies	Normal 46,XY or 46,XX
Familial occurrence	Exceptional, except in some identical twins	Frequent
Inheritance	None	Autosomal dominant, multifactorial and polygenic?

Modified from Zellweger H. Down syndrome. In: Vinken PJ, Bruyn GW, eds. Congenital malformations of the brain and skull, part II, vol 31, Handbook of clinical neurology. Amsterdam: North Holland; and Summitt RL. Turner syndrome. In: Bergsma D, ed. Birth defects compendium, 2nd ed. The National Foundation-March of Dimes. New York: Alan R Liss, 1979.

Nerve deafness, either present at time of birth or appearing later, occurs in approximately 50% of patients. Partial impairment of taste and smell has also been described.

Dermatoglyphics. Dermatoglyphic abnormalities consist of high total ridge count, deep palmar and sole crease present at birth, and other minor deviations from normal.

Cytogenetics. No established correlation exists between Turner syndrome and advanced parental age. The frequency of complete monosomy X is approximately 50% to 70% [Coco and Bergada, 1977]. Of the anomalous karyotypes, 30% are structural rearrangements, and 50% of these consist of an isochromosome Xq. Remaining rearrangements consist of ring chromosome, isodicentric X chromosome, centric fragment deletions, and X/autosomal translocation (Table 25-16). These latter defects are accompanied by less delayed growth, less pronounced somatic anomalies, and occasionally, normal menstrual physiology for several years [Bockowski et al., 1978]. Patients with partial or complete 45,X patterns often have mosaicism (10% to 20%); some particular mosaic types facilitate neoplastic transformation or abnormal gonadal development [Davidoff and Federman, 1973]. Approximately 80% of patients are sex chromatin negative, and the remainder are chromatin positive.

Differential diagnosis. In affected girls, Turner syndrome must be distinguished from mixed or pure gonadal dysgenesis, the Klippel-Feil syndrome and the Noonan-Ehmke syndrome (Figure 25-15 and Table 25-17). A comprehensive review of the changing phenotype of Noonan syndrome is available [Allanson et al., 1985, Allanson, 1987; Bawle and Black, 1986; Mendez and Opitz, 1985; Opitz, 1985; Sharland et al., 1992]. The clinical relationship between Noonan syndrome, Watson syndrome (pulmonary valvular stenosis, café-au-lait spots, dull intelligence, and short stature), and neurofibromatosis type 1 is being studied at the molecular level [Allanson, 1991].

REFERENCES

Aase JM, Smith DW. Congenital anemia and triphalangeal thumbs: a new syndrome. J Pediatr 1969; 74:417.

Aase JM, Wilson AC, Smith DW. Small ears in Down's syndrome: a helpful diagnostic aid. J Pediatr 1973; 82:845.

Aase JM. Diagnostic dysmorphology. New York: Plenum Medical Book, 1990.

Aase JM. Dysmorphologic diagnosis for the pediatric practitioner. Pediatr Clin North Am 1992; 39:135.

Agbata IA, Kovi J, Parshad R, et al. Holoprosencephaly and trisomy 13 in a cyclops. JAMA 1979; 241:1109 (letter).

Albert B, Bray D, Lewis J, et al. Molecular biology of the cell. New York: Garland Publishing, 1983.

Aleck K, Willisman J, Mongkolsmai C, et al. Partial trisomy 11p with interatrial septal aneurysm: case report and literature review. Ann Genet 1985; 28:102.

Allanson JE, Hall JG, Hughes HE, et al. Noonan syndrome: changing phenotype. Am J Med Genet 1985; 21:507.

Allanson JE. Noonan syndrome. J Med Genet 1987; 24:9.

Allanson JE, Upadhyaya M, Watson GH, et al. Watson syndrome: is it a subtype of type 1 neurofibromatosis? J Med Genet 1991; 28:752.

Allen JC, Venecia G, Opitz JM. Eye findings in the 13 trisomy syndrome. Eur J Pediatr 1977; 124:179.

Alvarez LA, Yamamoto T, Wong B, et al. Miller-Dieker syndrome: a disorder affecting specific pathways of neuronal migration. Neurology 1986; 36:489.

Angelman H. Puppet children. Dev Med Child Neurol 1965; 7:681.

Anneren G, Gustavoon KH. Trisomy 22 syndrome in a 26-year-old female: a follow-up examination. *Hereditas* 1981; 94:67.

Antonarakis SE, and the Down Syndrome Collaborative Group. Parental origin of the extra chromosome in trisomy 21 as indicated by analysis of DNA polymorphisms. N Engl J Med 1991; 324:872.

Arena J, Lubs H. A computerized approach to X-linked mental retardation syndrome. Am J Med Genet 1991a; 38:190a.

Arena JF, Lubs HA. Other disorders with X-linked mental retardation: a review of thirty-three syndromes. In: Hagerman RJ, Cronister-Silverman AC, eds. Fragile X syndrome diagnosis, treatment and research. Baltimore: Johns Hopkins University Press, 1991b.

Arias D, Passarge E, Engle MA, et al. Human chromosomal deletion: two patients with the 4p− syndrome. J Pediatr 1970; 76:82.

Arinami T, Sato M, Nakajima S, et al. Auditory brain-stem responses in the fragile X syndrome. Am J Hum Genet 1988; 43:46.

Auerback AL, Adler B, Chagani RSK. Pre- and post-natal diagnosis and carrier detection of Fanconi anemia by a cytogenetic method. Pediatrics 1981; 67:128.

Aughton DJ, Cassidy SB. Physical feature of Prader-Willi syndrome in neonates. Am J Dis Child 1990; 144:1251.

Aughton DJ, Cassidy SB, Whiteman DAH, et al. Chromosone 7p− syndrome: craniosynostosis with preservation of region 7p2. Am J Med Genet 1991; 40:440.

Aurias A. Aspects cytogenetiques de l'Ataxie telangiectasie. Med Sci 1986; 2:298.

Austin KD, Hall JG. Nontraditional inheritance. Pediatr Clin North Am 1992; 39:335.

Balazs R, Brooksband BWL. Neurochemical approaches to the pathogenesis of Down's syndrome. J Ment Defic Res 1985; 29:1.

Balazs R, Brooksband BWL. Certain neurochemical aspects of the pathogenesis of Down's syndrome. In: Epstein CJ, ed. The neurobiology of Down syndrome. New York: Raven Press, 1986.

Balkany TJ, Downs MP, Jafew BW, et al. Hearing loss in Down's syndrome: a treatable handicap more common than generally recognized. Clin Pediatr 1979a; 18:116.

Balkany TJ, Mischke RE, Downs MP, et al. Ossicular abnormalities in Down's syndrome. Otolaryngol Head Neck Surg 1979b; 87:372.

Ball MJ, Shapiro MB, Rapoporti JI. Neuro-pathological relationships between Down syndrome and senile dementia, Alzheimer type. In: Epstein CJ, ed. Neurobiology of Down syndrome. New York: Raven Press, 1986.

Barabas G, Wardell B, Sapiro M, et al. Coincident Down's and Tourette syndrome: three case reports. J Child Neurol 1986; 1:358.

Barch MJ, (ed). The ACT cytogenetics laboratory manual, 2nd ed. New York: Raven Press, 1991.

Bartley JA, Patel S, Davenport S, et al. Duchenne muscular dystrophy, glycerokinase deficiency and adrenal insufficiency associated with Xp21 interstitial deletion. J Pediatr 1986; 1908:189.

Bartsch O, Kalbe U, Ngo TKN, et al. Clinical diagnosis of partial duplication 7q. Am J Med Genet 1990; 37:254.

Bass HN, Sparkes RS, Miller AA. Features of trisomy 18 and 18p-syndromes in an infant with 45,XY,i(18q). Clin Genet 1979; 16:163.

Bawle EV, Black V. Nonimmune hydrops fetalis in Noonan's syndrome. Am J Dis Child 1986; 140:758.

Beck B, Mikkelsen M. Chromosomes in the Cornelia de Lange syndrome. Hum Genet 1981; 59:172.

Becker LE, Armstrong DL, Chan F. Dendritic atrophy in children with Down's syndrome. Ann Neurol 1986; 20:520.

Beemer F, Veene MA, de Pater JM. Cerebral gigantism (Sotos syndrome) in two patients with fra (x) chromosomes. Am J Med Genet 1986; 23:221.

Bell JA. The epidemiology of Down's syndrome. Med J Aust 1991; 155:115.

Bellugi U, Bihrle A, Jernigan T, et al. Neuropsychological, neurological, and neuroanatomical profile of Williams syndrome. Am J Med Genet 1990; (suppl): 6:115.

Benda CE. Mongolism. In: Minckler J, ed. Pathology of the nervous system. New York: McGraw-Hill, 1972.

Bender B, Fry E, Pennington B. Speech and language development in 41 children with sex chromosome anomalies. Pediatrics 1983; 71:262.

Bender B, Puck M, Salbenblatt J, et al. Cognitive development of unselected girls with complete and partial X monosomy. Pediatrics 1984; 73:175.

Bensen JT, Steele MW. A mildly retarded woman with 46,XX/47,XX, + 18 mosaicism. Am J Med Genet 1985; 22:343.

Berger R, Bloomfield CD, Sutherland GR. Report of the committee on chromosome rearrangements in neoplasia and on fragile sites. Human gene mapping 8. Cytogenet Cell Genet 1985; 40:490.

Berger R, Larsen CJ. Cytogenetique et cancer. Med Sci 1986; 2:246.

Bergsma D. Birth defects compoendium, 2nd ed. New York: Alan R. Liss, 1979.

Bernheim A. La cytogénétique: du microscope à la cartographie du génome humain. Bull Cancer (Paris) 1991; 78:41.

Bernheim A, Berger R, Vaugier G, et al. Partial trisomy 6p. Hum Genet 1979; 48:13.

Berry AC, Mutton DE, Lewis DG. Mosaicism and the trisomy 8 syndrome. Clin Genet 1978; 14:105.

Berry AC, Whittingham AJ, Neville BGR. Chromosome 15 in floppy infants. Arch Dis Child 1981; 56:882.

Berry-Kravis E, Huttenlocher PR. Cyclic adenosine monophosphate metabolism in fragile X syndrome. Ann Neurol 1992; 31:22.

Birnholz JC. Ultrasonic studies of human fetal brain development. Trends Neurosci 1986; 9:329.

Bishop JM. Molecular themes in oncogenesis. Cell 1991; 64:235.

Blomquist HK, Bohman M, Edninson SO, et al. Frequency of the fragile X syndrome in infantile autism. Clin Genet 1985; 27:113.

Bockowski K, Mikkelsen M, Poulsen H. Turner's syndrome with rare karyotypes. Clin Genet 1978; 13:409.

Boltshauser E, Meyer M, Deonna T. Klinefelter syndrome and neurological disease. J Neurol 1978; 219:253.

Boraz RA, Schimke RN, Collins D. Partial 15q trisomy: report of three siblings. J Pedod 1985; 10(1):89.

Borgaonkar DS. Chromosomal variation in man. A catalog of chromosomal variants and anomalies, 6th ed. New York: Alan R. Liss, 1991.

Borghgraef M, Fryns JP, Dielkens A, et al. Fragile (X) syndrome: a study of the psychological profile in 23 prepubertal patients. Clin Genet 1987; 32:179.

Borghgraef M, Fryns JP, Van den Berghe H. The female and the fragile X syndrome: data on clinical and psychological findings in 7 fra(X) carriers. Clin Genet 1990; 37:341.

Boué J, Vignal P, Aubry JP, et al. Ultrasound movement patterns of fetuses with chromosome anomalies. Prenat Diagn 1982; 2:61.

Boyd SG, Harlen A, Patton MA. The EEG in early diagnosis of the Angelman (happy puppet) syndrome. Eur J Pediatr 1988; 147:508.

Bray GA, Dahms WT, Swerdloff R, et al. The Prader-Willi syndrome: a study of 40 patients and a review of the literature. Medicine 1983; 62:59.

Breakefield XO, Stern DF. Oncogenes in neural tumors. Trends Neurosci 1986; 9:150.

Breemer FA, Von Doorne JM, Gorlin RJ, et al. Diagnostic measurements in T8m: report of three cases. J Craniofac Genet Dev Biol 1984; 4:233.

Breg WR. Abnormalities of chromosomes 4 and 5. In: Gardner LL, ed. Endocrine and genetic diseases of childhood and adolescence, 2nd ed. Philadelphia: WB Saunders, 1975.

Breg WR. Down syndrome: a review of recent progress in research. Pathobiol Ann 1977; 7:257.

Breg WR, Steele MW, Miller OJ, et al. The "cri du chat" syndrome in adolescents and adults: clinical findings in 13 older patients with partial deletion of the short arm of chromosome No. 5(5p-). J Pediatr 1970; 77:782.

Brice A, Mallet J. La génétique moléculaire: une nouvelle approche des neurosciences cliniques. Rev Neurol 1991; 147:1.

Bridge J, Sanger W, Mosher G, et al. Partial duplication of distal 17q. Am J Med Genet 1985a; 22:229.

Bridge J, Sanger W, Mosher G, et al. Partial deletion of distal 17q. Am J Med Genet 1985b; 21:225.

Brook DN, Wooley H, Kenpital GC. Hearing loss and middle ear disorders in patients with Down's syndrome (mongolism). J Ment Defic Res 1972; 16:21.

Brooke MH. A clinician's view of neuromuscular diseases, 2nd ed. Baltimore: Williams & Wilkins, 1986.

Brown WT. Invited editorial: the fragile X: progress toward solving the puzzle. Am J Hum Genet 1990; 47:175.

Brown WT, Jenkins EC, Cohen IL, et al. Fragile X and autism: a multicenter study. Am J Med Genet 1986; 23:341.

Bühler EM, Nasseem JM. The tricho-rhino-phalangeal syndrome(s): chromosome 8 deletion. Are they separate entities? Am J Med Genet 1984; 19:113.

Burge DM, Middleton AW, Kamatch R, et al. Intestinal haemorrhage in Turner's syndrome. Arch Dis Child 1981; 56:557.

Burnell RH, Stern LM, Sutherland GR. A case of ring 20 chromosome with cardiac and renal anomalies. Aust J Paediatr 1985; 21:285.

Butler MG. Hypopigmentation: a common feature of Prader-Labhart-Willi syndrome. Am J Hum Genet 1989; 45:140.

Butler MG. Prader-Willi syndrome: current understanding of cause and diagnosis. Am J Hum Genet 1990; 35:319.

Butler MG, Brunschwig A, Miller LK, et al. Standards for selected anthropometric measurements in males with the fragile X syndrome. Pediatrics 1992; 89:1059.

Butler MG, Kaler SG, Yu PL, et al. Metacarpophalangeal pattern profile analysis in Prader-Willi syndrome. Clin Genet 1981; 22:315.

Butler MG, Mangrum T, Gupta R, et al. A 15-item checklist for screening mentally retarded males for the fragile X syndrome. Clin Genet 1991; 39:347.

Calderon JP, Chess J, Borodic G, et al. Intraocular pathology of trisomy 18 (Edwards' syndrome): report of a case and review of the literature. Br J Ophthalmol 1983; 67:162.

Caldwell PD, Smith DW. The XXY (Klinefelter's) syndrome in childhood: detection and treatment. J Pediatr 1972; 80:250.

Caputo A, Wagner RS, Reynolds DR, et al. Down syndrome: clinical review of ocular features. Clin Pediatr (Phila) 1989; 28:355.

Carey JC. The spectrum of DiGeorge syndrome. J Pediatr 1980; 96:955.

Carlock LR, Wasmuth JJ. A molecular approach to analysing the human 5p deletion syndrome, cri du chat. Somat Cell Mol Genet 1985; 11:267.

Carney RG Jr. Incontinentia pigmenti: a world statistical analysis. Arch Dermatol 1976; 4:535.

Carr DH, Gedeon M. Population cytogenetics of human abortuses. In: Hook EB, Porter IH, eds. Population cytogenetics: studies in human. New York: Academic Press, 1977.

Carrano AV, Dilla MA, van Gray JW. Flow cytogenetics: a new approach to chromosome analysis. In: Melamed MR, Mullaney PF, Mendelsohn ML, eds. Flow cytometry and sorting. New York: John Wiley & Sons, 1979.

Carter PE, Pearn JH, Bell J, et al. Survival in trisomy 18: life tables for use in genetic counselling and clinical pediatrics. Clin Genet 1985; 28:59.

Casanova MF, Walker LC, Whitehouse PJ, et al. Abnormalities of the nucleus basalis in Down's syndrome. Ann Neurol 1985; 18:310.

Case ME, Sarnat HB, Monteleone P. Type II Arnold-Chiari malformation with normal spine in trisomy 18. Acta Neuropathol 1977; 37:259.

Caskey CT, Pizzuti A, Fu YH, et al. Triplet repeat mutations in human disease. Science 1992; 256:784.

Caspersson T, Zech L, Johansson C. Analysis of human metaphase chromosome set by aid of DNA-binding fluorescent agents. Exp Cell Res 1970; 62:490.

Cassidy SB, Ledbetter DH. Prader-Willi syndrome. Neurol Clin 1989; 7:37.

Cassidy SB, Thuline HC, Holm VA. Deletion of chromosome 15 (q11-13) in a Prader-Labhart-Willi syndrome: clinic population. Am J Med Genet 1984; 17:485.

Cavenee WK, Hansen MF, Nordenskjold M, et al. Genetic origin of mutations predisposing to retinoblastoma. Science 1985; 228:501.

Cavenee WK, Murphree AL, Shull MM, et al. Prediction of familial predisposition to retinoblastoma. N Engl J Med 1986; 314:1201.

Chamberlin J, Magenis RE. Parental origin of de novo chromosome rearrangements. Hum Genet 1980; 53:343.

Chandley AC, Hargreave TB, Fletcher JM, et al. Trisomy 8 report of a mosaic human male with near normal phenotype and normal IQ, ascertained through infertility. Hum Genet 1980; 55:31.

Chaves-Carballo E, Frank LM, Rary J, et al. Neurologic aspects of the 9p- syndrome. Pediatr Neurol 1985; 1:57.

Chen H, Faigenbaum D, Weiss H. Psychosocial aspects of patients with the Ullrich-Turner syndrome. Am J Med Genet 1981; 8:191.

Chitayat D, Davis EB, McGillivray C. Perinatal and first year follow-up of patients with Prader-Willi syndrome: normal size of hands and feet. Clin Genet 1989; 35:161.

Chudley AE, Hagerman RJ. Fragile X syndrome. J Pediatr 1987; 110:821.

Chung RV, Seizinger BR. Molecular genetics of neurological tumours. J Med Genet 1992; 29:361.

Citoler P, Gropp A, Gullotta F. Cytogenetics and pathological observations in the (4p-) syndrome (Wolf-syndrome). Beitr Pathol 1971; 143:84.

Coco R, Bergada C. Cytogenetic findings in 125 patients with Turner's syndrome and abnormal karyotypes. J Genet Hum 1977; 25:95.

Cohen MM, Jr. Syndromology's message for craniofacial biology. J Maxillofac Surg 1979; 7:89.

Collacott RA, Ismail IA. Tourettism in a patient with Down syndrome. J Ment Def Res 1988; 32:163-6.

Colomb D, Vittori F, Zonca C. Les manifestations cutanees de la trisomie 21. Sem Hop Paris 1977; 53:801.

Connor JM. Cloning of the gene for the fragile X syndrome: implications for the clinical geneticist. J Med Genet 1991; 28:811.

Conneally PM, ed. Molecular genetics in clinical medicine. Oxford: Blackwell, 1992.

Cooley WC, Graham JM Jr. Common syndromes and management issues for primary care physicians. Clin Pediatr 1991; 30:233.

Cooper DN, Schmidtke J. Diagnosis of genetic disease using recombinant DNA. Hum Genet 1991; 87:519.

Cowen JM, Walker S, Harris F. Trisomy 13 and extended survival. J Med Genet 1979; 16:155.

Cowie V. Chromosomal abnormalities and mental disorders. Postgrad Med 1972; 48:212.

Cox DM, Ray M. The human chromosomes and their aberrations. In: Vinken PJ, Bruyn GW, eds. Congenital malformation of the brain and skull, part 2. In: Handbook of clinical neurology, vol 31. Amsterdam: North Holland Publishing, 1977.

Crapper DR, Dalton AJ, Skoptik M, et al. Alzheimer degeneration in Down's syndrome: electrophysiologic alterations and histopathologic findings. Arch Neurol 1975; 32:618.

Creel DJ, Bendel CM, Wiesner GL, et al. Abnormalities of the central visual pathways in Prader-Willi syndrome associated with hypopigmentation. N Engl J Med 1986; 314:1606.

Crippa L, Marcoz JP, Klein D, et al. Do all cases of trisomy 18 with long survival (beyond 10 years) show mosaicism in fibroblasts? (author's translation). J Genet Hum 1978; 26:145.

Crnic KA, Sulzbacher S, Snow J, et al. Preventing mental retardation associated with gross obesity in the Prader-Willi syndrome. Pediatrics 1980; 66:787.

Croce CM, Klein G. Chromosomes translocation and human cancer. Sci Am 1985; 252:54.

Cronk C, Crocker AC, Pueschel SM, et al. Growth charts for children with Down syndrome: 1 month to 18 years of age. Pediatrics 1988; 81:102.

Cutler AT, Benezra-Obeiter R, Brink SJ. Thyroid function in young children with Down syndrome. Am J Dis Child 1986; 140:479.

D'Alton ME, DeCherney AH: Prenatal diagnosis. N Engl J Med 1993; 328:114.

Daly RF. Neurological abnormalities in XYY males. Nature 1969; 221:472.

Daniel A. Clinical implications and classification of the constitutive fragile sites. Am J Med Genet 1986; 23:419.

Davidoff F, Federman DD. Mixed gonadal dysgenesis. Pediatrics 1973; 52:725.

Davies KE, ed. Human genetic diseases: a practical approach. Ithaca, NY: ILR Press, 1986.

Davies KE, ed. The fragile X syndrome. Oxford: Oxford Univsity Press, 1989.

De Arce MA, Kearns A. The fragile X syndrome: the patients with their chromosomes. J Med Genet 1984; 21:84.

De Arce MA, Hecht F, Sutherland GR, et al. Guidelines for the diagnosis of fragile X. Clin Genet 1986; 29:95.

de France HF, Beemer FA, Senders RC, et al. Partial trisomy 11q due to paternal T(11q;18p): further delineation of the clinical picture. Clin Genet 1984; 25:195.

de Grouchy J. Les microdeletions chromosomiques. Arch Fr Pediatr 1983; 40:1.

de Grouchy J, Turleau C. Clinical atlas of human chromosomes. New York: John Wiley & Sons, 1984.

de Grouchy J, Turleau C, Leonard C. Etude en fluorescence d'une trisomie C mosaïque, probablement 8:46, XY-47, XY:8 + . Ann Genet 1971; 14:69.

de la Chapelle A. Sex chromosome abnormalities. In: Emery AH, Rimion DL, eds. Principles and practice of medical genetics, 2nd ed. New York: Churchill Livingstone, 1990.

Delozier-Blanchet CD, Pitwon D, Schorderet D, et al. Cri-du-chat syndrome and two other deformed children in a family carrying a pericentric inversion or insertion of chromosome 5. J Genet Hum 1985; 33:371.

DeMyer W. Orbital hypertelorism. In: Vinken PJ, Bruyn GW, eds. Congenital malformations of the brain and skull, vol 30. Handbook of clinical neurology. Amsterdam: North Holland Publishing, 1977.

Dicks-Mireaux MJ. Mental development of infants with Down's syndrome. Am J Ment Defic 1972; 77:26.

Dobbing J. Undernutrition and the developing brain: the relevance of animal models to the human problem. Am J Dis Child 1970; 120:411.

Dobyns WB, Curry CJR, Hoyme HE, et al. Clinical and molecular diagnosis of Miller-Dieker syndrome. Am J Hum Genet 1991; 48:584.

Dobyns WB, Dewald GW, Carlson RO, et al. Deficiency of chromosome 8q21.1 →8pter: case report and review of the literature. Am J Med Genet 1985a; 22:125.

Dobyns WB, Gilbert EF, Opitz JM. Further comments on the lissencephaly syndromes. Am J Med Genet 1985b; 22:97.

Donlon TA. Similar molecular deletions on chromosome 15q11.2 are encountered in both the Prader-Willi and Angelman syndromes. Hum Genet 1988; 80:322.

Donis-Keller. Human gene mapping techniques: a laboratory manual. New York: Stockton Press, 1991.

Down JLH. Observations on an ethnic classification of idiots. Lond Hosp Rep 1866; 3:259.

Duncan AMU, Hough CA, White BN, et al. Breakpoint location of the marker chromosome associated with the cat eye syndrome. Am J Hum Genet 1986; 38:978.

Dunger DB, Davies KF, Pembrey M, et al. Deletion of the X-chromosome detected by direct DNA analysis in one of two unrelated boys with glycerokinase deficiency, adrenal hypoplasia and Duchenne muscular dystrophy. Lancet 1986; 15:585.

Dunn HG, Ford DK, Auersperg N, et al. Benign congenital hypotonia with chromosomal anomaly. Pediatrics 1961; 28:578.

Dyer K, Meyne J. Molecular cytogenetics: use of DNA probes as an adjunct to classical clinical cytogenetics. In: Barch MJ, ed. The ACT Cytogenetics Laboratory Manual, 2nd ed. New York: Raven Press, 1991.

Dyken PR, Miller MD. Facial features of neurologic syndromes. St. Louis: Mosby, 1980.

Editorials. Imprinting makes an impression. Lancet 1991; 338:413.

Edwards JH. Chromosomal abnormalities in mendelian disorders. Lancet 1982; 7:322.

Edwards J, Harnden JDG, Cameron AH, et al. A new trisomic syndrome. Lancet 1960; 1:787.

Egli F, Stalder G. Malformations of kidney and urinary tract in common aberrations. Hummangenetik 1973; 18:16.

Ehrlich S, Bustos T, Paika IJ, et al. Brief clinical report: duplication 18q syndrome. Am J Med Genet 1983; 15:261.

Einfeld S, Molony H, Hall W. Autism is not associated with the fragile X syndrome. Am J Med Genet 1989; 34:187.

Ellingson RJ. EEG in disorders associated with chromosomal anomalies. In: Remond A, ed. Handbook of EEG and clinical neurophysiology. Amsterdam: Elsevier/Excerpta Medical/North Holland (Associated Scientific Publishers), 1972.

Ellingson RJ, Eisen JD, Ottersberg G. Clinical electroencephalographic observations on institutionalized mongoloids confirmed by karyotype. Electroencephalogr Clin Neurophysiol 1973; 34:193.

Elliott D, Weeks DJ, Elliott CL. Cerebral specialization in individuals with Down syndrome. Am J Ment Retard 1987; 92:263.

Ellis WG, McCulloch JR, Corley CL. Presenile dementia in Down's syndrome: ultrastructural identity with Alzheimer's disease. Neurology 1974; 24:101.

Emanuel BS. Invited editorial: molecular cytogenetics: toward dissection of contiguous gene syndrome. Am J Hum Genet 1988; 43:575.

Emerit I, Cerutti P. Clastogenic activity from Bloom syndrome fibroblast cultures. Proc Natl Acad Sci USA 1981; 78:1868.

Emery AEH, Rimoin DL, eds. Principles and practice of medical genetics, 2nd ed. New York: Churchill Livingstone, 1990.

Engel E, DeLozier-Blanchet CD. Uniparental disomy, isodisomy, and imprinting: probable effects in man and strategies for their detection. Am J Med Genet 1991; 40:432.

Epstein CJ. The consequences of chromosome imbalance: principles, mechanisms, and models. In: Developmental and cell biology. New York: Cambridge University Press, 1986a.

Epstein CJ. Neurobiology of Down syndrome. New York: Raven Press, 1986b.

Epstein CJ. Down syndrome. In: Scriver CR, Beaudet AL, Sly WS, et al., eds. The metabolic basis of inherited disease, 6th ed. New York: McGraw-Hill, 1989.

Epstein LB, Spencer HS, Lee SHS, et al. Enhanced sensitivity of trisomy 21 monocytes to the maturation-inhibiting effect of interferon. Cell Immunol 1980; 50:191.

Escobar V, Cantu JM, Martin AD. Familial holoprosencephaly. Clin Genet 1979; 15:203 (letter).

Evenhuis HM. The natural history of dementia in Down syndrome. Arch Neurol 1990; 47:263.

Eydoux P, Choiset A, Le Porrier N, et al. Chromosomal prenatal diagnosis: study of 936 cases of intrauterine abnormalities after ultrasound assessment. Prenat Diagn 1989; 9:255.

Farge P, Dallaire L, Potier M, et al. Prenatal diagnosis of trisomy 10p in a twin pregnancy. Prenat Diagn 1985; 5:199.

Felsenfeld G. DNA. Sci Am 1985; 253:58.

Ferguson-Smith MA. Sex chromatin, Klinefelter's syndrome and mental deficiency. In: Moore KL, ed. The sex chromatin. Philadelphia: WB Saunders, 1966.

Ferguson-Smith MA. Chromosomal abnormalities. II. Sex chromosome defects. In: McKusick VA, Claiborne R, eds. Medical genetics. New York: Hospital Practice Publishing, 1973.

Ferguson-Smith MA. Invited editorial: putting the genetics back into cytogenetics. Am J Hum Genet 1991; 48:179.

Ferrante E, Vignetti P, Antonelli M, et al. Partial monosomy for a 21 chromosome: report of a new case of r(21) and review of the literature. Hum Genet 1983; 63:305.

Ferrier PE, Ferrier SA, Pescia G. The XXXY Klinefelter syndrome in childhood. Am J Dis Child 1974; 127:104.

Finelli P, Pueschel SM, Padre-Mendoza T, et al. Neurological findings in patients with the fragile-X syndrome. J Neurol Neurosurg Psychiatry 1985; 48:150.

Fineman RM, Buyse M, Morgan M. Variable phenotype associated with duplication of different regions of 2p. Am J Med Genet 1983; 15:451.

Finerman GA, Sakai D, Weingarten S. Atlanto-axial dislocation with spinal cord compression in the mongoloid child: a case report. J Bone Joint Surg [Am] 1976; 58:408.

Finidori G, Rigault P, de Grouchy J, et al. Osteoarticular abnormalities and orthopedic complications in children with chromosomal aberrations. Ann Genet 1983; 26:150.

Fishler K, Koch R, Donnell GN. Comparison of mental development in individuals with mosaic and trisomy 21 Down's syndrome. Pediatrics 1976; 58:744.

Flint J. Editorial: Implications of genomic imprinting for psychiatric genetics. Psychol Med 1992; 22:5.

Ford CE, Jones KW, Polani PE, et al. Sex chromosome anomaly in case of gonadal dysgenesis (Turner's syndrome). Lancet 1959; 1:711.

Francke U. Chromosome 20: trisomy, partial of short arm: chromosomal aberration syndrome with neurological involvement. In: Vinken PJ, Bruyn GW, eds. Handbook of clinical neurology, vol 43. Amsterdan: North Holland Publishing, 1982.

Francke U, Arias DE, Nyhan WL. Proximal 4p deletion: phenotype differs from classical 4p syndrome. J Pediatr 1977; 90:250.

Francke U, Brown MG, Jones KL. Immediate chromosome diagnosis on bone marrow cells: an aid to management of the malformed newborn infant. J Pediatr 1979a; 94:289.

Francke U, Holmes LB, Atkins L, et al. Aniridia-Wilms' tumor association: evidence for specific deletion of 11p13. Cytogenet Cell Genet 1979b; 24:185.

Francke U, Ocho HD, de Martinville B, et al. Minor Xp21 chromosome deletion in a male associated with expression of Duchenne muscular dystrophy, chronic granulomatous disease, retinitis pigmentosa and McLeod syndrome. Am J Hum Genet 1985; 37:250.

Francke U, Harper JF, Darras BT, et al. Congenital adrenal hypoplasia, myopathy, and glycerol kinase deficiency : molecular genetic evidence for deletions. Am J Hum Genet 1987; 40:212.

Frangoulis M, Taylor D. Corneal opacities: a diagnostic feature of the trisomy 8 mosaic syndrome. Br J Ophthalmol 1983; 67:619.

Freund L, Reiss AL. Cognitive profiles associated with fragile X syndrome in males and females. Am J Med Genet 1991; 38:542.

Friedman JM, Howard-Peebles PN. Inheritance of fragile X syndrome: an hypothesis. Am J Med Genet 1991; 23:701.

Friedmann T. Opinion: the human genome project — some implications of extensive "reverse genetic" medicine. Am J Hum Genet 1990; 46:407.

Friend SH, Bernards R, Rogelj S, et al. A human DNA segment with properties of the gene that predisposes to retinoblastoma and osteosarcoma. Nature 1986; 323:643.

Froster-Iskenius U, Bodeker K, Oepen T, et al. Folic acid treatment in males and females with fragile (X) syndrome. Am J Med Genet 1986a; 23:273.

Froster-Iskenius U, Felsch G, Schirren C, et al. Screening for fra (x) in a population of mentally retarded males. Hum Genet 1983; 63:153.

Froster-Iskenius UG, Hayden MR, Wang HS, et al. A family with Huntington disease and reciprocal translocation 4;5. Am J Hum Genet 1986b; 38:759.

Fryns JP. The fragile-X syndrome. Clin Genet 1984; 2:497.

Fryns JP, Dereymaeker A, Hoefnagels M, et al. Partial fra (X) phenotype with megalotestis in fra (X)–negative patients with acquired lesions of the central nervous system. Am J Med Genet 1986; 23:213.

Fryns JP, Kleczkowska A, Dereymaker AM, et al. Partial 8p trisomy due to interstitial duplication: karyotype: 46,XX, inv dup(8)(p21.1--p22). Clin Genet 1985a; 28:546.

Fryns JP, Kleczkowska A, Vandenberghe K, et al. Cystic hygroma and hydrops fetalis in dup (11p) syndrome. Am J Med Genet 1985b; 22:287.

Fu YH, Kohl DP, Pizzuti A, et al. Variation of the CGG repeat at the fragile X site results in genetic instability: resolution of the Sherman paradox. Cell 1991; 67:1047.

Fujimoto A, Lin MS, Korula SR, et al. Trisomy 14 mosaicism with t(14;15)(q111) in offspring of a balanced translocation carrier mother. Am J Med Genet 1985; 22:333.

Fukushima Y, Kondo Y, Kuroki Y, et al. Are Down syndrome patients predisposed to moyamoya disease? Eur J Pediatr 1986; 144:516.

Gagliardi AR, Tajara EH, Varella-Garcia M, et al. Trisomy 8 syndrome. J Med Genet 1978; 15:70.

Galbraith GC. Unique EEG and evoked response patterns in Down syndrome individuals. In: Epstein CJ, ed. Neurobiology of Down syndrome. New York: Raven Press, 1986.

Gandi S, Duncan MC. Angelman's syndrome: clinical CT scan and serial electroencephalographic study. Clin Electroencephalogr 1989; 20:128.

Gardner RJ, Rudd NL, Stevens LJ, et al. Autosomal imbalance with a near normal phenotype: the small effect of trisomy for the short arm of chromosome 18. Birth Defects 1978; 14:359.

Gardner RJM, Sutherland GR. Chromosome abnormalities and genetic counseling. New York: Oxford University Press, 1989.

Garron DC, Vander Stoep LR. Personality and intelligence in Turner's syndrome: a critical review. Arch Gen Psychiatry 1969; 21:339.

Garvey M, Mutton DE. Sex chromosome aberrations and speech development. Arch Dis Child 1973; 48:937.

Gatti RA, Boder E, Vinters HV, et al. Ataxia-telangiectasia: an interdisciplinary approach to pathogenesis. Medicine 1991; 70:99.

Gerald PS. Sex chromosome disorders: current concepts in genetics. N Engl J Med 1976; 294:706.

Gershwin ME, Crinella FM, Castles JJ, et al. Immunologic characteristics of Down's syndrome. J Ment Defic Res 1977; 21:237.

Gilbert F. Chromosomes, genes and cancer: a classification of chromosome abnormalities in cancer. J Nat Cancer Inst 1983; 71:100.

Gilbert LA, Dudley AW Jr, Meisner L, et al. New neurological findings in trisomy 13. Arch Pathol Lab Med 1977; 101:540.

Glass IA. X-linked mental retardation. J Med Genet 1991; 28:361.

Vinken PJ, Bruyn GW. Neurogenetic directory, part 2. In: Vinken PJ, Bruyn GW. Handbook of clinical neurology, vol 43. Amsterdam: North Holland Publishing, 1982.

Vladutiu AO, Chun TC, Victor A, et al. Down's syndrome and hypothyroidism: a role for thyroid autoimmunity. Lancet 1984; 1:1416.

Voelckel MA, Philip N, Piquet C, et al. Study of a family with a fragile site of the X chromosome at Xq27-28 without mental retardation. Hum Genet 1989; 81:353.

Vogel F, Motulsky AG. Human genetics, 2nd ed. Berlin: Springer-Verlag, 1986.

Waber DP. Neuropsychological aspects of Turner's syndrome. Dev Med Child Neurol 1979; 21:58.

Wagstaff J, Knoll JHM, Fleming J, et al. Localization of the gene encoding the GABA$_A$ receptor β_3 subunit to the Angelman/Prader-Willi region of human chromosome 15. Am J Hum Genet 1991; 49:330.

Wald NJ, Cuckle HS, Densem JW, et al. Maternal serum screening for Down syndrome in early pregnancy. Br Med J 1988; 297:883.

Walker HA. Incidence of minor physical anomalies in autistic patients. In: Coleman M, ed. Autistic syndrome. New York: Elsevier-North Holland, 1976.

Walzer S, Wolff PH, Bowen D, et al. A method for the longitudinal study of behavioral development in infants and children: the early development of XXY children. J Child Psychol Psychiatry 1978; 19:213.

Warkany J. Syndromes associated with mental retardation. In: Frederiks JAM, ed. Handbook of clinical neurology, vol 2. Neurobehavioural disorders. New York: Elsevier Science Publishing, 1985.

Warkany J, Passarge E, Smith LB. Congenital malformations in autosomal trisomy syndrome. Am J Dis Child 1966; 112:502.

Warkany J, Lemire R, Cohen MM. Mental retardation and congenital malformations of the central nervous system. Chicago: Year Book Medical Publishers, 1981.

Watt JL, Olson IA, Johnston AW, et al. A familial pericentric inversion of chromosome 22 with a recombinant subject illustrating a pure partial monosomy syndrome. J Med Genet 1985; 22:287.

Waziri M, Patil SK, Hanson JW, et al. Abnormality of chromosome 11 in patients with features of Beckwith-Wiedemann syndrome. J Pediatr 1983; 102:873.

Webb TP, Bundey SE, Thake AI, et al. Population incidence and segregation ratios in the Martin-Bell syndrome. Am J Med Genet 1986; 23:573.

Webb T. The epidemiology of the fragile X syndrome. In: Davies KE, ed. The fragile X syndrome. Oxford: Oxford University Press, 1989.

Weber JL, May PE. Abundant class of human DNA polymorphisms which can be typed using the polymerase chain reaction. Am J Hum Genet 1989; 44:388.

Weemaes CMR, Hustinx TWJ, Scheres JMJC, et al. A new chromosomal instability disorder: the NIJMEGEN breakage syndrome. Acta Paediatr Scand 1981; 70:557.

Wertelecki W, Graham JM, Sergovich FR. The clinical syndrome of triploidy. Obstet Gynecol 1976; 47:69.

Wertelecki W, Breg WR, Graham JM Jr, et al. Trisomy 22 mosaicism syndrome and Ullrich-Turner stigmata. Am J Med Genet 1986; 23:739.

Whorton RH, Bresnan MJ. Neonatal respiratory depression and delay in diagnosis of Prader-Willi syndrome. Dev Med Child Neurol 1989; 32:231.

Wilcox LM Jr, Bercovitch K, Howard RO. Ophthalmic features of chromosome deletion 4p− (Wolf-Hirschhorn syndrome). Am J Ophthalmol 1978; 86:834.

Wilkins LE, Brown JA, Wolf B. Psychomotor development in 65 home-reared children with cri-du-chat syndrome. J Pediatr 1980; 97:401.

Wilks J, Wilks E. Bernard: bringing up our mongol son. London: Routledge & Kegan Paul, 1974.

Williams CA, Zori RT, Stone JW, et al. Maternal origin of 15q11-13 deletions in Angelman syndrome suggests a role for genomic imprinting. Am J Med Genet 1990; 35:350.

Williams JP, Somerville GM, Miner ME, et al. Atlanto-axial subluxation and trisomy 21: another perioperative complication. Anesthesiology 1987; 67:253.

Wilson GN, Sauder SE, Bush M, et al. Phenotypic delineation of ring chromosome 15 and Russell-Silver syndromes. J Med Genet 1985a; 22:233.

Wilson GN, Dasouki M, Barr M Jr. Further delineation of the dup(3q) syndrome. Am J Med Genet 1985b; 22:117.

Wilson M, Mulley J, Gedeon A, et al. New X-linked syndrome of mental retardation, gynecomastia, and obesity is linked to DXS255. Am J Med Genet 1991; 40:406.

Wisniewski KE. Down syndrome children often have brain with maturation delay, retardation of growth, and cortical dysgenesis. Am J Med Genet (Supp) 1990; 7:274.

Wisniewski KE, Dambska M, Jenkins EC, et al. Monosomy 21 syndrome: further delineation including clinical neuropathological, cytogenetic and biochemical studies. Clin Genet 1983; 23:102.

Wisniewski KE, Dalton AJ, McLachlan DRC, et al. Alzheimer's disease in Down's syndrome: clinico-pathologic studies. Neurology 1985a; 35:957.

Wisniewski KE, French JH, Brown WT, et al. The fragile X syndrome and developmental disabilities. In: French J, Harels CP, eds. Child neurology and development disabilities: selected proceedings of the Fourth International Child Neurology Congress. Baltimore: PH Brookes Publishing, 1989; 11-20.

Wisniewski KE, French JH, Fernando S, et al. Fragile X syndrome: associated neurological abnormalities and developmental disabilities. Ann Neurol 1985b; 18:665.

Wisniewski KE, Laura-Kamionowska M, Connell F, et al. Neuronal density and synaptogenesis in the post-natal stage of brain maturation in Down's syndrome. In: Epstein CJ, ed. Neurobiology of Down's syndrome. New York: Raven Press, 1986.

Wisniewski KE, Segan SM, Miezejeski CM, et al. The fra X syndrome: neurological, electrophysiological, and neuropathological abnormalities. Am J Med Genet 1991; 38:476.

Wolfe LS, Ng Ying Kin NMK, Palo J, et al. Dolichols are elevated in brain tissue from Alzheimer's disease, but not in urinary sediment from Alzheimer's disease and Down's syndrome. Neurochem Pathol 1985; 3:213.

Wolf U, Reinwein H, Porsch R, et al. Defizienz an den kurzen Armen eins Chromosoms Nr.4. Humangenetik 1965; 1:397.

Wright CG, Brown OE, Meyerhoff WL, et al. Inner ear anomalies in two cases of trisomy 18. Am J Otolaryngol 1985; 6:392.

Young RS, Bader P, Palmer CG, et al. Brief clinical report: two children with de novo del (9p). Am J Med Genet 1983; 14:751.

Young RS, Weaver DD, Kukolich MK, et al. Terminal and interstitial deletions of the long arm of chromosome 7: a review with five new cases. Am J Med Genet 1984; 17:437.

Young RS, Fidone GS, Reider-Garcia PA, et al. Deletions of the long arm of chromosome 6: two new cases and review of the literature. Am J Med Genet 1985; 20:21.

Yu S, Mulley J, Loesch D, et al. Fragile X syndrome : unique genetics of the heritable unstable element. Am J Med Genet 1992; 50:968.

Yu S, Pritchard M, Kremer E, et al. Fragile X genotype characterized by an unstable region of DNA. Science 1991; 252:1179.

Yunis E, Gonzales J, Zunigo R, et al. Direct duplication 2p14--- 2p23. Hum Genet 1979; 48:241.

Yunis JJ. The chromosomal basis of human neoplasia. Science 1983; 221:227.

Table 2

| Ovulati |
| (da |

1
2
2

2
2
3

4
4

5
11
15
18

Data fro

tube fc
the ad
microfi
tracell
modify

Neura

The
goes c
fusion
neural
tions s
three e
cavitie
and ac
three
mantle
the ro
brain)
(midb
(hindb
the pi
which
sphere
proser
which
the op
cepha
cepha
(rostra
bellun
the m

Yunis JJ. Mid-prophase human chromosomes. The attainment of 2000 bands. Human Genet 1981; 56:293.

Yunis JJ, Chandler ME. The chromosomes of man: clinical and biologic significance. Am J Pathol 1977; 88:446.

Yunis JJ, Lewandowski RC. High-resolution cytogenetics. Birth Defects 1983; 19:11.

Zellweger H. Down syndrome. In: Vinken PJ, Bruyn GW, eds. Congenital malformations of the brain and skull, part II, vol 31. Handbook of clinical neurology. Amsterdam: North Holland Publishing, 1977.

Zellweger H, Ionasescu V, Simpson J, Waziri M. Chromosomal aneuploidies excluding Down syndrome. In: Vinken PJ, Bruyn GW, eds. Congenital malformations of the brain and skull, part II, vol 31. Handbook of clinical neurology. Amsterdam: North-Holland Publishing, 1977.

Zellweger H, Patil SR. Chromosomal anomalies excluding Down syndrome. In: Myrianthopoulos NC, ed. Handbook of clinical neurology, vol 6, Malformations. New York: Elsevier Science Publishing, 1987a.

Zellweger H, Patil SR. Down sydrome. In: Myrianthopoulos NC, ed. Handbook of clinical neurology, vol 6, Malformations. New York: Elsevier Science Publishing, 1987b.

Zellweger H, Simpson J. Chromosomes of man. Philadelphia: JB Lippincott, 1977.

Zellweger H, Soper RT. The Prader-Willi syndrome. Med Hygiene 1979; 37:3338.

Zollinger H. XXXY syndrome: two new observations of early age and review of literature. Helv Paediatr Acta 1969; 24:589.

Zonana J, Brown MG, Magenis RE. Distal 19q duplication. Hum Genet 1982; 60:267.

Zori RT, Hendrickson J, Woolven S et al. Angelman syndrome: clinical profile. J Child Neurol 1992; 7:270.

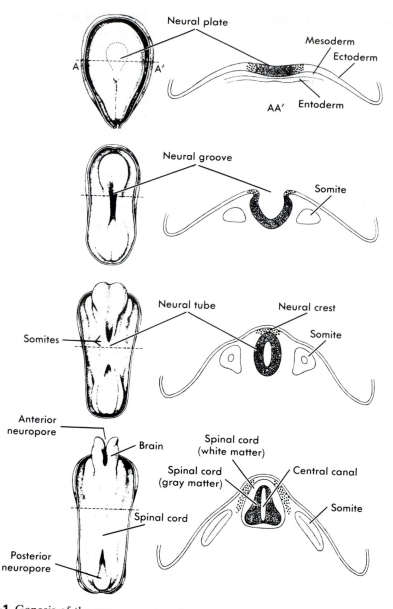

Figure 26-1 Genesis of the nervous system from the ectoderm, or outer cell layer, of a human embryo during the third and fourth weeks after conception. An external view of the developing embryo *(left)* and a corresponding cross-sectional view at about the middle of the future spinal cord *(right)* are shown. The CNS begins as the neural plate, a flat sheet of ectodermal cells on the dorsal surface of the embryo. The plate subsequently folds into a hollow structure—the neural tube. The head end of the central canal widens to form the ventricles, or cavities, of the brain. The peripheral nervous system is derived largely from the cells of the neural crest and from motor-nerve fibers that leave the lower part of the brain at each segment of the future spinal cord. (From Cowan WM. Sci Am 1979; 241:112.)

plate is columnar or vertical. This cellular arrangement within the neocortex is predetermined by radial (centrifugal) migration of cells. Immature neurons are guided to the distant cortex by the radially oriented glial fibers. At the cortical plate the neurons become aligned in a single vertical column. The migrating neurons follow an inside-out pattern of location, with each neuron along a given radial guide and settling external to its predecessor. The radial elongated glial cells eventually disappear, probably transformed into astrocytes. This radial guide hypothesis suggests a plausible mechanism by which migrating neurons reach the cortex. The final

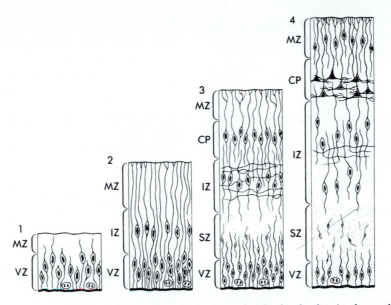

Figure 26-2 Progressive thickening of the wall of the developing brain. At the earliest stage *(1)* the wall consists only of a "pseudostratified" epithelium, in which the ventricular zone *(ZV)* contains the cell bodies and the margin zone *(MZ)* contains only the extended outer cell processes. When some cells lose their capacity for synthesizing DNA and withdraw from the mitotic cycle *(2)*, they form a second layer, the intermediate zone *(IZ)*. In the forebrain the cells that pass through this zone aggregate to form the cortical plate *(CP)*, the region in which the various layers of the cerebral cortex develop *(3)*. At the latest stage *(4)* the original ventricular zone remains as the ependymal lining of the cerebral ventricles. The comparatively cell-free region between this lining and the cortex becomes the subcortical white matter, through which nerve fibers enter and leave the cortex. The subventricular zone *(SZ)* is a second proliferative region where many glial cells and some neurons in the forebrain are generated. (From Cowan WM. Sci Am 1979; 241:112.)

location of the neuron may be designated by the structural and chemical interactions among migrating cells.

As part of the process of neuronal migration, selective cell aggregation occurs and is important in the formation of selective nuclear groups and the complex cortical laminations. Neuronal cytodifferentiation then begins with the appearance of neuronal processes, the development of specific neuronal cell membrane properties, and a designation toward a specific type of cell-to-cell transmission. As part of this process, further morphologic differentiation occurs, as does the process of more complex cell molecular and physiologic differentiation and the development of more complex synaptic interconnections [Cowan, 1992].

The histologic and gross morphologic approach to explain malformations is a simple beginning. The basic mechanisms of CNS maturation are overwhelmingly complex [Cowan, 1992; Williams and Caviness, 1984]. Studies on cell adhesion molecules, cell-surface complex glycoproteins, and models of teratogenesis in embryo culture offer new insights into the molecular embryology of the malformations of the nervous system [Edelman, 1983; Freinkel et al., 1984; McLone and Knepper, 1985].

DEVELOPMENTAL NEURAL TUBE DEFECTS

Spinal dysraphism and associated malformations

Spinal dysraphism may involve multiple germ layers and the ectoderm and mesoderm, with variable clinical manifestations. The condition includes lesions varying from a flat dermal aberration to a gross malformation of a region of the spinal canal and cord [French, 1983]. The subtlest defect, spina bifida occulta, arises when the vertebral arches fail to fuse. When this abnormality is associated with an underlying malformation of the spinal cord, the condition is known as *occult spinal dysraphism*; accompanying abnormalities of the overlying skin and soft tissue usually occur (e.g., dermal sinus or dimple, skin tag, tuft of hair, port-wine stain) [Anderson, 1975]. When the meninges alone protrude through the defect, the malformation is termed a *meningocele*. Myelomeningocele, in which a portion of the spinal cord or nerve roots are displaced through the spina bifida defect into a sac, is the most complex and usually symptomatic condition.

Pathogenesis. Two hypotheses have been suggested to explain the evolution of myelodysplasia. The most plausible theory is that the neural tube fails to close during embryogenesis [Laurence, 1964; Osaka et al.,

1978]. Lack of closure of the posterior neuropore, the terminal location of normal neural tube fusion, may explain the reason lumbosacral malformations frequently accompany the disorder. Primary failure of neural tube closure does not account for other dysplastic characteristics of myelodysplasia unless an associated defect of neural induction in the mesoderm is involved.

Another theory ascribes the deformity to a faulty primary hydrodynamic sequence [Gardner, 1965]. The roof of the fourth ventricle fails to become patent, preventing spinal fluid egress. The ensuing elevated pressure and attendant pulsations create distortion along the neuraxis, with eventual rupture of the neural tube. No substantiating evidence exists for this hypothesis.

Spinal dysraphism may be caused by a teratogenic agent acting before neural tube closure, which occurs during the fourth week of gestation. Teratogens capable of inducing myelodysplasia in experimental animals or human beings include radiation, maternal hyperthermia, gestational diabetes mellitus, vitamin A deficiency or excess, d-mannose, excess glucose in embryo culture, valproic acid, and folic acid deficiency.*

Spina bifida occulta

Spina bifida occulta occurs in at least 5% of the population but is most often asymptomatic. The diagnosis is confirmed by a radiograph of the spine that documents an incomplete vertebral arch. Accompanying associated features may include dermal hyperpigmentation, a patch of hair, a lump, or a dermal sinus. This defect is located most often in the lower lumbar area involving the lamina of L_5 and S_1. When associated neurologic involvement is present, the condition is occult spinal dysraphism.

Occult spinal dysraphism

The spectrum of occult spinal dysraphism includes distortion of the spinal cord or roots by fibrous bands and adhesions, intraspinal lipomas, dermoid or epidermoid cysts, fibrolipomas, subcutaneous lipomas (lipomyelomeningoceles), tethered cord, and diastematomyelia [Anderson, 1975]. A tethered cord is the most common condition.

Symptoms of an occult spinal dysraphism may be absent, minimal, or severe, depending on the degree of neural involvement. The patient may exhibit static or slowly progressive weakness or sensory loss in the legs or feet, gait difficulty, and foot deformity. Bowel and bladder dysfunction, such as incontinence, repeated bladder infection, and enuresis, may also occur. Symptoms are caused by abnormally formed neural tissue or pressure on the spinal cord or nerve roots. Common findings include diminished Achilles tendon reflexes, contracted heel cords, high arches, equinovarus deformity of the feet, decreased rectal sphincter tone, unequal leg or foot length, scattered sensory loss, Babinski signs, and trophic ulcers. Because many of these patients have associated posterior fossa or cervical cord malformations, neurologic involvement of the upper extremities may also occur [Jansen et al., 1991]. Ophthalmologic complications, usually observed when hydrocephalus is present, are also common and require careful evaluation and follow-up [Biglan, 1990]. Ultrasonography and MRI have greatly facilitated the diagnosis and management of these occult lesions (Figure 26-3) [Brunberg et al., 1988]. A tethered spinal cord or lipoma can be detected without invasive myelography. Ultrasonography can demonstrate a poorly pulsatile, low-lying, or thickened conus medullaris in infants [Raghavendra et al., 1983; Scheible et al., 1983]. Surgery is indicated in symptomatic patients; prophylactic intervention has become the standard treatment in asymptomatic children, partly because of technical advances [McLone and Naidich, 1986].

Recurrent meningitis from external contamination of CSF may result from occult congenital malformations along the spinal canal and neuraxis. These external connections include midline dermal sinus; temporal bone fistula to the middle ear, eustachian tube, or nasopharynx; neurenteric fistula; and basal encephalocele or meningocele involving the cribriform plate, sphenoid bone, or clivus [Hemphill et al., 1982]. A metrizamide myelogram with CT should be obtained, followed by appropriate surgical treatment.

Meningocele

Meningocele, a protrusion of meninges without accompanying nervous tissue, is not associated with neurologic deficit. The mass is usually evident as a fluid-filled protrusion covered by skin or membrane in the midline. Membranous lesions are found rostrally, and skin-covered lesions are more evenly distributed along the neuraxis. Very small subcutaneous lesions may remain undetected for prolonged periods.

When careful examination of patients with suspected meningocele reveals significant neurologic abnormality (e.g., equinovarus deformity, gait disturbance, abnormal bladder function) [Laurence, 1964], the diagnosis of myelomeningocele is appropriate. These patients have entrapped nerve roots within the defect, which can be identified during surgery.

A meningocele in the cranial or high cervical area may coexist with aqueductal stenosis, hydromyelia, and an Chiari malformation. Membrane-covered meningoceles are more likely to be accompanied by severe abnormalities; lesions covered with normal skin are often free of associated abnormalities (Figure 26-4). Elective surgi-

---

*Freinkel et al., [1984]; Holmes et al., [1976]; Layde et al., [1980]; Miller et al., [1981]; Pleet et al., [1981]; Shiota [1982]; Speidel [1973].

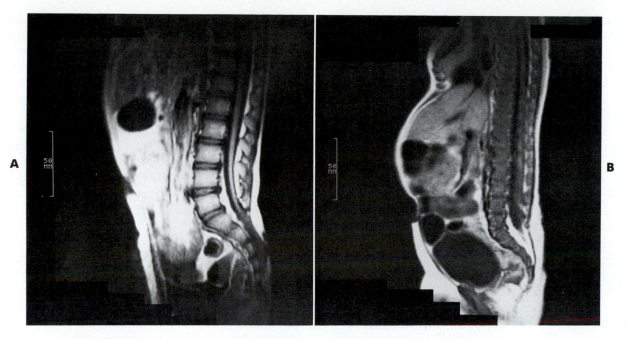

Figure 26-3 A, Tethered spinal cord. MRI scan demonstrates a low-lying spinal cord that ends at S_1-S_2. A normal spinal cord terminates at L_1-L_2. (Courtesy Westchester County Medical Center, Valhalla, NY.) **B,** Intraspinal lipoma. This MRI scan demonstrates a tethered spinal cord associated with a lipoma. (Courtesy Division of Neurosurgery, New York Medical College, New York, NY.)

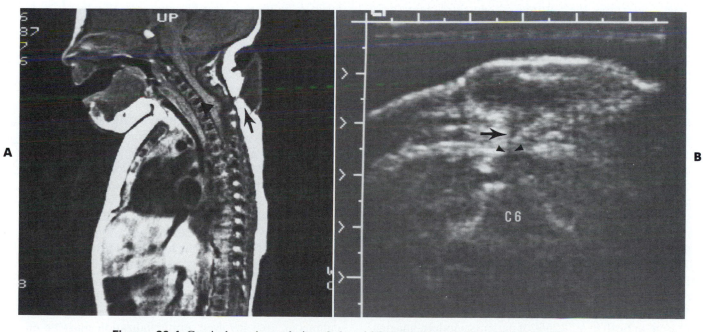

Figure 26-4 Cervical meningocele in a 3-day-old female infant. **A,** C_6 meningocele *(arrow)* extending through small dorsal rachischisis, which is demonstrated on this T_1 weighted sagittal MRI scan. Spinal cord is deformed *(arrowhead)* within focally widened thecal sac but does not extend into the dorsal cyst. **B,** Small meningocele tract *(arrow)* and overlying meningocele are well shown with transaxial sonogram. Note how the cord is tented towards dorsal opening *(arrowheads)*. (Courtesy Joseph R. Thompson, Department of Radiation Sciences, Loma Linda University School of Medicine, Loma Linda, California.)

cal treatment is recommended except for very small lesions [Steinbok and Cochrane, 1991].

Myelomeningocele

Myelomeningocele, the most complex of congenital spinal deformities, involves all underlying layers (i.e., spinal cord, nerve roots, meninges, vertebral bodies, skin). The spinal cord may be exposed because of complete failure of neural closure (myeloschisis). The incidence of myelomeningocele has been estimated to be 2 to 3 cases per 1000 live births. The incidence has steadily declined because of improved methods of prenatal diagnosis [Welch and Winston, 1987].

Clinical characteristics. The mortality rate of myelomeningocele is approximately 50% in the absence of therapy; surgical intervention is required because death results from hydrocephalus, meningitis, and renal failure. The last complication is induced by chronic urinary tract infections, abnormal urodynamic function, and genitourinary tract abnormalities such as progressive hydronephrosis [Liptak et al., 1988]. Recent studies have suggested that daily oral supplementation with folic acid before conception and during early pregnancy substantially reduces the recurrence risk of neural tube defects [MMWR, 1991].

Myelomeningoceles may be situated at any longitudinal level of the neuraxis. The location and extent of the defect determine the nature and degree of neurologic impairment. Lumbosacral involvement is most common. Thoracic defects are the most complex and are frequently associated with serious complications. The protuberant and fluctuant lesion is readily observable and palpable. Varying degrees of paresis of the legs, usually profound, and sphincter dysfunction are the major clinical manifestations. Congenital dislocation of the hips or deformities of the feet may also occur. Severe sensory loss and accompanying trophic ulcers may complicate the condition. Occasionally, only sphincter disturbances are present. Radiographs reveal the primary defect of the vertebral arch.

Hydrocephalus, a frequently associated defect, is the result of the Chiari malformation; there may be associated aqueductal stenosis. Hydrocephalus, present in 73% of patients with myelomeningocele, occurs most frequently when the lesion is situated in the thoracolumbar area, which is the case in 90% of patients [Lorber, 1971]. Although hydrocephalus was believed to be present at birth in only 25% of patients, modern imaging techniques almost always reveal the lesion to be present at birth. Lesions located more rostrally than others produce less lower motor unit paralysis and sphincter involvement. Caudal lesions in the neuraxis are typically associated with bladder and sphincter involvement. The profound paralysis that accompanies caudal involvement often prevents the patient from walking.

Genetics. Myelomeningocele may be transmitted as an autosomal-recessive trait, although recurrence risk statistics suggest a polygenic or environmental etiology. The recurrence risk of neural tube defects after the birth of an affected child is approximately 4% to 8% and increases to at least 10% after the birth of two affected children [McKusick, 1990]. The recurrence risk in children who have an affected parent is about 3%.

Antenatal diagnosis. The presence of abnormally high levels of alpha-fetoprotein in the amniotic fluid signals myelomeningocele [Milunsky and Albert, 1974]. Alpha-fetoprotein is a component of fetal CSF, and it probably leaks into the amniotic fluid from the open neural tube defect. Elevated amniotic alpha-fetoprotein concentrations correlate with the type of defect; closed lesions often do not cause increased alpha-fetoprotein concentration [Macri et al., 1974, 1979]. An amniotic fluid alpha-fetoprotein determination for myelomeningocele has a false-positive rate of less than 0.5% and a false-negative rate of 2%. Alpha-fetoprotein is synthesized by the yolk sac, hepatic cells, and the gastrointestinal tract of the fetus [Gitlin et al., 1972]. It is normally excreted into amniotic fluid in fetal urine [Brock et al., 1975].

Maternal serum alpha-fetoprotein levels are also elevated during pregnancy with affected fetuses after the second trimester [Seller et al., 1974]; thus screening low-risk mothers is feasible and cost effective [Chamberlain, 1978; Milunsky and Alpert, 1978]. The detection rate for open neural tube defects using maternal serum screening is approximately 80%, with a low false-positive rate [Ferguson-Smith et al., 1978; Richards et al., 1988]. Ultrasonography can detect or confirm the extent of the neural tube defect [Watson et al., 1991].

Management and prognosis. Management of a myelomeningocele requires the efforts of many specialists [Colgan, 1981; Liptak et al., 1988]. Treatment includes prevention of infection, surgical reduction and covering of the myelomeningocele, control of hydrocephalus, management of urinary dysfunction, and treatment of the paralysis and abnormalities of the hips and feet. The value of immediate correction of the defect within 24 hours of birth has been established [McLone and Naidich, 1989]. However, when no CSF leaks, a delay in closure for up to 48 hours does not increase the risk of infection or worsen the neurologic deficit. When primary closure is impossible because of the large cutaneous area involved, epithelialization must be encouraged and surgery performed later.

Cranial ultrasonography should be performed at birth and will determine the presence of hydrocephalus. Ultrasonography of the mother's uterus during pregnancy will often indicate the diagnosis of both myelomeningocele and hydrocephalus. Hydrocephalus may be present even though the infant's head is not enlarged.

Placement of a ventriculoperitoneal shunt alleviates the pressure problems engendered by hydrocephalus.

Bladder dysfunction and urinary incontinence pose major management problems and may be present at birth [Greig et al., 1991]. Interruption of sacral nerve roots and fiber connections between the brainstem and sacral cord causes the dysfunction. Normal bladder control occurs in 10% of children with myelomeningocele [Rink and Mitchell, 1984]. Prevention of bladder infection requires intermittent catheterization to maintain low residual urine volumes and prophylactic antibacterial drugs. Vesicoureteral reflux often develops during the second and third year of life and must be evaluated. Reimplantation of the ureters into the bladder or external drainage of the ureters either directly or through an ileal conduit may be helpful. Transurethral resection of the external sphincter has been recommended when ureteral dilatation occurs. The use of prosthetic devices emulating sphincters holds some promise [Cass et al., 1984].

Orthopedic defects may be severe and necessitate early intervention [Kupka et al., 1978]. Hip subluxation is usually treated with prosthetic splints or plaster casting. Sensory deficits of the casted skin areas frequently enhance the likelihood of skin ulcers. Clubfeet may also be treated with splinting or casting. Physical therapy may help to preserve and extend the range of motion of the joints [Carroll, 1987].

In infants and children, progressive leg or foot deformity, weakness, pain, or deterioration of gait or bladder function suggest restricted growth of the spinal cord. Stridor, retrocollis, and apnea suggests a brainstem malformation, and evidence of brainstem dysfunction may be recorded using brainstem auditory-evoked response testing [Davidson-Ward et al., 1986; Docherty et al., 1987]. These signs and symptoms indicate the possibility of a tethered spinal cord or Chiari malformation. The differential diagnosis of delayed deterioration in a child with repaired meningomyelocele includes a malfunctioning or infected shunt, seizures, scoliosis, progressive Chiari malformation, hydrocephalus, hydromyelia, or an undetected second lesion of occult spinal dysraphism. Surgical repair of a tethered spinal cord can prevent decline of function [Charney et al., 1987; McLone and Naidich, 1986; Sakamoto et al., 1991].

Optimal medical management should be provided at birth, including aseptic techniques. Results of extensive studies have indicated that 85% of infants not surgically treated die by 1 year of age [Laurence, 1966]. Routine early closure of myelomeningoceles became common practice in many medical centers in the 1960s. Unfortunately, more than half of the infants died, often after a long succession of procedures [Lorber, 1971]. Many survivors were severely paralyzed and incontinent and developed scoliosis. In other studies the best results were

obtained in patients with caudal lesions, either lumbar or lumbosacral, who did not require a shunt to treat hydrocephalus; 90% were ambulatory and had a normal range of intelligence [Ames and Schut, 1972].

As a result of the poor prognosis and poor results associated with high cord lesions accompanied by hydrocephalus, criteria were formulated to exclude infants from active treatment, with only routine nursing care provided [Lorber, 1973]. A very poor prognosis was associated with gross paralysis of the legs, thoracolumbar or thoracolumbosacral lesions, kyphosis or scoliosis, increased head circumference, and accompanying severe congenital birth defects; however, because of the medicolegal climate prevailing in the United States and increasing evidence that children who would have been excluded from treatment using Lorber criteria are doing reasonably well after medical management, there has been no concentrated effort not to provide surgical care. Virtually all infants and children born with such defects are being provided surgical and medical treatment. Recent studies reported that the 5-year survival rate for children with sacral lesions was 97%; for lumbar lesions, 93%; and for thoracic lesions, 75% [Welch and Winston, 1987]. These data suggest that selective criteria for surgical treatment offer the optimal outcome for the less severely affected child and less suffering and distress for the more handicapped patients with myelomeningocele.

Counseling is essential to ensure that parents understand the nature and severity of the deformities and the necessary surgical and long-term rehabilitative efforts [Liptak et al., 1988]. The parents should also be aware of the patient's potential for intellectual and physical development.

The decision for vigorous therapy for the most severely affected infants with myelomeningocele is beset by moral and medical considerations; restricted therapy is often associated with survival but poor outcome. Appropriate treatment of newborns with myelomeningocele increases the number of survivors and perhaps the quality of survival. Early surgical repair is appropriate for most newborns with myelodysplasia [McLaughlin et al., 1985]. Each patient must be assessed individually in the context of advances in technology and medical care.

Diastematomyelia

In diastematomyelia a midline septum divides the spinal cord longitudinally into two usually unequal portions extending up to 10 thoracolumbar segments [Bradford et al., 1991]. The septum may span the entire width of the spinal canal and is anchored to the ventral dura mater on the posterior aspect of the vertebral bodies. It may be attached posteriorly to the vertebral arch or dura mater. The septum is derived from mesoderm and it is composed of fibrous tissue, cartilage, or bone. Patients with diastematomyelia may have deformities of the feet, scoliosis, kyphosis, or discrepancy in leg length.

Diplomyelia

Diplomyelia is a side-by-side or anteroposterior duplication or splitting of the spinal cord, often accompanied by spina bifida and diastematomyelia. Two central canals are usually present, each surrounded by gray and white matter arranged in the normal pattern. The two cords are often completely reunited caudally but may remain separated to the tip of the conus medullaris. A bony septum may partly intervene. The two cords, which may be equally developed but are often unequal, may be side by side (the most common position), or one may be dorsal to the other. These malformations are compatible with normal function; deterioration suggests the presence of diastematomyelia.

Sacral agenesis (caudal regression syndrome)

Sacral agenesis, or caudal regression syndrome, is the complete or partial absence of the sacrum, hemisacrum, or coccyx and often includes genitourinary anomalies [Towfighi and Housman, 1991]. Maternal diabetes mellitus is associated with sacral agenesis in 16% of patients. Good diabetic control early in pregnancy decreases the incidence of congenital anomalies, thus demonstrating the effect of maternal carbohydrate metabolism on spinal cord embryogenesis [Fuhrmann et al., 1983; Miller et al., 1981].

The neurologic findings are similar to those of myelomeningocele, ranging from a minimal deficit to equinovarus deformity of the feet to more extensive sensory and motor deficits of the lower extremities. Most patients have neurogenic urinary tract and bowel impairment, flattened buttocks, and prominent iliac crests.

Treatment is similar to that for patients with myelodysplasia, particularly for the problems of urinary incontinence, constipation, progressive urinary tract and renal dysfunction, and orthopedic abnormalities. Some patients experience progressive neurologic deficits, demonstrating that sacral agenesis is not always a static disability. Slow deterioration of neurologic function may masquerade as an orthopedic or urologic problem unless the potential for progressive lesions is appreciated. Dural sac stenosis, tethered spinal cord, diastematomyelia, and cauda equina lipomas and dermoids have also been associated with sacral agenesis [Brooks et al., 1981; Pang and Hoffman, 1980]. Although plain radiographs demonstrate the degree of sacral agenesis, CT, MRI, or myelography is necessary to delineate the underlying spinal cord anomalies (Figure 26-5) [Cerisoli et al., 1983]. Surgical intervention is indicated in patients with progressive neurologic deficits associated with occult spinal cord lesions.

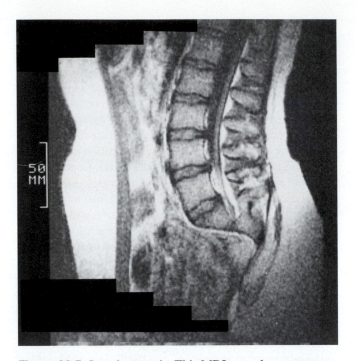

Figure 26-5 Sacral agenesis. This MRI scan demonstrates a tethered spinal cord that ends at L_5 and is associated with sacral agenesis. (Courtesy Westchester County Medical Center, Valhalla, NY.)

Chiari malformation

Four variations of the Chiari malformation exist [Caviness, 1976]. In type 2, the most frequently encountered, the cerebellum and medulla oblongata are shifted caudally; resultant packing into the cervical spinal canal results in deformation. Because of kinking, the thinned and elongated medulla may actually be positioned side-by-side with the upper segments of the dwarfed and deformed cervical spinal cord. Curiously, the abnormal positioning causes the upper cervical roots to course upward before leaving the vertebral foramina (Figures 26-6 and 26-7). The pons is thin and narrow. By definition, type 2 Chiari malformation is associated with myelomeningocele. Hydrocephalus occurs in most patients secondary to aqueductal stenosis or obstruction to CSF flow around the medulla. The precise mechanism is unknown [Gilbert et al., 1986]. Some authors have suggested that aqueductal stenosis is secondary to hydrocephalus [Masters, 1978]. Multiple cysts form inferior to the medulla in 40% of patients [Emery and Lendon, 1972]. Vascular lesions, including hemorrhage and infarcts, are often present in the tegmentum of the medulla in children, with resultant altered respiratory control [Papasozomenos and Roessman, 1981]. Other CNS defects, such as polymicrogyria, heterotropias, syringomyelia, hydromyelia, Klippel-Feil syndrome, craniolacunia, and bony anomalies at the base of the skull, often accompany Chiari malformation.

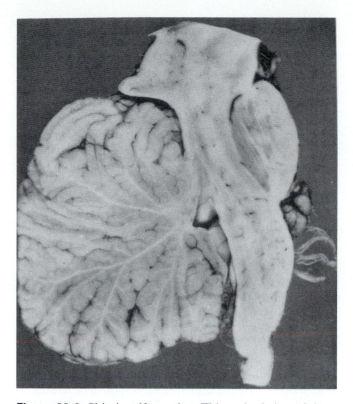

Figure 26-6 Chiari malformation. This sagittal view of the cerebellum and brainstem shows elongation of the pons and medulla, with notching at the junction of the medulla and spinal cord. The fourth ventricle is displaced downward.

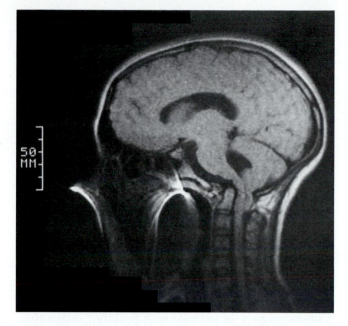

Figure 26-7 Chiari malformation and basilar impression. This MRI scan demonstrates moderate hydrocephalus, an enlarged fourth ventricle, the cerebellar tonsils and medulla displaced into the crowded cervical canal, and a superiorly placed odontoid process.

Type 1 Chiari malformation is similar to type 2, but the malformation is milder. The cerebellum is displaced into the cervical spinal canal. Although it is characteristically long and thin, the medulla does not have a side-by-side relationship with the cervical cord. No associated myelomeningocele exists. Type 3 is essentially an occipital encephalocele and consists of spina bifida over the cervical area with protrusion of the cerebellum through the opening. Type 4 consists of a single abnormality, hypoplasia of the cerebellum, and may be a variation of the Dandy-Walker syndrome [Caviness, 1976].

Clinical characteristics. Type 1 Chiari malformation may not be associated with clinical manifestations for many decades [Archer et al., 1977]. The initial symptoms are recurrent occipital and frontal headaches, neck pain, unsteady gait, progressive ataxia, and difficulty in swallowing. Various functions of cranial nerves IX to XII are compromised. The gag reflex may be unelicitable and the soft palate paretic. Cerebellar impairment, evidenced by ataxia and nystagmus, may be apparent. Downbeat nystagmus and periodic alternating nystagmus are characteristic of craniocervical anomalies, such as the Chiari malformation. Extensor toe signs and deep tendon reflexes are present, and the latter are pathologically increased. The posterior columns are usually involved with compromised vibration and position

sense. Increased intracranial pressure may also develop.

Management. Careful monitoring of infants with known Chiari malformations is advocated [Charney et al., 1987; Venes et al., 1986]. Evaluation with MRI is now the procedure of choice [Gammal et al., 1987]. Suboccipital craniectomy to decompress the suboccipital and cervical areas is the recommended treatment to alleviate the progressive compression of neural and vascular structures. Incision of the dura mater allows sectioning of the arachnoid bands. No resection of the cerebellar tonsils is advocated. Adequate treatment of hydrocephalus usually requires placement of a ventriculoperitoneal shunt. Failure of decompressive surgery in some infants with progressive symptoms suggests a primary brainstem etiology, such as infarction or hypoplasia of brainstem nuclei [Gilbert et al., 1986].

Encephalocele

An encephalocele is a protrusion of a portion of the cerebral hemisphere or meninges through a skull defect. The occipital area is involved most often (75%), followed by the frontal area (25%). The latter condition occurs most frequently among Asians. Basal and transsphenoidal encephaloceles are rare; they may appear between the ethmoid and sphenoid bones and extend into the upper pharynx [Harley, 1991]. Encephaloceles that extend from the area of the orbit, nose, or forehead are termed *sincipital encephaloceles*; those in the occipital region are termed *notencephaloceles*. Exencephaly consists of a large outpouching of brain tissue with surrounding thick walls. This defect may involve the spinal cord, forming an encephalomyelocele. Cranial encephalocele may contain a combination of meninges, ventricles, and brain parenchyma.

Clinical characteristics. A fluctuant, round, balloon-like mass that protrudes from the cranium, usually posteriorly, is the most common characteristic of encephaloceles. The mass may pulsate and be covered by an erythematous, translucent, or opaque membrane or by normal skin. The covering may not be uniform throughout its surface. The amount of compromised and deformed neural tissue determines the extent of cerebral dysfunction [Mealey et al., 1970]. Brain tissue not extending into the encephalocele may be deformed and functionally impaired.

Severe intellectual and motor delays typically occur in association with microcephaly; motor delay is accompanied by weakness and spasticity. Intellectual impairment is more common in patients with posterior rather than anterior encephaloceles [Hockley et al., 1990]. Occipital lobe destruction is associated with various degrees of visual impairment. When the deformity includes a ventricle, hydrocephalus is almost inevitable. Because of increased pressure, the encephalocele may become stretched until the covering is infarcted, with resultant infection and rupture. Other malformations may accompany encephaloceles, including Dandy-Walker syndrome, Klippel-Feil syndrome, Chiari malformation, porencephaly, agenesis of the corpus callosum, myelodysplasia, optic nerve dysplasia, and cleft palate [Cohen and Lemire, 1982]. Although ultrasonography may be helpful, the clinical diagnosis is confirmed by CT or MRI (Figure 26-8).

Neuroendocrine disturbance occurs, particularly with basal encephaloceles involving the sella turcica and sphenoid sinus [Ellyn et al., 1980]. These conditions may be undetectable by gross inspection. Intranasal mass or endocrine dysfunction is the cardinal feature.

Encephaloceles, which are usually associated with other defects, can be inherited in an autosomal-recessive mode [Cohen and Lemire, 1982]. Occipital encephalocele, microcephaly, cleft palate or lip, polydactyly, holoprosencephaly, and polycystic kidneys constitute Meckel syndrome [McKusick, 1990]. Retinal degeneration with detachment and occipital encephalocele is another autosomal-recessive condition [Knobloch and Layer, 1971].

Nasal glioma, a congenital tumor, appears as a frontonasal mass that mimics an encephalocele [Lemire et al., 1975; Younus and Coode, 1986]. The tumor is derived from herniated brain tissue that has lost its connection to the brain; this relationship can be demonstrated by neuroimaging techniques.

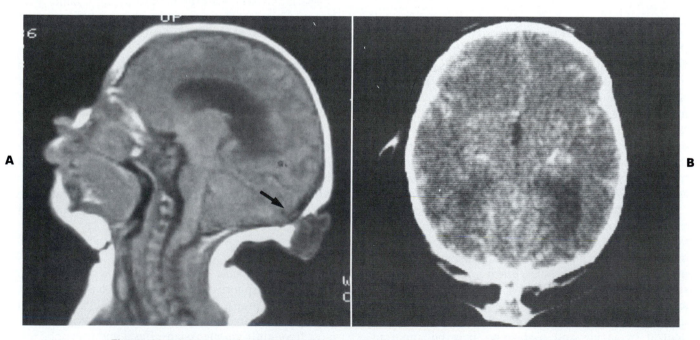

Figure 26-8 Meningoencephalocele in a 4-day-old female infant. **A,** Small nubbin of brain tissue *(arrow)* extending into small occipital meningoencephalocele; these defects are better demonstrated with this T_1 weighted sagittal MRI than with axial CT. **B,** Features of accompanying Chiari malformation are also seen because of better soft tissue resolution with MRI. (Courtesy Joseph R. Thompson, Department of Radiation Sciences, Loma Linda University School of Medicine, Loma Linda, Calif.)

Management. Prenatal diagnosis of encephaloceles may be established with determination of increased amniotic alpha-fetoprotein content and ultrasound studies [Goldstein et al., 1991]. Treatment is ineffective when the sac contains a significant mass of neural tissue; however, closure of the defect is necessary. Accompanying hydrocephalus may require ventriculoperitoneal shunting.

Anencephaly

Anencephaly is a congenital malformation in which both cerebral hemispheres are absent. The cranial vault defect is an extensive cranioschisis [Medical Task Force on Anencephaly, 1990]. Most anencephalic infants are stillborn. Those infants born alive die shortly after birth [Botkin, 1988].

Epidemiologic studies demonstrate a striking variation in prevalence rates. The highest incidence is in Great Britain and Ireland, and the lowest is in Asia, Africa, and South America. Other countries have intermediate rates of incidence. Anencephaly occurs six times more frequently in whites than in blacks. Females are more often affected than males.

Pathogenesis. Anencephaly follows failure of closure of the anterior neural tube [Lemire, 1987]. The critical period during which the neural tube closes is from approximately day 21 to day 26 of gestation; the embryonic defect probably occurs before closure of the anterior neuropore on day 26. A less plausible hypothesis posits that anencephaly is established after a reopening of the prosencephalic portion of the neural tube; the covering mesoderm and ectoderm subsequently incur injury.

The cause of the neural tube defect is unknown. Various agents have been incriminated, including perinatal infections, folic acid antagonists, drinking water minerals, maternal hyperthermia, chromosomal abnormalities, and an unidentified agent in blighted potato tubers [Hibbard and Smithells, 1965; Kurent and Sever, 1973; Miller et al., 1978; Renwick, 1972]. These allegations of causal relationship remain unproven.

Pathology. The cranial vault is defective over the vertex, exposing a soft, angiomatous mass of neural tissue covered by a thin membrane continuous with the skin [Lemire et al., 1978]. The cranial abnormality may extend inferiorly to the cervical region with formation of a complete spina bifida. The extremely thin and flattened spinal cord (craniorachischisis) is readily observed. The optic globes are usually protuberant because of inadequate bony orbits.

Clinical characteristics. Anencephaly is a lethal condition [Lemire et al., 1978; Melnick and Myriantho-poulous, 1987]. No specific treatment is available. Term infants with anencephaly who live for several days may respond to auditory, vestibular, and painful stimuli [Ashwal et al., 1990]. Neuroendocrine defects are frequent, with failure of endocrine end-organ development secondary to a hypoplastic pituitary. Adrenal insufficiency may be associated with adrenocortical hypoplasia. The posterior pituitary is also hypoplastic and may cause clinical diabetes insipidus.

Antenatal diagnosis is possible using assays of alpha-fetoprotein, which is increased in maternal serum and amniotic fluid [Brock et al., 1975; Seller et al., 1974]. Antenatal diagnosis is also feasible through the use of fetal ultrasonography [Goldstein and Filly, 1988].

In the United States, regulations do not permit organ donation from anencephalic infants because brain death criteria are not fulfilled [Peabody et al., 1989]. This policy is controversial, and future regulations would be necessary to modify this policy to allow organ donation [Medical Task Force on Anencephaly, 1990].

CLEAVAGE AND DIFFERENTIATION DEFECTS
Holoprosencephaly

Holoprosencephaly results from failure of separation of the embryonic forebrain, or prosencephalon, into symmetric cerebral hemispheres. The defect arises before day 23 of gestation. Only a single lobe is present (holosphere). There is no distinct sagittal division of the brain by an interhemispheric fissure in either the anlage of the telencephalon or of the diencephalon [Leech and Shuman, 1986; Peach, 1965]. The prosencephalic ventricle remains undivided and persists as a single ventricle.

The cleavage defects vary in severity. Manifestations range from a minor change, such as a single central incisor or a choroid fissure coloboma, to holoprosencephaly, a devastating structural aberration. The deformities in holoprosencephaly are categorized into three major types: alobar, semilobar, and lobar [DeMyer, 1971], in order of decreasing severity. The failure of prosencephalon division and subsequent formation of paired hemispheres determine the extent of the abnormality and the level of classification.

Clinical characteristics. The majority of patients with holoprosencephaly have severe delayed development, spastic quadriplegia, failure to thrive, and seizures. Neuroendocrine dysfunction results from defects of the anterior and posterior pituitary and secondary hypoplasia of endocrine end organs [Romshe and Sotos, 1973]. Cranial ultrasonography and CT demonstrate the malformation. EEG is suppressed over the holoprosencephalic region.

Holoprosencephaly occurs more commonly in infants born to diabetic mothers. Chromosome abnormalities detected in some patients with holoprosencephaly include trisomies 13 and 18, deletions 18p- and 13q-, ring 18, and triploidy. Autosomal-dominant and recessive inheritance may occur, but most cases are sporadic [Cohen, 1982a, 1982b]. More recently, holoprosencephaly has been reported in association with the "pseudotrisomy 13 syndrome" [Cohen and Gorlin, 1991]. Holoprosencephaly may also occur secondary to intrauterine infection from toxoplasmosis and syphilis, and from exposure to alcohol [Freide, 1989; Ronen and Andrews, 1991].

Alobar holoprosencephaly. Alobar holoprosencephaly arises from rudimentary development of the prosencephalon, which includes lack of delineation of an interhemispheric fissure. The undivided telencephalon persists as a solitary lobe without olfactory bulbs or tracts [DeMyer, 1975].

Various combinations of median facial defects are associated with the holoprosencephalic brain. The precordial mesoderm is the anlage of the median facial bones. Facial anomalies accompany holoprosencephaly because the induction process that eventually shapes the neural ectoderm and precordial mesoderm is flawed. When the precordial mesoderm is defective, the midline bones may be deformed. Division of the prosencephalon may be discontinued at various points during the process of formation. Conditions subsumed under alobar holoprosencephaly, such as cyclopia, ethmocephaly, cebocephaly, and premaxillary agenesis, are associated with identifiable facial abnormalities, thus the concept, "the face predicts the brain" [DeMyer, 1975].

Cyclopia. Cyclopia, a condition incompatible with life, is characterized by a single median eye and a small, grotesquely shaped nose (proboscis) that arises from the supraorbital area. No optic chiasm exists. A single optic nerve traverses a solitary optic foramen to reach the brain; it may then separate into right and left branches.

Ethmocephaly. Ethmocephaly is associated with exaggerated orbital hypotelorism; however, there are two orbits. The proboscis protrudes from the region between the eyes.

Cebocephaly. In cebocephaly the facial features include orbital hypotelorism and a proboscis with a single midline, nasal opening. No cleft lip is present. Although the karyotype is virtually always normal, the condition has accompanied trisomies 13 to 15.

Premaxillary agenesis. Facial features in premaxillary agenesis consist of hypotelorism, a flat nose, and a midline cleft upper lip. The hard palate is normally developed. There is no nasal septum. A median angle–like protrusion of the frontal bones may occur. The calvarium may be microcephalic.

Failure to thrive, delayed development, poor temperature control, and seizures are common symptoms of premaxillary agenesis. Poor visual acuity, synophrys, colobomas, and spastic quadriparesis are also evident. Most infants do not survive the first year of life.

Semilobar holoprosencephaly. In semilobar holoprosencephaly, prosencephalic cleavage is discernible, mostly posteriorly, with a hypoplastic intermaxillary segment. However, the separated cerebral lobes are grossly underdeveloped. The uncleaved cerebral neocortex is continuous from one side to the other, and the olfactory bulbs and tracts are undeveloped.

Facial abnormalities include a flattened nose, bilateral cleft lip and palate, a midline protrusion (the remnant of the premaxillary anlage), and orbital hypotelorism. Both trigonocephaly and microcephaly have been reported. Profound intellectual retardation usually occurs. Occasionally, patients live beyond infancy.

Lobar holoprosencephaly. Frontal lobes that are well developed and of normal weight are associated with lobar holoprosencephaly. Normal cleavage implements formation of a normal interhemispheric fissure; however, when the frontal neocortex continues across the midline, the interhemispheric fissure is foreshortened anteriorly. Olfactory bulbs and tracts are sometimes present. Complete or partial agenesis of the corpus callosum may be present. Facial distortion may be absent or subtle. Trigonocephaly and cleft lip and palate have been described, and severe mental retardation is usually present. Neuroimaging techniques confirm the diagnosis.

Klippel-Feil syndrome

The cardinal feature of the Klippel-Feil syndrome, a congenital malformation, is a decreased number and partial or complete fusion of the cervical vertebrae [Gunderson et al., 1967]. The anomaly is the result of failure of segmentation of cervical vertebrae and mesodermal somites before the fourth week of gestation.

Clinical characteristics. The neck is extremely short, and the head appears to extend upward from the shoulders. Head and neck movements are limited except for some flexion and extension. Scapulas are elevated and/or discrepant in size. Reported characteristics include facial asymmetry often associated with torticollis, fused and anomalous ribs including cervical ribs, hemivertebra, scoliosis or kyphosis, platybasia, Sprengel deformity, myelodysplasia, Chiari malformation, syringomyelia, and hydrocephalus. Additional abnormalities include cardiopulmonary, urogenital, and gastrointestinal anomalies; congenital deafness; absent ulna; and absent vagina [Chemke et al., 1980; Helmi and Pruzansky, 1980; McKusick, 1990].

Weakness and atrophy of arm muscles may be profound. Paraplegia may result from bony impingement on the spinal cord. Sympathetic dysfunction may also be prominent. Mirror movements (synkinesias) of the extremities, particularly the arms and hands, may be subtle or so overt that they are disabling. These movements have been ascribed to abnormalities of pyramidal decussation [Farmer et al., 1990]. Klippel-Feil syndrome frequently occurs sporadically, but autosomal-dominant transmission has been reported. Wildervanck syndrome (cervicooculoacoustic syndrome), a disease of girls, is characterized by fused cervical vertebrae, congenital sensorineural deafness, and abducens palsy with retracted optic globes (Duane syndrome).

Sprengel deformity

Sprengel deformity consists of rotation and elevation of the scapulas and is present at birth. The scapulas fail to migrate from the fetal neck site to the final shoulder location during the ninth gestational week. The deformity may follow abnormal shortening of the scapular muscles, which, in turn, retards downward scapular migration. An upward displacement of the scapulas, asymmetry and lack of elevation of the shoulder girdle, and compromised abduction of the shoulder are usually evident. No muscle weakness exists. Cervical ribs, hemivertebra, scoliosis, Klippel-Feil syndrome, or syringomyelia may accompany this condition.

Some cases of Sprengel deformity are genetically transmitted as an autosomal-dominant trait [McKusick, 1990]; however, it usually occurs sporadically. Treatment consists of surgical correction at 4 to 7 years of age.

NEURONAL MIGRATION DEFECTS

Disorders of neuronal migration are perhaps the most common of the CNS malformations, yet they remain poorly understood and difficult to classify. A relatively simple division into disorders of cell proliferation and cell migration provides a framework for understanding these disorders, although substantial overlap occurs. Many other conditions are related to disturbances in neuronal organization, synaptogenesis, programmed cell death, myelination, and gliogenesis. Alternatively, these disorders have been divided into two major groups: (1) abnormal cytogenesis and histiogenesis in the first half of gestation, which includes disorders of neuronal proliferation and migration, and (2) abnormal growth and differentiation in the second half of gestation, which is more typically associated with destructive events to the developing nervous system [Evrard et al., 1989a].

Disorders of neuronal proliferation

Megalencephaly. Megalencephaly is a disorder of neuronal proliferation in which the brain weight and size are greater than two standard deviations above the mean. Associated with this cell and volume proliferation is the presence of neuronal heterotopias and other neuronal migration abnormalities. Megalencephaly occurs in a wide variety of clinical disorders and syndromes, may be bilateral or unilateral, and is associated with an enormous spectrum of cognitive and motor symptoms. (This disorder is comprehensively reviewed in Chapter 14.)

Microcephaly. Microcephaly is present when the head circumference is greater than two standard deviations below the mean for gestational or chronologic age (whichever is appropriate) and gender. The circumference and volume of the skull are abnormally decreased because of inadequate growth and development of the brain.

In general, below-average intelligence is associated with the presence of microcephaly [Dolk, 1991; Nelson and Deutschberger, 1970]. Nevertheless, a head circumference two to three standard deviations below the mean is not inevitably linked with intellectual retardation; 7.5% of a large group of microcephalic children had normal intelligence [Martin, 1970; Sells, 1977].

Disruption of cellular induction, multiplication, growth, or migration during the first 4 months of gestation is the presumed cause of familial microcephaly. During pregnancy, maternal, fetal, and environmental factors may cause microcephaly. Many cases of microcephaly are sporadic, and no underlying cause is identifiable. Pathologic conditions that retard brain growth after birth and during the first year or two of life also may lead to microcephaly. Microcephaly may also be associated with other brain malformations or heterotopic brain growth. In some patients with profound microcephaly a decrease in the number of radial neuronal–glial units accounts for the development of this disorder [Evrard et al., 1989a].

Genetic and malformation syndromes associated with microcephaly

Familial microcephaly. Familial microcephaly is an autosomal-recessive, dominant, X-linked, or polygenic disorder [McKusick, 1990; Volpe, 1987]. The exceedingly small cerebrum contrasts with the normal cerebellum. Accompanying aberrations of cellular migration include agenesis of the corpus callosum, agyria, disrupted cortical lamination, gray matter heterotopias, macrogyria, polymicrogyria, and schizencephaly (Figure 26-9). Examination reveals obvious microcephaly, a narrow forehead, and a flat occiput. The face and ears may be of disproportionate normal size. Intellectual retardation is usually profound, and overactivity may dominate the patient's behavior. Visual impairment is common, and subtle to mild spasticity is often present. Epilepsy occurs in one third of patients. There is a 6% risk of a family having a second microcephalic child. In families with a known pattern of inheritance, the recurrence risk may be 25% to 50%.

Various chromosomal anomalies, including trisomies (i.e., 21, 18, 13) and deletion syndromes, are associated with microcephaly (see Chapter 23).

Several nonchromosomal hereditary syndromes, such as Rubinstein-Taybi, Smith-Lemli-Opitz, Cornelia de Lange, Hallermann-Streiff, and Prader-Willi, are associated with microcephaly [Jones, 1988; Opitz and Holt, 1990].

Maternal and prenatal disorders associated with microcephaly. The developing nervous system is highly vulnerable to infections, including toxoplasmosis, rubella, cytomegalovirus, herpes simplex, and group B coxsackievirus, which often cause microcephaly [Evrard et al., 1989b;

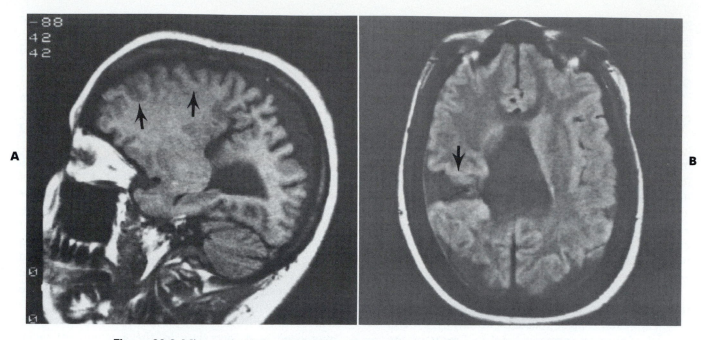

Figure 26-9 Microcephaphaly with heterotopia and schizencephaly in a 19-year-old female. **A,** Heterotopic gray matter *(arrows)* shown on the T_1 weighted parasagittal MRI. **B,** Axial spin–density weighted MRI also demonstrating heterotopic gray matter lining the schizencephalic cleft and extending in white matter anterior to the cleft *(arrow).* (Courtesy Joseph R. Thompson, Department of Radiation Sciences, Loma Linda University School of Medicine, Loma Linda, Calif.)

Johnson, 1972]. Microcephaly has also been reported in infants of women exposed to ionizing radiation from the atomic bomb [Wood et al., 1967] or radium implantation in the cervix during the first trimester [Dekaban, 1968].

Maternal metabolic disorders that coexist with pregnancy, such as diabetes mellitus, uremia, and undiagnosed or inadequately treated phenylketonuria, have been associated with neonatal microcephaly [Lenke and Levy, 1982]. Malnutrition, hypertension, and placental insufficiency may result in microcephaly and intrauterine growth retardation. Maternal carbon monoxide poisoning results in offspring with microcephaly, polymicrogyria, mental retardation, seizures, and occasionally hydrocephalus [Longo, 1977].

Maternal alcoholism during pregnancy has also been linked with microcephaly as part of the fetal alcohol syndrome [Clarren and Smith, 1978; Ouellette et al., 1977]. Clinical features include growth and mental retardation, midfacial hypoplasia, short palpebral fissures, epicanthal folds, and behavioral disturbances [Rosett and Weiner, 1984]. Neuropathologic findings include heterotopias, microcephaly, widespread cortical and white matter dysplasias, and defects of neuronal and glial migration [Wisniewski et al., 1983]. Maternal cigarette smoking, as well as maternal substance abuse of cocaine and other illegal drugs are common causes of microcephaly [Dominquez et al., 1991].

Postnatal disorders associated with microcephaly. A variety of

neurologic insults to the developing nervous system in neonates and infants results in microcephaly. These insults include hypoxic-ischemic encephalopathy, intracranial hemorrhage, CNS infections, malnutrition, and inherited metabolic disorders. Pathologic findings include encephalomalacia, porencephaly, gliosis, abnormal myelination, and atrophy.

Acquired immunodeficiency syndrome in infants causes microcephaly associated with encephalopathy, delayed development, incoordination, and basal ganglia calcifications. Acquired microcephaly is a major feature of xeroderma pigmentosa; cutaneous photosensitivity, carcinomas, dementia, deafness, cerebellar dysfunction, and short stature complete the clinical picture [Mimaki et al., 1988]. Chronic systemic diseases during infancy such as uremia may be associated with microcephaly [Rotundo et al., 1982].

Two syndromes that have gained increasing attention and that are associated with postnatal development of microcephaly include Rett and Angelman syndromes. Dementia, ataxia, autism, and hand-wringing movements in girls comprise Rett syndrome [Hagberg et al., 1983]. Angelman syndrome is associated with seizures, hypotonia, hyperreflexia, hyperkinesis, and growth failure [Fryburg et al., 1991]. These children have an unusual facies and personality; the term *happy puppet syndrome* has been used to describe them.

Children with microcephaly display a wide variety of

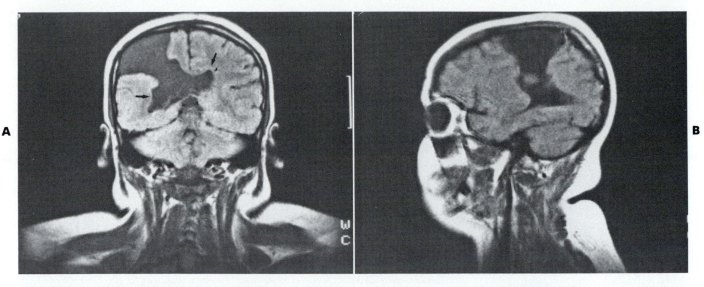

Figure 26-10 Unilateral schizencephaly in a 17-year-old girl. **A,** Unilateral frontoparietal open cleft schizencephalic defect without hydrocephalus. Coronal T_1 weighted MRI showing tissue of cortical signal *(arrows)* lining the cleft all the way to the ependymal surface. **B,** T_1 weighted MRI in parasagittal plane through the cystic defect. (Courtesy Joseph R. Thompson, Department of Radiation Sciences, Loma Linda University School of Medicine, Loma Linda, Calif.)

handicaps. Many infants have mental retardation, seizures, incoordination, movement disorders, and spasticity [Dorman, 1991].

Investigation of patients with microcephaly includes evaluation for prenatal exposure to teratogens, especially alcohol, drugs, and isotretinoin (a vitamin A analog), and assessment of the family history, birth history, and associated dysmorphic conditions. Laboratory studies should include titers for toxoplasmosis, syphilis, rubella virus, cytomegalovirus, and herpes simplex viruses; neuroimaging, evaluation of maternal and childhood metabolic disorders; and chromosome analysis.

Disorders of neuronal migration

Schizencephaly. The term *schizencephaly* designates the presence of clefts in the cerebral hemispheres that results from flawed development of the cortical mantle during cell migration in the first trimester of pregnancy [Yakovlev and Wadsworth, 1946]. The clefts are almost invariably located in the area of the sylvian fissures. The fluid-filled brain cavity is covered by normal dura or a thin pia-arachnoid membrane. The gyral pattern of the neighboring gyri is abnormal.

Clinical characteristics. Schizencephaly is associated with profound intellectual retardation, epilepsy, and generalized spasticity. Clinical findings are usually commensurate with the size of the lesion [Aniskiewicz et al., 1990], and although typically sporadic, a familial form has been described [Robinson, 1991]. Neuroimaging techniques may demonstrate symmetric or unilateral defects in the sylvian regions (Figure 26-10).

Porencephaly. An entity that is sometimes confused with schizencephaly is porencephaly. It results from one of two abnormal processes; in one there is disruption of normal brain tissue, and in the other a faulty induction process and aberrant neuronal migration occur. The terms *encephaloclastic porencephaly* and *pseudoporencephaly* indicate circumscribed defects in the cerebral mantle that rarely communicate with the ventricles and that result from destruction of cerebral tissue. Porencephaly may follow periventricular intracerebral hemorrhage with ensuing encephalomalacia in premature infants [Pasternak et al., 1980].

Porencephalic cysts may be attended by an overlying encephalocele, alopecia, or other cranial defects [Yokota and Matsukado, 1979]. Linear sebaceous nevi and developmental failure of cerebral venous sinuses may also accompany porencephaly [Chalhub et al., 1975]. Motor dysfunction ranges from spastic monoparesis to hemiplegia. Supranuclear bulbar palsy is associated with bilateral lesions. Basal ganglia compromise may lead to hypotonia during the neonatal period; abnormal involuntary movements, usually athetosis, may appear during the first year of life. Delayed or impaired growth and development, epilepsy, and hydrocephalus are also often present [Nixon et al., 1974]. If the cyst dilates, the ensuing increased intracranial pressure will cause progressive neurologic impairment and hydrocephalus [Tardieu et al., 1981]. Neuroimaging techniques, including cranial ultrasonography, reveal the cyst or cysts (Figure 26-11). In some patients, instilled contrast medium in conjunction with CT is necessary to determine whether

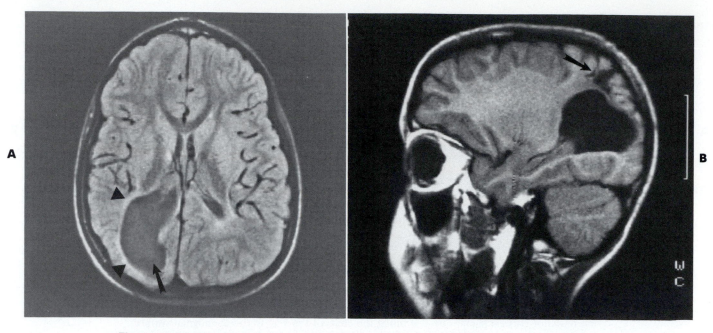

Figure 26-11 Porencephaly in a 9-year-old girl. **A,** Dilated occipital horn *(arrow)* is surrounded by tissue with bright signal *(arrowheads)* on this spin-density weighted axial MRI. **B,** In addition to the bright signal about the cystic occipital horn shown in **A,** this parasagittal T₁ weighted magnetic image shows another sign of parenchymal insult, a focally dilated sulcus *(arrow).* (Courtesy Joseph R. Thompson, Department of Radiation Sciences, Loma Linda University School of Medicine, Loma Linda, Calif.)

the cyst communicates with the ventricular system. A ventriculoperitoneal shunt is indicated for progressive enlargement of the porencephalic cyst. Furthermore, a progressive neurologic deficit may be an indication for surgical removal or shunting. In these patients, special neuroradiologic evaluation is necessary to determine the relation of the cyst to the ventricular system [Kolawole et al., 1987]. Most patients have static neurologic deficits that require rehabilitation and antiepileptic drugs if seizures occur.

Lissencephaly. Lissencephaly is a brain malformation manifested by a smooth cerebral surface, thickened cortical mantle, and microscopic evidence of incomplete neuronal migration [Barth, 1987; Dobyns et al., 1992]. It comprises the agyria-pachygyria spectrum of malformations, thus excluding polymicrogyria and other cortical dysplasias.

Type I or classical lissencephaly results from abnormal neuronal migration between about 10 and 14 weeks gestation [Dobyns, 1987]. The brain is often small, and the ventricles are enlarged posteriorly. The corpus callosum may be small or absent. The structural pattern of the cerebral hemispheres and ventricles is distinctly immature, reminiscent of fetal brain. The superficial cellular layer resembles an immature cortex, with some separation into zones similar to layers III, V, and VI of normal cortex, although the cell population is decreased. The

heterotopic neurons are separated from the superficial layer by an acellular zone, although this varies in thickness and may be absent. Gray matter heterotopias may be present in the white matter, which is much thinner than normal. Atypical forms of lissencephaly comprising agyria, pachygyria, and other changes such as polymicrogyria, porencephaly, and intracerebral calcifications also occur. Rare variants include lissencephaly with extreme micrencephaly (head circumference at birth of 24 to 28 cm; brain weight less than 100 g), and lissencephaly with cerebellar hypoplasia.

Type I lissencephaly occurs in several syndromes. Miller-Dieker syndrome consists of severe type I lissencephaly, abnormal facial appearance, and sometimes other birth defects. The facial changes include prominent forehead, bitemporal hollowing, short nose with upturned nares, protuberant upper lip, thin vermillion border of the upper lip, and small jaw. Some patients have an unusual midline calcification in the region of the septum. Visible deletions of chromosome band 17p13.3 are observed in about half of all patients, whereas the remainder have submicroscopic deletions of the same region [Dobyns et al., 1991]. Isolated lissencepahly sequence consists of type I or atypical lissencephaly and minor facial changes such as small jaw and bitemporal hollowing. Nongenetic causes include intrauterine infections such as cytomegalovirus and intrauterine perfusion failure. About 15% to 20% of patients with lissencephaly have submicroscopic deletions of 17p13.3 that are usually smaller than those observed in Miller-Dieker syndrome [Ledbetter et al., 1992]. Autosomal-recessive inheritance has been observed in a few families with "pure" isolated lissencephaly, in isolated lissencephaly with neonatal death due to respiratory insufficiency, and in at least one family with Norman-Roberts syndrome, which consists of lissencephaly, severe congenital microcephaly, and wide nasal bridge [Norman et al., 1976]. X-linked recessive lissencephaly with small penis has been observed in one family [Berry-Kravis and Israel, 1992].

Type II lissencephaly is a more complex malformation that consists of agyria, pachygyria, or even polymicrogyria with a pebbled surface, thickened cortex, edematous or cystic white matter, and often hydrocephalus. The cortex is severely disorganized, with no recognizable layers and widespread disruption by abnormal vascular channels and fibroglial bands. The latter often extends to the subarachnoid space, which may be partly obstructed. The white matter is poorly myelinated with large numbers of heterotopic neurons. Associated malformations include absent septum pellucidum, absent corpus callosum, vermis hypoplasia, Dandy-Walker malformation, and brainstem hypoplasia. These changes reflect a protracted process beginning as early as 6 weeks gestation and continuing as late as 24 weeks [Evrard et al., 1989a; Dobyns et al., 1989]. Type II lissencephaly has been observed in two syndromes, both of which have associated congenital muscular dystrophy. Fukuyama congenital muscular dystrophy is the least severe, although all patients are severely retarded. Eye and cerebellar malformations are minimal or absent. Walker-Warburg syndrome includes severe eye malformations and either vermian hypoplasia or Dandy-Walker malformation. The eye malformations may consist of microphthalmia, cataracts, Peter anomaly, congenital glaucoma, and retinal malformations, although the last malformations are the most constant. Another rare syndrome, proliferative vasculopathy with hydranencephaly-hydrocephaly, may be related [Norman and McGillivray, 1988].

Clinical characteristics. Gestation is usually of normal duration, although many infants with lissencephaly are small for gestational age and experience severe failure to thrive. Polyhydramnios is often present but is a nonspecific feature. Appearance may be normal or abnormal, depending on the particular lissencephaly syndrome. For example, the facial appearance is always abnormal in children with Miller-Dieker syndrome and is usually abnormal in children with Walker-Warburg syndrome. Bitemporal hollowing and small jaw are common in all syndromes. Only a minority of children have microcephaly at birth, although virtually all become microcephalic within the first year of life. Many children with Walker-

Warburg syndrome have congenital hydrocephalus, and the head size is often large. Poor feeding and hypotonia are commonly observed in neonates, and some have apnea. Seizures may occur during the first few days of life, but it is much more typical for them to begin later in the first year of life. A large majority of patients have seizures during the first year, including myoclonic, tonic, and tonic-clonic types. In over half the patients seizures consist of or include infantile spasms. Other neurologic manifestations include severe or profound mental retardation, hypotonia that evolves to spastic quadriplegia, and opisthotonus. Many patients require a gastrostomy because of poor nutrition and repeated aspiration pneumonias.

CT and especially MRI imaging reveal the smooth surface, thickened cortex, thin white matter, lack of the normal interdigitations between cortex and white matter, and enlargement of the posterior portions of the lateral ventricles. Some patients also have agenesis or thinning of the corpus callosum (Figure 26-12)[Byrd et al., 1988]. Cerebellar malformations, especially vermian hypoplasia or Dandy-Walker malformation, are seen in Walker-Warburg syndrome.

The various clinical subtypes have different risks of recurrence in siblings. Isolated lissencephaly is causally heterogenous. The empiric recurrence risk is 5% to 7% [Dobyns et al., 1992]. The recurrence risk for Miller-Dieker syndrome depends on results of chromosome and DNA analysis; it is not inherited as an autosomal-recessive trait. The recurrence risk is 25% for isolated lissencephaly with neonatal death, Norman-Roberts syndrome, Fukuyama congenital muscular dystrophy, and Walker-Warburg syndrome. The recurrence risk for unusual types of lissencephaly such as lissencephaly with extreme micrencephaly and lissencephaly with cerebellar hypoplasia may be as high as 25%. The recurrence risk is 50% for brothers of boys with X-linked lissencephaly with microphallus. Genetic evaluation and counseling are always indicated for families of children with lissencephaly.

Macrogyria (pachygyria). Macrogyria indicates a simplified convolutional pattern with widened gyri and a decreased number of sulci; only one hemisphere may be involved. This disorder is caused by a defect in neuronal migration in the fourth month of gestation, and children with this disorder share many of the same clinical symptoms as children with lissencephaly. The abnormal cortical areas undergo dense gliosis and contain large, unusual neurons. Clinical findings consist of spasticity and weakness. In some patients, central rolandic and sylvian macrogyria have been associated with epilepsy, pseudobulbar palsy, and mental retardation [Kuzniecky et al., 1989].

Neuronal heterotopias. Neuronal heterotopias are now a commonly recognized form of neuronal migration disorder. Resulting from the arrested migration along radial glial elements before the fifth month of gestation, clusters of subcortical neurons can be demonstrated pathologically and more recently by MRI imaging. Neuronal heterotopias occur in myotonic dystrophy [Garcia-Alix et al., 1991], neurofibromatosis, and Duchenne muscular dystrophy [Volpe, 1987] and are believed to account for the intellectual impairment observed in these disorders. Subtle disturbances of neuronal migration and postmigratory organization — neuronal microdysgenesis — have recently been implicated in patients with partial complex and other forms of focal epilepsy [Kuzniecky et al., 1991], and developmental dyslexia [Humphreys et al., 1990].

Two forms of this migrational disorder have been reasonably well characterized, laminar and nodular heterotopias [Friede, 1989]. Laminar heterotopias are usually diffuse and symmetric and separated from the normal-appearing cortex by a thick layer of white matter [Barkovich et al., 1989; Palmini et al., 1991a]. These heterotopias form symmetric ribbons of gray matter in the centrum semiovale. Patients with these disorders display a wide variety of symptomatology from mild cognitive and behavioral disorders to severe retardation and uncontrolled seizures. Nodular heterotopias are more common and consist of masses of gray matter deep in the periventricular subcortical white matter. Microscopic examination reveals disorganized arrays of both neuronal and glial cells. These heterotopias may be seen in conjunction with other malformations such as microcephaly, agenesis of the corpus callosum, septo-optic dysplasia, and chromosomal malformations. Neurologic symptoms in these patients vary from mild-to-severe impairment and frequently are associated with epilepsy. Recent studies suggest that patients with nodular heterotopias or other focal neuronal migration defects and uncontrolled seizures benefit from epilepsy surgery [Palmini et al., 1991b].

Agenesis of corpus callosum. The corpus callosum, a forebrain commissure, originates from the primitive lamina terminalis (terminal plate). The first callosal fibers form at day 74 of gestation, and formation is complete by 115 days; however, myelination continues after birth [Yakovlev and LeCours, 1967]. The extent of the malformation varies from partial to complete agenesis.

Pathologic findings. The lateral ventricles are shifted laterally, with the resultant formation of a large, midline interhemispheric subarachnoid space. The foramina of Monro are malformed and elongated to reach the lateral ventricles, and the third ventricle is enlarged, its roof

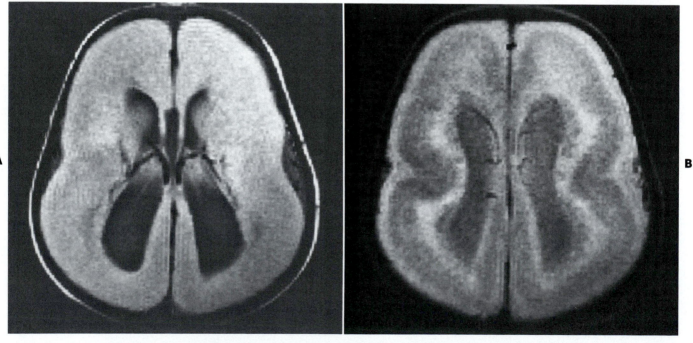

Figure 26-12 Lissencephaly in a 3-month-old female. **A,** Smooth brain surface and dilated ventricles resulting from early arrest in neuronal migration are evident on this spin-density axial MRI. **B,** Note the three-layer appearance from the primitive cortex peripherally, the darker matrix centrally, and the nonmigrating neurons that have proliferated in the periventricular region on a more T_2 weighted image at a slightly higher level. (Courtesy Joseph R. Thompson, Department of Radiation Sciences, Loma Linda University School of Medicine, Loma Linda, Calif.)

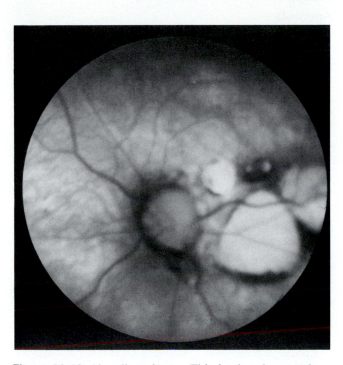

Figure 26-13 Aicardi syndrome. This fundus photograph depicts the retinal lacunae characteristic of the syndrome. (Courtesy the Division of Pediatric Neurology, University of Minnesota Medical School, Minneapolis, Minn.)

extending dorsally [Friede, 1989]. Accompanying abnormalities may include heterotopias, microgyria, abnormal cerebral fissures, porencephalic cysts, and hydrocephalus. The sulci over the medial surface of the hemisphere may manifest an unusual radial pattern. Failure of decussation causes the fiber tracts to form large ipsilateral bundles of Probst. More profound pathologic deviations from normal have been typical of either the X-linked hereditary type or Aicardi syndrome.

Clinical characteristics. The extent and nature of neurologic compromise results from associated brain abnormalities and congenital absence of the corpus callosum. Absence of the corpus callosum alone may be accompanied by very mild or subtle clinical manifestations [Parrish et al., 1979]. Normal intelligence is not unusual. Mild compromise of skills requiring matching of visual patterns and crossed tactile localization have been described. Severe compromise may be present, including intellectual retardation, epilepsy, failure to thrive, spasticity, and hydrocephalus; these findings are particularly likely to occur in children with extensive malformations [Lacey, 1985].

Agenesis of the corpus callosum occurs in about 1 to 3 infants per 1000 births, is usually sporadic, and may be transmitted as sex-linked or autosomal-dominant traits [Lynn et al., 1980]. It has also been associated with approximately 25 different syndromes [Chevrie and

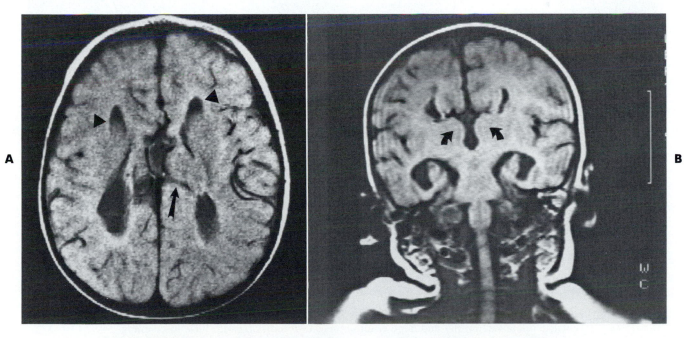

Figure 26-14 Agenesis of the corpus callosum in a 4-month-old female. **A,** Axial spin–density weighted MRI showing classic findings of widespread frontal horns *(arrowheads)* and longitudinal fissure into third ventricle *(arrows)*. **B,** T₁ weighted coronal MRI shows characteristic "viking hat" sign *(arrows)*. (Courtesy Joseph R. Thompson, Department of Radiation Sciences, Loma Linda University School of Medicine, Loma Linda, Calif.)

Aicardi, 1986], as well as several inborn errors of metabolism, including nonketotic hyperglycinemia and fetal alcohol syndrome [Kolodny, 1989]. The genetically determined sex-linked type of partial agenesis of the corpus callosum is associated with seizures that are evident during the first hours of life, with subsequent profound developmental retardation [Menkes et al., 1964]. In girls, Aicardi syndrome, a sex-linked dominant condition, is associated with agenesis of the corpus callosum, infantile spasms, intellectual retardation, vertebral anomalies, and chorioretinal lacunae (Figure 26-13) [Chevrie and Aicardi, 1986]. The condition is probably lethal in males. Gray matter heterotopias are common. Hypsarrhythmia and burst suppression are often visualized by EEG.

Patients with agenesis of the corpus callosum often have asynchronous sleep spindles, and the hemispheral electrical activity may appear to be independent of the other side [Lynn et al., 1980]. Neuroimaging techniques document the unique pattern resulting from the abnormal space between the lateral ventricles and the upward displacement and enlargement of the third ventricle (Figure 26-14). Chromosome analysis is recommended for patients with abnormal neurologic findings. Intrauterine diagnosis by ultrasound is also technically feasible [Bertino et al., 1988].

CEREBELLAR MALFORMATIONS
Agenesis

Isolated agenesis of the cerebellum is distinctly uncommon and often asymptomatic. The dentate nuclei, vermis, and cerebellar peduncles are poorly developed [Macchi and Bentivoglio, 1987]. This condition and related conditions are diagnosed more frequently since the advent of modern neuroimaging techniques. Cerebellar agenesis has been associated with chromosomal defects such as trisomies 13 and 18.

Unilateral cerebellar defects are more common and are also usually asymptomatic. Hemiagenesis is accompanied by poor development of the red nucleus, contralateral inferior olive, and ipsilateral brachium conjunctivum.

Agenesis of the vermis. Agenesis of the vermis is usually partial but may be complete. In partial agenesis the posterior vermis is absent, which is consistent with its embryologic development; the anterior part of the vermis is formed before the posterior area. In cases of complete vermian agenesis the insult occurs earlier than in partial agenesis.

Clinical characteristics. Agenesis of the vermis may be asymptomatic. Neurologic findings result from abnormalities in cerebellar hemispheres and nuclei and associated brainstem pathways. Neurologic features

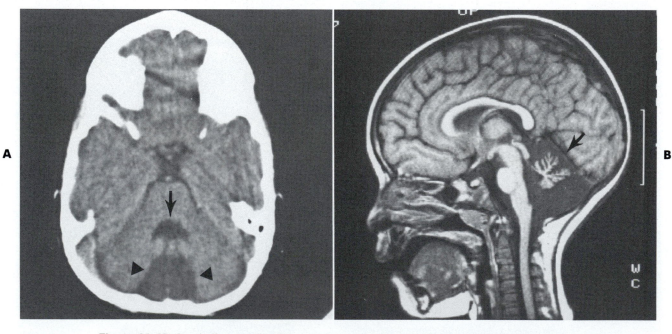

Figure 26-15 Cerebellar vermian hypoplasia in a 3½-year-old boy. **A,** Moderate fourth ventricle dilatation *(arrow)* and large cisterna magna *(arrowheads)* with little intervening vermian tissue seen on this axial CT scan. **B,** Midsagittal T₁ weighted MRI showing leaf-like small cerebellar vermis *(arrow)* surrounded by CSF. (Courtesy Joseph R. Thompson, Department of Radiation Sciences, Loma Linda University School of Medicine, Loma Linda, Calif.)

include hypotonia in infants and incoordination, tremor, and truncal ataxia in children. Delayed fine and gross motor milestones, nystagmus, and decreased deep tendon reflexes may occur. Mild neurologic symptoms may even improve with maturation. Agenesis of the vermis may be an associated finding with myelomeningocele, agenesis of the corpus callosum, heterotopias, and holoprosencephaly.

An autosomal-recessive form of agenesis of the cerebellar vermis has been reported [Joubert et al., 1969; King et al., 1984]. Joubert syndrome consists of episodic hyperpnea and apnea, rotatory nystagmus, ataxia, and mental retardation. The respiratory abnormality worsens with stimulation and improves with maturation. Neuroimaging techniques reveal an enlarged fourth ventricle and dilated cisterna magna (Figure 26-15).

Cerebellar hypoplasia has also been reported in association with Werdnig-Hoffmann disease, although the relationship between these two disorders is uncertain [DeLeon et al., 1984].

Dandy-Walker syndrome

Dandy-Walker syndrome consists of a malformation of the fourth ventricle and cerebellum and occurs in approximately 1 in 30,000 live births. The malformation is most likely a developmental cerebellar defect that originates before embryologic differentiation of the foramina of the fourth ventricle [Golden et al., 1987]. The cystic transformation of the fourth ventricle and attendant hydrocephalus have been ascribed to atresia of the foramina of the fourth ventricle, the foramen of Magendie, and the lateral paired foramina of Luschka [Epstein and Johanson, 1987]. Postmortem studies often reveal intact foramina [Hart et al., 1972]. The massive cystic formation may originate from compromised absorption of ventricular fluid and subsequent increased pressure because of failure of the normal perforation of the superior coverings of the third and fourth ventricles [Gardner, 1977]. Dandy-Walker syndrome or cerebellar hypoplasia may be associated with maternal exposure to isotretinoin in the first trimester and can be detected prenatally [Nyberg et al., 1988].

Pathologic findings. The fourth ventricle is grossly misshapen and is a large, ependymal-lined cyst that extends into the spinal canal [Pascual-Castroviejo et al., 1991]. The cerebellar hemispheres are rudimentary and displaced superiorly, and the posterior vermis is hypoplastic or absent. Rostral fluid-containing spaces, including the aqueduct of Sylvius, third ventricle, and lateral ventricles, are grossly enlarged. The posterior fossa is enlarged with upward displacement of the lateral sinuses, tentorium, and torcular.

Numerous brain abnormalities accompany the Dandy-Walker malformation, including agenesis of the corpus callosum, polymicrogyria, agyria, gray matter heterotopias, aqueductal stenosis, Klippel-Feil syndrome, microcephaly, posterior fossa lymphomas, hamartomas of the infundibulum, and syringomyelia [Hart et al., 1972]. Other nonneural-associated abnormalities include polydactyly, syndactyly, cleft palate, polycystic kidneys, and abnormal lumbar vertebrae.

Clinical characteristics. Clinical manifestations are often evident during infancy. Delayed motor development, hydrocephalus, nystagmus, spasticity, titubation, and apnea are common features. The posterior portion of the head is enlarged, and a flattened protuberance is present in the inferior occipital area [Tal et al., 1980]. Difficulties in older children and adults may be manifestations of increased intracranial pressure and ataxia [Maria et al., 1987]. Normal intellectual functioning is rare.

Cranial ultrasonography accurately defines the posterior fossa cyst and hydrocephalus. Lateral plain radiographs may prove diagnostic; the posterior fossa is enlarged, with superior placement of the torcular herophili and lateral sinus grooves. CT and cranial ultrasonography best demonstrate the characteristic

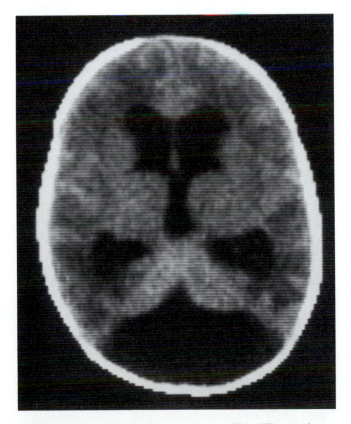

Figure 26-16 Dandy-Walker syndrome. This CT scan demonstrates hydrocephalus and cystic dilatation of the fourth ventricle with cerebellar hypoplasia. (Courtesy D. Munson.)

pattern of hydrocephalus and cystic enlargement of the fourth ventricle (Figure 26-16).

Familial forms of Dandy-Walker syndrome have been described with autosomal-recessive inheritance [McKusick, 1990]. The familial cases are associated with either polycystic kidneys or cataracts, retinal dysgenesis, and choroid coloboma [Chemke, et al., 1975].

The presence of an arachnoid cyst may prove confounding because clinical findings may be similar [Arai and Sato, 1991]. The condition must be distinguished from Dandy-Walker syndrome [Haller et al., 1971; Menezes et al., 1980]. Neuroimaging techniques reveal a normal-sized fourth ventricle that is displaced anteriorly by the arachnoid cyst (Figure 26-17) [Rock et al., 1986]. If necessary, metrizamide CT will demonstrate whether the cyst communicates with the ventricular system.

Management. A shunt from the ventricles, cyst, or both has replaced removal of the cyst wall as the primary treatment for Dandy-Walker or posterior fossa cysts. Surgery may be indicated when occipital bossing is evident, with distortion or obliteration of CSF cisterns of the posterior fossa, compression and deformity of the brain surrounding the cyst, disturbed CSF circulation, or a noncommunicating cyst [Arai and Sato, 1991]. When

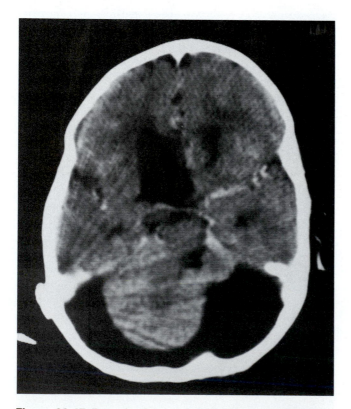

Figure 26-17 Posterior fossa cyst. This CT scan demonstrates hydrocephalus and a large posterior fossa cyst displacing the fourth ventricle. (Courtesy the Division of Pediatric Neurology, University of Minnesota Medical School, Minneapolis, Minn.)

the ventricles and cyst communicate, a cystoperitoneal shunt may suffice [Sawaya and McLaurin, 1981].

Intracranial arachnoid cysts

Intracranial arachnoid cysts are benign, nongenetic developmental cysts that contain spinal fluid and occur within the arachnoid membrane (intraarachnoid cysts) [Rengachary and Watanabe, 1981]. The mechanism of formation during embryogenesis is uncertain [Naidich et al., 1985-1986]. The cysts occur in proximity to arachnoid cisterns, most often in the sylvian fissure (Table 26-2). Arachnoid cysts occur most often in males and in patients with Marfan syndrome. Common neurologic features are headache, seizures, hydrocephalus, focal enlargement of the skull, and signs and symptoms of elevated intracranial pressure, developmental delay, and specific signs or symptoms resulting from neural compression. Some arachnoid cysts may remain asymptomatic; progressive enlargement and intracystic or subdural hemorrhage are potential complications. Suprasellar arachnoid cysts may produce neuroendocrine dysfunction, hydrocephalus, and optic nerve compression.

Skull radiographs may suggest the diagnosis; CT or MRI is the definitive diagnostic procedure [Weiner et al., 1987] (Figure 26-18). Injection of contrast medium into the cyst to document communication with the ventricular system is seldom necessary.

Management. When symptoms warrant, surgical intervention to decompress the cyst, including shunting procedures, is required [Harsh et al., 1986; Raffel and McComb, 1988].

POSTNEURONAL MIGRATION DEFECTS
Hydrocephalus

Hydrocephalus results from obstruction of CSF egress from the ventricular system, reduced absorption from arachnoid villi, or rarely, excess production of CSF within an abnormal choroid plexus. The excess CSF enlarges the cerebral ventricles and elevates intracranial

Table 26-2 Distribution of arachnoid cysts

Location	Percentage
Sylvian fissure	49
Cerebellopontine angle	11
Quadrigeminal area	10
Vermian area	9
Sellar-suprasellar area	9
Interhemispheric fissure	5
Cerebral convexity	4
Clival area	3

Modified from Rengachary SS, Watanabe I. J Neuropathol Exp Neurol 1981; 40:61.

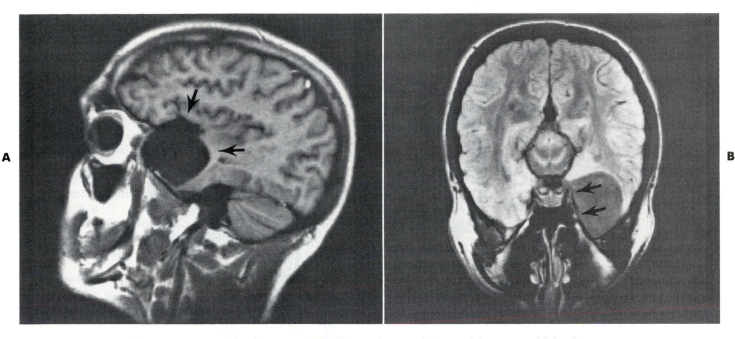

Figure 26-18 Arachnoid cyst. **A,** CSF-like cystic mass deforms right temporal lobe *(arrows)* as shown on this T_1 weighted parasagittal MRI. **B,** Note the eroded appearance of the greater sphenoid wing *(arrows)* from the arachnoid cyst on this axial spin–density weighted MRI. (Courtesy Joseph R. Thompson, Department of Radiation Sciences, Loma Linda University School of Medicine, Loma Linda, Calif.)

pressure, which produces the clinical manifestations of hydrocephalus.

Pathophysiology. Most CSF (70%) is secreted by the choroid plexus within the cerebral ventricles. Extrachoroidal CSF production in subarachnoid sites and by way of a transependymal route also has been documented [Fishman, 1980].

The process of CSF formation by the choroid plexus includes plasma ultrafiltration and secretion. Secretion, an energy-dependent process, is initiated by hydrostatic pressure in the choroidal capillaries and by active transport of sodium. The enzymes sodium-potassium ATPase and carbonic anhydrase partly regulate CSF secretion [Fishman, 1980].

After formation, CSF exits from the lateral ventricles through the foramina of Monro into the third ventricle (Figure 26-19). CSF then traverses the aqueduct of Sylvius into the fourth ventricle and enters the subarachnoid space through the foramina of Luschka and Magendie. Information gained from MRI analysis of CSF movement demonstrates pulsatile to-and-fro motion of CSF within the lateral ventricles, produced from a brain-pumping motion that ejects the CSF, causing a net downward flow [Feinberg and Mark, 1986.] CSF is absorbed into the vascular system through the arachnoid villi within the arachnoid granulations covering the brain and spinal cord leptomeninges [Alksne and Lovings, 1972; Welch, 1975]. A layer of endothelium within the

arachnoid villi separates the subarachnoid CSF space from the vascular system. Water and electrolytes pass freely across these arachnoid membranes. Larger proteins and macromolecules cannot pass through intercellular junctions but are selectively transported across the cytoplasm of endothelial cells by an active process involving micropinocytosis [Alksne and Lovings, 1972]. CSF is also absorbed by the choroid plexus, leptomeninges, ventricular ependyma, and lymphatics [Fishman, 1980]. Increased absorption through the arachnoid villi protects the brain from transient increases in intracranial pressure [Mann et al., 1978]. Normally, rates of production (0.35 ml per minute) and absorption of CSF are equal. Total CSF volume is 65 to 140 ml in children and 90 to 150 ml in adults.

Classification. Because many processes and structures affect CSF dynamics [Davson, 1972], hydrocephalus results from multiple causes. Inadequate absorption of CSF is the prime mechanism producing hydrocephalus. A blockage of CSF circulation at any point from the site of production to the site of absorption through the arachnoid villi enlarges the proximal cerebral ventricles because of excessive CSF accumulation.

Hydrocephalus is classified as either noncommunicating or communicating. In the noncommunicating form, ventriculomegaly occurs rostral to the site of obstructed CSF flow. Vulnerable blockage sites include the foramina of Monro, aqueduct of Sylvius, third and

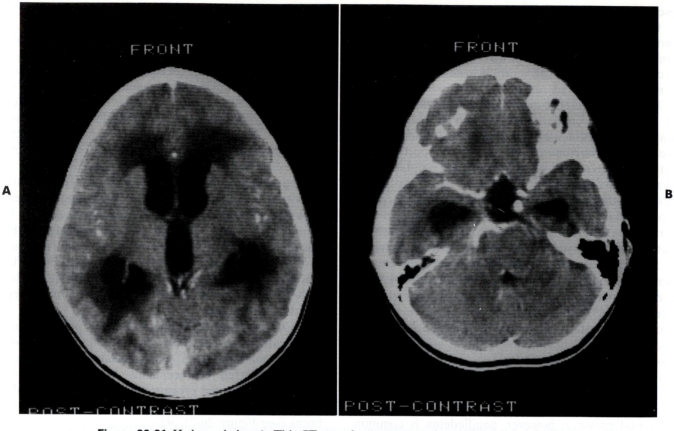

Figure 26-21 Hydrocephalus. **A,** This CT scan demonstrates enlarged lateral and third ventricles caused by obstruction of the aqueduct of Sylvius by a venous angioma. Note the lucency in the periventricular white matter indicating transependymal edema. **B,** This CT scan of the posterior fossa reveals a small fourth ventricle, which confirms the diagnosis of aqueductal stenosis in **A.** Note the vascular malformation. (Courtesy the Division of Pediatric Neurology, University of Minnesota Medical School, Minneapolis, Minn.)

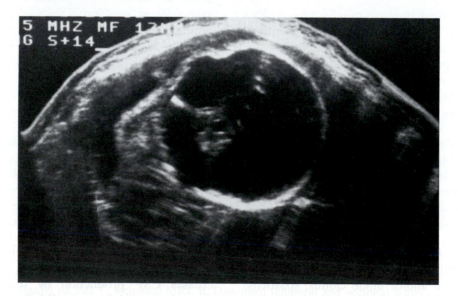

Figure 26-22 Hydrocephalus detected in utero. This fetal ultrasonogram demonstrates massive ventricular dilatation during the third trimester of pregnancy. (Courtesy the Division of Pediatric Neurology, University of Minnesota Medical School, Minneapolis, Minn.)

removal of the obstruction is preferred. This situation occurs infrequently when compared with the incidence of communicating hydrocephalus.

Most hydrocephalic patients require placement of an extracranial shunt. These shunts redirect CSF flow or circulation into the peritoneal or pleural cavity. Refinements of the Holter, Pudenz, and Hakim valves continue to be used [McLaurin et al., 1989]. Shunts cause CSF to flow unidirectionally under the aegis of a valve system. Pressures required to overcome valve resistance are preset and can be used in patients with different pressure requirements. Ventriculoperitoneal shunting is the most accepted initial procedure.

Common complications of ventricular shunts include meningitis, ventriculitis, and repeated surgical procedures for shunt obstruction. The incidence of these complications has been greatly reduced in recent years. Shunt malfunction caused by disconnection, kinking, or obstruction of the tubing results in typical signs and symptoms of increased intracranial pressure. Fever may occur if infection is present.

Other complications of ventriculoperitoneal shunts include peritonitis, CSF ascites, inguinal hernia, intraabdominal cysts, intracranial granulomas, gastrointestinal obstruction, migration of the shunt within the peritoneal cavity, headache, and perforation of abdominal viscera. Abdominal pseudocysts manifest with nausea, vomiting, and abdominal distention and pain; abdominal ultrasonography may demonstrate the cysts [Hann et al., 1985-1986]. Thromboembolic phenomena, cardiac arrhythmias, cardiovascular perforation, endocarditis, catheter embolization, pulmonary thromboembolism, and immune complex shunt nephritis are special complications of ventriculoatrial shunts [Bell and McCormick, 1978; McLaurin et al., 1989; Wyatt et al., 1981]. Correction of longstanding hydrocephalus may cause subdural hematomas.

Staphylococcus epidermidis and *S. aureus* are the most common causes of shunt-related infection, which usually occur within 2 months of shunt placement. The infection rate varies but is less than 5% [Quigley et al., 1989]. Organisms that are ordinarily nonpathogenic may cause infection in the presence of shunt tubing in the ventricles, body cavities, or circulation. Whenever suppurative infection is suspected, appropriate blood and CSF cultures must be obtained, the organism isolated, and sensitivities determined to facilitate effective antimicrobial therapy. Most shunts can be tapped to obtain CSF cultures and assess CSF dynamics. If infection impairs the shunt mechanism, removal and replacement are usually required; temporary insertion of an external ventriculostomy may be necessary until the infection is controlled. Prophylactic antibiotics during shunt placement have significantly reduced the incidence of early-onset shunt infections [Venes, 1976]; however, this

conclusion is not universally accepted [Shurtleff et al., 1985-1986; Slight et al., 1985].

Because fetal hydrocephalus can be detected with ultrasonography, medical and surgical managements of the condition have evolved. Temporary placement of a ventriculoamniotic shunt offers a surgical treatment [Clewell et al., 1982]; however, fetal surgery remains controversial, and the initial enthusiasm for this procedure has waned [Manning et al., 1986; Pinckert and Golbus, 1988]. In fetuses older than 32 weeks gestation with ventriculomegaly, early delivery and ventriculostomy after determining fetal lung maturity may be of benefit. In fetuses younger than 32 weeks gestation the likelihood of fetal lung immaturity substantially increases the risks of early delivery. Serial ultrasounds and use of corticosteroids to accelerate lung maturity may provide a greater potential for long-term survival with lower morbidity.

The neurologic and intellectual disabilities among patients with hydrocephalus depend on many factors, including etiology and degree of hydrocephalus, thickness of the cortical mantle, requirement for a shunt, and presence of other brain anomalies [Dennis et al., 1981; Laurance, 1969]. Associated conditions such as intraventricular hemorrhage, CNS infection [McLone et al., 1982], and hypoxia may dictate the ultimate prognosis more than the hydrocephalus. The predictive value of cortical mantle thickness remains controversial [Hunt and Holmes, 1976].

Intellectual sequelae include significant scatter among WISC-R subtest scores, often with greater impairment of performance and motor tasks. Normal intellectual function is present in 40% to 65% of treated patients [Dennis et al., 1981]. The probability of normal intelligence is enhanced if shunts are placed early and proper function maintained.

Aqueductal stenosis

Aqueductal stenosis leads to a form of noncommunicating hydrocephalus. Partial or complete obstruction of the aqueduct of Sylvius is associated with congenital structural malformations, hemorrhage, infection, neoplasms, and vascular malformations. Concomitant occlusion of the subarachnoid space may occur. Specific pathologic types of aqueductal stenosis, including congenital narrowing, aqueductal forking, septum formation, and aqueductal gliosis, are difficult to differentiate clinically [Drachman and Richardson, 1961]. The inflammatory process subsequent to neonatal meningitis and intraventricular hemorrhage can cause aqueductal gliosis. Hereditary aqueductal stenosis is transmitted as a gender-linked recessive trait [Edwards, 1961].

Aqueductal stenosis may accompany Chiari malformations, myelomeningocele, and neurofibromatosis. Aqueductal stenosis may also be secondary to an existing communicating hydrocephalus [Nugent et al., 1979].

In experimental animals, vitamin A excess, mumps encephalitis, and other viruses cause aqueductal gliosis with associated aqueductal stenosis and hydrocephalus [Johnson, 1972]. In humans, mumps encephalitis has been associated with acquired aqueductal stenosis and hydrocephalus after a latent period of 3 months to 4 years [Spataro et al., 1976]. The pathogenesis in experimental animals and humans may be the propensity for selective infection of ependymal cells by the mumps virus [Johnson, 1972].

Patients with congenital aqueductal stenosis are hydrocephalic at birth. Cranial ultrasonography demonstrates enlarged lateral and third ventricles with a normal or small fourth ventricle. Other neuroimaging techniques may detect tumor, vascular malformation, and associated congenital anomalies (see Figures 26-20 and 26-21).

Remarkably, some patients with congenital and even early acquired aqueductal stenosis are asymptomatic until later childhood or early adult life; some remain free of symptoms. When they become apparent, manifestations include findings consistent with chronic increased intracranial pressure, such as an enlarged head, headache, seizures, gait disturbance, decreased visual acuity, dementia, and occasionally CSF rhinorrhea [Little et al., 1975].

Hypothalamic-pituitary disturbance may occur, including precocious or delayed puberty, impotence, short stature, obesity, hypothyroidism, temperature instability, diabetes insipidus, and amenorrhea. Abnormalities of growth hormone, antidiuretic hormone, thyroid-stimulating hormone, gonadotropins, and gonadotropin-releasing hormone have been documented [Fiedler and Krieger, 1975; Hier and Wiehl, 1977]. Treatment is similar to that for progressive hydrocephalus. After shunting procedures, patients with hypothalamic-pituitary disturbance often improve.

Hydranencephaly

Hydranencephaly is a devastating CNS malformation consisting of nearly complete absence of the cerebral hemispheres. A variety of destructive or developmental abnormalities occurring after the fourth month of gestation may lead to hydranencephaly [Evrard et al., 1989a; Halsey et al., 1971].

Pathologic findings. The cranium is intact and therefore does not suggest anencephaly. Only small portions of the frontal, temporal, and occipital cortex are identifiable. A well-formed and somewhat thickened sac consists of an outer leptomeningeal layer and a rudimentary representation of the cerebral cortex; no suggestion of normal ventricular configuration or ependymal lining can be delineated. The optic nerves are attenuated. The brainstem is also involved, as evidenced by underdeveloped cerebellar peduncles, pons, and medulla.

Compromise of blood flow within the fetal internal carotid arteries or toxoplasmosis may be the basis of the extensive CNS malformation [Altschuler, 1973; Vogel and McClenahan, 1952]. Hydranencephaly has also been reported as a result of maternal cocaine use [Rais-Bahrami, 1990].

Hydranencephaly may develop in neonates and older infants after widespread cerebral infarction associated with extensive meningitis, intracerebral hemorrhage, and ischemia [Lindenberg and Swanson, 1967].

Clinical characteristics. Neonates may appear normal and behave appropriately in the perinatal period. The head circumference is usually within normal limits. After a few weeks, abnormal neurologic findings become apparent, including spasticity, myoclonic seizures, and an enlarged head circumference from hydrocephalus.

Cranial ultrasonography readily demonstrates this malformation (Figure 26-23, A). Transillumination of the skull is startling because the islands of tissue, sagittal sinus, and meningeal blood vessels are quite visible. Islands of preserved cortical tissue are seen as small opacities. Other neuroimaging techniques provide detailed documentation of the extent of the malformation (Figure 26-23, B) and may be required to distinguish severe hydrocephalus or severe subdural effusions from hydranencephaly. EEG reveals suppressed or absent activity corresponding to the loss of brain tissue.

Although an infant may occasionally survive for 1 or 2 years, most die before 1 year of age. Ventriculoperitoneal shunting may be necessary in selected patients with associated progressive hydrocephalus.

Polymicrogyria

Cytoarchitectonic analysis of the microgyric layers and their continuity with the layers of normal cortex allow some understanding of the mechanism that underlies microgyria formation [Evrard et al., 1989a; Richman et al., 1974]. The superficial and deep cellular layers of microgyri appear as normal cortical layers II (the most superficial layer), III, IV, and VI. The defect in microgyria is in the middle cortical layer, which has a reduced cellular population. Because the last cells to migrate form the superficial cortex, the presence of a normal superficial cortical layer documents normal neuronal migration. Microgyria, which most likely results from a postmigratory encephaloclastic injury presumably due to perfusion failure, produces laminar destruction of the middle layers of the cerebral cortex rather than an arrest of neuronal migration (Figure 26-24).

Polymicrogyria may be caused by intrauterine hypoxia or ischemia [Evrard et al., 1989a], maternal cytomegalic inclusion disease [Crome and France, 1959], maternal

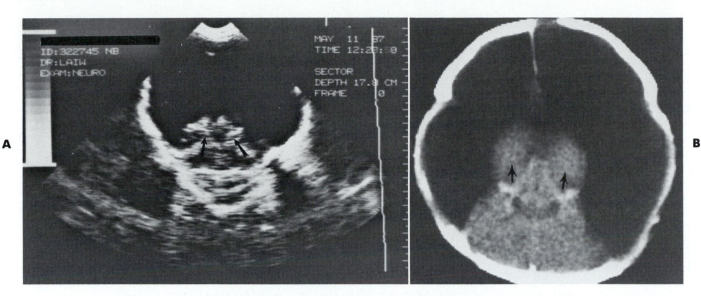

Figure 26-23 Hydranencephaly in a 1-day-old female. **A,** CSF-filled cranial cavity with posterior fossa and diencephalic structures *(arrows)* shown on coronal, transbregmatic cranial sonogram. **B,** Axial CT scan showing CSF-filled supratentorial compartment except for thalamic nuclei *(arrows)* and small residuum of medial right occipital lobe tissue *(arrowheads)*. (Courtesy Joseph R. Thompson, Department of Radiation Sciences, Loma Linda University School of Medicine, Loma Linda, Calif.)

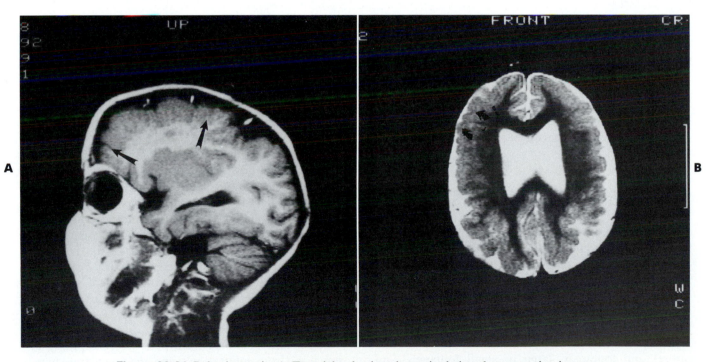

Figure 26-24 Polymicrogyria. **A,** T_1 weighted spin echo sagittal view demonstrating irregular, closely spaced small frontal gyri *(arrows)*. Note normal occipital lobe gyri for comparison. **B,** T2-weighted spin echo axial view at level of body of lateral ventricles. Note closely spaced, small gyri of right frontal lobe *(arrows)*. Note normal occipital lobe gyri for comparison.

Congenital Abnormalities of Ossification of the Skull

Decreased Ossification

Associated major neural defect
Anencephaly
Cranium bifidum
Dandy-Walker syndrome
Encephalocele
Holoprosencephaly
Hydranencephaly
Hydrocephalus
Porencephaly
Bone disorder or variation
Biparietal thinning
Cleidocranial dysostosis
Fibrous dysplasia (monostotic, polyostotic)
Hypophosphatasia
Large sinus grooves
Metopic fontanel
Neurofibromatosis (sphenoid bone and lamboid suture defects)
Osteogenesis imperfecta
Pacchionian granulations
Parietal foramina
Persistent emissary foramina
Persistent fontanels
Pyknodysostosis
Sinua pericranii
Venous lakes

Increased Esnity and/or Thickness of the Skull (Sclerosis, Hyperostosis)

Craniotubular bone-modeling disorders
Craniodiaphyseal dysplasia
Craniometaphyseal dysplasia
Dysosteosclerosis
Osteopetrosis
Sclerosteosis
Van Bucehm syndrome
Other disorders
Aminopterin embryopathy
Craniosynostosis
Fibrous dysplasia (monostotic, polyostotic)
Myotonia congenita (Thomsen disease)
Myotonic dystrophy
Neurofibromatosis
Pyknodysostosis
Thickened normal cranial vault
Tuberous sclerosis

Deformity of the Cranial Base

Achondroplasia
Basilar impression
Osteogenesis imperfecta
Skeletal dysplasia

Modified from Jacobson RI. Neurol Clin 1985; 3:117.

---

carbon monoxide poisoning [Ginsberg and Myers, 1978], or an associated finding with the type II Chiari malformation.

CONGENITAL ABNORMALITIES OF THE SKULL
Classification

The congenital abnormalities of skull ossification listed in the box above include primary skull or bone disorders and skull abnormalities associated with CNS and systemic disorders. Neurologic features of these disorders may include abnormal head size and shape, hydrocephalus, localized scalp mass or skull deformity, headache, proptosis, pulsating exopthalmos (Figure 26-25), premature or delayed closure of the cranial sutures and fontanels, large or small fontanels, and progressive compression of neural and vascular structures leading to elevated intracranial pressure and cranial nerve or spinal cord injury. Many bone diseases that affect the skull cause or are associated with skeletal abnormalities. Other noteworthy features include short stature, syndactyly, polydactyly, and frequent fractures of long bones.

The examination of the skull includes determination of the greatest head circumference; palpation to detect ridging or separation of sutures, size of the fontanels, and skull defects or softening; and assessment of skull configuration and symmetry. The head circumference should be recorded sequentially and compared with appropriate growth charts [Nellhaus, 1968].

The skull radiograph is often diagnostic. Skull disorders can be classified into abnormalities of sutures or ossification. The terminology used to describe skull abnormalities [Burrows and Leeds, 1981] includes *sclerosis* (increased density), *hyperostosis* (increased thickness), *erosion* (thinning from pressure resorption), *destruction* (from infiltration), and *deformity* (misshapen skull).

Normal development and anatomy

The skeletal system develops from the mesodermal germ layer during the third week of gestation. The

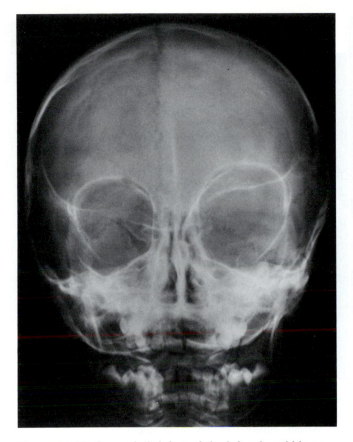

Figure 26-25 Congenital defect of the left sphenoid bone. This skull radiograph shows the dysplastic sphenoid bone, enlarged orbit, and harlequin appearance of the sphenoid wing that occur in neurofibromatosis. Pulsating exophthalmos is the associated clinical phenomenon.

mesenchyme or embryonic connective tissue, a mesodermal derivative, forms the fibroblasts, chondroblasts, and osteoblasts. The large surface bones of the skull ossify directly from the mesenchymal tissues (membranous ossification) to form the cranial vault, or membranocranium. The smaller bones of the base of the skull and part of the occipital bone change from mesenchyme to cartilage before ossification (endochondral ossification) and compose the chondrocranium. The cranial vault and chondrocranium encase the brain and are collectively called the *neurocranium*. The term *viscerocranium* refers to the remaining bones of the skull and face, which are derived partly from the neural crest cells in the head region. The base of the skull, including the foramen magnum, is prone to developmental defects, probably as a result of the more complex intrinsic control of endochondral bone formation.

The membranous skull bones are joined by connective tissue at the sagittal, coronal, lambdoidal, metopic, and squamosal sutures (Figure 26-26). These sutures are easily palpated in neonates and may be overriding as a

consequence of normal cranial molding during delivery. The anterior fontanel is the soft spot at the junction of the frontal and parietal bones, the intersection of the metopic, coronal, and sagittal sutures. Normal closure of the anterior fontanel occurs between 6 and 20 months with fibrous suture union. The oblique diameter of the anterior fontanel in neonates ranges from 0.6 to 3.6 cm [Duc and Largo, 1986]. A large, persistent anterior fontanel may constitute a normal variation or a pathologic feature of many disorders (see box on p. 457) [Tan, 1976]. The posterior fontanel located at the junction of the lambdoidal and sagittal sutures closes by the age of 3 months. A third fontanel, actually a defect in ossification, may occur 2 cm anterior to the posterior fontanel in 6.3% of normal preterm and term infants and is common in infants with Down syndrome and congenital rubella [Chemke and Robinson, 1969]. Mature suture closure occurs by age 12 years, but completion of bony fusion continues at least through the third decade of life. Elevated intracranial pressure may separate the sutures, especially the sagittal suture, until ages 10 to 12 years.

Many developmental skull variations exist. Wormian bones are small, multiple bones that occur in sutures, particularly in the lambdoidal suture (Figure 26-27). They may be a normal variation but often occur in hydrocephalus and other skull disorders (see box on p. 457). Parietal foramina are symmetric, full-thickness congenital defects in the parietal bones close to the midline (see Figure 26-31, *A*). They are often familial and may have no pathologic significance.

Abnormalities of cranial sutures

Craniosynostosis

Pathogenesis. Primary craniosynostosis results from premature fusion of single or multiple cranial sutures that deforms the skull or face. The process of premature fusion begins in utero and can be detected in neonates. The primary pathologic bony defect restricts normal growth across the affected sutures and consequently may limit adequate brain growth, resulting in neurologic deficits.

The shape and size of the skull depend on adequate brain growth without restriction. Inadequate brain growth, such as that occurring in microcephaly or after surgical shunting of severe hydrocephalus, may also result in premature closure of cranial sutures—secondary craniosynostosis. Secondary craniosynostosis does not further compromise the already impaired brain growth.

The etiology of primary craniosynostosis may be a defect in the mesenchymal layer of the ossification centers within the skull. Pathologic examination reveals obliterated sutures that can be distinguished from normal suture closure [Albright and Byrd, 1981]. Evidence for a systemic disorder of mesenchymal tissue and

Table 26-3 Classification of craniosynostosis

Type	Disorder	Sutures affected
Primary—head shape syndrome	Scaphocephaly	Sagittal
	Brachycephaly	Coronal
	Plagiocephaly	Coronal, lambdoidal, or both (unilateral)
	Trigonocephaly	Metopic
	Oxycephaly	Multiple
	Apert sydnrome	Coronal and basal skull
	Carpenter syndrome	Coronal and basal skull
	Crouzon disease	Coronal and basal skull
Associated conditions	Chromosomal abnormality	
	Endocrine—hyperthyroidism (endogenous and exogenous), hypophosphatasia, hypercalcemia, rickets	
	Hematologic diseases with bone marrow hyperplasia	
	Inadequate brain browth—microcephaly, post-shunted hydrocephalus	

Modified from Jacobson RI. Neurol Clin 1985; 3:117.

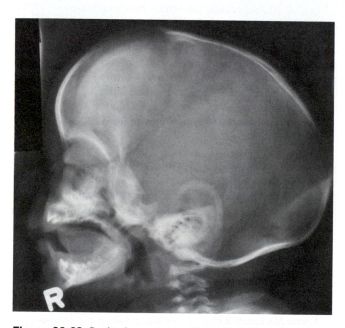

Figure 26-28 Sagittal synostosis. Plain skull film of a 6-week-old infant demonstrates premature fusion and sclerosis of the sagittal suture. Note the elongated skull— scaphocephaly. (Courtesy the Division of Pediatric Neurology, University of Minnesota Medical School, Minneapolis, Minn.)

Sagittal synostosis. Premature fusion of the sagittal suture (scaphocephaly) is the most common form of craniosynostosis, comprising approximately 60% of all types. Most patients are boys; the defect may be familial. The anteroposterior diameter of the skull is elongated and the transverse diameter decreased (Figure 26-28).

This abnormal head shape is present at birth, with palpable ridging over the sagittal suture. The neurologic examination is normal in most patients. Scaphocephaly (dolichocephaly) in premature infants results from positional molding and not from premature suture closure.

Coronal synostosis. Coronal synostosis (brachycephaly) comprises about 20% of cases of craniosynostosis and is more common in females. The skull is shorter in the anteroposterior diameter but is widened with a high vault; the occiput and forehead are flattened. The anterior fontanel is displaced anteriorly, and ridging may be palpated over the prematurely closed coronal sutures. Neurologic features, especially in untreated cases, include proptosis, strabismus, and papilledema or optic atrophy. The skull radiograph may document an elliptic orbit or harlequin eye sign on the side of the coronal synostosis (Figure 26-29).

Single synostosis. Single synostosis, or plagiocephaly, describes the asymmetric skull without indicating which suture is involved. Unilateral closure of a coronal suture, lambdoidal suture, or both causes an asymmetric skull. In lambdoidal synostosis the ipsilateral ear is displaced anteriorly, one frontal bone is larger than the other, and the occipital bones manifest a similar but contralateral asymmetry [Hinton et al., 1984]. The head shape is skewed to resemble a parallelogram. A similar head shape occurs in infants with congenital torticollis but without craniosynostosis. Congenital muscular torticollis, or congenital wryneck, consists of head tilt and unilateral shortening and contracture of the sternocleidomastoid muscle. During early infancy the head and face become progressively deformed, producing

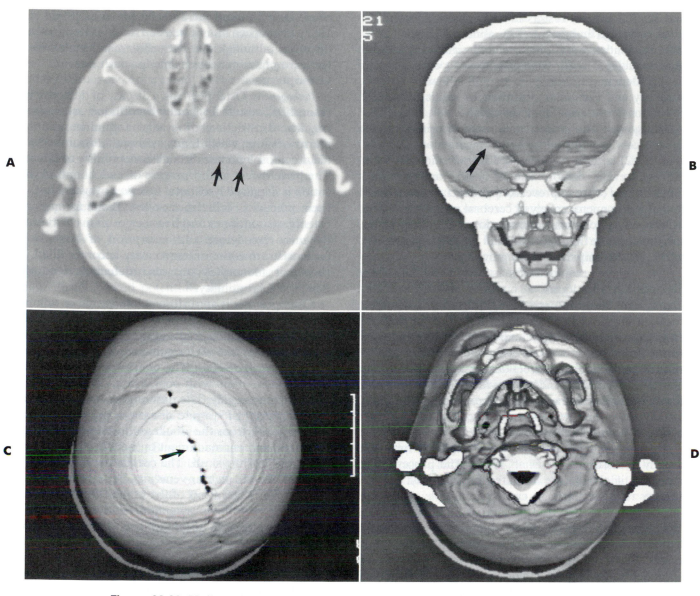

Figure 26-29 Unilateral coronal synostosis in a 1-year-old male. **A,** Axial CT with bone windowing showing "contraction" of skull base on the left side of the synostosis *(arrows)*. **B,** Cut away ventral view of inner calvarium from same study as **A** using CT with three-dimensional reconstructions. Note elevated left sphenoidal wing *(arrow)*. **C,** Viewing skull from above, same three-dimensional data, the sagittal suture *(arrow)* can be seen to be rotated away from the synostotic suture and the flattened contour of the skull around it. **D,** Flattened skull deformity is well demonstrated looking from below. (Courtesy Joseph R. Thompson, Department of Radiation Sciences, Loma Linda University School of Medicine, Loma Linda, Calif.)

asymmetry of the head that may mimic plagiocephaly from craniosynostosis—that is, flat contralateral occiput and ipsilateral face and frontal area. The characteristic clinical features are the head tilted toward the side of the affected muscle and the chin turned to the opposite side.

Metopic synostosis. Premature closure of the metopic suture (trigonocephaly) results in a pointed forehead with a prominent ridge in the midforehead area. The eyes are close together, the forehead is narrow, and the anterior skull appears triangular when viewed from above. Some patients may have related abnormalities, including mental retardation, cleft palate, coloboma, anomalies of the urinary tract, and holoprosencephaly [Anderson and Geiger, 1965].

Multiple synostosis. Premature closure of both coronal

to cerebral palsy over and above their contribution to low birth weight and predict cerebral palsy in term infants. Maldevelopment and infection apparently predispose to preterm birth and may contribute to neurologic morbidity either via, or independently of, prematurity.

Another factor associated with low birth weight that predisposes to cerebral palsy is twinning. In addition to their tendency to be low in birth weight, twins, especially monozygotic twins, are also subject to other problems, including excesses of congenital malformations and anastomotic connections in placental vessels. The death of a co-twin is a situation of special risk for neurologic and other complications in the surviving twin [Szymonowicz et al., 1986]. The most common pathologic brain condition in the vascular disruption sequence in twins when one has died is multicystic encephalomalacia accompanied by disruption in other organ systems as well, with such problems as intestinal atresia, renal cortical defects, horseshoe kidney, terminal limb defects, aplasia cutis, and a range of other abnormalities [Hoyme et al., 1981; Paludetto, 1991]. Other cerebral defects, including anencephaly, holoprosencephaly, hydraencephaly, and periventricular leukomalacia, have been reported as part of the vascular disruption sequence. A syndrome of optic nerve hypoplasia with encephalopathy, reported in the ophthalmic literature, has been associated with the twin transfusion syndrome [Burke et al., 1991]. Twins, who constitute about 2% of the population, contributed 10% the incidence of cerebral palsy in a recent American study [Grether et al., 1992].

Cerebral palsy in sick term infants

Term infants whose brains have been irreversibly injured during delivery are ill, neurologically and systemically, in the newborn period. The progression of illness often includes low Apgar scores, persisting hypotonia, difficulty in initiating and maintaining respiration, and depression of other reflexes, with subnormal level of consciousness and often with early seizures. Infants whose neurologic illness in the newborn period arises as a result of birth asphyxia also show evidence of asphyxial injury in other organ systems, including renal, intestinal, myocardial, and pulmonary. However, this clinical picture is not specific to asphyxial states, and the proportion of neonatal encephalopathy that is asphyxial in origin remains unclear [Nelson and Leviton, 1991].

Whether defined by cardiac arrest in the neonate, by lengthy delay in first breath or cry, or by very low Apgar score, the natural history of severe neonatal depression has been consistent in a variety of studies. The mortality is high. The cerebral palsy rate increases among survivors, but except at the rare extreme, the risk of cerebral palsy is not high in absolute terms [Nelson and Ellen-

berg, 1981]. Infants at special risk of later neurologic disability are those with low Apgar scores, other neurologic signs in the early hours of life, and seizures in the 48 hours after birth. Term infants with neonatal depression without seizures and those with seizures but no depression are much less at risk. The subgroup who are seriously depressed and neurologically symptomatic from birth and later have seizures accounts for an important but small sector of total cerebral palsy—16% in one series [Ellenberg and Nelson, 1988]. Among children who survive severe clinical depression without cerebral palsy, there is no increase in the rate of mental retardation [Seidman et al., 1991] or epilepsy.

The few large studies of acid-base metabolism in unselected populations suggest that these measures are not better than Apgar scores and may be inferior to them as predictors of cerebral palsy [Ruth and Raivio, 1988; Dennis et al., 1989].

Electronic fetal monitoring in labor, although it was introduced in part in the hope of reducing the cerebral palsy rate, is not known to predict cerebral palsy [Colditz and Henderson-Smart, 1990; Melone et al., 1991].

Most clinical predictors in the period of labor and delivery have very high rates of false-positive identification. For meconium in the amniotic fluid, severe fetal bradycardia (60 beats/min), delayed first cry, and low Apgar scores, the false-positive rate is at least 95%. This finding indicates that there are important problems in using these factors as a basis for making clinical decisions because any risk or expense of an intervention based on the known predictors will not have counterbalancing benefits for most of the mothers and infants to whom it is applied.

Population-based studies indicate that most persons with cerebral palsy—about 80%—did not have serious asphyxia in the perinatal period. Studies that consider factors present before labor, such as intrauterine infection and malformation, suggest that even fewer cases of cerebral palsy, perhaps in the range of 3%, are the result of birth asphyxia. The form of cerebral palsy most convincingly linked with birth asphyxia, although not specific to it, is spastic quadriparesis with movement disorder. Hemiparesis may often be related to strokes before birth or in the perinatal period [Nelson, 1991].

In term infants a course that includes low 5-minute Apgar score, continuing abnormal neurologic signs in the hours and days thereafter, and seizures occurring in the first 2 days of life mark a tiny group of newborns who are at high risk for death or cerebral palsy [Ellenberg and Nelson, 1988]. These signs are compatible with birth asphyxia but not specific to it. It is necessary to seek other possible diagnoses (e.g., syndromes of malformation, metabolic disorders). It is necessary to consider that when long-term neurologic abnormality follows neonatal depression, the latter may have been the first postnatally recognizable manifestation of a brain abnormality present since fetal life.

If an individual was not seriously ill in the newborn period neurologically and systemically, the cause of a later-discovered defect is probably not birth asphyxia. The consistency of the evidence and the magnitude of the differences in risk based on early clinical evolution make it reasonable to apply this criterion to individual patients.

Infants with congenital malformations outside the CNS are more likely to demonstrate clinical signs commonly interpreted as indicating perinatal asphyxia. Bacterial infection of placental membranes can produce decreases in umbilical arterial pH and significant base excess, even in the absence of clinical evidence of chorionitis in the mother and the absence of prolonged rupture of the fetal membranes [Peevy and Chalhub, 1983; Meyer et al., 1992]. Because both maldevelopment and infection can themselves underlie adverse outcome, with or without asphyxia, caution is necessary in assuming that any later-identified neurologic abnormality was caused by birth asphyxia.

The presence of malformations or dysmorphic features in an individual patient may be helpful in suggesting early maldevelopment, particularly if a specific diagnosis can be made. However, these malformations are markers of maldevelopment that apply to groups, rather than causes in themselves of neurologic morbidity, and interpretation of their relationship to neurologic outcome in the individual case is not necessarily obvious. To assess causation requires a balancing of the probabilities, and no consensus has yet been reached regarding a straightforward approach. Fenichel et al. [1989] have used a bayesian approach to assess the probability of causation of neurologic injury in individual cases evaluated for any relationship with immunization procedures. Unless a similar approach is accepted as relevant in cerebral palsy, it is unlikely that a confident assessment of causation can be made in most individual children with cerebral palsy.

Because the cause of most cerebral palsy is unknown, and of known predictors prenatal characteristics predominate over birth factors, the occurrence of cerebral palsy in an individual is not a reliable tool for the assessment of the quality of obstetric care given that person. Expert testimony that strives to take into account the circumstances of the individual case may be inferior to epidemiologic-statistical information in predicting outcome and therefore in recognizing causal relationship [Faust and Ziskin, 1988].

The most convincing way to examine the hypothesis that medical management can prevent an outcome is to change something in that management and examine whether the outcome changes. To date, the track record for guesses as to what will prevent cerebral palsy has not been good. There will not be convincing answers to questions about the obstetric preventability of cerebral palsy until those questions have been addressed by controlled clinical trials.

Cerebral palsy arising without obvious postnatal insult in term infants who were well as newborns

These children are seen and examined by their obstetric and neonatal caregivers without special note or anxiety. Although the other two groups are clearly identifiable in the newborn period and have a natural history known through studies that follow high-risk newborns, this third group was brought to our awareness relatively recently by the emergence of the large population studies. It was the appearance of these studies that accounts for a substantial part of the recent change in perception concerning the causes of cerebral palsy.

A recent MRI study included 15 persons with cerebral palsy who were born at term without neurologic depression in the neonatal period; of these, two had migration defects (lissencephaly and schizencephaly), two were normal, and nine had evidence suggestive of white matter necrosis [Krageloh-Mann et al., 1992].

Factors other than prematurity and birth asphyxia that predispose to cerebral palsy

As a group, children with cerebral palsy have an excess of congenital malformations both within and outside the brain. MRI suggests that about one third of cerebral palsy in term infants is related to cortical dysgenesis secondary to abnormal neuronal migration [Volpe, 1992].

In the past, athetosis was a more common form of cerebral palsy than today because of the frequency of exposure of infants to marked hyperbilirubinemia caused by Rh incompatibility. Jaundiced newborns often began to exhibit signs by the third day of life, beginning with weak suck, poor cry, and listlessness, which progressed to deepening hypotonia, depressed level of consciousness, and other manifestations of toxic encephalopathy. Over the months, hypotonia gave way to hypertonia and opisthotonus, and eventually to choreoathetosis, tremors, and rigidity.

Sensorineural deafness was commonly associated with this condition, and mental retardation was often present. Pathologically, the basal ganglia, cerebellum, and brainstem nuclei were stained yellow, and late findings in severe cases included gliosis, demyelination, and decreased neuronal numbers. Techniques to prevent sensitization and phototherapy or exchange transfusion to prevent a marked rise in unconjugated bilirubin have made this form of cerebral palsy, kernicterus, very uncommon. Within the limits of values of neonatal bilirubin permitted before exchange transfusion in modern neonatal care units, bilirubin does not appear to threaten motor or cognitive function, even in infants of low birth weight [Scheidt et al., 1990].

Ingestion of methyl mercury by pregnant women in the Minamata Bay disaster resulted in the birth of children who were spastic, microcephalic, and mentally retarded. Few other toxic exposures are known to have accounted for many cases of human cerebral palsy, but a few agents used in the neonatal nursery [Benda et al., 1986] have come under serious suspicion. Certainly alertness for exposure to potential neurotoxins by either parent or infant is necessary.

Toxoplasmosis and certain viral agents can infect the fetus or neonate and can produce serious encephalitides with motor sequelae. Sever [1985] reviewed the diagnostic procedures for documenting such infections. Other infections, intrauterine and neonatal, such as rubella and cytomegalovirus, have been linked with cerebral palsy. Maternal conditions, including unusual menstrual cycles and thyroid disorders and administration of thyroid hormone and estrogen, have also been associated with cerebral palsy [Nelson and Ellenberg, 1985a], but maternal diabetes has not.

To date, the range of hypotheses explored in the causation of cerebral palsy has been narrow.

GENERAL PATHOLOGY

In preterm infants, subependymal and intraventricular hemorrhages, sometimes accompanied by ischemic events, may be precursors of long-term motor disability. Of hemorrhages invading the parenchyma, only large ones may be associated with motor problems in surviving infants. Perhaps of even greater pathogenetic influence is the occurrence of severe cystic damage to white matter in immature infants [de Vries et al., 1987; Bejar et al., 1986]. Decreases in blood flow through the distal vessels to paraventricular white matter and/or metabolic disturbance related to infection appear to be important antecedents [Leviton and Gilles, 1984]. In term, asphyxiated infants, an impairment of the blood flow in parasagittal areas has been observed on positron emission tomography by Volpe et al. [1985], an occurrence that had previously been postulated on pathologic grounds. Volpe [1992] has recently summarized the literature on MRI studies relating to cerebral palsy.

In studies that have considered persons with established motor disabilities, rather than compromised newborns, clinical neuropathologic correlative studies have been scattered, variously selective, and different in methods of evaluation, vocabulary, and interpretation. Little use has been made of newer quantitative techniques of neuropathology, stains for cell processes, or examination of fine structure in brains not demonstrating obvious perinatal destructive lesions. Malamud et al. [1964] considered the causes of cerebral palsy to be about equally divided between malformations and perinatal destructive pathologic conditions. Gross et al. [1968] stressed the marked lack of correlation between the clinical symptoms and the neuropathologic findings. The discrepancy between clinical impression and pathologic findings was also striking. Gross et al. observed, "In less than half the cases with reports of abnormal deliveries, was the morphological brain damage reasonably referable to birth injury. On the other hand, perinatal accidents were reported in one-third of all morphologically confirmed cerebral malformations." They remarked that, "From this striking fact it may be concluded that organic cerebral damage is often only the sequel but may even be the cause of a birth complication or apparent perinatal accident."

Evaluation of cause

Parents of children with cerebral palsy, and others, often are interested in establishing the cause of cerebral palsy in a child. How is it possible to reach a rational conclusion about whether cerebral palsy developed in a child because of intrapartum asphyxia? In many cases it is not possible to be confident about the cause of the disorder in an individual child. That factor is consistent with the observation that it is not possible to predict whether cerebral palsy will be present in a given child, given neonatal characteristics; if one truly understands the etiology of a condition, one can predict the occurrence of that condition. Currently, the best that is feasible is to ask a series of questions as follows:

1. Was there good and consistent evidence of a marked degree and substantial duration of intrapartum asphyxia? A positive response would require an extreme and severe degree of asphyxia, such as fetal bradycardia of 60 beats/min or below (which by itself is not associated with a high, absolute degree of risk, as has been observed), delay for at least 5 minutes in the establishment of independent respiration, and other evidence of marked intrapartum compromise. It is difficult to accept any particular alteration in fetal heart pattern on electronic fetal monitoring equipment as an indicator of degree of asphyxia because although it is often assumed—and asserted—that abnormal fetal heart patterns are indicators of impending brain damage, there is no evidence linking electronic fetal heart patterns with long-term adverse neurologic outcome. There is also no evidence to demonstrate a superiority of electronic fetal monitoring over auscultation with respect to the frequency of later cerebral palsy.

2. Was the newborn course consistent with moderate

or severe hypoxic-ischemic encephalopathy as described above; that is, did disturbance of feeding, tone, and consciousness occur, and was there evidence of anoxic injury in other organ systems? Early and hard-to-control seizures may be an especially indicative marker, although they are not specific to hypoxic-ischemic encephalopathy. Indeed, it remains uncertain how much of neonatal encephalopathy is asphyxial in origin [Nelson and Leviton, 1991], and the question gains in significance as the possibilities for new treatments for birth asphyxia can be contemplated.

3. Is the outcome one that intrapartum asphyxia could explain? The form of cerebral palsy most convincingly related to intrapartum asphyxia (although not specific to it) is spastic quadriplegia with athetosis and severe mental retardation. Mental retardation, seizure disorders, and learning disorders are not likely to have been caused by intrapartum asphyxia in the absence of motor findings [Paneth and Stark, 1983; Nelson and Ellenberg, 1981]. Pure ataxic syndromes, especially those accompanied by mental retardation, are unlikely to have been caused by birth asphyxia.

4. Can other plausible explanations be excluded? Children with the tone abnormalities of Prader-Willi or Rett syndromes or myotonic dystrophy sometimes are diagnosed initially as having cerebral palsy caused by birth asphyxia. Findings such as microcephaly at birth, dysmorphic features, and congenital anomalies outside the nervous system suggest early development defects. Because the cause of cerebral palsy probably is unknown in most cases, the failure to find a positive alternative explanation does not strengthen an assumption that birth asphyxia was causal.

General prognosis for motor function

A number of factors affect the prognosis of a child: the clinical type of cerebral palsy; the degree of delay in meeting milestones present at evaluation; the pathologic reflexes present; and, most importantly, the degree of associated deficits in intelligence, sensation, and emotional adjustment. Molnar [1979] has discussed these factors. Cognitive level is difficult to assess in the young child with motor impairments, but it is possible to gauge even in the severely affected child [McCarty et al., 1986]. It is necessary to consider the cognitive level despite the difficulty because the level of mental function may be the factor that really determines the quality of life the child will enjoy.

Some kinds and degrees of early motor abnormalities tend to resolve without leaving significant motor disability. Overall, about 50% of children who met the criteria for cerebral palsy diagnoses at the age of 1 year did not have cerebral palsy at early school age. However, nonfebrile seizures, abnormalities in the articulation of speech and in extraocular movements, and mental retardation all were more common among these children than in the general population. Resolution of clinically detected physical findings does not necessarily imply the disapperance of the underlying neuropathologic lesions. Some forms of cerebral palsy resolve much more reliably than others. Monoparesis observed at 1 year of age is almost always resolved; however, mixed cerebral palsy, which involves both spastic and dyskinetic elements, is almost never resolved.

Children with hemiplegia but with no other major problems almost always walk by the age of about 2 years; some benefit from use of a short leg brace, often needed only as a temporary assistance. The presence of a small hand on the hemiplegic side, with a thumbnail that is narrower than that of the other thumb, may be associated with sensory dysfunction of parietal origin, and the sensory defect may limit the development of fine motor skills in that hand. About 25% of children with hemiplegias have hemianopia, recognition of which allows the clinician to advise placing the children in an area of the classroom that maximizes their useful vision. Because most daily activities can be accomplished with only one hand, using the affected hand only as a "helper" and being aided by small adaptations such as shoes that do not require lacing and tying means that hemiplegic children of reasonable intelligence can achieve independence in daily living. Seizures may be a problem in children with hemiplegia.

More than 50% of children with spastic diplegia learn to walk, commonly by the age of about 3 years, but gait is often abnormal, and some children require assistive devices such as crutches. Hand activities commonly are involved to some degree, although the impairment may be subtle. Abnormalities of extraocular movement are relatively common.

Of children with spastic quadriplegia, 25% require total care; approximately 33% walk, usually after the age of 3 years. Intellectual function often is the most life-limiting concomitant problem, and involvement of the bulbar musculature may add further difficulties. Marked truncal hypotonia with pathologic reflexes or persisting rigidity have unfavorable outlooks. Most such children have grave intellectual limitations.

Most children who do not have serious accompanying spasticity with athetosis eventually walk. Balance and skillful use of the hands may remain difficult. Most children who sit by 2 years of age learn to walk. Conversely, the child who still has a Moro reflex, an asymmetric tonic neck reflex, extensor thrust, and no parachute reflex is unlikely to learn to walk. Few children who do not sit by the age of 4 years will learn to walk.

Specific cerebral palsy syndromes
Kenneth F. Swaiman

Spastic hemiplegia

Clinical findings. Although children may have obvious hemiplegia in the second year of life, their difficulties may not be observed during the first 3 to 5 months of life. The arm is usually affected more than the leg, and hypotonia may be the most prominent finding [Byers, 1941]. For unexplained reasons the left hemisphere (right side) is affected in two thirds of patients [Crothers and Paine, 1959]. The parents may observe that the child has prematurely developed right or left handedness during the first 2 years of life.

During the examination the child exhibits impaired gross and fine motor coordination, has difficulty moving the hand quickly, and is frequently unable to grasp small items with a pincer grasp. The obligate palmar grasp reflex, which is usually absent by age 6 months and frequently rudimentary after age 4 months, may be obligate. Weakness of the wrist and forearm is often associated with limitation of range of motion of supination. The range of elbow extension may be restricted. Attempts at reaching for objects may be accompanied by athetotic posturing with flexion of the wrist and hyperextension of the fingers (avoidance reaction).

Facial involvement is unusual. Only 10% of these patients, including those with extensive hemiplegia, have homonymous hemianopia [Black, 1988]. Children with hemiparesis have a circumductive gait that is present in varying degrees. Most commonly the child walks on the toes and swings the affected leg over a nearly semicircular arc during the course of each step. In contrast to the leg the affected arm usually moves less than normal and does not participate in a normal reciprocal motion during ambulation. There is an equionvarus positioning of the foot, and weakness and lack of full range of motion of dorsiflexion are often present. Further evidence of upper motor neuron involvement on the hemiplegic side includes hyperreflexia of the deep tendon reflexes, ankle clonus, and extensor toe signs. It is noteworthy that such children usually have intact cremasteric and abdominal reflexes.

Growth retardation of the abnormal side, usually more prominent in the distal arm and hand, or distal leg and foot, may be manifest. An indication of the presence of growth impairment may be obtained when the thumb and thumbnail of the affected side are compared to their normal opposite members and found to be smaller. Growth discrepancy of the leg may prove a significant problem during walking and may cause orthopedic difficulties of the proximal leg and the lower spinal vertebrae.

Although frequently overlooked, corticosensory impairment of the affected side is common. Examination for the integrity of stereognosis and graphesthesia usually reveals varying degree of compromise [Skatvedt, 1960; Brown et al., 1987].

Perlstein and Hood [1955] reported that approximately 28% of patients with infantile hemiplegia have some degree of mental retardation. Seizures occur in approximately one third of patients who have spastic hemiplegia. Mental retardation is highly correlated with epilepsy in hemiplegic patients [Uvebrandt, 1988; Aicardi, 1990]. Prognosis is difficult to establish in patients with hemiplegic cerebral palsy. Review of birth histories, EEGs, and CT scans in 52 children was performed by Cohen and Duffner [1981]. They concluded that the birth history was of little value in judging prognosis. EEG and neuroimaging provide a better correlation with the development of seizures and mental impairment. Furthermore, if anatomic abnormalities of the cerebral cortex, commissural pathways, or association pathways are present, these children are more likely to experience seizures and mental retardation.

Pathology. Because there are varying underlying conditions that lead to spastic hemiplegia, the neuropathology varies. The development of infarction with subsequent cystic formation in the distribution of the middle cerebral artery is a common concomitant. The pathogenesis of the vascular insult is rarely deducible (i.e., thrombosis, embolism, hemorrhage) [Uvebrandt, 1988; Asindi et al., 1988; Guzetta et al., 1986]. The vascular insult may be prenatal [Asindi et al., 1988] or perinatal [Baumann et al., 1987; Wiklund et al., 1991]. The degree of involvement varies. In an extreme form the white and gray matter overlying the lateral ventricle may be so greatly thinned that the ventricle may extend into the area with the development of a porencephalic cyst.

Gross examination of the brain demonstrates generalized atrophy in the affected hemisphere. Although the affected areas may be small and few in number, there may be large areas of gross cortical thinning with loss of underlying white matter and extensive dilatation of the adjoining lateral ventricle. Microscopic examination confirms disruption of the neuronal laminar pattern, neuronal loss, and associated gliosis of variable extent.

Asymmetric periventricular leukomalacia with resultant loss of white matter and ventricular dilatation in preterm infants may be the underlying cause [Uvebrandt, 1988; Wiklund et al., 1991].

In one report of CT scans of 111 children with hemiplegia, scans were normal in 29%, periventricular atrophy was present in 42%, maldevelopment in 17%, cortical-subcortical atrophy in 12%, and miscellaneous findings in 3% [Wiklund et al., 1991].

Spastic quadriplegia

Clinical findings. Little [1861] first described cerebral palsy. He used the term "spastic rigidity" in place of the modern term spasticity. As part of his original treatise he wrote:

Both lower extremities are more or less generally involved. Sometimes the affection of one limb only is observed by the parent, but examination usually shows a smaller degree of affection in the limb supposed to be sound. The contraction in the hips, knees, and ankles is often considerable. The flexors and adductors of thighs, the flexors of knees, and the gastrocnemii, preponderate. In most cases, after a time, owing to structural shortening of the muscles and of the articular ligaments, and perhaps to some change of form of articular surface, the thighs cannot be completely abducted or extended, the knees cannot be straightened, nor can the heels by properly applied to the ground. The upper extremities are sometimes held down by preponderating action of pectorals, teres major and teres minor, and latissimus dorsi; the elbows are semiflexed, the wrists partially flexed, pronated, and the fingers incapable of perfect voluntary direction. Sometimes the upper extremities appear unaffected with spasm or want of volition, sometimes a mere awkwardness in using them exists.

Spastic quadriplegia is characterized by generalized increase in muscle tone. The legs are involved more than the arms, and there is paucity of limb movement. Opisthotonic posturing may be evident in early infancy and may persist through the first year of life. Movement of the head often initiates forced extension of the arms and legs similar to the position of decerebrate rigidity. Accompanying supranuclear bulbar palsy, the result of bilateral corticospinal tract impairment, may produce difficulties with swallowing and articulation. The incoordination of the oropharyngeal muscles may predispose the patient to recurrent pneumonia during the first years of life. Almost 50% of children with spastic quadriplegia have generalized tonic-clonic seizures [Ingram, 1964]. In addition, a large, but indeterminant, number are grossly retarded [Crothers and Paine, 1959].

Neurologic examination demonstrates marked spasticity and accompanying signs of corticospinal tract involvement, including hyperactive deep tendon reflexes, ankle clonus, and extensor toe signs. Weakness of dorsiflexion of the feet associated with equinovarus deformities is very common. Marked spasticity of the hip muscles may lead to subluxation of the hip and associated acetabular pathologic conditions. Radiographs may be necessary to exclude the abnormal positioning of the head of the femur. Flexion contractures of the wrists and elbows of various degrees and spasticity of the arm muscles are readily evident.

Ophthalmologic evaluation of children with spastic quadriplegia reveals visual impairment more commonly in these children than in children with athetoid cerebral palsy [Preakey et al., 1974]. There is a much higher incidence of auditory, visual, motor, and learning disability in children with spastic quadriplegia than in

children with spastic hemiplegia, spastic diplegia, and ataxic cerebral palsy [Robinson, 1973].

Pathology. Brains of these children exhibit cystic degeneration as the final outcome of softening, necrosis, edema, and cystic formation of the central white matter. Although cortical abnormalities are almost always present, involvement is not as great as that found in the white matter. Multicystic encephalomalacia and brain malformations are commonly present [Benda, 1952; Chutorian et al., 1979].

Mantle sclerosis may be found in patients with mild to moderate quadriplegia. Necrosis of the subcortical white matter is accompanied by degeneration of the overlying cortical laminar pattern. Underlying status spongiosus may be the endstage of a grouping of numerous small subcortical cysts. Gliosis is prominent in the area usually occupied by neurons, and the meninges are grossly thickened. The extent of the lesions varies from involvement of an entire hemisphere to an entire lobe to portions of one lobe. Mantle sclerosis may be bilateral, but is almost always more profound in one hemisphere. The distribution of these pathologic changes indicates that they are most likely the result of vascular impairment (e.g., occlusion of main arterial branches, venous thrombosis, and sinus thrombosis) [Benda, 1952].

Alterations in brainstem structure are also commonly present [Wilson et al., 1982].

Spastic diplegia

Clinical findings. Spastic diplegia is characterized by bilateral leg involvement and commonly some degree of upper extremity impairment. Premature infants are particularly prone to spastic diplegia. It is noteworthy that 80% of premature infants who manifest motor abnormalities have spastic diplegia [McDonald, 1963]. In recent years the survival of very small preterm infants has led to a group of more severely neurologically impaired survivors than before [Hagberg et al., 1989].

Some infants with spastic diplegia manifest ataxia after further maturation (see the discussion of ataxic cerebral palsy). These infants have a great increase of tone of the leg muscles and accompanying difficulties in coordination and strength. Impairment may be asymmetric. When a small child is held in the vertical position by the examiner and the plantar surfaces of the feet are lightly bounced on the examining table, there is adduction of the legs (scissoring) and obligatory extension (extensor thrust). The feet are also kept in an equinovarus posture. Further examination reveals weakness of dorsiflexion of the feet. In older children, this same phenomenon causes them to toewalk. As expected, signs of upper motor unit involvement are easily demonstrable in the legs (e.g., hyperactive deep tendon reflexes, bilateral ankle clonus, extensor toe signs). Striking spasticity of the hip muscles may lead to subluxation of the hip and associated acetabular pathologic conditions and further restriction of motion. Radiographs may be necessary to exclude the abnormal positioning of the femoral head. The arms may be affected but usually only to a mild degree. The child may hold the arms in unusual fixed postures, either extended or flexed during walking, and may have clumsy, reciprocating, swinging arm movements or hold both arms flexed at the elbows. Affected children may extend their arms, pronate their hands, and clench their fists during running. Associated athetosis makes this latter posturing more likely.

Vasomotor instability, often manifested by cold extremities and variable and sometimes unpredictable patterns of sweating, may prove troublesome for the patient.

For reasons that are unclear—either disuse or probably hemispheric (parietal) lobe dysfunction—there may be marked retardation of growth of leg length.

After a variable period, usually 18 months to 2 years in children with moderate involvement, spasticity is increasingly accompanied by contractures that maintain the hips in flexion, knees in flexion, and the feet in an equinovarus position.

In one series, seizures (usually generalized tonic-clonic) were present in 27% of the children with spastic diplegia [Ingram, 1955]. Strabismus is also common, manifested by 43% of spastic diplegia patients [Ingram, 1995]. Approximately 30% have been retarded in the past [Hagberg et al., 1975a; 1975b], but the rate of retardation is increasing with the survival of extremely small preterm infants [Hagberg et al., 1989].

Pathology. Gross examination of the brain of infants with spastic diplegia may reveal porencephalic cysts and abnormalities of gyrus size (microgyria). Periventricular leukomalacia at the site of the germinal matrix in the path of the fibers subserving the legs as they course through the internal capsule serves to explain the clinical symptomatology in many of these infants [Benda, 1952; Christensen and Melchior, 1967]. Preterm infants are particularly susceptible to these periventricular lesions in the germinal matrix, although both the pathologic and clinical pattern develop in term infants [Hagberg et al., 1975a; 1975b].

CT confirms the presence of periventricular leukomalacia and varying degrees of ventricular dilatation. The presence of atrophy, abnormal gray matter configuration, and marked leukomalacia is correlated with severe impairment [Hagberg et al., 1991; Yokochi et al., 1989]. MRI studies appear to be more sensitive than CT studies and correlate well with clinical impairment [Yokochi et al., 1990].

Extrapyramidal cerebral palsy

This classification is rather broad based, but for all practical purposes there is little in the way of patho-genetic lesions or specific involvement of gray matter masses that can be uniformly associated with each type of individual movement abnormality or a specific combination of these movements. The patients are unable to smoothly perform meaningful movements because of interfering movements and involvement of inappropriate agonist and antagonist muscles (see Chapter 18).

Extrapyramidal cerebral palsy involves defects of posture and involuntary movement (e.g., athetosis, ballismus, chorea, dystonia); increased tone is usually associated with these conditions and is of the leadpipe or rigid variety.

Extrapyramidal cerebral palsy can be divided arbitrarily into two primary clinical subtypes: choreoathetotic and dystonic. Each may be accompanied by other extrapyramidal movements. Other classifications and subdivisions have been proposed [Kyllerman, 1983]. No classification is fundamentally satisfactory.

Choreoathetotic cerebral palsy

Clinical findings. Choreoathetotic cerebral palsy is characterized by large-amplitude, involuntary movements. The most obvious and dominating movement component is athetosis. Chorea is present in varying degrees. Tremor, myoclonus, and even some element of dystonia also may be evident.

Athetosis usually involves the distal limbs. Athetosis results in slow, writhing involuntary movements. Often there is finger and toe extension with rotation of the limb and its long axis. The resultant pattern of these movements culminates in bizarre transient positions of the limbs.

Choreiform movements may occur in the face, limbs, and rarely the trunk. These movements can be characterized as asymmetric, fleeting, incoordinated, involuntary contractions of individual muscle groups.

The combination of athetoid and choreiform movements results in a pattern of distal extremity movement, ongoing hypertonia, and rotary writhing movements of the limbs.

Athetotic posturing may be evident in the first year of life when the child begins to reach for objects. The movements, as is generally true of most involuntary movements, are not present during sleep. Movements are more prominent during stress or illness, and their intensity changes from day to day.

As expected from the pathologic findings described below, evidence of upper motor neuron unit impairment (e.g., hyperactive deep tendon reflexes, ankle clonus, positive extensor toe signs), as well as seizures, spasticity, and mental retardation, may be present.

Children with choreoathetosis may have marked difficulty with speech that is characterized by great variability in rate and explosive changes in volume.

Ballismus, a movement disorder in which the arms and legs are violently flung about, may be an extreme form of choreoathetotic cerebral palsy. Most of the activity takes place at the shoulders and hips. Although patients with balismus are said to have a shortened life expectancy and do not survive beyond the second decade, few data are available, and clinical pathologic correlation is undefined.

Dystonic cerebral palsy

The dystonic form of cerebral palsy is uncommon. Indeed, the patient with the dystonic form may be misdiagnosed as having athetosis. The underlying pathophysiology is poorly explained.

The dystonic movements are not unlike other conditions exhibiting dystonia. The trunk muscles and proximal portions of the limbs are predominantly affected. Movements may be slow and persistent, particularly of the head and neck, which may be pulled to one side or the other, or there may be retrocollis. At times the movements may consist of rapid and repetitive retractions of the head. The trunk may be literally twisted into many fixed positions that may appear bizarre.

Pathology. The extrapyramidal form of cerebral palsy is often, but not always, preceded by birth asphyxia and anoxia. Requirement for respiratory support and hypoxic-ischemic encephalopathy at birth is usually historically documented. Patients also may have had unusual presentations at the time of delivery.

Neighboring the ependyma of the lateral ventricles is the head of the caudate nucleus, which contains both lenticular striate arteries and veins. The veins become congested and the adjacent perivascular tissue necrotic. Examination of the caudate nucleus reveals cystic changes. Small punctate areas of hemorrhage are found in the putamen. The venous congestion and obstruction result in status marmoratus [Benda, 1945]. When these areas are examined grossly, they appear marbled. Light microscopic examination demonstrates many myelin fibers but also neuronal loss, laminar cortical necrosis, microgyria, gliosis, and cystic degenerations of the adjacent periventricular areas [Vogt and Vogt, 1928; Volpe, 1987].

Corticospinal tract findings may be evident in children who have choreoathetosis. On pathologic examination the brains of these children may reveal large areas of patchy necrosis of the cortical laminar pattern, venous congestion in the cortex, ventricular dilatation, and accompanying white matter loss that may be related to demyelination and central necrosis. Fibrosis in the meninges may also be present. Thus both cortex and basal ganglia may be jointly involved in these patients. Furthermore, cortical lesions associated with necrosis in areas adjacent to the ventricles may be the result of occlusion of the vein of Galen. Obstruction of this major vessel triggers a chain of events, including rupture of blood vessels, primarily veins, with ensuing mutiple hemorrhages in the areas served by the branches of the internal cerebral veins. The hemorrhages result in subependymal necrosis and subsequent pathologic dilatation of the lateral ventricles and associated atrophy of the basal ganglia. If obstruction is extremely widespread, the internal capsule may be involved, and further symptoms and signs of corticospinal tract involvement arise.

In one report, patients with severe athetoid cerebral palsy originating perinatally were divided into two groups neuropathologically, the "globo-Luysian group" and the "thalamoputaminal group." The major abnormal sites in the globo-Luysian group were the pallidum and subthalamic nucleus, and in the thalamoputaminal group the thalamus and putamen. The causative pathologic condition in the globu-Luysian group was primarily perinatal severe jaundice, and the cause of the thalamoputaminal group was predominantly neonatal asphyxia. The patients in the thalamoputaminal group demonstrated lower mental ability and suffered from more intractable convulsions than those in the globo-Luysian group. In the globo-Luysian group, rigidospasticity was frequently demonstrated with fluctuation of athetoid movements, whereas in the thalamoputaminal group, various abnormalities of muscle tone and rather restricted athetosis were observed [Hayashi et al., 1991].

MRI studies of 22 children with athetotic cerebral palsy frequently revealed high-intensity areas in the thalamus and putamen in T_2 weighted images. In 16 children with known perinatal asphyxia, 14 had lesions in the basal ganglia, thalamus, and/or cerebral white matter. Seven of the 22 children had normal scans [Yokochi et al., 1991].

Atonic (hypotonic) cerebral palsy

Infants with atonic cerebral palsy have hypotonicity and associated leg weakness. Although hypotonic, the arms may manifest near-normal strength and coordination. In the past, this combination of clinical findings has led to the use of the term *atonic diplegia* by some authors to describe such children.

Diagnosis is difficult because of the plethora of possibilities. Most children with generalized hypotonia have so-called central hypotonia (see Chapter 16) resulting from inadequate control of the motor pathways and subsequent disruption of gamma loop function. Others, with absent or hypoactive deep tendon reflexes, may have involvement of the lower motor neuron unit (i.e., anterior horn cell, peripheral nerve, neuromuscular junction, muscle). Extrapyramidal (choreoathetotic and dystonic) cerebral palsy may be preceded by a hypotonic phase.

The condition atonic cerebral palsy is relatively uncommon compared with other forms of cerebral palsy; it is often associated with slow attainment of motor milestones and the presence of normal or hyperactive deep tendon reflexes. Children with atonic cerebral palsy, when suspended while held under the arms, flex both legs at the hips (Förster's sign).

Although in the past it has been thought that tone almost always increases with maturation in these children [Ingram, 1964], experience has taught that a sizable number do not develop spasticity but remain hypotonic.

The cause and anatomic location of involvement of the brain that leads to this condition are unknown. It is through their effect on the gamma motor neuron that portions of the CNS (e.g., motor cortex, thalamus, basal ganglia, vestibular nuclei, reticular formation, and cerebellum) modify tone, with ensuing hypotonia.

Ataxic cerebral palsy

The last common form of cerebral palsy is the ataxic form. It is sometimes associated with spastic diplegia [Hagberg et al., 1975b]. This form is usually associated with other motor abnormalities; however, the diagnosis is applied only when the predominant manifestations are those of cerebellar dysfunction. Patients with this form of cerebral palsy may have some impairment of intellectual ability, but they are rarely grossly retarded [Clement et al., 1984]. The motor difficulties are often not apparent until late in the first year of life. Early manifestations include hypotonia, truncal ataxia while sitting, dysmetria, and gross incoordination. The motor involvement results in delayed attainment of motor skills; independent walking may not occur until age 3 or 4 years and then with great difficulty and frequent falling. Compromise of writing skills and other skills that demand good fine motor coordination often adversely affects educational endeavors.

Examination often reveals nystagmus, dysmetria, hypotonia, and a wide-based gait. The Romberg test is positive with the eyes open. Likely sites of involvement are the cerebellum and adjacent brainstem.

Because of the large number of conditions associated with slowly progressive ataxia, the clinician must exclude conditions in which ataxia predominates in early childhood (see Chapter 19). Ataxia, especially if accompanied by mental retardation, may not be included properly among cerebral palsy conditions but may be the result of one of many inherited conditions [Hagberg et al., 1984].

Pathology. The pathology of ataxic cerebral palsy is poorly defined and inconstant. The discussion of the pathology of ataxic cerebral palsy is confounded by the fact that the total absence of the vermis may not give rise to cerebellar symptoms in certain congenital conditions, whereas aplasia of the vermis may be associated with nonprogressive ataxia [Bordarier and Aicardi, 1990]. Cerebellar hemispheral lesions may or may not be present in patients with ataxic cerebral palsy. The lack of correlation of evident structural changes is epitomized by CT studies. In one report, CT evaluation of patients

with ataxic cerebral palsy revealed that the posterior fossa was normal in 38% and abnormal in 28%. In contrast, the cerebral hemispheres were abnormal in 55% of the patients [Miller and Cala, 1989].

Mixed cerebral palsy

Mixed cerebral palsy includes manifestations of both spastic and extrapyramidal types. Patients with predominantly spastic quadriplegia may have a mild to marked degree of choreoathetosis. Conversely, frequently patients who have predominant choreoathetosis as their symptomatology may also manifest upper motor neuron unit involvement. These patterns of motor impairment are the result of compromise of large areas of brain with sequelae of basal ganglia, cortex, and subcortical disruption. Characteristics of these patients are discussed in the sections describing individual types. Most patients can be categorized into the types discussed on the basis of predominant manifestations.

Treatment of cerebral palsy
Barry S. Russman

General principles

Before discussing specific treatment programs for cerebral palsy, some important general principles should be stated as follows:

1. Long-term treatment objectives must be defined, taking into consideration not only the patient's motor deficits, but also his or her cognitive abilities, social skills, emotional status, vocational potential, and, most importantly, the availability of family support. Will the patient be able to accomplish his or her own daily living needs? Will the patient be independent in all areas, or just some? Will the patient need public or private transportation to reach his or her place of employment? Will leisure activities be accessible? These questions should be considered at all times as the treatment program is being developed.
2. The effects of the patient's growth and development on his or her problem, with and without the proposed treatment, should be evaluated.
3. Valid alternatives, which look at risk/benefit ratios and humane/ethical dilemmas, and which might include nontreatment, should be considered.
4. The goals of a treatment program vary with the individual's age.

Because cerebral palsy is the result of a brain injury/dysfunction, several of these problems may not be treatable, and others can only be partially remedied. Any treatment approach should be based on the functional abnormality of the patient. When the treatment is completed, it should be critically evaluated to optimize the outcome and to prevent perpetuation of errors in future cases. The motor deficits can be analyzed in four distinctive ways: (1) loss of selective motor control and dependence on primitive reflex patterns for ambulation; (2) abnormal muscle tone that is strongly influenced by body posture and/or position and/or movement; (3) imbalance between muscle agonists and antagonists; and (4) impaired body balance mechanisms.

Loss of selective motor control and dependence on primitive reflex patterns for ambulation. A remedy does not exist that can significantly alter selective motor loss, such as lack of control of lower extremity muscle, whether the problem is related to spasticity or dystonia. Physical and occupational therapy programs can provide help. Various schools of therapy promote programs that superficially vary greatly, but nevertheless have certain common principles, including development of sequence learning, normalization of tone, training of normal movement patterns, inhibition of abnormal patterns, and prevention of deformity. Schools use different stimuli and facilitation techniques to accomplish these goals. In general, because a child learns motor control in a cephalocaudal direction, the therapist works in the same way by first trying to establish trunk control and then working toward control of the lower extremities.

Early programs [Weiss and Betts, 1967] emphasized passive range of motion and use of braces to prevent contractures and to inhibit abnormal muscle function, a program developed by Phelps. Once these objectives were met, it was expected that the normal muscles would provide the necessary functions for the child to attain normal milestones. In the 1940s, Deaver promoted a program that emphasized functional abilities rather than movement patterns. Extensive bracing was used to prevent abnormal motor movements from interfering with function. At about the same time, Fay developed the prototype of what became known as the Doman-Delacato or "patterning" program. Other therapeutic approaches in vogue at that time included providing sensory input, for example, stroking, icing, and heat, to promote a motor output, a program developed by Rood. In the late 1950s the Bobaths [Bobath, 1967] developed the neurodevelopmental treatment program for this patient population. The methods used in this program attempt to inhibit abnormal infantile reflexes, such as the tonic neck and Moro reflex, and to promote or facilitate more normal movement patterns, such as the righting reflex.

Studies suggest that, for some patients, certain therapy programs may make a difference in the patient's outcome. Paine [1962] noted that individuals who received intensive physical therapy had fewer contractures compared with those who did not receive a therapy program but that both treated and untreated patients required a similar number of surgical procedures. In 1973, Wright and Nicholson reported that treatment programs did not affect range of motion or influence the retention or loss of developmental reflexes. Conversely, some possible benefit was found for children who had quadriparesis in the first year of life. Scherzer et al. [1976] reported a strong trend toward improvement in motor status and social motivation after treatment of children with cerebral palsy who had normal IQs compared with those who were retarded. Many studies of therapy programs have reached negative conclusions regarding the benefit of such programs on the eventual motor outcome of the patient [Scherzer et al., 1976]. However, when reviewing the benefits of any program, more than the motor outcome must be considered. The psychologic impact of rearing a disabled child can be devastating. This subject has been the focus of several studies. In a study addressing the issue of psychologic stress in mothers whose children are disabled, Breslaw et al. [1982] concluded that the specific diagnosis did not cause as much stress as expected among mothers; however, the dependency of the disabled child on the mother in helping accomplish activities of daily living was significantly correlated with maternal stress. A therapy program might be helpful in these cases, not necessarily to stimulate development but to offer parents easier ways to work with their child.

The therapist should serve as a coach to the parents, who implement much of the actual treatment on a daily basis at home. Realistic expectations must be articulated firmly. Rather than cautiously attempting to correct a dysfunction that cannot be corrected, the therapist should help the patient develop compensation techniques, recognizing that the severity of the disability mitigates against the development of "normal" motor control.

Abnormal muscle tone that is strongly influenced by body posture and/or position and/or movement. In a child with spasticity, fixed muscle contractures occur with growth. A child whose bones are growing stretches his muscles daily during normal activities and thus maintains muscle growth in proportion to bone growth. The inability of the child with cerebral palsy to adequately stretch spastic muscles favors static muscle contracture of certain muscle groups. Anything that normalizes or at least reduces tone helps to prevent contracture. Even if tone cannot be normalized, spastic muscles still grow, provided they receive adequate stretch. Thus a program to prevent muscle contracture should logically be designed that reduces or normalizes tone, adequately stretches muscles that need to be elongated, and removes the stimulus of stretch from the muscles that need to be shortened. Unfortunately, this is easy to conceive but difficult to accomplish.

Medication has been used to alter muscle tone

[Young, 1987; Davidoff, 1985]. The three agents used most often can be outlined as follows:

1. Diazepam appears to act on the CNS at the level of the limbic system (i.e., the thalamus and hypothalamus). It is also a mild sedative.
2. Baclofen acts through the inhibition of monosynaptic and polysynaptic reflexes at the spinal cord level. It is an analog of the inhibitory neurotransmitter gamma-aminobutyric acid but does not appear to have any central action on spasticity, although it can act as a CNS depressant.
3. Dantrolene acts on skeletal muscle beyond the myoneural junction, probably by inhibiting the release of calcium ions from the sacroplasmic reticulum. Dantrolene can be hepatotoxic in selected individuals, and liver function tests must be monitored at regular intervals when the drug is used.

Although baclofen has been used to alter muscle tone in patients with cerebral palsy, experience suggests that it only alters spasticity in very high doses because it does not readily cross the blood-brain barrier. Conversely, intrathecal baclofen, in the short term, can decrease spasticity in patients with cerebral palsy [Albright et al., 1991]. Botulinum toxin has been used in patients with spastic cerebral palsy [Narayan et al., 1991]. Studies of the short-term and long-term results of this intervention have not been published.

Inhibition casting as advocated by Sussman [1978] and Watt et al. [1986] and appropriate use of orthotics can modify tone to some degree. For example, a hinged ankle-foot orthosis with a plantar flexion stop may be useful to prevent excessive extensor thrust. In addition, it will control foot position throughout the gait cycle, which may also provide a significant reduction in extensor tone. Physical therapy also attempts to lower tone, mainly through positioning and/or facilitation techniques; however, the effects of facilitation therapy on tone are relatively transitory.

Occasionally, alcohol "washes" of contracted muscles, as advocated by Bleck [1987], can be used to regain adequate control of an early static deformity. This usually results in approximately 6 weeks of relative weakness of the treated muscle or muscle group, and during this time an appropriate program of therapy, casting, or bracing can be performed to regain muscle length without resorting to surgery.

In the mid-1970s, chronic cerebellar stimulation, accomplished by the surgical implantation of electrodes on the superior surface of the cerebellum, was proposed as a way of decreasing spasticity, which, in turn, would allow functional improvement in patients with spastic cerebral palsy [Cooper et al., 1976]. A subsequent study, controlled for placebo effect, could not confirm the initial findings [Gahm et al., 1981]. A second neurosur-

gical procedure that has been proposed to alter either tone or movement disorders is stereotaxic thalamotomy [Broggi et al., 1983]. To date, this procedure has been effective in decreasing hemiparetic tremors only.

Recently, Peacock and Staudt [1990] have advocated selective, partial dorsal root rhizotomy as a method of deafferentiating the muscle spindles and thereby obtaining a true reduction in muscle tone. This procedure is performed on the dorsal roots of L_2 through S_1 bilaterally and, according to these authors, produces a permanent reduction of tone without significantly altering sensation or strength. If effective, this procedure will represent a major advance in the treatment of cerebral palsy. However, many concerns have been raised about the efficacy of this treatment for the child with spastic cerebral palsy [Landau, 1990].

Imbalance between muscle agonists and antagonists. Static contracture of muscle related to spasticity is a common problem for which surgical lengthening of the musculotendinous unit is frequently performed. Fixed muscle contractures are almost never seen in patients with pure dyskinesias, but when they do occur, surgical intervention is considered, but with extreme caution. Given the absence of a constant kinematic baseline, the results of surgery are difficult to predict. Furthermore, if the agonist is surgically weakened in the dyskinetic patient, the result is often a postoperative deformity that favors the antagonist. For example, if the adductors are lengthened or released, a fixed abduction deformity of the hips is likely to occur postoperatively. Consequently, if possible, it is best to avoid surgery in athetoid patients. They are unlikely to benefit, and it is very likely to be that their condition will worsen because of the intervention.

Surgical lengthening of tendons and/or muscles is probably the most effective way of restoring balance once static contracture of muscle has developed. Unfortunately, the lengthened muscle is also weakened. Currently, there is no way to strengthen the antagonist. In general, lengthening is not a problem with isometric muscles (stabilizers) because they are usually weak in spastic cerebral palsy and rarely require elongation. In most cases, eccentric muscles (decelerators and shock absorbers) can be lengthened without significant loss of function. However, lengthening is a major problem with concentric muscles (accelerators) because these muscles are necessary to initiate movement of the part on which they are acting. Because a hip flexion contracture is usually present in spastic cerebral palsy, the iliopsoas is a prime example of this dilemma. If lengthening of the musculotendinous unit is sufficient to correct the contracture, the iliopsoas is often weakened to the point that the patient has difficulty in initiating hip flexion. In this particular problem, performing an intramuscular lengthening of the tendinous portion of the psoas and accepting some contracture of the iliacus in exchange for better muscle strength is recommended.

Rang et al. [1986] and Bleck [1987] have both argued cogently that the overall result is much better if all contracted muscles are lengthened simultaneously rather than staging the procedures. Not only is morbidity lessened by accomplishing all surgery during the course of a single procedure, but by simultaneously balancing all major lower extremity joints, much better function is possible. Because many of the muscles that require lengthening are biarticulate, surgical lengthening of muscles to correct imbalance at any one joint is likely to cause imbalance at the joint above or below. For example, if the hamstrings are lengthened in a patient with knee flexion contractures, the result is likely to be better extension at the knee but at a cost of increased flexion contracture at the hips. This outcome occurs because the hamstrings, in addition to being knee flexors, are also hip extensors. Thus hamstring lengthening also lessens hip extensor power, and in cases with spastic hip flexors, the hips move into a more fixed flexion deformity.

It is useful to think of the low back, hip, knee, and ankle as four weights on the corners of a suspended balance board. Unless weight is subtracted or added evenly at all four corners, the board will tip. Unfortunately, the more muscles that are lengthened at one time, the more likely the possibility of making a judgment error. Therefore the muscle imbalance must be precisely defined. In addition, primary abnormalities must be differentiated from adaptive or "coping" mechanisms. A simple example of this is a circumduction gait in a child who does not have sufficient knee flexion for foot clearance during swing. This is a simple example, but the coping mechanisms can be extremely subtle. Unfortunately, if the surgeon focuses on the coping mechanism rather than the primary abnormality, the patient's condition is often worsened by the procedure rather than helped. The differentiation between primary and secondary abnormalities often cannot be accomplished without dynamic gait analysis.

Gait analysis is a method by which the walking pattern of an individual is examined in detail [Gage, 1991]. It is based on the gait cycle, which is the basic unit of walking. The gait cycle begins at initial contact when the foot strikes the ground and ends when the same foot strikes the ground again. As such, it consists of a period of stance, when the foot is on the ground, and a period of swing, when the foot is off the ground. For normal walking to occur, more than 30 major muscles in each lower extremity must act precisely with respect to both timing and power during each gait cycle.

Computerized gait analysis has made rapid progress in recent years, and several commercial systems are currently available. The modern gait analysis laboratory usually consists of three major measurement systems: motion analysis, force plate, and electromyography. The laboratory's software outputs integrate these three measurement parameters to provide information regarding the specific abnormalities at each of the major joints of the lower extremity throughout the gait cycle, as well as the electromyographic activity of the muscles controlling the joint. With the aid of this information a much more precise definition of the gait abnormality is possible. Treatment can then be tailored specifically to the child's abnormality. Furthermore, more extensive treatment is possible at one time with less risk of error (e.g., surgical lengthening of all contracted musculature at hips, knee, and ankles bilaterally during the course of a single operation). After convalescence, postoperative gait analysis allows accurate assessment outcome.

Impaired body balance mechanisms. The child with cerebral palsy invariably has abnormalities of balance to some degree. In spastic diplegia, posterior balance is affected most severely. A child with only disturbances in posterior equilibrium is usually able to walk without the use of external aids. If anterior balance is also affected, crutches are necessary for ambulation. Children with deficiencies in lateral equilibrium usually require a walker or, if the lateral equilibrium reactions are severely deficient, may be unable to walk independently. The deficiencies in equilibrium are related to an irreparable neurological lesion and are lifelong. However, a good physical therapy program in early childhood may help the child to improve his or her equilibrium responses to some degree. If there is instability in the stance phase of gait, appropriate orthotics and/or surgery can be used to provide a stable plantigrade foot that will, in turn, have a beneficial overall effect on balance. Independent ambulation without crutches demands that the mass of the head and upper trunk be maintained over the base of support. When fixed contractures at the hips, knees, and/or ankles prevent this alignment, surgical lengthening of contracted musculature may allow independent ambulation if the child's equilibrium reactions are adequate.

Summary of treatment protocol for spastic cerebral palsy

It is now possible to formulate a rational treatment protocol for the child with cerebral palsy. Although each patient is unique and treatment must be individualized, the method of approach can be similar. There are four major tenets of treatment as follows:

1. Avoid surgery to improve ambulation until after the gait has matured. Generally, a program of physical therapy should be started early in conjunction with a good home maintenance program. Parents should be taught to place the child in positions that prevent the deformities and favor

recovery, for example, lying prone to stretch the hip flexors and long sitting to elongate the hamstrings. Night splinting is often effective but must not interfere with normal nocturnal movements or the child will not tolerate the splints. For example, an Ilfield abduction splint provides stretch to the hip adductors while still allowing the hips to move in the sagittal and transverse planes. This splint can often be used in conjunction with ankle-foot orthoses that maintain the triceps surae on stretch but still allow the child sufficient freedom to turn in bed. If hamstrings and heel cords are contracted, a knee immobilizer on one limb and an ankle-foot orthosis on the contralateral limb, reversing them every other night, can be effective. In that way the child is not overly encumbered by the splinting. Inhibition casts, as advocated by [Watt et al., 1986] are useful in controlling dynamic spasticity and hence maintaining length of the posterior tibial musculature; however, the long-term benefit of their use has not been established. Meanwhile, function should be maximized with appropriate orthotics, physical therapy, and a home maintenance program. Various modalities that alter muscle tone may be attempted, including medication, transcutaneous stimulation, and selective posterior rhizotomy. The latter two modalities are experimental at this time.

2. When the gait is mature, usually sometime between the age of 6 and 10 years, gait analysis should be performed. These data are used in conjunction with the clinical examination to determine an appropriate course of treatment, which is usually some combination of surgery and orthotics.

3. If surgery is elected, staging should be avoided. The surgeon should lengthen and/or transfer all muscles necessary to obtain balance during the course of a single surgical procedure. If this is not possible, two procedures are staged closely so that only one extended period of recovery is necessary.

4. After surgery, casting should be minimized, and the patient should be remobilized rapidly. An active physical therapy program should be maintained, provided the gait is improving (usually about 12 months). Recurrence of contractures is prevented throughout the remaining years of growth with appropriate night splinting and a good home maintenance program designed to stretch tight musculature adequately.

REFERENCES

Aicardi J. Epilepsy in brain-injured children with cerebral palsy. Dev Med Clin Neurol 1990; 32:191.

Albright AL, Cervi A, Singletary J. Intrathecal Baclofen for spasticity in cerebral palsy. JAMA 1991; 265:1418.

Asindi AA, Stephenson JBP, Young DG. Spastic hemiparesis and presumed prenatal embolisation. Arch Dis Child 1988; 63:68.

Barabas G, Taft LT. The early signs and differential diagnosis of cerebral palsy. Pediatr Ann 1986; 15:203.

Baumann RJ, Carr WA, Shuman RM. Patterns of cerebral arterial injury in children with neurological disabilities. J Child Neurol 1987; 2:298.

Bejar R, Coen RW, Merritt TA, et al. Focal necrosis of the white matter (periventricular leukomalacia): sonographic, pathologic and electroencephalographic features. Am J Neuroradiol 1986; 7:1073.

Benda CE. Late effects of cerebral birth injuries. Medicine 1945; 24:71.

Benda CE. Developmental disorders of mentation and cerebral palsies. New York: Grune & Stratton, 1952.

Benda GI, Hiller JL, Reynolds JW. Benzyl alcohol toxicity: impact on neurologic handicaps among surviving very low birthweight infants. Pediatrics 1986; 77:507.

Black PD. Ocular defects in children with cerebral palsy. Br Med J 1988; 281:487.

Blair E, Stanley F. Interobserver reliability in the classification of cerebral palsy. Dev Med Child Neurol 1985; 27:615.

Bleck EE. Orthopedic management in cerebral palsy. Oxford: Mac-Keith Press, 1987:190.

Bobath B. The very early treatment of cerebral palsy. Dev Med Child Neurol 1967; 9:373.

Bordarier C, Aicardi J. Dandy-Walker syndrome and agenesis of the cerebellar vermis: diagnostic problems and genetic counseling. A review. Dev Med Child Neurol 1990; 32:285.

Breslaw N, Starvch KS, Mortimer EA. Psychological stress in mothers of disabled children. Am J Dis Child 1982; 136:682.

Broggi G, Angelini L, Bono R, et al. Long-term results of stereotactic thalmotomy for cerebral palsy. Neurosurgery 1983; 12:195.

Brown JK, Van Rensburg F, Walsh G, et al. A neurological study of hand function of hemiplegic children. Dev Med Child Neurol 1987; 29:287.

Burke JP, O'Keefe M, Bowell R. Optic nerve hypoplasia, encephalopathy, and neurodevelopmental handicap. Br J Ophthalmol 1991; 75:236.

Byers RK. Evolution of hemiplegias in infancy. Am J Dis Child 1941; 61:915.

Capute AJ, Palmer FB, Shapiro BK, et al. Primitive reflex profile: a quantitation of primitive reflexes in infancy. Dev Med Child Neurol 1984; 26:375.

Christensen E, Melchior J. Cerebral palsy—a clinical and neuropathological study. Clin Dev Med 1967; 25:1.

Chutorian AM, Michener RC, Defendini R, et al. Neonatal polycystic encephalomalacia: four new cases and review of the literature. J Neurol Neurosurg Psychiatry 1979; 42:154.

Clement MC, Briard JL, Ponsot G, et al. Ataxies cerebelleuses congenitales nonprogressives. Arch Fr Pediatr 1984; 41:685.

Cohen ME, Duffner, PK. Prognostic indicators in hemiparetic cerebral palsy. Ann Neurol 1981; 9:353.

Colditz PB, Henderson-Smart DJ. Electronic fetal heart rate monitoring during labour: does it prevent perinatal asphyxia and cerebral palsy? Med J Aust 1990; 153:88.

Cooper IS, Riklan M, Amin I, et al. Chronic cerebellar stimulation in cerebral palsy. Neurology 1976, 26:744.

Crothers B, Paine RS. The natural history of cerebral palsy. Cambridge: Harvard University Press, 1959.

Davidoff, RA. Antispasticity drugs: mechanism of action. Ann Neurol 1985; 17:107.

Dennis J, Johnson MA, Mutch LMM, et al. Acid-base status at birth in term infants and outcome at 4.5 years. Am J Obstet Gynecol 1989; 161:213.

de Vries LS, Connell JA, Dubowitz LMS, et al. Neurological, electrophysiological and MRI abnormalities in infants with extensive cystic leukomalacia. Neuropediatrics 1987; 18:61.

Ellenberg JH, Nelson KB. Cluster of perinatal events identifying infants at high risk for death or disability. J Pediatr 1988; 113:546.

Ellison PH. Neurologic development of the high-risk infant. Clin Perinatol 1984; 11:41.

Evans PM, Evans SJW, Alberman E. Cerebral palsy: why we must plan for survival. Arch Dis Child 1990; 65:1329.

Eyman RK, Grossman HJ, Chaney RH, et al. The life expectancy of profoundly handicapped people with mental retardation. N Engl J Med 1990; 323:584.

Faust D, Ziskin J. The expert witness in psychology and psychiatry. Science 1988; 239:31.

Fenichel GM, Lane DA, Livengood JR, et al. Adverse events following immunization: assessing probability of causation. Pediatr Neurol 1989; 5:287.

Gage JR. Gait analysis in cerebral palsy. Oxford: MacKeith Press, 1991.

Gahm NH, Russman BS, Cerciello RL, et al. Chronic cerebellar stimulation for cerebral palsy: a double-blind study. Neurology 1981; 31:87.

Grether JK, Cummins SK, Nelson KB. The California Cerebral Palsy Project. Paediatr Perinat Epidemiol 1992.

Gross H, Jellinger K, Kaltenback E, et al. Infantile cerebral disorders: clinical neuropathological correlations to elucidate the aetiological factors. J Neurol Sci 1968; 7:551.

Guzzetta F, Shackelford GD, Volpe S, et al. Periventricular intraparenchymal echodensities in the premature newborn: critical determinant of neurologic outcome. Pediatrics 1986; 78:995.

Hagberg B, Hagberg G, Olow I. The changing panorama of cerebral palsy in Sweden 1954-1970. I. Analysis of the general changes. Acta Paediatr Scand 1975a; 64:187.

Hagberg B, Hagberg G, Olow I. The changing panorama of cerebral palsy in Sweden 1954-1970. II. Analysis of the various syndromes. Acta Paediatr Scand 1975b; 64:193.

Hagberg B, Hagberg G, Olow I. The changing panorama of cerebral palsy in Sweden: IV. Epidemiological trends 1959-78. Acta Paediatr Scand 1984; 73:433.

Hagberg B, Hagberg G, Olow I, et al. The changing panorama of cerebral palsy in Sweden: V. The birth year period 1979-52. Acta Paediatr Scand 1989; 78:283.

Hagberg B, Hagberg G, Zetterstrom R. Decreasing perinatal mortality—increase in cerebral palsy morbidity? Acta Paediatr Scand 1989; 78:664.

Hayashi M, Satoh J, Sakamoto K, et al. Clinical and neuropathological findings in severe athetoid cerebral palsy: a comparative study of globo-Luysian and thalamo-putaminal groups. Brain Dev 1991; 13:47.

Hoyme HE, Higginbottom MC, Jones KL. Vascular etiology of disruptive structure defects in monozygotic twins. Pediatrics 1981; 67:288.

Ingram T. A study of cerebral palsy in the childhood population of Edinburgh. Arch Dis Child 1955; 117:395.

Ingram TTS. Paediatric aspects of cerebral palsy. Edinburgh: Churchill-Livingstone, 1964.

Koeda T, Suganuma I, Kohno Y, et al. MR imaging of spastic diplegia: comparative study between preterm and term infants. Neuroradiology 1990; 32:187.

Krageloh-Mann I, Hagberg B, Petersen D, et al. Bilateral spastic cerebral palsy—pathogenetic aspects from MRI. Neuropediatrics 1992; 23:46.

Kyllerman M. Reduced optimality in pre- and perinatal conditions in dyskinetic cerebral palsy. Distribution and comparison to controls. Neuropediatrics 1983; 14:29.

Landau WM, Hunt CC. Dorsal rhizotomy, a treatment of unproven efficacy. J Child Neurol 1990; 5:174.

Leviton A, Gilles FH. Acquired perinatal leukoencephalopathy. Ann Neurol 1984; 16:1.

Leviton A, Paneth N. White matter damage in preterm newborns—an epidemiologic perspective. Early Hum Dev 1990; 24:1.

Little WJ. On the influence of abnormal parturition, difficult labours, premature birth, and asphyxia neonatorum on the mental and physical condition of the child, especially in relation to deformities. Trans Obstet Soc London 1861; 3:293.

Malamud N, Itabashi HH, Castor J, et al. An etiologic and diagnostic study of cerebral palsy. J Pediatr 1964; 65:270.

McCarty SM, St. James P, Berninger VW, et al. Assessment of intellectual functioning across the life span in severe cerebral palsy. Dev Med Child Neurol 1986; 28:364.

McDonald AD. Cerebral palsy in children of very low birth weight. Arch Dis Chil 1963; 38:579.

Melone PJ, Ernest JM, O'Shea MD, et al. Appropriateness of intrapartum fetal heart rate management and risk of cerebral palsy. Am J Obstet Gynecol 1991; 165:272.

Meyer BA, Dickinson JE, Chambers C, et al. The effect of fetal sepsis on umbilical cord blood gases. Am J Obstet Gynecol 1992; 166:612.

Miller G, Cala LA. Ataxic cerebral palsy—clinico-radiologic correlations. Neuropediatrics 1989; 20:84.

Molnar GE. Cerebral palsy: prognosis and how to judge it. Pediatr Ann 1979; 8:43.

Narayan RK, Loubser PG, Jankovic J, et al. Intrathecal Bacolfen for intractable axial dystonia. Neurology 1991; 41:1141.

Nelson KB. Prenatal origin of hemiparetic cerebral palsy: how often and why? Pediatrics 1991; 88:1059.

Nelson KB, Leviton A. How much of neonatal encephalopathy is due to birth asphyxia? Am J Dis Child 1991; 145:1325.

Nelson KB, Ellenberg JH. Apgar scores as predictors of chronic neurologic disability. Pediatrics 1981; 68:36.

Nelson KB, Ellenberg JH. Antecedents of cerebral palsy. 1. Univariate analysis of risks. Am J Dis Child 1985a; 139:1031.

Nelson KB, Ellenberg JH. Predictors of low and very low birth weight and the relation to these to cerebral palsy. JAMA 1985b; 254:1473.

Paine RS. On the treatment of cerebral palsy: the outcome of 177 patients, 74 totally untreated. Pediatrics 1962; 29:605.

Paine RS. The evolution of infantile postural reflexes in the presence of chronic brain syndromes. Dev Med Child Neurol 1964; 6:345.

Paludetto R. Neonatal complications specific to twin (multiple) births (twins transfusion syndrome, intrauterine death of cotwin). J Perinat Med 1991; 19(suppl 1):246.

Paneth N, Stark RI. Cerebral palsy and mental retardation in relation to indicators of perinatal asphyxia, an epidemiologic overview. Am J Obstet Gynecol 1983; 147:960.

Peacock W, Staudt LA. Spasticity in cerebral palsy and the selective posterior rhizotomy procedure. J Child Neurol 1990; 5:179.

Peevy KJ, Chalhub EG. Occult group B streptococcal infection: an important cause of intrauterine asphyxia. Am J Obstet Gynecol 1983; 146:989.

Perlstein M, Hood P. Infantile spastic hemiplegia. Am J Med 1955; 34:391.

Pharoah POD, Cooke T, Cooke RWI, et al. Birthweight specific trends in cerebral palsy. Arch Dis Child 1990; 65:602.

Preakey A, Wilson J, Wilson B. Sensory and perceptual function in the cerebral palsied; III. Some visual perceptual relationships. J Nerv Ment Dis 1974; 158;70.

Rang M, Silver R, Garza J. Cerebral palsy. In: Lovell WW, Winter RB, eds. Pediatric orthopedics. Philadelphia: JB Lippincott, 1986.

Robinson R. The frequency of other handicaps in children with cerebral palsy. Dev Med Child Neurol 1973; 15:305.

Ruth VJ, Raivio KO. Perinatal brain damage: predictive value of metabolic acidosis and the Apgar score. Br Med J 1988; 297:24.

Scheidt PC, Bryla DA, Nelson KB, et al. NICHD phototherapy clinical trial: six year follow-up. Pediatrics 1990; 85:455.

Scherzer AL, Mike V, Ilson J. Physical therapy as a determinant of change in the cerebral palsied infant. Pediatrics 1976; 58:47.

Seidman DS, Paz I, Laor A, et al. Apgar scores and cognitive performance at 17 years of age. Obstet Gynecol 1991; 77:875.

Sever JL. TORCH tests and what they mean. Am J Obstet Gynecol 1985; 152:495.

Skatvedt M. Sensory, perceptual and other non-motor defects in cerebral palsy. Little Club Clin Dev Med 1960; 1:115.

Steer PJ. Premature labour. Arch Dis Child 1991; 66:1167.

Sussman MD. The use of casts as an adjunct to physical therapy management of cerebral palsy patients. Proceedings: Orthopedic aspects of developmental disabilities. School of Medicine, University of North Carolina, Chapel Hill, 1978:47.

Swaiman KF. Muscular tone. In: Swaiman KF, ed. Pediatric neurology: principles and practice. St. Louis: Mosby, 1989b; 196.

Szymonowicz W, Preston H, Yu VY. The surviving monozygotic twin. Arch Dis Child 1986; 61:454.

Uvebrant P. Hemiplegic cerebral palsy aetiology and outcome. Acta Paediatr Scand 1988; 345(suppl):5.

Vogt C, Vogt O. Zur psychiatrischen wurdingung der anatonschen entdeckung und wertung des status marmoratus striat. J Psychol Neurol 1928; 37:387.

Volpe JJ. Neurology of the newborn, 2nd ed. Philadelphia: WB Saunders, 1987.

Volpe JJ. Value of MR in definition of the neuropathology of cerebral palsy in vivo. Am J Neuroradiol 1992; 13:79.

Volpe JJ, Herscovitch P, Perlman JM, et al. Positron emission tomography in the asphyxiated term newborn: parasagittal impairment of cerebral blood flow. Ann Neurol 1985; 17:287.

Watt J, Sims D, Harchom F. A controlled study of inhibition casting as an adjunct to physiotherapy for cerebral-palsied children. Dev Med Child Neurol 1986; 28:480.

Weiss H, Betts HB. Methods of rehabilitation in children with neuromuscular disorders. Pediatr Clin North Am 1967; 14:1009.

Wiklund LM, Uvebrant P, Flodmark O. Computed tomography as an adjunct in etiological analysis of hemiplegic cerebral palsy. I: Children born preterm. Neuropediatrics 1991; 22:50.

Wilson ER, Mirra S, Schwartz JF. Congenital diencephalic and brain stem damage: neuropathologic study of three cases. Acta Neuropathol 1982; 57:70.

Wright T, Nicholson J. Physiotherapy for the spastic child and evaluation. Dev Med Child Neurol 1973; 15:146.

Yokochi K, Hosoe A, Shimabukuro S, et al. Gross motor patterns in children with cerebral palsy and spastic diplegia. Pediatr Neurol 1990; 6:245.

Yokochi K, Aiba K, Kodama M, et al. Magnetic resonance imaging in athetotic cerebral palsied children. Acta Paediatr Scand 1991; 80:818.

Young RR. Physiologic and pharmachologic approaches to spasticity. Neurol Clin 1987; 5:529.

28

Hypoxic-ischemic Cerebral Injury in the Newborn

Alan Hill and Joseph J. Volpe

Hypoxic-ischemic cerebral injury in the newborn is a major cause of mortality or long-term morbidity (e.g., cerebral palsy, mental retardation, and seizures) [Volpe, 1987; Hill 1991]. In this chapter, we discuss the clinical features, diagnostic techniques, pathogenesis, management, and prognostic features of hypoxic-ischemic cerebral injury in both premature and term newborns.

PATHOGENESIS

Hypoxic-ischemic cerebral injury in the newborn is caused by a combination of hypoxemia and ischemia that results in a decreased supply of oxygen to cerebral tissue. The term *hypoxic-ischemic* is preferred because the extent and significance of each individual insult is often difficult to determine precisely. In the context of perinatal asphyxia, hypercapnia and acidosis may contribute further to the cerebral insult [Volpe, 1987].

At a cellular and biochemical level, hypoxic-ischemic cerebral insult results in increased glycolysis, increased production of lactic acid, decreased production of high-energy phosphate compounds (e.g., adenosine triphosphate and phosphocreatine), accumulation of extracellular potassium and intracellular calcium, generation of injurious free radicals, as well as alterations in neurotransmitter and excitatory amino acid metabolism [Engelson, 1986; Johnston, 1983; Volpe, 1987; Hill, 1991]. The latter appear to be the critical final common pathway of hypoxic-ischemic neuronal injury [Hill, 1991; Volpe, 1987].

TIMING OF INSULT

In infants in whom hypoxic-ischemic cerebral injury develops the insult occurs most frequently during the antepartum or intrapartum periods [Volpe, 1987]. Two large epidemiologic studies (i.e., the National Collabo-

rative Perinatal Project [Freeman and Nelson, 1988; Nelson and Ellenberg, 1986] and the Western Australian Cerebral Palsy Register [Blair and Stanley, 1988]) suggest that the significance of antepartum events may have been underestimated previously. Thus in these studies, only approximately 10% to 15% of children with cerebral palsy had a history of severe intrapartum hypoxic-ischemic cerebral insult. Approximately one third of the children had at least one congenital anomaly involving another organ outside the CNS, which raises the possibility that an unrecognized insult earlier during gestation may have predisposed these infants to subsequent intrapartum hypoxic-ischemic insult.

CLINICAL FEATURES

Term newborns who sustain acute, intrapartum hypoxic-ischemic insult that is severe enough to result in long-term neurologic sequelae invariably demonstrate a recognizable clinical encephalopathy during the first days of life. Conversely, the absence of such encephalopathy does not support the diagnosis of significant intrapartum hypoxic-ischemic cerebral injury. It is important to realize that infants exposed to earlier intrauterine hypoxic-ischemic insult do not necessarily either sustain cerebral injury or display neurologic abnormalities during the neonatal period.

Although there is a complete spectrum of hypoxic-ischemic encephalopathy, it is often advantageous to classify the severity of encephalopathy as mild, moderate, or severe for purposes of accurate prognosis (Table 28-1) [Sarnat and Sarnat, 1976]. Clinical features of encephalopathy are more difficult to define in the premature newborn. It is important to emphasize that neurologic findings must be interpreted in the context of the stage of maturation of the immature brain at the time of insult.

Table 28-1 Correlation of severity of clinical abnormalities and outcome

Severity of encephalopathy	% with abnormal outcome
Mild	
Jitteriness, increased irritability and tendon reflexes, exaggerated Moro response	0
Moderate	
Lethargy, hypotonia, suppressed reflexes ± seizures	20-40
Severe	
Coma, hypotonia, seizures, brainstem, and autonomic dysfunction ± elevated intracranial pressure	100

±, With or without.
Based on Finer et al., 1981; Sarnat and Sarnat, 1976.

There is a recognizable progression of clinical features of acute, severe hypoxic-ischemic encephalopathy in the term newborn that is outlined in detail. Initially, during the first 12 hours, there is evidence of bilateral hemispheric dysfunction with decreased level of consciousness [Sarnat and Sarnat, 1976; Hill, 1991]. Subsequently, between 12 and 24 hours, there may be "apparent" improvement in the level of consciousness, which may be distinguished from genuine improvement by concomitant worsening of other aspects of cerebral function (e.g., seizures, apnea). Seizures, which are recognized in at least 50% of newborns with hypoxic-ischemic encephalopathy, denote moderate or severe encephalopathy. Infants with all degrees of encephalopathy may exhibit jitteriness, which may be misdiagnosed as seizures. Seizures usually begin on the first day of life and are often difficult to control with anticonvulsants.

Signs of brainstem dysfunction (e.g., impaired extraocular eye movements, abnormal pupillary responses, apnea and bulbar deficits) often worsen during the first 3 days of life and may result in respiratory arrest or death, most commonly at about 72 hours of age.

Increased intracranial pressure is uncommon and occurs only in severely asphyxiated term newborns. It is usually maximal between 24 and 96 hours of age. It may be diagnosed clinically by palpation of a tense anterior fontanel. Alternatively, quantitative measurements of intracranial pressure may be obtained by either a noninvasive technique, such as the Ladd intracranial pressure monitor, or invasive methods, such as the subarachnoid bolt [Levene and Evans, 1985; Levene et al., 1987; Lupton et al., 1988; Clancy et al., 1988b]. In a

study of 32 asphyxiated term newborns, we documented increased intracranial pressure in only seven infants, all of whom had severe encephalopathy and abnormal CT scans and who subsequently died or had severe neurologic abnormalities [Lupton et al., 1988]. Autopsy of infants who died demonstrated extensive cerebral necrosis. Similar findings have been reported in experimental models of neonatal hypoxic-ischemic injury in newborn rats [Muscje et al., 1987].

After 3 or 4 days, gradual improvement in neurologic status is usually observed during subsequent weeks. In severely affected infants, there are invariably persistent neurologic abnormalities that include diminished level of consciousness, feeding problems related to abnormalities of sucking and swallowing, and abnormal muscle tone [Hill, 1991; Volpe, 1987].

DIAGNOSIS
History and physical examination

The diagnosis of hypoxic-ischemic encephalopathy in the newborn is based principally on a detailed history and neurologic examination. The history should include details of complications of pregnancy, labor and delivery (e.g., results of electronic fetal heart rate monitoring, acid-base status of the fetus, Apgar scores, presence of meconium, and placental pathologic condition) that may support the notion that the intrapartum asphyxia was severe enough to explain the subsequent neonatal encephalopathy [Low, 1989; Schiffrin, 1989]. It is important to remember that the clinical features of neonatal encephalopathy are nonspecific and may occur after other types of insult (e.g., infection, metabolic derangements). Thus adjunctive studies may be required, such as EEG, evoked responses, neuroradiologic techniques, and biochemical parameters, such as CSF hypoxanthine and creatine kinase BB determinations.

Electrodiagnostic techniques

A characteristic sequence of EEG abnormalities may be observed after severe hypoxic-ischemic cerebral insult, especially in the term newborn [Holmes et al., 1982; Sarnat and Sarnat, 1976]. Initially there is marked suppression of amplitude and slowing of electrical activity that is followed within 24 to 48 hours by a discontinuous pattern characterized by marked voltage suppression, interposed with bursts of high-voltage sharp and slow waves. Because of the grave implications of this "burst suppression" pattern, care must be taken to distinguish it from normal variants, for example, the periodic EEG patterns of the premature infant and the normal trace alternant pattern observed during quiet sleep in the term newborn. During the few days after severe hypoxic-ischemic insult, the periodicity may become more pronounced and deteriorate further to an isoelectric recording. Conversely, rapid resolution of EEG abnormalities and/or a normal interictal EEG suggest a good prognosis [Sarnat and Sarnat, 1976; Werner et al., 1977]. In infants who have been paralyzed by neuromuscular blockers for the purpose of ventilatory management the diagnosis of frequent electrical seizures by continuous EEG monitoring permits early intervention with antiepileptic medications [Clancy et al., 1988a, b; Eyre et al., 1983; Goldberg et al., 1982]. It is not clear whether medical intervention is beneficial in electrical seizures without recognizable associated clinical accompaniments.

The value of other electrodiagnostic techniques — brainstem auditory-evoked potentials, visual-evoked potentials, and somatosensory-evoked potentials — for the assessment of hypoxic-ischemic brain injury is less well established. However, brainstem auditory evoked potentials may permit evaluation of the integrity of brainstem structures [Hakamada et al., 1981; Hecox and Cone, 1981; Stockard et al., 1983]. Preliminary studies with visual-evoked potentials [Hakamada et al., 1981; Hrbek et al., 1977; Whyte et al., 1986] and somatosensory-evoked potentials [Hrbek et al., 1977] demonstrate the potential value of these techniques. However, their routine clinical application has been limited in the newborn by technical difficulties.

Imaging techniques

Radionuclide scanning. The largest experience with technetium brain scanning is provided by the work of O'Brien et al. [1979]. Scans obtained 2 to 4 hours after radionuclide injection were abnormal in approximately 50% of 85 asphyxiated infants, reflecting disturbance of the blood-brain barrier. Distinct neuropathologic patterns of injury, including selective cortical necrosis, parasagittal injury [Volpe and Pasternak, 1977], focal cerebral injury, and periventricular leukomalacia, have been identified by means of technetium scanning. The development of new tracers that are able to cross the intact blood-brain barrier (e.g., single photon emission CT) has resulted in renewed interest in radionuclide scanning techniques [Denays et al., 1989]. The principle approach with single photon emission CT is to use tracers for the measurement of cerebral perfusion; areas of cerebral injury are marked by decreased radioactivity.

CT. In premature newborns the role of CT is limited to the documentation of hypoxic-ischemic brain injury. Thus cranial ultrasonography is considered the technique of choice for the diagnosis of germinal matrix/intraventricular hemorrhage, although other types of intracranial hemorrhage may be visualized better with CT (e.g., extradural, subdural, or subarachnoid hemorrhage). Fitzhardinge et al. [1981a] demonstrated a lack of correlation between parenchymal hypodensities on CT and outcome in 145 infants with birth weights less

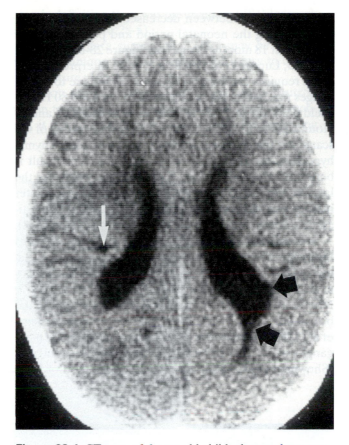

Figure 28-1 CT scan of 6-year-old child who was born prematurely and had spastic diplegia and visual impairment. Note the reduction in quantity of periventricular white matter posteriorly *(black arrows)* and the deep prominent sulci *(white arrow).*

than 1500 g, presumably as a result of the normally high water content of the premature brain. However, CT scans obtained later in infancy in infants born prematurely may demonstrate features of hypoxic-ischemic cerebral injury (e.g., periventricular leukomalacia) [Chow et al., 1985; Flodmark et al., 1987; Schellinger et al., 1984]. The characteristic abnormalities that are considered diagnostic of periventricular leukomalacia on CT scans performed during late infancy include (1) ventriculomegaly with irregular outline of the body and trigone of the lateral ventricles; (2) deep and prominent cortical sulci, which are directly adjacent to the ventricles without interposed white matter; and (3) reduction of quantity of periventricular white matter, particularly at the trigone [Flodmark et al., 1987] (Figure 28-1).

CT is of major importance for assessment of hypoxic-ischemic cerebral injury in the term newborn.* There is

---

* References Adsett et al., 1985; Clancy et al., 1985; Fitzhardinge et al., 1981b; Flodmark et al., 1980; Lipp-Zwahlen et al., 1985a; Lipp-Zwahlen et al., 1985b; Lupton et al., 1987; Mannino and Trauner, 1983; Naidich and Chakera, 1984; Pasternak, 1987.

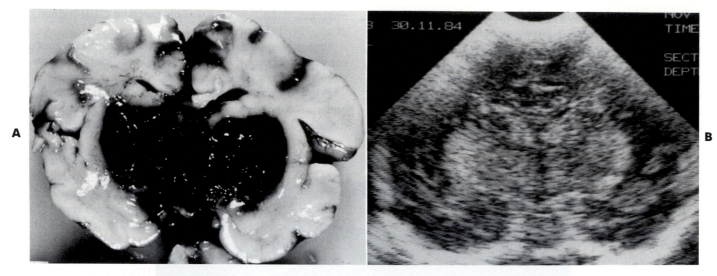

Figure 28-4 **A,** Coronal section of brain of term infant who died on the first postnatal day. Note hemorrhagic infarction in thalami and basal ganglia. **B,** Coronal cranial ultrasound scan at 1 day of age. Note increased echoes in region of thalami and basal ganglia.

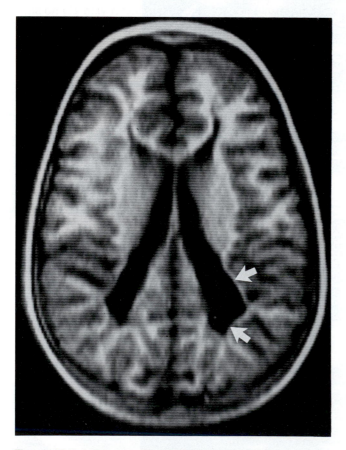

Figure 28-5 MRI scan (T_1 weighted image) of the patient shown in Figure 28-1, a 6-year-old child with spastic diplegia and visual impairment who was born prematurely. Note the decreased quantity of white matter posteriorly *(arrows)* and deep sulci.

regional cerebral perfusion and metabolism after intraventricular hemorrhage in premature infants [Volpe et al., 1983] and hypoxic-ischemic cerebral injury in term infants [Volpe et al., 1985].

Monitoring of intracranial pressure

Continuous or frequent serial measurements of intracranial pressure are of value for diagnosis of brain swelling in the severely asphyxiated term newborn [Hill and Volpe, 1981b; Hill, 1985; Lupton et al., 1988; Levene et al., 1987; Clancy et al., 1988] and in posthemorrhagic hydrocephalus in premature infants [Hill and Volpe, 1981c; Kreusser et al., 1985]. Recent data in both human newborns and experimental animals demonstrate a relative resistance to the development of cerebral edema in the immature brain [Lupton et al., 1988; Mujsce et al., 1987; Levene et al., 1987]. Severe CT abnormalities and increased intracranial pressure (maximum at 2 to 4 days) are associated with poor outcome. The temporal profile of elevated intracranial pressure and CT abnormalities suggest that the principal cause of clinically recognizable brain swelling is previous tissue necrosis. On the basis of these data, antiedema agents are unlikely to play a major role in the practical management of the asphyxiated term newborn [Muscje 1987; Levene et al., 1987; Lupton et al., 1988].

Biochemical markers

A variety of biochemical disturbances may accompany hypoxic-ischemic insult and contribute to the neurologic syndrome, including hypoglycemia, hypocalcemia, hyponatremia, hyperammonemia, and acidosis [Volpe, 1987]. Other metabolic derangements (e.g., elevated braintype isoenzyme of creatine kinase (CK-BB) [Walsh et al., 1982], hypoxanthine, aspartate aminotransferase, lactate, lactate dehydrogenase, hydroxybutyrate dehydrogenase, and fibrin-fibrinogen degradation products) produce identifiable enzymes or metabolites that may serve as "markers" of hypoxic-ischemic injury and permit rough quantification of the injury.

Cerebral blood flow

The circulatory abnormalities that occur after perinatal asphyxia include initial redistribution of cardiac output with increased regional and total cerebral blood flow and loss of cerebrovascular autoregulation. Subsequently there may be a decrease in cardiac output resulting in systemic hypotension which, in turn, results in decreased cerebral perfusion.

Evidence for impaired cerebrovascular autoregulation after perinatal asphyxia is provided by experimental human studies that demonstrate a pressure-passive relationship between systemic blood pressure and the cerebral circulation occurring after an even relatively mild hypoxic-ischemic cerebral injury [Lou et al., 1979a, 1979b; Barkovich, 1992].

NEUROPATHOLOGY AND CLINICOPATHOLOGIC CORRELATION

The patterns of clinical and neuropathologic abnormalities observed after neonatal hypoxic-ischemic cerebral injury are determined principally by the nature of the insult and by the gestational age of the affected infant. Thus the patterns of cerebral injury in term and premature infants are discussed separately (see box above right).

Term newborn

The clinicopathologic correlations of the major categories of hypoxic-ischemic cerebral injury are listed in Table 28-2.

Selective neuronal necrosis

Neuropathology. Selective neuronal necrosis, a common type of hypoxic-ischemic injury, involves principally the cerebral cortex (Sommer sector), cerebellar cortex (Purkinje cells), thalamus, brainstem, and anterior horn cells of the spinal cord.* The ability to recognize neuronal injury is influenced by the gestational age of the infant and by the length of survival after the insult. Prolonging survival by means of mechanical ventilation may result in cerebral autolysis, which obscures previous focal areas of cellular necrosis. The chronic neuropathologic changes include neuronal loss and astrocytosis that result in cerebral atrophy and multicystic encephalomalacia.

Our ability to define the precise extent of selective neuronal injury in the term newborn has improved with the use of imaging techniques, such as ultrasound, CT

Predominant Neuropathologic Patterns of Hypoxic-ischemic Cerebral Injury in the Newborn
Premature Newborn
Selective neuronal necrosis
Periventricular leukomalacia
Focal and multifocal ischemic cerebral necrosis
Periventricular hemorrhagic infarction
Term Newborn
Selective neuronal necrosis
Status marmoratus of basal ganglia and thalamus
Parasagittal cerebral injury
Focal and multifocal ischemic cerebral necrosis

(Figure 28-6), MRI [Johnson et al., 1987; McArdle et al., 1987b; Barkovich, 1992], and positron emission tomography [Volpe et al., 1985]. The pathogenesis of this pattern of injury relates in part to circulatory factors, with particular vulnerability of vascular border zones. Furthermore, it is postulated that the rapid rate of differentiation and metabolism of neurons in the thalamus and brainstem nuclei may account for the susceptibility of this area to injury. More recent experimental evidence strongly suggests that the topography of injury may relate to the anatomic distribution of glutamatergic nerve terminals [Hill, 1991; Greenamyre et al., 1987; Silverstein et al., 1986b].

Clinicopathologic correlation

Short-term effects. Injury to the cerebral hemispheres, reticular activating system, or both may result in a decreased level of consciousness. Seizures (subtle, tonic, or myoclonic) reflect injury to the cerebral cortex, diencephalic, or perhaps even midbrain structures. Abnormalities of muscle tone may reflect dysfunction of the cortex, cerebellum, or spinal cord. Direct brainstem injury may result in extraocular muscle dysfunction or disturbances of respiration, sucking, or swallowing [Hill and Volpe, 1981a]. Similar clinical features may represent corticobulbar dysfunction (i.e., pseudobulbar palsy).

Long-term effects. Long-term neurologic sequelae include varying degrees of intellectual impairment, motor deficits, and seizures (see Table 28-2). Intellectual handicap results principally from injury to the cerebral cortex. Motor deficits (cerebral palsy) may reflect injury at any level of the motor system including the cerebral cortex, subcortical white matter, midbrain, cerebellum,

---

* References Griffiths and Laurence, 1974; Grunnet et al., 1974; Hall, 1962, 1963; Leech and Alvord, 1977; Norman, 1972, 1974; Salford et al., 1973; Schneck and Neuberger, 1962; Schneider et al., 1975.

Table 28-2 Patterns of hypoxic-ischemic cerebral injury in the newborn: clinicopathologic correlation

Pattern	Topography	Neurologic features	
		Newborn	Long-term
Selective neuronal necrosis	Cerebral cortex, thalamus, reticular formation, brainstem nuclei	Diminished level of consciousness, seizures, hypotonia, cranial nerve dysfunction	Intellectual deficits, seizures, spastic quadriparesis, ataxia, bulbar and pseudobulbar palsy, attention deficits
Status marmoratus	Basal ganglia, cerebral cortex	Unknown	Choreoathetosis, spastic quadriparesis, intellectual impairment
Parasagittal injury	Parasagittal cerebral cortex/subcortical white matter—posterior more than anterior	Proximal limb weakness, upper more than lower	Spastic quadriparesis, intellectual impairments
Focal/multifocal injury	Cerebral cortex/subcortical white matter, usually in distribution of vascular territory	Hemiparesis, focal seizures	Spastic hemiparesis, focal seizures, intellectual deficits
Periventricular leukomalacia	Periventricular white matter (motor, optic, and acoustic radiation)	Unknown, perhaps lower limb weakness	Spastic diplegia, ± visual impairment, intellectual deficits
Periventricular hemorrhagic infarction	Unilateral periventricular white matter, often with intraventricular hemorrhage	Hypotonia	Hemiparesis, intellectual deficits, quadriplegia

±, With or without.

brainstem, and spinal cord. Seizures develop in approximately 10% to 30% of infants. Disorders of sucking and swallowing may reflect localized brainstem dysfunction that is associated with poor long-term survival [Roland et al., 1986b]. The anatomic substrate of attention-deficit disorders and hyperactivity may relate to injury involving the reticular activating system.

Status marmoratus of the basal ganglia and thalamus

Neuropathology. Status marmoratus of the basal ganglia and thalamus may be considered a variety of selective neuronal necrosis. The neuropathologic features include neuronal loss, gliosis, and hypermyelination, which occur principally in the basal ganglia and cerebral cortex and are associated with a marbled appearance of these regions [Friede, 1989; Malamud, 1950].

The pathogenesis of this pattern is now considered to correspond directly to the transient, extensive glutamatergic innervation of basal ganglia in the newborn [Greenamyre et al., 1987; Barks et al., 1988] and the rapid differentiation of neurons in this age group [Silverstein et al., 1986a, 1987]. Decreased uptake of glutamate has been documented after hypoxic-ischemic insult, which may relate to high dopamine levels that are released at the time of insult [Hill, 1991; Silverstein et al., 1986b].

Clinicopathologic correlation

The clinical features in the newborn are unknown. The long-term sequelae of status marmoratus include intellectual impairment, choreoathetosis, dystonia, and tremor [Malamud, 1950].

Parasagittal cerebral injury

Neuropathology. Parasagittal cerebral injury implies necrosis of the cerebral cortex and subcortical white matter located in the superomedial (parasagittal) regions of the cerebral convexities. The lesions are in watershed zones of blood supply located between the anterior, middle, and posterior cerebral arteries [Volpe, 1987; Hill, 1991]. Impaired cerebrovascular autoregulation may result in marked ischemia in these watershed zones, with only minor reduction of cerebral perfusion pressure [Lou et al., 1979a]. Although they are usually bilateral and symmetric, occasionally the lesions are asymmetric (Figure 28-7).

Clinicopathologic correlation. The clinical features of parasagittal injury in the newborn include hypotonia and weakness in the proximal limbs (greater in upper than in lower limbs). This specific pattern of weakness correlates with the anatomic location of the lesion in the motor cortex. This lesion has been recognized in newborns on technetium scans [O'Brien et al., 1979; Volpe and Pasternak, 1977] and more recently on CT [Pasternak, 1987], positron emission tomography scans

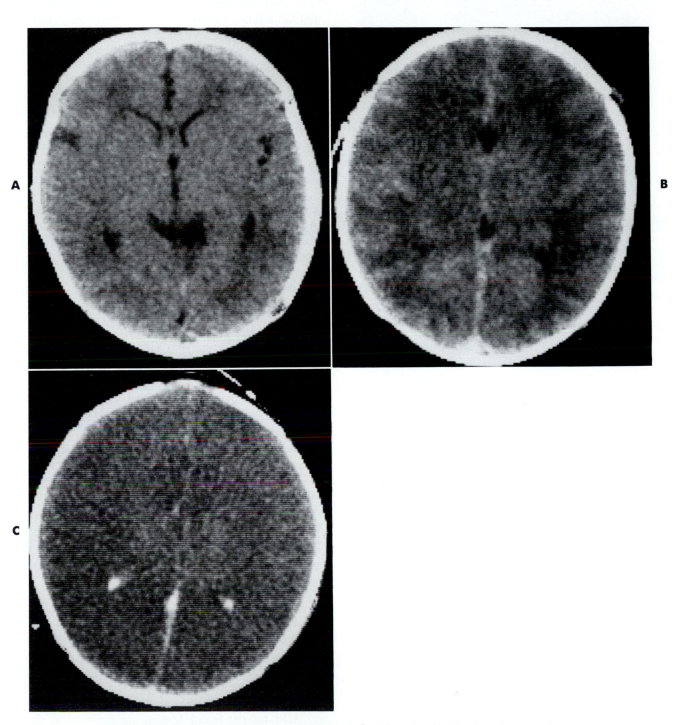

Figure 28-6 A, CT scan of a normal term newborn. Note the distribution of gray and white matter. **B,** CT scan of a moderately asphyxiated term newborn at 3 days of age. Note the patchy area of decreased attenuation, with extension of white matter hypodensities into cortex. **C,** CT scan of a severely asphyxiated term newborn at 3 days of age. Note the generalized decreased densities, with total loss of gray matter and white matter differentiation.

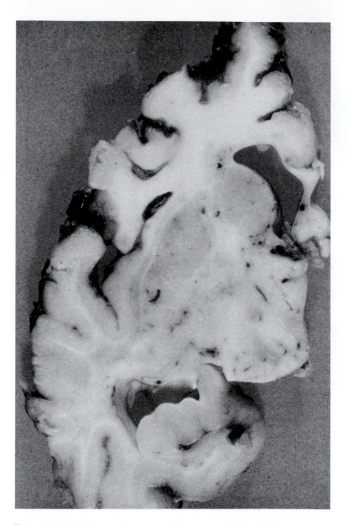

Figure 28-7 Coronal section of the hemisphere of a 6-month-old infant who had sustained perinatal hypoxic-ischemic insult at term. Note the cortical atrophy (pale area in parasagittal region).

[Volpe et al., 1985] and single photon emission CT scans [Denays et al., 1989].

The long-term sequelae of parasagittal necrosis almost certainly include spastic quadriparesis. In addition, specific deficits of language and visual/spatial perception may be a consequence of more posterior parasagittal injury.

Focal ischemic brain injury

Neuropathology. Focal necrosis is presumed to result from focal vascular occlusion. A review of 592 autopsies over a 4-year period by Barmada et al. [1979] suggests that 5.4% had arterial occlusion. More recent data suggest that focal brain injury may occur much more commonly than suspected previously and may occur in up to 15% to 20% of asphyxiated newborns [Hill, 1991]. In term newborns the territory of the middle cerebral artery is involved most commonly, and the cerebral infarction is usually extensive. The chronic lesion in-

volves cystic cavitation, which may or may not communicate with the lateral ventricles. There may be associated unilateral dilatation of the ventricle related to localized neuronal loss and cerebral atrophy [Nadich and Chakera, 1984; Raybaud, 1983; Schmitt, 1984]. The propensity for cystic cavitation of the necrotic lesions relates to the high water content [Suzuki, 1981], paucity of myelin, and poor astroglial response [Friede, 1989] of the immature brain. In addition to arterial occlusion, it has been demonstrated by MRI studies and by angiography that cortical venous thrombosis may result in focal cerebral injury [Wong et al., 1987; Konishi et al., 1987; Roland et al., 1990].

Thromboembolism is considered the most probable cause of focal brain injury because of the distribution of the lesions within vascular territories.* Possible sources of emboli include placental infarction, involuting placental vessels [Friede 1989; Larroche, 1977], and injured or catheterized vessels [Prian et al., 1978; Roessman and Miller, 1980; Yates, 1959]. Developmental abnormalities of cerebral vessels occurring early in gestation are considered less common causes [Myers, 1976; Stewart et al., 1978; Barmada et al., 1979]. Hematologic derangements may include polycythemia and other hypercoagulable states (e.g., antithrombin III or protein C deficiency) or isoimmune thrombocytopenia. Disseminated intravascular coagulation has been reported in as many as 60% of newborns with cerebral infarction [Barmada et al., 1979].

Interestingly, in many instances, it is not possible to document a specific vascular lesion. Furthermore, generalized systemic circulatory insufficiency, occurring either in utero or during the neonatal period, may result in focal infarction. In the absence of infection or dehydration, there often is no identifiable cause for venous thrombosis [Wong et al., 1987; Konishi et al., 1987).

Clinicopathologic correlation. Newborn infants with focal injury may be asymptomatic. Focal seizures may occur in infants with relatively large unilateral lesions. Hemiparesis may be recognized on the basis of decreased spontaneous movement or asymmetric Moro reflex. Because of the frequent involvement of the middle cerebral artery, more upper than lower limb weakness is present [Volpe, 1987].

The long-term clinical correlates relate to the extent of brain injury. Focal lesions may result in spastic hemiparesis, whereas multifocal lesions result more commonly in quadriparesis. When the lesion becomes cystic and communicates with the lateral ventricle, there

---

* References Aicardi et al., 1972; Amit and Camfield, 1980; Banker, 1961; Clark and Linnell, 1954; Cocker et al., 1965; Gross, 1945; Harvey and Alvord, 1972; Mannino and Trauner, 1983; Ment et al., 1984; Miller et al., 1981; Moore et al., 1969; Mueh et al., 1980; Norman, 1974.

may be progressive enlargement of the porencephalic cyst which, in turn, may produce progressive focal neurologic deficits. Surgical drainage may be required [Milhorat, 1978; Tardieu et al., 1981]. Involvement of cerebral cortex may be associated with intellectual impairment and seizures.

Premature infant

The high incidence of cardiorespiratory problems (related to hyaline membrane disease, patent ductus arteriosus, apnea, and bradycardia) combined with impaired cerebrovascular autoregulation and other postnatal disturbances predispose the premature infant to hypoxic-ischemic injury [Volpe, 1987]. The patterns of cerebral injury are summarized in Table 28-2.

Selective neuronal necrosis

Neuropathology

Diffuse neuronal necrosis. Diffuse neuronal necrosis after hypoxic-ischemic cerebral insult is recognized more commonly in term infants (see previous section). Neuronal injury in premature infants is more difficult to detect, principally because of the close packing of cortical neurons and the relative lack of Nissl substance [Volpe, 1987]. Neuronal injury usually progresses to neuronal necrosis, with microglial proliferation and the appearance of hypertrophic astrocytes.

Diencephalic neuronal necrosis. Infants who probably experienced hypoxic-ischemic cerebral insult during the third trimester may demonstrate neuronal injury restricted to the thalamus and brainstem [Parisi et al., 1983; Wilson et al., 1982]. Neurons of the hypothalamus and lateral geniculate bodies may also be affected. These lesions reflect transient, increased glutamatergic innervation in these regions [Hill, 1991; Silverstein et al., 1986b].

Pontosubicular necrosis. Premature infants who experience a period of hypoxia and acidosis followed by hyperoxia demonstrate a unique pattern of neuronal injury that involves primarily the pontine nuclei and the subiculum of the hippocampus [Barmada et al., 1980; Friede, 1989]. Lesions are most extensive in infants born between 26 and 36 weeks' gestation. It is unknown whether pontosubicular necrosis results from decreased cerebral blood flow resulting from hyperoxemia, from direct toxicity of high blood oxygen content, or from an unrelated factor (e.g., hypoglycemia).

Clinicopathologic correlation. Severely affected newborns may demonstrate decreased level of consciousness, seizures, impaired primitive reflexes, and abnormal brainstem function. Long-term sequelae include spastic quadriplegia, mental retardation, microcephaly, seizures, blindness, and deafness. Milder forms of diffuse injury may explain the learning disabilities and attention deficit disorders observed commonly in children who were born prematurely.

Periventricular leukomalacia

Neuropathology. Hypoxic-ischemic cerebral insult in the premature infant results in coagulation necrosis and infarction of periventricular white matter, which is a border-zone of arterial blood supply in the immature brain located between the ventriculofugal choroidal arteries and the ventriculopedal–penetrating branches of anterior, middle, and posterior cerebral arteries [Banker and Larroche, 1962; Dereuck et al., 1972; Leech and Alvord, 1974; Pape and Wigglesworth, 1979; Volpe, 1987; Takashima et al., 1978]. The two most common locations of periventricular leukomalacia are in the watershed regions in the posterior white matter involving the occipital radiations at the trigone of the lateral ventricles and, more anteriorly, in the white matter around the foramen of Monro [Shuman and Selednick, 1980]. In addition to the peculiar anatomic vascular factors and the intrinsic vulnerability of actively myelinating glia, other recognized pathogenetic factors include impaired cerebrovascular autoregulation and the limited vasodilatory capacity of the periventricular region of the premature brain when responding to hypoxic-ischemic insults. These insults cause increased substrate use by means of anaerobic glycolysis, which, especially in the periventricular region, may exceed substrate supplies. A role for endotoxin also has been suggested in the pathogenesis of perinatal telencephalic leukoencephalopathy, which most probably represents an early form of periventricular leukomalacia [Gilles et al., 1976, 1977]. Relative sparing of the cerebral cortex in the premature infant has been considered a consequence of the location of rich interarterial anastomoses among meningeal branches of the anterior, middle, and posterior arteries in the premature brain [Vander-Eecken, 1959]. Hemorrhage into areas of periventricular infarction occurs in approximately 25% of patients and often coexists with severe intraventricular hemorrhage [Armstrong and Norman, 1974].

The pathologic result of periventricular leukomalacia depends on the size of the lesion, which ranges from small areas of gliosis and reduction of myelin with ventricular dilatation in mild cases to multicystic encephalomalacia in more severe cases.

Clinicopathologic correlation. The neurologic manifestations of periventricular leukomalacia in the neonatal period have not been clearly defined. This lack of definition is partially related to difficulties in assessment caused by interference from complex life support systems and by concomitant occurrence of other forms of cerebral injury, such as intraventricular hemorrhage. However, in some instances, decrease of tone and muscle power in the lower extremities may be recognized.

Classic, long-term sequelae include motor handicap, usually spastic diplegia or quadriplegia, with greater involvement of the lower limbs [Bowerman et al., 1984;

Commey and Fitzhardinge, 1979; Hagberg et al., 1984; Larroche, 1977; McDonald, 1967]. These abnormalities relate to the anatomic location of the lesion. Fibers from the motor cortex that subserve lower limb function descend medially in the periventricular white matter in close proximity to the lateral ventricles. Severe lesions may cause upper limb dysfunction and intellectual deficits [McDonald, 1967]. Involvement of the optic radiations [Larroche, 1977] may result in visual impairment [Roland et al., 1986a].

Focal and multifocal ischemic brain necrosis

Neuropathology. Focal ischemic cerebral lesions associated with arterial occlusion are less common in premature than in term newborns. In the series by Barmada et al. [1979], no such lesions occurred in infants less than 28 weeks' gestation, and 5% of infants between 28 and 32 weeks' gestation and 10% of infants of 32 to 37 weeks' gestation had these lesions. Multiple, small, scattered infarcts resulting from occlusion of multiple small vessels are more common in premature infants.

Focal cerebral necrosis in premature infants most commonly results in cavitation, which may lead to porencephaly, hydranencephaly, or multicystic encephalomalacia [Manterola et al., 1966]. The factors that predispose to cavitation of the premature brain are similar to those discussed previously in the term infant.

Clinicopathologic correlation. Both short-term and long-term neurologic sequelae correspond to the ana-tomic location and extent of focal injury. Unilateral lesions may be demonstrated by unilateral decrease in spontaneous movements or by focal seizures. Long-term sequelae include hemiparesis, quadriplegia, mental retardation, and/or seizures.

Periventricular hemorrhagic infarction

Neuropathology. Hemorrhagic periventricular parenchymal injury occurs commonly in association with severe intraventricular hemorrhage in the premature infant. Hemorrhagic intracerebral lesions are usually unilateral and located dorsal and lateral to the lateral ventricles in 15% to 25% of patients [Dolfin et al., 1984; Dubowitz et al., 1985; Guzzetta et al., 1986; Levene et al., 1983; McMenamin et al., 1984; Nwaesei et al., 1984]. Neuropathologic observations and positron emission tomography scanning data [Volpe et al., 1983] suggest that the intracerebral hemorrhagic component is part of a more widespread ischemic lesion of periventricular white matter and therefore should be regarded as hemorrhagic infarction, most probably of venous origin. Venous infarction may result from obstruction of the medullary and terminal veins by large subependymal germinal matrix hemorrhage [Guzetta et al., 1986; Volpe, 1987; Volpe 1989]. Figure 28-8 demonstrates both hemorrhagic and ischemic lesions in the premature infant.

Clinicopathologic correlation. The short-term and long-term clinical correlates of hemorrhagic intracere-

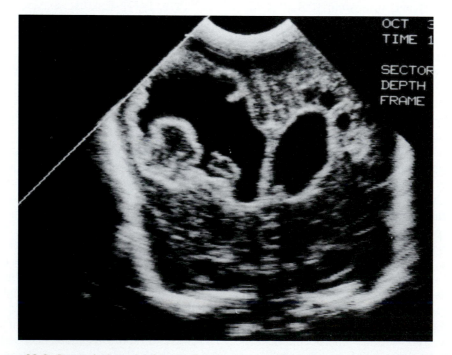

Figure 28-8 Coronal ultrasound scan of a premature infant after hypoxic-ischemic insult. Note the resolving intraventricular hemorrhage (clot in right lateral ventricle), the porencephalic cyst on the right, the cystic periventricular leukomalacia on the left, and the ventriculomegaly.

bral involvement associated with intraventricular hemorrhage are similar to clinical features observed with other focal ischemic lesions in the premature infant [Guzzetta et al., 1986; Levene et al., 1983; McMenamin et al., 1984]. In addition, there may be associated posthemorrhagic ventriculomegaly or hydrocephalus, which may require ventriculoperitoneal shunting [Guzzetta et al., 1986; McMenamin et al., 1984; Volpe, 1987]. Neurologic outcome correlates more closely with the extent of the ischemic cerebral injury than with the size of the intracerebral hemorrhage.

MANAGEMENT

Infants with hypoxic-ischemic encephalopathy, especially if severe, frequently have dysfunction of multiple organs, including heart, lungs, kidneys, and liver. Although the diagnosis and intervention are clearly important, specific management of these problems is not covered in this section. Discussion is limited to prevention and supportive care of CNS involvement.

Prevention

In the majority of infants with hypoxic-ischemic encephalopathy the primary insult originates in utero. Thus prevention of intrauterine asphyxia is of major importance, which is accomplished by recognition of maternal risk factors and close monitoring of the high-risk fetus during labor and delivery [Volpe, 1987; Low et al., 1984].

Supportive care

Maintenance of adequate ventilation. The importance of adequate ventilation and cerebral perfusion cannot be overemphasized. Although the primary hypoxic-ischemic cerebral insult often occurs before delivery, affected infants are especially vulnerable to additional insult. Recent studies have demonstrated that hypoxemia may be associated with a variety of normal activities and standard management techniques in the premature infant (Long et al., 1979, 1980; Lou et al., 1979a). Conversely, hyperoxemia should be avoided because of the possible association with retinopathy of prematurity, pontosubicular necrosis [Barmada et al., 1980], and vasoobliterative cerebral changes [Hannah and Hannah, 1980; Kennedy et al., 1971]. Increased cerebral perfusion may provoke intraventricular hemorrhage.

Maintenance of adequate cerebral perfusion. Impairment of cerebrovascular autoregulation and the presence of a pressure-passive relationship between systemic blood pressure and cerebral blood flow emphasizes the importance of avoiding systemic hypotension [Lou et al., 1979a, 1979b]. Values for normal blood pressure in the newborn have been reported [Versmold et al., 1981]. Decreased cerebral perfusion may result

from patent ductus arteriosus, with possible steal from the cerebral circulation [Lipman et al., 1982; Martin et al., 1982; Perlman et al., 1981]. In addition, apneic episodes associated with bradycardia have been demonstrated to cause a decrease in cerebral blood flow velocity [Perlman and Volpe, 1985]. Conversely, systemic hypertension should be avoided to decrease the likelihood of intracranial hemorrhage.

Polycythemia occurs commonly in the newborn [Black and Lubchenco, 1982; Hathaway, 1983] and relates rarely to cerebral infarction [Amit and Camfield, 1980; Black et al., 1985; Hathaway, 1983]; thus careful surveillance and treatment of increased hematocrit are indicated.

Maintenance of adequate blood glucose. The optimal blood glucose level to be achieved at the time of hypoxic-ischemic cerebral insult is controversial. Data are available that suggest both a beneficial and a detrimental effect of hyperglycemia at the time of insult [Ginsberg et al., 1980; Myers, 1976; Plum, 1983; Pulsinelli et al., 1982, 1985; Rehncrona et al., 1980, 1981; Vannucci et al., 1985]. Data in neonatal animals generally indicate a beneficial effect from glucose administration [Vannucci et al., 1985; Holowach-Thurston et al., 1973, 1974]. The beneficial effect may relate to maintenance of cerebral glucose and adenosine triphosphate concentrations. The detrimental effect may relate to excessive accumulation of lactic acid (secondary to tissue injury). Our current practice is to maintain normoglycemia.

There is increasing experimental evidence that even relatively moderate levels of hypoglycemia may be associated with neurologic impairment [Lucas et al., 1988].

Control of seizures. Seizures occur commonly after hypoxic-ischemic cerebral injury, especially in the term infant. Vigorous treatment is recommended because of the potential for additional brain injury [Soderfield et al., 1981]. Seizures may compromise ventilation and result in increased systemic blood pressure, with increased cerebral perfusion [Gado et al., 1976; Kuhl et al., 1980; Perlman and Volpe, 1983; Perlman et al., 1985] related to impaired cerebrovascular autoregulation [Howse et al., 1974; Kreisman et al., 1983; Plum et al., 1968], which may cause intraventricular hemorrhage, hemorrhagic infarction, or both. Furthermore, seizures may result in exhaustion of cerebral glucose and high-energy phosphate compounds, accumulation of excitotoxic amino acids, or both. Experimental studies have demonstrated that seizures result in a decrease in brain protein, cholesterol, deoxyribonucleic acid, ribonucleic acid, and cell content [Wasterlain and Vert, 1990; Younkin et al., 1985].

Antiepileptic treatment should begin with phenobarbital in a loading dose of 20 mg/kg administered intravenously. If seizures persist, an additional dose of 5 to 20 mg/kg is given intravenously in 5 mg/kg aliquots every 5 min, for a total dose of 40 mg/kg if necessary. The use of phenobarbital in this manner has been demonstrated to control seizures in 88% of infants [Gal et al., 1984]. Careful monitoring of cardiorespiratory function is essential. When seizures persist, phenytoin is used in a dose of 20 mg/kg intravenously (given slowly in 10-mg/kg doses) [Volpe, 1987]. Cardiac function should be monitored carefully during administration of this drug because of its potential to cause cardiac arrhythmias. Other antiepileptic medications, such as paraldehyde, diazepam, primidone, and lorazepam, have not been used consistently.

The maintenance dose of both phenobarbital and phenytoin is approximately 3 to 4 mg/kg per day. Although phenobarbital can be given orally, phenytoin should be administered intravenously because of its variable bioavailability when used orally and the propensity to precipitate in muscle when administered intramuscularly. Because of increasing rates of drug elimination in the first weeks of life, blood levels should be monitored frequently and drug doses adjusted appropriately.

The duration of antiepileptic therapy is governed by the likelihood of seizure recurrence. Factors such as the severity of hypoxic-ischemic encephalopathy and the persistence of neurologic and EEG abnormalities assist with decisions concerning duration of treatment [Volpe, 1987]. It is important to aim for brief durations of therapy.

Control of brain swelling. The management of brain swelling in the neonatal period is controversial [Lupton et al., 1988; Volpe, 1987]. However, avoidance of fluid overload appears appropriate in the asphyxiated term infant. Careful surveillance of serum electrolytes, osmolality, urine output, and body weight is important. Current data on the human newborn do not provide convincing evidence that the use of antiedema agents (e.g., glucocorticoids, hyperosmolar agents, and hyperventilation) improves ultimate neurologic outcome [Lupton et al., 1988; Levene and Evans, 1985; Levene et al., 1987; Whitelaw, 1989].

Other methods of brain preservation. Various experimental methods of brain preservation are currently under investigation, such as barbiturates [Goldberg et al., 1986; Vannucci, 1990; Hill, 1991], glutamate receptor antagonists [Germono et al., 1989; Silverstein et al., 1986a; Gunn et al., 1989], opiate antagonists (e.g., naloxone) [Baskin et al., 1982; Chernick and Craig, 1982; Fallis et al., 1983; Faden, 1984; Young et al., 1984; Zambramski et al., 1984], phenytoin [Artu and Michenfelder, 1980], free radical scavengers and inhibitors (e.g., indomethacin, allopurinol) [Hallenbeck et al., 1982; Rosenberg et al., 1989; Sasaki et al., 1988; Martz et al., 1989], and hypothermia [Cordey et al., 1983].

Principal research interest has focused on calcium channel blockers and excitatory amino acid antagonists. Thus high levels of cytosolic calcium lead to a wide variety of deleterious metabolic events, including particular generation of toxic free radicals. Preliminary results in animals suggest that at least pretreatment with calcium channel blockers (e.g., flunarizine and nifedipine) may be effective for reduction of hypoxic-ischemic cerebral injury [Germano et al., 1989; Silverstein et al., 1986a; Gunn et al., 1989]. The efficacy of treatment with such agents after the insult has occurred is not clear. There is increasing experimental evidence to suggest that the use of excitatory amino acid antagonists (e.g., phencyclidine, dextromethorphan, ketamine, MK-801) may be useful for reduction of hypoxic-ischemic cerebral injury [Albers et al., 1989; Hill, 1991; McDonald et al., 1989a, 1989b; Hattori et al., 1989; Vannucci, 1990]. There are insufficient data for human infants. Currently the benefit of none of the experimental methods outlined above has been proved sufficiently to warrant recommendation for routine clinical use in the asphyxiated newborn [Volpe, 1987; Hill, 1991; Vannucci, 1990].

PROGNOSIS

An accurate prognosis after hypoxic-ischemic encephalopathy is difficult to determine because of the

---

Useful Prognostic Factors in Hypoxic-ischemic Encephalopathy

Electronic fetal heart monitoring—late decelerations, prolonged bradycardia
Fetal blood gas sampling/cord pH
Low extended Apgar scores <5 at 5 minutes
Thick meconium
Neonatal neurologic syndrome
  Moderate/severe
  Occurrence of seizures
  Duration more than 1 week
  Systemic abnormalities
Abnormal neurophysiologic parameters
  EEG
  Evoked responses
  Magnetic spectrophotometry
Neuroimaging data
  Radionuclide studies—technetium, single photon emission CT
  Cranial ultrasonography
  CT
  MRI
Cerebral blood flow studies
  Doppler, positron emission tomography
  Near-infrared spectroscopy
Biochemical derangements (e.g., creatine kinase BB, hypoxanthine)

inability to establish precisely the extent and location of the cerebral insult and injury. Useful prognostic factors are listed in the box on p. 502. During recent years, there has been an overall improvement in outcome [Brown et al., 1974; Brown, 1976; DeSouza and Richards, 1978; Finer et al., 1981, 1983; 1985a, 1985b; Mulligan et al., 1980; Robertson and Finer, 1985; Robertson and Grace, 1992]. Because most insults appear to occur before delivery, electronic fetal monitoring and fetal blood gas sampling may be useful [Low et al., 1985b, Low, 1989; Niswander et al., 1984; Volpe, 1987]. The value of Apgar scores, which have been used traditionally for immediate postpartum assessment and prognosis, is limited by observer variability, the effects of maternal drugs, and the reversible stress of delivery. The National Collaborative Perinatal Project has demonstrated the value of extended Apgar scores. Apgar scores between 0 and 3 at 10, 15, and 20 minutes have been associated with mortality rates of 18%, 48%, and 59%, respectively. The morbidity of the group studied (percentage with cerebral palsy in survivors in whom the outcome was known) was 5%, 9%, and 59%, respectively [Nelson and Ellenberg, 1981, 1984, 1986; Freeman and Nelson, 1988].

The most useful prognostic factors relate to the severity and duration of hypoxic-ischemic encephalopathy. Four major studies, which involved principally term infants, provided useful data regarding prognosis [Brown et al., 1974; DeSouza and Richards, 1978; Finer et al., 1981; Sarnat and Sarnat, 1976]. Over a period of 15 years we have not yet observed a child with documented perinatal asphyxia who had no neonatal neurologic syndrome and subsequently developed major neurologic sequelae. Specific aspects of the clinical neurologic syndrome that may be particularly useful are the severity of the syndrome, the occurrence of seizures, and the duration of the syndrome. Robertson and Finer [1985] have demonstrated that, with respect to the severity of the neonatal syndrome, infants with only mild encephalopathy experienced no sequelae, whereas infants with severe encephalopathy experienced neurologic sequelae or died. The overall incidence of sequelae at 3½ years of age was 17% in this study. Our own observations are consistent with these data [Lupton et al., 1988]. More recent data on follow-up of the above cohort of infants at 5 years of age revealed that more than 40% of infants with moderate encephalopathy had *school-readiness* delay [Robertson and Grace, 1992].

The likelihood of neurologic sequelae is increased twofold to fivefold when there are neonatal seizures [Brown, 1974; Finer et al., 1981, 1983; Robertson and Finer, 1985; Sarnat and Sarnat, 1976]. Seizures that occur early, are difficult to control, or both are generally associated with a poorer prognosis.

The relationship between duration of encephalopathy and outcome has been clearly demonstrated. Infants in whom the neurologic examination was normal at discharge had normal outcomes [Robertson and Finer 1985; Sarnat and Sarnat, 1976; Robertson and Grace, 1992]. Our experience is similar.

As an adjunct to careful neurologic assessment, EEG and imaging techniques discussed previously may assist with prognosis, especially in the term infant. CT scans demonstrate a relationship between the extent of areas of decreased tissue attenuation and poor outcome [Adsett et al., 1985; Fitzhardinge et al., 1981b; Flodmark et al., 1980, 1987; Lipp-Zwahlen et al., 1985a, 1985b; Lupton et al., 1988; Barkovich, 1992]. In the premature infant the interpretation of changes in attenuation is more difficult. Ultrasound scanning may demonstrate hemorrhagic lesions or focal ischemic lesions.

REFERENCES

Adsett DB, Fitz CR, Hill A. Hypoxic-ischemic cerebral injury in the term newborn: correlation of CT findings with neurological outcome. Dev Med Child Neurol 1985; 27:155.

Aicardi J, Goutieres F, de Verbois AH. Multicystic encephalomalacia of infants and its relation to abnormal gestation and hydranencephaly. J Neurol Sci 1972; 15:357.

Albers G, Goldberg MP, Choi DW. *N*-methyl-D-aspartate antagonists: ready for a clinical trial in brain ischemia? Ann Neurol 1989; 25:398.

Amit M, Camfield P. Neonatal polycythmia causing multiple cerebral infarcts. Arch Neurol 1980; 37:109.

Armstrong D, Norman MG. Periventricular leukomalacia in neonates: complications and sequelae. Arch Dis Child 1974; 49:367.

Artru AA, Michenfelder JD. Cerebral protective, metabolic and vascular effects of phenytoin. Stroke 1980; 11:377.

Babcock DS, Ball W Jr. Postasphyxial encephalopathy in full-term infants: ultrasound diagnosis. Radiology 1983; 148:417.

Banker BQ. Cerebral vascular disease in infancy and childhood. I. Occlusive vascular disease. J Neuropathol Exp Neurol 1961; 20:127.

Banker BQ, Larroche JC. Periventricular leukomalacia of infancy. Arch Neurol 1962; 7:386.

Barkovich AJ. MR and CT abnormalities in newborn and infantile asphyxia. AJNR Am J Neuroradiol 1992; 13:959.

Barks JD, Silverstein FS, Simms K, et al. Glutamate recognition sites in human fetal brain. Neurosci Lett 1988; 84:131.

Barmada MA, Moosy J, Painter M. Pontosubicular necrosis and hyperoxema. Pediatrics 1980; 66:840.

Barmada MA, Moosy J, Shuman RM. Cerebral infarcts with arterial occlusion in neonates. Ann Neurol 1979; 6:495.

Baskin DS, Kieck CF, Hosobuchi Y. Naloxone reversal of ischemic neurologic deficits in baboons is not mediated by systemic effects. Life Sci 1982; 31:2201.

Black VD, Lubchenco LO. Neonatal polycythemia and hyperviscosity. Pediatr Clin North Am 1982; 29:1137.

Black VD, Lubchenco LO, Koops BL, et al. Neonatal hyperviscosity: randomized study of effect of partial plasma exchange transfusion on long-term outcome. Pediatrics 1985; 75:1048.

Blair E, Stanley FJ. Intrapartum asphyxia: a rare cause of cerebral palsy. J Pediatr 1988; 112:515.

Bowerman RA, Donn SM, DiPietro MA, et al. Periventricular leukomalacia in the pre-term newborn infant: sonographic and clinical features. Radiology 1984; 151:383.

Brown JK. Infants damaged during birth—perinatal asphyxia. In: Hull D, ed. Recent advances in pediatrics. London: Churchill Livingstone, 1976.

autonomous in the genesis of seizures and may develop characteristic histologic and biochemical changes. Clusters of neurons may become epileptogenetically unstable because of either disinhibition or denervation hypersensitivity to neurotransmitters. Propagation of an abnormal discharge, which can be detected by electrodiagnostic means from the depth or surface of the brain, results in a concomitant clinical seizure. Abnormal polarization at the immediate site and surrounding area of the focus is partially linked to changes in extracellular potassium concentration. Although the neuron undoubtedly plays the major role in this mechanism, the control that glial cells exert over extracellular potassium ion concentration is probably a factor in the focal abnormality.

Developing a focus of epileptic activity leads to the possibility of kindling. Kindling is the development of spontaneous epilepsy after the delivery of repeated subconvulsive stimuli. Kindling occurs in experimental situations, but its human counterpart has not been defined.

Experimentally, applying subepileptic electrical or chemical stimulation ultimately results in the development of an afterdischarge; seizures that ultimately become autonomous are the result of repeated stimulation. It appears that the substantia nigra can regulate the threshold of motor seizures in the kindling model because, in one study, gamma-aminobutyric acid (GABA) agonists injected into this region suppressed kindled motor and limbic seizures [McNamara et al., 1984]. Continuing subclinical focal seizure activity is probably an epileptogenic factor in kindling when considering its induction experimentally, and such activity may account for the intractability that develops in situations when repetitive focal discharges persist. An epileptic discharge may evoke an inhibitory response through hyperpolarization occurring at the site. This response may result from inhibitory interneurons discharged by an axonal-spike discharge [Prince, 1985]. This hyperpolarization may account for the partial discharge that remains localized by promoting a limitation of the activity spread into adjacent brain areas. Todd paralysis is a focal, postictal paralysis resulting from either enhanced focal inhibitory activity or neuronal absorption, and it frequently follows partial seizures.

CLASSIFICATION OF PARTIAL SEIZURES

Two general schemes of classification of seizures and epilepsy are presented in the boxes on pp. 511 to 514. The current official classification of seizures was created by the International League Against Epilepsy Commission on Classification, 1981. Common classification and use standardization allow individual investigators to utilize the same terms for the same seizure phenomena. These practices also make it possible to recognize underlying pathologic and physiologic alterations and common characteristics among seizure types. Unfortunately, phenomenologic descriptions, although extremely helpful in accurately classifying outward manifestations, do not indicate that similar underlying pathophysiologic mechanisms exist. Furthermore, seizures that outwardly manifest differently may not be pathophysiologically separate.

It cannot be sufficiently stressed that seizures classified in the same category by generally accepted standards may be associated with different anatomic substrates, pathogenetic causes, and mechanisms of propagation. One classification of focal (partial) seizures is illustrated in the box on p. 515.

Simple partial seizures

With motor signs. Any body part may be activated during partial seizure activity; the anatomic location within the motor strip in which the abnormal discharge occurs is the determining factor. There is disproportionate representation of the tongue, lips, and hands (particularly the thumbs and forefingers) in the motor strip, thus enhancing the likelihood that focal seizures will affect these areas [Penfeld and Jasper, 1954].

Although partial motor seizures may remain localized, they may be disseminated to adjacent subcortical and cortical areas, resulting in sequential motor movements of body parts. Body parts are often initially involved distally and then more proximal portions are involved in an epileptic march; this phenomenon is a Jacksonian seizure.

Adversive seizures are focal motor phenomena during which the eyes and head are turned to the contralateral side in relation to the discharging cortical focus. At times the patient may be forced to gaze at the hand contralateral to the discharging hemispheral focus; furthermore, the hand may be tonically raised concurrently with the adversive movements of the eyes and head. These seizures probably originate in the supplementary motor strip. In another variation the patient experiences a hallucination in the contralateral visual field, then the head and eyes move in that direction. Such seizures originate in a temporal lobe focus. Although not explained, several patients report the abortion or termination of an epileptic seizure by engaging in volitional forced thinking or by placing concerted pressure on the limb proximal to the area of clonic movement. The terminated or aborted seizure is often followed by Todd paralysis.

With special sensory or somatosensory symptoms. The homunculus of sensory distribution within the cortex is similar to the motor homunculus. Somatosensory seizures originate from these sensory cortical areas, primarily in the region of the postcentral gyrus.

Partial sensory seizures can take many forms and are

International Classification of Seizure Disorders

I. Partial (focal, local) seizures

Partial seizures are those in which, in general, the first clinical and EEG changes indicate initial activation of a system of neurons limited to part of one cerebral hemisphere. A partial seizure is classified primarily on the basis of whether or not consciousness is impaired during the attack. When consciousness is not impaired, the seizure is classified as a simple partial seizure. When consciousness is impaired, the seizure is classified as a complex partial seizure. Impairment of consciousness may be the first clinical sign, or simple partial seizures may evolve into complex partial seizures. In patients with impaired consciousness, aberrations of behavior (automatisms) may occur. A partial seizure may not terminate, but instead progress to a generalized motor seizure. Impaired consciousness is defined as the inability to respond normally to exogenous stimuli by virtue of altered awareness and/or responsiveness.

There is considerable evidence that simple partial seizures usually have unilateral hemispheric involvement and only rarely have bilateral hemispheric involvement; complex partial seizures, however, frequently have bilateral hemispheric involvement.

Partial seizures can be classified into one of the following three fundamental groups:
A. Simple partial seizures
B. Complex partial seizures
    1. With impairment of consciousness at onset
    2. Simple partial onset followed by impairment of consciousness
C. Partial seizures evolving to generalized tonic-clonic convulsions
    1. Simple evolving to generalized tonic-clonic convulsions
    2. Complex evolving to generalized tonic-clonic convulsions (including those with simple partial onset)

Clinical seizure type	EEG seizure type	EEG interictal expression
A. *Simple partial seizures* (consciousness not impaired)	Local contralateral discharge starting over the corresponding area of cortical representation (not always recorded on the scalp)	Local contralateral discharge

    1. With motor signs
       a. Focal motor without march
       b. Focal motor with march (jacksonian)
       c. Versive
       d. Postural
       e. Phonatory (vocalization or arrest of speech)
    2. With somatosensory or special-sensory symptoms (simple hallucinations, e.g., tingling, light flashes, buzzing)
       a. Somatosensory
       b. Visual
       c. Auditory
       d. Olfactory
       e. Gustatory
       f. Vertiginous
    3. With autonomic symptoms or signs (including epigastric sensation, pallor, sweating, flushing, piloerection, and pupillary dilatation)
    4. With psychic symptoms (disturbance of higher cerebral function). These symptoms rarely occur without impairment of consciousness and are much more commonly experienced as complex partial seizures
       a. Dysphasic
       b. Dysmnesic (e.g., déjà-vu)
       c. Cognitive (e.g., dreamy states, distortions of time sense)
       d. Affective (fear, anger, etc.)
       e. Illusions (e.g., macropsia)
       f. Structured hallucinations (e.g., music, scenes)

International Classification of Seizure Disorders—cont'd

Clinical seizure type	EEG seizure type	EEG interictal expression
B. *Complex partial seizures* (with impairment of consciousness; may sometimes begin with simple symptomatology)	Unilateral or, frequently bilateral discharge, diffuse or focal in temporal or frontotemporal regions	Unilateral or bilateral generally asynchronous focus; usually in the temporal or frontal regions
1. Simple partial onset followed by impairment of consciousness		
a. With simple partial features (A1–A4 above) followed by impaired consciousness		
b. With automatisms		
2. With impairment of consciousness at onset		
a. With impairment of consciousness only		
b. With automatisms		
C. *Partial seizures evolving to secondarily generalized seizures* (this may be generalized tonic-clonic, tonic, or clonic)	Above discharges become secondarily and rapidly generalized	
1. Simple partial seizures (A) evolving to generalized seizures		
2. Complex partial seizures (B) evolving to generalized seizures		
3. Simple partial seizures evolving to complex partial seizures evolving to generalized seizures		

II. Generalized seizures (convulsive or nonconvulsive)

Generalized seizures are those in which the first clinical changes indicate initial involvement of both hemispheres. Consciousness may be impaired and this impairment may be the initial manifestation. Motor manifestations are bilateral. The ictal EEG patterns initially are bilateral and presumably reflect neuronal discharge, which is widespread in both hemispheres.

Clinical seizure type	EEG seizure type	EEG interictal expression

A. 1. *Absence seizures*
  a. Impairment of consciousness only
  b. With mild clonic components
  c. With atonic components
  d. With tonic components
  e. With automatisms
  f. With autonomic components
  (b through f may be used alone or in combination)
	Usually regular and symmetric 3 Hz but may be 2 to 4 Hz spike-and-slow-wave complexes and may have multiple spike-and-slow-wave complexes. Abnormalities are bilateral.	Background activity usually normal although paroxysmal activity (such as spikes or spike-and-slow-wave complexes) may occur. This activity is usually regular and symmetric.

International Classification of Seizure Disorders—cont'd

2. *Atypical absence* May have: a. Changes in tone that are more pronounced than in A1 (above) b. Onset and/or cessation that is not abrupt	EEG more heterogeneous; may include irregular spike-and-slow-wave complexes, fast activity, or other paroxysmal activity. Abnormalities are bilateral but often irregular and asymmetric.	Background usually abnormal; paroxysmal activity (such as spikes or spike-and-slow-wave complexes) frequently irregular and asymmetric.
B. *Myoclonic seizures* Myoclonic jerks (single or multiple)	Polyspike-and-wave, or sometimes spike-and-wave or sharp and slow waves	Same as ictal
C. *Clonic seizures*	Fast activity (10 c/sec or more) and slow waves; occasional spike-and-wave patterns	Spike-and-wave or polyspike-and-wave discharges
D. *Tonic seizures*	Low-voltage, fast activity or a fast rhythm of 9 to 10 c/sec or more decreasing in frequency and increasing in amplitude	More or less rhythmic discharges of sharp-and-slow waves, sometimes asymmetric; background is often abnormal for age
E. *Tonic-clonic seizures*	Rhythm at 10 or more c/sec decreasing in frequency and increasing in amplitude during tonic phase, interrupted by slow waves during clonic phase	Polyspike-and-waves or spike-and-wave, or, sometimes, sharp-and-slow-wave discharges
F. *Atonic seizures* (Astatic) (combinations of the above may occur (e.g., B and F, B and D)	Polyspikes-and-wave or flattening or low-voltage fast activity	Polyspike and slow wave

III. Unclassified epileptic seizures

Includes all seizures that cannot be classified because of inadequate or incomplete data and some that defy classification in hitherto described categories. This includes some neonatal seizures: for example, rhythmic eye movements, chewing, and swimming movements.

IV. Addendum

Repeated epileptic seizures occur under a variety of circumstances:

1. As fortuitous attacks, coming unexpectedly and without any apparent provocation; 2. as cyclic attacks, at more or less regular intervals (e.g., in relation to the menstrual cycle, or the sleep-waking cycle); 3. as attacks provoked by: (a) nonsensory factors (fatigue, alcohol, emotion, etc.), or (b) sensory factors, sometimes referred to as "reflex seizures."

Prolonged or repetitive seizures (status epilepticus). The term "status epilepticus" is used whenever a seizure persists for a sufficient length of time or is repeated frequently enough that recovery between attacks does not occur. Status epilepticus may be divided into partial (e.g., jacksonian), or generalized (e.g., absence status or tonic-clonic status). When very localized motor status occurs, it is referred to as epilepsia partialis continua.

Modified from International League Against Epilepsy. Epilepsia 1981; 22:489.

often unaccompanied by concomitant motor phenomena. The patient may describe numbness or dysesthesias, such as a pins-and-needles sensation in the body part. Less frequently, abnormalities of proprioception that interfere with the appreciation of spatial position of the arms or legs may occur. A sensory epileptic march, analogous to a motor seizure march, usually begins in the distal limb and spreads proximally. Such sensory seizures involving the arms may propagate to the face or to the leg on the ipsilateral side. Partial sensory seizures may

---

Proposed Classification of Epilepsies and Epileptic Syndromes

A. Localization-related (focal, local, partial) epilepsies and syndromes
  1. *Idiopathic with age-related onset*
     At present, two syndromes are established, but more may be identified in the future.
     a. Benign childhood epilepsy with centrotemporal spike
     b. Childhood epilepsy with occipital paroxysms
  2. *Symptomatic*
     This category comprises syndromes of great individual variability, which will mainly be based on anatomic localization, clinical features, seizure types, and etiologic factors (if known).
B. Generalized epilepsies and syndromes
  1. *Idiopathic, with age-related onset, listed in order of age*
     a. Benign neonatal familial convulsions
     b. Benign neonatal convulsions
     c. Benign myoclonic epilepsy in infancy
     d. Childhood absence epilepsy (pyknolepsy)
     e. Juvenile absence epilepsy
     f. Juvenile myoclonic epilepsy (impulsive petit mal)
     g. Epilepsy with grand mal seizures (generalized tonic-clonic seizures) on awakening
        Other generalized idiopathic epilepsies, if they do not belong to one of the above syndromes, can still be classified as generalized idiopathic epilepsies.
  2. *Idiopathic and/or symptomatic, in order of age of appearance*
     a. West syndrome (infantile spasms, Blitz-Nick-Salaam-Krämphe)
     b. Lennox-Gastaut syndrome
     c. Epilepsy with myoclonic-astatic seizures
     d. Epilepsy with myoclonic absences
  3. *Symptomatic*
     a. Nonspecific etiology (early myoclonic encephalopathy)
     b. Specific syndromes (epileptic seizures may complicate disease states)
        Included here are those diseases in which seizures are an initial or predominant feature.
C. Epilepsies and syndromes undetermined as to whether they are focal or generalized.
  1. *With both generalized and focal seizures*
     a. Neonatal seizures
     b. Severe myoclonic epilepsy in infancy
     c. Epilepsy with continuous spike-waves during slow-wave sleep
     d. Acquired epileptic aphasia (Landau-Kleffner syndrome)
  2. *Without unequivocal generalized or focal features*
     This heading covers all cases with generalized tonic-clonic seizures where clinical and EEG findings do not permit classification as clearly generalized or localization-related, such as in many cases of sleep grand mal.
D. Special syndromes
  1. *Situation-related seizures (Gelegenheitsanfälle)*
  a. Febrile convulsions
  b. Seizures related to other identifiable situations, such as stress, hormonal changes, drugs, alcohol, or sleep deprivation
  2. *Isolated, apparently unprovoked epileptic events*
  3. *Epilepsies characterized by specific modes of seizure precipitation*
  4. *Chronic progressive epilepsia partialis continua of childhood*

Modified from Dreifuss FE, Martinez-Lage M, Roger J, et al. Epilepsia 1985; 26:268.

become generalized to involve both cerebral hemispheres, resulting in unconsciousness. It is common for these sensory seizures to remain localized. If the partial sensory seizure spreads to affect the motor function of the same limb, Todd paralysis may result. Seizures that initially affect the visual system are uncommon but well known. The complexity of the alteration in the visual pattern depends on the locale of the involved cortex. Organized hallucinations are the most complex form of visual seizures and are initiated in the temporal lobe

Classification of Focal Seizures

A. Simple partial seizures
Clinical seizure type: Simple partial seizures: consciousness not impaired.
EEG seizure type: Local contralateral discharge starting over the corresponding area of cortical representation (not always recorded on the scalp).
EEG interictal expression: Local contralateral discharge.
1. With motor signs
   a. Focal motor without march
   b. Focal motor with march (jacksonian)
   c. Versive
   d. Postural
   e. Phonatory (vocalization or arrest of speech)
2. With autonomic symptoms (including epigastric sensation, pallor, sweating, flushing, piloerection, and pupillary dilatation)
3. With somatosensory or special sensory symptoms (simple hallucinations; e.g., tingling, light flashes, buzzing)
   a. Somatosensory
   b. Visual
   c. Auditory
   d. Olfactory
   e. Gustatory
   f. Vertiginous
4. With psychic symptoms (disturbance of higher cerebral function). These rarely occur without impairment of consciousness and are more commonly seen as complex partial seizures.
   a. Dysphasic
   b. Dysmnesic (e.g., déjà vu)
   c. Cognitive (e.g., dreamy states, distortions of time sense)
   d. Affective (i.e., fear, anger, and other emotional states)
   e. Illusions (e.g., macropsia)
   f. Structured hallucinations (e.g., music, scenes)

B. Complex partial seizures
Clinical seizure type: Complex partial seizures: with impairment of consciousness, may sometimes begin with simple symptoms.
EEG seizure type: Unilateral or frequently bilateral discharge, diffuse or focal in temporal or fronto-temporal regions.
EEG interictal expression: Unilateral or bilateral, generally asynchronous focus; usually in the temporal regions.
1. Simple partial onset followed by impairment of consciousness
   a. With simple partial features (A-1 — A-4, above) followed by impaired consciousness
   b. With automatisms
2. With impairment of consciousness at onset
   a. With impairment of consciousness only
   b. With automatisms

C. Partial seizures evolving to generalized tonic-clonic seizures
Clinical seizure type: Generalized tonic-clonic seizures with partial or focal onset.
EEG seizure type: Discharges like those for complex partial seizures, becoming secondarily and rapidly generalized.
1. Simple partial seizures evolving to generalized tonic-clonic seizures
2. Complex partial seizures evolving to generalized tonic-clonic seizures
3. Simple partial seizures evolving to complex partial seizures evolving to generalized tonic-clonic seizures

area, where more complex integration of visual functions occurs. The simplest visual seizures are initiated in the primary areas in the occipital cortex. Visual seizures initiating in the occipital lobe may include flashing lights or scotomas in the homonymous field contralateral to the focus. The positive or flashing-light sensations may take the form of teichopsias (zigzag lines) or fiery, circumscribed circles. Discharges emanating from associated areas result in more highly complex visual sensations ranging from geometric shapes, such as squares and stars, to animal forms; the hallucinations may be so well formed and recognizable that vivid visual memories remain.

Hallucinations of objects that appear smaller than actual size (lilliputian hallucinations or micropsia) may result from temporal lobe discharges. Many characteristics of auditory seizures parallel the characteristics of visual seizures. Auditory seizures range from primitive auditory perceptions, such as loud swishing noises, to easily recognized, complex auditory hallucinations. Loss of consciousness frequently follows the onset of auditory seizures, which primarily represent an epileptic aura. Other special sensory seizures, including vertigo, are known. Vertiginous seizures have been termed *tornado fits* and may arise from suprasylvian parietal cortex. Olfactory and gustatory sensations are usually unpleasant and difficult to categorize. Olfactory sensations may become associated with a dreamy state, and this alteration of consciousness then characterizes the attack as a complex partial seizure. These attacks frequently arise from the uncus region and are known as *uncinate fits*.

Seizures with autonomic phenomena may involve pupillary dilatation, which accompanies many seizure types. Rarely, transient Horner syndrome may be observed on the side contralateral to a discharging parietal lobe focus. Seizure manifestations may include recurrent abdominal discomfort and vomiting, as well as unilateral piloerection, pallor, flushing, or salivation; the latter may be so profuse as to gush from the mouth.

With psychic symptoms (disturbances of higher cerebral function). Although psychic symptoms occur frequently in complex partial seizures, they may be observed in focal disturbances of temporal lobe function that do not lead to alteration in consciousness and therefore manifest as simple partial seizures. These features may include dysmnesic symptoms in which there is distortion of memory or time, flashback experiences, or déjà vu. Occasionally, as a form of forced thinking the patient may experience a rapid recollection of episodes from his or her life, known as *panoramic vision*.

Cognitive disturbances may include sensations of extreme pleasure or displeasure. Such disturbances frequently involve feelings of fear and intense depression accompanied by attacks of unworthiness and rejection that last a few minutes. Anger or rage is rare. Unlike temper tantrums, these episodes are unprovoked and abate as rapidly as they begin. Illusions may be distorted perceptions in which objects appear deformed in size or shape. Distortions may also affect sound and body image (corporeal awareness); thus altered perception of limb size or weight may be experienced.

Structured hallucinations. Structured hallucinations may occur as perceptions without a corresponding stimulus and may be sensory, visual, auditory, olfactory, or gustatory. Usually the hallucinations are quite prim-itive, but when visual association areas are affected, they may become elaborate, including scenes, sounds of voices, or music.

Specific simple partial seizure syndromes

Benign childhood partial (rolandic) seizures. First described by Nayrac and Beaussart [1958], benign childhood partial seizures are now recognized as a frequent childhood seizure type beginning during the first decade of life and usually ending spontaneously during the second decade. Characteristically the seizures are nocturnal, last a few minutes, and result in unilateral facial grimacing and twitching, saliva swallowing, and inability to speak. Sometimes they occur only during sleep; in some instances they may manifest during either sleep or the waking state. The seizures are characterized on EEG by midtemporal or centrotemporal spike activity that is usually unilateral, although it occasionally can be bilateral. These attacks respond well to most antiepileptic drugs and have a benign outcome. By virtue of their genetic inheritance and prognosis, these seizures are classified under the primary epilepsies despite being focal.

Epileptic aphasia. Several types of speech difficulties, such as a cry or speech arrest, may occur during a focal motor seizure. Seizures arising from the dominant hemisphere are more likely to be associated with speech arrest. Seizures arising from a nondominant hemisphere may be accompanied by repetitive ictal utterances. In addition to transient ictal phenomena, speech disturbance may take the form of prolonged acquired aphasia, which is associated with an epileptic disturbance. It may precede or follow the occurrence of seizures and may persist for months to years, even though seizures may be rare or controlled. This syndrome is the Landau-Kleffner syndrome [Landau and Kleffner, 1957]. Although its etiology is not well understood, Landau-Kleffner syndrome may be caused by a form of focal encephalitis.

A developmental expressive aphasia may rarely occur, resulting from a bilateral epileptic cerebral hemispheric dysfunction. Improvement may occur after administering antiepileptic drugs.

Unilateral seizures. Unilateral seizures account for various childhood epileptic syndromes. Some infants and young children have unilateral clonic seizures that may shift from side to side during different attacks, producing seesaw seizures. Gastaut et al. [1974] regarded these attacks as a unilateral manifestation of a generalized condition.

Unilateral epileptic seizures associated with infantile hemiplegia are a frequently observed clinical syndrome. Onset usually occurs with a convulsive seizure that is followed by flaccid hemiplegia. In other instances, hemiplegia may develop first, followed by convulsions.

Such conditions may be caused by vascular occlusions, encephalitis, vasculitis, sickle cell disease, retropharyngeal abscess, moyamoya disease, or congenital heart disease.

Initial seizures usually subside rapidly but frequently recur and then are usually confined to the hemiparetic side.

Radiographically, porencephaly is often present, as well as unilateral ventricular dilatation. The limbs on the side of the hemiparesis are frequently hypoplastic.

There is a special variety of this syndrome associated with Sturge-Weber malformation in which a cutaneous angioma is part of a congenital ectodermal disorder along with a shrunken hemisphere, telangiectasa of the meninges, and intracranial cortical calcifications.

Epilepsia partialis continua (Kozhevnikoff disease). Although epilepsia partialis continua is considered to be the result of chronic encephalitis, the cause is unknown [Rasmussen and McCann, 1968]. Partial motor seizures are often associated with myoclonus, which may appear early in the course of the illness. Progressive motor deficit develops during the illness, as does mental retardation. The seizures are extremely resistant to treatment, and the condition usually progresses to complete hemiplegia with progressive unilateral brain atrophy [Andermann, 1991].

Complex partial seizures

The primary feature that separates complex partial seizures from simple partial seizures is impairment, distortion, or loss of consciousness. These manifestations are the result of the epileptic discharge involving a region where structures subserving memory, consciousness, emotion, and vision are affected; thus a different order of sensation supervenes and can effect a dreamy state, visual symptoms, autonomic manifestations, affective disturbances, and frequently automatic behavior. All the psychic symptoms referred to previously are based in the temporal lobe and limbic cortex; however, an alteration of consciousness in complex partial seizures occurs either near the beginning or during the attack.

As in simple partial seizures, hallucinatory phenomena may characterize seizure onset. These phenomena may affect various systems, and their complexity depends on the association areas involved. Unlike simple partial seizures, most complex partial seizure hallucinatory phenomena are elaborate and realistic. As with simple partial seizures, there may be affective symptoms, particularly fear, loneliness, depression, sadness, anger, joy, or ecstasy. At times, fear during a seizure is pervasive and leads to running away; if consciousness is impaired, the patient may end up located a long distance from where the seizure began.

Psychomotor automatisms are the most prominent aspect of complex partial seizures. Automatisms are activities occurring during a period of altered consciousness for which the patient is amnesic. While engaged in these episodes, the patient may respond perfunctorily to the immediate milieu or may execute complex motor activities that are inappropriate. A distinction has been made between forced automatisms, such as mastication or swallowing, and reactive motor activities, such as scratching or fumbling with clothes or objects; the former are believed to result from epileptic discharge, and the latter from unrecalled psychosensory manifestations. Automatisms that have been identified include oroalimentary automatisms, such as chewing, lip-smacking, and swallowing; automatisms of mimicry, such as fear, anger, anxiety, and joy; gestural automatisms, such as clapping, scratching, and stereotyped hand movements; ambulatory automatisms, such as walking or riding a bicycle in which the activity may appear to be either goal-directed or completely disorganized; and verbal automatisms, which may be in response to stimulation or may be a stereotyped repetitive utterance. Some automatisms may represent the continuation of ongoing activities (perseverative automatisms), whereas others may provoke seizures and thus are regarded as reactive to external or internal environmental stimuli [Penry and Dreifuss, 1969].

Postictal disorientation is a prominent feature in psychomotor automatisms. Automatisms have little localization significance; they may emanate not only from temporal regions but also from the frontal lobes, and they can be produced experimentally by stimulating the fornix, circuminsular cortex, amygdala, hippocampal gyrus, and anterior part of the sylvian fissure.

Delgado-Escueta et al. [1982] reported that complex partial seizures emanating from the frontal lobe begin with automatic behavior; conversely, those seizures emanating from temporal regions are initially associated with cessation of activities and a blank stare, which is followed by the development of automatisms. It is unknown whether such a distinction is valid on clinical grounds. Occasionally, complex partial seizures occur in the form of status epilepticus as "continuous aura," or as an episodic dreamy state with a prolonged confusional state; such seizures may be difficult to distinguish from absence status or spike-and-wave stupor. Sometimes psychomotor status is not continuous, with periods of relatively good orientation interspersed with periods of confused, restless, and disoriented behavior.

Complex partial seizures may occasionally manifest as impaired consciousness only; this temporal lobe absence may closely simulate the absence exhibited petit mal seizures. However, temporal lobe absence is usually more prolonged, is unaccompanied by the expected 3-Hz spike-and-wave EEG activity, and terminates in postictal confusion.

Intensive monitoring in association with patient evaluation for epilepsy surgery has revealed much information about complex partial seizures arising from the frontal lobes. The syndrome of frontal lobe epilepsy is of special interest because of the ease with which it is confused with pseudoepileptic seizures by virtue of the varied behavioral repertoire and the frequently difficult-to-detect EEG concomitant. Complex gestural automatisms, prominent tonic or postural mode of manifestations, and the frequent absence of postictal confusion contribute to diagnostic difficulty.

Interictal manifestations of complex partial seizures. Many authors have described the personality characteristics, the relationship of epilepsy to intelligence, the changes in mood and affect, and the prevalence of psychosis in patients with complex partial seizures. Most of these reports, however, poorly document the relationships between cause and effect and specifically between localized and generalized cerebral dysfunctions.

Interference with intellectual functions may result from the same process that is responsible for the epilepsy rather than from a cause-and-effect relationship. However, a disparity between verbal and visual spatial function in subtest scores tends to be related to the site of seizure focus, regardless of whether the focus occurs in the left or right hemisphere. Similarly, disorders of the limbic system and temporal lobe cortex may interfere with memory recording and retrieval functions. This relationship is not nearly as frequently encountered in children as in adults. Personality characteristics that have been reported include irritability, loss of libido, self-recrimination, circumstantiality, hypergraphia, and religiosity, but the patient's sociopsychologic background is probably more important than the site or nature of the epileptic process. In addition, most of these reports have emanated from institutional rather than outpatient clinic practice. There has been little study of patients who do not exhibit personality changes despite having seizures identical to those in patients who do exhibit such alleged changes. Patients with cerebral lesions who have no seizures may have characteristics similar to those described in patients with seizures. However, an inverse relationship appears to exist between affective disorders and complex partial seizures. When seizures are controlled, the affective disorder tends to be more prominent in some patients [Landolt, 1960]; onset usually occurs at puberty. More females are affected than males.

Partial seizures secondarily generalized. Whether the discharge that initiates a partial seizure becomes propagated from its focal cortical site depends on the intensity of the epileptiform discharges; the individual, innate threshold; and inhibition. The evolution of a focal (partial) seizure into a generalized seizure probably requires dissemination to the thalamic, diencephalic, and mesencephalic areas, which subsequently results in discharges that invade the cortex of both hemispheres.

It is known that brainstem structures are unnecessary for developing bilateral synchrony. In addition, the belief that involvement of so-called centrencephalic structures in humans is required for the development of bilateral synchrony is not yet firmly supported by demonstration. Orbital frontal and parasagittal lesions enhance the likelihood of resultant bilateral synchrony [Tukel and Jasper, 1952]. There is little question that some seizures believed to be generalized are the result of focal cortical discharges with secondary bilateral synchrony [Stewart and Dreifuss, 1967]. In fact, this method of propagation probably underlies many seizures that are considered to be generalized (see Chapter 31). It is likely that some generalized seizures are subsequent to a focal cortical discharge, even though the only symptoms evident—amnesia or alteration of consciousness—are not focal symptoms [Bancaud et al., 1965; Williams, 1965]. Before generalization of a focal seizure, the manifestation of the episode that precedes loss of consciousness is the aura. The patient is not amnesic but remains aware during this event. By convention, if there is no loss of consciousness and the epileptic episodes continue to be focal, the result is similar, but the experience is not termed an aura.

Status epilepticus

Status epilepticus is rapidly recurrent or continuous (more than 20 minutes) generalized or focal seizures during which the patient remains unconscious or has two or more sequential seizures without full recovery of consciousness between seizures. Ventilation is embarrassed, and life is threatened. Status epilepticus is always a medical emergency, and all measures should be taken to curtail its duration. In many instances, status epilepticus is the first indication of an epileptic disorder, or it may occur in a known epileptic patient and results from noncompliance with antiepileptic drug administration or abrupt discontinuation of medication. On other occasions, status epilepticus is associated with acute intercurrent infection.

The differential diagnosis of the conditions responsible for status epilepticus includes meningitis, depressed skull fracture, subarachnoid hemorrhage, subdural hematoma, anoxia, hypoxic ischemia, meningitis, encephalitis, electrolyte disturbances, hypoglycemia, lead intoxication, and hyperpyrexia (greater than 40° C) [Aicardi and Chevrie, 1970; Grand, 1974]. If untreated, many of these conditions may result in death or permanent neurologic impairment. Therapy is directed toward circulatory and ventilatory support, terminating the seizures, and counteracting the underlying cause.

The airways should be cleared immediately by suctioning, and a plastic airway should be inserted. Suctioning should be gentle to avoid enhancing seizure activity by overstimulation. After the patient's clothing is loosened, the patient should be turned to the side to prevent aspiration of saliva or gastric contents. Soft objects, such as pillows, carpeting, or cloth, should be placed under the head to prevent head injury during the seizures. Oxygen administration should be initiated by standard inhalation techniques. If these techniques are insufficient, quick initiation of general anesthesia with endotracheal intubation may prove necessary.

An intravenous line (or preferably two, one with normal saline solution) must be placed, and blood must be obtained for laboratory study of routine electrolytes, calcium, glucose, and antiepileptic blood concentrations. Procuring a sample for blood culture is often appropriate. At this point, intravenous glucose (25%) l g/kg may be injected together with thiamine 1 mg/kg.

Several therapeutic schemes can be used to terminate seizures. The physician should be familiar with a few of these techniques. Instituting intravenous diazepam is a commonly accepted approach. Lorazepam usually acts quickly, and side effects are uncommon when it is used as the initial drug; it has a better duration of effectiveness than diazepam. If a benzodiazepine is administered after the patient has received parenteral barbiturates, then cardiac rhythm and rate, blood pressure, and respiration must be monitored on an ongoing basis. Lorazepam should be administered in a dose of 0.05 to 0.2 mg/kg at a rate of no greater than 2 mg/min diluted in an equal volume of intravenous solution. The appropriate dose for infants is 0.05 mg/kg, with a maximum dose of 2 mg. Intravenous administration of benzodiazepines may be complicated by apnea, cardiac arrest, hypertension, bradycardia, and thrombophlebitis [Schneider and Mace, 1974]. After seizures are controlled an epileptic drug with more prolonged activity should be administered, preferably phenytoin 18 mg/kg at no greater than 2 mg/kg/min in infants or 30 mg/min in older children or slower if hypertension or arrhythmias occur.

If phenytoin does not control status, consideration should be given to barbiturate coma induction in an intensive care unit setting and an intubated patient. Pentobarbital is usually given in a dose of 12 mg/kg intravenously at 50 mg/min or less to control seizures and obtain a specific EEG pattern of burst suppression. Thereafter pentobarbital can be continued at 0.25 to 1 mg/kg/hr for a minimum of 12 hours and possibly considerably longer, although the patient should from time to time be allowed to emerge sufficiently to determine whether seizures remain controlled. As soon as seizures are controlled, oral therapy with phenytoin, carbamazepine, valproate, or phenobarbital should be started.

GENETICS

Hippocrates theorized that epilepsy was hereditary. Over the centuries, inhumane eugenic methods have been instigated ostensibly to prevent genetic transmission of epilepsy.

The multifactorial causation of epilepsy has proved confounding, and the subject has proved confusing for both professionals and lay people. The dissimilarity among posttraumatic seizures, febrile seizures, and absence seizures associated with 3-Hz spike-and-wave EEG discharges discourages comparison of genetic factors among them. Nevertheless, a common genetic skein underlies these conditions and may even underlie traumatic seizures, establishing an epileptogenic threshold level below that expected. Specific syndromes have been investigated for their possible underpinnings in addition to those known hereditary conditions, such as the sphingolipidoses, mucopolysaccharidoses, and other inherited conditions of lipid, glucose, and amino acid metabolism.

Generalized seizures

Metrakos and Metrakos [1961] studied the genetics of absence seizures. They reported a 12% incidence of seizures in siblings, parents, and offspring of probands who have epilepsy associated with spike-and-wave EEG discharges. This incidence is quadruple that found in relatives of control subjects. The incidence of spike-and-wave discharges among siblings and offspring of probands was approximately 35%, and 10% among parents. The incidence in relatives of the control group was 3%. The characteristic EEG discharge is associated with age, is usually found in the 5- to 15-year age range, and often vanishes with maturation. Therefore there is a lower incidence of the electrical discharge in parents than in siblings. This particular constellation of clinical and EEG abnormalities most likely results from an autosomal-dominant trait, although other factors are likely to enhance the incidence of seizures in individuals who have inherited the trait.

Photosensitive epilepsy

Epilepsy induced by flickering lights or unusual light patterns is photosensitive epilepsy. Original studies by Doose et al. [1969] and later by Jeavons [1985] have delineated the condition. Photosensitive epilepsy appears to be inherited as an autosomal-dominant trait. Its onset is partly related to age. Curiously, degree of penetrance can be demarcated by varying either frequencies or intensities of stimulation. Although absence and photosensitive seizures are accompanied by EEG generalized spike-and-wave patterns, it appears that inheritance of hyperventilation-sensitive absence seizures and photosensitive epilepsy is genetically distinct.

Primary generalized myoclonic seizures

Tsuboi [1977] described genetic studies of primary generalized myoclonic seizures. There was a family history in 30% of the probands. This study, similar to others, demonstrated a tendency for a particular age distribution; the age at onset was somewhat later than that in patients with absence seizures.

Juvenile myoclonic epilepsy

There has been much interest recently in the inheritance of juvenile myoclonic epilepsy. This syndrome is characterized by the occurrence of myoclonic jerks (usually in the morning hours), occasional generalized tonic-clonic convulsions (usually on awakening), and occasional juvenile absence seizures. Photic sensitivity may be present. The syndrome usually begins in adolescence, and symptoms are frequently precipitated by sleep deprivation, alcohol intake, and noncompliance with an antiepileptic drug regimen. There is increasing evidence that this condition is associated with a gene defect on the short arm of chromosome 6 (tightly linked to the human leukocyte antigen region on this chromosome) [Greenberg et al., 1988].

Benign neonatal convulsions (third-day episodes). This condition is characterized by dominant inheritance, and very large pedigrees have been reported. Leppert et al. reported linkage to chromosome 20 in this condition in 1989.

Progressive myoclonic epilepsy. Evidence is accruing that Baltic myoclonus (Unverricht-Lundborg disease) is the result of a gene deletion on chromosome 21.

Partial seizures

The most studied group among the partial epilepsies is the group of complex partial seizures subjected to temporal lobectomy. The results of Falconer et al. [1964], Ounsted [1955], Bray and Wiser [1965], and Andermann and Metrakos [1969] all suggest that a genetic factor is involved, although the evidence is considerably less persuasive than that in the primary generalized epilepsies. EEG findings in first-degree relatives strongly suggest an underlying genetic factor. The likelihood of immature brain convulsions appears to be an age-dependent characteristic of the convulsive genome. Children with complex partial seizures suffered severe febrile seizures during early childhood; it is likely that these children were genetically predisposed to febrile convulsions. Children with convulsions that lasted longer suffered mesiotemporal sclerosis. Benign partial seizures of childhood with centrotemporal spikes (rolandic epilepsy) have a dominant inheritance pattern similar to that of absence seizures. The number of children who bear the EEG trait exceeds the number of those with clinical seizures [Lerman, 1985].

ETIOLOGY

Although partial seizures are more likely to be associated with focal hemispheric lesions than are generalized seizures, such structural causes are rarely identified. In children, approximately 30% to 50% of patients have an unknown cause, and others have vague putative causes, such as a difficult birth, and various degrees of head trauma in early childhood that cannot be substantiated. Moreover, there appears to be a genetic factor that determines whether a focal lesion becomes epileptogenic. Benign focal rolandic childhood seizures frequently demonstrate an apparently dominant mode of inheritance; these seizures should be regarded separately as a focal form of primary or idiopathic epilepsy.

Prenatal and perinatal complications constitute most of the causative factors for seizures during the first few years of life. Thereafter trauma becomes most important, followed later by brain tumors and vascular lesions.

Inborn errors of metabolism

Metabolic errors may result in partial seizures associated with mental retardation. At other times the seizures are generalized. Their onset may be early or delayed. Maple syrup urine disease, phenylketonuria, galactosemia, hyperglycinemia, and other major conditions may manifest with seizures early in life, whereas progressive heritable familial degenerative disorders, which are characterized by storage abnormalities, such as GM1 and GM2 gangliosidoses and neuronal ceroid lipofuscinosis, occur later in infancy or early in childhood. In those conditions where gray matter disease is predominant, seizures begin earlier and myoclonus occurs frequently. Seizures are less prominent in the leukodystrophies and spasticity with progressive paresis being more evident. All of these inborn errors of metabolism are most frequently associated with partial seizures of the focal or multifocal variety.

Other metabolic diseases

Hypoglycemic seizures. There are many causes of hypoglycemia and hypoglycemic seizures. Among the causes are several glycogen storage diseases, idiopathic hypoglycemia, islet cell tumors, nesidioblastomas, fructose intolerance, leucine sensitivity, ketotic hypoglycemia, and maple syrup urine disease.

Disorders of sodium concentration. Hyponatremia resulting from water intoxication may manifest after excessive water intake, including inappropriate dilution of infant formula, inappropriate secretion of antidiuretic hormone subsequent to an intracranial pathologic condition, or too vigorous and rapid intravenous fluid replacement after dehydration in the adrenogenital syndrome. Sudden onset of salt loss without proper intervention may be fatal.

Hypertonic dehydration and diabetes insipidus, whether primarily pituitary or nephrogenic, may lead to hypernatremia. On rare occasions, massive salt intake related to improper formula preparation has resulted in hypernatremia. General shrinkage of the brain and subsequent cortical vein stretching and thrombosis of these veins as they enter the superior sagittal sinus may result in permanent neurologic impairment. Multifocal cortical seizures are often engendered by both hypernatremia and hyponatremia.

Hypocalcemia. Neonatal seizures are occasionally associated with hypocalcemia. The highest incidence of occurrence is after the third day of life [Brown et al., 1972]. The seizures are frequently multifocal and usually are not accompanied by alteration of consciousness. Although primary neonatal tetany is the most common cause of hypocalcemia, there are other causes, including hypoxic-ischemic encephalopathy, birth trauma, maternal diabetes mellitus, exchange transfusions, intermittent positive-pressure respiration, tracheoesophageal fistula repair, magnesium absorption abnormalities, hypoparathyroidism, maternal steatorrhea, and renal impairment. Other than seizures, manifestations that are frequently observed include increased extensor tone and jittery movements both at rest and during movement. Neonatal hypocalcemia is associated with hypomagnesemia in more than 50% of affected infants. In the older child, hypocalcemia may occur as a result of primary hypoparathyroidism and manifests as muscle irritability. CT may reveal calcification of the basal ganglia. Pseudohypoparathyroidism differs from hypoparathyroidism because of end-organ unresponsiveness to parathormone and unusual physical characteristics, including brachydactyly.

Congenital and perinatal factors

Chromosomal pathologic conditions may result in malformations. Intrauterine infections, specifically cytomegalic body disease, toxoplasmosis, and rubella, are well known for their ability to cause abnormal brain development. Syphilis, now rare in many parts of the world, may also cause intrauterine brain infection with severe neurologic residuals. Maternal exposure to radiation during pregnancy or ingestion by the mother of teratogenic drugs may also lead to gross cerebral malformations. In addition to other manifestations, all of these etiologic conditions may also result in focal and multifocal seizures. An unusual seizure type, myoclonic spasms, sometimes results from intrauterine infections. Tuberous sclerosis may manifest during the first few months of life and may be accompanied by focal seizures or infantile myoclonic spasms. Other causes of seizures in the perinatal period are discussed in Chapter 33.

Infectious diseases

Seizures are often the first indication of bacterial meningitis in infants and children; moreover, seizures are frequently associated with established bacterial meningitis. The simultaneous presence of generalized seizures and fever generally suggests bacterial meningitis. Mechanisms of seizure production in bacterial meningitis include cortical vein and sagittal sinus thrombosis, primary involvement of the cortical tissue, cerebritis and subsequent abscess formation, and subdural effusions. Hydrocephalus and seizures may result from ependymitis, ventriculitis, or involvement of the meninges with subsequent impairment of spinal fluid absorption.

Focal or multifocal seizures may be associated with viral encephalitis. Many patients with viral encephalitis have only minor neurologic impairment, and their seizures may be transient. Conversely, severe encephalitis, such as herpes simplex virus or Epstein-Barr virus instigated with a predilection for the temporal lobes, may result in severe sequelae with intractable seizures and permanent intellectual and memory dyusfunction. Subacute sclerosing panencephalitis is associated with rubeola infection. This condition is often heralded by multifocal myoclonic seizures and focal and multifocal seizures. Diphtheria-pertussis-tetanus immunization may be followed by focal or generalized seizures. It is generally believed that these seizures are fever induced and that pertussis encephalopathy is exceedingly rare. Conversely, it is recommended that persons with epilepsy or other neurologic diseases, particularly if progressive, should have pertussis inoculation deferred.

Parasitic infestation may result in focal seizures. In particular, cysticercosis infection is accompanied by circumscribed cortical cysts and ventricular blockage. Echinococcosis is another parasitic infection that results in focal brain lesions. Tuberculosis with tuberculoma formation in the brain continues to be a problem in some parts of the world [Dastur and Desai, 1965].

Trauma

One the most important consequences of head injury is the development of convulsions, although the incidence depends on many factors, including injury severity. Epilepsy occurs more frequently after penetrating wounds [Jennet, 1975]. In closed-head injuries, which constitute most of the wounds suffered by the general population, the incidence of traumatic epilepsy is relatively small. Cerebral damage during or near the time of birth may be manifested by early or late seizures. The effect of closed-head injuries depends on the mechanical factors involved. In children the most frequent causes of epilepsy are associated with linear or depressed skull fractures. Except for some instances of early traumatic epilepsy after relatively trivial injury, the incidence of epilepsy after head trauma is generally proportional to the duration of posttraumatic amnesia.

Early epilepsy is usually associated with simple partial seizures and motor signs. In more than 50% of patients, it arises within 24 hours of injury. Children younger than 5 years of age frequently manifest status epilepticus after severe injuries. Patients suffering early-onset posttraumatic epilepsy have favorable outcomes compared with those in whom late-onset epilepsy develops. Late-onset posttraumatic epilepsy represents most posttraumatic seizures. Generally, these seizures occur within 3 years of injury and are more frequently generalized tonic-clonic than partial seizures, in contrast to early-onset traumatic epilepsy. The pathogenesis of posttraumatic epilepsy remains unknown despite the standard explanation of meningocerebral cicatrix and focal ischemic factors. Experimental animal models suggest that neurons in affected regions are structurally abnormal, with changes in dendritic spin density and electrical hyperexcitability. Extravasation of blood and deposition of hemoglobin may stimulate peroxidation of microsomal lipids; this process may be epileptogenic.

Although epilepsy develops in nearly 50% of patients with penetrating head wounds and dural tears, seizures develop in only about 5% of patients after closed-head injury [Jennett, 1975].

Brain tumors

Tumors are an uncommon cause of seizures during childhood. Tumors occur less frequently in children than in adults and are more commonly found in regions of the brain that are not predisposed to developing epileptogenic activity (e.g., thalamus, cerebellum, brainstem). Nevertheless, focal seizures in children can be caused by tumors [Backus and Millichap, 1962; Dreifuss and Mushet, 1966]. In a study of 100 patients with seizures of focal origin, four had associated hemispheric gliomas and two had arteriovenous malformations. During the subsequent 10 years, temporal lobe tumors were discovered in three additional patients. MRI has greatly facilitated the diagnosis of cryptic tumors, which occur more frequently than previously believed. Tumors that are relatively less malignant and slow growing are more often associated with seizures than are malignant tumors. Furthermore, tumors located close to the brain surface have a greater propensity to cause seizures than do deep subcortical neoplasms. Although arteriovenous malformations are usually near the surface, they generally cause intracerebral or subarachnoid hemorrhage as the initial clinical event and are less likely to cause seizures in children than in adults. Nevertheless, focal seizures accompanied by a history of headaches may be caused by such a tumor. The diagnosis of arteriovenous malformation may be confounded by the fact that bruits are frequently heard over the skull or orbits in normal children younger than 10 years of age and are therefore of less significance than those heard in adults.

Focal seizures may result from subdural hematomas in childhood; multifocal seizures can result from bilateral subdural hematomas. Bilateral subdural hematomas are frequently found in infants. Unless acute, an associated increase in the occipitofrontal circumference along with increased tension of the anterior fontanel is common.

Cerebrovascular disease

Focal seizures in children rarely result from cerebrovascular disease. Sturge-Weber syndrome (i.e., encephalofacial angiomatosis) usually manifests with a port-wine nevus in the distribution of one or more divisions of cranial nerve V. The associated angiomatosis is found over the ipsilateral cortex in the pia-arachnoid. The associated gyri are atrophied, and linear calcifications may be present, most often in the occipital lobes. There may be accompanying brain hypoplasia and focal seizures, and hemiparesis may compromise the contralateral extremities.

Hemispherectomy is often indicated and should probably be undertaken early in life when seizures are intractable and particularly when learning is impaired and a hemiplegia exists [Dreifuss, 1987]. Congenital heart lesions or bacterial endocarditis may cause emboli that flow to the brain and instigate seizures. Unfortunately, hemiplegia beginning in infancy that results from hemispheral infarction is not only likely to be associated with early-onset seizures, but the seizures may persist for years and be difficult to manage. The association of such hemiplegia with early-onset seizures in patients is about 50% [Solomon et al., 1970]. The differential diagnosis of early-onset hemiplegia includes fibromuscular hyperplasia, intraoral trauma to the internal carotid artery, carotid dissection, and arteritis (both autoimmune and associated with the use of intravenous amphetamines), and with cocaine, which may produce consequences if used by the mother. Moyamoya disease and mitochondrial disorders, sickle cell disease, circulating lupus anticoagulant, and homocystinuria may produce similar insults.

Other etiologic factors

The neuropathologic effect of early-onset epilepsy is of great interest in considering the possible cause of complex partial seizures. The best recognized of these is mesiotemporal sclerosis. This condition involves Ammon horn of the hippocampus. This pathologic pattern has frequently been found in patients who have undergone temporal lobectomy for uncontrolled complex partial seizures [Corellis and Meldrum, 1976]. Such sclerosis may also affect the amygdala and the parahippocampal gyrus. Patients undergoing temporal lobectomy with subsequent pathologic documentation of mesiotemporal sclerosis frequently experience prolonged febrile convulsions in infancy and early childhood. Ounsted et al. [1966] stressed that early-onset seizures and severe generalized tonic-clonic seizures accompanied by a high frequency of temporal lobe attacks were associated with an adverse prognosis. Meldrum [1978] stressed the metabolic process by which neuronal hippocampal changes could be produced by recurrent seizures. It is generally believed that prolonged febrile convulsions in early life may cause hippocampal sclerosis, which subsequently results in complex partial seizures. A primate model of hippocampal sclerosis induced by epilepsy has been produced by administering bicuculline or allylglycine to baboons [Meldrum, 1983]. The initiation of such seizures is associated with ischemic changes in cerebellar Purkinje cells, a finding that is also observed in patients with long-standing epilepsy. Therefore repeated generalized seizures probably result in focal pathologic changes.

PRECIPITATING FACTORS

A discussion of the theoretic aspects of precipitating factors is found elsewhere [Newmark, 1983]. Some specific factors are mentioned in the following sections.

Reflex seizures

Photosensitive seizures. Attacks triggered by photic stimulation are almost always generalized. The underlying mechanism that precipitates these episodes in the presence of repetitive light flashes is unknown [Bickford and Klass, 1969]. Although the phenomenon may be characterized as a heightened evoked-potential response, this appears insufficient to explain the frequent perpetuation of seizures after the light stimuli have been terminated; therefore the subcortical structures are probably involved. Children may trigger seizures by waving their fingers rhythmically while staring at a bright light source [Chao, 1962]. The frequency of this stimulation appears to be critical. Such self-stimulation most frequently occurs in children with intellectual retardation. Photosensitive seizures occur predominantly in adolescent females, and they may occasionally complicate juvenile myoclonic epilepsy where they may be part of the differential diagnosis. A common precipitating factor is sunlight flickering between trees when seen from a moving vehicle and light flickering from video games.

In a large cooperative study, Mattson et al. [1985] reported that approximately 80% of partial seizures could be controlled by monotherapy. Administration of carbamazepine, phenytoin, phenobarbital, or primidone were all effective, but carbamazepine and phenytoin were better tolerated. More recently, a subsequent study indicated that use of valproate was also effective in the treatment of partial seizures.

Sound-sensitive seizures. The most common sound-sensitive seizures are those engendered by music and are referred to as *musicogenic epilepsy*. This type of epilepsy has also been reported to be triggered by church bells. The seizures usually originate in one temporal lobe and give rise to the complex symptoms that characterize seizures originating from this area. Occasionally, these seizures may become generalized.

Other forms of reflex epilepsy. On rare occasions, paretic patients attempting movements of the hemiparetic limbs initiate a jacksonian seizure, which disseminates rapidly and may not terminate until a generalized seizure occurs. In some patients a startle response may evolve into a full-fledged focal or generalized seizure, particularly in patients who have hyperacusis.

Emotional stimulation

Epileptic episodes may be precipitated by emotional stress associated with either negative or positive events. The clinician must be cognizant of these problems and not erroneously assume the presence of a conversion reaction. When ongoing adverse conditions are present, consideration should be given to removing the patient from the area.

Menstruation

Patients and clinicians have long known that the menstrual cycle has an effect on seizure control; however, the mechanism is unknown. The time of greatest risk is the several days preceding the onset of menstruation [Mattson and Cramer, 1985].

Hyperventilation

Hyperventilation is commonly used during EEG examinations to potentiate the appearance of abnormal discharges. Hyperventilation may also lead to focal seizures and, more commonly, to generalized seizures, particularly absence.

Sleep deprivation

Sleep deprivation followed by sleep during EEG recording is another method of enhancing the possible occurrence of abnormal electrical discharges. Sleep is also associated with precipitation of seizures. Differentiating between myoclonic seizures occurring during early sleep and normal myoclonic sleep jerks may be difficult and require the use of sophisticated monitoring techniques.

MANAGEMENT

Principles of management

Therapy should not be initiated before an attempt is made to determine the cause of the seizures. The underlying cause is more readily recognized in seizures of neonates than in seizures of older children. Identifying an etiologic agent, such as certain metabolic states or space-occupying masses, should lead to specific treatment when possible, such as drug therapy or excision.

Although surgery is infrequently indicated in most seizures, some types of seizures, such as those originating from a unilateral temporal lobe site, can be successfully treated by surgery. However, surgery is not indicated until appropriate drug therapy has proved unsuccessful. Selection of an antiepileptic drug should be based on the evaluation of the characteristics of the seizures, as discussed in the following sections on individual drugs. The selected antiepileptic drug is used alone until the seizures terminate, until adequate therapeutic epileptic blood concentrations have been achieved, or until toxicity prevents dosage increase. At this point, combination drug therapy may be required.

Emotional, social, educational, or vocational considerations may preclude successful therapy, and a multidisciplinary approach, such as that available in a specialized epilepsy treatment center, is an aid to initiation of optimal therapy.

When antiepileptic drug administration requires change from one drug to another, such changes should be as gradual as possible; the administration and/or dosage of only one drug should be altered at any given time. Therefore sound judgment is required as to whether to withdraw the currently administered drug and then replace it, or to decrease the dosage of the currently administered drug and add a different drug. Dosage requirements may fluctuate for individuals because of illness, pregnancy, or medication side effects.

Drug therapy

Drug therapy for epilepsy commenced in 1857 when Locock discovered the beneficial effect of potassium bromide on seizures. Bromide was the preferred drug for more than 70 years; then phenobarbital was found to be effective by Hauptmann in 1912. Although many agents have since been introduced, phenobarbital remains the most commonly used agent in the world. A major advance in antiepileptic drug therapy was the introduction of phenytoin by Merritt and Putnam in 1938.

Laboratory evaluation of antiepileptic drugs considers their ability to abort or mute maximal electroshock seizures, minimal threshold seizures, pentylenetetrazol-induced seizures, photic seizures in the Senegalese baboon, and audiogenetic seizures in mice, as well as inhibition of kindling both electrical and pharmacologic.

Newer antiepileptic drugs are more specific for particular seizure forms. This more sophisticated pharmacologic approach has required more precise classification of seizures. For example, newer antiepileptic drugs intended for absence seizures are ineffective in managing complex partial seizures, which may clinically resemble absence seizures.

Recent pharmacologic refinements have allowed a more effective use of older antiepileptic drugs. These refinements include the ability to ascertain rapidly drug concentrations in serum and, when necessary, other body fluids. Furthermore, these newly available techniques have greatly facilitated the understanding of pharmacokinetics and drug interactions, which allows for more knowledgeable antiepileptic drug therapy.

Frequently used antiepileptic drugs

Phenytoin

Pharmacologic actions. Laboratory studies demonstrate that phenytoin (Dilantin, Epanutin) is effective against maximal tonic-clonic electroshock seizures, decreases the propagation of seizure discharges by diminishing afterdischarge, and limits posttetanic potentiation. All of these actions may contribute to limitation of dissemination of neuronal epileptic discharges. Phenytoin apparently facilitates expulsion of sodium ions through reinforcement of the sodium pump action, probably by Na^+-K^+-ATPase activity. Phenytoin is also believed to have an inhibitory effect on calcium-mediated neurotransmitter release.

Phenytoin is readily absorbed from the gastrointestinal tract. Several days are required for therapeutic blood concentrations to be attained. Intravenous administration greatly enhances this process. Hepatic degradation in the form of parahydroxylation results in a product that is excreted in the bile, reabsorbed into the gut, and then primarily excreted in the urine. A small amount of phenytoin is secreted by the salivary glands into the saliva. Gingival hypertrophy probably results from contact with the saliva containing phenytoin.

Side effects. Side effects may be attributed to hypersensitivity, overdosage, and effects unrelated to dose [Dreifuss, 1983a].

Hypersensitivity reactions may be acute or may not manifest until several months of therapy have elapsed. Lymphadenopathy, fever, maculopapular skin rash, splenomegaly, and hyperbilirubinemia may occur. The entire clinical pattern may be confused with infectious mononucleosis. Acute reactions related to overdosage usually manifest as brainstem and cerebellar impairment with vomiting, diplopia, ataxia, and occasionally alteration of consciousness. When overdosage associated with intravenous administration occurs, bradycardia or asystole may occur as a result of interference with cardiac conduction. This situation may be phenytoin mediated or may be the effect of the solvent, propylene glycol.

Symptoms of chronic drug toxicity include ataxia, diplopia, and nausea, as described in relation to acute overdosage. In addition, seizure frequency rarely may be increased, particularly of generalized seizures. Impaired intellectual functioning, including the development of dementia, has been reported. Aberrations in calcium and phosphorus metabolism, as well as osteomalacia and rickets, have been reported in association with ongoing phenytoin therapy [Crosley et al., 1975; Tolman et al., 1975].

Untoward effects unrelated to dosage or blood concentration include folate deficiency (which may be accompanied by macrocytic anemia), hirsutism, gum hyperplasia, and rarely lymphadenopathy, which has a subsequent clinical course inseparable from lymphoma. However, lymphadenopathy may be reversed by discontinuing phenytoin therapy.

Dosage. The oral dose of phenytoin is approximately 5 mg/kg/day; the maximum dose for adults is 200 to 400 mg/day. The range of therapeutic blood concentrations is 10 to 20 µg/ml. Phenytoin is manufactured in capsules (30 to 100 mg), chewable tablets (50 mg), and as a suspension (20 or 120 mg/5 ml). Use of the suspension is not suggested because the material tends to settle, thus the suspension strength is often less than expected in the full bottle and greater than expected in the nearly empty bottle. Intravenous phenytoin is one of the mainstays of status epilepticus management.

Phenobarbital

Pharmacologic actions. Phenylethylbarbituric acid *(phenobarbital; Luminal)* inhibits multisynaptic and spinal monosynaptic circuitry, probably as a result of enhancement of presynaptic inhibition. The drug also suppresses posttetanic potentiation.

Phenobarbital is absorbed rapidly and well from the gastrointestinal tract and is distributed in many organs. Blood concentrations peak approximately 12 hours after oral administration.

Metabolic degradation of phenobarbital occurs in the liver, where it is oxidized and then conjugated with glucoronic acid. A small portion of the drug remains unmetabolized and is excreted by the kidneys.

Side effects. Phenobarbital produces fewer serious side effects than most antiepileptic drugs. Hypersensitivity occurs in the form of periorbital edema, urticaria, maculopapular rashes, and other dermal reactions. Responses to overdosage include sedation, ataxia, impaired fine motor coordination, and irritability. In small children, hyperactivity may be induced or enhanced by phenobarbital. Hyperactivity is often accompanied by a decreased attention span and subsequent interference with learning skills.

Dosage. Phenobarbital remains the barbiturate of choice because of the disparity between the concentration required for antiepileptic effect and the concentration that produces toxicity. The usual dose is 4 to 6 mg/kg in children; the maximum adult dose is 120 to 200 mg/day. The recommended therapeutic blood concentration is between 20 and 40 µg/ml. Phenobarbital is supplied in tablets (15, 30, 60, and 100 mg) and as an elixir (20 mg/5 ml).

Carbamazepine

Pharmacologic actions. Carbamazepine (Tegretol) has been used since 1962. It is an iminostilbene derivative that is fully absorbed from the gut; peak blood levels are usually attained 3 hours after ingestion. Blood concentrations after administration of the same oral dose vary widely among individuals. Because most drugs require five half-lives to reach steady-state kinetics, the carbamazepine half-life of 12 hours necessitates administration over 2 to 4 days before a steady state is attained. The 12-hour half-life is comparatively short and necessitates divided daily doses.

Urinary excretion is in the form of carbamazepine-10-11-epoxide and iminostilbene. The epoxide metabolite possesses antiepileptic capabilities.

Although the precise mechanism of carbamazepine action is unknown, studies demonstrate that it inhibits maximal electroshock seizures. It is also an effective inhibitor of polysynaptic pathways while permitting the spinal monosynaptic reflex to remain intact. It probably inhibits ion conductance through fast sodium channels.

Side effects. The clinical pattern associated with overdosage includes ataxia, diplopia, dizziness, nausea, and vomiting. The symptoms may not be related to blood concentration and often manifest at the initiation of therapy; they may be most pronounced during the first hour after ingestion. Untoward effects may be modified by taking the medication during meals. During therapy initiation, it is often best to increase gradually the dosage over 1 to 2 weeks to decrease side effects. Evidence indicates that some side effects are the result of the epoxide metabolite.

Bone marrow suppression and impaired hepatic function may occur during therapy. These side effects should be monitored by appropriate studies biweekly during the first month of treatment, then bimonthy for 6 months, and every 3 to 6 months thereafter. Induced decrease in the granulocyte count frequently occurs and usually relents without altering therapy; however, leukocyte counts below 3500/mm^3 or a granulocyte count of less than 25% of the total should be managed by a decrease in carbamazepine dosage. Inappropriate antidiuretic hormone secretion may occur and lead to hyponatremia.

Carbamazepine is unlike other antiepileptic drugs and has a chemical configuration similar to tricyclic antidepressants. Psychotropic effects have occasionally been reported. These effects, usually beneficial, may not be related to administration of carbamazepine but rather to the decrease and discontinuation of other drugs, such as phenytoin and phenobarbital.

Dosage. Carbamazepine is usually administered in doses of 20 to 40 mg/kg/day (200 to 1600 mg/day). The therapeutic range of blood concentration is between 6 and 12 µg/ml. The drug is useful in managing simple partial seizures, complex partial seizures, and generalized tonic-clonic seizures. It has been particularly useful in managing complex partial seizures. Simultaneous administration of carbamazepine with phenobarbital, phenytoin, or valproic acid results in blood concentrations less than expected; therefore periodic determination of blood concentration is necessary to monitor the drug properly.

Valproic acid

Pharmacologic actions. Valproic acid (Depakene, Epilim, Atemporator, dipropylacetate), a short, branched-chain dicarboxylic acid, increases the brain concentration of gamma-aminobutyric acid by an unknown mechanism. Evidence suggests that this antiepileptic drug impairs degradation of gamma-amionobutyric acid; moreover, it may also inhibit synaptic reuptake of gamma-aminobutyric acid.

Valproic acid is particularly effective in treating generalized seizures and is one of the best drugs directed against absence seizures. It is also highly effective in myoclonic seizures (see Chapter 30). Valproic acid appears to have some effect on partial seizures, but its therapeutic effect is variable. The medication appears as efficacious as ethosuximide for absence seizures and may prove beneficial when ethosuximide therapy has been unsuccessful.

Side effects. Gastrointestinal upset and somnolence may accompany initiation of therapy; however, these symptoms usually dissipate after several days.

Simultaneous administration with phenobarbital may result in increased phenobarbital blood concentrations and subsequent drowsiness. Phenobarbital blood concentrations should be assessed frequently. When phenytoin is also administered, blood levels are highly variable because of competitive protein binding between the two drugs. Therefore the free phenytoin blood concentration may be increased and side effects may occur, even though total phenytoin concentration is relatively low. Unusual alertness, transient hair loss, and some weight gain with associated increase in appetite have been described. Thrombocytopenia may occur as a dose-related phenomenon.

Hepatotoxicity and occasionally pancreatitis may occur and may be fatal. Hepatic toxicity is most frequent in children younger than 3 years of age, especially when they are receiving valproate as a medication in multiple antiepileptic drug therapy. The risk of fatal hepatotoxicity declines with age and is very low for all patients receiving monotherapy [Dreifuss and Santilli, 1986].

Liver function studies should be performed frequently; symptoms such as nausea, vomiting, lethargy, edema, and jaundice are particularly significant.

Dosage. Valproic acid is a highly water-soluble and rapidly absorbed compound that provides peak blood levels within 1 hour after administration. It is taken in three or four divided doses per day because of its short half-life (6 to 13 hours). The daily dosage is 20 to 60 mg/kg; the expected blood concentrations range from 50 to 100 µg/ml. Dosage forms include sodium valproate (250 mg/5 ml), valproic acid capsules (250 mg), and divalproex sodium tablets (125, 250, and 500 mg) and sprinkles (125 mg). Epilim is dispensed in 200 mg tablets, and Atemporator as magnesium valproate in 250 and 500 mg tablets.

Primidone

Pharmacologic actions. Primidone (Mysoline) is a pyrimidine and is structurally similar to phenobarbital, a major product of primidone degradation. Phenylethylmalonic acid is the other major metabolite and has an antiepileptic effect. Primidone is readily absorbed from the gastrointestinal tract. The phenobarbital metabolite, as expected, is further metabolized by conjugation with glucuronic acid and is partly excreted in the urine as phenobarbital.

Side effects. Acute overdosage results in nausea, ataxia, vertigo, and somnolence. Initiation of primidone therapy should be very gradual.

Personality changes, hyperkinetic activity, and reduced attention span have been reported. Personality changes may include aggressive behavior and extreme irritability. These untoward effects may be rapidly evident when the drug is discontinued.

Dosage. Primidone is available in tablets (50 to 200 mg) and as a suspension (250 mg/5 ml). The maximum tolerated dosage is 25 mg/kg/day. Blood levels of primidone should be maintained between 6 and 8 µg/ml.

Clonazepam

Pharmacologic actions. Clonazepam (Klonopin, Rivotril) is a benzodiazepine that is rapidly absorbed after ingestion, and peak blood concentrations occur in 1 hour. The drug is degraded in the liver and is excreted as oxazepam in the free and conjugate form of the 7-amino-acid derivative.

Benzodiazepines depress electrically induced afterdischarges in the limbic system, in brainstem reticular formation, and in seizures initiated by pentylenetetrazol (Metrazol), strychnine, and electrical stimulation. This action suggests that inducement or enhancement of an inhibitory mechanism occurs. Benzodiazepines facilitate gamma-aminobutyric acid–mediated inhibition through the effect of the benzodiazepine receptor on the chloride channel.

Clonazepam is of value in managing absence seizures that are unresponsive to ethosuximide or valproic acid, or when ethosuximide or valproic acid is not tolerated. Clonazepam has some value in managing myoclonic seizures that accompany mixed minor motor seizures, such as those found in Lennox-Gastaut syndrome or some of the progressive myoclonic epilepsies.

Side effects. Clonazepam often causes somnolence. Tolerance to the drug results from activation of hepatic degradation enzymes and from adaptation of the nervous system to the drug. Seizures are common because adaptation occurs comparatively quickly, and increasing the dosage of the drug may be only temporarily effective. Unfortunately, during the process of drug discontinuation, generalized tonic-clonic seizures may occur and prove difficult to manage, and at times status epilepticus may occur.

Dosage. The half-life of clonazepam is approximately 18 hours; therefore the drug is administered in divided doses. The recommended dose is 0.05 to 0.2 mg/kg/day administered in three divided doses. The therapeutic blood level range is 13 to 72 ng/ml.

New antiepileptic drugs

Vigabatrin (gamma-vinyl-gamma-aminobutyric acid, Sabril) Vigabatrin is a structural analog of gamma-aminobutyric acid and a selective enzyme-activated, irreversible inhibitor of gamma-aminobutyric acid transaminase.

Vigabatrin is rapidly and completely absorbed after oral administration and rapidly enters the brain and CSF. It is not protein bound and does not induce hepatic metabolism. It interacts with phenytoin, resulting in a 25% decrease in the latter drug's plasma concentrations.

Vigabatrin appears to be particularly effective in complex partial seizures and has been found to be effective in infantile spasms that occur as a result of tuberous sclerosis.

Side effects include drowsiness, irritability, dizziness, headache, and confusion at times, although only drowsiness has occurred with any significant frequency. In animal studies, microvacules were found in white matter, which apparently are reversible when the drug is stopped; they have not been found clinically or pathologically in humans.

The elimination half-life of vigabatrin is between 6½ and 12 hours. The dosage is 50 mg/kg, with an upper limit in children of 150 mg/kg.

Vigabatrin is not yet approved for use in the United States.

Oxcarbazepine (Trileptal). Oxcarbazepine is the keto-analog of carbamazepine and differs from carbamazepine in that it is converted to 10-hydroxy-carbazepine, bypassing the epoxide that is believed to be more toxic than the parent carbamazepine. The active metabolite has a half-life of 8 to 13 hours and appears to be the active principal agent.

Although the dose of oxcarbazepine is approximately 50% greater than carbamazepine to produce the same effectiveness, there appear to be fewer allergic effects than with carbamazepine. The spectrum of activity and indications are similar to those for carbamazepine.

Oxcarbazepine is not yet approved for use in the United States.

Felbamate. Felbamate is a dicarbamate, and its mode of action as an antiepileptic drug has not been clearly identified. Preliminary testing in the antiepileptic drug development program suggests that it has a broad spectrum of antiepileptic activity in that it is effective in suppressing maximal electroshock and pentylenetetrazol seizures. It also has a high protective index. Its elimination half-life is approximately 19 hours. The drug is poorly soluble in water. Felbamate has little toxicity up to 45 mg/kg in children and an upper limit dose of 3600 mg in adults, although insomnia and anorexia may be seen. In experimental studies, it appears to be effective against complex partial seizures and appears to have some efficacy against the manifestations of the Lennox-Gastaut syndrome.

There are some interesting interactions with other drugs in that it raises phenytoin and valproate levels by 25% and appears to hasten the metabolism of carbamazepine to carbamazepine epoxide, thus being conducive to the side effects of the latter, while lowering the blood level of the parent drug.

Felbamate has been approved for use in the United States.

Other agents. Other drugs under investigation include lamotrigine (Lamictal) and Gabapentin, but to date there has been no significant documentation of these drugs in the treatment of childhood epilepsies.

Common errors in management

Inaccurate classification of an epileptic type may lead to administration of inappropriate drugs, such as administering phenobarbital or phenytoin for absence seizures, ethosuximide for partial complex seizures that generalize secondarily, or high doses of antiepileptic drugs for seizures resulting from metabolic aberrations, such as hyperosmolality and diabetes mellitus. A misdiagnosis of conversion reaction when the patient has bona fide seizures also results from inaccurate classification.

The clinician must not substitute one drug for another prematurely. Attainment of steady-state blood levels is directly related to the half-life of the individual drug. Other discrete factors related to absorption, bioavailability, and concomitant use of other drugs—including nonantiepileptic drugs—may alter the period necessary to attain a steady state. At the least, days and sometimes weeks may be required until the drug's effect can be ascertained. Increasing or decreasing the dose of a drug without allowing adequate time for evaluation, or adding other drugs before a reasonable time has elapsed, should be avoided. Evaluating clinical effect without concomitant knowledge of antiepileptic blood levels is illogical.

The clinician should not discontinue drug therapy too quickly after seizure control has been achieved. Although there is no consensus, most clinics observe a seizure-free period of 2 to 4 years before drugs are withdrawn. In one study, 4 years of seizure control were observed before the medication was gradually discontinued over a 3-month period. When more than one antiepileptic drug was being administered concurrently, each drug was gradually withdrawn sequentially over a 3-month period. The relapse rate in this study was 24% [Todt, 1984].

Identifying the child who will have exacerbation of seizures after discontinuing antiepileptic drugs remains difficult. Seizure frequency, seizure severity, family history of epilepsy, sex, and race appear not to influence the likelihood of further seizure activity after drug withdrawal [Holowach et al., 1982]. Seizure types with favorable remission patterns include febrile seizures, absence seizures, and tonic-clonic seizures. Other favorable factors include early onset (younger than 8 years of age) and early control. Conversely, jacksonian seizures (relapse rate: 40%), onset after 9 years of age, interictal neurologic impairment, and a paroxysmal, profoundly abnormal EEG pattern do not bode well. It may be exceedingly difficult to decide whether drugs should be withdrawn, and the factors surrounding each child's condition must be carefully assessed.

Ongoing epilepsy has always been a major obstacle in living a normal life. Social, psychologic, and medical aspects of epilepsy are often overwhelming. Furthermore, it appears that the longer time between onset of seizures and control, the more intractable the seizures become. When seizure control is not attained within a reasonable period, it is in the best interests of the patient to refer the patient to an epilepsy center, where the most advanced equipment for intense monitoring, cumulative experience in managing intractable seizures, and skilled physiologic and pharmacologic consultations are available. These centers are often engaged in evaluating new drugs, and personnel are experienced in evaluating patients for possible surgical intervention.

Surgical management

Surgical management of epilepsy can be divided into two categories—restorative or ablative. The former consists of clipping aneurysms, excising tumors, aspirating cysts and removing cyst walls, evacuating subdural hematomas and stripping their membranes, shunting to circumvent ventricular and aqueductal obstructions, and evacuating abscesses.

Ablative surgery is directed at excising the brain tissue in either circumscribed or large involved areas that serve as the epileptogenic foci. Lesions that are ablated include gliotic scars, small cryptic tumors, and poren-cephalic cysts. Sometimes tissues that appear grossly normal but that can be identified as containing a consistently abnormal and well-delineated EEG focus may be excised. Hemispherectomy, first described by Krynauw [1950], has been used for intractable seizures and malignant behavioral disturbances in children with early acquired or congenital hemiplegia. Although this operation has been of benefit for some patients, long-term evaluation indicates that this approach should be reserved only for the most intransigent situations.

Temporal lobectomy has been used for temporal lobe seizures that are refractory to drug therapy and in which EEG abnormalities reside entirely or predominantly in one temporal lobe. Preliminary studies obtained before surgery is undertaken are vital. If possible, the site of the seizure focus should be delineated by positron emission tomography. The epileptogenic focus should be further demarcated by using depth electrodes. Recordings taken during seizure activity are necessary for accurate localization of the discharges. It is essential that hemispheric dominance be determined by appropriate tests for speech and memory; intracarotid amytal sodium injection may prove necessary. Innovative surgical techniques now allow removal of small areas of the temporal lobe (amygdalohippocampectomy).

Assessing the advisability of surgical therapy for children with epilepsy should include the knowledge that severe and uncontrollable epilepsy may improve spontaneously during maturation and by using both currently available and future drugs. Nevertheless, the disruption of emotional and cognitive development and function by uninterrupted epileptic episodes may be so great that surgery is justified. Patients who need surgical therapy are best managed by a planning team that includes a neurosurgeon, neurologist, clinical neurophysioloigst, neuropsychologist, and psychiatrist [Dreifuss, 1983b].

When epileptiform activity appears to be present in small, delimited cortical areas, focal cortical excision may be indicated. In selective cases, corpus callosotomy may be performed to relieve distressing and dangerous drop attacks that are intractable and may damage children suffering from secondarily generalized epilepsies, such as the Lennox-Gastaut syndrome and secondarily generalized tonic-clonic and atonic seizures arising from a unilateral frontal focus.

REFERENCES

Aicardi J, Chevrie JJ. Convulsive status epilepticus in infants and children: a study of 239 cases. Epilepsia 1970; 11:187.

Andermann F. Chronic encephalitis and epilepsy: Rasmussen's syndrome. Stoneham, Mass: Butterworth-Heineman, 1991.

Andermann E, Metrakos JD. EEG studies of relatives of probands with focal epilepsy who have been treated surgically. Epilepsia 1969; 10:415.

Backus RE, Millichap JG. The seizure as a manifestation of intracranial tumor in children. Pediatrics 1962; 29:978.

Bancaud J, Talairch J, Boris A, et al. La stereoelectroencephalographie dans l'epilepsie. Paris: Charles Masson et Cie, 1965.

Bickford RG, Klass DW. Sensory precipitation and reflex mechanisms: In: Jasper HH, Ward AA, Pope A, eds. Basic mechanisms of the epilepsies. Boston: Little Brown, 1969.

Bray PF, Wiser WC. The relation of focal to diffuse epileptiform EEG discharges in genetic epilepsy. Arch Neurol 1965; 13:223.

Brown JK, Cockburn F, Forfar JO. Clinical and chemical correlates in convulsions of the newborn. Lancet 1972; 1:135.

Chao D. Photogenic and self-induced epilepsy. J Pediatr 1962; 61:733.

Commission on Classification, International League Against Epilepsy. Proposed revisions of clinical and electroencephalographic classification of epileptic seizures. Epilepsia 1981; 22:480.

Corellis JAN, Meldrum BS. Epilepsy. In: Blackwood W, Corsellis JAN, eds. Greenfield's neuropathology, 3rd ed. London: Edward Arnold (Publishers), 1976.

Crosley CJ, Chee C, Berman PH. Rickets associated with long-term anticonvulsant therapy in a pediatric outpatient population. Pediatrics 1975; 56:52.

Dastur HM, Desai AD. A comparative study of brain tuberculomas and gliomas based upon 107 case records of each. Brain 1965; 88:375.

Delgado-Escueta AV, Bascal FE, Treiman DM. Complex partial seizures in closed-circuit television and EEG: a study of 691 attacks in 79 patients. Ann Neurol 1982; 11:292.

Doose H, Gerken H, Hien-Volpek KF, et al. Genetics of photosensitive epilepsy. Neuropaediatrie 1969; 1:56.

Dreifuss FE. Adverse effects of antiepileptic drugs. In: Ward AA Jr, Penry JK, Purpura D, eds. Epilepsy. New York: Raven Press, 1983a.

Dreifuss FE, ed. Pediatric epileptology. Boston: John Wright/PSG, 1983b.

Dreifuss FE. Goals of surgery for epilepsy. In: Engel J Jr, ed. Surgical treatment of the epilepsies. New York: Raven Press, 1987.

Dreifuss FE, Mushet GR. Unpublished observations, 1966.

Dreifuss FE, Santilli N. Fatal hepatotoxicity with valproate: analysis of 37 cases. Neurology 1986; 36:175.

Falconer MA, Serafetinides EA, Corsellis JAN. Etiology and pathogenesis of temporal lobe epilepsy. Arch Neurol 1964; 10:232.

Ferrier D. Experimental researchs in cerebral physiology and pathology. West Riding Lunatic Asylum Med Rep 1873; 3:30.

Fisher RS. Animal models of the epilepsies. Brain Res Rev 1989; 14:245.

Fritsch G, Hitzig E. Uker die elecktrische Erregbarkeit des Grosshirs. Arch Anal Physiol 1870; 37:300.

Gastaut H, Broughton R, Tassinari CA, et al. Unilateral seizure. In: Vinkin PJ, Bruyn GW, eds. Handbook of clinical neurology. Amsterdam: North Holland Publishing, 1974.

Grand W. Significance of posttraumatic status epilepticus in childhood. J Neurol Neurosurg Psychiatry 1974; 37:178.

Greenberg DA, Delgado-Escueta AV, Widelitz H, et al. Juvenile myoclonic epilepsy (JME) may be linked to the Bf and HLA foci on human chromosome 6. Am J Genet 1988; 31:85.

Hauptmann A. Luminol bei epilepsie. Munch Med Wochenschr 1912; 59:107.

Holowach J, Thurston DL, Hixon B et al. Prognosis in childhood epilepsy: additional follow-up of 148 children 15-23 years after withdrawal of anticonvulsants. N Engl J Med 1982; 306:831.

Jeavons PM. Photosensitive epilepsies. In: Roger J, Dravet C, Bureau M, et al., eds. Epileptic syndromes in infancy, childhood and adolescence. Paris and London: John Libbey, 1985.

Jennet B. Epilepsy after non-missile head injuries. 2nd ed. London: William Heinemann Medical Books, 1975.

Krynauw RA. Infantile hemiplegia treated by removing one cerebral hemisphere. J Neurol Neurosurg Psychiatry 1950; 13:243.

Landau WM, Kleffner FR. Syndrome of acquired aphasia with convulsive disorder in children. Neurology 1957; 7:523.

Landolt H. Die temporallappenepilepsie und ihre Psychopathologie. Basel, Switzerland: S Karger AG, Medical & Scientific Publishers, 1960.

Leppert M, Anderson VE, Wuattelbaum T, et al. Benign familial neonatal convulsions linked to genetic markers on chromosome 20. Nature 1989; 337:647.

Lerman P. Benign partial epilepsy with centro-temporal spikes. In: Roger J. Dravet C, Bureau M, et al., eds. Epileptic syndromes in infancy, childhood and adolescence. Paris and London: John Libbey, 1985.

Locock C. Contribution to discussion on paper by E.H. Sieveking. Lancet 1857; 1:528.

Loescher W, Schmidt D. Which animal models should be used in the search for new antiepileptic drugs? A proposal based on experimental and clinical considerations. Epilepsy Res 1988; 2:145.

Lothman EW, Bertram EH, Stringer JL. Functional anatomy of hippocampal seizures. Neurobiol 1991; 37:1.

MacDonald RL, Meldrum BS. Principles of antiepileptic drug action. In: Levy R, Mattson RH, Meldrum BS, et al., eds. Antiepileptic drugs, 3rd ed. New York: Raven Press, 1989.

Mattson RH, Cramer JA. Epilepsy, sex hormones, and antiepileptic drugs. Neurology 1985; 26:S40.

Mattson RH, Cramer JA, Collins JF, et al. Comparison of carbamazepine, phenobarbital, phenytoin and primidone in partial and secondary generalized tonic-clonic seizures. N Engl J Med 1985; 313:145.

McNamara JO, Galloway MT, Rigsbel LC, et al. Evidence implicating substantia nigra in regulation of kindled seizure threshold. J Neurosci 1984; 4:2410.

Meldrum BS. Metabolic factors during prolonged seizures and their relation to cell death. In: Delgado-Esceuta AV, Wasterlain CJ, Treiman DM, et al., eds. Advances in neurology, vol 34. New York: Raven Press, 1983.

Meldrum BS. Physiological changes during prolonged seizures and epileptic brain damage. Neuropaediatrie 1978; 9:203.

Merritt HH, Putnam TJ. Sodium diphenylhydantoinate in treatment of convulsive disorders. JAMA 1938; 111:1068.

Metrakos JD, Metrakos K. Genetics of convulsive disorders: genetic and electroencephalographic studies in centrencephalic epilepsy. Neurology 1961; 11:474.

Morrell F. Secondary epileptogenesis in man. Arch Neurol 1985; 42:318.

Nayrac P, Beaussart M. Les pointes-ondes prerolandiqnes: expression EEG treis particuliere. Etude electroclinique de 21 cas. Rev Neurol (Paris) 1958; 99:201.

Newmark ME. Sensory evoked seizures. In: Dreifuss FE, ed. Pediatric epileptology. Boston: John Wright/PSG, 1983.

Noebels JL, Qiao X, Bronson RT, et al. Stargazer: a new neurological mutant on chromosome 15 in the mouse with prolonged cortical seizures. Epilepsy Res 1990; 7:129.

Ounsted C. Genetic and social aspects of epilepsies of childhood. Eugen Rev 1955; 47:33.

Ounsted C, Lindsey J, Norman R. Biological factors in temporal lobe epilepsy. London: William Heinemann Medical Books, 1966.

Penfield W, Jasper H. Epilepsy and functional anatomy of the human brain. Boston: Little, Brown, 1954.

Penry JK, Dreifuss FE. Automatisms associated with the absence of petit mal seizures. Arch Neurol 1969; 21:142.

Prince DA. Physiological mechansims of focal epileptogenesis. Neurology 1985; 26:S3.

Rasmussen T, McCann W. Clinical studies of patients with focal epilepsy due to "chronic encephalitis," Trans Am Neurol Assoc 1968; 93:89.

tisms. In a study of 926 absence seizures in 54 children, automatisms occurred more frequently in typical absence seizures than in atypical ones, whereas decreases in postural tone or tonic activity occurred more frequently in atypical ones. Atypical absence seizures lasted significantly longer [Holmes et al., 1987]. These findings make the differentiation of complex absence from partial complex seizures virtually impossible on purely clinical grounds and necessitate clinical and EEG analysis.

In absence seizures with autonomic phenomena the alterations in pupil size, skin color, and heart rate suggest sympathetic nervous system effect. Urinary incontinence can also occur.

The effect of absence seizures (and the associated EEG discharge) on cognitive function has been elucidated. In 14 patients with absence seizures who were investigated by use of a computer-assisted reaction time measurement triggered by the onset of EEG paroxysms, 56% of the reaction times measured were distinctly abnormal [Porter et al., 1973]. Later-onset stimuli yielded even more abnormal reaction times. In a study of 26 patients [Browne et al., 1974], 413 auditory reaction times were determined; they were normal during the 1 second before the EEG paroxysms. A total of 43% of the reaction times were normal at the onset of paroxysms, but only 20% were normal after a delay of 0.5 second into the paroxysm. It appeared that the spike-and-wave paroxysm impaired consciousness regardless of duration, and therefore treatment should attempt to control all spike-and-wave paroxysms.

Whether to pursue further diagnostic studies or treatment in the asymptomatic patient with 3 Hz spike-and-wave activity observed incidentally on EEG has not been determined, although some impairment of function has been presumed [Browne and Mirsky, 1983].

CLINICAL LABORATORY TESTS

In both typical and atypical absence seizures the diagnosis is confirmed by EEG. During the seizure the EEG exhibits the sudden onset of bilaterally synchronous, frontally predominant 3 Hz spike-and-slow-wave activity. After the discharge the record returns to its preictal appearance, with no intervening voltage depression or postictal slowing. The interictal EEG is usually normal. Brief bursts of spike-and-wave activity without obvious clinical seizures are found in up to 33% of patients.

Electrical and clinical seizures can be precipitated by activation, particularly hyperventilation (and sometimes photic stimulation). In the usual technique the patient takes about 60 deep breaths/min for 3 to 4 minutes, which often precipitates a typical clinical seizure with concomitant EEG paroxysms. Hyperventilation has been found more effective than prolonged monitoring in predicting clinical seizure frequency [Adams and Lueders, 1981], and prolonged monitoring is more effective than parent or teacher observation [Browne et al., 1983; Keilson et al., 1987]. Hyperventilation also is useful when assessing the efficacy of pharmacotherapy.

GENETICS

Since the appearance of an early report [Metrakos and Metrakos, 1961] that indicated a strong family tendency toward the spike-and-wave pattern in siblings (37%), particularly between the ages of 4 to 7 years (50%), there has been speculation about the genetic transmission of absence seizures. A high concordance rate in twins for 3 Hz spike-and-wave discharges (84%) and absence seizures (75%) has also been reported [Lennox, 1960]. The observation that generations are not skipped suggests a dominant mode of inheritance [Metrakos and Metrakos, 1970], but the precise genetic mechanism has not yet been determined [Andermann, 1982]. The large contribution of genetic susceptibility has been further enhanced by the demonstration of spike-and-wave complexes in 72% of 50 siblings of patients with idiopathic absence; both waking and sleep recordings were obtained [Degen et al., 1990]. In comparing the risk for unprovoked seizures in the offspring of patients with partial or generalized epilepsy, no difference was found between the two except for generalized absence in which the risk was three times greater [Ottman et al., 1989].

PATHOLOGIC CONDITIONS

There is no well-documented, common underlying pathologic lesion in patients with typical absence seizures. In the rare reports of brain lesions, including tumors, in patients with "absence seizures" the clinical features are highly atypical [Farwell and Stuntz, 1984; Page et al., 1969]. In several large series of patients with both epilepsy and brain tumor, none had primary, generalized, nonconvulsive epilepsy [Gastaut and Gastaut, 1976; McGahan et al., 1979; Page et al., 1969].

BIOCHEMISTRY

The biochemical basis for absence seizures, although suggested by the strong genetic tendency, is unknown. Particular attention has been directed toward the excitatory amino acid neurotransmitters, glutamate and aspartate. A hyperfunctioning glutamate system has been reported in both experimental [Van Gelder et al., 1983] and clinical [Janjua et al., 1982] circumstances. The role of gamma-aminobutyric acid (GABA) in absence seizures is also under study. The role of GABAergic transmission within the thalamus in the control of absence seizures in genetic absence epileptic rat models has been shown in a number of studies [Liu et al., 1991a; 1991b]. In the rat model, injection into the substantia nigra of

GABA agonists (e.g., muscimol or THIP) significantly decreases the EEG-recorded spike-and-wave activity [Depaulis et al., 1988]. In Wistar rats with spontaneous absence seizures, THIP abolishes, or even reverses, the antiepileptic effectiveness of valproate, but not of ethosuximide, which is still effective when coadministered [Vergnes et al., 1985]. Valproate and the benzodiazepines stimulate GABA activity, although through different mechanisms, and are effective in generalized seizures. Conversely, in all experimental animal studies, the administration of GABA agonists promotes the clinical and electrical concomitants of corticoreticular epilepsy [Fariello, 1985]. In vitro studies of membrane binding in some experimental models of generalized epilepsy suggest an alteration of the high-affinity benzodiazepine binding site [Meldrum and Chapman, 1986]. During absence attacks there is a striking increase in the cortical fluorodeoxyglucose uptake in gray matter, demonstrated by positron emission tomography [Engel et al., 1985].

During seizures in the genetic rat model of absence epilepsy, a diffuse increase in cerebral energy metabolism has been demonstrated using the 2-[^{13}C]deoxyglucose autoradiographic method; similar increases have been found in humans using positron emission tomography scanning [Nehlig et al., 1991].

Conversely, blood flow decreased in the middle cerebral artery 7 to 9 seconds after the onset of 3 Hz spike-and-wave activity in two patients during absence seizures as measured by transcranial Doppler blood flow-meter. It reached a trough 0 to 8 seconds after the disappearance of the bursts, rebounded, and returned to preictal value within 1 minute [Sanada et al., 1988]. The administration of gamma-hydroxybutyrate provides a useful model of absence epilepsy in animals [Snead, 1988]. In the tottering mouse, an electrophysiologic model of human absence epilepsy, there is an abnormality of opioid receptors. In this model, methionine-enkephalin, but not beta-endorphin or dynorphin, is increased in the striatum, cortex, pons, and medulla [Patel et al., 1991].

More recently, in the lethargic mouse model of spontaneous absence, antagonists of the GABA$_B$ receptor suppressed the seizures, whereas agonists exacerbated them [Hosford et al., 1992]. In this interesting model, medications effective against human absence episodes were also effective, whereas phenytoin and carbamazepine were not. The number of GABA$_B$ receptors is apparently increased in these mice, and the synaptic response to stimulation enhanced.

PATHOPHYSIOLOGY

The role of sucortical areas in initiating, promoting, and terminating generalized seizures has been examined for many years. The concept of centrencephalic seizures embraces the importance of subcortical areas [Sarnat, 1977]. Penfield and Jasper [1954] promulgated the concept of a "centrencephalic system that integrates the functions of the two hemispheres." It has been found that 3 Hz spike-and-wave activity occurring diffusely over the cortex can be elicited by rhythmic stimulation of the medial interlaminar region of the thalamus [Jasper and Droogleever-Fortuyn, 1946] or the mesencephalic reticular formation [Wier, 1964]. Implanting aluminium oxide in the interlaminar nuclei of kittens produced 3 Hz spike-and-wave activity and behavioral absence seizures, results that could not be elicited in older animals [Guerriro-Figueroa et al., 1963]. Other studies suggested that the thalamic-induced activity actually originated in the cortex [Pollen, 1964]. In patients, electrical stimulation of the mesiofrontal cortex produced 3 Hz spike-and-wave activity and clinical absence seizures [Bancaud et al., 1974]. It has also been suggested that absence seizures result from paroxysmal activity in cortical inhibitory pathways [Fromm and Kohli, 1972]. Among the structures that have influenced absence seizures are the brainstem, diencephalon, less well-defined areas in the reticular formation, and areas such as the hypothalamus, certain thalamic nuclei, and the substantia nigra. Recent studies of pentylenetetrazol-induced seizures, a model for human absence epilepsy, have implicated the mamillary bodies [Mirski and Ferrendelli, 1986] and suggest that ethosuximide may exert antiepileptic action through inhibition of an efferent pathway. The mechanism of action of ethosuximide is unknown. One possible explanation is the reduction of low threshold calcium current in ventrobasal thalamic neurons; this calcium current is important in thalamic oscillatory behavior [Coulter et al., 1989a].

Ethosuximide and dimethadione, antiepileptic drugs effective against absence seizures, reduced this current, whereas phenytoin and carbamazepine had minimal effects [Coulter et al., 1989b].

MANAGEMENT

Treatment with a single antiepileptic drug (monotherapy) is preferred. Ethosuximide has been the drug of choice for almost 30 years [O'Donohoe, 1964]. Ethosuximide probably acts by increasing the activity of certain inhibiting systems rather than by direct general membrane depression [Englander et al., 1977; Nowack et al., 1979]. Ethosuximide can be effectively administered once daily to patients who do not develop gastrointestinal side effects [Dooley et al., 1990].

More recently, valproate has been demonstrated to be equally effective [Sato et al., 1982], but the higher incidence of side effects, some of which are serious, and the need to monitor hematologic and liver function make it a second choice for treatment of absence seizures. Its action has been reported to be related to increasing GABA effect and to hyperpolarizing neuronal membranes. In a series of seven children the response to valproate was dose dependent, with a level of 440 to 660 μM needed to achieve at least 50% reduction of seizure activity [Braathen et al., 1988].

Absence seizures can be exacerbated by administration of carbamazepine [Horn et al., 1986; Snead and Hosey, 1985]. Atypical absence also can be exacerbated [Snead et al., 1985].

PROGNOSIS

About 50% of patients with absence seizures become seizure-free, and medication may be withdrawn after 2 to 4 years. For the remainder, either the absence seizures persist or tonic-clonic seizures develop. In a prospective study of 48 patients with absence seizures [Sato et al., 1976], 90% of patients with normal or better intelligence and no tonic-clonic seizures or family histories of seizure disorders became seizure-free. A prospective study reported on 90 patients with typical absence seizures [Loiseau et al., 1983], with follow-up to 15 years, and concluded that those patients with myoclonic or atonic absence seizures had poor prognoses. Patients with typical absence seizures or absence seizures with automatisms often experienced remission. The overall remission rate with absence seizures was only 57.5%, and tonic-clonic seizures developed in 36% of the patients. These figures are in general agreement with older retrospective studies. More recently a follow-up study of 83 patients followed for an average of 9½ years found that prognoses were better for male patients with normal IQs and normal neurologic examination but without hyperventilation-induced spike-and-wave activity [Sato et al., 1983]. Seizures stopped in more than 90% of patients who had three or more of these findings. Relapse is most likely to occur in the first year after treatment is discontinued [Thurston et al., 1982]. Absence seizures may be a harbinger of juvenile myoclonic epilepsy, appearing on average 4½ years before the myoclonic jerks and tonic-clonic seizures [Panayiotopoulos et al., 1989].

Typical absence seizures and absence seizures with automatisms are not necessarily benign conditions, and the prognosis is guarded. Current pharmacologic management, although often effective in controlling clinical seizures, does not appear to influence significantly the long-term outcome.

REFERENCES

Adams DJ, Lueders H. Hyperventilation and 6-hour EEG recording in evaluation of absence seizures. Neurology 1981; 31:1175.

Aicardi J. Epilepsy in children. New York: Raven Press, 1986.

Andermann F. Chronic encephalitis and epilepsy: Rasmussen's syndrome. Stoneham, Mass: Butterworth-Heinemann, 1991.

Andermann E. Multifactorial inheritance of generalized and focal epilepsy. In: Anderson VE, Hauser WA, Penry JK, et al., eds. Genetic basis of the epilepsies. New York: Raven Press, 1982.

Bancaud J, Talairach P, Morel M, et al. "Generalized" epileptic seizures elicited by electrical stimulation of the frontal lobe in man. Electroencephalogr Clin Neurophysiol 1974; 37:275.

Braathen G, Theorell K, Persson A, et al. Valproate in the treatment of absence epilepsy in children: a study of dose-response relationships. Epilepsia 1988; 29:548.

Browne TR, Dreifuss FE, Penry JK, et al. Clinical and EEG estimates of absence seizure frequency. Arch Neurol 1983; 40:469.

Browne TR, Mirsky AF. Absence (petit mal) seizures. In: Browne TR, Feldman RG, eds. Epilepsy, diagnosis and management. Boston: Little, Brown, 1983.

Browne TR, Penry JK, Porter RJ et al. Responsiveness before, during and after spike wave paroxysms. Neurology 1974; 24:659.

Cavazzuti GB, Ferrari F, Galli V, et al. Epilepsy with typical absence seizures with onset during the first year of life. Epilepsia 1989; 30:802.

Commission on Classification and Terminology of the International League Against Epilepsy. Proposal for revised clinical and electroencephalographic classification of epileptic seizures. Epilepsia 1981; 22:489.

Commission on Classification and Terminology of the International League Against Epilepsy. Proposal for classification of the epilepsies and epileptic syndromes. Epilepsia 1985; 26:268.

Coulter DA, Huguenard JR, Prince DA. Characterization of ethosuximide reduction of low-threshold calcium current in thalamic neurons. Ann Neurol 1989a; 25:582.

Coulter DA, Huguenard JR, Prince DA. Specific petit mal anticonvulsants reduce calcium currents in thalamic neurons. Neurosci Lett 1989b; 98:74.

Dalby MA. Epilepsy and 3 per second spike wave rhythms. A clinical, EEG and prognostic analysis of 346 patients. Acta Neurol Scand 1969; 40(suppl):1.

Degen R, Degen HE, Roth C. Some genetic aspects of idiopathic and symptomatic absence seizures: waking and sleep EEGs in siblings. Epilepsia 1990; 31:784.

DeMarco P. Reflex petit mal absence? Clin Electroencephalogr 1990; 21:74.

Depaulis A, Vergnes M, Marescaux C, et al. Evidence that activation of GABA receptors in the substantia nigra suppresses spontaneous spike-and-wave discharges in the rat. Brain Res 1988; 448:20.

Dooley JM, Camfield PR, Camfield CS, et al. Once-daily ethosuximide in the treatment of absence epilepsy. Pediatr Neurol 1990; 6:38.

Engel J, Lubens P, Kuhl DE, et al. Local cerebral metabolic rate for glucose during petit mal absences. Ann Neurol 1985; 17:121.

Englander RN, Johnson RN, Brickley JJ, et al. Effects of antiepileptic drugs on thalamocortical excitability. Neurology 1977; 27:1134.

Fariello RG. Biochemical approaches to seizure mechanisms: the GABA and glutamate systems. In: Porter RJ, Morselli PL, eds. The epilepsies. London: Butterworth, 1985.

Farwell JR, Stuntz JT. Frontoparietal astrocytoma causing absence seizures and bilaterally synchronous epileptiform discharges. Epilepsia 1984; 26:695.

Fromm GH, Kohli CM. The role of inhibitory pathways in petit mal epilepsy. Neurology 1972; 22:1012.

Gastaut H, Gastaut JL. Computerized transverse axial tomography in epilepsy. Epilepsia 1976; 17:325.

Guerriro-Figueroa R, Barros A, de Balbian VM, et al. Experimental "petit mal" in kittens. Arch Neurol 1963; 9:297.

Holmes GL, McKeever M, Adamson M. Absence seizures in children: clinical and electroencephalographic features. Ann Neurol 1987; 21:268.

Horn CS, Ater SB, Hurst DL. Carbamazepine-exacerbated epilepsy in children and adolescents. Pediatr Neurol 1986; 2:340.

Hosford DA, Clark S, Cao Z, et al. The role of GABA$_B$ receptor activation in absence seizures of lethargic (lh/lh) mice. Science 1992; 257:398.

Janjua NA, Metrakos JD, Van Gelder NM. Plasma amino acids in epilepsy. In: Anderson VE, Hauser WA, Penry JK, et al., eds. Genetic basis of the epilepsies. New York: Raven Press, 1982.

Jasper HH, Droogleever-Fortuyn J. Experimental studies on the functional anatomy of petit mal epilepsy. Res Publ Assoc Res Nerv Ment Dis 1946; 26:272.

Keilson MJ, Hauser A, Magrill JP, et al. Ambulatory cassette EEG in absence epilepsy. Pediatr Neurol 1987; 3:273.

Lennox WG. Epilepsy and related disorders. Boston: Little, Brown, 1960.

Liu Z, Snead OC III, Vergnes M, et al. Intrathalamic injections of gamma-hydroxybutyric acid increase genetic absence seizures in rats. Neurosci Lett 1991a; 125:19.

Liu Z, Vergnes M, Depaulis A, et al. Evidence for a critical role of GABAergic transmission within the thalamus in the genesis and control of absence seizures in the rat. Brain Res 1991b; 545:1.

Livingston S, Torres I, Pauli LL, et al. Petit mal epilepsy. Results of a prolonged follow-up study of 117 patients. JAMA 1965; 194:227.

Loiseau P, Pestre M, Dartigues JF, et al. Long-term prognosis in two forms of childhood epilepsy: typical absence seizures and epilepsy with Rolandic (centrotemporal) EEG foci. Ann Neurol 1983; 13:642.

McGahan JP, Dublin AB, Hill RP. The evaluation of seizure disorders by computerized tomography. J Neurosurg 1979; 50:328.

Meldrum BS, Chapman AG. Benzodiazepine receptors and their relationship to the treatment of epilepsy. Epilepsia 1986; 27(suppl 1):3.

Metrakos JD, Metrakos K. Genetic factors in epilepsy. In: Niedermeyer E, ed. Epilepsy. Modern problems in pharmacopsychiatry. Basel: Karger, 1970.

Mirski MA, Ferrendelli JA. Selective metabolic activation of the mammalary bodies and their connections during ethosuximide-induced suppression of pentylenetetrazol seizures. Epilepsia 1986; 27:194.

Nehlig A, Vergnes M, Marescaux C, et al. Local cerebral glucose utilization in rats with petit mal-like seizures. Ann Neurol 1991; 29:72.

Nowack WJ, Johnson RN, Englander RN, et al. Effects of valproate and ethosuximide on thalamocortical excitability. Neurology 1979; 29:96.

O'Donohoe NV. Treatment of petit mal with ethosuximide. Dev Med Child Neurol 1964; 6:498.

Ottman R, Annegers JF, Hauser WA, et al. Seizure risk in offspring of parents with generalized versus partial epilepsy. Epilepsia 1989; 30:157.

Page LK, Lombroso CT, Matson DD. Childhood epilepsy with late detection of cerebral glioma. J Neurosurg 1969; 32:253.

Panayiotopoulos CP, Obeid T, Waheed G. Absences in juvenile myoclonic epilepsy: a clinical and video-electroencephalographic study. Ann Neurol 1989; 25:391.

Patel VK, Abbott LC, Rattan AK, et al. Increased methionine-enkephalin levels in genetically epileptic (tg/tg) mice. Brain Res Bull 1991; 27:849.

Penfield W, Jasper H. Epilepsy and the functional anatomy of the human brain. Boston: Little, Brown, 1954.

Penry JK, Dreifuss FE. Automatisms associated with the absence of petit mal epilepsy. Arch Neurol 1969; 21:142.

Penry JK, Porter RK, Dreifuss FE. Simultaneous recordings of absence seizures with videotape and EEG. Brain 1975; 98:427.

Penry JK, So E. Refractoriness of absence seizures and phenobarbital. Neurology 1981; 31(suppl):158.

Pollen DA. Intracellular studies of cortical neurons during thalamic-induced wave and spike. Electroencephalogr Clin Neurophysiol 1964; 17:398.

Porter R, Penry JK, Dreifuss FE. Responsiveness at the onset of spike-wave bursts. Electroencephalogr Clin Neurophysiol 1973; 34:239.

Roger J. Prognostic features of petit mal absences. Epilepsia 1974; 15:433.

Sanada S, Murakami N, Ohtahara S. Changes in blood flow of the middle cerebral artery during absence seizures. Pediatr Neurol 1988; 4:158.

Sarnat HB. Changing concepts of the absence seizure: a review of the pathogenesis of petit mal epilepsy. Aust Paediatr J 1977; 13:158.

Sato S, Dreifuss FE, Penry JK. Prognosis factors in absence seizures. Neurology 1976; 26:788.

Sato S, Dreifuss FE, Penry JK, et al. Long-term follow-up of absence seizures. Neurology 1983; 33:1590.

Sato S, White BG, Penry JK, et al. Valproic acid versus ethosuximide in the treatment of absence seizures. Neurology 1982; 32:157.

Snead OC III. gamma-Hydroxybutyrate model of generalized absence seizures: further characterization and comparison with other absence models. Epilepsia 1988; 29:361.

Snead OC III, Hosey LC. Exacerbation of seizures in children by carbamazepine. N Engl J Med 1985; 313:916.

Thurston JH, Thurston DL, Hixon BB, et al. Prognosis in childhood epilepsy: additional follow-up of 148 children 15 to 23 years after withdrawal of anticonvulsant therapy. N Engl J Med 1982; 306:831.

Van Gelder NM, Siaitas I, Menini C, et al. Feline generalized penicillin epilepsy; changes in glutamic acid and taurine parallel the progressive increase in excitability of the cortex. Epilepsia 1983; 24:200.

van Luijtelaar EL, de Bruijn SF, Declerck AC, et al. Disturbances in time estimation during absence seizures in children. Epilepsy Res 1991; 9:148.

Vergnes M, Marescaux C, Micheletti G, et al. Blockade of "antiabsence" activity of sodium valproate by THIP in rats with petit mal-like seizures. Comparison with ethosuximide. J Neural Transm 1985; 63:133.

Wier B. Spike-wave from stimulation of reticular core. Arch Neurol 1964; 11:209.

31

Nonabsence Generalized Seizures

Lawrence A. Lockman

Several epileptic syndromes with generalized seizures and bilateral EEG discharges have been described; these include impulsive petit mal seizures, juvenile absence seizures with myoclonic phenomena, and atonic-astatic seizures. Tonic-clonic seizures are also included in this category.

MYOCLONIC-ASTATIC SEIZURES (LENNOX-GASTAUT SYNDROME)

The essential diagnostic features of the Lennox-Gastaut syndrome are early onset of epilepsy; multiple seizure types in the same patient, including absence seizures, myoclonic jerks, and atonic seizures; impaired development and intellect; and generalized, pseudo-rhythmic, slow spike-and-wave discharges on EEG. This form of epilepsy has also been called static seizures, akinetic epilepsy, minor epileptic status, minor motor epilepsy, propulsive petit mal, akinetic petit mal, myoclonic-astatic petit mal, and severe myokinetic epilepsy of early childhood with slow spike-and-wave activity. The use of the term *minor motor seizure* has been abandoned by contemporary epileptologists. Lennox [1945] described the "petit mal triad," which included petit mal (absence), myoclonic, and astatic seizures. Massive myoclonic jerks were added later, expanding the seizure variety to the "petit mal quartet" [Lennox, 1950]. Lennox also reported a greater variety of seizures, earlier onset, and more evidence of "brain damage" in patients with the petit mal quartet. Gastaut et al. reported in detail on patients with epileptic encephalopathy with diffuse slow spike-waves [1966]. Their criteria for diagnosis included: onset between the ages of 1 to 6 years; frequent seizures, almost always including tonic seizures, atonic seizures, and a variant of absence seizures; and pronounced mental retardation. Seizures resembling infantile spasms have also been observed [Donat and Wright, 1991]. Onset after 7 years of age has been described, but is unusual, and carries a worse prognosis. Many patients had periods of relative freedom from seizures interspersed with periods of distressingly frequent seizures and sometimes even absence status. The frequent and often forceful falls caused recurrent injury, particularly to the face and head, resulting in lacerations and often subsequent disfiguring scars.

These falls have been categorized into four types by careful monitoring: (1) tonic; (2) flexor spasms; (3) myoclonic-atonic; and (4) atonic. Atonic or myoclonic-atonic falls are not commonly observed unless the patient has a history of infantile spasms [Ikeno et al., 1985]. The patient's wearing of a football helmet or hockey helmet is of some benefit in reducing the severity of injury.

Differential diagnosis

An erroneous diagnosis of Lennox-Gastaut syndrome may be made in patients with "atypical benign partial epilepsy" as described by Aicardi and Chevrie [1982] because of atonic or myoclonic falls and the occurrence of slow spike-and-wave complexes during drowsiness and slow-wave sleep. The outlook is generally favorable.

A rare form of myoclonic-astatic epilepsy occurring in patients 1 to 5 years of age, with male preponderance and normal intelligence evident, was described by Doose et al. [1970]. Tonic seizures are not usually observed in this rare type. A genetic predisposition to this form may exist, and the prognosis is much better than in the Lennox-Gastaut syndrome. Nolte et al. [1988] found in follow-up of 27 patients who had epileptic drop attacks that 13 had Lennox-Gastaut syndrome and 14 had primary generalized myoclonic-astatic epilepsy as described by Doose [1970].

Other causes of drop attacks to be considered are narcolepsy-cataplexy syndrome, breath-holding episodes, syncope, orthostatic collapse, and a variety of cardiac conditions, including long-QT syndrome, complete atrioventricular block, sick sinus syndrome, progressive familial left bundle branch block, congenital aortic stenosis, obstructive cardiomyopathy, and corrected transposition of the great vessels.

EEG

Gibbs et al. [1939] described the slow (about 2 Hz) spike-and-wave discharge, later referring to it as the "petit mal variant" pattern [Gibbs et al., 1943]. It has been emphasized by many authors that the slow spike-and-wave discharges are an interictal EEG phenomenon and are activated by sleep [Markand, 1977]. Ictally the same discharge may be observed during an atypical absence attack, one in which there is less abrupt but complete loss of consciousness. Other findings may supervene during seizures, such as desynchronization of the EEG record [Gibbs and Gibbs, 1952; Gastaut et al., 1966; Blume et al., 1973; Gastaut and Tassinari, 1975], which is especially associated with tonic seizures [Markand, 1977], and brief bursts of polyspikes or rapid spikes [Niedermeyer, 1972]. The interictal EEG contains generalized bursts of 1.5- to 2.5-Hz spike-and-wave activity that does not respond to activation procedures [Markand, 1977]. Runs of rapid rhythmic spikes at about 10 to 25 Hz usually occur during sleep. This lack of a one-to-one relationship between the epileptiform discharges and the clinical seizures is in marked contrast to other generalized seizures, especially simple absence seizures. The slow spike-and-wave pattern is abundant, not influenced by hyperventilation, but increased by sleep, not regularly accompanied by decreased level of consciousness, and usually persists unchanged for many years, regardless of the age of the subject. Depth recordings from the centromedian thalamic nuclei of the thalamus correlated well with clinical events [Velasco et al., 1991]. Conversely, Dreifuss [1983] stated that some children with Lennox-Gastaut syndrome are in absence status for years at a time, suggesting that the slow spike-and-wave discharge may correlate with a clinical seizure state. Recent studies suggest that a subgroup of these patients has markedly abnormal sleep patterns, with severe reduction in the amount of rapid eye movement observed during polysomnography [Amir et al., 1986]. The differential diagnosis of epileptic syndromes with slow spike-and-wave discharges is listed in the box above right.

Etiology

A specific cause can be found in 50% to 90% of children with myoclonic-astatic epilepsy [Markand, 1977; Kurokawa et al., 1980], a marked contrast to the

---

Differential Diagnosis of Slow Spike-and-Wave Complexes*

Frontal Maximum (frontal midline, superior frontal regions)

Lennox-Gastaut syndrome (common)
Posttraumatic epilepsy with slow spike-and-wave pattern (rare)
Frontal lobe epileptogenic foci with secondary bilateral synchrony (moderately common)

Occipital Maximum

Benign occipital lobe epilepsy (rare)
Posterior variant of Lennox-Gastaut syndrome (very rare)

Midtemporal Maximum

Aphasia-convulsion syndrome (rare)

Temporooccipital Maximum

Occasionally in children (girls) with Rett syndrome and epileptic seizures (rare)

Undetermined Maximum

Epileptic seizure disorder related to radiation necrosis in children—mostly deep tumors (rare)
Electrical status epilepticus of sleep—no real spike-and-wave formation (rare)

---

*From Niedermeyer E. The electroencephalogram in the differential diagnosis of the Lennox-Gastaut syndrome. In: Niedermeyer E, Degen R, eds. The Lennox-Gastaut syndrome. New York: Alan R. Liss, 1988.

---

usual lack of success in finding a cause for generalized absence and impulsive petit mal seizures, in which genetics probably plays a major role. The most commonly attributed cause of myoclonic-astatic epilepsy is perinatal neurologic insult. A significant number of patients have a history of infantile spasms. A variety of other causes has been implicated in individual patients, including tuberous sclerosis, lysosomal storage disease, and aminoacidopathies. A high frequency of cerebral atrophy occurs, particularly subcortical, on CT [Gastaut et al., 1980]. Migrational defects can be detected by MRI [Palmini et al., 1991; Ricci et al., 1992]. Numerous authors have reported a much higher incidence of epilepsy in the families of patients with myoclonic-astatic epilepsy than in the general population, but the seizures in the relatives are rarely of the myoclonic-astatic type. Males predominate in most series, comprising up to 71% of patients. Four metabolic subtypes were delineated using 2-deoxyglucose positron emission tomography [Chugani et al. 1987]: unilateral focal hypometabolism, unilateral diffuse hypometabolism, bilateral diffuse hypometabolism, and normal. General hypometabolism was noted in some patients using the same technique in 10 patients who had normal imaging studies [Theodore et al., 1987].

Management

Patients with myoclonic-astatic epilepsy are notoriously resistant to treatment. Many of these patients are subjected to polypharmaceutic regimens, with no detectable difference in seizure frequency or severity. Indeed, some agents may worsen seizures or the patient's overall condition [Shields and Saslow, 1983; Lerman, 1986]. Use of sedative antiepileptics probably should be avoided. Phenobarbital almost never influences seizures and may cause cognitive and behavioral aberrations. Carbamazepine can exacerbate the seizures and even cause absence status [Horn et al., 1986]. Treatment failure greater than 80% is to be expected with all otherwise useful antiepileptic drug regimens, including phenytoin, phenobarbital, carbamazepine, valproic acid, benzodiazepines, adrenocorticotropic hormone, or corticosteroids [Erba and Browne, 1983; Aicardi, 1986].

In a prolonged study of 16 patients, Papini et al. [1984] found that the average number of seizures was about 25 per day. About 31% of the seizures occurred during drowsiness, and 54% occurred during inactive wakefulness. Only 6% occurred during sleep, and 1% during active wakefulness. The authors suggested that secondary effects of sedative antiepileptic drugs may increase seizure frequency by decreasing active alertness in these patients. Patients taking clonazepam, originally believed to be effective in these seizures, often exhibit tolerance, thus necessitating a dosage increase and eventually resulting in sedation. Other benzodiazepine drugs that have also been used successfully in some patients include nitrazepam and, more recently, clobazam [Farrell, 1986]. In addition, clobazam (1 mg/kg orally in a single dose) may abolish secondary bilateral synchrony in about 30 to 40 minutes and allow the differentiation of secondary bilateral synchrony from Lennox-Gastaut syndrome [Gastaut and Zifkin, 1988]. Monotherapy with valproic acid is as likely to benefit the patient as any other therapy, but early reports of its efficacy and its enabling some patients to discard their protective helmets, resulted in slight overenthusiasm. The ketogenic diet, originally proposed by Wilder [1921] and later modified by Huttenlocher et al. [1971; Huttenlocher, 1976] to permit a more normal nutritional state, has been extraordinarily effective in an occasional otherwise intractable patient. Unpalatability, expense, and social isolation imposed by such a stringent diet are the major drawbacks to its use. More recently, administration of adrenocorticotropic hormone has been found effective for seizure control in up to 80% of patients in an uncontrolled study [Snead et al., 1983].

Surgical ablation of part or essentially all of the corpus callosum may lead to a reduction in seizures, particularly the falls [Purves et al., 1988]. In an uncontrolled study, intravenous gamma-globulin was believed to be helpful in some patients [Illum et al., 1990]. Recently, felbamate has been reported to be an effective treatment for seizures in Lennox-Gastaut syndrome. In the 73 patients treated, there was a 34% decrease in the number of atonic seizures and a 19% decrease in total seizure frequency [New Engl J Med, 1993].

IMPULSIVE PETIT MAL SEIZURES

The term *impulsive petit mal,* coined in 1955 by Janz and Christian [1957], refers to a specific syndrome of epileptic seizures that occurs in the second decade of life. For a complete discussion of this syndrome, see Chapter 30. Tsuboi and Christian [1973] reported a high family incidence of myoclonic events. About 41% of patients' relatives had these abnormalities, with a peculiar propensity among female relatives; 15% of relatives without clinical myoclonus demonstrated the EEG findings.

OTHER RARE FORMS OF GENERALIZED SEIZURES

Delgado-Escueta et al. [1982] and Janz et al. [1981] described several other varieties of absence seizures. Juvenile absence seizures are clinically identical to classic absence seizures and have an EEG signature of 8 to 12 Hz "diffuse rhythms." Myoclonic absence seizures are characterized by brief unconsciousness with staring, stereotyped automatisms, and bilateral, symmetric clonic jerks. Myoclonus absence seizures differ in that the clonic jerks are asymmetric and the automatisms are reactive. These seizures all reportedly respond to valproic acid.

TONIC-CLONIC SEIZURES

The tonic-clonic seizure, formerly called a grand mal seizure, is the prototype of the epileptic seizure and exemplifies epilepsy to the general population. Patients with any other type of seizure fear having such a convulsion. In a large cohort of children examined subsequently for 7 years, tonic-clonic seizures were more common than all other seizure types combined [Ellenberg et al., 1984]. These seizures occurred in 25% of patients with seizures in another large study [Juul-Jensen and Foldsprang, 1983]. Although tonic-clonic seizures may be the most common type of seizure to occur in childhood, surprisingly few studies have been reported.

The tonic-clonic seizure begins with a tonic phase that is accompanied by immediate loss of consciousness and an abrupt fall. Forced expiration against a partially closed glottis often leads to a hoarse cry. There is usually limb extension, back arching, trismus, and apnea. The tonic phase lasts from several seconds to several minutes, and cyanosis develops. Swallowing ceases and may be accompanied by hypersalivation. The tonus is replaced by clonic jerking, with the head retroflexed, the arms usually flexed, and the lower extremities extended. The clonic phase can continue for minutes, waxing and waning, or may not stop at all, as in status epilepticus. In most instances the clonic phase gradually subsides as the jerks decrease in frequency. The patient regains consciousness for a few minutes, and often experiences a severe headache and some confusion. Deep postictal sleep ensues, which lasts from 30 minutes to several hours. In tonic-clonic epilepsy the tonic-clonic convulsion is the only type present; no obvious predisposing pathologic cause is manifest except possibly a genetic one. Tonic-clonic seizures may also occur after focal (or multifocal) epileptic discharges, a situation referred to as *secondary generalization*. At times the spread of the paroxysmal electrical activity can be so rapid that the focal signature is not apparent clinically, and it may even be difficult to ascertain with EEG. The tonic-clonic seizure is also the type most likely to be recognized as a manifestation of metabolic derangements, such as hypoglycemia, hypocalcemia, electrolyte imbalance, uremia, or hepatic failure. Tonic-clonic seizures can also occur immediately after head trauma.

Subclassification

The primary tonic-clonic epilepsies have been subdivided by the age of onset of the recurrent seizures. Although a distinct group of younger children, younger than age 15 years and with an approximate 2:1 male predominance, was reported by Gastaut et al. [1973], other authors have suggested that these tonic-clonic episodes in young children represent a variant of childhood myoclonic seizures [Aicardi, 1986]. Older children are more likely to have impulsive petit mal, which is improperly diagnosed as tonic-clonic epilepsy.

Clinical laboratory tests

In patients with tonic-clonic epilepsy, the interictal EEG is normal or reveals bilateral epileptiform bursts of varying frequencies. At the beginning of the seizure the EEG record discloses bilaterally synchronous and generalized bursts of spikes, which correlate with the tonic phase of the seizure. The electrical activity is sometimes difficult to see because it is obscured by the muscle artifact. The trains of spikes decrease in frequency and are replaced by bilaterally synchronous, generalized spike-and-slow-wave activity, which is phase-locked to the clonic movements observed clinically. As the frequency of these discharges slows and the clinical seizure ends, the EEG records generalized voltage suppression, followed by very slow, high-voltage slowing.

The major use of the EEG in tonic-clonic seizures is to help differentiate a physiologic seizure from a pseudoseizure. It is useful interictally to display focal or multifocal epileptiform discharges, which suggests that the seizures are localized in origin, with secondary generalization. To be certain that epilepsy is primarily generalized, long-term monitoring and recording of the clinical and electrical aspects of several clinical seizures are sometimes necessary. Because tonic-clonic seizures are commonly the result of other abnormalities, a number of other laboratory tests must be used to establish cause, particularly with the first or first several seizures. Direct infection of the nervous system, as in meningitis or encephalitis, can be established by examination of the cerebrospinal fluid. Assay of blood electrolytes can help detect abnormalities of calcium, sodium, and magnesium concentrations, as well as alterations of osmolality and acid-base balance. Hypoglycemia and kidney or hepatic failure should be considered. Possible toxic exposure can be explored through taking a history and performing laboratory screens for common toxins, particularly lead and drugs. Certain medications may cause seizures, most notably insulin, theophylline, and diuretics.

Management

Of the commonly used antiepileptic drugs, only ethosuximide has demonstrated no effect in controlling tonic-clonic seizures. Choosing among carbamazepine, phenobarbital, phenytoin, and valproic acid as the initial therapy rests as much on potential side effects and cost as on efficacy. Either carbamazepine or valproic acid is currently recommended initially, and, in patients with impulsive petit mal or morning generalized tonic-clonic seizures, valproic acid is the current drug of choice. Excellent control can be achieved in up to 75% of patients, and some improvement is expected in another 10% to 20% [Delgado-Escueta et al., 1982]. Prognosis for remission after 4 to 5 years of therapy is good.

REFERENCES

Aicardi J. Epilepsy in children. New York: Raven Press, 1986.
Aicardi J. Lennox-Gastaut syndrome and myoclonic epilepsies of infancy and early childhood. In: Aicardi J, ed. Epilepsy in children. New York: Raven Press, 1986.
Aicardi J, Chevrie JJ. Atypical benign epilepsy of childhood. Dev Med Child Neurol 1982; 24:281.
Amir N, Shalev RS, Steinberg A. Sleep patterns in the Lennox-Gastaut syndrome. Neurology 1986; 36:1224.
Blume WT, David RB, Gomez MR. Generalized sharp and slow wave complexes. Brain 1973; 96:289.
Chugani HT, Mazziotta JC, Engel J Jr, et al. The Lennox-Gastaut syndrome: metabolic subtypes determined by 2-deoxy-2[18F]fluoro-D-glucose positron emission tomography. Ann Neurol 1987; 21:4.

Delgado-Escueta AV, Treiman DM, Enrile-Bascal FE. Phenotypic variations of seizures in adolescents and adults. In: Anderson VE, et al., eds. Genetic basis of the epilepsies. New York: Raven Press, 1982.

Donat JF, Wright FS. Seizures in series: similarities between seizures of the west and Lennox-Gastaut syndromes. Epilepsia 1991; 32:504.

Doose H, Gerken H, Leonhardt R, et al. Centrecephalic myoclonic-astatic petit mal. Clinical and genetic investigation. Neuropaediatrie 1970; 2:59.

Dreifuss FE. Pediatric epileptology: classification and management of seizures in the child. Boston: John Wright-PSG, 1983.

Ellenberg JH, Hirtz DG, Nelson KB. Age at onset of seizures in young children. Ann Neurol 1984; 15:127.

Erba G, Browne TR. Atypical absence, myoclonic, atonic, and tonic seizures and the Lennox-Gastaut syndrome. In: Browne TR, Feldman RG, eds. Epilepsy, diagnosis and management. Boston: Little, Brown, 1983.

Farrell K. Benzodiazepines in the treatment of children with epilepsy. Epilepsia 1986; (suppl 1):45.

Gastaut H, Gastaut JA, Gastaut L, et al. Epilepsie generalisee primaire grand mal. In: Lugaresi E, Pazzaglia P, Tassinari CA, eds. Evolution and prognosis of epilepsies. Bologna: Aulo Gaggi, 1973.

Gastaut H, Pinsard N, Genton P. Electrical correlations of CT scans in secondary generalized epilepsies. In: Canger R, Angeleri F, Penry JK, eds. Advances in epileptology. New York: Raven Press, 1980.

Gastaut H, Roger J, Suolayrol R, et al. Childhood epileptic encephalopathy with diffuse slow spike-waves (otherwise known as "petit mal variant") or Lennox syndrome. Epilepsia 1966; 7:139.

Gastaut H, Tassinari CA. Epilepsies. In: Remond A, ed. Handbook of electroencephalography and clinical neurophysiology. Amsterdam: Elsevier-North Holland, 1975.

Gastaut H, Zifkin BG. Secondary bilateral synchrony and Lennox-Gastaut syndrome. In: Niedermeyer E, Degen R, eds. The Lennox-Gastaut syndrome. New York: Alan R. Liss, 1988.

Gibbs FA, Gibbs EL. Atlas of electroencephalography, vol II. Epilepsy. Reading, Mass.: Addison-Wesley, 1952.

Gibbs FA, Gibbs EL, Lennox WG. Influence of the blood sugar level on the spike-and-wave formation in petit mal epilepsy. Arch Neurol Psychiatry 1939; 41:1111.

Gibbs FA, Gibbs EL, Lennox WG. Electroencephalographic classification of epileptic patients and control subjects. Arch Neurol Psychiatry 1943; 50:111.

Horn CS, Ater SB, Hurst DL. Carbamazepine-exacerbated epilepsy in children and adolescents. Pediatr Neurol 1986; 2:340.

Huttenlocher PR. Ketonemia and seizures: metabolic and anticonvulsant effects of two ketogenic diets in childhood epilepsy. Pediatr Res 1976; 10:536.

Huttenlocher PR, Wilbourn AJ, Signore JM. Medium-chain triglycerides as a therapy for intractable childhood epilepsy. Neurology 1971; 21:1097.

Ikeno T, Shigematsu H, Miyakoshi M. An analytic study of epileptic falls. Epilepsia 1985; 26:612.

Illum N, Taudorf K, Heilmann C, et al. Intravenous immunoglobulin: a single-blind trial in children with Lennox-Gastaut syndrome. Neuropediatrics 1990; 21:87.

Janz D, Christian W. Impulsive-petit mal. Dtsch Z Nervenheilk 1957; 176:346.

Janz D, Kern A, Mossinger JH, et al. Ruckfall-prognoses warend und nach reduktion der medikamente bei epilepsiebehandlung. In: Remschmidt H, Rentz R, Jungmann J, eds. Epilepsie 1981. Stuttgart: Georg Thieme, 1981.

Juul-Jensen P, Foldspang A. Natural history of epileptic seizures. Epilepsia 1983; 24:297.

Kurokawa T, Goya N, Fukuyama Y, et al. West syndrome and Lennox-Gastaut syndrome: a survey of natural history. Pediatrics 1980; 65:81.

Lennox WG. The petit mal epilepsies, their treatment with tridione. JAMA 1945; 129:1069.

Lennox WG. Epilepsy and related disorders. Boston: Little, Brown, 1950.

Lerman P. Seizures induced or aggravated by anticonvulsants. Epilepsia 1986; 27:706.

Markand ON. Slow spike-wave activity in EEG and associated clinical features: often called "Lennox" or "Lennox-Gastaut" syndrome. Neurology 1977; 27:746.

New Engl J Med. Efficacy of felbamate in childhood opileptic encelphalopathy (Lennox-Gastaut syndrome). 1993; 328:29.

Niedermeyer E. The generalized epilepsies. Springfield, Ill: Charles C. Thomas, 1972.

Niedermeyer E. The electroencephalogram in the differential diagnosis of the Lennox-Gastaut syndrome. In: Niedermeyer E, Degen R, eds. The Lennox-Gastaut syndrome. New York: Alan R. Liss, 1988.

Nolte R, Wolff M, Krägeloh-Mann I. The atonic (astatic) drop attacks and their differential diagnosis. In: Niedermeyer E, Degen R, eds. The Lennox-Gastaut syndrome. New York: Alan R. Liss, 1988.

Palmini A, Andermann F, Aicardi J, et al. Diffuse cortical dysplasia, or the 'double cortex' syndrome: the clinical and epileptic spectrum in 10 patients. Neurology 1991; 41:1656.

Papini M, Pasquinelli A, Armellini M, et al. Alertness and incidence of seizures in patients with Lennox-Gastaut syndrome. Epilepsia 1984; 25:161.

Purves SJ, Wada JA, Woodhurst WB, et al. Results of anterior corpus callosum section in 24 patients with medically intractable seizures. Neurology 1988; 38:1194.

Ricci S, Cusmai R, Fariello G, et al. Double cortex. A neuronal migration anomaly as a possible cause of Lennox-Gastaut syndrome. Arch Neurol 1992; 49:61.

Shields WD, Saslow E. Myoclonic, atonic, and absence seizures following institution of carbamazepine therapy in children. Neurology 1983; 33:1287.

Snead OC, Benton JW, Myers GJ. ACTH and prednisone in childhood seizure disorders. Neurology 1983; 33:966.

Theodore WH, Rose D, Patronas N, et al. Cerebral glucose metabolism in the Lennox-Gastaut syndrome. Ann Neurol 1987; 21:14.

Tsuboi T, Christian W. On the genetics of the primary generalized epilepsy with sporadic myoclonias of the impulsive petit mal type: a clinical and electroencephalographic study of 399 probands. Humangenetik. 1973; 19:155.

Velasco M, Velasco F, Alcala H, et al. Epileptiform EEG activity of the centromedian thalamic nuclei in children with intractable generalized seizures of the Lennox-Gastaut syndrome. Epilepsia 1991; 32:310.

Wilder RM. The effect of ketonuria on the course of epilepsy. Mayo Clin Bull 1921; 2:307.

32

Myoclonic Seizures

Dinesh Talwar and Kenneth F. Swaiman

Myoclonus consists of sudden, brief, involuntary contractions or inhibitions of a single muscle or, more often, of muscle groups and is caused by a functional disturbance of the CNS [Fahn et al., 1986]. The movement can be characterized electrophysiologically as nonepileptic or epileptic. The terms *epileptic* versus *nonepileptic myoclonus* are primarily used to indicate the electrophysiologic origin of myoclonus. The term *myoclonic seizure* refers to a form of primary generalized seizure typically characterized by bilaterally synchronous jerks of the body or synchronous jerks of a segment of the body associated with a bilaterally synchronous spike-polyspike discharge on EEG. *Myoclonic epilepsy* refers to a clinical syndrome in which myoclonic seizures form a major component.

Etiologic classification is also possible because myoclonus occurs in various physiologic and pathologic conditions. Myoclonus may be a manifestation of a benign condition or a prominent component of progressive neurologic syndromes. Myoclonus epilepsy has been used to denote certain clinical syndromes that are characterized by both myoclonus and seizures and that often lead to significant disability and death. (e.g., Lafora disease, Unverricht-Lundborg disease).

Pathologic myoclonus occurs in conditions that are accompanied by hyperexcitability of the gray matter of many parts of the CNS including the cerebral cortex, basal ganglia, brainstem, and spinal cord.

Myoclonus or myoclonic seizures can result from encephalopathic disorders or focal brain lesions such as hypoxic-ischemic encephalopathy, viral encephalitis, bacterial meningitis, metabolic derangement, degenerative disease, vasculitis, and neoplasm. Myoclonic epilepsy may occur independently without explanation.

CLASSIFICATIONS

Electroencephalographic and electromyographic classification

Myoclonus may be classified electrophysiologically into nonepileptic or epileptic. Nonepileptic myoclonus includes normal physiologic and pathologic entities. Categories encompass common physiologic phenomena (e.g., hiccups, sneezing, sleep jerks, periodic movements of sleep, exaggerated startle reflex); myoclonus triggered in the basal ganglia; involuntary movements associated with an electromyographic pattern similar to that seen with a rapid (ballistic) voluntary movement, possibly with accompanying tics; and segmental myoclonus, including spinal myoclonus and palatal myoclonus [Hallet, 1985].

Epileptic myoclonus is defined electrophysiologically as myoclonic jerks related temporally to an EEG discharge and accompanied by a short burst duration on electromyography (50 ms and occasionally 50 to 100 ms), in contrast to a longer electromyographic burst duration (50 to 300 ms) in nonepileptic myoclonus. In addition, muscle contraction during a single jerk is synchronous in epileptic myoclonus, whereas muscle contraction can be nonsynchronous, alternating, or synchronous in nonepileptic myoclonus [Hallet, 1985].

Pathophysiologic classification

The 3 types of epileptic myoclonus are cortical reflex (epileptic) myoclonus, reticular reflex (epileptic) myoclonus, and primary generalized (epileptic) myoclonus. These conditions have been identified and classified with detailed electrophysiologic (both EEG and electromyographic) recording.

Cortical reflex (epileptic) myoclonus. Cortical re-

543

choice; however, great disparity exists in the literature concerning the therapeutic schedule and dosage [Hrachovy et al., 1989; Riikonen, 1984]. Studies have demonstrated better developmental outcome with early treatment; therefore infantile spasms should be managed aggressively and promptly at diagnosis [Singer et al., 1980]. Adrenocorticotropic hormone therapy administered within the first month of onset of the spasms is reported to be more effective than treatment begun after infantile spasms had persisted for more than 1 month [Riikonen, 1982].

Before initiation of adrenocorticotropic hormone (or adrenocorticosteroid) therapy, the physician should be cognizant of the possible side effects, which include marked irritability, hyperglycemia, hypertension, sodium and water retention, potassium depletion, weight gain, gastric ulcers, occult gastrointestinal bleeding, and diabetic ketoacidosis. The following laboratory tests should first be performed: serum electrolytes, blood urea nitrogen and creatinine, blood glucose, complete blood count, urinalysis, chest radiography, and tuberculin skin test. During adrenocorticotropic hormone therapy, serum electrolytes, blood glucose, stool guaiac, weight, and blood pressure should be closely monitored. Attendant management should include administration of foods high in potassium and antacid gel and/or H_2 blockers such as ranitidine. Natural adrenocorticotropic hormone is reported to have fewer side effects than the synthetic form.

Currently, opinions vary considerably on the appropriate adrenocorticotropic hormone dose and duration of treatment. Response to adrenocorticotropic hormone (or prednisone), when present, is frequently dramatic. Although some authors have recommended high-dose adrenocorticotropic hormone (up to 160 units/m^2/day) [Singer et al., 1980; Snead, 1990], others have suggested low-dose therapy (40 units/day) [Hrachovy et al., 1989; Ito et al., 1990; Riikonen, 1982]. Duration of therapy has also been quite varied, but most studies report 6 to 12 weeks; however, significantly shorter and longer courses have been used. Although proponents of high-dose therapy claim higher frequency of seizure control (90% of patients) [Snead et al., 1983], no prospective, controlled, and blinded studies comparing high-dose adrenocorticotropic hormone with low-dose adrenocorticotropic hormone have been performed, particularly in reference to long-term outcome. With adrenocorticotropic hormone, seizures can generally be controlled within 2 weeks [Hrachovy et al., 1989]; when infantile spasms persist beyond this time on adrenocorticotropic hormone therapy, control is unlikely.

In a double-blind, crossover study, Hrachovy et al. [1983; 1989] demonstrated equal effectiveness of 20 to 30 units/day of adrenocorticotropic hormone for 2 to 6 weeks, compared with prednisone 2 mg/kg/day for 2 to 6 weeks. Response rate was 60% to 70%. In a retrospective analysis, Riikonen [1982] compared high-dose adrenocorticotropic hormone (120 to 160 units/m^2/day) with low-dose adrenocorticotropic hormone (20 to 40 units/m^2/day) and found no significant difference in outcome. In a recent study, Ito et al. [1990] reported an optimal seizure response to adrenocorticotropic hormone doses greater than 0.6 units/kg/day; however, adrenocorticotropic hormone doses of 1.6 to 2.4 units/kg/day resulted in better mental development. Side effects increased with increasing doses; too small or too large a dose did not result in better mental development. The doses used in this study were significantly lower than those in most studies in the United States. Snead et al. [1983; 1990] reported control of spasms in 90% of patients with very high-dose adrenocorticotropic hormone gel (150 units/m^2/day), in contrast to control in 40% of patients with prednisone (2 mg/kg). This group recommended high-dose adrenocorticotropic hormone (150 units/m^2/day) administered intramuscularly divided twice a day for 1 week, 75 units/m^2/day in the morning for the second week, and 75 units/m^2 on alternating days for the third week. Adrenocorticotropic hormone is gradually withdrawn over the next 9 weeks.

The authors' current recommendation is to use 90 to 100 units/m^2/day (approximately 5 units/kg/day for a child weighing 8 kg). Treatment with the full dose is continued for approximately 2 to 3 weeks, but this duration may be shorter if a positive clinical appearance and EEG response occur earlier. A subsequent EEG 1 to 2 weeks after treatment aids in evaluating the degree of response. If the patient's episodes have ceased after 3 weeks, adrenocorticotropic hormone should be gradually withdrawn over the next 6 to 9 weeks. This decrease may be implemented by continuing adrenocorticotropic hormone every other morning for 3 additional weeks and then reducing it by 20% per week. If a relapse occurs during the withdrawal period, the dose should again be increased to the previous effective dose for 2 weeks and gradually withdrawn after that. If no substantial improvement has occurred after 3 weeks, therapy administered every other morning should be instituted for 1 week. The dosage should then be reduced in 20% decrements per week until it is discontinued. Prednisone (2 to 3 mg/kg/day) is substituted when adrenocorticotropic hormone cannot be administered for technical reasons (e.g., the parents cannot or will not learn to give injections). Again the full dose is generally continued for 3 weeks and gradually withdrawn in a schedule similar to the adrenocorticotropic hormone withdrawal. Some authors also recommend a trial of prednisone when there is no response to adrenocorticotropic hormone [Hrachovy, 1983; 1989].

The initiation of adrenocorticotropic hormone therapy should occur in the hospital; during hospitalization the parents should be taught proper injection techniques and use of systematic rotation of injection sites. Most parents can be taught intramuscular injection easily. Because various dosage regimens have been reported in the literature, the actual dosage chosen will depend on the experience and preference of the treating pediatric neurologist. High doses have the potential for serious, adverse effects, including hypertension, cardiomyopathy [Bobele et al., 1991], and potentially reversible cerebral atrophy [Lyen et al., 1979], in addition to the side effects previously mentioned.

Of all antiepileptic drugs, valproic acid [Dyken et al., 1985; Ito et al., 1991; Prats et al., 1991], clonazepam, and nitrazepam [Dreifuss et al., 1986] reportedly have some effectiveness against infantile spasms and can be used if no effect on the spasms has occurred with adrenocorticotropic hormone or prednisone therapy. Valproic acid is usually begun at a dosage of 20 to 30 mg/kg/day in three divided doses. Drug dosage is modified according to blood concentration and clinical response. Blood concentrations should be maintained between 75 and 125 mg/dl, although higher concentrations may be required in many cases. Clonazepam has been reported to be of help in some infants. It may be administered using a 0.03 mg/kg/day dosage administered in two to three divided doses and gradually increased to 0.1 mg/kg/day. Extreme somnolence may prove to be a limiting factor; most children cannot tolerate more than 0.15 mg/kg/day. Nitrazepam has been reported to be effective in the treatment of infantile spasms in some trials [Dreifuss, 1986]; however, the studies have predominantly evaluated the effects on seizure frequency and have not addressed the dramatic effect that may accompany adrenocorticotropic hormone therapy. In addition, effects on the EEG pattern have not been adequately reported. Reports on its benefits in this condition are hopeful, but past experience fosters skepticism that nitrazepam is of greater value than clonazepam or valproic acid. Nitrazepam is not commercially available in the United States. Several anecdotal reports appear in the literature on the effect of vitamin B_6 in the treatment of infantile spasms [Blennon and Starck, 1986; Prats et al., 1991]; however, well-designed studies to evaluate effectiveness of this vitamin have not been performed.

Partly based on early reports concerning the value of fasting for epilepsy [Geylin, 1921], Peterman [1924a; 1924b] introduced the ketogenic diet in the treatment of seizures. Treatment of infantile spasms with the ketogenic diet sometimes has gratifying results. The diet must be administered meticulously, or failure is likely. The patient should be hospitalized for initiation of the diet. A plan using a 3:1 ratio of fat-to-carbohydrate calories is first used (see box above right) [Swaiman, 1982], with medium-chain triglyceride oil as a source of lipid [Huttenlocher et al., 1971]. Protein needs are first

---

Sample Ketogenic Diet for 3-Year-Old Boy Weighing 15 kg

Calories needed daily:
  100 cal/kg = 1500
Protein needed daily:
  3 g/kg = 45
  Calories as protein: 45 × 4 = 180
Calories to be divided between fat and carbohydrate:
  1500 − 180 = 1320
  Fat to carbohydrate ratio:
  3 g:1 gm = 27 cal fat to 4 cal carbohydrate
$$\frac{1{,}320 \text{ cal}}{31 \text{ cal}} = 42.6$$
Total daily dietary needs:
  Fat: 3 × 42.6 = 127.8 g
  Carbohydrate: 1 × 42.6 g
  Protein: 45 g

---

ascertained, and the calories to be administered as protein are subtracted from the total daily caloric intake before the fat-to-carbohydrate ratio is translated into actual meal planning. The patient fasts only on the night before the diet is begun. The urine is tested for ketone bodies with chemically treated cardboard sticks every morning and afternoon, and the results are recorded. When ketosis cannot be maintained at the "small level," a 4:1 ratio diet is instituted. Hypoglycemia, vomiting, and dehydration are the most likely problems engendered by the diet.

The success of the ketogenic diet may mitigate the need for other medication or may reduce the dose of medication to less than usual and therefore avoid side effects. The disadvantages consist of the need for the parents' ability and motivation to prepare the diet and the psychologic difficulties of the child in adjusting to the necessary restrictions. When the diet is effective in controlling seizures, every effort should be made to maintain it for at least 1 year. Recurrences of seizures following effective management with drugs or diet are possible, and second remissions are common after reinstitution of therapy.

Success in controlling infantile spasms and consequently improving developmental outcome with regional excisional surgery in children with infantile spasms intractable to medical therapy has been reported. Surgery is performed on a region of a cortical abnormality (parietooccipitotemporal region) defined by EEG, MRI, and positron emission tomography [Chugani et al., 1990]. In the patients studied by Chugani et al. [1990], postoperative neuropathologic examination revealed microscopic cortical dysgenesis. The role of surgical treatment, if any, is likely to be better defined in the future.

Prognosis

Gibbs et al. [1954] originally reported that 87% of children with infantile spasms were or became retarded. The outlook for normal mental development continues to be poor. Etiology of infantile spasms, whether idiopathic (cryptogenic) or symptomatic, is the most important determinant of prognosis [Glaze et al., 1988]. Over 30% and perhaps up to 70% of cryptogenic cases are expected to have a good outcome with treatment [Cowan, 1991; Glaze et al., 1988]. Prognosis is significantly worse for children with a preexisting neurologic condition and is more likely determined by their underlying brain abnormalities. However, the question of whether infants who are neurologically impaired before seizure onset will enjoy preservation of abilities when seizures are treated promptly and successfully is not definitively addressed in the literature.

Prompt recognition of the syndrome and subsequent timely therapy may have some effect on the prognosis, particularly when treatment is initiated within 1 month of onset [Lombroso, 1983; Riikonen et al., 1982]. This concept, however, is not uniformly accepted [Hrachovy, 1989]. The spectrum ranging from normal mental development to mild retardation occurs more frequently when the infantile spasms are controlled soon after onset in infants who were apparently normal before the seizures appeared. A review of the prognosis of 150 children with infantile spasms indicated that normal development before the onset of spasms, short duration of seizures before control, and absence of abnormal physical findings are favorable prognostic indicators [Jeavons et al., 1973]. Unfortunately, success in the control of infantile spasms does not ensure that the patient will enjoy reasonable intellectual and motor growth.

EARLY MYOCLONIC ENCEPHALOPATHY

Early myoclonic encephalopathy [Aicardi and Goutieres, 1978; Dalla Bernardina et al., 1983] is characterized by the following:
1. Erratic (multifocal, random) myoclonus with onset early in infancy
2. Burst-suppression pattern on EEG
3. Profound neurologic impairment

Onset of this condition is typically in the neonatal period. Other seizure types are usually present. Often an etiology is not determined, although inborn errors of metabolism (particularly nonketotic hyperglycinemia), hypoxic-ischemic encephalopathy, and dysgenetic brain disorders should be excluded [Lombroso, 1990]. Familial cases have also been described. Prognosis is very poor, with many children ultimately dying early and others being left with profound neurologic impairment. Seizures are usually resistant to the available antiepileptic drugs.

EARLY INFANTILE EPILEPTIC ENCEPHALOPATHY

This syndrome has been described by Ohtahara et al. [1987b]. Its main features include onset very early in infancy, often in the neonatal period; tonic spasms similar to infantile spasms occurring singly or in clusters; and burst-suppression pattern on EEG, often evolving into some form of hypsarrhythmia. Severe neurologic impairment is the usual outcome. Other seizure types may be present. Various etiologies include perinatal difficulties and cerebral dysgenesis. This syndrome differs from early myoclonic encephalopathy in that there is no erratic myoclonus, although there are other common features. Some authors consider this syndrome to be an early variant of West syndrome [Lombroso, 1990]. Seizures are often very resistant to pharmacotherapy. As in early myoclonic encephalopathy the prognosis is dismal.

INFANTILE MYOCLONIC EPILEPSIES

Benign infantile myoclonic epilepsy, which occurs before 2 years of age, was first described in the literature by Dravet et al. [1985a]. Some children manifested febrile seizures before onset of their more typical seizures. Other than this history of febrile seizures, children with benign infantile myoclonic epilepsy are apparently normal neurologically until they develop myoclonic and subsequently generalized tonic-clonic seizures. EEG characteristically demonstrates generalized bursts of spike-polyspike-and-wave activity. A positive family history of epilepsy or febrile convulsions is present in up to one third of patients. According to the early descriptions of this syndrome, seizures respond well to treatment, although this has not been a universal experience. Atonic seizures are also described in some of these patients. Dravet et al. [1985a] describe a benign outcome (i.e., the epilepsy ultimately subsides as the child gets older), although neuropsychologic and behavioral abnormalities persist in many children.

Severe infantile myoclonic epilepsy has also been well delineated [Dravet et al., 1985b]. Onset of this syndrome also occurs before 2 years of age. Characteristically, previously normal children first exhibit frequent febrile seizures. Subsequently, nonfebrile myoclonic and generalized tonic-clonic seizures develop. As in benign infantile myoclonic epilepsy, although the EEG may be normal at the time when only febrile seizures are evident, it later shows the characteristic spike-polyspike-and-wave activity exacerbated by drowsiness and sometimes photic activation. Myoclonic seizures occur very frequently with varying degrees of intensity. Children may develop other seizure types, including atonic, absence, and partial seizures. As children grow older, neurologic abnormalities become evident, including ataxia, developmental delay, and mental retardation. Family history of epilepsy or febrile convulsions can be obtained in about 25% of patients with severe infantile myoclonic epilepsy. Both benign infantile myoclonic epilepsy and severe infantile myoclonic epilepsy are idiopathic, primary generalized epileptic syndromes with no identifiable etiology. Tonic seizures are characteristically absent in both.

Except for a more favorable response to treatment and neurologic outcome in benign infantile myoclonic epilepsy, there appears to be little differentiation between these two syndromes. In a series of patients with infantile myoclonic seizures described by Lombroso [1990], myoclonic seizures followed an initial period of febrile convulsions in all patients. Febrile convulsions were often prolonged, repetitive, and resistant to treatment. Lombroso [1990] proposed that benign infantile myoclonic epilepsy and severe infantile myoclonic epilepsy may be a continuum of the same epileptic syndrome and suggested that they should be combined under the common title of *infantile myoclonic epilepsy following febrile convulsions*.

Treatment of the two conditions is often difficult. Febrile convulsions occur despite phenobarbital prophylaxis. Myoclonic and generalized tonic-clonic seizures do not respond to and may be exacerbated by phenytoin, carbamazepine, and phenobarbital. Seizure frequency may decrease with high-dose valproic acid, but daily myoclonic seizures with or without other seizures types will often continue. Lombroso [1990] has reported success with high-dose valproic acid in combination with lorazepam, nitrazepam, or the ketogenic diet. Ethosuximide as a supplementary drug may also be useful in some patients [Hurst, 1987].

MYOCLONIC-ASTATIC EPILEPSY

Myoclonic-astatic epilepsy, which usually manifests during the first 5 years of life, has been described [Doose, 1985]. Children typically manifest myoclonic, atonic, and atypical absence seizures. Generalized tonic-clonic seizures may also occur. Characteristically, tonic seizures are absent [Maton et al., 1990]. The patients exhibit slow spike-and-wave (1 to 3 Hz) and polyspike-and-wave discharges on EEG. Due to the frequent and multiple seizure types and the markedly abnormal EEG pattern, there is some resemblance to Lennox-Gastaut syndrome. However, unlike Lennox-Gastaut syndrome, tonic seizures are typically not observed, and although most patients have neurologic impairment, prognosis has been reported to be significantly better than in Lennox-Gastaut syndrome. Recent reports indicate good seizure control with a combination of valproic acid and ethosuximide [Maton et al., 1990; Sheth and Talwar, 1991].

JUVENILE MYOCLONIC EPILEPSY

Juvenile myoclonic epilepsy, which is sometimes termed *benign juvenile myoclonic epilepsy* or *impulsive petit mal epilepsy* [Janz, 1973; Janz and Christian, 1957], has only in the last decade been recognized in the English medical literature [Asconape and Penry, 1984; Delgado-Escueta and Enrile-Bacsal, 1984]. Juvenile myoclonic epilepsy has been classified as a primary generalized epilepsy characterized by myoclonic jerks on awakening, generalized tonic-clonic and absence seizures, normal neurologic examination, and typical EEG abnormalities [Dreifuss, 1989; Janz, 1989].

Demographics

The incidence of juvenile myoclonic epilepsy has been underestimated for many years. It most likely accounts for about 4% to 11% of all childhood-onset epileptic syndromes [Dreifuss, 1989; Janz, 1973; Panayiotopoulos et al., 1991]. In the adolescent age group, it probably constitutes more than 20% of all new onset epilepsies. Juvenile myoclonic epilepsy characteristically occurs in the second decade, with approximately 50% manifesting the condition between 13 to 16 years of age and 25% each before and after this age [Asconape and Penry, 1984; Dreifuss, 1989].

Clinical characteristics

Myoclonic jerks (seizures), the hallmark of this epileptic syndrome, occur primarily on awakening in the morning but may also occur after an afternoon nap or at times of rest. They typically involve the upper extremities in a symmetric distribution, although the legs may also be affected. The entire body is rarely involved. Myoclonic jerks may be mild enough so as to be only perceived by the patient without the manifestation of an overt jerk. At other times, they may be severe enough to knock objects out of the hands. Consciousness is preserved during the myoclonic jerks unless repetitive myoclonic jerks ensue, representing a form of myoclonic status epilepticus. Myoclonic jerks may occasionally be unilateral [Panayiotopoulos et al., 1991]. The diagnosis of juvenile myoclonic epilepsy primarily depends on the presence of myoclonic jerks on awakening [Janz, 1989]. A history of myoclonic jerks is usually not volunteered by the patient, necessitating careful history taking on the part of the examining physician. Myoclonic jerks are often believed to represent "a nervous personality" or "clumsiness." Occasionally, despite the best attempt to obtain this history during the first clinic visit, the patient will deny experiencing myoclonic jerks [Panayiotopoulos et al., 1991].

Another characteristic feature of juvenile myoclonic epilepsy is generalized tonic-clonic seizures, which occur in perhaps all patients at some time during the course of untreated epilepsy. Over 80% of the patients manifested generalized tonic-clonic seizures at presentation in one study [Asconape and Penry, 1984]; generalized tonic-clonic seizures are usually the symptom for which patients seek medical attention. The myoclonic seizures will invariably precede the onset of generalized tonic-clonic seizures by a mean duration of 2 years [Asconape and Penry, 1984; Janz, 1989]. Although they most often occur on awakening, generalized tonic-clonic seizures can occur at other times, particularly at times of relaxation or rest. Nocturnal generalized tonic-clonic seizures may also occur and do not conflict with the diagnosis of juvenile myoclonic epilepsy [Panayiotopoulos et al., 1991]. Sleep deprivation, anxiety and stress, and alcohol intake are common precipitating factors for generalized tonic-clonic seizures, factors commonly a part of life for many adolescents. Approximately 33% of patients suffer from or have experienced absence seizures [Asconape and Penry, 1984; Janz, 1989]. These are characteristically typical absence seizures and manifest before the myoclonic jerks, often in the first decade of life. Some atypical features of the absence seizures include brief duration, low frequency, and the EEG accompaniment of a faster spike-and-wave discharge (3.5 to 4 Hz).

The neurologic examination is typically normal in juvenile myoclonic epilepsy patients [Janz, 1989]. Mental status examination and intellect in the interictal period is normal. CT and MRI scans usually do not demonstrate any abnormalities. Personality disturbances in some patients have been described. Juvenile myoclonic epilepsy is considered an idiopathic, genetic epilepsy. Microdysgenesis was reported on an autopsy study [Meencke and Janz, 1984]. However, the number of patients studied have been very few and the changes described very mild.

Many patients (17% to 49%) with juvenile myoclonic epilepsy have a family history that is positive for seizures [Janz, 1989]. In first-degree relatives of patients with juvenile myoclonic epilepsy the incidence of nonfebrile seizures has been reported to be 4.1% to 5.5% [Janz, 1989; Tsuboi and Christian, 1973]. Preliminary linkage studies have shown that the gene for juvenile myoclonic epilepsy is linked to the blastogenic factor and human leukocyte antigen loci on the short arm of chromosome 6 [Greenberg et al., 1988].

Clinical laboratory tests

EEG is the most useful test in the accurate diagnosis of juvenile myoclonic epilepsy. EEG abnormalities are best displayed by sleep deprivation. EEG background is usually normal, with no evidence of slowing or disorganization. The characteristic EEG abnormality is bursts of bifrontal or generalized, bilaterally synchronous, spike-polyspike-and-wave activity [Janz, 1989]. Fast spike-and-wave activity of 4 to 6 Hz is also frequently observed [Dreifuss, 1989]. During absence seizures the typical spike-and-wave activity is visualized but is usually faster than 3 Hz [Asconape and Penry, 1984]. Focal polyspike-and-wave activity accompanied by focal jerks has also been reported [Panayiotopoulos et al., 1991]. Photoparoxysmal response composed primarily of generalized or frontally predominant polyspike-and-wave activity occurs in approximately 30% to 35% of patients [Janz, 1989]. The myoclonic jerks are associated on the EEG with a burst of polyspikes at a frequency of 10 to 16 Hz, followed by high-amplitude slowing at a frequency of 2 to 5 Hz [Janz, 1989]. This complex of polyspikes followed by slow waves will often outlast the duration of the myoclonic jerk or jerks.

Management

Ancillary measures, such as adequate and regular sleep and adequate rest, avoidance of sudden awakening, and abstinence from alcohol intake are as important as pharmacologic treatment. The drug of choice for managing juvenile myoclonic epilepsy is valproic acid [Delgado-Escueta and Enrile-Bacsal, 1984]. Many patients enjoy complete or significant seizure control of myoclonic, generalized tonic-clonic, and absence seizures on valproic acid. Valproic acid is effective in controlling seizures in 85% to 90% of patients with juvenile myoclonic epilepsy. Relapses may occur if ancillary measures are not carefully followed [Penry et al., 1989]. Primidone and phenobarbital are also effective in controlling generalized tonic-clonic seizures but are less effective against myoclonic and absence seizures and also cause more significant cognitive and behavioral side effects. Treatment with an antiepileptic drug such as valproic acid is probably required throughout life; initial studies indicate a relapse rate of 75% to 100% when medication is withdrawn [Delgado-Escueta and Enrile-Bascal, 1984; Penry et al., 1989].

OTHER MYOCLONIC EPILEPSIES OF CHILDHOOD

A universally accepted classification encompassing all forms of myoclonic epilepsies remains elusive and controversial. Several patients with predominantly myoclonic seizures cannot be assigned to a category in the international classification. For example, some patients who have had myoclonic and generalized tonic-clonic seizures between the ages of 2 and 4 years, were neurologically normal, and demonstrated an excellent response to valproic acid were reported [Sheth and Talwar, 1991]. Presently, the varieties of seizure patterns, etiologic origins, and prognoses make a complete classification difficult.

Myoclonic seizures combined with absence activity that manifests after 2 years of age but usually during the first decade of life has also been described [Tassinari and Bureau, 1985]. Mental retardation is a prominent aspect of the clinical pattern. The EEG pattern consists of 3 Hz spike-and-wave discharges.

Progressive myoclonus epilepsy (Baltic myoclonus or Unverricht-Lundborg disease) is a progressive, inherited seizure disorder that is accompanied by the development of dementia. Despite its name, it is unclear whether this disorder should be classified with degenerative brain diseases or with the epilepsies. (This condition and some allied conditions are discussed in Chapter 55).

MANAGEMENT OF MYOCLONIC EPILEPSIES OF CHILDHOOD

Management of myoclonic seizures is often difficult. The underlying epileptic syndrome often determines the response. Valproate and clonazepam are among the antiepileptic drugs that have been most beneficial. Ethosuximide may have some role. Using 5-hydroxytryptophan in managing myoclonic epilepsy has not received adequate study. The ketogenic diet may occasionally prove useful. Using adrenocorticotropic hormone or prednisone in patients who have myoclonic epilepsy but not of the infantile spasm type has been of value on rare occasions.

REFERENCES

Aicardi J, Goutieres F. Encephalopathie myoclonique neonatale. Rev EEG Neurophysiol Clin 1978; 8:99.

Asconape J, Penry JK. Some clinical and EEG aspects of benign juvenile myoclonic epilepsy. Epilepsia 1984; 25:108.

Bertoni JM, Von Loh S, Allen RJ. The Aicardi syndrome: report of 4 cases and review of the literature. Ann Neurol 1979; 5:475.

Blennon G, Starck L. High-dose vitamin B6 treatment in infantile spasms. Neuropediatrics 1986; 17:7.

Bobele GB, Ward KE, Bodensteiner JB. Hypertrophic cardiomyopathy from adrenocorticotropic hormone in treatment of infantile spasms. Ann Neurol 1991; 30:460.

Chugani HT, Shields WD, Shewmon DA, et al. Infantile spasms: I. PET identifies focal cortical dysgenesis in cryptogenic cases of surgical treatment. Ann Neurol 1990; 4:406.

Cody CL, Baraff LJ, Cherry JD, et al. Nature and rates of adverse reactions associated with DPT and DT immunizations in infants and children. Pediatrics 1981; 68:650.

Commission on Classification and Terminology of the International League Against Epilepsy. Proposal for revised clinical and electroencephalographic classification of epileptic seizures. Epilepsia 1981; 22:489.

Commission on Classification and Terminology of the International League Against Epilepsy. Proposal for the classification of the epilepsies and epileptic syndromes. Epilepsia 1985; 26:268.

Commission on Pediatric Epilepsy of the International League Against Epilepsy. Workshop on infantile spasms. Epilepsia 1992; 33:195.

Cowan LD, Hudson LS. The epidemiology and natural history of infantile spasms. J Child Neurol 1991; 6:355.

Dalla Bernardina B, Dulac O, Fejerman N, et al. Early myoclonic epileptic encephalopathy (E.M.E.E.). Eur J Pediatr 1983; 140:248.

Delgado-Escueta AV, Enrile-Bacsal F. Juvenile myoclonic epilepsy of Janz. Neurology 1984; 34:285.

Doose H. Myoclonic astatic epilepsy of early childhood. In: Roger J, Dravet C, Bureau M, et al., eds. Epileptic syndromes in infancy, childhood and adolescence. London: Eurotext, 1985.

Dravet C, Bureau M, Roger J. Benign myoclonic epilepsy in infants. In: Roger J, Dravet C, Bureau M, et al., eds. Epileptic syndromes in infancy, childhood and adolescence. London: Eurotext, 1985a.

Dravet C, Bureau M, Roger J. Severe myoclonic epilepsy in infants. In: Roger J, Dravet C, Bureau M, et al., eds. Epileptic syndromes in infancy, childhood and adolescence. London: Eurotext, 1985b.

Dreifuss FE. Juvenile myoclonic epilepsy: characteristics of a primary generalized epilepsy. Epilepsia 1989; 30(suppl):S1.

Dreifuss FE, Farwell J, Holmes G, et al. Infantile spasms: comparitive trial of nitrazepam and corticotropin. Arch Neurol 1986; 43:1107.

Dyken PR, DuRant RH, Minden DB, et al. Short term effects of valproate on infantile spasms. Pediatr Neurol 1985; 1:34.

Fahn S, Marsden CD, Van Woert MH. Definition and classification of myoclonus. In: Fahn S, Marsden CD, Van Woert MH, eds. Myoclonus: adv neurol, vol 43. New York: Raven Press, 1986.

Gastaut H, Gastaut JL, Goncalves e Silva GE, et al. Relative frequency of different types of epilepsy: a study employing the classification of the International League Against Epilepsy. Epilepsia 1975; 16:457.

Geylin HR. Fasting as a method for treating epilepsy. Med Rec 1921; 99:1037.

Gibbs EL, Flemming MM, Gibbs FA. Diagnosis and prognosis of hypsarrhythmia and infantile spasms. Pediatrics 1954; 13:66.

Gibbs FA, Gibbs EL. Atlas of electroencephalography, vol 2. Cambridge: Addison-Wesley, 1952.

Glaze DG, Hrachovy RA, Frost JD Jr, et al. Prospective study of outcome of infants with infantile spasms treated during controlled studies of adrenocorticotropic hormone and prednisone. J Pediatr 1988; 112:389.

Greenberg DA, Delgado-Escueta AV, Widelitz H, et al. Juvenile myoclonic epilepsy (JME) may be linked to the BF and HLA loci on human chromosome 6. Am J Med Genet 1988; 31:185.

Hallet M. Myoclonus: relation to epilepsy. Epilepsia 1985; 26(suppl):S67.

Hallet M, Chadwick D, Marsden CD. Cortical reflex myoclonus. Neurology 1979; 29:1107.

Hallet M, Chadwick D, Adam J, et al. Reticular reflex myoclonus. J Neurol Neurosurg Psychiatry 1977; 40:253.

Hrachovy RA, Frost JD Jr. Infantile spasms. Pediatr Clin North Am 1989; 36:311.

Hrachovy RA, Frost JD Jr, Kellaway PR. Sleep characteristics in infantile spasms. Neurology 1981; 31:688.

Hrachovy RA, Frost JD Jr, Kellaway PR. Hypsarrhythmia: variations on the theme. Epilepsia 1984; 25:317.

Hrachovy RA, Frost JD Jr, Kellaway PR, et al. Double-blind study of adrenocorticotropic hormone vs prednisone therapy in infantile spasms. J Pediatr 1983; 103:641.

Hurst DL. Severe myoclonic epilepsy of infancy. Pediatr Neurol 1987; 12:21.

Huttenlocher P, Wilbourn AJ, Signore JM. Medium-chain triglycerides as a therapy for intractable childhood epilepsy. Neurology 1971; 21:1097.

Ito M, Okuno T, Fujii T, et al. Adrenocorticotropic hormone therapy in infantile spasms: relationship between dose of adrenocorticotropic hormone and initial effect and long term prognosis. Pediatr Neurol 1990; 4:240.

Ito M, Okuno T, Hattori H, et al. Vitamin B6 and valproic acid in treatment of infantile spasms. Pediatr Neurol 1991; 7:91.

Janz D. The natural history of primary generalized epilepsies with sporadic myoclonias of the impulsive petit mal. In: Lugareshi E, Pazzaglia P, Tassinari CA, eds. Evolution and prognosis of epilepsies. Bologna, Italy: Aulo Gaggi, 1973.

Janz D. Juvenile myoclonic epilepsy. Cleve Clin J Med 1989; 56:23.

Janz D, Christian W. Impulsiv-petit mal. Dtsch Z Nervenheilk 1957; 176:348.

Jeavons PM, Bower BD, Dimitrakoudi M. Long-term prognosis of 150 cases of "West syndrome." Epilepsia 1973; 14:153.

Kellaway P. Neurologic status of patients with hypsarrhythmia. In: Gibbs FA, ed. Molecules and mental health. Philadelphia: JB Lippincott, 1959.

Kellaway P, Hrachovy RA, Frost JD Jr, et al. Precise characterization and quantification of infantile spasms. Ann Neurol 1979; 6:214.

King DW, Dyken PR. Spinks IL Jr, et al. Infantile spasms. Pediatr Neurol 1985; 1:213.

Lacy JR, Penry JK. Infantile spasms. New York: Raven Press, 1976.

Livingston S, Eisner V, Pauli L. Minor motor epilepsy. Pediatrics 1958; 21:916.

Lombroso CT. A prospective study of infantile spasms: clinical and therapeutic correlations. Epilepsia 1983; 24:135.

Lombroso CT. Early myoclonic encephalopathy, early infantile epileptic encephalopathy, and benign and severe infantile myoclonic epilepsies: a critical review and personal contributions. J Clin Neurophysiol 1990; 7:380.

Lyen KR, Holland IM, Lyen YC. Reversible cerebral atrophy in infantile spasms caused by corticotrophin. Lancet 1979; 2:237.

Maton B, Hirsch E, Finck S. Benign form of childhood epilepsy with astatomyoclonic seizures. Epilepsia 1990; 31:607.

Matsumoto A, Wantanabe K, Negoro T, et al. Long term prognosis after infantile spasms: a statistical study of prognostic factors in 200 cases. Dev Med Child Neurol 1981; 23:51.

Meencke HJ, Janz D. Neuropathologic findings in primary generalized epilepsy: a study of eight cases. Epilepsia 1984; 25:8.

Melchior JC. Infantile spasms and early immunization against whooping cough: Danish Survey from 1970 to 1975. Arch Dis Child 1977; 52:134.

Mizrahi EM, Kellaway P. Characterization and classification of neonatal seizures. Neurology 1987; 37:1837.

Ohtahara S, Ohtsuka Y, Yamatogi Y. The West syndrome: developmental aspects. Acta Pediatr Jpn 1987a; 29:61.

Ohtahara S, Ohtsuka Y, Yamatogi Y, et al. The early-infantile epileptic encephalopathy and suppression-burst. Brain Dev 1987b; 9:371.

Panayiotopoulos CP, Tahan R, Obeid T. Juvenile myoclonic epilepsy: factors of error involved in the diagnosis and treatment. Epilepsia 1991; 32:672.

Penry JK, Dean JC, Riela AR. Juvenile myoclonic epilepsy: long-term response to therapy. Epilepsia 1989; 30(suppl):S19.

Peterman MG. The ketogenic diet in the treatment of epilepsy. Minn Med 1924a; 27:708.

Peterman MG. The ketogenic diet in the treatment of epilepsy: a preliminary report. Am J Dis Child 1924b; 28:28.

Prats JM, Garaizar C, Rua MJ, et al. Infantile spasms treated with high doses of sodium valproate: initial response and follow-up. Dev Med Child Neurol 1991; 33:617.

Riikonen R. A long-term follow-up study of 214 children with the syndrome of infantile spasms. Neuropediatrics 1982; 13:14.

Riikonen R. Infantile spasms: modern practical aspects. Acta Paediatr Scand 1984; 73:1.

Sheth R, Talwar D. Idiopathic myoclonic epilepsies of early childhood onset. Ann Neurol 1991; 30:496.

Singer WD, Rabe EF, Haller JS. The effect of adrenocorticotropic hormone therapy upon infantile spasms. J Pediatr 1980; 96:485.

Snead OC III. Treatment of infantile spasms. Pediatr Neurol 1990; 6:147.

Snead OC III, Benton JW, Myers GJ. Adrenocorticotropic hormone and prednisone in childhood seizure disorders. Neurology 1983; 33:966.

Sorel L, Dusaucy-Bauloye A. A propos de 21 cas d'hypsarhythmie de Gibbs, traitement spectaculaire par l'adrenocorticotropic hormone. Rev Neurol 1956; 99:136.

Swaiman KF. Absence seizures. In: Swaiman KF, Wright FS, eds. The practice of pediatric neurology, 2nd ed. St. Louis: Mosby, 1982.

Tassinari C, Bureau M. Epilepsy with myoclonic absences. In: Roger J, Dravet C, Bureau M, et al., eds. Epileptic syndromes in infancy, childhood and adolescence. London: Eurotext, 1985.

Tsuboi T, Christian W. On the genetics of the primary generalized epilepsy with sporadic myoclonias of the impulsiv petit mal type. Humangenetik 1973; 19:155.

Watanabe K, Iwase K, Hara K. The evolution of EEG features in infantile spasms. Dev Med Child Neurol 1973; 15:584.

West WJ. On a peculiar form of infantile convulsions. Lancet 1841; 1:724.

Wilkins DE, Hallet M, Erba G. Primary generalized epileptic myoclonus: a frequent manifestation of minipolymyoclonus of central origin. J Neurol Neurosurg Psychiatry 1985; 48:506.

Yamatogi Y, Ohtahara S. Age-dependent epileptic encephalopathy: a longitudinal study. Folia Psychiatr Neurol Jpn 1981; 35:321-32.

33

Neonatal Seizures

Michael Painter

DIAGNOSIS AND SIGNIFICANCE

The diagnosis of neonatal seizures is frequently difficult and is usually based on clinically described activity that is stereotyped, repetitive, and usually associated with abnormal eye movements. Concomitant EEG recording is ideal and sometimes essential for diagnosis. Five clinical seizure patterns have been described [Volpe, 1977]. Tonic seizures are characterized by extension of the arms and legs resembling decerebrate posturing. Subtle seizures are isolated abnormal eye movements, sucking, and rowing, pedaling, or swimming movements. Multifocal clonic seizures are characterized by random migration of movements from limb to limb. Focal clonic seizures are repetitive and localized to a single limb. Myoclonic seizures are single or multiple flexion movements of the extremities.

These seizure pattern types are more fragmentary than those observed in older children. The reason for this difference lies in the cellular organization of the immature and mature brains. Glial proliferation, migration of neurons, establishment of complex axonal and dendritic contacts, and myelin deposition are incomplete in the neonatal brain. Electrical discharges are incompletely spread, tend to remain localized to one hemisphere, and are slow to diffuse from the point of origin [Purpura, 1964]. Bilateral synchronous epileptic discharges are rare.

Not all repetitive neonatal movements are epileptic. Some are due to drug withdrawal [Desmond et al., 1972], impaired cerebral inhibition [Kellaway and Hrachovy, 1983], or normal sleep activity [Prechtl, 1975; Roffwarg, 1966; Emde and Metcalf, 1970]. Jitteriness, or neonatal clonus, can be distinguished from seizures by being stimulus provoked, ablated with change in posture or restraint, and unaccompanied by abnormal eye movements. Recurrent apnea may be a seizure manifestation, especially if associated with tonic posturing, but more often it is due to pulmonary, cardiovascular, or gastrointestinal disturbance.

The use of video EEG monitoring has prompted the re-evaluation of several clinical patterns previously classified as seizures. Tonic "seizures" are not usually associated with cortical electrical discharges and may be caused by lack of cerebral inhibition [Kellaway and Hrachovy, 1983]. Swimming, pedaling, and rowing movements, often called *subtle seizures*, are frequently normal movements not associated with paroxysmal electrical discharges. Generalized clonic activity associated with eye deviation in term infants correlates best with cortical electrical discharge [Mizrahi and Kellaway, 1984]. EEG correlates manifest differently in preterm infants in whom clonic activity is less predictably accompanied by electrical seizure activity [Scher et al., 1989]. Convulsive apnea occurs most frequently in the rapid eye movement phase of sleep [Watanabe et al., 1982], is most often represented on EEG by paroxysmal alphalike activity, and is usually not associated with a change in heart rate [Fenichel et al., 1980].

The frequent use of neuromuscular paralyzing agents in the treatment of neonatal cardiorespiratory disorders complicates the task of detecting seizure activity. Paroxysmal activity occurs in a significant number of infants paralyzed to facilitate pulmonary ventilation [Tharp and Laboyrie, 1983].

Although a significant percentage of neonatal paroxysmal discharges may emanate from subcortical gray matter [Ferguson et al., 1974] and are not reflected in scalp electrode monitoring, the degree to which continuous EEG monitoring will influence the diagnosis and management of neonatal seizures is undetermined. Wider use of concomitant EEG monitoring has already raised significant questions, and its use will undoubtedly be expanded to more routine detection and treatment of neonatal seizure activity. The fact that not all seizures are accompanied by concomitant EEG discharges complicates diagnosis and management. Identical seizure activity has been noted with and without EEG concomitants in the same infant during the same recording [Weiner et al., 1991]. As in adults, foci not always detected by surface EEG recordings are probably responsible for seizure propagation in newborns.

The diagnosis and treatment of neonatal seizures are important. Neonatal seizures are an adverse predictor of neurologic outcome in asphyxiated newborns [Mulligan et al., 1980] and reliably predict children who will develop cerebral palsy in high-risk populations [Nelson and Broman, 1977; Nelson and Ellenberg, 1979; Amiel-Tison, 1969]. Although outcome depends mostly on the underlying etiology and extent of brain injury, experimental evidence suggests that seizures themselves may be damaging to the developing brain. Moreover, changes in systemic blood pressure and increases in the anterior cerebral blood flow velocity during seizures may be harmful to premature neonates. These changes may result in hemorrhage and elevations of intracranial pressure [Perlman and Volpe, 1983].

The hypothesis that prevention of neonatal seizures or early, accurate detection followed by prompt, efficacious treatment will result in improved outcome of neonates treated in an intensive care unit is important to those who manage problems of neonates.

EEG characteristics

EEG patterns mature with increasing gestational age [Dreyfus-Brisac 1962, 1964; Samson-Dollfus et al., 1964]. Premature infants younger than 32 weeks gestation have recordings that are discontinuous with high-amplitude (100 mV) frontal sharp waves, rhythmic theta activity, and isolated sharp waves seen in sleep. The duration of continuous background activity increases with gestational age, so by 36 weeks gestation the EEG is continuous during wakefulness and active sleep. The background remains discontinuous during non–rapid eye movement sleep. Because background and ictal patterns vary with different gestational ages and sleep states, the clinical state of the infant is important. EEG patterns that have been recorded during neonatal seizure activity include migratory sharp waves, rhythmic 1 to 4 Hz delta [Eyre et al., 1983; Harris and Tizard, 1960], positive and negative 2 to 6 Hz spike-and-slow-wave complexes and runs of 6 to 10 Hz alphalike activity with amplitudes of 25 to 30 mV. Discharges tend to remain confined to a hemisphere, and bilaterally synchronous spike-and-wave complexes are unusual [Dreyfus-Brisac 1962, 1964]. Certain ictal patterns correlate with specific seizure types. Tonic seizures are often accompanied by rhythmic delta activity, whereas repetitive focal spikes are associated with clonic seizures. Periodic disturbances of respiration are often accompanied by rhythmic alphalike activity.

The value of EEG is not confined to the diagnosis of seizures; it also provides prognostic information [Engel, 1975; Monod et al., 1972; Rose and Lombroso, 1970]. In term infants, normal EEG patterns tend to predict normal development, whereas flat and burst-suppression recordings imply neurologic handicap [Prichard, 1964]. The prognostic value of EEG is greatest in the first few days of life, and recordings tend to normalize thereafter, even in infants with severe neurologic sequelae [Rose and Lombroso, 1970]. In newborns with asphyxia an EEG that remains abnormal for more than 2 weeks always predicts a poor neurologic outcome.

ETIOLOGY AND APPROACH

The differential diagnosis of neonatal seizures is listed in the box on p. 557. Rational treatment is based on an accurate diagnosis. An accurate history may be difficult to obtain. The mother is usually remote from the intensive care unit, often on another floor and sometimes in another hospital. Infant transportation teams do not always have time to obtain the complete details regarding labor and delivery. The individual responsible for the infant's care should review historical details with all other appropriate individuals. The most common cause of neonatal seizures is hypoxic-ischemic encephalopathy [Bergman et al., 1983; Tibbles and Prichard, 1965], but other entities that masquerade as hypoxic-ischemic encephalopathy can be missed without a proper history. Blood pressure should not be overlooked because hypertensive encephalopathy may cause seizures in neonates; appropriate treatment includes control of blood pressure and not antiepileptic drugs. Indirect funduscopy should be carefully performed, because retinal hemorrhages are a clue to trauma and chorioretinitis is a clue to infection. Skin lesions can indicate infection or neurocutaneous syndromes.

Metabolic abnormalities may occur in combination or in conjunction with structural disease. Every infant with neonatal seizures should have a CSF examination. Figure 33-1 is a flow diagram of the key aspects that should be stressed in evaluation.

Metabolic abnormalities

The two most common and most treatable metabolic abnormalities that cause seizures are hypoglycemia and hypocalcemia. Every newborn with seizures should have a blood glucose determination using a Dextrostix screen, followed by a standard glucose oxidase determination. Hypoglycemia is present when glucose concentration in whole blood is below 20 mg/dl in a preterm infant or 30 mg/dl in a term newborn. After the newborn is 72 hours of age, blood glucose concentrations should be above 40 mg/dl. Neonates with seizures have brain metabolic rates that require higher blood glucose concentrations than these minimum values. Although hypoglycemia is not a

---

Differential Diagnosis of Neonatal Seizures

Trauma
  Subdural hematoma
  Intracortical hemorrhage
  Cortical vein thrombosis
Asphyxia—subependymal hemorrhage
Congenital abnormalities (cerebral dysgenesis)
Hypertension
Metabolic
  Hypocalcemia
    Hypomagnesemia
    High phosphate load
    Infant of a diabetic mother
    Hypoparathyroidism
    Maternal hyperparathyroidism
    Idiopathic
  Hypoglycemia
    Galactosemia
    Intrauterine growth retardation
    Infant of a diabetic mother
    Glycogen storage disease
    Idiopathic
  Electrolyte imbalance
    Hypernatremia
    Hyponatremia
Infections
  Bacterial meningitis
  Cerebral abscess
  Herpes encephalitis

Coxsackie meningoencephalitis
Cytomegalovirus
Toxoplasmosis
Syphilis
Drug withdrawal
  Methadone
  Heroin
  Barbiturate
  Propoxyphene
Pyridoxine dependency
Amino acid disturbances
  Maple syrup urine disease
  Urea cycle abnormalities
  Nonketotic hyperglycinemia
  Ketotic hyperglycinemia
Toxins
  Local anesthetics
  Isoniazid
  Bilirubin
Familial seizure disorders
  Neurocutaneous syndromes
    Tuberous sclerosis
    Incontinentia pigmenti
  Genetic syndromes
    Zellweger
    Smith-Lemli-Opitz
    Neonatal adrenoleukodystrophy
  Benign familial epilepsy

---

primary cause of seizures when blood glucose concentrations are 20 mg/dl in premature infants or 30 mg/dl in term infants, part of the treatment approach in neonatal seizures is to achieve blood glucose concentrations in the 100 to 150 mg/dl range [Wasterlain, 1972, 1974; Wasterlain and Dwyer, 1983; Wasterlain and Plum, 1973]. The treatment of hypoglycemia consists of 5 to 10 mg/kg of 10% to 15% dextrose solution intravenously followed by 8 to 10 mg/kg/min (e.g., 80 ml/kg/24 hours of 15% dextrose solution). When hypoglycemia is refractory to usual therapy, more hypertonic glucose solutions may be required. Prednisone (2 mg/kg/day) or cortisone acetate (10 mg/kg/day) may also be of value. Infants who are low birth weight for gestational age are at particular risk for symptomatic hypoglycemia. Infants of diabetic mothers frequently have low blood glucose concentrations but are rarely symptomatic. Hypoglycemia may occur in conjunction with asphyxia, maple syrup urine disease, methylmalonic acidemia, and propionic acidemia.

Definitions of hypocalcemia vary, but most clinicians agree that it is present when blood concentrations are below 7 mg/dl and ionized calcium is below 3 mg/dl. EKG determination of Q-oTc intervals has been found unreliable. The most reliable means of diagnosing hypocalcemia is by determination of ionized calcium concentrations [Nelson and Illes, 1989]. A slow intravenous infusion of 200 mg/kg of calcium gluconate is the treatment of choice. This dose may need to be repeated every 5 hours for a day. Serum magnesium concentrations should also be obtained. Hypocalcemia accompanying hypomagnesium will respond only when hypomagnesium is treated. A magnesium level of less than 1.5 mg/dl suggests the diagnosis. Treatment consists of 0.2 ml/kg of 50% magnesium sulfate given intramuscularly.

Hypocalcemia occurring in low birth weight infants, infants of hyperparathyroid mothers, infants of diabetic mothers, and infants with DiGeorge syndrome tends to occur in the first 72 hours after delivery. Hypocalcemia occurring between 4 and 7 days is associated with high phosphate feedings (now of historic interest), immature renal and parathyroid function, and perhaps relative maternal vitamin D deficiency. Diabetic mothers and mothers with hyperparathyroidism have parahormone levels that suppress fetal parathyroid activity, rendering

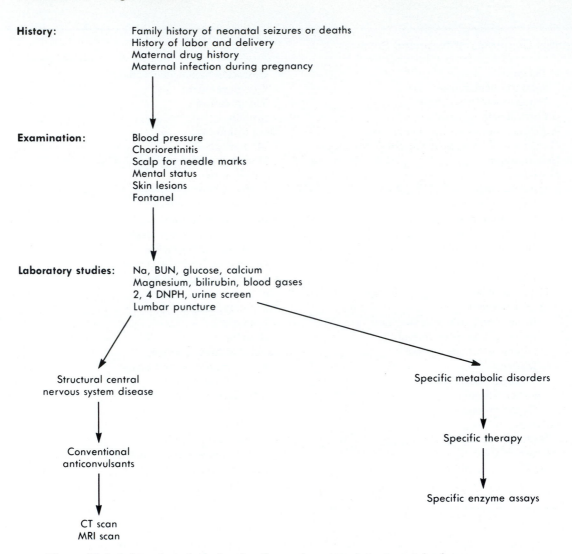

History: Family history of neonatal seizures or deaths
               History of labor and delivery
               Maternal drug history
               Maternal infection during pregnancy

Examination: Blood pressure
               Chorioretinitis
               Scalp for needle marks
               Mental status
               Skin lesions
               Fontanel

Laboratory studies: Na, BUN, glucose, calcium
                      Magnesium, bilirubin, blood gases
                      2, 4 DNPH, urine screen
                      Lumbar puncture

Structural central
nervous system disease   Specific metabolic disorders

Conventional
anticonvulsants   Specific therapy

CT scan
MRI scan   Specific enzyme assays

Figure 33-1 A flow chart depicting the diagnostic approach to neonatal seizures.

these infants susceptible to hypocalcemia following delivery. Infants with seizures caused by hypocalcemia are usually alert between episodes, and the seizures are most often multifocal. Hypocalcemia is frequently associated with but not the cause of neonatal seizures. The apparent beneficial response to intravenous calcium infusions and low blood calcium levels should not exclude consideration of such primary causes as asphyxia and/or hemorrhage [Volpe, 1977].

In the event of a family history of neonatal seizures, a peculiar odor of the infant, milk intolerance, acidosis, or alkalosis, other primary metabolic disorders should be considered.

Pyridoxine dependency. Pyridoxine dependency is inherited as an autosomal-recessive trait. Intractable, generalized clonic seizures occur shortly after birth [Clarke et al., 1979]. It has been suspected as a cause of intrauterine seizures, and infants with pyridoxine depen-

dency are commonly born meconium stained. Meconium staining, flaccidity, and early neonatal seizures frequently lead to the misdiagnosis of perinatal asphyxia. Seizures due to asphyxia, however, are usually delayed for 4 to 6 hours.

Glutamic acid decarboxylase is necessary for the synthesis of the inhibitory neurotransmitter γ-aminobutyric acid, and infants with pyridoxine dependency require very high levels of pyridoxine as a cofactor of this enzyme. The diagnosis of pyridoxine dependency is confirmed when 100 mg of pyridoxine is given intravenously with EEG monitoring. The seizures respond within minutes, and the EEG, which is characterized by generalized spike, polyspike, and burst-suppression patterns, reverts to normal in hours. Pyridoxine supplementation is maintained for life.

Maple syrup urine disease. Maple syrup urine disease is inherited as an autosomal-recessive trait. It is

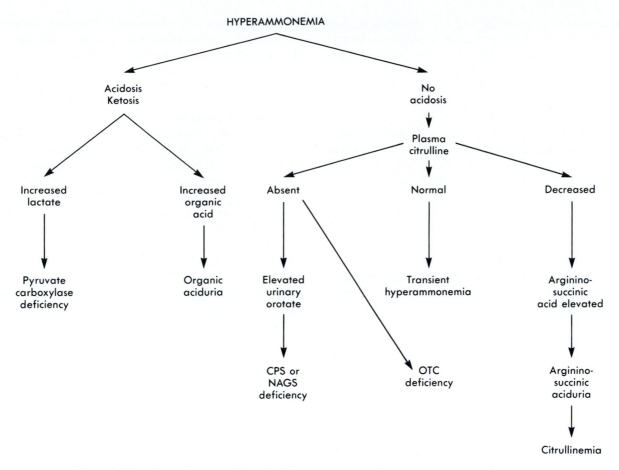

Figure 33-2 A flow chart depicting the diagnostic approach to hyperammonemia.

caused by the inability to decarboxylate the amino acids leucine, isoleucine, and valine [Hammersen et al., 1978]. The keto derivatives of these amino acids are excreted in the urine, imparting the odor of maple syrup, but also circulate in plasma, causing a severe metabolic acidosis. Newborns with maple syrup urine disease may appear healthy until protein feeding is instituted or they become catabolic. The clinical characteristics include vomiting, convulsions, and hypertonia. A variant form presents later in life as intermittent ataxia. A rapid screen for maple syrup urine disease consists of boiling urine briefly to remove nonspecific ketones and then mixing it with an equal volume of 2,4 dinitrophenylhydrazine. In the presence of the keto derivatives a fluffy, yellow precipitate forms. Plasma amino acid chromatography and the absence of the decarboxylase enzyme in cultured fibroblasts confirm the diagnosis.

Treatment consists of peritoneal dialysis, exchange transfusion, and intravenous infusion of hypertonic glucose to treat the accompanying hypoglycemia. After acute treatment a high caloric intake (150 cal/kg/day) must be used to reduce elevated plasma leucine levels and correct hypoglycemia. A thiamine-responsive form

of maple syrup urine disease has been recognized, and vitamin B_1 is administered at a dose of 10 mg/day to all infants with this disorder.

Urea cycle enzyme defects. Infants with urea cycle abnormalities may present shortly after birth or later in childhood [Batshaw and Brusilow, 1980]. Protein feeding or a catabolic state precipitates the clinical symptoms. These infants vomit, are lethargic, have seizures, lose muscle tone, and often develop a bulging fontanel. Cerebral edema, presumably caused by hyperammonemia, is another feature [Shih, 1976].

Hyperammonemia is common to all urea cycle enzyme deficiencies and other conditions. Uncomplicated hyperammonemia is associated with respiratory alkalosis. Figure 33-2 is a flow diagram of the approach to the diagnosis or causes of neonatal hyperammonemia.

Treatment consists of peritoneal dialysis, which is superior to exchange transfusion in the removal of ammonia under these conditions [Batshaw and Brusilow, 1980], and arginine supplementation. Other than those with argininemia, all patients with urea cycle abnormalities are hypoargininemic, and arginine infusions maintain functioning segments of the urea cycle. In the case of argininosuccinic aciduria, arginine supplementation may be the only treatment needed to maintain normal blood ammonia values. Sodium benzoate has also been found to decrease blood ammonia levels by increasing nitrogen removal through hippurate synthesis. During the acute phase of treatment, protein is withheld and hypertonic glucose infusions are used.

Hyperglycinemias. Glycine encephalopathy (nonketotic hyperglycinemia) presents in the newborn period with hypotonia, lethargy, and myoclonic seizures [Dalla Bernardina et al., 1979]. The infant is usually deeply comatose and has a burst-suppression EEG pattern with long periods of background attenuation. Glycine levels in plasma and CSF are markedly elevated. This disorder is caused by lack of a glycine cleavage enzyme that prevents glycine from metabolizing to carbon dioxide, ammonia, and a one-carbon tetrahydrofolate fragment. This metabolic defect has been demonstrated in liver fibroblasts and brain tissue. Treatment with exchange transfusions and strychnine sulfate has been attempted but not proved to be useful [MacDermot et al., 1980]. This disorder is usually fatal in the neonatal period, but several infants have survived for months with severe neurologic impairment.

The ketotic hyperglycinemias, including propionic and methylmalonic acidemia, may present early in the neonatal period and are characterized by vomiting, dehydration, coma, and seizures. A vitamin B_{12}-dependent form of methylmalonic acidemia and a biotin-dependent form of propionic acidemia have been reported, and these disorders may respond to dietary therapy. The presence of ketone bodies in the urine associated with acidosis and thrombocytopenia in newborns with seizures are clues to the diagnosis, but not all infants are acidotic. Hyperammonemia is commonly associated with these disorders. The finding of elevated urinary levels of the appropriate organic acid confirms the diagnosis.

Isovaleric acidemia. Isovaleric acidemia is a very rare disorder that may present with seizure activity, vomiting, acidosis, and ketosis in the newborn period. Infants with this disorder have an offensive body odor described as "cheesy" or like "sweaty feet." The diagnosis is confirmed by detecting urinary and plasma elevations of isovaleric acid. Treatment should include controlling episodes of acidosis and limitation of leucine intake.

Drug-withdrawal seizures

Seizures in the newborn may be caused by withdrawal of medications taken by the mother during the last trimester of pregnancy. Hypnotics and analgesics are the primary offenders. Seizures have been noted in newborns whose mothers have used propoxyphene as an analgesic and barbiturates as hypnotics [Clarke et al.,

1979]. Seizures are uncommon following withdrawal from longer-acting barbiturates such as phenobarbital but have been noted during withdrawal from shorter-acting barbiturates such as secobarbital. Maternal heroin addiction frequently results in a neonatal syndrome of jitters, sneezing, and gastrointestinal symptoms. Seizures are uncommon; 1.4% follow heroin withdrawal, and 7.8% follow methadone withdrawal [Herzlinger et al., 1977]. Close observation of the infant of a drug-addicted mother is important. The most common time of onset of neonatal seizures in this condition is 10 days, but the range may be 3 to 34 days and depends on the time of the mother's last dose of heroin or methadone. The longer the time interval between birth and the last dose, the shorter the interval from birth to the onset of neonatal seizures. Other researchers have not confirmed this observation.

In recent years, neonatal seizures, particularly those accompanied by stroke, associated with maternal cocaine use, have become more frequent.

Local anesthetic toxicity

The newborn may inadvertently receive substantial amounts of local anesthetic intended for the mother during labor and delivery. Direct injection of procaine substances into newborns has been described following saddle block, paracervical, and pudendal anesthesia. Newborns with local anesthetic toxicity are often misdiagnosed as being asphyxiated. Meconium staining, flaccidity, and apnea are characteristic findings. Cranial nerve abnormalities and cardiac arrhythmias, which are uncommon in asphyxia, also occur. Determination of local anesthetic blood levels in the newborn confirms the diagnosis. Levels must be determined shortly after birth because procaine derivatives are rapidly metabolized. Treatment consists of diuresis and acidification of the urine [Hillman et al., 1979]. Conventional antiepileptic drugs may be of some benefit, but measures to promote drug elimination are of greater importance. Seizures caused by local anesthetic poisoning are self-limited and occur when local anesthetic blood levels are highest.

Hypoxia-ischemia and/or intracranial hemorrhage

Asphyxia and/or intracranial hemorrhage are the most common causes of neonatal seizures. In an evaluation of 131 neonates with seizures, this combination of entities accounted for 58% of the total [Bergman et al., 1983]. This finding is consistent with other estimates in the literature [Volpe, 1977]. In asphyxiated newborns, in whom asphyxia was defined as the need for positive-pressure ventilation for more than 1 minute before the onset of spontaneous respiration, the incidence of seizures was 14%, and the mean time of onset of seizures was 13 hours [Mulligan et al., 1980]. The mean time of onset of spontaneous respirations is greater for newborns who develop seizures (14.2 ± 1.7 min), compared with those who do not (6.0 ± 0.7 min) [Mulligan et al., 1980]. Neonatal stroke has recently drawn attention as an etiology of neonatal seizures, but its prevalence is unknown [Levene and Trounce, 1986].

Seizures caused by asphyxia and/or hemorrhage may be generalized clonic or multifocal in type. They are most severe in the first 72 hours after delivery and then subside irrespective of therapy. Tonic seizures are frequently seen with subependymal hemorrhage but may be the result of brainstem release phenomena rather than cerebral cortical discharge [Kellaway and Hrachovy, 1983].

Both pyridoxine-dependent seizures and local anesthetic toxicity may mimic postasphyxic seizures and should be considered in the differential diagnosis. Hyponatremia due to inappropriate antidiuretic hormone secretion, hypocalcemia, and hypoglycemia is known to complicate asphyxia. Cardiac involvement in asphyxia may also compromise cerebral blood flow.

With improved obstetric delivery techniques, trauma as a cause of neonatal seizures has largely disappeared. When present, subdural and epidural hematomas are associated with a bulging fontanel, retinal hemorrhages, and irritability. Large newborns delivered by primigravida mothers with difficult labors and small newborns delivered precipitously are at greatest risk for trauma to the nervous system.

Neurocutaneous syndromes

Incontinentia pigmenti and tuberous sclerosis may cause seizures in the newborn. Incontinentia pigmenti is characterized by a vesicular, crusting rash, mimicking herpes simplex. The vesicular rash heals, leaving a lightly pigmented, whorled, cutaneous lesion. Seizures are usually generalized clonic and respond readily to anticonvulsant therapy. Two neonates with tuberous sclerosis and symptomatic subependymal giant cell tumors have been described [Painter et al., 1984]. One had patches of unusually pigmented hair and refractory generalized seizures.

Neonatal adrenoleukodystrophy

Neonatal adrenoleukodystrophy is a progressive neurodegenerative disorder with onset within days of birth and death by 5 years. Unlike the later childhood variant of this disease, which is transmitted as a sex-linked trait, neonatal adrenoleukodystrophy is transmitted by autosomal-recessive inheritance. The clinical features are hypotonia and refractory generalized clonic and myoclonic seizures [Jaffe et al., 1982]. These newborns have the phenotypic appearance of Zellweger syndrome but are biochemically distinct. They are deficient in the oxidation of long-chain fatty acids, resulting in the accumulation of these substances in plasma and cultured fibroblasts.

Benign familial neonatal convulsions

Several families are described with seizures of the generalized and focal clonic variety that occur during the first 2 weeks of life [Carton, 1978]. These seizures are relatively refractory to antiepileptic medication, but the outcome is usually good. A metabolic defect has not been elucidated, but the defect has been localized to the long arm of chromosome 20.

ANTIEPILEPTIC TREATMENT

Despite experimental data suggesting an adverse effect of many antiepileptic drugs on brain growth [Diaz et al., 1977; Diaz and Shields, 1978; Swaiman et al., 1980], most pediatric neurologists and neonatologists agree that neonatal seizures should be vigorously and effectively treated. The choice of antiepileptic drugs in neonates is based on tradition rather than proved efficacy. No studies demonstrate the superiority of phenobarbital, phenytoin, or the benzodiazepines, but at present, phenobarbital is the initial drug chosen in almost all neonatal units [Boer and Gal, 1982]. Loading doses of at least 20 mg/kg of phenobarbital should be given intravenously to achieve efficacious but nontoxic levels [Jalling, 1975; Lockman et al., 1979; Painter et al., 1978, 1981, 1983] (Figure 33-3). Seizure control is attained in 85% of newborns when loading doses of up

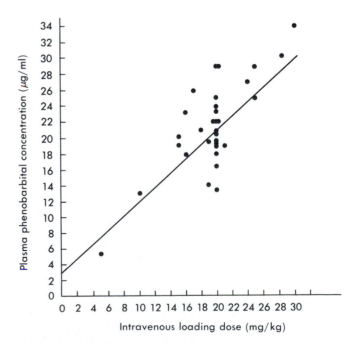

Figure 33-3 A graph demonstrating that 20 mg/kg of phenobarbital is the most effective loading dose in the management of neonatal seizures.

to 40 mg/kg are used [Gal et al., 1982]. The study of Gal et al. [1982], however, reported seizure control in a much higher proportion of neonates with plasma levels of approximately 20 µg/ml of phenobarbital. Comparison of series is hampered by inadequate control for population differences and unspecified diagnostic criteria. Because the volume of distribution of phenobarbital in the newborn is approximately 0.9 ± 0.1 L/kg, a significant number should achieve blood levels above 50 µg/ml with these high loading doses. The consequences of such high blood concentrations are an invariable decrease in heart rate below 100 and a decreased heart rate variability [Svennissen et al., 1982]. Although data regarding the effects of plasma levels of phenobarbital above 40 µg/ml on the newborn are limited, significant cardiovascular compromise and impaired cerebral blood flow probably occur.

Because the half-life of phenobarbital is relatively long in newborns, maintenance doses of 2 to 4 mg/kg/day are sufficient. After 2 weeks, metabolism and/or clearance of phenobarbital increases, and maintenance doses must be increased to approximately 5 mg/kg/day. Seizure control is unusual below a level of 16 µg/ml [Lockman et al., 1979].

Phenytoin is the second agent selected when phenobarbital fails. As with phenobarbital, loading doses of 20 mg/kg must be used to obtain plasma levels in the 15 to 20 µg/ml range (Figure 33-4). Intravenous maintenance dosages are within the range of 4 to 6 mg/kg/day. Careful monitoring is necessary when plasma levels of 20 mg/ml are achieved because drug accumulation may

begin at these levels. The brain/plasma ratios reflecting distribution of phenobarbital and phenytoin to brain are approximately 1.0 and 1.2, respectively, values comparable with those reported in adults [Sherwin et al., 1973; Vajda et al., 1974]. Using phenobarbital and phenytoin at loading doses of 20 mg/kg controls approximately 70% of neonatal seizures.

Primidone may be of value in treating newborns whose seizures are refractory to phenobarbital and phenytoin [Powell et al., 1984]. Primidone is not converted to phenobarbital as in older children but does impair phenobarbital clearance and may cause a precipitous rise in phenobarbital levels after primidone loading. Primidone loading doses of 15 to 20 mg/kg and maintenance doses of 12 to 20 mg/kg/day are recommended. The lowest effective primidone level is 6 µg/ml.

Diazepam is an effective antiepileptic drug when administered as a continuous intravenous infusion diluted in isotonic saline at a rate of 0.3 mg/kg/hour [Gamstrop and Sedin, 1982]. It causes somnolence but does not compromise respiration. Effective blood levels range from 35 to 80.5 µmol/L. Other benzodiazepines, clonazepam, and lorazepam have similar efficacy.

Paraldehyde has been advocated as an effective antiepileptic drug in the newborn and may be administered as a 4% solution intravenously. This agent, however, has produced pulmonary edema, pulmonary hemorrhage, and hypotension in older children [Sinai and Crowe, 1976] and should be used with caution in the neonate with respiratory disease. The intravenous form of this drug is no longer manufactured. Loading doses of 200 mg/kg of paraldehyde followed by infusion of 16 to 20 mg/kg/hr or infusions of 200 mg/kg/hr for 2 hours can be expected to produce effective plasma levels (greater than 10 mg/dl) [Koren et al., 1986].

The reported efficacy of anticonvulsant agents in the treatment of neonatal seizures is based only on clinical observations. Most investigators have noted far less improvement in associated electrical discharges. Current treatment regimens are far from optimal.

OUTCOME OF NEONATES WITH SEIZURES

A review of 1667 neonates with seizures demonstrated an improvement in the neurologic outcome of infants born after 1969, but the morbidity and mortality together remained at about 50% [Bergman et al., 1983]. Studies of infants in the National Collaborative Perinatal Project report 70% normal outcome, but these studies contain no information regarding etiology, and the infants were observed before neonatal intensive care was established [Coen, 1983; Holden et al., 1980]. A total of 53% of newborns with seizures due to hypoxia ischemia and/or intracranial hemorrhage had severe or moderate neurologic impairment at follow-up. Most newborns who have seizures for 4 or more days or require more than

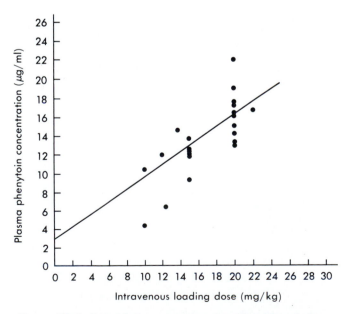

Figure 33-4 A graph demonstrating that 20 mg/kg of phenytoin is the most effective loading dose in the management of neonatal seizures.

two antiepileptic drugs for control will have severe neurologic impairment. The unexpected late recurrence rate of frequent seizures was 8% within this population, leading to the recommendation that antiepileptic drugs be discontinued after 2 seizure-free weeks in the neonate [Bergman et al., 1983]. Neonatal convulsions are not a risk factor for later epilepsy unless the epilepsy is part of a chronic brain syndrome that includes cerebral palsy, mental retardation, or both [Holden et al., 1980].

REFERENCES

Amiel-Tison C. Cerebral damage in full-term newborn: etiological factors, neonatal status and long-term follow-up. Biol Neonate 1969; 14:234-250.

Ballard RH, Vinocur B, Reynolds JW, et al. Transient hyperammonemia of the preterm infant. N Engl J Med 1978; 299:920-925.

Batshaw ML, Brusilow SW. Treatment of hyperammonemic coma caused by inborn errors of urea synthesis. J Pediatr 1980; 97:893-900.

Bergman I, Painter MJ, Hirsch RP, et al. Outcome in neonates with convulsions treated in an intensive care unit. Ann Neurol 1983; 14:642-647.

Boer HR, Gal P. Neonatal seizures: a survey of current practice. Clin Pediatr 1982; 21:453-457.

Carton D. Benign familial neonatal convulsions. Neuropaediatrie 1978; 9:167-171.

Clarke TH, Saunders BS, Feldman B. Pyridoxine-dependent seizures requiring high doses of pyridoxine for control. Am J Dis Child 1979; 133:963-965.

Coen RW. Neonatal seizures. Pediatrics 1983; 71:467-468.

Dalla Bernardina B, Aicardi J, Goutileres F, et al. Glycine encephalopathy. Neuropaediatrie 1979; 10:209-225.

Desmond MM, Schwanecke RP, Wilson GS, et al. Maternal barbiturate utilization and neonatal withdrawal symptomatology. J Pediatr 1972; 80:190-197.

Diaz J, Schain RJ, Bailey BG. Phenobarbital-induced brain growth retardation in artificially reared rat pups. Biol Neonate 1977; 32:77-82.

Diaz J, Shields WD. Chronic administration of dipropylacetate early in life: effects on brain development and behavior. Ann Neurol 1978; 4: 198 (abstract).

Dodson WE. Antiepileptic drug utilization in pediatric patients. Epilepsia 1984; 25 (suppl):132-139.

Dreyfus-Brisac C. The electroencephalogram of the premature infant. World Neurol 1962; 3:5-15.

Dreyfus-Brisac C. The electroencephalogram of the premature infant and full-term newborn. In: Kellaway P, Petersen I, eds. Neurological and electroencephalographic correlative studies in infancy. New York: Grune & Stratton, 1964; 186-207.

Dreyfus-Brisac C, Monod N. Electroclinical studies of status epilepticus and convulsions in the newborn. In: Kellaway P, Petersen I, eds. Neurological and electroencephalographic correlative studies in infancy. New York: Grune & Stratton, 1964; 250-252.

Emde RN, Metcalf DR. An electroencephalographic study of behavioral rapid eye movement states in the human newborn. J Nerv Ment Dis 1970; 150:376-386.

Engel RC. Abnormal electroencephalograms in the neonatal period. Springfield, Ill: Charles C Thomas, 1975.

Eyre JH, Dozeer RC, Wilkinson AR: Diagnosis of neonatal seizure by continuous recording and rapid analysis of the electroencephalogram. Arch Dis Child 1983; 58:785-790.

Fenichel GM, Olson BJ, Fitzpatrick JR. Heart rate changes in convulsive and nonconvulsive neonatal apnea. Ann Neurol 1980; 7:577-582.

Ferguson JH, Levinsohn MW, Derakshan I. Brainstem seizures in hydranencephaly. Neurology 1974; 24:1152-1157.

Fujikawa DG, Vannucci RC, Dwyer BE, et al. Cerebral energy metabolism during generalized seizures in newborn primates. Neurology 1985; 35(suppl 1):196.

Gal P, Toback J, Boer HR, et al. Efficacy of phenobarbital monotherapy in treatment of neonatal seizures—relationship to blood levels. Neurology 1982; 32:1401-1404.

Gamstrop I, Sedin G. Neonatal convulsions treated with continuous intravenous infusion of diazepam. Ups J Med Sci 1982; 87:143-149.

Hammersen G, Wille L, Schmidt H, et al. Maple syrup urine disease: emergency treatment of the neonate. Monogr Hum Genet 1978; 9:84-89.

Harris R, Tizavd JP. The electroencephalogram in neonatal convulsions. J Pediatr 1960; 57:501-520.

Herzlinger RH, Kandall SR, Vaughan HG Jr. Neonatal seizures associated with narcotic withdrawal. J Pediatr 1977; 91:638-641.

Hillman LS, Hillman RE, Dodson WE. Diagnosis, treatment and follow-up of neonatal mepivacaine intoxication secondary to paracervical and pudendal blocks during labor. J Pediatr 1979; 95:472-477.

Holden KR, Freeman JM, Mellits ED. Outcomes of infants with neonatal seizures. In: Wada JA, Perry JK, eds. Advances in epileptology: The Xth Epilepsy International Symposium. New York: Raven Press, 1978; p. 155.

Jaffe R, Crumrine P, Hashida Y, et al. Neonatal adrenoleukodystrophy: clinical, pathologic, and biochemical delineation of a syndrome affecting both males and females. Am J Pathol 1982; 108:100-111.

Jalling B. Plasma concentrations of phenobarbital in the treatment of seizures in newborns. Acta Paediatr Scand 1975; 64:514-524.

Kellaway P, Hrachovy RH. Status epilepticus in newborns: a perspective on neonatal seizures. Ann Neurol 1983; 34:93-99.

Koren G, Butt W, Rajchgot P, et al. Intravenous paraldehyde for seizure control in newborn infants. Neurology 1986; 36:108-111.

Kuromori N, Arai H, Ohkubo O, et al. A prospective study of epilepsy following neonatal convulsions. Folia Psychiatr Neurol Jpn 1976; 30:379-388.

Levene MI, Trounce JQ. Causes of neonatal convulsions: towards a more precise diagnosis. Arch Dis Child 1986; 61:78-79.

Lockman LA, Kriel R, Zaske D, et al. Phenobarbital dosage for control of neonatal seizures. Neurology 1979; 29:1445-1449.

Lou HC, Friis-Hansen B. Arterial blood pressure elevations during motor activity and epileptic seizures in the newborn. Acta Paediatr Scand 1979; 68:803-806.

MacDermot KD, Nelson W, Reichert CM, et al. Attempts at use of strychnine sulfate in the treatment of nonketotic hyperglycinemia. Pediatrics 1980; 65:61-64.

Mace S, Hirschfeld S. Hypertensive encephalopathy: a cause of neonatal seizures. Am J Dis Child 1983; 137:32-33.

Mizrahi EM, Kellaway P. Characterization of seizures in neonates and young infants by time-synchronized electroencephalographic/ polygraphic/video monitoring. Ann Neurol 1984; 16:383.

Monod N, Dreyfus-Brisac C, Sfaelo A. Detection and prognosis of the neonatal male according to the electroclinical study of 150 cases. Arch Fr Pediatr 1969; 26:1085-1102.

Monod N, Pajot N, Guidasci S. The neonatal EEG: statistical studies and prognostic value in full-term and pre-term babies. Electroencephalogr Clin Neurophysiol 1972; 32:529-544.

Mulligan JC, Painter MJ, O'Donoghue PH, et al. Neonatal asphyxia. II. Neonatal mortality and long-term sequelae. J Pediatr 1980; 96:903-907.

Nelson KB, Broman SH. Perinatal risk factors in children with serious motor and mental handicaps. Ann Neurol 1977; 2:371-377.

Nelson KB, Ellenberg JH. Neonatal signs as predictors of cerebral palsy. Pediatrics 1979; 64:225.

Nelson N, Illes L. The Q-oTc and oTc interval and ionized calcium in newborns. Clin Physiol 1989; 9:39-45.

Painter MJ, Alvin JD, David R. Use of a nonradioactive isotope to study phenobarbital metabolism in the neonate. Ann Neurol 1983; 14:380 (abstract).

Painter MJ, David R, Alvin JD. The use of a stable isotope to study phenytoin metabolism in the newborn. Ann Neurol 1984; 16:379.

Painter MJ, Pang D, Ahdab-Barmada M, et al. Connatal brain tumors in patients with tuberous sclerosis. Neurosurgery 1984; 14:570-573.

Painter MJ, Pippenger C, MacDonald H, et al. Phenobarbital and diphenylhydantoin levels in neonates with seizures. J Pediatr 1978; 92:315-319.

Painter MJ, Pippenger C, Wasterlain C, et al. Phenobarbital and phenytoin in neonatal seizures: metabolism and tissue distribution. Neurology 1981; 31:1107-1112.

Passouant P, Cadilhac J. EEG and clinical study of epilepsy during maturation in man. Epilepsia 1962; 3:14-43.

Perlman JM, Volpe JJ. Seizures in the preterm infant: effects on cerebral blood flow velocity, intracranial pressure, and arterial blood pressure. J Pediatr 1983; 102:288-293.

Powell C, Painter MJ, Pippenger CE. Primidone therapy in refractory neonatal seizures. J Pediatr 1984; 105:651-654.

Prechtl JF. The behavioral states of the newborn infant: a review. Brain Res 1975; 76:185-212.

Prichard JS. The character and significance of epileptic seizures in infancy. In: Kellaway P, Petersen I, eds. Neurological and electroencephalographic correlative studies in infancy. New York: Grune & Stratton, 1964; 273-276.

Purpura DP. Relationship of seizure susceptibility to morphologic and physiologic properties of normal and abnormal immature cortex. In: Kellaway P, Peterson I, eds. Neurological and electroencephalographic correlative studies in infancy. New York: Grune & Stratton, 1964; 117-157.

Roffwarg HP, Muzio JN, Dement WC. Ontogenetic development of the human sleep-dream cycle. Science 1966; 152:604-619.

Rose AL, Lombroso CT. Neonatal seizure states: a study of clinical, pathological and electroencephalographic features in 137 full-term babies with a long-term follow up. Pediatrics 1970; 45:404-425.

Samson-Dollfus C, Forthomme J, Capron E. EEG of the human infant during sleep and wakefulness during the first year of life: normal patterns and their maturational changes; abnormal patterns and their prognostic significance. In: Kellaway P, Petersen I, eds. Neurological and electroencephalographic correlative studies in infancy. New York: Grune & Stratton, 1964; 208-229.

Scher M, Painter MJ, Bergman I, et al. EEG diagnosis of neonatal seizures: clinical correlations and outcome. Pediatr Neurol 1989; 5:17-24.

Sherwin AL, Wisen AA, Sogolowski CD. Anticonvulsant drugs in human epileptogenic brain: correlation of phenobarbital and diphenylhydatoin levels with plasma. Arch Neurol 1973; 29:73-77.

Shih VE. Congenital hyperammonemic syndromes. Clin Perinatal 1976; 3:3-14.

Sinai SH, Crowe JE. Cyanosis, cough and hypotension following intravenous administration of paraldehyde. Pediatrics 1976; 57:158-159.

Svennissen NW, Blennow G, Lindroth M, et al. Brain-oriented intensive care treatment in severe neonatal asphyxia: effects of phenobarbitone protection. Arch Dis Child 1982; 57:176-183.

Swaiman KF, Schrier BK, Neale EA, et al. Effects of chronic phenytoin and valproic acid exposure on fetal mouse cortical cultures. Ann Neurol 1980; 8:230.

Tharp BR, Laboyrie PM. The incidence of EEG abnormalities and outcome of infants paralyzed with neuromuscular blocking agents. Crit Care Med 1983; 11:926-929.

Tibbles JA, Prichard JS. The prognostic value of the electroencephalogram in neonatal convulsions. Pediatrics 1965; 35:778-786.

Vajda F, Williams FM, Davidson S, et al. Human brain, cerebrospinal fluid, and plasma concentrations of diphenylhydantoin and phenobarbital. Clin Pharmacol Ther 1974; 15:597-603.

Volpe JJ. Management of neonatal seizures. Crit Care Med 1977; 5:43-49.

Wasterlain CG. Breakdown of brain polysomes in status epilepticus. Brain Res 1972; 39:278-284.

Wasterlain CG. Inhibition of cerebral protein synthesis by epileptic seizures without motor manifestations. Neurology 1974; 24:175-180.

Wasterlain CG, Dwyer BE. Brain metabolism during prolonged seizures in neonates. Adv Neurol 1983; 34:241-260.

Wasterlain CG, Plum F. Vulnerability of developing rat brain to electroconvulsive seizures. Arch Neurol 1973; 29:38-45.

Watanabe K, Hara K, Miyazaki S, et al. Apneic seizures in the newborn. Am J Dis Child 1982; 136:980-984.

Weiner S, Painter MJ, Geva D, et al. Neonatal seizures: electroclinical dissociation. Pediatr Neurol 1991; 7:363-368.

34

Febrile Seizures

Karin B. Nelson and Deborah G. Hirtz

Vulnerability to seizures with high fevers is an age-related phenomenon. Febrile seizures are rare after 5 years of age, and most commonly begin before 2 years of age. Children who have these seizures are usually normal before and after the seizure. The more typical the clinical picture, the greater the probability of a good outcome. A primary responsibility of the clinician is to educate and reassure the family and prepare them to cope optimally should there be a recurrence in the affected child or a sibling.

Febrile seizures are common in early childhood, occurring in 2% to 5% of young children. A consensus statement by the National Institutes of Health [1980] states the following:

A febrile seizure is an event in infancy or childhood, usually occurring between 3 months and 5 years of age, associated with fever but without evidence of intracranial infection or defined cause. Seizures with fever in children who have suffered a previous nonfebrile seizure are excluded. Febrile seizures are to be distinguished from epilepsy, which is characterized by recurrent nonfebrile seizures.

Convulsions and fever can occur together in meningitis, electrolyte imbalance, lead encephalopathy, and other specific conditions that affect the CNS directly; by definition, these are not febrile seizures.

CLINICAL CHARACTERISTICS AND SUBCLASSIFICATIONS

Febrile seizures may be of any type but are most often generalized tonic-clonic convulsions. They are usually self-limiting and continue for only a few minutes. The average age of onset is 18 to 22 months. Febrile seizures occur more frequently in boys than in girls and slightly more frequently in black than white children. Most febrile seizures occur in children who are normal, but children with pre-existing neurologic or developmental abnormalities may be more vulnerable. The neurologic

and developmental conditions of the patient before the first seizure are important determinants of long-term outcome.

Febrile seizures are often classified as simple or complex, the latter being characterized by a duration of more than 15 min, focal features, or the occurrence of more than a single seizure within a 24-hour period. "Simple" febrile seizures are far more common than "complex" (85% versus 15%) and are brief and generalized. In general, pregnancy and birth histories have not been related to the occurrence or prognosis of febrile seizures. A British national cohort study [Verity et al., 1985a; 1985b] indicated that breech delivery was marginally more frequent in children with febrile seizures, but an American study [Nelson and Ellenberg, 1990] did not observe a relationship between any pregnancy or birth factors and febrile seizures. This study did not reveal any potentially preventable risk factor that could account for an important proportion of febrile seizures.

Febrile seizures usually manifest in the first hours of acute infectious illness. Except for the common situation in which acute otitis media supervenes during an upper respiratory infection, the occurrence of a seizure more than a day after the onset of febrile illness should lead the clinician to consider other diagnostic possibilities such as meningitis and electrolyte imbalance. The illnesses most often associated with febrile seizures are upper respiratory infection, otitis media, roseola, urinary tract infection, and gastrointestinal infection. Viral and bacterial infections and fever resulting from other causes such as immunizations can contribute to a reduction of the seizure threshold. Some seasonal variation has been observed in the occurrence of febrile seizures: peaks occur in November and January, perhaps related to respiratory infections, and peaks also occur from June through August, when gastrointestinal illnesses are most prevalent.

GENETICS

Febrile seizures tend to be familial. The exact pattern of inheritance is uncertain, but many authors favor a multifactorial model. The possible contribution of environmental factors shared by families has not been excluded; twin studies that examined this possibility have not been conclusive. About 10% of parents of children with febrile seizures have had seizures themselves, chiefly febrile, and van den Berg [1974] observed that 9% of younger siblings of children with febrile seizures have at least one convulsion.

Assuming that vulnerability to febrile seizures is at least partly genetically determined, it is unknown which characteristic is inherited: a specific susceptibility to seizure with fever when young or a more general lowering of the convulsive threshold. Most studies reveal nonfebrile seizure disorders to be more frequent in the siblings of children with febrile seizures than in the general population. Hauser et al. [1985] observed an increased risk for febrile seizures and epilepsy (recurrent nonfebrile seizures) among siblings of children with febrile seizures. A synergistic increase in risk occurred for siblings of children who had both febrile and subsequent nonfebrile seizures, suggesting that the underlying susceptibility was not the same for both conditions. A British national cohort study observed that children with a positive family history were more likely to have a complex first febrile seizure than those with a negative history [Verity et al., 1985a, 1985b].

NATURAL HISTORY

The best sources of information concerning the natural history of febrile seizures are studies of populations rather than of samples from referral clinics or hospitals [Hauser and Kurland, 1975; Nelson and Ellenberg, 1978; van den Berg and Yerushalmy, 1969; Verity and Golding, 1991; Verity et al., 1985a; 1985b;]. The results of these studies are similar on several points.

Neither death nor permanent motor disability appears to be a consequence of febrile seizures. The British National Child Development Study documented that children with febrile seizures perform as well in school as children with no seizures at the ages of 7 and 11 years [Ross et al., 1980]. The NINDS Collaborative Perinatal Project revealed no difference between children with febrile seizures and their seizure-free siblings in intelligence quotient results or performance results on the wide range achievement test at 7 years of age [Ellenberg and Nelson, 1978]. In the more recent British cohort study, Verity et al. [1985a; 1985b] indicated no difference between 5-year-old children with febrile seizures and their peers in head circumference or performance on either the English picture vocabulary test or the copying designs test. Furthermore, children with complex febrile seizures did not differ from those with simple febrile seizures. In the latter study "an extensive series of questions about behavior failed to show any significant differences between patients with febrile convulsions and the rest of the population" [Verity et al., 1985b].

About 33% of children with febrile seizures had at least 1 recurrence, and 9% had 3 or more seizures; 15 was the maximum number of recurrent seizures in the British study. The number of subsequent seizures was not different in the patients whose initial seizures were complex. Of recurrences, 75% occurred within the first year after the initial episode; 90% occurred within 2 years. The best predictor of recurrence was an early age at the time of the initial seizure. Of the children with an initial seizure in the first year of life, 50% experienced at least one recurrence, whereas only 10% to 15% of those with onset after 4 years of age had another seizure. A family history of febrile seizures has been associated with an increase in risk of febrile seizure recurrence; data on risk with family history of nonfebrile seizures are less consistent [Berg et al., 1990]. In a recent Dutch study, a fever of more than 40° C at the time of an initial seizure was associated with a reduced risk of recurrence [Offringa et al., 1992].

The risk of epilepsy in children who have had febrile seizures is increased, but that risk was below 5% in most population-based series. Risk factors for nonfebrile seizures were a complex initial seizure, a developmental or neurologic abnormality present before the first seizure, and a history of nonfebrile seizures in a parent or sibling. A single risk factor was not accompanied by much increase in risk, but the increase was appreciable in the presence of two or more factors. Up to 10% of children with two or more risk factors later developed epilepsy [Nelson and Ellenberg, 1978; Verity and Golding, 1991]. If nonfebrile seizures developed, they usually began fairly soon; 75% began within the first 3 years after the initial febrile seizure. In the Rochester, Minnesota, study [Annegers et al., 1979], in which the investigators were able to follow probands longer than in other studies, some increase in the risk of epilepsy occurred when the subjects were compared with controls until the third decade of life, but the magnitude of the increase was small after the first few years. Controversy continues concerning whether there is a disproportionate increase in risk of complex partial seizures (as opposed to other types of seizures), because a history of febrile seizures may be more common in adults with this type of epilepsy. However, for this and other types of later epilepsy the sequence of febrile seizures leading to brain damage and then to epilepsy has not been proved. Febrile seizures may simply be the initial expression of a seizure disorder, or both febrile and nonfebrile seizures may be indicators of an underlying and preexisting brain abnormality.

MANAGEMENT

Acute treatment

For the child receiving medical attention while the convulsion is occurring, acute treatment is identical to that for other seizure types: establishment and maintenance of a clear airway and termination of the seizure (see Chapter 36). Diazepam, administered 0.2 to 0.4 mg/kg intravenously at a maximum rate of 1 mg/min, is often used initially and may be repeated. Provisions for ventilatory assistance should be available. If the seizure is not controlled in a reasonable time, the child should be transferred to (if not already at) a facility that can provide more aggressive treatment. Fever should be reduced by uncovering the child and administering antipyretics. Once the seizure has ended, clinicians should obtain a detailed history and perform a physical examination. Although a febrile and convulsing young child is a likely candidate for a diagnosis of febrile seizure, that conclusion can be reached only after meningitis, encephalitis, serious electrolyte imbalance, heat stroke, and other acute neurologic illnesses requiring rapid and specific treatment have been excluded.

The need for a lumbar puncture in young children with febrile seizures has been discussed frequently. A history of previous febrile seizures or febrile seizures in a sibling is an important element in the history, but a positive personal or family history does not exclude meningitis as the cause of the current episode. Attention must be directed toward the level of consciousness, evidence of meningismus, and the presence of a tense or bulging fontanel. In the very young child, meningeal signs may frequently be absent, and if any uncertainty exists, lumbar puncture should be performed promptly. In the absence of suspicious physical findings and when the child is older than 18 months of age, a period of observation may clarify the clinical situation and permit clearer judgment regarding the need for a lumbar puncture and further examination; a reassuring second physical examination and supportive family members who live near the medical care facility permit a minimum of invasive procedures. If doubt exists, a lumbar puncture should be performed. A very sick young infant often requires blood cultures and hospitalization; an older child who is alert and responsive on awakening is probably better observed at home if the family's lifestyle permits such an arrangement.

When the site of infection can be identified and the child is alert and responsive, further investigation may not be needed. Depending on the specific situation a hemogram, urinalysis, and serum electrolyte, glucose, and calcium tests may be warranted. Skull radiographs are almost never useful in diagnosing febrile seizures, and CT or MRI is indicated only when an underlying structural lesion is suspected. EEG is not generally useful except in children who have had lengthy focal seizures to identify evidence of underlying structural abnormality. Paroxysmal features of the EEG tend to occur more frequently in older children with febrile seizures [Sofijanov et al., 1992]; however, EEG is probably not helpful in predicting later epilepsy or recurrent febrile seizures.

There is no evidence that antipyretic treatment influences the recurrence of febrile seizures. However, fever should be treated to prevent dehydration and increase the comfort of the child. Tepid sponging may be useful, but cold bathing and ice packs should be avoided.

Long-term treatment

Chronic administration of phenobarbital, usually given in a dosage of 4 to 5 mg/kg/day, has been believed to be effective in preventing recurrences [Herranz et al., 1984; Mamelle et al., 1984; Wolf et al., 1977]. Studies that examined populations of children at higher risk for subsequent seizures and analyzed results according to the intention to treat, did not find that the treatment was effective [Farwell et al., 1990; Newton, 1988]. Although it is inexpensive, familiar, and not commonly associated with major hypersensitivity reactions and medical side effects, phenobarbital does have disadvantages. Experimental and clinical studies have suggested adverse effects on the developing nervous system. Parents frequently report negative effects on behavior and mood. A recent randomized clinical trial reported lower scores on intelligence quotient testing in the group assigned to phenobarbital compared with the group assigned to placebo [Farwell et al., 1990]. Chronic daily sodium valproate has been reported to reduce the risk of febrile seizure recurrences [Herranz et al., 1984, Mamelle et al., 1984], but very rare, life-threatening reactions can occur. Thus long-term chronic prophylaxis with either phenobarbital or valproic acid is rarely justified when the side effects of the drugs are compared against the favorable prognosis, even with recurrences.

Whether prophylaxis of febrile seizure recurrences can prevent the later occurrence of nonfebrile seizures is not known. The development of nonfebrile seizures has occurred in some children who receive continuous prophylactic therapy with antiepileptic drugs and who have serum levels in the therapeutic range [Hirata et al., 1985; Takizawa and Sumi, 1984]. A more recent alternative to chronic antiepileptic drug therapy is the treatment of febrile episodes or actual seizures with administration of a benzodiazepine, usually diazepam [Rosman, 1993; Knudsen, 1985; Thorn, 1981; Ventura et al., 1982]. In most reports, rectal administration has been employed, but oral administration at onset of fever decreased the recurrence rate in a study of children with febrile seizures ans was not associated with any major side effects

[Rosman, 1993]. This intermittent treatment with diazepam and nitrazepam has been about as effective as chronic treatment with phenobarbital and has generally been safe. Knudsen [1985] administered diazepam per rectum (5 mg in children ages 3 years or younger and 7.5 mg in older children) when the child had a fever of 38.5° C or higher and repeated doses every 12 hours to a maximum of four doses. Caution is necessary concerning respiratory depression and the masking of evolving illness, especially in the very young child or in the child treated with concurrent phenobarbital therapy. Intermittent therapy with a rapid-acting agent is appealing because the child is treated at the time of greatest risk: the onset of febrile illness. The same strategy can be used at the beginning of a seizure to terminate it rapidly and to prevent immediate recurrence [Camfield et al., 1989].

The more typical the seizure history in the individual child, the more likely that the generally reassuring clinical studies of febrile seizures are expected to apply. However, no study has followed enough children who had extraordinary frequency, prolonged duration, onset with marginal fever, or Todd paralysis to engender confidence that the studies also apply to such atypical cases. Although the vast majority of children with febrile seizures do not require any treatment, a clearly atypical history may be the basis for a different conclusion.

Long-term treatment with antiepileptic drugs to prevent febrile seizure recurrences is rarely justified considering the side effects and favorable prognosis [Knudsen, 1991]. However, for some patients, preventing recurrences with benzodiazepines at the time of febrile illness or abbreviating a recurrence may be a useful although not completely effective approach. Not all recurrences can be predicted or prevented, but many can, with minimal side effects and risks.

IMMUNIZATIONS IN CHILDREN WITH FEBRILE SEIZURES

Many childhood immunizations can trigger fever, and many are administered during the age of susceptibility to febrile seizures. The physician should discuss this issue with parents of the child with a personal or family history of febrile seizures, weighing the advantage of illness protection against the disadvantage of possibly precipitating a seizure. Regardless of the conclusion, results of the discussion should be included in the child's record. Parents should be counseled to be alert for fever and to give antipyretics if it occurs. Highest susceptibility is on the first or second day after diphtheria-tetanus-pertussis immunization and during the seventh through tenth day after measles immunization.

PARENT COUNSELING

Although they are usually benign, febrile seizures can be extremely frightening to parents and other observers. Even after the initial panic has subsided, parents often are anxious about their child's future. Providing opportunity for discussion, often requiring more than a single session, is mandatory. There is a risk of subsequent seizures in the child who has had a febrile seizure and also in younger siblings, regardless of whether treatment is prescribed. The parents must be instructed in the management of febrile illness, in first-aid treatment in the event of a seizure, and in summoning medical care when a seizure does not cease quickly. This information should be provided to babysitters and other caretakers. Informed and responsive counseling of the parents is probably the most important contribution the clinician can make to the care of the child with febrile seizures.

REFERENCES

Annegers JF, Hauser WA, Elveback LR, et al. The risk of epilepsy following febrile convulsions. Neurology 1979; 29:297-303.

Berg AT, Shinnar S, Hauser WA, et al. Predictors of recurrent febrile seizures: a metaanalytic review. Pediatrics 1990; 116:329-337.

Camfield CS, Camfield PR, Smith E, et al. Home use of rectal diazepam to prevent status epilepticus in children with convulsive disorders. J Child Neurol 1989; 4:125-126.

Consensus statement. Febrile seizures: long-term management in children with fever-associated seizures. Pediatrics 1980; 66:1009-1012.

Ellenberg JH, Nelson KB. Febrile seizures and later intellectual performance. Arch Neurol 1978; 35:17-21.

Farwell JR, Lee YJ, Hirtz DG, et al. Phenobarbital for febrile seizures—effects on intelligence and on seizure recurrence. N Engl J Med 1990; 322:364-369.

Hauser WA, Kurland LT. The epidemiology of epilepsy in Rochester, Minnesota, 1935 through 1967. Epilepsia 1975; 16:1-66.

Hauser WA, Annegers JF, Anderson VE, et al. The risk of seizure disorders among relatives of children with febrile convulsions. Neurology 1985; 35:1268-1273.

Herranz JL, Armijo JA, Arteaga R. Effectiveness and toxicity of phenobarbital, primidone, and sodium valproate in the prevention of febrile convulsions controlled by plasma levels. Epilepsia 1984; 25:89-95.

Hirata Y, Mizuno Y, Nakano M, et al. Epilepsy following febrile convulsions. Brain Dev 1985; 7:75.

Knudsen FU. Recurrence risk after first febrile seizure and effect of short term diazepam prophylaxis. Arch Dis Child 1985; 60:1045-1049.

Knudsen FU. Intermittent diazepam prophylaxis in febrile convulsions. Pros and cons. Acta Neurol Scand 1991; 135(suppl):1-24.

Mamelle N, Mamelle, JC, Plasse JC, et al. Prevention of recurrent febrile convulsions—a randomized therapeutic assay: sodium valproate, phenobarbital and placebo. Neuropediatrics 1984; 15:37-42.

Nelson KB, Ellenberg JH. Prognosis in children with febrile seizures. Pediatrics 1978; 61:720-727.

Nelson KB, Ellenberg JH. Prenatal and perinatal antecedents of febrile seizures. Ann Neurol 1990; 27:127-131.

Newton RW. Randomized controlled trials of phenobarbitone and valproate in febrile convulsions. Arch Dis Child 1988; 63:1189-91.

Offringa M, Derksen-Lubsen, G, Bossuyt, PM, et al. Seizure recurrence after a first febrile seizure: a multivariate approach. Dev Med Child Neurol 1992; 34:15-24.

Rosman NP, Colton T, Labazzo J, et al. A controlled trial of diazepam administered during febrile illness to prevent recurrence of febrile seizures. New Engl J Med 1993; 329:79-84.

Ross EM, Peckham CS, West PB, et al. Epilepsy in childhood: findings from the National Child Development Study. Br Med J 1980; 1:207-210.

Sofijanov N, Emoto S, Kuturec M, et al. Febrile seizures: clinical characteristics and initial EEG. Epilepsia 1992; 1:52-57.

Takizawa K, Sumi K. Prophylactic therapy for febrile convulsions— recurrence of febrile convulsions and occurrence of subsequent non-febrile convulsions on continuous prophylactic medication. Brain Dev 1984; 6:69.

Thorn I. Prevention of recurrent febrile seizures: intermittent prophylaxis with diazepam compared with continuous treatment with phenobarbital. In: Nelson KB, Ellenberg JH, eds. Febrile seizures. New York: Raven Press, 1981; 119-126.

van den Berg BJ. Studies on convulsive disorders in young children. IV. Incidence of convulsions among siblings. Dev Med Child Neurol 1974; 16:457-464.

van den Berg BJ, Yerushalmy J. Studies on convulsive disorders in young children. I. Incidence of febrile and nonfebrile convulsions by age and other factors. Pediatr Res 1969; 3:298-304.

Ventura A, Basso T, Bortolan G, et al. Home treatment of seizures as a strategy for the long-term management of febrile convulsions in children. Helv Paediatr Acta 1982; 37:581-587.

Verity CM, Butler NR, Golding J. Febrile convulsions in a national cohort followed up from birth. I. Prevalence and recurrence in the first five years of life. Br Med J 1985a; 290:1307-1310.

Verity CM, Butler NR, Golding J. Febrile convulsions in a national cohort followed up from birth. II. Medical history and intellectual ability at 5 years of age. Br Med J 1985b; 290:1311-1315.

Verity CM, Golding G. Risk of epilepsy after febrile convulsions: a national cohort study. Br Med J 1991; 303:1373-1376.

Wolf SM, Carr A, Davis DC, et al. The value of phenobarbital in the child who has had a single febrile seizure: a controlled prospective study. Pediatrics 1977; 59:378-385.

35

Nonepileptic Paroxysmal Disorders

Lawrence A. Lockman

Hughlings-Jackson [1888] wrote, "the great thing as to the diagnosis of epilepsy is not the quantity of the symptoms, nor the severity of the fits, but the paroxysmalness." However, a variety of conditions are characterized by abrupt onset, stereotypic course, and spontaneous cessation that affect children but appear not to depend on paroxysmal electrical discharges of brain and therefore cannot be considered to represent forms of epilepsy.

Jeavons [1983] indicated that up to 25% of patients in his epilepsy clinics did not have epilepsy. Of the 200 children studied, 44% had syncope, 20% had psychiatric illness, 11% had breath-holding spells, 6% had migraine, 6% had night terrors, 5% had daydreams, and 11% were accounted for by other causes.

SYNCOPE

Fainting or syncope is a transient loss of consciousness resulting from inadequate cerebral perfusion. The patient commonly experiences lightheadedness, nausea, anxiety, and visual changes, including either constriction of the visual fields or a sensation of diminishing or darkening vision. Falling and unconsciousness then ensue. When the attack is prolonged, a tonic motor seizure is likely to occur; tonic-clonic convulsions are less commonly observed. Among adult blood donors, up to 42% of those with syncope had some sort of convulsive movement [Lin et al., 1982]. Examination during the attack frequently discloses a thready pulse and bradycardia that return to normal before the patient awakens.

Syncope almost always occurs in the upright and usually standing position and is frequently associated with overheating, emotional upset, and fright. An inherited tendency to faint appears to exist, as evidenced by 27 of 30 children referred with this complaint having a first-degree relative with syncope as compared with only 8 of 24 best-friend controls [Camfield and Camfield, 1990]. Syncope may also occur in patients with pre-existing cardiac rhythm abnormalities.

Of 77 patients appearing in an emergency room complaining of "fainting," 20 had not had a syncopal or near-syncopal attack, 40 had had syncope, and 17 had near-syncope. Vasovagal (50%) and orthostatic hypotension (20%) were the most common causes in patients with syncope. In the near-syncopal episodes, diagnoses included lightheadedness (29%), seizure (18%), tension headache (12%), and migraine (6%) [Pratt and Fleisher, 1989].

Adolescents may induce syncope by stretching with the neck hyperextended; cardiovascular events and Valsalva response do not appear to be the mechanism [Pelakanos et al., 1990].

In patients with recurrent episodes, appropriate diagnosis and treatment may require detailed testing, including cardiac evaluation for congenital heart disease, electrocardiographic abnormalities (particularly Wolff-Parkinson-White syndrome), and prolonged QT syndrome, which has been associated with sudden death [Villain et al., 1992]. Autonomic function testing may identify patients with β-adrenergic hypersensitivity, who usually respond well to β-adrenergic blocking agents, particularly atenolol [Perry and Garson, 1991]. Tilt-table testing is particularly useful, with an isoprotorenol infusion being used as a provocative agent in some cases [Grubb et al., 1992a; 1992b; Lerman-Sagie et al., 1991; Ross et al., 1991; Thilenius et al., 1991].

BREATH-HOLDING SPELLS

The common features of breath-holding spells include apnea and an alteration in the state of consciousness, often in the form of unresponsiveness. The initial event is always crying, which is provoked by pain, fear, or

Classification of Seizure Type
Generalized Status Epilepticus Convulsive seizures 1. Tonic-clonic status epilepticus 2. Tonic status epilepticus 3. Clonic status epilepticus 4. Myoclonic status epilepticus Nonconvulsive generalized status epilepticus, including absence status or spike-and-wave stupor **Partial Status Epilepticus** Simple partial status, including somatomotor status epilepticus 1. Epilepsy partialis continua 2. Condition characterized by paroxysmal, lateralized, epileptic discharges 3. Possible dysphasic status epilepticus [Sato and Dreifuss, 1973] Complex partial status epilepticus or "psychomotor status" characterized by nonconvulsive confusional state with automatisms Modified from Dreifuss, 1983.

Childhood Conditions Meeting the Definition of Status Epilepticus
1. West syndrome (infantile spasms with hypsarrythmia) 2. Lennox-Gastaut syndrome 3. Landau-Kleffner syndrome 4. Pyknoepilepsy 5. Continuous spike-and-wave during sleep 6. Continuous occipital spike-and-wave during sleep

grim prognosis; diagnosis can be aided by neuroimaging studies [Tien et al., 1992].

Electrical status epilepticus during slow-wave sleep is characterized by the presence of continuous spike-and-slow-wave activity on EEG during non-rapid eye movement sleep. It is associated with partial motor seizure during sleep, and progressive neuropsychologic regression often occurs [Jayakar and Seshia, 1991]. Few patients have been reported from North America. Sudden death occurs in about 10% of patients with epilepsy; status epilepticus may be one cause [Earnest et al., 1992].

Incidence

Most of the 50,000 to 60,000 individuals in the United States who experience status epilepticus are children. The patients make up approximately equal-sized groups: those with status as the presenting symptom of an initial unprovoked seizure or with epilepsy, those with established epilepsy, and those with no history of epilepsy [Hauser, 1990].

Shinnar et al. [1992] prospectively studied 95 children who presented with their first episode of status epilepticus; 17% eventually had at least two episodes of status epilepticus. These two episodes occurred in 44% of the patients who had a identifiable antecedent cause, in 67% with an acute cause, and in 67% with progressive neurologic disease. All children with three or more episodes had been neurologically abnormal.

NEONATAL STATUS EPILEPTICUS

Classification of seizures in the newborn is different from that for older patients and is being reevaluated. Because of the immature neuronal interconnections and the lack of myelination at this age, seizures are apt to be fragmentary, and multiple seizure types may be seen in the same patient. Subtle manifestations of seizures are most common [Volpe, 1977].

The diagnosis of neonatal seizures and decisions about the efficacy of therapy depend on the use of frequent if not continuous electrographic monitoring. Three major factors contribute to this need: First, focal, multifocal, and generalized clonic movements are frequently related to abnormal cortical discharges, as are certain more complex activities such as chewing, lip smacking, and bicycling [Mizrahi and Kellaway, 1987]. Conversely, evidence is accumulating that recurrent tonic posturing is usually not accompanied by paroxysmal electrical activity and is usually caused by brainstem release phenomena that are unresponsive to antiepileptic drugs and perhaps made worse by sedative drugs such as barbiturates [Kellaway and Hrachovy, 1983]. Second, many neonates who have undergone the insults that lead to seizures require respiratory support and are therefore paralyzed with neuromuscular blocking agents. Paroxysmal electrical activity occurs in a significant number of these infants [Tharp and Laboyre, 1983]. Third, even the most skilled observer will frequently have difficulty distinguishing between normal motor activity and activity that represents seizure.

When frequent or prolonged EEG monitoring is used, electrical seizures are often documented unaccompanied by clinical events. In humans, it is unclear whether neonatal seizures cause brain damage as they do in experimental animals or whether the subsequent neurologic impairments, including epilepsy, are the result of the underlying provoking problem. Before the use of loading doses of antiepileptic drugs became common, neonatal seizures frequently "did not respond to treatment for 3 or 4 days" [Lockman et al., 1979]. This sequence of events represents the natural history of neonatal seizures; even untreated, they frequently remit

+---+
| **Approach to Status Epilepticus** |
| **in the Newborn** |
+---+
| 1. Seek a specifically treatable cause |
| 2. Treat for hypoglycemia and sepsis |
| 3. Use antiepileptic drugs |
+---+

Table 36-1 Antiepileptic drugs commonly used in newborns

Drug	Route	Loading dose (mg/kg)	Maintenance dosage (mg/kg/day)
Phenobarbital	IV	20 (+20)	4-8
Phenytoin	IV	20 (+10)	4-8
Diazepam	IV or R	0.3	—
Paraldehyde	R	0.3	—

IV, Intravenous; *R*, rectal.

toward the end of the first week of life. Two forms of "benign" neonatal convulsions have been identified: familial and nonfamilial ("fifth-day fits"); neither requires therapy, and the prognosis is good [Miles and Holmes, 1990].

Nonetheless, neonatal seizures are commonly treated as if they represented status epilepticus (see box above). Because hypoglycemia is relatively frequent in the newborn, the blood glucose level is always determined, and supplemental glucose (1 g/kg) is administered intravenously to ameliorate seizures and stave off brain damage. Calcium should also be measured, but neonatal hypocalcemia is no longer seen very often in the United States. Pyridoxine dependency, an autosomal recessively inherited disorder, is characterized by intractable, generalized clonic seizures beginning shortly after birth [Clarke et al., 1979]. An intravenous dose (100 mg) of pyridoxine administered during EEG monitoring stops the seizures within minutes and reverses the EEG abnormality in several hours. Appropriate blood and urine screening may suggest other metabolic causes of neonatal seizures that require specific therapy. In the absence of a specifically treatable cause, pharmacologic management is usually initiated with loading doses of antiepileptic drugs. Commonly used drugs are listed in Table 36-1. Drug therapy is stopped as soon as the offending agents are eliminated.

EEG monitoring

Patients with status epilepticus are difficult to stabilize because of the motor activity that frequently leads to hypoventilation and complicates starting and maintaining intravenous lines. These patients are frequently treated with neuromuscular blocking agents to achieve paralysis. Clinical recognition of seizures is impossible in this circumstance, and electrical monitoring is needed [Hellström-Westas et al., 1985; Stidham et al., 1980]. However, using a standard EEG is frequently not satisfactory because of the need for sophisticated bedside interpretation. In addition, the volume of paper record generated is immense. When therapy proceeds to barbiturate coma, methods to monitor the depth of suppression of electrical activity and detect the occurrence of electrical seizures must be used. A combination of the cerebral function monitor and the compressed spectral array can be used for this purpose [Altafullah et

al., 1991; Talwar and Torres, 1988]. The cerebral function monitor was engineered by Maynard et al. [1969]. Briefly, this device displays data derived from a single channel of EEG (usually between P_3 and P_4 of the International 10-20 System), although any location suitable for recording an abnormality can be used. The printout is in the form of a thick band that represents an amplitude distribution plot. In a recent model of the cerebral function monitor the component frequencies of 0 to 16 Hz are plotted along the upper edge of the paper.

With this device, epileptiform discharges are usually detected as a striking increase in amplitude. The appearance of burst suppression depends on the relative contributions of periods of burst activity and periods of suppression.

The compressed spectral array [Bickford et al., 1972] records a power-frequency spectrum over time. The analog signal undergoes spectral analysis using the fast Fourier transform [Cooley and Turkey, 1965] and is displayed (and printed) as partly overlapping epochs. During seizures a frequency band different from background and usually at higher frequencies abruptly appears.

In all cases of status epilepticus the choice of monitor and the selection of the electrodes from which to record are determined by routine EEG. The routine EEG is also recorded at intervals during therapy to verify the findings seen on the prolonged monitoring device.

These devices have proved to be valuable additions to the management of patients in status because they permit more precise control of barbiturate coma and signal the appearance of electrical seizures that occur between the times of routine EEG recording.

PHARMACOTHERAPY

Drugs commonly used for treating status epilepticus in infants and older children are listed in Table 36-2. More vigorous therapy is sometimes needed.

The successful use of pentobarbital in two pediatric patients was reported by Young et al. [1983]. Their seizures were refractory to loading doses of both phenobarbital and phenytoin with additional intrave-

Table 36-2 Antiepileptic drugs commonly used during infancy and childhood

Drug	Route	Loading dose (mg/kg)	Maintenance dosage (mg/kg/day)
Sedative			
Barbiturates			
Phenobarbital	IV	20 (+20)	4-8
Pentobarbital	IV	20	24 (1 mg/kg/hr)
Paraldehyde	R or IV*	0.3	—
Benzodiazepines			
Diazepam	IV or R	0.3	—
Lorazepam	IV or IM	0.1-0.2	—
Midazolam	IV or IM	0.2	—
Clonazepam*	IV	0.25-0.75	?
Nonsedative			
Phenytoin	IV	20 (+10)	4-8
Valproate	R	60	30-60
Lidocaine	IV	2-3	—

IV, Intravenous; *R*, rectal; *IM*, intramuscular.
*Not available in the United States.

nous diazepam. A loading dose of 8 mg/kg of pentobarbital as a bolus led to abolition of seizures and conversion of the EEG pattern from continuous high-voltage spike-and-wave to burst suppression. The patients received a continuous pentobarbital infusion at 3 mg/kg/hr for 3 days with intermittent EEG monitoring. The authors describe the toxicities of pentobarbital (e.g., respiratory and cardiac depression) and report that after 5 or more days of continuous infusion, mild pulmonary edema, skin edema, and ileus regularly occurred in their patients. The use of "pentobarbital coma" is now one of the standard therapies for refractory status epilepticus in children.

A total of 50 children with status epilepticus refractory to initial therapy were given very high doses of phenobarbital without a predetermined maximum blood level limit [Crawford et al., 1988]. In 47 of these patients, seizures were controlled. A total of 40 patients were intubated before phenobarbital administration but recovered their respiratory drive despite high serum levels and could be removed from the ventilator. Hypotension did not present an insurmountable problem.

Knudsen [1979] found diazepam rectal administration to be effective in the acute therapy of convulsions in children. Hoppu and Santavuori [1981] used diazepam rectal solution in treating 17 children with prolonged seizures at home. In 65 episodes, 67% of the seizures were stopped in less than 15 min. Only 1 patient had respiratory difficulties that did not require intervention; this patient, a 16-year-old male, was receiving phenobarbital. In addition, 1 child complained of dizziness, and 2 had mild, transient skin reactions. The authors used a beginning dose of about 0.5 mg/kg with a maximum dose per episode of 20 mg.

Midazolam, a benzodiazepine, has rapid and nearly complete absorption after intramuscular administration and may be useful if venous access is not practical [Bell et al., 1991].

Camfield et al. [1989] reported that of 30 children whose families were taught how to administer rectal diazepam to treat prolonged afebrile seizures (12 patients) or prolonged or repeated febrile seizures, 17 had episodes that required this treatment. Seizures stopped within an average of 5 min after diazepam administration. This treatment was ineffective in 2 patients. They used a dose of 0.5 mg/kg and a maximum of 15 mg. Each child received a test dose under medical supervision to ascertain whether side effects would prevent safe home use.

A few pediatric patients have status epilepticus as the sole manifestation of a seizure disorder. The frequency of status epilepticus episodes is often not altered by daily administration of antiepileptic drugs. The best approach to management of these patients may be to withhold medication between episodes and treat the acute seizure at home with rectal diazepam [Lombroso, 1989].

Although lorazepam has also been administered rectally to treat seizures in children [Dooley et al., 1985], studies of pharmacokinetics in adult volunteers indicated that peak concentrations attained are significantly lower and later than concentrations attained after the same dose given intravenously [Graves et al., 1987]; doses two to four times higher than the IV dose, which are necessary to achieve early, effective serum concentrations, may pose the risk of prolonged toxicity.

The Lennox-Gastaut syndrome may represent a special situation. This syndrome consists of multiple seizure types (usually any combination of atonic, tonic, absence, myoclonic, and possibly tonic-clonic), mental retardation, and an EEG with prominent slow spike-and-wave pattern. The essentially continuous slow spike-and-wave activity on EEG and the innumerable seizures suffered by these patients imply that they may be in status epilepticus for hours to weeks at a time. Using sedative antiepileptic drugs, particularly barbiturates, does not ameliorate the seizures and may further dull the intellect—a situation in which the patient gets worse while the seizures do not get better. In addition, benzodiazepines usually do not help the seizures and may precipitate tonic seizures in these children [Bittencourt and Richens, 1981; Livingston and Brown, 1987].

Conversely, low morbidity and mortality were found in the large series reported by Maytal et al. [1989]. Of 193 subjects, 97 were recruited prospectively. All deaths (7 patients) and 15 of 17 patients with sequelae occurred in the 56 subjects with acute or progressive neurologic insults. The precise seizure manifestations were not detailed, although the authors indicated that the majority were generalized. Details of treatment were also not presented.

Prolonged confusion lasting up to 10 days can occasionally occur, particularly after tonic-clonic status epilepticus [Biton et al., 1990].

The outcome of tonic-clonic status epilepticus appears to be related to the underlying cause rather than the duration of the seizure or the response to treatment in children. Conversely, the more subtle, nonconvulsive status epilepticus episode, in which an etiology is found only rarely, is more likely to be associated with a poor developmental outcome.

REFERENCES

Altafullah I, Asaikar S, Torres F. Status epilepticus: clinical experience with two special devices for continuous cerebral monitoring. Acta Neurol Scand 1991; 84:374-381.

Bell DM, Richards G, Dhillon S, et al. A comparative pharmacokinetic study of intravenous and intramuscular midazolam in patients with epilepsy. Epilepsy Res 1991; 10:183-190.

Bickford RG, Billinger TW, Fleming N, et al. The compressed spectral array (CSA): a pictorial EEG. Proc San Diego Biomed Symp 1972; 11:365-370.

Biton V, Gates JR, dePadua Sussman L. Prolonged postictal encephalopathy. Neurology 1990; 40:963-966.

Bittencourt PRM, Richens A. Anticonvulsant-induced status epilepticus in Lennox-Gastaut syndrome. Epilepsia 1981; 22:129-134.

Brett EM. Minor epileptic status. J Neurol Sci 1966; 3:52-75.

Camfield CS, Camfield PR, Smith E, et al. Home use of rectal diazepam to prevent status epilepticus in children with convulsive disorders. J Child Neurol 1989; 4:125-126.

Clarke TH, Saunders BS, Feldman B. Pyridoxine-dependent seizures requiring high doses of pyridoxine for control. Am J Dis Child 1979; 133:963-965.

Cooley JW, Turkey JW. An algorithm for machine calculation of complex Fourier series. Math Comput 1965; 19:297-301.

Crawford TO, Mitchell WG, Fishman LS, et al. Very-high-dose phenobarbital for refractory status epilepticus in children. Neurology 1988; 38:1035-1040.

Dooley JM, Tibbles JAR, Rumney G, et al. Rectal lorazepam in the treatment of acute seizures in children. Ann Neurol 1985; 18:412-413.

Doose H, Volzke E. Petit mal status in early childhood and early dementia. Neuropaediatrie 1979; 10:10-14.

Dreifuss FE. Pediatric epileptology: classification and management of seizures in the child. Boston: John Wright, 1983.

Earnest MP, Thomas GE, Eden RA, et al. The sudden unexplained death syndrome in epilepsy: demographic, clinical, and postmortem features. Epilepsia 1992; 33:310-316.

Gastaut, H. Dictionary of epilepsy. Part 1. Definitions. Geneva: World Health Organization, 1973.

Graves NM, Kriel RL, Jones-Saete C. Bioavailability of rectally administered lorazepam. Clin Neuropharm 1987; 10:555-559.

Hauser WA. Status epilepticus: epidemiologic considerations. Neurology 1990; 40(suppl 2):9-13.

Hellström-Westas L, Rosén I, Svenningsen NW. Silent seizures in sick infants in early life: diagnosis by continuous cerebral function monitoring. Acta Paediatr Scand 1985; 74:741-747.

Hoppu K, Santavuori P. Diazepam rectal solution for home treatment of acute seizures in children. Acta Paediatr Scand 1981; 70:369-372.

Jayakar PB, Seshia SS. Electrical status epilepticus during slow-wave sleep: a review. J Clin Neurophysiol 1991; 8:299-311.

Kellaway P, Hrachovy RH. Status epilepticus in newborns: a perspective on neonatal seizures. Adv Neurol 1983; 34:93-99.

Knudsen FU. Rectal administration of diazepam in solution in the acute treatment of convulsions in infants and children. Arch Dis Child 1979; 54:855-857.

Livingston JH, Brown JK. Non-convulsive status epilepticus resistant to benzodiazepines. Arch Dis Child 1987; 62:41-44.

Lockman LA, Kriel R, Zaske D, et al. Phenobarbital dosage for control of neonatal seizures. Neurology 1979; 29:1445-1449.

Lombroso, CT. Intermittent home treatment of status and clusters of seizures. Epilepsia 1989; 30[suppl.] 2:S11-4.

Manning DJ, Rosenbloom L. Non-convulsive status epilepticus. Arch Dis Child 1987; 62:37-40.

Maynard DE, Prior PF, Scott DF. Device for continuous monitoring of cerebral activity in resuscitated patients. Br Med J 1969; 4:545-546.

Maytal J, Shinnar S, Moshé SL, et al. Low morbidity and mortality of status epilepticus in children. Pediatrics 1989; 83:323-331.

Miles DK, Holmes GL. Benign neonatal seizures. J Clin Neurophysiol 1990; 7:369-379.

Mizrahi EM, Kellaway P. Characterization and classification of neonatal seizures. Neurology 1987; 37:1837-1844.

Ohtahara S, Oka E, Yamatogi Y, et al. Non-convulsive status epilepticus in childhood. Folia Psychiatr Neurol Jpn 1979; 33:345-351.

Phillips SA, Shanahan RJ. Etiology and mortality of status epilepticus in children: a recent update. Arch Neurol 1989; 46:74-76.

Sato S, Dreifuss FE. Electroencephalographic findings in a patient with developmental expressive aphasia. Neurology 1973; 23:181-185.

Shinnar S, Maytal J, Krasnoff L, et al. Recurrent status epilepticus in children. Ann Neurol 1992; 31:598-604.

Stidham GL, Nugent SK, Rogers MC. Monitoring cerebral function in the ICU. Crit Care Med 1980; 8:519-523.

Talwar D, Torres F. Continuous electrophysiologic monitoring of cerebral function in the pediatric intensive care unit. Pediatr Neurol 1988; 4:137-147.

Tharp BR, Laboyre PM. The incidence of EEG abnormalities and outcome of infants paralyzed with neuromuscular blocking agents. Crit Care Med 1983; 11:926-929.

Tien RD, Ashdown BC, Lewis DV Jr, et al. Rasmussen's encephalitis: neuroimaging findings in four patients. Am J Roentgenol 1992; 158:1329-1332.

Volpe JJ. Neonatal seizures. Clin Perinatol 1977; 4:43-63.

Young RSK, Ropper AH, Hawkes D, et al. Pentobarbital in refractory status epilepticus. Pediatr Pharmacol 1983; 3:63-67.

37

Antiepileptic Drug Therapy in Children: Pharmacokinetics, Adverse Effects, and Monitoring

Robert L. Kriel and James C. Cloyd

Rational management of drug therapy in children requires an understanding of pharmacokinetics, pharmacodynamics, and toxicology. Pharmacokinetics is the study of drug absorption, distribution, metabolism, and elimination, or what the body does with a drug. Pharmacodynamics is the study of a drug's biochemical and physiologic effects, or what the drug does to the body. Children much more than adults have widely varying abilities to absorb, distribute, metabolize, and eliminate drugs [Rane and Wilson, 1976]. Evidence also exists that antiepileptic drugs (AEDs) pharmacodynamics in children differ from those in adults [White et al., 1983]. Application of basic pharmacokinetic and pharmacodynamic principles to AED therapy facilitates the attainment and maintenance of targeted serum concentrations, interpretation of clinical response, and control of drug interactions.

Adverse reactions often dictate the choice of an AED and subsequent adjustment of therapy. An understanding of these reactions, including their differences and similarities among various AEDs, and the application of appropriate clinical and laboratory monitoring provide the tools needed for the clinician to prescribe drug therapy rationally.

PHARMACOKINETIC PRINCIPLES

AED pharmacokinetics differ qualitatively and quantitatively between children and adults. Children, particularly neonates, have greater variability than adults in their ability to absorb and eliminate AEDs. Infants have the greatest capacity to metabolize AEDs, resulting in the largest doses relative to body weight to attain targeted plasma concentrations. After infancy, drug clearance progressively declines until adult values are reached around 12 to 15 years of age. Other than age-related differences, drug-specific pharmacokinetics such as saturable metabolism, protein binding, and enzyme induction are similar for children and adults.

An overview of pharmacokinetic principles and the most clinically relevant features of specific AED pharmacokinetics are presented. A comprehensive list of absorption characteristics is provided in Table 37-1, and other pharmacokinetic data are presented in Tables 37-2 through 37-4.

Absorption

Absorption, along with elimination, determines the amount of drug in the body. Formulation or age-dependent variations in absorption are often overlooked as causes for changes in plasma AED concentrations.

Absorption is a complex phenomenon controlled by the physical-chemical properties of the drug, the formulation, and the physiologic conditions at the site of absorption. A solid formulation must first disintegrate into small particles, which are then dissolved in gastrointestinal fluid. Once the drug is dissolved, it is available for absorption, usually by passive diffusion of the unionized form. Absorption is influenced by physiologic variables such as gastric emptying time, pH, absorptive area, and gastrointestinal transit time.

Absorption is described in terms of rate and extent. An absorption half-life is commonly used to describe the rate at which drug reaches the blood. An indirect measure of absorption rate is the time to maximum

The preparation of this chapter was supported in part by a grant from the National Institute of Neurological Disorders and Stroke, NIH P50 NS 16308.

Table 37-1 Formulations, routes of administration, and bioavailability of AEDs

Medication	Available formulations	Possible routes (primary and alternates)	Tmax (hr)	Fraction absorbed	Special problems
Acetazolamide	tablets	PO			
	slow-release capsules	PO			
	injection	IV, IM			
Carbamazepine	tablet	PO	3-8	.7-.9 estimate	Has prolonged absorptive phase with variable time to maximum plasma concentration. Induction results in earlier time to maximum plasma concentration
	chewable tablet	PO	2	.7-.9 estimate	
	suspension	PO, PR	0.5-3.0	.7-.9 estimate	Earlier time to maximum plasma concentration results in higher maximum concentration, possibly producing transient side effects
Clonazepam	tablet	PO	1-8	0.85	
Clorazepate	tablet	PO			
Diazepam	tablet	PO	0.5-2.0	0.8-1.0	
	solution	PO	0.1-0.5	0.8-1.0	
	injection	IM, IV, PR	1.0-1.5	0.8-1.0	IM absorption is slow and variable
Ethosuximide	capsules	PO	1.5-4.0		
	syrup	PO	3.7		
Ethotoin	tablet	PO			
Felbamate	tablets	PO	1-4		
	suspension	PO	2.5-7.5		
Gabapentin	capsule	PO	2-4	0.6	
Lamotrigine	tablets	PO	1-3		
Lorazepam	tablets	PO	1.0-2.5	0.85-1.0	
	injection	IM, IV, PR	0.75-2.0	0.85-1.0	
Methsuximide	tablet	PO			
Paraldehyde	solution	PR, PO			Do not use discolored solution; will cause bonding of plastic plunger to syringe barrel
Phenacemide	tablets	PO			
Phenobarbital	syrup	PO (PR)	1	1	Has unpleasant taste, is rejected by many
	tablet	PO	0.5-8.6	1	
	injection	IM, IV	0.5-4.0	1	
Phenytoin	suspensions (phenytoin acid) of 30 mg/5 ml 125 mg/5 ml	PO	6-12	0.9-1.0	Patients should use accurate measuring device; dosing errors possible if suspension not adequately resuspended; strength of suspension must be clearly emphasized when prescribing
	suspension-unit foil 125 mg/5 ml	PO			Minimizes errors from inadequate resuspension of suspension
	chewable tablet (phenytoin acid)	PO	4-8	0.9-1.0	
	prompt release capsules (phenytoin sodium)	PO	2-6	0.9-1.0	Time to maximum plasma concentration depends on maximum concentration
	extended-release capsules (phenytoin sodium) 30 and 100 mg	PO	2-10	0.9-1.0	Time to maximum plasma concentration depends on maximum concentration
	injection (phenytoin sodium) 50 mg/ml	IM, IV	15-25	0.9-1.0	IM injection is not recommended: absorption is slow and erratic, injection is painful and must be diluted with normal saline without glucose and slowly administered

PO, by mouth; *PR*, by rectum; *IM*, intramuscular; *IV*, intravenous.

Table 37-1 Formulations, routes of administration, and bioavailability of AEDs—cont'd

Medication	Available formulations	Possible routes (primary and alternates)	Tmax (hr)	Fraction absorbed	Special problems
Primidone	suspension	PO	4-6	NA	
	tablet	PO	4-6	NA	
Trimethadione	tablets	PO			
	capsules	PO			
	solution	PO			
Valproate	capsules	PO	0.5-4.0	0.9-1.0	Capsule is filled with a bitter liquid, should be swallowed whole
	enteric-coated tablet	PO	2-6	0.9-1.0	Food delays time to maximum plasma concentration
	sprinkle caps	PO	4-6	0.9-1.0	
	syrup	PO, PR	0.5-2.0	0.9-1.0	Has an objectional aftertaste

plasma concentration, which is useful when comparing the rate of absorption of different brands or formulations of the same drug. An earlier time to maximum plasma concentration is usually an indication of a faster rate of absorption. When all other pharmacokinetic parameters are constant, a faster rate of absorption will result in a higher maximum concentration.

The extent of absorption defines the amount of drug that reaches the blood. Bioavailability is the fraction of the dose that reaches the systemic circulation after crossing the gastrointestinal wall and liver. Absolute bioavailability of a drug is determined by comparing the area under the concentration-time curve after an oral (or rectal, intramuscular, and so on) dose with the area under the concentration-time curve (AUC) obtained after intravenous administration of the same drug. Relative bioavailability can be determined by comparing the area under the concentration-time curve from a test brand or formulation with a reference product. For example, the relative bioavailability of a generic brand of phenytoin sodium 100 mg capsule is measured by comparing its area under the concentration-time curve with that from a Dilantin 100 mg capsule.

Bioavailability, along with the rate of elimination, determines average plasma concentration as follows:

$$\text{Average plasma concentration} = \frac{\text{Fraction absorbed} \times \text{Daily dose}}{\text{Clearance}}$$

Changes in bioavailability due to alteration in drug, dosage form, gastrointestinal physiology, or interactions can result in clinically significant increases or decreases in plasma drug concentration.

Profiles of absorption, including the maximum concentration, the time of maximum concentration, and even the total bioavailability, may vary considerably among formulations of the same drug. The rate of absorption generally proceeds in the following order: solutions greater than suspensions greater than capsules greater than tablets greater than extended-release formulations [Garnett and Cloyd, 1992]. Formulation-related differences in absorption characteristics are determined by the composition of the nondrug ingredients (e.g., filler, particle size of drug, nature of capsule or tablet, coating).

Absorption characteristics of AEDs

Benzodiazepines. As a group these drugs are rapidly (time to maximum plasma concentration of 30 to 180 minutes) and completely absorbed when given orally. Intramuscular administration of diazepam or lorazepam is not recommended because of slow or erratic absorption.

Carbamazepine. Carbamazepine is a water-insoluble, neutral compound with a slow dissolution rate in gastrointestinal fluid. The relative bioavailability is similar for all three formulations (i.e., suspension, chewable tablet, regular tablet), ranging from 65% to 75%, although there is marked intrapatient and interpatient variability [Leppik et al., 1984; Maas et al., 1987]. In children on maintenance therapy the suspension displays a much faster rate of absorption than tablet formulations, resulting in a significantly earlier time to maximum plasma concentration and a higher maximum concentration (Figure 37-1), which occasionally produces transient concentration-dependent CNS side effects. Administering the same daily dose in smaller amounts given more frequently will usually correct this problem. Recent studies conducted by the Food and Drug Administration have demonstrated that carbamazepine tablets are significantly less well absorbed when exposed to high humidity [Meyer et al., 1992; Wang, 1990]. These reports emphasize the importance of storing all AEDs at room temperature in a dry location.

Table 37-2 Pharmacokinetics of phenytoin

Age	Volume of distribution (L/kg)	Protein binding (%)	Vmax (mg/kg/day)	Km (µg/ml)	$T_{1/2}$ (hr)	Routes of elimination	Active metabolites	Initial maintenance dose	Comments
Neonates	0.7-1.2	74-90			3-140	Hepatic, 95%; renal, 5%	No	4-6	$T_{1/2}$ varies with concentrations
3 mo-3 yr		85-91	13.9	4.0-6.6	1.2-31.5			6-10	
4-6 yr			11	4.0-6.8				5-7	
7-9 yr			9.75	3.6-6.5				4-7	
>10 yr	0.7-0.8	87-93	8.1	3.0-5.7	6-60			4-6	

Vmax, Maximum capacity of the enzyme system to metabolize phenytoin; *Km*, plasma concentration at which the rate of metabolism is 50% of maximum capacity; $T_{1/2}$, elimination half-life.

Table 37-3 Pharmacokinetics of other AEDs

Drug	Age group	Volume of distribution (L/kg)	Protein binding (%)	$T_{1/2}$ (hr)	Routes of elimination	Active metabolites	Initial maintenance dose (mg/kg)	Comments
Carbamazepine	Neonate	1.1-2.6	65-70	7.2-27.0	Hepatic	Carbamazepine epoxide	5-20	Therapy should be initiated at 30%-50% of initial dose and increased as autoinduction occurs
	Children	0.8-2.0	75-85	5-26				
Clonazepam	Children	1.5-4.4	80-90	22-33	Hepatic	None	0.05-0.2	Tolerance to antiepileptic effect frequently occurs
Ethosuximide	Neonate			32-41	Hepatic	None	20-40	
	Children	0.7	<10	15-68				
Phenobarbital	Neonate	0.8-1.0	32	82-199	Hepatic, 50%-80%; renal, 20%-50%	None	3-4	
	Infants	0.6-0.9	40-55	37-73			4-5	
	Children	0.7	20	21-75			2-3	
Primidone	Children			4.4-11.0	Hepatic, 60%-70%; renal, 30%-40%	PB, PEMA	10-15	Therapy should be initiated at 30%-50% of initial dose
Valproic acid	Neonate	0.28-0.43	68-89	17-40	Hepatic, 95%; renal, 5%	2-en-valproic acid, 4-en-valproic acid, 2,4-dien-valproic acid	5-10	
	Infants	0.2-0.34		6-8			10-20 (monotherapy), 20-30 (induced)	
	Children	0.1-0.3	80-95	4-15			10-20 (monotherapy), 20-30 (induced)	

Table 37-4 Pharmacokinetics of recently approved and investigational AEDs

Drug	Age group	Volume of distribution (L/kg)	Protein binding (%)	$T_{1/2}$ (hr)	Routes of elimination	Active metabolites	Initial maintenance dose (mg/kg)
Felbamate	Adults	0.7-0.8	<10	20-24; induced, 14	Hepatic, 50%-60%; renal, 40%-50%	None	15
Gabapentin	Adults	0.7	0	4-6	Renal, >95%;	None	4-25
Lamotrigine	Adults	1.3	55	21-50; induced, 7-21	Hepatic	None	0.7-5.7?

$T_{1/2}$, Elimination half-life.
?, Not fully established.

Phenytoin Phenytoin is a poorly soluble acid that is slowly absorbed. Available formulations include suspensions, chewable tablets, and capsules. Important differences exist among the dosage forms with regard to amount of phenytoin and rate of absorption (see Table 37-1). The chewable tablet and suspensions contain phenytoin acid, whereas the capsules contain phenytoin sodium, which yields 92% phenytoin acid. Thus two 50 mg chewable tablets will deliver 9% more phenytoin than a 100 mg phenytoin sodium capsule. The nonlinear, saturation pharmacokinetics of phenytoin make even these small differences clinically significant. Differences in phenytoin content may make dose adjustment necessary when formulations are changed. Alternatively, monitoring plasma concentration is advisable. The suspensions are available in both pediatric (30 mg/5 ml) and adult (125 mg/5 ml) strengths. Occasionally these formulations are inadvertently interchanged with serious consequences. In the past the reliability of the suspensions has been questioned because of their tendency to settle [Pellock, 1984]. Recently it has been demonstrated that minimal agitation (i.e., one inversion of the bottle) is sufficient to deliver the specified amount of drug [Sarkar et al., 1989]. Unexpected fluctuations in plasma phenytoin concentrations associated with the use of suspensions have probably been the result of nonlinear pharmacokinetics rather than formulation problems.

Phenytoin capsules are available in prompt- or extended-release form. Extended-release forms (Dilantin Kapseals) may be particularly useful in some children who rapidly eliminate phenytoin because the slower rate of absorption may permit fewer daily doses. Patient and family education about the differences in phenytoin dosage forms is important to maintain optimal therapy.

Bioavailability, time to maximum plasma concentration, and maximum plasma concentration are altered when large amounts of phenytoin are given as a single loading dose, presumably because of the formation of a multicapsule concretion. In a study involving 6 healthy adults, absorption was reduced by 10% to 15% and time to maximum plasma concentration increased to 18 to 32 hours when phenytoin sodium capsules were given in a single dose of 10 mg/kg or more [Jung et al., 1980]. Dividing the total loading dose into 5 mg/kg doses given every 2 to 3 hours overcomes this problem. The most rapid way to attain therapeutic plasma concentrations after oral loading is to use prompt-release phenytoin sodium capsules or the suspension form [Goff et al., 1984].

Some reports have suggested that phenytoin is poorly absorbed in newborns because of irregular gastric emptying time, relatively high gastric pH (greater than 4), or decreased absorptive surface [Morrow and Richens, 1989; Morselli, 1983; Painter et al., 1978]. More recent evidence indicates that formulation-related differences in absorption, nonlinear pharmacokinetics, and age-dependent changes in elimination account for much of the variability in plasma concentrations [Dodson, 1984].

Intramuscular injection of the parenteral solution (pH 11) results in precipitation of drug that is then slowly and erratically absorbed [Kostenbauder et al., 1975]. Injection is painful and occasionally causes muscle necrosis [Serrano and Wilder, 1974]. An investigational formulation of phenytoin—fosphenytoin—is well tolerated when given intramuscularly [Leppik et al., 1989].

Valproic acid. Valproic acid appears to be completely absorbed from all the available products, but the rate of absorption varies significantly with dosage form (see Table 37-1). Maximum plasma concentration occurs 30 to 60 minutes after syrup, 30 minutes to 2 hours after the capsule, 1 to 6 hours after the enteric-coated tablet, and 3 to 6 hours after sprinkle [Cloyd et al., 1983; 1985; 1992]. Absorption after ingestion of the enteric coated tablet is delayed for several hours; as a result a lag phase occurs, during which plasma concentrations may continue to decline. Food further delays but does not decrease valproic acid absorption from the enteric-coated tablet [Fischer et al., 1988].

Generic formulations. Absorption may differ between similar formulations (such as tablets) from various manufacturers (e.g., carbamazepine) [Kauko and Tammisto, 1974; Pynnönen et al., 1978; Sillanpää, 1981].

Patient 002

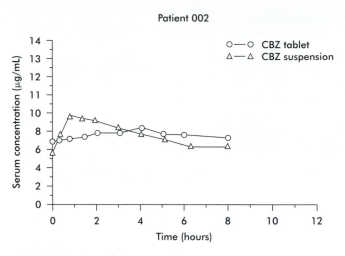

Figure 37-1 Comparison of serum concentration-time curves following administration of carbamazepine tablets and suspension. Crossover study in a child with epilepsy on steady-state, maintenance therapy.

Significant increase in serum phenytoin concentrations has been observed when the same maintenance doses of medication are taken from different sources. For drugs with nonlinear kinetics such as phenytoin, this can lead to clinical toxicity [Mikati et al., 1992]. Substitution of drugs made by differing manufacturers may lead to problems, especially when drugs with narrow therapeutic ranges or nonlinear pharmacokinetics are used. Therefore counseling patients to keep taking medication prepared by the same pharmaceutical source whenever possible is usually advisable [Nuwer et al., 1990].

Distribution volume and protein binding

Volume of distribution in its simplest form is the ratio of amount of drug in the body to blood concentration and is expressed in terms or liters or liters per kilogram. Mathematically, the ratio is expressed as the following:

$$\text{Volume of distribution} = \frac{\text{Intravenous dose}}{\text{Plasma concentration immediately after injection}}$$

Because calculation of the distribution volume is based on plasma concentration, volume usually does not directly relate to a physiologic space. For example, drugs that concentrate in certain tissues and have relatively low plasma concentrations may have distribution volumes measured in hundreds of liters. Changes in body composition such as increases or decreases in fat, muscle, or water can alter distribution volume. For drugs that are highly bound to plasma proteins, distribution volume may vary when total plasma concentration is altered because of changes in protein binding. In such cases a distribution volume based on the unbound

plasma concentration may be a better indicator of a drug's distribution in the body.

The value of distribution volume in drug therapy is its use in calculating loading doses. The concept of a loading dose is to rapidly fill body compartments to reach a targeted plasma concentration and thus a targeted concentration at the site of action. The equation for calculating a loading dose is the following:

$$\text{Loading Dose} = \text{Volume of distribution (L/kg)} \times \text{Body weight} \times \text{Desired change in plasma concentration}$$

The change in plasma concentration denotes the desired increase after administration of the loading dose. For example, if a patient has a plasma concentration of 5 µg/ml and the target concentration is 20 µg/ml, the change in concentration is 15 mg/l. When loading doses are administered intramuscularly, orally, or rectally, resultant maximum plasma concentrations are usually less than after intravenous administration due to slower and incomplete absorption and the elimination of some drug during the absorption phase. Table 37-5 presents loading dose information for four major AEDs.

Several AEDs are highly bound to one or more plasma proteins, most commonly albumin or alpha-1-acid glycoprotein. Drug assays usually measure the total concentration of drug, which is a combination of the bound and unbound concentrations. The free fraction is the ratio of unbound to total plasma drug concentration:

$$\text{Free fraction} = \frac{\text{Unbound concentration}}{\text{Total concentration}}$$

Generally, only unbound drug is free to cross the blood-brain barrier and correlates best with brain and spinal fluid concentrations (Figure 37-2). Theoretically the unbound drug should correlate best with clinical response and toxicity. For drugs that have limited protein binding (less than 50%) or a constant ratio of unbound to total concentration, total plasma concentration is equally reliable. In situations where drug is highly protein bound (greater than 75%) and the unbound to total concentration ratio varies, the unbound concentration is a better measure of the amount of drug at the site of action.

Disruptions in protein binding, such as those due to hypoalbuminemia or drug interactions, alter total concentrations but do not affect the concentration of unbound drug. When alterations in protein binding are suspected, measuring the unbound concentration and determining the free fraction may be useful responses. Dosing adjustments are generally not necessary when protein binding is altered but the unbound concentrations remain unchanged.

Table 37-5 Loading doses of AEDs

Drug	Distribution volume (L/kg)	Loading dose (mg/kg)	Route/formulation	Cmax (μg/ml)	Tmax (hr)
Carbamazepine	0.8	10	Oral/suspension	6-9	1-6
Phenobarbital	0.8	20	Intravenous	15-25	Immediate
Phenytoin	0.75	20	Intravenous	20-30	Immediate
	0.75	20	Oral/prompt-release cap*	15-25	8-12
	0.75	20	Oral/extended-release cap*	10-20	10-24
Valproic acid	0.2	15	Oral/syrup	60-100	0.5-2.0

Cmax, Maximum concentration; *Tmax*, time to maximum plasma concentration.
*Fastest and most complete absorption occurs when the loading dose is divided into several smaller doses given every 2 to 3 hours.

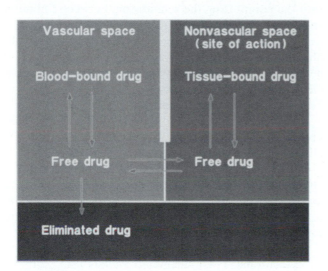

Figure 37-2 Relationship of unbound drug in vascular and nonvascular compartments.

Distribution and protein binding of AEDs

Benzodiazepine. The benzodiazepines rapidly cross the blood-brain barrier. Brain concentrations reach equilibrium with plasma within seconds after intravenous administration. The highly lipid-soluble nature of diazepam and lorazepam causes them to redistribute to other body tissues, resulting in a decrease in brain concentrations. This redistribution, which takes place in minutes, is responsible for the short duration of action.

Carbamazepine. The volume of distribution for carbamazepine ranges from 0.8 to 1.4 L/kg. Carbamazepine and its active metabolite, carbamazepine-10,11-epoxide, are both bound to several plasma proteins. Approximately 65% to 85% of carbamazepine and 30% to 60% of the epoxide are bound to albumin. Both compounds also bind to the reactant protein alpha-1-acid glycoprotein. Protein binding varies with the concentration of these proteins. In particular, binding to alpha-1-acid glycoprotein increases after physiologic stress, such as burn injuries, inflammatory diseases (e.g., juvenile rheumatoid arthritis), and concurrent drug therapy with enzyme-inducing drugs. Increased binding to alpha-1-acid glycoprotein can increase total carbamazepine and carbamazepine epoxide concentrations without necessarily increasing unbound concentrations. In such situations, patients may have total concentrations above the desired range but have no side effects. Adjusting dosage is not necessary; plasma concentrations will return to baseline as alpha-1-acid glycoprotein declines.

Phenytoin. Phenytoin distribution volume in children and adolescents is approximately 0.7 ± 0.1 L/kg. The relatively small variability in phenytoin distribution volume permits the precise calculation of loading doses. For example, a 15 mg/kg loading dose given intravenously will result in a postinfusion mean concentration of 20 μg/ml with a range of 15 to 25 μg/ml.

Phenytoin is highly protein bound to albumin. In healthy children the percentage bound ranges from 87% to 93% and is usually stable within a patient. Hypoalbuminemia, uremia, and certain drugs can decrease binding.

Valproic acid. Valproic acid distribution volumes vary more than those of carbamazepine, phenobarbital, and phenytoin, ranging from 0.12 to 0.49 L/kg. When loading doses are calculated, a distribution volume of 0.2 L/kg is recommended.

Valproic acid protein binding to albumin is saturable. At concentrations below 40 to 50 μg/ml the bound fraction averages 90% to 95%. As total concentration rises to the upper boundary of the therapeutic range, the percentage bound decreases to 80% to 85%. Saturable protein binding results in a nonlinear relationship between total valproic acid concentration and dose. Unbound valproic acid concentrations, however, remain linear with dose.

Metabolism and Elimination

AEDs are primarily eliminated from the body through hepatic metabolism, although the kidney is an important route of elimination for several agents. *Clearance* and *elimination half-life* are the pharmacokinetic terms that quantitatively describe drug elimination. Clearance is the more useful of the two in describing the rate of elimination and dosage requirements; half-life is useful in determining time to steady state and dosing intervals. Clearance is the volume of blood from which drug is removed (cleared) in some unit of time. It is identical conceptually and mathematically to the physiologic parameter creatinine clearance. The major AEDs are cleared primarily by liver metabolism via hepatic microsomal and related enzymes. Clearance, with the amount of drug reaching systemic circulation, determines steady-state, total plasma drug concentration:

$$\text{Total Concentration} = \frac{\text{Fraction absorbed} \times \text{Daily dose}}{\text{Clearance}}$$
$$= \frac{\text{Fraction absorbed} \times \text{Daily dose}}{\text{Free fraction} \times \text{Unbound clearance}}$$

For AEDs that are eliminated by the liver, clearance is determined by the free fraction of drug and the intrinsic ability of hepatic enzymes to metabolize unbound drug. This intrinsic drug metabolism is known as *unbound clearance*.

In contrast, the steady-state, unbound serum concentration is determined only by the amount of drug absorbed and unbound clearance:

$$\text{Unbound concentration} = \frac{\text{Fraction absorbed} \times \text{Daily dose}}{\text{Unbound clearance}}$$

The following points are important to remember:
1. Clearance and absorption determine the amount of drug a patient requires to maintain a targeted plasma concentration.
2. Changes in unbound clearance result in changes in unbound concentration and potentially the resultant pharmacologic response.
3. Changes in protein binding affect total but not unbound concentration.

Changes in total drug concentration without a corresponding change in unbound concentration therefore do not require a dosage adjustment.

Elimination half-life is the time required for the amount of drug in the body or plasma concentration to decline by 50%. Half-life is determined by both distribution volume and clearance:

$$\text{Elimination half life} = \frac{0.693 \times \text{Distribution of volume}}{\text{Clearance}}$$

Thus half-life is not a direct measure of metabolizing capacity but is useful in calculating the time to reach steady state or the time required for drug elimination. After initiation or modification of therapy or any change in clearance, five half-lives must elapse to reach a new steady-state plasma concentration. After therapy is discontinued, five half-lives must elapse before drug is completely eliminated from the body.

Active metabolites

Active metabolites can contribute significantly to the desired and toxic effects of the parent drug. Metabolites exist in both bound and unbound states. Only the unbound metabolite is available for elimination or biotransformation to an inactive metabolite. As with unbound parent drug, the unbound plasma metabolite concentration most closely correlates with the concentration of metabolite at the site of action. The presence of active metabolites complicates the interpretation of plasma drug concentrations and clinical response. As with the parent drug the relationship between unbound and total metabolite concentrations can be disrupted by displacement from serum proteins or changes in metabolism. In fact, parent or metabolite concentrations may be altered independently by drug interaction or physiologic change in metabolism.

Elimination pharmacokinetics of AEDs

AEDs display a variety of elimination patterns (Figure 37-3). The most clinically relevant aspects of AED elimination pharmacokinetics are discussed.

Benzodiazepines. The benzodiazepines follow a linear elimination pattern via hepatic metabolism. Some of the metabolites possess antiepileptic activity and contribute to toxicity. Pharmacologically active metabolites are formed from diazepam and chlorazepate.

Carbamazepine. Carbamazepine is primarily eliminated by cytochrome P-450–mediated metabolism, forming an active metabolite. Carbamazepine displays dose-dependent elimination pharmacokinetics, in which dosage increases produce a less than proportionate increase in steady-state total concentration (see Figure 37-3). Carbamazepine undergoes autoinduction, in which clearance increases over time following exposure to the drug. Within 30 days after therapy begins, carbamazepine clearance increases by 300%. Recent evidence suggests that further increases in maintenance doses may result in further induction [Koudriakova, 1992]. In some children, induction causes plasma carbamazepine concentrations to remain unchanged or even decline despite increasing dosages to 40 to 50 mg/kg/day [Curatolo et al., 1988]. Carbamazepine epoxide metabolism can also be induced by phenytoin or phenobarbital, resulting in a 100% increase in clearance [Kerr and Levy, 1989]. Initial carbamazepine half-life ranges from 10 to 20 hours but decreases with autoinduction to 4 to 12 hours. Consequently, many children require 3 to 4 doses daily to maintain targeted plasma concentrations.

Phenytoin. Phenytoin is primarily eliminated by hepatic metabolism, with a small fraction, 5% or less, excreted unchanged. It is metabolized by a saturable, cytochrome P-450 enzymatic pathway. Phenytoin follows Michaelis-Menton or saturable elimination kinetics (see Figure

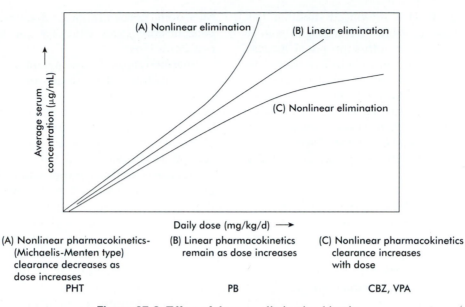

Figure 37-3 Effect of dose on elimination kinetics.

37-3). As the plasma concentration rises, phenytoin clearance decreases because of saturation of enzymatic metabolism; therefore, increases in dose result in disproportionately greater increases in steady-state plasma concentration:

$$\frac{\text{Daily}}{\text{dose}} = \frac{\text{Vmax} \times \text{Steady-state plasma concentration}}{\text{KM} + \text{Steady-state plasma concentration}}$$

The rate of phenytoin metabolism is defined by the enzyme kinetic terms *Vmax* (the maximum capacity of the enzyme system to metabolize phenytoin) and *Km* (the plasma concentration at which the rate of metabolism is 50% of maximum capacity). As the plasma phenytoin concentration approaches the latter value, a nonlinear relationship between dose and concentration appears.

Phenytoin half-life also varies with plasma concentration. As plasma concentration rises, the half-life is prolonged. Half-life ranges from 8 to 12 hours at low concentrations to longer than 60 hours at concentrations greater than 20 μg/ml. At concentrations within or above the therapeutic range, 1 to 4 weeks may be required to reach steady state.

Phenytoin metabolism in neonates is reduced compared with that of older children. Within days to weeks after birth, the rate of metabolism accelerates, reaching a maximum in the 6-month to 3-year age range. Children in this age group require the highest mg/kg daily doses (Figure 37-4). Thereafter, metabolism and dosage requirements decline gradually, reaching adult values during adolescence.

Figure 37-4 illustrates that even minor alterations in

dosage produce disproportionately large changes in plasma concentration. Therefore small adjustments in daily dose are indicated as the plasma concentration approaches or exceeds the plasma concentration at which the rate of metabolism is 50% of maximum capacity, which usually ranges from 5 to 10 μg/ml. Use of the scored, 50-mg chewable tablet, the 30-mg phenytoin sodium capsule, or the suspensions facilitates making such adjustments in dose.

Valproic acid. Valproic acid is extensively metabolized to both active and inactive metabolites. Principal pathways include glucuronidation, beta oxidation in the mitochondria, and oxidation through cytochrome P-450. The monounsaturated metabolites, 2-ene-valproic acid and 4-ene-valproic acid, possess anticonvulsant activity; the 2-ene-valproic acid achieves pharmacologically relevant concentrations in brain. In brain, 2-ene-valproic acid accumulates more slowly than valproic acid and may account for the slow onset and offset of anticonvulsant activity of valproic acid. The diunsaturated metabolites, 2,4 diene and 4-ene-valproic acid, are potent hepatotoxins; however, their role in valproic acid hepatoxicity remains unclear.

The elimination half-life of valproic acid is short. In the first few weeks after birth, elimination half-life ranges from 17 to 40 hours but rapidly declines to 3 to 20 hours in infants and young children. Evidence suggests that the full antiepileptic effect of valproic acid occurs days to weeks after reaching steady state and continues for some time after the drug is discontinued. This lingering effect may be partly the result of its inhibitory effect on the enzymes responsible for the degradation of γ-aminobutyric acid or the accumulation of 2-ene-valproic acid. This prolonged duration has prompted some to propose single daily dosing [Stefan et al., 1984]; however, there are other proposed mechanisms of action in which seizure control is related to plasma valproic acid concentrations. Under these circumstances, dosing at least every half-life is indicated to minimize fluctuations in plasma concentrations. Monotherapy with long half-lives maintains therapeutic concentrations for up to 24 hours in some children. Such children may be able to tolerate valproic acid once a day [Cloyd et al., 1985].

Recently Approved and Investigational AEDs

Several investigational AEDs are now under review by the Food and Drug Administration [Graves and Leppik, 1991]. These drugs may be useful in the treatment of children with epilepsy.

Felbamate. Felbamate is a dicarbamate closely related to the the antianxiety agent meprobamate. In animal studies, felbamate is effective against maximal electroshock and pentylenetetrazol-induced seizures and exhibits very low toxicity. No pharmacokinetic studies have included children. In adult controls and patients, felbamate pharmacokinetics appear to be linear. Coadministration of carbamazepine or phenytoin appears to decrease plasma felbamate concentrations, presumably by inducing clearance. Felbamate increases

phenytoin concentrations, decreases carbamazepine concentration, and increases carbamazepine-epoxide concentrations.

Fosphenytoin. Fosphenytoin is a prodrug that is rapidly hydrolyzed by tissue and erythrocyte alkaline phosphatases to phenytoin. It is water soluble, thus permitting formulation in nontoxic, parenteral solutions. The pharmacokinetics of phenytoin derived from fosphenytoin are identical to phenytoin given directly [Leppik et al., 1989].

Gabapentin. Gabapentin is an amino acid structural analog to γ-aminobutyric acid. Clinical studies indicate that it may be useful in the treatment of partial and generalized tonic-clonic and absence seizures.

Dosages used in clinical trials vary from 300 to 1800 mg/day, which result in plasma concentrations of 1 to 8 μg/ml. Over a dose range of 25 to 1200 mg, gabapentin pharmacokinetics are linear. Unique among AEDs, gabapentin is primarily eliminated by the kidney, with renal clearance of 100 to 160 ml/min. Gabapentin neither alters antipyrine pharmacokinetics—a marker of liver metabolism—nor affects phenytoin concentrations. Gabapentin pharmacokinetics are not affected by coadministration of phenytoin.

Lamotrigine. Lamotrigine appears to exert anticonvulsant activity by inhibiting the release of glutamate. Lamotrigine pharmacokinetics are linear up to dosages

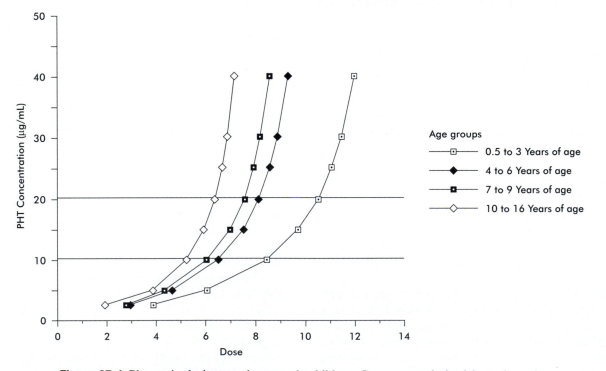

Figure 37-4 Phenytoin dosing requirements in children. Curves were derived from data of maximum capacity of the enzyme system to metabolize phenytoin (Vmax) and the plasma concentration at which the rate of metabolism is 50% of maximum capacity for children (Km) (see Table 37-2).

of 240 mg/day. It is extensively metabolized to an inactive glucuronide. Dosages used in clinical trials range from 50 to 300 mg/day, producing plasma concentrations of 0.5 to 5 µg/ml. Lamotrigine elimination half-life decreases by 40% to 50% in patients on carbamazepine or phenytoin, presumably because of induction of metabolism. Coadministration of valproate inhibits the elimination of lamotrigine, prolonging its half-life from 30.5 to 89 hours. The effect of lamotrigine on other AEDs is unknown.

PHARMACODYNAMICS

Pharmacologic and many toxicologic responses are determined by a drug's intrinsic activity and the amount of drug at the site of action. Generally, seizure control and side effects are related to drug concentration; the exceptions include hypersensitivity and idiosyncratic adverse reactions.

Dose or concentration-response concepts

Substantial evidence exists that the number of patients experiencing seizure control increases and the degree of seizure control for a given patient improves with greater AED concentrations [Porter, 1989; Schmidt, 1984]. The minimum effective concentration defines the concentration at which the desired pharmacologic response is observed initially. The intensity of response increases in direct proportion to drug concentration until a response is maximized. This result is the maximum pharmacologic effect for that drug. In some cases such as phenytoin, further increases in concentration may reduce response (e.g., phenytoin-induced exacerbation of seizures) [Troupin and Ojemann, 1975]. It is unknown whether other AEDs share this property. The incidence and severity of side effects also increase in direct proportion to drug concentration. The concentration at which side effects appear is usually but not always greater than the concentration needed to achieve seizure control. The difference between concentrations that produce desired and toxic responses defines the therapeutic range. Therapeutic ranges for commonly used AEDs are listed in Table 37-6.

Table 37-6 Therapeutic ranges for commonly prescribed AEDs

Drug	Range (µg/ml)
Carbamazepine	4-12
Ethosuximide	50-100
Phenobarbital	10-40
Phenytoin	10-25
Primidone	5-15
Valproic acid	40-120

Tolerance

Tolerance is a phenomenon in which pharmacologic or toxicologic effect diminishes with repeated doses even at the same or increasing plasma concentrations. Different mechanisms exist for the development of tolerance [Froscher and Engels, 1986; Koella, 1986]. One is the result of biochemical adaptation (e.g., up or down regulation of receptor sites). The effectiveness of benzodiazepine therapy diminishes over time, necessitating ever larger doses. Animal studies have demonstrated that chronic exposure to benzodiazepines causes a down regulation of benzodiazepine receptors, which reduces the anticonvulsant effect [Miller et al., 1989].

Another mechanism of tolerance is behavioral: The patient becomes progressively insensitive to drug effect without any apparent biochemical change [Siegel, 1986]. For example, many patients initiated on phenobarbital or primidone exhibit mild neurotoxicity, even at low plasma concentrations [Leppik et al., 1984]. Neurotoxicity clears within hours to a few days even as plasma concentrations increase.

Tolerance can produce changes in clinical response that mimic certain drug interactions. For example, loss of seizure control may result from either tolerance, as in the case of clonazepam, or enzyme induction, which decreases carbamazepine or valproate concentrations. Differentiating between these phenomena is important when considering adjustments in drug therapy.

PHYSIOLOGIC FACTORS AFFECTING DRUG DISPOSITION IN CHILDREN

AED pharmacokinetics and dosage requirements are influenced by the changing physiology of children as they age. Table 37-7 summarizes the effect of various developmental stages on absorption, protein binding, metabolism, and excretion.

Neonates

Gastric emptying time is irregular, absorption area is reduced, and biliary function is underdeveloped for

Table 37-7 Drug disposition at different ages

	Neonates	Infants	Adolescents
Absorption	↓	↑	A
Plasma protein binding	↓	↓	↓ →A
Metabolism	↓	↑	↑ →A
Excretion	↓	A	A

↑ Increased from adult levels; ↓ decreased from adult levels; *A*, equivalent to adult levels.
From Morrow JI, Richens A. Clin Pharmacokin 1989; 17(suppl 1):89-104.

several months or more after birth, factors that can contribute to erratic drug absorption [Morselli, 1983]. In addition, gastric pH is elevated, which may reduce the absorption of certain drugs such as clonazepam [Meyer and Straughn, 1993]. In contrast to the oral route, rectal absorption is reliable and efficient. Protein binding is reduced because of lower plasma albumin concentrations, whereas greater extracellular water and less adipose tissue can either increase or decrease distribution volume. Neonatal drug metabolism and renal excretion are reduced. Reactions mediated by hepatic cytochrome P-450 enzymes reach and then exceed adult values within a few weeks after birth. In contrast, renal elimination of drugs and active metabolites may be lower than adult values until 6 months of age.

Infants and children

Gastric emptying time and intestinal motility are increased. Absorptive area, microbial flora, and biliary function approach those of the adult. Conversely, gastrointestinal blood flow is greater than in adults. These physiologic characteristics contribute to faster absorption of most drugs, resulting in earlier maximum plasma concentrations. Plasma albumin remains less than adult values, particularly in infancy, resulting in an increased free fraction. Infants and children are capable of synthesizing alpha-1-acid glycoprotein, which alters the free fraction of drug bound to this protein. Metabolism remains elevated for the first 2 years of life; in some cases, drug clearances may be two to three times the values observed in adults. Thereafter, metabolism slowly declines, reaching adult values at puberty. After the first 6 months of life, renal excretion is comparable to that of adults.

DRUG INTERACTIONS

Interactions involving AEDs may alter pharmacokinetics, pharmacodynamics, or both. The clinical significance of pharmacokinetic and pharmacodynamic interactions is determined by several factors, including concentration of the interacting drugs, degree of seizure control, and presence of toxicity.

Pharmacokinetic interactions

Pharmacokinetic interactions involve an increase or decrease in plasma concentration of one or both interacting drugs as a result of alteration in absorption, protein binding, metabolism, or elimination. Interactions affecting absorption can alter the rate and amount of drug absorbed. Protein-binding interactions usually involve displacement of a drug from a binding site. Interactions that alter elimination can increase or decrease clearance. Drugs that alter AED metabolism do so by either inhibiting drug-metabolizing enzymes or

inducing the synthesis of additional enzyme. Inhibition and induction interactions occur over very different periods. Inhibition of metabolism occurs as soon as the inhibiting drug reaches the hepatocyte; maximal inhibition occurs after the inhibiting drug achieves steady state. The degree of inhibition depends on the concentration of the inhibiting drug and its affinity to the enzyme. Clearance of the affected drug is reduced, plasma concentration accumulates, and elimination half-life is often prolonged. A new steady-state plasma concentration is reached approximately five half-lives after the inhibiting drug is added. In contrast, induction interactions have a longer time course. Synthesis of new enzyme begins after the inducer is added to the regimen. The full inducing effect is not realized until the inducing drug reaches steady state. Approximately five half-lives of the enzyme must then elapse before the maximum increase in clearance of the affected drug occurs. The increase in clearance results in a reduction in steady-state plasma concentration and usually a faster half-life. Once induction is complete, five half-lives of the affected drug must elapse before a new steady state is attained.

The reverse of enzyme inhibition and induction interaction also have clinical importance. Once an inhibiting drug is withdrawn, the clearance of the affected drug increases to its preinteraction value. In this case, plasma concentrations of the affected drug decline to a new, lower steady state after five half-lives. Conversely, once an enzyme inducer is discontinued, enzyme synthesis returns to its preinteraction rate (deinduction). Clearance of the affected drug decreases, resulting in a longer half-life and a rise in plasma concentration, which reaches a new steady state five half-lives after clearance stabilizes.

AED pharmacokinetic interactions

A summary of AED interactions is presented in Table 37-8. Aspects of clinically significant interactions are discussed below in this section. To date, there are no known effects of lamotragine and gabapentin on other AEDs. A more complete characterization of the interaction profile for these two drugs awaits further clinical experience.

Absorption. Concomitant therapy may influence the absorption of AEDs. For example, continuous tube feedings interfere with phenytoin absorption [Maynard et al., 1987]. Calcium- and magnesium-containing antacids appear to complex with phenytoin, thus affecting the rate and extent of absorption. They should not be administered concurrently [Cacek, 1986]. Gastric pH affects the rate and extent of benzodiazepine absorption; thus use of antacids and H_2 blockers may decrease the plasma concentration of these drugs [Meyer and Straughn, 1993].

Protein Binding. Concurrent administration of either

Table 37-8 AED pharmacokinetic interactions

Interacting drug/ drugs	Affected drug(s)	Absorption	Protein binding	Induction	Inhibition
Antacids	Phenytoin	*			
Carbamazepine	Coumadin			†	
	Carbamazepine			†	
	Felbamate			†	
	Lamotrigine				
	Theophylline			†	
	Valproic acid			†	
Cimetidine	Carbamazepine				*
	Carbamazepine epoxide				*
	Phenytoin				*
Chloramphenicol	Phenytoin				*
Diltiazem	Carbamazepine				*
Erythromycin	Carbamazepine				†
Ethanol	Phenytoin			*Chronic	*Acute
Felbamate	Carbamazepine				‡
	Carbamazepine epoxide				*
	Phenytoin				§
	Phenytoin				†
	Valproic acid				†
Fluoxetine	Carbamazepine				*
Phenobarbital	Coumadin			†	
Phenytoin	Cyclosporine			†	
	Carbamazepine			†	
	Carbamazepine epoxide			†	
	Lamotrigine			†	
	Primidone			*	
	Theophylline			†	
	Valproic acid			†	
Propoxyphene	Carbamazepine				*
	Phenytoin				*
	Primidone				*
Valproic acid	Carbamazepine		*		*
	Carbamazepine epoxide				*
	Phenytoin		†		*
	Felbamate				*
	Phenobarbital				†
Verapamil	Carbamazepine				*

*Occasionally clinically significant.
†Usually clinically significant.
‡Carbamazepine concentrations may decrease 20%-25% by undetermined mechanism.
§Epoxide concentrations increase by undetermined mechanism.

aspirin or valproic acid may decrease phenytoin binding. When this occurs, unbound phenytoin briefly rises, possibly leading to clinical toxicity. Total phenytoin concentration decreases; however, unbound phenytoin rapidly reequilibrates to the original concentration, which can be confusing to the clinician who may be only monitoring total phenytoin concentrations. In general, phenytoin dosing does not have to be adjusted when valproic acid or aspirin is administered even though total

phenytoin levels decrease, unless indicated by clinical response [Scheyer and Cramer, 1990].

Induction of metabolism. Carbamazepine, phenobarbital, phenytoin, and primidone are potent inducers of the microsomal enzymes, including the hepatic cytochrome P-450 system. As such, they can have significant effects on drugs metabolized by these enzymes. Adding an AED inducer to a patient's regimen increases clearance of the benzodiazepines and valproic acid by as much as 100%, which may result in the need for increased doses. The clearance of carbamazepine is further increased with the addition of phenobarbital or phenytoin. AED enzyme inducers also increase the metabolism of other drugs, such as theophylline, chloramphenical, coumadin, cyclosporine, antipsychotics, and oral contraceptives, with resultant alteration in response [Kutt, 1989a; 1989b; Perucca, 1982; Pitlick and Levy, 1989].

Inhibition of Metabolism. Valproate inhibits phenobarbital, causing a 30% to 50% increase in plasma phenobarbital concentrations. Valproate weakly inhibits carbamazepine epoxide, which may produce side effects in some patients.

Cimetidine inhibits carbamazepine and carbamazepine epoxide metabolism; the effect, however, is generally transient. Patients should be advised that symptoms of carbamazepine toxicity may occur for 3 to 5 days after beginning cimetidine. Long-term adjustment of maintenance carbamazepine doses are not generally necessary [Dalton et al., 1986]. Erythromycin, fluoxetine (Prozac), verapamil, and diltiazem inhibit carbamazepine metabolism and can produce carbamazepine toxicity [Grimsley et al., 1991; Miles and Tennison, 1989; Pitlick and Levy, 1989; Wrobleski et al., 1986]. The interaction between phenobarbital and phenytoin is complex: phenytoin rarely alters phenobarbital concentrations; phenobarbital both induces the enzymes involved in phenytoin metabolism and competes as a substrate with phenytoin for those enzymes. This dual effect often leads to a variable effect on plasma phenytoin concentrations, although there is a tendency toward a decrease in phenytoin concentrations [Kutt, 1989a].

Pharmacodynamic interactions

Pharmacodynamic interactions occur when one drug alters the pharmacologic or toxicologic activity of another drug. The interaction can produce an additive or synergistic effect on activity, in which clinical response is magnified, or an antagonistic effect, in which the interacting drug diminishes clinical response. An additive pharmacodynamic interaction exists between phenobarbital and benzodiazepines, both of which enhance γ-aminobutyric acid activity and depress CNS function. The most common complication of this interaction is increased sedation. A potentially serious interaction is severe respiratory depression, which occurs with high phenobarbital concentrations and the bolus intravenous administration of diazepam. The addition of carbamazepine, which stimulates secretion of antidiuretic hormone, to a thiazide diuretic is an example of an antagonistic pharmacodynamic interaction. CNS stimulants such as theophylline, amphetamines, and cocaine and certain antipsychotics and antibiotics can lower seizure threshold and may compromise the success of AED therapy [Alldredge and Simon, 1992].

PHYSIOLOGIC AND PATHOPHYSIOLOGIC VARIABLES INFLUENCING AED PHARMACOKINETICS

A number of physiologic and pathophysiologic processes can alter AED pharmacokinetics. Gastrointestinal disorders, particularly those that increase transit time, can alter the endothelial lining and decrease absorption. AEDs that are slowly absorbed such as carbamazepine and phenytoin are most likely to be affected. Physiologic stress such as that associated with myocardial infarction, burns, traumatic injury, chronic inflammation, and surgery increases alpha-1-acid glycoprotein levels, resulting in greater binding with carbamazepine and carbamazepine epoxide [MacKichan, 1992]. Febrile illnesses may produce increases in phenytoin clearance that persist for several weeks, resulting in as much as a 50% lowering of plasma concentrations [Leppik et al., 1986b]. Renal failure can affect the excretion of AEDs, for which the kidney is the primary route of elimination. Among the AEDs, acetazolamide, bromides, and to a lesser extent, primidone and phenobarbital can accumulate in both acute and chronic renal failure. Gabapentin, an investigational AED that is 95% eliminated by the kidney, also accumulates. The binding of phenytoin is reduced in uremic patients, which is apparently the result of a decrease in albumin concentration and the accumulation of endogenous substances that compete with phenytoin for binding sites. The displacement of phenytoin results in lower total plasma concentration, but unbound concentrations are usually unaffected. Whether other highly bound AEDs are affected in a similar manner is unknown. Both clinical response and plasma AED concentrations should be carefully assessed in patients with renal disease.

Severe liver disease can alter the metabolism of AEDs, resulting in an accumulation of the parent drug [Kutt, 1983]. However, AED metabolism appears to be well preserved in mild to moderate liver disease. Clinical response may vary depending on the particular AED.

Plasma AED concentrations can fluctuate in a predictable manner over a 24-hour cycle. Reports have described a day-night cycle in which both valproic acid and carbamazepine concentrations decreased at night [Lockard and Levy, 1990; Pisani et al., 1990]. The mechanism for this alteration is presumably an increase in clearance. More recently, it has been found that absorption of enteric-coated valproate tablets may be reduced at night [Cloyd, 1991]. In either case evaluating night time plasma AED concentrations in patients with poorly controlled seizures may be helpful.

DOSAGE FORMULATIONS AND ROUTES OF ADMINISTRATION

The formulations available and possible routes of administration for the AEDs are listed in Table 37-1.

Rectal administration

Patients may occasionally be unable to take medications orally. Unfortunately, most AEDs do not have parenteral formulations because of their poor water solubility, and therefore AED administration is difficult after surgical procedures or during gastrointestinal illnesses when the oral route is not available. At those times, alternative routes of administration are highly desirable. The rectal route of administration has been extremely useful in these situations [Graves and Kriel, 1987].

When given as a solution, diazepam is also rapidly absorbed rectally, reaching maximum plasma concentration within 5 to 20 minutes in children [Lombroso, 1989]. In contrast, rectal administration of lorazepam is relatively slow, with a time to maximum plasma concentration of 1 to 2 hours [Graves et al., 1987]. Table 37-9 provides a comprehensive list of AEDs available for rectal administration and recommendations for use.

CLINICAL AND LABORATORY MONITORING DURING THERAPY

Clinical monitoring of therapeutic efficacy

The clinical assessment of patients on anticonvulsant therapy is of paramount importance. The clinician must assess the effectiveness of therapy with regard to seizure control and determine the existence of adverse effects and whether they are tolerable. A satisfactory clinical response to AED therapy includes a substantial reduction or elimination of seizures and/or reduction of adverse effects. Complete seizure control with no adverse effects of medication is ideal; however, this response usually does not occur.

An accurate record of seizure frequency and severity must be obtained both before and during therapy to assess whether there has been an improvement in seizure control. Seizures may be eliminated, reduced in frequency, or be less severe. Patients with epilepsy often have varying seizure frequency even before therapy. The length of time a patient must remain seizure free to establish that a significant response to therapy has occurred varies inversely with the frequency of seizures observed before therapy begins. Patients who have relatively infrequent seizures need a longer period of observation to assess clinical response. Changes in seizure frequency can be statistically interpreted based on a modified sequential analysis [Leppik et al., 1989].

One of the most common clinical errors is the attempt

to interpret clinical response prematurely. The drug must be at steady state to determine whether a medication has been given an adequate clinical trial. The time to achieve steady state varies considerably depending on the half-life, but in every case, five half-lives must elapse to attain a new steady state.

The interpretation of clinical response during multiple drug therapy is especially difficult. As an example, clinical improvement (or deterioration) with the addition of a second AED could be caused by many factors, including the additive or synergistic effect of the two medications, the effect of the second drug itself, and the effect that the second drug may have on the metabolism and displacement of the initial drug. Again, clinical conclusions should be attempted only after a steady state is reached. When improvement with the addition of a second medication has occurred, the clinician should then attempt to discontinue the first medication to determine whether the clinical improvement is an effect of synergistic therapy or that of the second medication itself. Withdrawal of comedication may affect the disposition of the remaining drug or drugs, which could influence clinical response.

Clinical monitoring of adverse effects

Clinical assessment is of primary importance in assessing adverse responses. Factors, such as steady state conditions and effects of drug interactions, are equally applicable in the clinical assessment of adverse effects.

The most frequent adverse effects are dose related and involve the nervous system. Common symptoms include decreased alertness or cognitive changes but may also include symptoms suggestive of attention-deficit disorders, especially in children. Impairment of coordination, ataxia, and diplopia are other commonly observed adverse effects.

Continuous monitoring of clinical states is possible, whereas laboratory tests are generally sampled at arbitrary points; therefore impending liver failure can usually be detected earlier by relying on clinical changes rather than laboratory tests. Anorexia, nausea, vomiting, lethargy, and abdominal pain are early, reliable clinical signs of liver failure during valproic acid therapy and should command the clinician's immediate attention [Dreifus et al., 1987; Scheffner et al., 1988].

Likewise, dermatologic manifestations are especially common idiosyncratic reactions to AEDs. Generally, medication should be discontinued when rashes develop. Recognizing specific dermatologic syndromes in children on AEDs is important because these conditons are often associated with catastrophic outcomes and are indications for promptly discontinuing therapy. Stevens-Johnson syndrome is a severe form of erythema multiforme involving the mucous membranes of the mouth,

Table 37-9 AEDs available for rectal administration

Drug	Treatment usefulness	Dosage (mg/kg/day)	Preparation	Pharmacokinetics	Comments
Carbamazepine	Maintenance	Same as oral	Oral suspension (dilute with equal volume of water) Suppository gel (carbamazepine powder dissolved in 20% alcohol and methyl hydroxy cellulose)*	Peak concentration 4-8 hr; 80% absorbed	Definite cathartic effect
Clonazepam	Acute (?)	0.02-0.1 mg	Suspension	Peak concentration 0.1-2.0 hr	Possibly too slow onset for acute use
Diazepam	Acute	0.2-0.5 mg	Parenteral solution	Effect in 2-10 min; peak concentration 2-30 min	Well tolerated; nordiazepam accumulation with repeated doses
Lorazepam	Acute	0.05-0.1 mg	Parenteral solution	Peak concentration 0.5-2.0 hr	Well tolerated
Paraldehyde	Acute	0.3 ml	Oral solution (dilute with equal volume of mineral oil)	Effect in 20 min; peak concentration 2.5 hr	Moderate cathartic effect; glass syringe needed
Phenobarbital	Acute (?)	10-20 mg	Parenteral solution	Peak concentration 4-5 hr; 90% absorbed	Possibly too slow onset for acute use
	Maintenance	Same as oral	Same as acute	Same as acute	
Secobarbital	Acute	5 mg	Parenteral solution	Peak concentration 0.5-1.5 hr	
Valproic Acid	Acute	5-25 mg	Oral syrup (dilute with equal volume of water)	Peak concentration 1-3 hr	Definite cathartic effect
	Maintenance	Same as oral	Valproic acid liquid from capsules mixed into Supocire C lipid base*	Peak concentration 2-4 hr; 80% absorbed	Well tolerated

Adapted from Graves NM, Kriel RL. Pediatr Neurol 1987; 3:321-326; and Garnett WR, Cloyd JC. Dosage form considerations in the treatment of pediatric epilepsy. In: Dotson WE, Pellock JM, eds. Pediatric epilepsy: diagnosis in therapy. New York: Demos, 1993; 241-252.
*Extemporaneously prepared using commercial; all other preparations are commercial products given rectally.

anal, and genital mucosa and is accompanied by constitutional symptoms and high fever. The mucous membrane lesions may form vesicles, bullae, and ulcers; the cutaneous lesions vary from red or purple macules to vesicles and may form "target" lesions with normal skin surrounded by a halo of erythema. Toxic epidermal necrolysis (scalded skin syndrome or Lyell syndrome) is manifested by the rapid development of flaccid bullae and fever, leading to exfoliation. Fatal outcomes are possible with both Stevens-Johnson and Lyell syndromes. Treatment of Stevens-Johnson syndrome with steroids is controversial. Recent reports imply that morbidity and mortality are improved with reverse isolation, meticulous skin care, and early detection of infection, without the use of systemic steroids [Prendiville et al., 1989].

Monitoring antiepileptic drug concentrations

The ability to measure plasma levels of AEDs has been a major advance in the medical management of epilepsy. The influence of periodic monitoring of blood levels during therapy has reduced the number of therapeutic failures by 50% [Kutt and Penry, 1974]. AED levels are generally obtained after each change of dosage. Drug levels are usually related to the dose administered except for drugs with nonlinear kinetics such as phenytoin and carbamazepine [Bochner et al., 1972]. Unless there is some overriding clinical decision to do otherwise (e.g., development of acute toxicity, deteriorating seizure control), waiting until steady state is obtained before drawing blood levels is reasonable and economical. With drugs such as phenytoin, the half-life increases with increasing plasma concentration, and therefore the steady state may not be attained at higher dosages of phenytoin until 3 to 4 weeks after the adjustment. The addition, reduction, or discontinuation of other AEDs during therapy can have a profound effect on concomitant AEDs [Cloyd et al., 1983; 1985; Duncan et al., 1991]. Therefore obtaining repeat drug concentrations when a second medication is added or discontinued is often useful.

Therapeutic ranges represent statistical averages based on relatively small numbers of patients, usually adults. Considerable variability exists among patients in responses to therapy due to patient sensitivity to medication, variabilities in protein binding, and the severity of the underlying seizure disorder. Therefore it is very useful to obtain AED levels periodically, even when the patient's condition is well controlled, to establish the therapeutic window. The clinician (and patient) should relate the therapeutic window to the AED plasma concentration as opposed to dosage because the amount of medication necessary to achieve a stated plasma concentration can vary in the same patient with changes in comedication, diet, and age.

Rechecking AED levels when clinical problems (e.g., interpretation of possible toxicity in the presence of other nonspecific illness, loss of seizure control) are present is also useful. The determination of blood levels in these circumstances enables the physician to determine whether problems with compliance, absorption, or drug interaction exist.

What to measure

Newer technologies are improving the ease and lowering the cost of making unbound determinations; however, most laboratories routinely perform only total drug concentrations. In addition, reference therapeutic ranges are available for total drug concentration. Until more information is available, the clinician may have difficulty interpreting unbound concentrations, even when they are obtained. Fortunately, the ratio of free to bound drug is relatively constant, at least for a particular patient, and therefore total drug concentrations are generally adequate.

Situations exist in which unbound drug concentrations may be especially helpful. Some patients develop clinical toxicity at either relatively low-dose or low-total drug levels. A higher than expected unbound drug level could explain clinical toxicity. These circumstances particularly arise during multiple drug therapy when a second drug may displace the first from protein binding sites. The percentage of unbound valproate increases with higher drug concentrations and comedication [Cloyd et al., 1993]. When the bound fraction is doubled, the valproate acid free fraction may be eight times higher [Fenichel, 1986].

The measurement of AED metabolites can also be useful. Many AED metabolites are clinically active and contribute to clinical response and toxicity. A noteworthy example is the appearance of phenobarbital during primidone therapy in therapeutic or even toxic concentrations. Although carbamazepine epoxide may contribute to the drug effect, the usefulness of monitoring carbamazepine epoxide remains controversial [Riva et al., 1984; Theodore et al., 1989].

Interpretation of drug levels

Numerous factors should be considered in the interpretation of drug levels. Drugs that have rapid absorption and clearance cause wide fluctuations between dosing intervals. For example, valproic acid syrup, especially when given to a child with an enzyme-inducing comedication, is rapidly absorbed and eliminated and may cause a twofold fluctuation during a dosing interval. Recording the time of the blood sample with regard to the last dose is frequently necessary to determine whether a trough, peak, or mid specimen dose is obtained. Unexpectedly high or low values may also arise from overzealous administration or poor compliance.

The clinician is often puzzled when obtaining phenytoin levels. Nonlinear kinetics for phenytoin may be responsible for large increases in blood levels with relatively small dosage increments. Conversely, autoinduction of carbamazepine metabolism can lead to a decrease in carbamazepine concentration while the patient is on the same (or an increasing) dosage. The addition or deletion of additional medication may result in increased clearance or hepatic metabolism of the initial drugs.

On occasion, unexpected plasma drug levels result from laboratory error. Most laboratories participate in quality control programs in which specimens of known drug concentrations are submitted to the participating laboratory. In one study, half the laboratories participating reported drug concentrations greater than one standard deviation above or below the mean of reference laboratories [Pippenger et al., 1976]. In subsequent years the availability of national quality assurance programs and greater proficiency with analytic technique has improved the reliability of AED measurements. The clinician should know whether the laboratory is participating in a national quality assurance program. At this point the most reliable determinations are generally made in hospital or commercial laboratories where AED levels are measured frequently. Kits have recently become available to determine AED levels in the physician's office or patient's home.

Laboratory monitory of adverse reactions

Although most adverse effects of medication in patients with epilepsy are tolerable and reversible, occasional idiosyncratic reactions can be serious or even life threatening. In an effort to identify patients at risk for these more serious adverse reactions, obtaining laboratory tests of serum chemistries, hematology, and even urine analysis routinely is standard clinical practice. Most pharmaceutical companies have recommended periodic laboratory tests during AED therapy. The costs for recommended laboratory monitoring would probably exceed those of medication by twofold to threefold [Hart and Easton, 1982]. Moreover, controversy exists about whether routine laboratory monitoring can actually identify the patient at risk for serious reactions. Routine monitoring of patients taking carbamazepine often identifies clinically irrelevant leukopenia and elevation of hepatic function. Identification of life-threatening reactions, however, is rarely made by routine laboratory screening of asymptomatic children [Camfield et al., 1986]. Likewise, fulminant and irreversible hepatic failure during valproate therapy is not reliably predicted by laboratory monitoring [Willmore et al., 1991]. Some researchers have reported that routine laboratory screening is of doubtful value [Camfield et al., 1989; Pellock and Willmore, 1991]. Others, however, still believe that it is prudent to obtain routine laboratory

monitoring during treatment with valproate, carbamazepine, and ethosuximide [Hart and Easton, 1982; Scheffner et al., 1988; Wyllie and Wyllie, 1991].

Before initiation of AED therapy, screening laboratory tests (e.g., complete blood count with differential, serum glutamic-oxaloacetic transaminase) have been suggested [Camfield et al., 1986]. Certain patients may be at higher risk for hepatotoxicity during valproate therapy. For example, some patients with hepatotoxicity during valproate therapy had metabolic diseases, including urea cycle defects, organic acidurias, multiple carboxylase deficiency, mitochondrial or respiratory-chain dysfunction, GM_2 gangliosidosis, spinocerebellar degeneration, Friedreich ataxia, Lafora body disease, Alper disease, and myoclonic epilepsy with ragged red fibers [Willmore et al., 1991]. It has been suggested that children at high risk for valproate-induced hepatotoxicity have additional screening tests before initiation of therapy. These high-risk patients are young (less than 3 years of age), are in need of polytherapy, and have presumptive metabolic disorders, neurodegenerative disease, or a history of previous adverse drug experiences (see Table 37-10). The recommendations of Pellock and Willmore [1991] may be followed with regard to prescreening tests.

Table 37-10 Blood monitoring in children with epilepsy

Low-risk children	High-risk children
Before therapy	
CBC, differential, platelets; serum chemistry profile (glucose, BUN, electrolytes, Ca, P, Mg, creatinine, urate, Fe, Cholesterol, bilirubin, alkaline phosphatase, AST, ALT, total protein, albumin, globulin, PT, PTT)	CBC with differential, platelets; serum chemistry profile; tests for underlying metabolic diseases (lactate, pyruvate, ABGs, ammonia, carnitine, urine metabolic screen, urine organic acids)*
On therapy	
Asymptomatic	
Not necessary	Annual CBC and serum chemistry profile
Symptomatic†	
Specific laboratory tests	Specific laboratory tests

CBC, Complete blood count; *BUN*, blood urea nitrogen; *AST*, angiotensin sensitivity test; *ALT*, alanine aminotransferase; *PT*, prothrombin time; *PTT*, partial thromboplastin time; *ABGs*, arterial blood gases.
Adapted from Pellock JM, Willmore LJ. Neurology 1991; 41:961-964.
*For high-risk children before valproic acid therapy.
†Bruising, bleeding, vomiting, nausea, lethargy, coma increasing, and seizures.

Patients who are unable to communicate adequately, especially those who are nonambulatory and institutionalized, should be monitored somewhat differently. These children should have blood monitoring yearly [Pellock and Willmore, 1991]. Conversely, asymptomatic ambulatory children probably do not need routine tests of blood and urine (see Table 37-10).

Children who develop specific symptoms should be promptly evaluated. Such symptoms would include bruising, bleeding, rash, abdominal pain, vomiting, jaundice, lethargy, coma, and marked increase in seizure frequency [Pellock and Willmore, 1991].

Certain tests require special handling to obtain reproducible results. For example, the clinician should inquire about the laboratory's procedures for proper equipment and handling before obtaining a specimen to measure blood ammonia.

ADVERSE EFFECTS

The most frequent adverse effects are dose-related and are mild and reversible. Less frequently observed but potentially more serious are the idiosyncratic adverse effects that are generally not related to dosage. Additional adverse effects of medication include drug interactions on the developing fetus (i.e., teratogenicity). The effects of AEDs on reproduction and fetal malformations are not reviewed in this chapter. The risk of adverse effects increases with the number of AEDs used. Complex drug interactions can be avoided when one drug is used [Wilder, 1987].

In addition to adverse effects of medication are unintended effects that nevertheless may have important therapeutic applications. For example, acetazolamide, originally developed as a diuretic, has antiepileptic potential and can also inhibit the production of spinal fluid.

Cognitive impairment

Although patients with epilepsy have a significantly higher incidence of impairment of cognitive function, the relative contributions of the underlying disorder, seizure type and frequency, and therapy are often difficult to assess. Reaction times, disordered attention, and impulsivity differ even in untreated children with epilepsy from those of controls. The differences in attention and reaction time, however, are small between children with very mild versus severe seizure disorders [Mitchell et al., 1992].

The effects of AEDs on cognitive function are generally concentration- and dose-dependent. Drug therapy is recognized to contribute to the cognitive deficits, especially treatment with multiple drugs [Thompson and Trimble, 1982]. Removal of AEDs frequently results in improved cognitive function and motor skills [Duncan et al., 1990].

Phenobarbital. During therapy with phenobarbital, sedation is common, especially during initiation of therapy and at higher dosages. Phenobarbital has been associated with a significant depression of cognitive function when used to treat children with febrile seizures. In a randomized, placebo-controlled prospective study, children had lower mean intelligence quotient scores both during and 6 months after stopping therapy with phenobarbital [Farwell et al., 1990]. Clinical tolerance does develop to some degree; however, an unacceptably high frequency of adverse effects of phenobarbital maintenance is commonly observed in children [Farwell et al., 1990; Wolf and Forsythe, 1978]. The adverse effects are reminiscent of the complaints often present in attention-deficit disorders, including overactivity, aggressiveness, inattention, and irritability. The behavioral disorders are observed in 20% to 50% of children treated with phenobarbital for febrile seizures and result in therapy being discontinued in 20% to 30% of children [Herranz et al., 1984]. Pre-existing behavioral problems, especially hyperactivity, are strongly predictive of adverse reactions during phenobarbital therapy. In a study of children treated with phenobarbital for febrile seizures, 80% of those with abnormal behavior before drug therapy reported worsening of behavior with phenobarbital, whereas only 20% of children with normal preseizure behavior exhibited increased problems [Wolf and Forsythe, 1978]. In some cases these adverse effects may improve with continuation or a lower dose of phenobarbital; however, discontinuation of therapy and consideration of alternative medication should be discussed.

Primidone. Sleepiness, incoordination, and vertigo are commonly observed during initiation of therapy with primidone but can be minimized by initiating the medication with a very low dose. Toxicity at this point is probably related to primidone itself, since the metabolites have not yet appeared. Much of the toxicity is transient with tolerance developing [Leppik et al., 1984]. In general, the dose-related adverse effects are the same as those with phenobarbital.

Phenytoin. Although considerable variability exists in the individual patient's susceptibility to phenytoin, a variety of clinical symptoms can be expected with increasing plasma levels. Whereas adverse effects with plasma levels below 14 μg/ml are difficult to detect, approximately 75% of patients with levels greater than 30 μg/ml reported adverse effects [Bucthal et al., 1960]. Initial signs of phenytoin intoxication may consist of diplopia or blurred vision, anxiety, and irritability, progressing to ataxia, dysarthria, vertigo, and depressed sensorium as plasma levels increase [Kutt et al., 1964].

Carbamazepine. Approximately 16% of adult patients with epilepsy report adverse effects with carbamazepine. Most were dose dependent and were ob-

from patients having hypersensitivity reactions with aromatic AED drugs (e.g., phenobarbital, phenytoin, carbamazepine) has suggested that the immunologic responses could be initiated by arene oxide AED metabolites [Shear and Spielberg, 1988]. In addition, Stevens-Johnson syndrome (erythyma multiforme exudativum), Lyell syndrome (toxic epidermal necrolysis), and purpura fulminans can occur during AED therapy (see Table 37-11) and are indications for prompt discontinuation of therapy. Exacerbation of acne is sometimes associated with treatment involving phenytoin and bromides.

Osteomalacia

Osteomalacia (rickets) is occasionally observed in patients taking AEDs. In a survey of institutionalized, mentally retarded patients from 3 to 26 years of age on AED therapy at least 2 years, 52 of 144 had serum alkaline phosphatase levels elevated more than two standard deviations above normal. Most were taking phenytoin and/or phenobarbital [Hunt et al., 1986]. The cause of osteomalacia during AED therapy appears multifactorial. Many AEDs presumably enhance hepatic conversion of 25-hydroxyvitamin D to biologically inactive metabolites; however, ambulatory children on AED therapy and institutionalized children who are not taking medication seldom develop clinically significant rickets. Conversely, clinically overt rickets was observed in 10% of institutionalized children on phenobarbital and/or phenytoin. In these patients, sunlight was more important for the maintenance of serum 25-hydroxyvitamin D than were supplements of vitamin D [Morijiri and Sato, 1981].

Prophylactic treatment of all patients taking AEDs is inadvisable because therapy is potentially toxic and, in most cases, changes in mineral content are minimal.

Screening all patients on AEDs for serum calcium and/or alkaline phosphatase levels would be costly and not likely of value [Christiansen et al., 1983]. Screening should be directed toward nonambulatory children on phenytoin, phenobarbital, primidone, or carbamazepine who are seldom exposed to sunlight.

Other effects

Hair changes have been associated with AED treatment. Hair changes (thinning or wavy hair) were observed in 12% of children during valproate therapy [Clark et al., 1980]. Additional dose-related adverse effects of phenytoin include hirsuitism, coarse facial features, and acne, especially in children and teenagers. Pancreatitis has also been associated with valproate therapy [Coulter and Allen, 1980; Wyllie et al., 1984].

Management

The clinician and patient are faced with adverse effects approximately 30% of the time AED is used, especially during the initiation of therapy. In many instances these adverse effects are acceptable, especially when the patient and physician mutually agree on which problems are most important to prevent. When there is no urgency, many adverse effects can be prevented during the initiation of therapy by gradually increasing dosages. In general, management of adverse effects depends on the problem (see Table 37-12). Most adverse effects are concentration dependent and are less prominent at lower dosages and blood concentrations. Seizure control may be maintained at the lower dosage; if not, the clinician and patient need to consider whether a compromise is acceptable with regard to either increased seizures or increased adverse effects or whether alternative medication should be considered.

Table 37-11 Idiosyncratic reactions

Medication	Rash	Other reactions
Valproate	Uncommon	Potentially fatal hepatotoxicity, pancreatitis, weight gain, benign essential tremor, hair loss, thrombocytopenia
Phenytoin	5%-8%	Exfoliative dermatitis, Stevens-Johnson syndrome, toxic epidermal necrolysis (Lyell syndrome), aplastic anemia, hepatotoxicity, peripheral neuropathy, lupus-like reaction
Carbamazepine	3%-4%	Aplastic anemia (1/200,000 patient years), agranulocytosis, neutropenia, thrombocytopenia, anemia, Stevens-Johnson syndrome, toxic epidermal necrolysis, hepatitis
Phenobarbital, primidone	1%-2%	Exfoliative dermatitis, Stevens-Johnson syndrome, agranulocytosis (bone marrow depression), megaloblastic anemia, lupus erythematosus syndrome
Acetazolamide	Uncommon	Aplastic anemia (1/18,000 patient years, less frequent in epilepsy), acute renal failure, agranulocytosis, thrombocytopenic purpura
Ethosuximide	1%	Stevens-Johnson syndrome, scleroderma, lupus-like syndrome, blood dyscrasias (leukopenia, pancytopenia)
Lamotrigine	2%	Stevens-Johnson syndrome, lupus erythematosus

Toxicity is sometimes encountered only with high drug concentrations observed at peak times; for these patients, frequent and lower doses may prevent toxicity. Gastric irritation is generally dose dependent and may be managed in several ways. The amount of drug can be reduced, the effective dosage to the gastric mucosa can be lowered by use of enteric-coated formulations, or the patient can be protected by use of H_2-receptor antagonists.

Idiosyncratic reactions pose another problem. Asymptomatic elevations of liver enzymes generally do not mandate discontinuation of therapy if they are not in excess of two to three times normal values. Conversely, Stevens-Johnson and Lyell syndromes, clinically symptomatic hepatotoxicity, pancreatitis, and most rashes are indications for immediate cessation of the responsible medication.

Comparative studies

A listing of adverse effects is useful for the patient and clinician when confronted with problems during AED therapy. When selecting a drug for initial therapy, however, the clinician should not only be aware of the adverse effects of medication, but also be able to compare one agent with another with regard to both efficacy and adverse effects.

Adults on phenytoin did less well on memory tasks than patients treated with carbamazepine and untreated patients [Andrewes et al., 1986]. However, in a double-blind, triple crossover design investigation, carbamazepine, phenobarbital, and phenytoin had comparable neuropsychologic function on most measures [Meador et al., 1990]. In another report, adult patients were randomly assigned to one of four medications (phenobarbital, phenytoin, primidone, carbamazepine) [Mattson et al., 1985]. As illustrated in Table 37-13, toxicity was a common reason for treatment failure in all drugs; it was especially common in patients receiving primidone. Fewer patients continued on primidone therapy than on the other three drugs (Figure 37-5). Phenobarbital was associated with the lowest incidence of motor disturbances and gastrointestinal complaints, and phenytoin had the highest incidence of dysmorphic and idiosyncratic reactions. In another double-blind, randomized study comparing carbamazepine with phenytoin, minor side effects and seizure control were the same. Rash and pruritus were the most common reasons for terminating therapy. Specific adverse effects differed for the two drugs (e.g., gum hypertrophy with phenytoin) [Ramsay et al., 1983]. Valproate has been compared with carbamazepine during a double-blind study for the treatment of complex partial and secondarily generated tonic-clonic seizures in adults. It was associated more frequently with weight gain, hair loss, and tremor, and

Table 37-12 Managing adverse effects

Type of adverse effect	Management
Dose-related concentration	
Sedation and other cognitive, tremor, motor/ataxia, gastric irritation, osteomalacia, gingival hyperplasia	More gradual introduction of drug, reduction of dose, more frequent and smaller doses, enteric-coated formulations, H_2-receptor antagonists, exposure to sunlight, vitamin D supplements, oral hygiene
Idiosyncratic	
Stevens-Johnson and Lyell syndromes, allergic rash, pancreatitis, clinical hepatotoxicity, aplastic anemia, agranulocytosis	Discontinuation of responsible drug

Table 37-13 Reasons for failure of AED therapy*

	Treatment group				
	Carbamazepine (n = 101)	Phenobarbital (n = 101)	Phenytoin (n = 110)	Primidone (n = 109)	All (n = 421)
Toxicity alone	12	19	18	36	85
Toxicity and seizures	30	33	29	35	127
Seizures alone	3	4	1	3	11
TOTAL Failures	45	56	48	74	223

From Mattson RH, Cromer JA, Collins JF, et al. N Engl J Med 1985; 313:145-151.
*Treatment failure because of seizures or without side effects was similar with all drugs. The inability to continue treatment because of adverse effects was greatest with primidone.

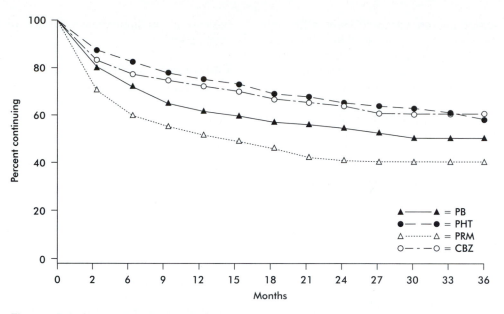

Figure 37-5 Percentage of patients continuing on drug therapy. Decreasing percentage over time is the result of either poor seizure control, adverse effects, or both. (From Mattson RH, Cramer JA, Collins JF, et al. N Engl J Med 1985; 313:145-151.)

carbamazepine was associated more with rash. Carbamazepine was superior as meaured by a composite score of seizure control and adverse effects [Mattson et al., 1992].

Few reports compare adverse effects in children. A retrospective, nonrandomized survey in 312 children in a hospital school with epilepsy found depression to be associated with therapy involving phenobarbital, valproic acid, and phenytoin. Conduct disorder was observed with phenobarbital and valproate therapy and a decrease in intelligence quotient with valproate, sulthiame, primidone, and phenytoin. Distractibility was least associated with carbamazepine [Trimble and Corbett, 1980]. In a double-blind, counterbalanced, crossover study in children, patients did less well on tests of neuropsychologic function and exhibited significantly worse behavior while on phenobarbital as compared with valproate [Vining et al., 1987]. One nonrandomized, nonblinded report of 392 children on monotherapy with febrile and epileptic seizures observed that the best tolerated drug was carbamazepine and the least tolerated, phenytoin. Adverse effects of sufficient severity to require withdrawal were phenytoin (10%), valproate (8%), primidone (8%), phenobarbital (4%), and carbamazepine (3%). Less severe side effects ranged from 29% for primidone to 71% for phenytoin [Herranz et al., 1988]. As expected the specific adverse effects observed differed with the medication used. For example, adverse behavioral effects were more frequently observed during phenobarbital therapy, digestive with valproic acid, and neurologic (ataxia) with phenytoin. In general, intoler-able adverse effects were dose-related and observed with high plasma levels.

Two reports compare valproic acid with ethosuximide in the treatment of absence seizures. One study used a double-blind, crossover design in which patients were stratified by their response to prior therapy [Sato et al., 1982]. Treatment periods were 6 weeks each, and response was assessed by 12-hour EEG telemetry. Overall response to valproic acid was 75% and to ethosuximide 50%; however, neither clinical response nor adverse effects differed statistically. The other study used a prospective, randomized design. Valproic acid and ethosuximide were equally effective. One child was taken off of valproic acid after developing pancreatitis and another because of uncontrolled obesity; no patients were withdrawn from ethosuximide [Callaghan et al., 1982].

Selection of drugs for initiation of AED therapy

The selection of a specific drug for the treatment of epilepsy is made primarily by the criteria of therapeutic efficacy expected for the patient and seizure type. Certain epileptic syndromes require specific therapy. For most patients and seizure types, however, efficacy differences are minimal, and the selection of the initial drug for AED therapy is guided equally by a consideration of potential adverse effects. Although highly effective, phenytoin is rarely a drug of first choice in children due to a higher incidence of dysmorphic effects. In children, especially those with preexisting tendencies for attention-deficit disorders, there is an unacceptable incidence of behavioral problems and cognitive dysfunction with barbiturate therapy. Use of valproic acid in very young children, especially those on other AEDs, carries a risk of fatal hepatotoxicity. The principles to be used during initiation and selection of AED therapy in children have been summarized by Fenichel [1986].

ACKNOWLEDGMENTS

We gratefully acknowledge Carolyn Jones-Saete, R.N., and Fatah Rahman, M.S., for their contributions to this chapter.

REFERENCES

Alldredge BK, Simon RP. Drugs that can precipitate seizures. In: Resor SR, Kutt H, eds. The medical treatment of epilepsy. New York: Marcel Dekker, 1992; 497-524.

Andrewes DG, Bullen JG, Tomlinson L, et al. A comparative study of the cognitive effects of phenytoin and carbamazepine in new referrals with epilepsy. Epilepsia 1986; 27:128-134.

Andrews J, Chadwick D, Bates D, et al. Gabapentin in partial epilepsy. Lancet 1990; 335:1114-1117.

Angelopoulos A. A clinicopathological review: diphenylhydantoin gingival hyperplasia: aetiology, pathogenesis, differential diagnosis and treatment. J Can Dent Assoc 1975; 41:275-277.

Babcock JR. Incidence of gingival hyperplasia associated with dilantin therapy in a hospital population. J Am Dent Assoc 1965; 71:1447-1450.

Betts T, Goodwin G, Withers RM, et al. Human safety of lamotrigine. Epilepsia 1991; 32(suppl 2):S17-S21.

Bochner F, Hooper WD, Tyrer JH, et al. Effect of dosage increments on blood phenytoin concentrations. J Neurol Neurosurg Psychiatry 1972; 35:873-876.

Bucthal F, Svensmark O, Schiller PJ. Clinical and electroencephalographic correlations with serum levels of diphenylhydantoin. Arch Neurol 1960; 2:624-630.

Butler RT, Kalkwarf KL, Kaldahl WB. Drug-induced gingival hyperplasia: phenytoin, cyclosporine, and nifedipine. J Am Can Assoc 1987; 114:56-60.

Cacek AT. Review of alterations in oral phenytoin bioavailability associated with formulation, antacids, and food. Ther Drug Monit 1986; 8:166-171.

Callaghan N, O'Hare J, O'Driscoll D, et al. Comparative study of ethosuximide and sodium valproate in the treatment of typical absence seizures (petit mal). Dev Med Child Neurol 1982; 24:830-836.

Camfield P, Camfield C, Dooley J, et al. Routine screening of blood and urine for severe anticonvulsant reactions in asymptomatic patients is of doubtful value. Can J Neurol Sci 1989; 16:361-364.

Camfield C, Camfield P, Smith E, et al. Asymptomatic children with epilepsy: little benefit from screening for anticonvulsant-induced liver, blood, or renal damage. Neurology 1986; 36:838-841.

Christiansen C, Rodbro P, Tjellesen L. Pathophysiology behind anticonvulsant osteomalacia. Acta Neurol Scand 1983; 94(suppl):21-28.

Clark JE, Covanis A, Gupta AK, et al. Unwanted effects of sodium valproate in children and adolescents. In: Parsonage MJ, Caldwell ADS, eds. The place of sodium valproate in the treatment of epilepsy. Royal Society of Medicine Series, International Congress and Symposium Series no 30. London: Academic Press, 1980.

Clark JE, Covanis A, Gupta AK, et al. Unwanted effects of sodium valproate in children and adolescents. In: Parsonage MJ, Caldwell ADS, eds. The place of sodium valproate in the treatment of epilepsy. London: Academic Press, 1980; 133-139.

Cloyd JC. Pharmacokinetic pitfalls of present antiepileptic medications. Epilepsia 1991; 32(suppl 5):S53-S65.

Cloyd JC, Fischer JH, Kriel RL, et al. Valproic acid pharmacokinetics in children. IV. Effects of age and antiepileptic drugs on protein binding and intrinsic clearance. Clin Pharmacol Ther 1993; 53:22-29.

Cloyd JC, Kriel RL, Fischer JH. Valproic acid pharmacokinetics in children. II. Discontinuation of concomitant antiepileptic drug therapy. Neurology 1985; 35:1623-1627.

Cloyd JC, Kriel RL, Fischer JH, et al. Pharmacokinetics of valproic acid in children. I. Multiple antiepileptic drug therapy. Neurology 1983; 33:185-191.

Cloyd JC, Kriel RL, Jones-Saete CM, et al. Comparison of sprinkle versus syrup formulations of valproate for bioavailability, tolerance, and preference. J Pediatr 1992; 120:634-638.

Commander M, Green SH, Prendergast M. Behavioural disturbances in children treated with clonazepam. Dev Med Child Neurol 1991; 33:362-363.

Coulter DL, Allen RJ. Pancreatitis associated with valproic acid therapy for epilepsy. Ann Neurol 1980; 7:92.

Covanis A, Gupta AK, Jeavons PM. Sodium valproate: monotherapy and polytherapy. Epilepsia 1982; 23:693-720.

Curatolo P, Bruni O, Cusmai R. Use of erythromycin to inhibit carbamazepine metabolism in children with partial complex seizures. Brain Dev 1988; 10:206.

Dalton MJ, Powell JR, Messenheimer JA Jr, et al. Cimetidine and carbamazepine: a complex drug interaction. Epilepsia 1986; 27:553-558.

Dean JC, Penry JK. Valproate. In: Resor SR Jr, Kutt H, eds. The medical treatment of epilepsy. New York: Dekker, 1992.

DeGiorgio CM, Rabinowicz AL, Olivas RD. Carbamazepine-induced antinuclear antibodies and systemic lupus erythematosus-like syndrome. Epilepsia 1991; 32:128-129.

Dodson WE. Antiepileptic drug utilization in pediatric patients. Epilepsia 1984; 25(suppl 2): S132-S139.

Dreifuss FE, Langer DH. Hepatic considerations in the use of antiepileptic drugs. Epilepsia 1987; 28:S23-S29.

Dreifuss FE, Langer DH, Moline KA, et al. Valproic acid hepatic fatalities. II. US experience since 1984. Neurology 1989; 39:201-207.

Dreifuss FE, Santilli N, Langer DH, et al. Valproic acid fatalities: a retrospective review. Neurology 1987; 37:379-385.

Duncan JS, Patsalos PN, Shorvon SD. The effects of discontinuation of phenytoin, carbamazepine, and valproate on concomitant antiepileptic medication. Epilepsia 1991; 32:101-105.

Duncan JS, Shorvon SD, Trimble MR. Effects of removal of phenytoin, carbamazepine, and valproate on cognitive function. Epilepsia 1990; 31:584-591.

Farwell JR, Lee YJ, Hirtz DG, et al. Phenobarbital for febrile seizures—effects on intelligence and seizure recurrence. N Engl J Med 1990; 322:364-369.

Faught E, Sachdeo RC, Remler MP, et al. Felbamate monotherapy for partial-onset seizures: an active-control trial. Neurology 1993; 43:688-692.

Fenichel GM. Anticonvulsant therapy in children. Int Pediatr, 1986; 1:231-235.

Fischer JH, Barr AN, Paloucek FP, et al. The effect of food on the serum concentration profile of enteric coated valproic acid. Neurology 1988; 38:1319-1322.

Froscher W, Engels HG. Tolerance to the anticonvulsant effect of clonazepam: tolerance to beneficial and adverse effects of antiepileptic drugs. New York: Raven Press, 1986; 127-136.

Ganick DJ, Sunder T, Finley JL. Severe hematologic toxicity of valproic acid: a report of four patients. Am J Pediatr Hematol/Oncol 1990; 12:80-85.

Garnett WR, Cloyd JC. Dosage form considerations in the treatment of pediatric epilepsy. In: Dotson WE, Pellock JM, eds. Pediatric epilepsy: diagnosis in therapy. New York: Demos, 1993; 241-252.

Gerson WT, Fine DG, Spielberg SP, et al. Anticonvulsant-induced aplastic anemia: increased susceptibility to toxic drug metabolites in vitro. Blood 1983; 61:889-893.

Goff DA, Spunt AL, Jung D, et al. Absorption characteristics of three phenytoin sodium products after administration of oral loading doses. Clin Pharmacol 1984; 3:634-638.

Graves NM, Kriel RL. Rectal administration of AEDs in children. Pediatr Neurol 1987; 3:321-326.

Graves NM, Kriel RL, Jones-Saete C. Bioavailability of rectally administered lorazepam. Clin Neuropharmacol 1987; 6:555-559.

Graves NM, Leppik IE. Antiepileptic medications in development. DICP Ann Pharmacother 1991; 25:978-986.

Grimsley SR, Jann MJ, Carter JG, et al. Increased carbamazepine plasma concentrations after fluoxetine coadministration. Clin Pharmacol Ther 1991; 50:10-15.

Hart RG, Easton JD. Carbamazepine and hematological monitoring. Ann Neurol 1982; 11:309-312.

Herranz JL, Armijo JA, Arteaga R. Effectiveness and toxicity of phenobarbital, primidone, and sodium valproate in the prevention of febrile convulsions controlled by plasma levels. Epilepsia 1984; 25:89-95.

Herranz JL, Armijo JA, Arteaga R. Clinical side effects of phenobarbital, primidone, phenytoin, carbamazepine, and valproate during monotherapy in children. Epilepsia 1988; 29:794-804.

Hunt PA, Wu-Chen ML, Handal NJ, et al. Bone disease induced by anticonvulsant therapy and treatment with calcitriol (1,25-dihydroxyvitamin D$_3$). Am J Dis Child 1986; 140:715-718.

Jung D, Powell JR, Walson P, et al. Effect dose on phenytoin absorption. Clin Pharmacol Ther 1980; 28:479-485.

Karas BJ, Wilder BJ, Hammond EJ, et al. Valproate tremors. Neurology 1982; 32:428-432.

Kauko K, Tammisto P. Comparison of two generically equivalent carbamazepine preparations. Ann Clin Res 1974; 11:21-25.

Keisu M, Wilholm BE, Ost A, et al. Acetazolamide-associated aplastic anemia. J Int Med 1990; 228:627-632.

Kerr BM, Levy RH. Carbamazepine-carbamazepine epoxide. In: Levy RH, Mattson R, Meldrum B, et al., eds. Antiepileptic drugs, 3rd ed. New York: Raven Press, 1989; 505-520.

Koella WP. Tolerance: its various forms and their nature. In: Frey HH, Froscher W, Koella WP, et al., eds. Tolerance to beneficial and adverse effects of antiepileptic drugs. New York: Raven Press, 1986; 1-7.

Kostenbauder HB, Rapp RP, McGovern JP, et al. Bioavailability in single-dose pharmacokinetics of intramuscular phenytoin. Clin Pharmacol Ther 1975; 18:449-456.

Koudriakova TB, Sirota LA, Rozova GI, et al. Autoinduction and steady-state pharmacokinetics of carbamazepine and its major metabolites. Br J Clin Pharmacol 1992; 33:611-615.

Kutt H. Effects of acute and chronic diseases on the disposition of antiepileptic drugs. In: Morselli PL, Pippenger CE, Penry JK, eds. Antiepileptic drug therapy in pediatrics. New York: Raven Press, 1983; 293-302.

Kutt H. Phenobarbital-interactions with other drugs. In: Levy RH, Mattson R, Meldrum B, et al., eds. Antiepileptic drugs, 3rd ed. New York: Raven Press, 1989a; 313-328.

Kutt H. Phenytoin-interactions with other drugs. In: Levy RH, Mattson R, Meldrum B, et al., eds. Antiepileptic drugs, 3rd ed. New York: Raven Press, 1989b; 215-232.

Kutt H, Penry JK. Usefulness of blood levels of antiepileptic drugs. Arch Neurol, 1974; 31:283-288.

Kutt H, Winters W, Kokenge R, et al. Diphenylhydantoin metabolism blood levels and toxicity. Arch Neurol 1964; 11:642-648.

Leppik IE, Boucher R, Wilder BJ, et al. Phenytoin prodrug: preclinical and clinical studies. Epilepsia 1989; 30(suppl 2):S22-S26.

Leppik IE, Brundage RC, Krall R. Double blind withdrawal of phenytoin and carbamazepine in patients treated with progabide for partial seizures. Epilepsia 1986a; 27:563-568.

Leppik IE, Cloyd JC, Miller K. Development of tolerance to side effects of primidone. Ther Drug Monit 1984; 6:189-191.

Leppik IE, Dreifuss FE, Pledger GW, et al. Felbamate for partial seizures: results of a controlled clinical trial. Neurology 1991; 41:1785-1789.

Leppik IE, Fischer JH, Kriel RL. Pharmacokinetics of carbamazepine suspension. Neurology 1984; 34(suppl):213.

Leppik IE, Fischer JH, Kriel RL, et al. Altered phenytoin clearance with febrile illness. Neurology 1986b; 36:1367-1370.

Little TM, Girgis SS, Masotti RE. Diphenyhydantoin-induced gingival hyperplasia: its response to changes in drug dosage. Dev Med Child Neurol 1975; 17:421-424.

Lockard JS, Levy RH. Valproate and paroxysmal cyclicity compared to other anticonvulsants in monkey model. In: Dreifuss FE, Meinardi H, Stefan H, eds. Chronopharmacology in therapy of the epilepsies. New York: Raven Press, 1990; 105-127.

Lombroso CT. Intermittent home treatment of status and clusters of seizures. Epilepsia 1989; 30(suppl 2):S11-S14.

Maas B, Garnett WR, Pellock JM, et al. A comparative bioavailability study of carbamazepine tablets in a chewable tablet formulation. Ther Drug Monit 1987; 9:28-33.

MacKichan JJ. Influence of protein binding and use of unbound (free) drug concentrations. In: Evans WE, Schentag JJ, Jusko WJ, eds. Applied pharmacokinetics, 3rd ed. Vancouver, Wash: Applied Therapeutics; 1992.

Marks WA, Morris MP, Bodensteiner JB, et al. Gastritis with valproate therapy. Arch Neurol 1988; 45:903-905.

Mattson RH, Cramer JA, Collins JF, et al. Comparison of carbamazepine, phenobarbital, phenytoin, and primidone in partial and secondarily generalized tonic-clinic seizures. N Engl J Med 1985; 313:145-151.

Mattson RH, Cramer JA, Collins JF, et al. A comparison of valproate with carbamazepine for the treatment of complex partial seizures and secondarily generalized tonic-clonic seizures in adults. N Engl J Med 1992; 327:765-771.

Maynard GA, Jones KM, Guidry JR. Phenytoin absorption from tube feedings. Arch Intern Med 1987; 147:1821.

Meador KJ, Loring DW, Huh K, et al. Comparable cognitive effects of anticonvulsants. Neurology 1990; 40:391-394.

Meyer MC, Straughn AB. Biopharmaceutical factors that could affect seizure control and toxicity. Am J Hosp Pharm 1993(suppl) (in press).

Meyer MC, Straugn AB, Jarvi EJ, et al. The bioinequivalence of carbamazepine tablets with a history of clinical failures. Pharm Res 1992; 9:1612-1616.

Mikati M, Bassett N, Schachter S. Double-blind randomized study comparing brand-name and generic phenytoin monotherapy. Epilepsia 1992; 33:359-365.

Miles MV, Tennison MB. Erythromycin effects on multiple-dose carbamazepine kinetics. Ther Drug Monit 1989; 11:47-52.

Miller LG, Greenblatt DJ, Barnhill JG, et al. Chronic benzodiazepine administration. I. Tolerance is associated with benzodiazepine receptor down regulation and decreased gamma-aminobutyric acid$_A$ receptor complex binding and function. J Pharmacol Exp Ther 1988; 266:170-176.

Mitchell WG, Zhou Y, Chavez JM, et al. Reaction time, attention, and impulsivity in epilepsy. Pediatr Neurol 1992; 8:19-24.

Modeer T, Dahllof G. Development of phenytoin-induced gingival overgrowth in non-institutionalized epileptic children subjected to different plaque control programs. Acta Odontol Scand 1987; 45:81-85.

Morijiri Y, Sato T. Factors causing rickets in institutionalized handicapped children on anticonvulsant therapy. Arch Dis Child 1981; 56:446-449.

Morrow JI, Richens A. Disposition of anticonvulsants in childhood. Clin Pharmacokin 1989; 17(suppl 1):89-104.

Morselli PL. Development of physiological variables important for drug kinetics. In: Morselli PL, Pippenger CE, Penry JK, eds. Antiepileptic drug therapy in pediatrics. New York: Raven Press, 1983; 1-12.

Nuwer MR, Browne TR, Dodson WE, et al. Generic substitutions for AEDs. Neurology 1990; 40:1647-1651.

Painter MJ, Pippenger CE, McDonald H, et al. Phenobarbitol and diphenylhydantoin levels in neonates with seizures. J Pediatr 1978; 92:315-319.

Pellock JM. Status epilepticus. In: Pellock JM, Meyer EC, eds. Neurologic emergencies in infancy and childhood. Philadelphia: Harper & Row, 1984.

Pellock JM, Willmore LJ. A rational guide to routine blood monitoring in patients receiving antiepileptic drugs. Neurology 1991; 41:961-964.

Perucca E. Pharmacokinetic interactions with antiepileptic drugs. Clin Pharmacokin 1982; 7:57-84.

Pihlstrom BL, Carlson JF, Smith QT, et al. Prevention of phenytoin associated gingival enlargement—a 15 month longitudinal study. J Peridontol 1980; 51:311-317.

Pippenger CE, Penry JK, et al. Inter-laboratory variability in determination of plasma antiepileptic drug concentrations. Arch Neurol 1976; 33:351-355.

Pisani F, Oteri G, Caputo M, et al. Diurnal fluctuations in plasma drug levels at steady-state: studies with valproic acid and carbamazepine. In: Dreifuss FE, Meinardi H, Stefan H, eds. Chronopharmacology in therapy of the epilepsies. New York: Raven Press, 1990; 129-144.

Pitlick WH, Levy RH. Carbamazepine-interactions with other drugs. In: Levy RH, Mattson R, Meldrum B, et al., eds. Antiepileptic drugs, 3rd ed. New York: Raven Press, 1989; 521-531.

Porter RJ. General principles—how to use antiepileptic drugs. In: Levy RH, Mattson R, Meldrom B, et al., eds. Antiepileptic drugs, 3rd ed. New York: Raven Press, 1989; 117-131.

Prendiville JS, Herbert AA, Greenwald MJ, et al. Management of Stevens-Johnson syndrome and toxic epidermal necrolysis in children. Pediatrics 1989; 115:881-887.

Pynnönen S, Mantyla R, Iisalo E. Bioavailability of four different pharmaceutical preparations of carbamazepine. Acta Pharmacol Toxicol 1978; 43:306-310.

Ramsay RE, Wilder BJ, Berger JR, et al. A double blind study comparing carbamazepine with phenytoin as initial seizure therapy in adults. Neurology 1983; 33:904-910.

Rane A, Wilson JT. Clinical pharmacokinetics in infants and children. Clin Pharmacoki 1976; 1:2-24.

Resor SR Jr, Resor LD. Acetazolamide. In: Resor SR Jr, Kutt H, eds. The medical treatment of epilepsy. New York: Dekker, 1992.

Riva R, Contin M, Albani F. Free and total plasma concentrations of carbamazepine and carbamazepine-10,11-epoxide in epileptic patients: diurnal fluctuations and relationship with side effects. Ther Drug Monit 1984; 6:408-413.

Sarkar MA, Garnett WR, Karnes HT. The effect of storage and shaking on the settling properties of phenytoin suspension. Neurology 1989; 39:207-209.

Sato S, White BG, Penry JK, et al. Valproic acid versus ethosuximide in the treatment of absence seizures. Neurology 1982; 32:157-163.

Scheffner D, Konig ST, Rauterberg-Ruland I, et al. Fatal liver failure in 16 children with valproate therapy. Epilepsia 1988; 29:530-542.

Scheyer RD, Cramer JA. Pharmacokinetics of AEDs. Semin Neurol 1990; 10:414-421.

Schmidt D. Adverse effects of anticonvulsant drugs. New York: Raven Press, 1982.

Schmidt D. Adverse effects of valproate. Epilepsia 1984; 25:S44-S49.

Schmidt D. How to use benzodiazepines. In: Morselli PL, Pippenger CE, Penry JK, eds. Antiepileptic drug therapy in pediatrics. New York: Raven Press, 1983.

Schmidt D, Haenel F. Therapeutic plasma levels of phenytoin, phenobarbitol, and carbamazepine: individual variation in relation to seizure frequency and type. Neurology 1984; 34:1252-1255.

Schmidt D, Rohrer E. Carbamazepine. In: Resor SP, Kutt H, eds. The medical treatment of epilepsy. New York: Dekker, 1992.

Serrano WE, Wilder BJ. Intramuscular administration of diphenylhydantoin: histologic follow-up. Arch Neurol, 1974; 31:276-278.

Shear NH, Spielberg SP. Anticonvulsant hypersensitivity syndrome: in vitro assessment of risk. J Clin Invest 1988; 82:1826-1832.

Sherwin AL. How to use ethosuximide. In: Morselli PL, Pippenger CE, Penry JK, eds. Antiepileptic drug therapy in pediatrics. New York: Raven Press, 1983.

Siegel S. Environmental modulation of tolerance: evidence from benzodiazepene research: tolerance to beneficial and adverse effects of antiepileptic drugs. New York: Raven Press, 1986; 89-100.

Silanpää M. Carbamazepine: pharmacology and clinical uses. Acta Neurol Scand 1981; 64(suppl):88.

Spielberg SP, Gordon GB, Blake DA, et al. Predisposition to phenytoin hepatotoxicity assessed in vitro. N Engl J Med 1981; 305:722-727.

Stefan H, Burr W, Fichsel H, et al. Intensive follow-up monitoring in patients with once daily and evening administration of sodium valproate. Epilepsia 1984; 25:152-160.

Theodore WH, Narang PK, Holmes MD, et al. Carbamazepine and its epoxide: relation of plasma levels to toxicity and seizure control. Ann Neurol 1989; 25:194-196.

Theodore WH, Raubertas RF, Porter RJ, et al. Felbamate: a clinical trial for complex partial seizures. Epilepsia 1991; 32:392-397.

Thompson PJ, Trimble MR. Anticonvulsant drugs and cognitive functions. Epilepsia 1982; 23:531-544.

Trimble MR, Corbett JA. Behavioural and cognitive disturbances in epileptic children. Irish Med J 1980; 73(suppl):21-28.

Trimble MR, Thompson PJ. Sodium valproate and cognitive function. Epilepsia 1984; 25:S60-S64.

Troupin AS, Ojemann LM. Paradoxical intoxication: a complication of anticonvulsive administration. Epilepsia 1975; 16:753-758.

Vining EPG, Mellits ED, Dorsen MM, et al. Psychological and behavioral effects of antiepileptic drugs in children: a double-blind comparison between phenobarbital and valproic acid. Pediatrics 1987; 80:165-174.

Wang JT, Shiu GK, Worsley W, et al. The effect of humidity and temperature on in vitro performance of carbamazepine tablets. Pharm Res 1990; 7(suppl):S143.

Wilder BJ. Treatment considerations in anticonvulsant monotherapy. Epilepsia 1987; 28(suppl 2):S1-S7.

Wilder BJ, Karas BJ, Penry JK, et al. Gastrointestinal tolerance of divalproex sodium. Neurology 1983; 33:808-811.

Willmore LJ, Triggs WJ, Pellock JM. Valproate toxicity: risk screening strategies. Child Neurol 1991; 6:3-6.

Wolf SM, Forsythe A. Behavior disturbance, phenobarbital and febrile seizures. Pediatrics 1978; 61:728-731.

Wrobleski BA, Singer WD, Whyte J. Carbamazepine-erythromycin interaction: case studies and clinical significance. JAMA 1986; 255:1165-1167.

Wyllie E, Wyllie R. Routine laboratory monitoring for serious adverse effects of antiepileptic medications: the controversy. Epilepsia, 1991; 32:S74-S79.

Wyllie E, Wyllie R, Cruse RP, et al. Pancreatitis associated with valproic acid therapy. Am J Dis Child 1984; 138:912-914.

ACUT

Bac

neuro

diagnc

influei

almost

therap

tality i

The

reflect

nation

commi

approx

The ra

cases p

5 years

per yea

the est

b meni

year. T

and 12

of the

Walling

a child

by age

disease

1991].

non-At

childre

1991].

inciden

United

Bact

months

spring a

likely t

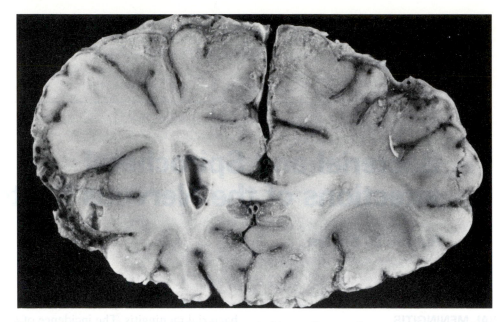

Figure 38-1 A 7-month-old child with congenital heart disease, *S. pneumoniae* meningitis, and sepsis. Patient died after 7 days of illness. Purulent exudate distends the subarachnoid space, particularly over the convexity. (Courtesy Dr. Mario Kornfeld, Albuquerque, NM.)

phages. The causative bacteria can be found free in the exudate and within cells of the exudate. During the second or third week of illness the exudate changes to mononuclear cells, mainly macrophages. Fibrosis of the leptomeninges begins, and thick strands of collagen are observed [Bell and McCormick, 1981].

Although the major pathologic effect is within the subarachnoid space and basilar cisterns, careful pathologic examination suggests widespread involvement. When death occurs during the acute illness, the superficial cortex is swollen with venous congestion. Inflammation is present in varying degrees in brain parenchyma (Figure 38-2) and within the ventricles (Figure 38-3). Pyknotic changes occur in cortical neurons, and areas of pallor are found in the cortex and white matter. These changes are attributed to infarcts that are secondary to inflammatory vasculitis of the arteries and veins (Figure 38-4) [Bell and McCormick, 1981; Snyder et al., 1981]. Segmental arteritis of meningeal and perforating branches and phlebitis of cortical veins contribute to clinical symptoms and sequelae (Figures 38-5 to 38-7). The inflammatory cell infiltrate involves the walls of vessels, with elevation of the endothelium and narrowing of the vessel or actual occlusion occurring (Figure 38-8). Segmental narrowing of major intracranial arteries has been demonstrated by angiography [Gado et al., 1973; Lyons and Leeds, 1967; Raimondi and DiRocco, 1979]. Brain edema with vascular compression add to the vascular difficulties, as does hypotension. Pathologically the areas of infarction are bland or hemorrhagic. Clinical

symptoms of meningitis, including seizures, may be present with minimal pathologic alteration.

The spinal cord and its structures are also involved, as evidenced by the recovery of purulent material from the lumbar subarachnoid space on lumbar puncture.

Pathogenesis

Many diverse factors contribute to the symptoms of bacterial meningitis, including virulence of the organism, inflammation, obstruction of subarachnoid pathways, interference with vessels entering and leaving the brain, irritation of brain parenchyma by toxic products of bacteria and leukocytes, breakdown of the blood-brain barrier, and the neurologic effects of anoxia, shock, fever, dehydration, and hyponatremia [Saez-Llorens et al., 1990; Sande et al., 1989; Tunkel et al., 1990].

Bacterial meningitis is commonly the result of the hematogenous spread of organisms from a remote focus of infection. The remote focus leads to septicemia, with resultant passage of organisms into the nervous system through the choroid plexus and deposition of organisms in ventricles and subarachnoid spaces. This septicemic phase explains the frequency with which organisms are found in blood cultures. Entry of bacteria into the subarachnoid pathways can also occur by direct spread from the external environment in cases of open head trauma, by spread from infected contiguous structures such as the ear and sinuses, and during neurosurgery. Infection does not spread along nerve roots in bacterial meningitis.

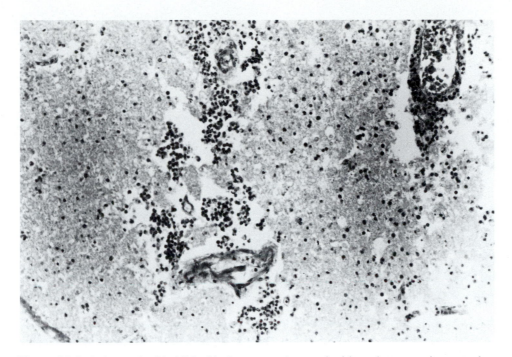

Figure 38-2 A 4-month-old child with *S. pneumoniae* meningitis and suppurative encephalitis. Inflammatory cells infiltrate perivascular parenchyma. Original magnification ×64. (Reduced to 70%.) (Courtesy Dr. Mario Kornfeld, Albuquerque, NM.)

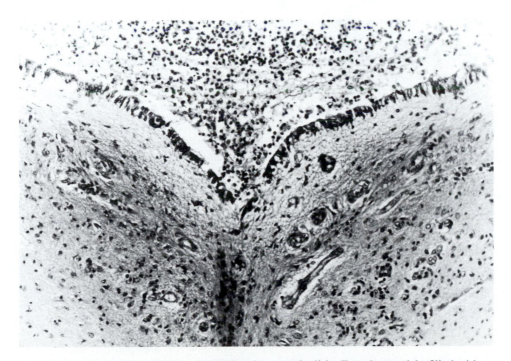

Figure 38-3 Same case as Figure 38-2, showing ventriculitis. Fourth ventricle filled with fibrinopurulent exudate. Original magnification ×40. (Reduced to 70%.) (Courtesy Dr. Mario Kornfeld, Albuquerque, NM.)

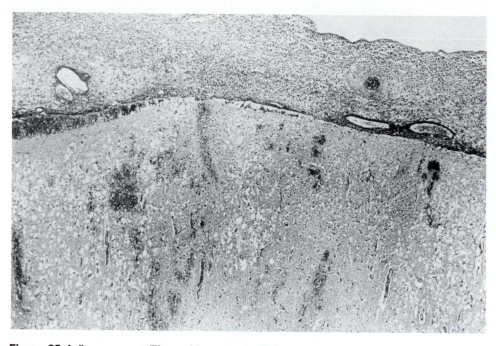

Figure 38-4 Same case as Figure 38-1, showing cortical infarct (central compact zone). Original magnification ×40. (Reduced to 70%.) (Courtesy Dr. Mario Kornfeld, Albuquerque, NM.)

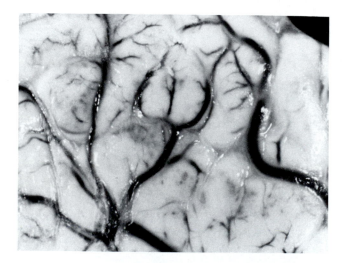

Figure 38-5 A 7-year-old chid with *S. pneumoniae* meningitis. Patient died after 3 days of illness. Close-up view of brain surface demonstrating exudate along blood vessels, two of which (*center* and *right*) are thrombosed. Discolored parenchyma in the vicinity of occluded vessels is infarcted. (Courtesy Dr. Mario Kornfeld, Albuquerque, NM.)

CSF supports the growth of most meningeal pathogens. When meningitis becomes established, polymorphonuclear cells migrate from the bloodstream into the CSF, and the leptomeninges become inflamed with a polymorphonuclear infiltrate. Acute inflammation of the leptomeninges and subarachnoid spaces results in decreased efficiency of the blood-brain barrier [Tunkel and Scheld, 1989]. Potentially undesirable substances that do not normally enter the brain have the opportunity to do so. The loss of efficiency has the advantage of providing easier access for antibiotics and resultant higher concentrations in the infected area. When the blood-brain barrier is injured, immunoglobulins and complement pass from the blood into the CSF. Immunoglobulins are also produced by the meninges during infections [Maida and Horvatis, 1986].

All vessels entering and leaving the brain must pass through the subarachnoid space. When a vessel passes through an area of inflammation, vasculitis becomes a potential problem, with possible occlusion of that vessel and ischemic infarction [Igarashi et al., 1984]. The permanent neurologic deficits occurring after meningitis are partly related to vasculitis and secondary infarction of brain substance. Other factors may lead to brain necrosis, including toxic products of bacteria or leukocytes, systemic shock, hypoxia, prolonged seizures, pressure hydrocephalus, extraaxial fluid collections, and acidosis.

In general, a capsule confers virulence on bacteria. Differences in capsular polysaccharide may cause differences in the virulence of organisms. Capsular polysaccharide, which is equated to endotoxin, appears to function in immunogenicity, the production of inflammatory effects within the CNS, and the response of CNS

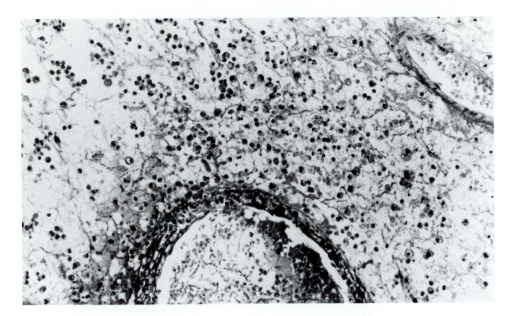

Figure 38-6 Same case as Figure 38-1, showing leptomeningeal exudate with a strong fibrinous component. The wall of a vein in the subarachnoid space *(lower border, center)* is infiltrated with inflammatory cells. Original magnification ×40. (Reduced to 70%.) (Courtesy Dr. Mario Kornfeld, Albuquerque, NM.)

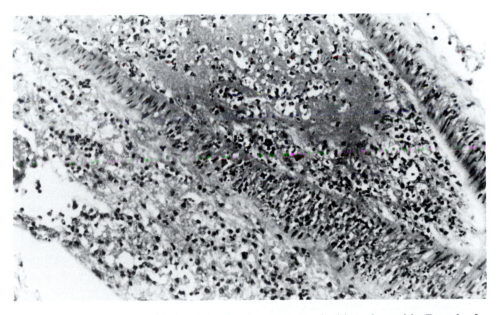

Figure 38-7 Same case as Figure 38-1, showing acute meningitis and arteritis. Branch of middle cerebral artery shows focal necrosis and inflammation. Lumen occluded by partially organized thrombus. Original magnification ×40. (Reduced to 70%.) (Courtesy Dr. Mario Kornfeld, Albuquerque, NM.)

defense mechanisms. Other surface antigens may also be important in virulence and immunity [Moxon, 1985].

Profound alterations in brain physiology occur. Cerebral blood flow is decreased, enhancing susceptibility to ischemia and infarction [Ashwal et al., 1990]. In-creased resistance to CSF outflow occurs, and CSF resorption is reduced. Cerebrovascular endothelial permeability increases, resulting in vasogenic edema, toxins resulting in cytotoxic edema, and interstitial edema probably resulting from obstructive hydrocephalus

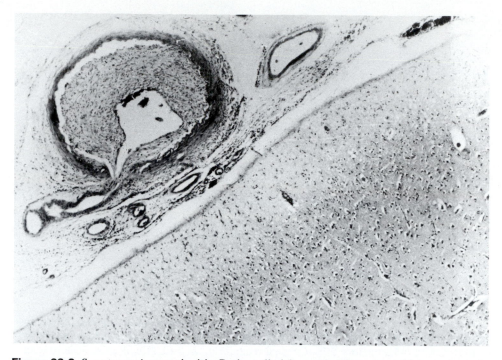

Figure 38-8 *S. pneumoniae* meningitis. Patient died 2 months after onset. Note endarteritis obliterans of a branch of middle cerebral artery. Original magnification ×10. (Reduced to 70%.) (Courtesy Dr. Mario Kornfeld, Albuquerque, NM.)

[Tauber, 1989]. Usual compensatory processes for increased intracranial pressure are disturbed. Edema results in further compromise of cerebral circulation. The early increase in intracranial pressure, which is often the first sign of meningitis, may stem from a different mechanism than the more serious increased pressure and brain edema that occur later [Fishman, 1975; Paulson et al., 1974]. Excitatory amino acid neurotransmitters may have a role in pathogenesis [Simon, 1989].

The use of highly bactericidal antibiotics and natural mechanisms facilitate the release of lipopolysaccharide endotoxin by the rapid lysis of the cell wall of gram-negative organisms. This process may detrimentally enhance the inflammatory response of the host [Arditi et al., 1989; Tauber and Sande, 1991]. Endotoxin probably damages the endothelium of brain capillaries, with subsequent vascular leakage exaggerating inflammation and brain edema [Tauber et al., 1987]. Endotoxin in the CSF induces the production of cytokines that can initiate an inflammatory response even in the absence of bacteria. These cytokines are found in increased amounts in the CSF in experimental and human meningitis after treatment with bacteriocidal antibiotics. Bacterial cell products in the CSF can initiate the arachidonic acid cascade [Niemoller and Tauber, 1989], the release of free radicals [Pfister et al., 1990], and the release of prostaglandins, interleukin 1-beta, and cachectin/tumor necrosis factor-alpha [Arditi et al., 1990; Mustafa et al., 1989; Tracy et al., 1989]. Interleukin 1-beta concentration in the CSF correlates with the number of days of CSF positive culture [McCracken et al., 1989]. All these substances are inflammatory mediators, and counteracting their effects may be an important aspect of therapy. The administration of steroids in children with *H. influenzae* meningitis and animals with experimental meningitis reduces levels of these cytokines [Jacobs and Tabor, 1990; Mustafa et al., 1990].

An episode of *H. influenzae* type b meningitis does not always confer lasting immunity. The risk of a second episode may be higher for affected individuals than is the risk of a first episode for healthy individuals. This phenomenon suggests a genetic predisposition [Granoff et al., 1986].

Clinical characteristics

The initial neurologic signs of meningitis are caused by leptomeningeal inflammation and increased intracranial pressure. Onset is frequently abrupt but may be gradual. Fever is usually present except in the small infant or debilitated child. An alteration of consciousness is present as either depression of consciousness or irritability. There may be fullness of the fontanel, stiff neck or other signs of meningeal irritation, seizures, headache, and focal neurologic deficits. Signs of meningeal irritation may be absent, especially in the

Signs and Symptoms of Bacterial Meningitis
Fever
Depression of consciousness
Full fontanel
Irritability
Stiff neck
Seizures
Headache
Focal neurologic deficits
Petechial skin rash

child younger than 1 year of age. A child younger than 3 years of age seldom complains of headache (box).

A history of a preceding upper respiratory or gastrointestinal infection with chills, fever, acute rhinitis, cough, vomiting, and anorexia is often revealed. The neurologic findings may be overshadowed by signs and symptoms of sepsis or of respiratory or gastrointestinal infection. Recognizing the point at which an upper respiratory or gastrointestinal infection has evolved into an infection of the nervous system is frequently difficult; there is never a definite moment of CNS involvement. One study concluded that bacterial meningitis was correctly diagnosed on first medical examination in only 58% of 130 childhood cases [Valmari, 1985]. An insidious course causes additional difficulty in diagnosis, and diagnostic delay may be unavoidable [Kilpi et al., 1991]. Experience and a high degree of clinical suspicion are essential.

The diagnosis of bacterial meningitis should be a major consideration when a febrile child develops neurologic signs such as seizures or a significant alteration of consciousness. Depending on the clinical situation, that diagnostic consideration should lead to further studies.

Purpuric skin lesions in a febrile child also suggest meningitis. Such lesions are especially common in *N. meningitidis* meningitis but can occur with other organisms. Skin lesions appear within the first several days after onset. The lesions are produced by direct embolization of organisms or by arteritis. Retinal hemorrhages seldom occur in children with bacterial meningitis; their presence should suggest head trauma. Likewise, papilledema is rare in meningitis and should suggest alternate causes of increased intracranial pressure.

In addition to stiff neck, other meningeal signs may be found, especially in older children. Kernig sign, or straight leg-raising sign, is obtained with the patient supine and is elicited when the child flexes the thigh on the chest with the knee flexed and then straightens the knee. When meningeal irritation is present, this maneuver produces resistance and pain. Brudzinski sign consists of a reflex flexion of the legs occurring on passive flexion of the neck and has the same significance as Kernig sign [Verghese and Gallemore, 1987]. Opisthotonus in meningitis is probably a sign of severe nuchal rigidity. Tripod posture, another sign of meningeal irritation, is evident when the patient sits with partial support from the arms, which are held back and straight with the hands on the sitting surface. Athetosis, chorea, and hemiballismus have been associated with meningitis. These movement disorders may have a sudden onset and can be mistaken for seizures [Burstein and Breningstall, 1986]. Ataxia has also been reported [King and Read, 1988].

Historically, bacterial meningitis was known as *spinal meningitis,* although this term has fallen into disuse. CSF obtained by lumbar puncture usually contains bacteria and manifests other abnormalities, indicating that the spinal cord is surrounded by the infectious process even though clinical spinal signs are rare. Encasement of the cord in purulent exudate has been reported [Bell and McCormick, 1981]. Spinal cord findings on clinical examination appear related to cord infarction and necrosis [Haupt et al., 1981; Tal et al., 1980]. Recovery from spinal cord involvement is poor [Seay, 1984].

Arthritis can precede or follow *H. influenzae, N. meningitidis,* and *Staphylococcus aureus* meningitis and confuses the neurologic examination by producing the superficial appearance of a monoparesis. Elbows and knees are commonly involved. Of the patients with *H. influenzae* type b septic arthritis, 30% have a concurrent meningitis [Rotbart and Glode, 1985]. About 2% of patients with *H. influenzae* meningitis have arthritis [Likitnukul et al., 1986]. Orbital cellulitis also occurs in *H. influenzae* meningitis.

EEG may be normal, slow, or epileptiform. Abnormalities are focal or generalized and are nonspecific.

The differential diagnosis of bacterial meningitis includes head trauma, subdural hematoma, viral CNS infection, febrile seizure, septicemia, brain abscess, metabolic derangement, Reye syndrome, poisoning or intoxication, subarachnoid hemorrhage, and neoplastic meningitis. In addition, unusual infectious agents, such as fungus, *Rickettsia* organisms, or tuberculosis, must be considered (box).

Complications occur during the acute illness even when diagnosis is prompt and appropriate therapy rapidly instituted. Patients with complications are more likely to have an unfavorable outcome. Major complications include increased intracranial pressure, seizures, extraaxial fluid collections, shock, brain infarction or necrosis, ventriculomegaly, cranial nerve involvement, and inappropriate secretion of antidiuretic hormone. Disseminated intravascular coagulation, subdural empyema, and brain abscess also occur but are rare. Persistence of fever for 4 to 6 days after the institution of

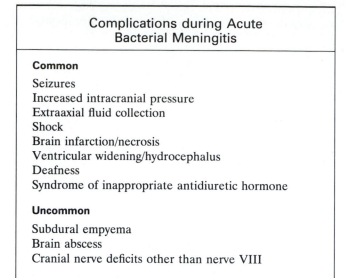

Differential Diagnosis of Bacterial Meningitis
Febrile seizure
Viral CNS infection
Head trauma
Subdural hematoma
Septicemia
Metabolic derangement/Reye syndrome
Poisoning/intoxication
Subarachnoid hemorrhage
Tuberculous/fungal meningitis
Brain/epidural abscess
Neoplastic meningitis

Complications during Acute Bacterial Meningitis
Common
Seizures
Increased intracranial pressure
Extraaxial fluid collection
Shock
Brain infarction/necrosis
Ventricular widening/hydrocephalus
Deafness
Syndrome of inappropriate antidiuretic hormone
Uncommon
Subdural empyema
Brain abscess
Cranial nerve deficits other than nerve VIII

antibiotics or a secondary fever is not cause for major concern in a patient with an otherwise uneventful clinical course [Daoud and Al-Saleh, 1989] (box).

Lumbar puncture

Lumbar puncture is an integral part of the initial work-up of suspected bacterial meningitis. The performance of a lumbar puncture engenders a certain amount of risk [Richards and Towu-Aghantse, 1986]. The risk of herniation after lumbar puncture is quite low in children, but the accurate prevalence is unknown [Marton and Gean, 1986]. The finding of increased intracranial pressure is a relative contraindication to lumbar puncture, but the diffuse increased pressure of meningitis in the infant or child seldom leads to difficulty. Only the minimum amount of CSF necessary for appropriate studies should be removed. The quantity of fluid removed varies with laboratory requirements and the clinical situation. Attention to depth of needle placement reduces the possibility of a traumatic tap [Bonadio et al., 1988]

Considering the frequency of fatal outcome from herniation, care should be exercised in selecting patients for lumbar punctures. When intracranial pressure is significantly elevated or other diagnoses are being ruled out, especially subdural hematoma and other intracranial mass lesions, cranial CT or MRI should be considered before lumbar puncture [Haslam, 1991]. Tonsillar herniation can produce a stiff neck indistinguishable from the nuchal rigidity of meningitis. Brain imaging before lumbar puncture provides some assurance that lumbar puncture can be safely performed. When blood culture, other relevant cultures, and blood and urine antigen studies are obtained immediately and if initial appropriate antibiotics are then instituted, the delay in lumbar puncture associated with the performance of a CT or MRI scan before the procedure results in no loss of therapeutic effectiveness. A short period of antibiotic therapy before lumbar puncture also results in

no significant alteration in CSF findings or inability to culture the organism [Wehrle, 1973]. CSF remains positive for culture for several hours after the initiation of antibiotics [Bonadio and Smith, 1990]; Gram stain and antigen studies remain positive for 24 to 48 hours. When imaging cannot be obtained immediately, the patient can be treated empirically with appropriate antibiotics until imaging is possible [Benjamin et al., 1988].

If malignant increased intracranial pressure develops as manifested by severe obtundation, pupillary irregularities or nonreactive pupils, irregular vital signs, and need for ventilator support, lumbar puncture may be of increased risk. Mannitol or a similar osmotic agent can be administered before and during the procedure when marked increased intracranial pressure is present and lumbar puncture must be performed.

The risk of producing meningitis by performing a lumbar puncture in a child with septicemia is insignificant and not a contraindication to the test [Shapiro et al., 1986]. A lumbar puncture should not be performed through an area of infected skin or infected underlying soft tissue. If a hypocoagulable state is present, that state can be corrected with appropriate blood products before performing the lumbar puncture.

When the child is quiet, as is often the situation in meningitis with a depressed level of consciousness, CSF pressure should be obtained. For the struggling child, sedation may be appropriate to perform a successful lumbar puncture, which includes measurement of CSF pressure. A brief period of sedation will not adversely affect outcome and may significantly enhance the accuracy of the findings.

Early in bacterial meningitis, CSF may be completely normal, only to become abnormal within hours. If lumbar puncture results are normal in a child in whom meningitis is suspected and that suspicion persists, repeat lumbar puncture is appropriate [Feigin and Shackelford, 1973]. Controversy surrounds the frequency with which a lumbar puncture should be performed following the initial examination. Lumbar puncture should not be repeated unless the findings will make a difference in the management of the patient. With an unfavorable clinical course, a repeat lumbar puncture may be indicated for repeat smear, culture, and pressure measurement.

Headache 1 to 6 hours after a lumbar puncture is a troublesome but benign complication. This complication occurs in 10% to 25% of adults, is less frequent in children before adolescence, and may be a cause of irritability in infants [Marton and Gean, 1986]. When present, the headache is frontal and is exaggerated by movement from a lying to a sitting or standing position. Lumbar puncture headache appears to be caused by continued leak of CSF from the site of the puncture, with resulting low CSF pressure and pulling of the brain on pain-sensitive structures. The problem can possibly be reduced by removal of a minimum amount of fluid and use of a small-bore needle, although the procedure's failure rate is higher with a small-bore needle [Lynch et al., 1992]. Pain in the low back or legs occurs occasionally after lumbar puncture. This pain is of uncertain etiology and resolves spontaneously in several days.

Laboratory findings

The value of the CSF examination in the diagnosis of bacterial meningitis has been well established. Typical findings are positive Gram stain, polymorphonuclear pleocytosis, low glucose concentration, and elevated protein levels. The fluid is often cloudy and is under increased pressure. The recovery of cloudy fluid under increased pressure alone is almost diagnostic of bacterial meningitis. Standard tests are always indicated. These tests include a smear with Gram staining, bacterial culture, sensitivities, cell count and differential count, and glucose and protein concentrations. A smear with Gram staining remains an excellent diagnostic tool [Martin, 1983]. Usually 3 ml or less of CSF suffices for testing. Tuberculous cultures, fungal cultures, India ink preparations, and serologic studies may be indicated in certain cases. Blood cultures are also essential because blood may be the only site from which the organism is cultured.

The cell count on initial CSF examination usually ranges from 300 to 10,000 cells/mm^3, predominantly polymorphonuclear cells. A predominance of polymorphonuclear cells may be found in bacterial or aseptic meningitis on initial lumbar puncture at the onset of illness [Baker and Lenane, 1989]. A predominance of lymphocytes or only a minimal cellular response is occasionally a confusing early finding in bacterial men-

ingitis, especially partially treated meningitis. Care must be exercised in attributing CSF lymphocytosis to viral meningitis [Powers, 1985]. Similar care must be exercised in excluding bacterial meningitis because of the absence of CSF cellular response [Onorato et al., 1980].

Contrary to usual perceptions, several polymorphonuclear cells in CSF are not always an abnormal finding [Portnoy and Olson, 1985]. When the significance of polymorphonuclear cells in CSF is uncertain, beginning treatment with antibiotics appropriate for bacterial meningitis is the best response. A repeat CSF examination at a later time frequently clarifies the problem, and in H. influenzae meningitis, CSF can change from normal to abnormal within 30 minutes [Bonadio, 1989; Onorato et al., 1980]. The damage to CNS structures produced by meningitis can cause erythrocytes to appear in CSF. Whenever erythrocytes are obtained, the possibility of a traumatic tap must be considered. A mildly traumatic tap is useful for culture and possibly useful for the comparison of erythrocyte/leukocyte ratios with the peripheral blood cell profile [Bonadio et al., 1990]. A significantly traumatic lumbar puncture is useful only for culture.

The normal CSF glucose level after the neonatal period is usually greater than 40 mg/dl. In bacterial meningitis, CSF glucose level is low, usually less than 20 mg/dl and sometimes undetectable. Low CSF glucose level may represent defective glucose transport across the blood-brain barrier or increased brain use of glucose [Menkes, 1969]. Common clinical practice dictates that simultaneous blood glucose samples be obtained and a ratio determined between blood and CSF glucose levels. However, blood glucose content fluctuates widely. The absolute value of CSF glucose content is probably of diagnostic importance, unless the patient has a concomitant condition leading to hyperglycemia or hypoglycemia. Low CSF glucose levels may rarely occur in other conditions such as viral CNS infection, subarachnoid hemorrhage, and neoplasm of the meninges.

CSF protein content is elevated, and the degree of elevation can be variable. Levels of CSF immunoglobulins are not usually elevated in acute bacterial meningitis. Seizures do not appear to change CSF cell count, glucose levels, or protein concentrations [Portnoy and Olson, 1985]. The concentrations of bacteria and bacterial antigen in CSF are related to morbidity and sequelae [Feldman, 1977]. In S. pneumoniae meningitis the degree of elevation of protein levels and depression of glucose levels correlates with an unfavorable outcome [Laxer and Marks, 1977].

Culture of bacteria requires 24 to 72 hours. Additional diagnostic tests are available for rapid determination of the bacteria involved. The studies become important when initial Gram stain studies are not diagnostic and decisions must be made regarding appropriate antibiotics. The studies include counterimmuno-electrophoresis, latex agglutination study, and limulus lysate assay. These studies use antisera to detect the presence of bacterial antigens in body fluids. Counter-immunoelectrophoresis can distinguish among the capsular polysaccharide of *H. influenzae, N. meningitidis,* group B streptococcus, and *S. pneumoniae,* thus providing rapid etiologic diagnosis; however, a lack of sensitivity and a high rate of false negatives occur. This study can be performed on CSF, serum, and urine. Latex agglutination is more sensitive, especially for *H. influenzae* and *N. meningitidis,* but can also identify *S. pneumoniae* and group B streptococcus. Latex agglutination can be performed on CSF or urine, requires only a small quantity of fluid, and provides results in about 30 minutes. Persistence of positive CSF latex agglutination results for longer than 7 to 9 days after the onset of antibiotic treatment suggests continued infection. Limulus lysate assay of CSF is useful in gram-negative bacterial meningitis but is nonspecific and does not discriminate among different types of gram-negative organisms [Martin, 1983]. When only a single test is performed, latex agglutination is appropriate.

Serum C-reactive protein assay is a nonspecific test for bacterial meningitis and bacterial infections in general. Most febrile children with a serum C-reactive protein concentration greater than 40 mg/dl have bacterial infection [Putto et al., 1986]. The test is not positive until an inflammatory response has occurred. In uncomplicated cases, C-reactive protein level decreases to normal in 1 to 2 days. If a secondary rise occurs, the possibility of bacterial complications should be considered.

The CSF findings of most value in determining whether a CNS infection is bacterial and not viral are a positive Gram stain, depressed glucose concentration, and positive latex agglutination. However, the total clinical and laboratory picture remains important in diagnosis. CSF findings should be used within the context of the patient's initial condition and clinical status. Rigid criteria for CSF abnormalities should be replaced by a flexible and individualized approach (box).

Within 48 to 72 hours after the institution of antibiotic therapy the CSF culture is negative [Bonadio and Smith, 1990]. Pleocytosis and hypoglycorrhachia persist in CSF for days or weeks, even in patients who respond favorably [Chartrand and Cho, 1976]. Thereafter complete clearing of CSF is not an appropriate end point for treatment. However, continued improvement in CSF parameters is expected.

Brain imaging

Cranial CT has been a major asset in managing bacterial meningitis. MRI provides improved resolution when compared with CT, provides additional insights

---

CSF Examinations in Suspected Bacterial Meningitis
Routine Tests
Gram stain
Bacterial culture and sensitivities
Cell count and differential
Glucose
Protein
Bacterial antigen
Special Tests
Culture for tuberculosis, fungus, virus
Additional bacterial antigen studies
Serology
Cryptococcus antigen
India ink
Coccidiodomycosis antibody

---

into the pathogenesis of the neurologic complications, and may eventually replace CT in all but the most acute clinical situations. Bacterial meningitis should be managed at facilities that offer noninvasive diagnostic imaging whenever possible.

CT or MRI should be obtained on patients with unfavorable clinical courses, such as the presence of prolonged depressed consciousness, persistent full fontanel, prolonged fever, focal neurologic deficits, apnea, and seizures [Stovring and Snyder, 1980]. Failure to display clinical improvement or sudden unexplained clinical deterioration are additional indications. Clinically significant extraaxial fluid collections occur less frequently than anticipated by studies performed before the advent of imaging. Abscesses are rarely found. Areas of infarction and necrosis are common in clinically complicated cases, especially when imaging is obtained late in the course of the acute illness (Figure 38-9). Care must be exercised in attributing ventriculomegaly to increased intracranial pressure. Imaging is of little value in children with prolonged fever alone [Kline and Kaplan, 1988].

Cortical enhancement may occur and is presumed to indicate cerebritis but may also indicate meningeal inflammation or brain infarction (Figure 38-10). Repeat imaging is useful in following the evolution of abnormalities [Bodino et al., 1982] and in determining the need for subsequent intervention. CT abnormalities are associated with unfavorable outcome [Packer et al., 1982].

Complications

Increased intracranial pressure. The presence of increased intracranial pressure early in the course of

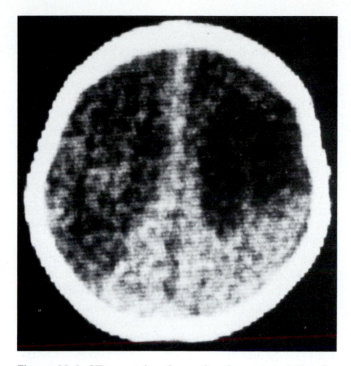

Figure 38-9 CT scan taken 2 months after onset of *H. influenzae* meningitis in a 3-month-old infant. Bilateral infarction of brain, verified by biopsy [Snyder et al., 1981]. Ventriculomegaly.

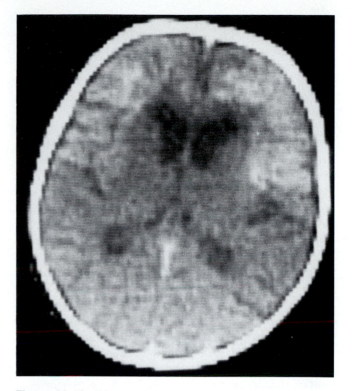

Figure 38-10 CT scan of 5-month-old infant with *H. influenzae* meningitis, seizures, and coma. Note bilateral cortical enhancement.

bacterial meningitis and the associated full fontanel are the features of the disease that often lead to the correct diagnosis in infants with open fontanels. In an uncomplicated case of meningitis the full fontanel disappears within several days and an uneventful recovery ensues. The pathogenesis of this initial increased intracranial pressure is not clear. Obstruction of CSF resorption over the convexities with communicating hydrocephalus is the most likely cause.

The early increased intracranial pressure may become malignant rather than resolve, leading to compromise of cerebral blood flow and herniation in the most severe cases. This type of situation is manifested by rapidly progressive clinical deterioration. Severe obtundation occurs, often preceded by seizures [Horwitz et al., 1980]. Pupillary irregularities are present. Unresponsive pupils are accompanied by varying degrees of dilatation. Other signs include posturing, abnormal respiratory patterns, bradycardia, elevated blood pressure, and irregular vital signs. Ventilatory support may be necessary. CT or MRI scans should be obtained to exclude the possibility of an extraaxial fluid collection. The pathogenesis of malignant increased intracranial pressure is usually diffuse cerebral edema, which is revealed by brain imaging.

Overhydration with intravenous fluids may predispose patients to or exaggerate existing cerebral edema; therefore fluids should be carefully administered to minimize the risk of developing cerebral edema. In the absence of hypertension and with normal serum sodium content, administering two thirds of the calculated daily maintenance fluids intravenously during the first 24 hours of illness is usual practice [Laine et al., 1991]. Usually the fluid is administered as one-quarter to one-third normal saline in 5% dextrose. Fluid restriction has a theoretic disadvantage because many patients are dehydrated on arrival at a medical facility. Fluid restriction in a volume-depleted child may maintain the dehydrated state, encourage intracranial vascular sludging and thrombosis, and enhance the likelihood of hypotension. In bacterial meningitis, maintaining a state of fluid balance as close to physiologically normal as possible is advisable [Prince and Neu, 1980; Trachtman, 1991].

About 20% of children with bacterial meningitis develop hyponatremia. The frequency of hyponatremia related to inappropriate hypothalamic release of antidiuretic hormone and secondary fluid retention is controversial [Laine et al., 1991]. In hyponatremia the symptoms are those of water intoxication (e.g., restlessness, irritability, lethargy, seizures, coma). With inappropriate secretion of antidiuretic hormone the serum sodium level is low, the serum hyposmolar, and the urine excessively concentrated with elevated urine sodium concentrations. Treatment for inappropriate release of antidiuretic hormone is fluid restriction. The recommendation has been made to institute fluid restriction only when serum sodium concentration decreases to less than 125 mEq/L [Powell, 1991; Powell et al., 1990]. Rapid correction of severe hyponatremia may be dangerous and should be avoided [Narins, 1986].

Appropriate management of increased intracranial pressure when symptoms are sufficiently threatening consists of tracheal intubation with controlled hyperventilation to maintain P_{CO_2} at about 30 torr. Mannitol can be administered intravenously, 0.25 to 0.5 g/kg, over 20 to 30 minutes. This dose can be repeated every 2 to 4 hours as necessary. Subsequent doses of mannitol are usually not as effective as the initial dose. Steroids such as dexamethasone are often administered intravenously because of the desperate nature of the clinical situation, although the benefit of steroids in this setting is not established. Sedation or administration of a neuromuscular blocking agent such as pancuronium bromide may be necessary to enhance controlled ventilation.

Ventriculomegaly developing during acute meningitis always leads to concern regarding hydrocephalus secondary to increased intraventricular pressure. However, surgical intervention with ventricular drainage should be approached with caution [Snyder, 1984a]. Ventriculomegaly is frequently transient and in some cases may represent the subacute development of hydrocephalus ex vacuo secondary to loss of brain parenchyma. When the clinical situation is sufficiently severe that surgical intervention is necessary, ventricular drainage to an external collection device should be considered initially to avoid the danger of shunting infected fluid into a body cavity. Surgical intervention should be limited to patients who manifest ventriculomegaly and persistent traditional signs of increased intracranial pressure, such as full fontanel, abnormally increasing head circumference, depressed consciousness, vomiting, and elevated intraventricular pressure by direct measurement.

The usefulness of intracranial pressure–recording devices in the prevention and management of increased pressure in bacterial meningitis is not well established. Insertion of a foreign body into an infected cavity is always a concern. Such devices are known to produce ventriculitis and meningitis [Aucoin et al., 1986]. The usefulness of a pentobarbital-induced coma is also not established.

Seizures. Seizures complicate 20% to 50% of cases of childhood bacterial meningitis as an initial symptom and a later complication, especially in infants. Seizures may be focal or generalized. They occur most frequently 2 to 3 days into the illness and cease 1 to 3 days later, sometimes irrespective of treatment. Seizures may be toxic in origin or secondary to vasculitis, cortical irritation, fever, electrolyte disturbance, or an immune process. Severe ventricular widening and parenchymal infarction or necrosis are associated with seizures (see box below) [Snyder, 1984b]. EEG may be normal or may reveal generalized or focal epileptiform abnormalities, focal slowing, or only background slowing. Seizures do not necessarily indicate a failure of antibiotic treatment. The overall clinical situation and laboratory results must be considered before a repeat lumbar puncture is undertaken because of seizures. Persistent seizures do not necessarily indicate extraaxial fluid collection.

Although seizures are frequently self-limited, vigorous treatment by standard methods is appropriate to prevent additional damage to an already compromised CNS. Adequate ventilation and cardiovascular support should be ensured. Phenobarbital, phenytoin, diazepam, and lorazepam appear useful in controlling seizures when administered individually or in combination. The most commonly used antiepileptic drug in this setting is phenobarbital (initial dose: 10 to 20 mg/kg), administered slowly intravenously. Phenytoin may be added when required (initial dose: 10 to 20 mg/kg), also administered slowly intravenously. Cardiac function should be monitored during the injection of phenytoin. Phenytoin has the advantage of causing less sedation than phenobarbital. When needed, diazepam may be administered intravenously (initial dose: 0.2 to 0.5 mg/kg; maximum dose: 5 mg) no faster than 1 to 2 mg/min for children younger than 5 years of age. Lorazepam is also useful in this situation (initial dose: 0.05 to 0.1 mg/kg) no faster than 1 to 2 mg/kg/min. Ventilator support may be indicated, especially during status epilepticus. Sedation or administration of pancuronium bromide may be required to ensure satisfactory ventilator function. Pancuronium bromide stops the motor manifestations of seizures, but antiepileptic drugs remain necessary to control abnormal electrical activity.

Chronic seizures are rare after recovery from meningitis [Annegers et al., 1988; Pomeroy et al., 1990]. The self-limited seizure disorder that occurs within the first several days after onset of bacterial meningitis may not require prolonged antiepileptic drug therapy. If the seizures cease within several days of onset, the subse-

---

Causes of Seizures in Bacterial Meningitis

Cytokine release/inflammation
Vasculitis
Infarction
Fever
Electrolyte imbalance
Extraaxial fluid

quent clinical course of the illness is benign, and an EEG obtained near the end of the course of antibiotics is not epileptiform, discontinuation of antiepileptic drug therapy (usually by gradual withdrawal) should be considered. A prolonged course of such therapy is avoided. If seizures recur after the acute illness, antiepileptic drugs can be restarted. Whether early treatment with antiepileptic drugs has an effect on the development of chronic seizures is unknown.

Extraaxial fluid collections. Brain imaging often cannot distinguish between a subdural fluid collection and a widened subarachnoid space. The fluid collection is properly referred to as an *extraaxial fluid collection.* There are two anatomic locations for fluid collections: the subdural space and the subarachnoid space. The collection in the subarachnoid space may represent loculated CSF, widening of the subarachnoid space in response to inflammation, or loss of brain parenchyma (Figure 38-11).

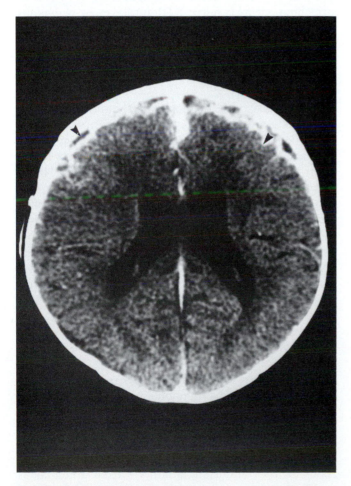

Figure 38-11 *H. influenzae* meningitis in a 10-month-old infant. CT was done without contrast. Extraaxial fluid collection with surrounding enhancement (possible membrane) *(arrows).* Ventriculomegaly.

A potential intracranial space is situated between the arachnoid and the dura [Schachenmayr and Friede, 1978]. For unexplained reasons, fluid can accumulate in this potential space in children with bacterial meningitis. The collection occurs more commonly in bacterial meningitis during the first year of life and is usually recognized during the first week of illness. Children with these collections have a rapid onset of meningitis, low peripheral white count, and high CSF protein [Snedeker et al., 1990]. The fluid is serosanguineous, has a high protein content, is usually sterile, contains polymorphonuclear cells, is usually situated over the convexities, and may accumulate bilaterally. With time the fluid collection follows one of several courses: (1) it resolves (most common course), (2) it continues to accumulate and acts as a mass, (3) it organizes into a fibrin network or becomes surrounded by a membrane (Figure 38-12), or (4) it becomes an empyema.

Extraaxial collections can be asymptomatic. The presence of persistent fever, persistent full fontanel, persistent clinical signs of meningitis, seizures, and focal neurologic deficits should alert the clinician to the possibility of a collection. Except for increased intracranial pressure and some focal deficits, it is seldom clear that the extraaxial collection is producing the symptoms observed. Brain damage and extraaxial fluid may be independent expressions of the same severe initial infection [Syrogiannopoulos et al., 1986].

When the collection is liquid, as it usually is initially, it can be partly removed by needle aspiration through the lateral aspect of an open fontanel. However, needle aspiration often cannot determine whether fluid is removed from the subdural or the subarachnoid space. In previous studies in which routine puncture through the fontanel was undertaken, fluid was recovered in about one third of patients [Benson et al., 1960]. In a more recent study, extraaxial fluid collections were found in 50% of children with bacterial meningitis who had cranial CT performed [Syrogiannopoulos et al., 1986].

Clinicians must exercise care when associating clinical symptoms, such as fever and seizures, to extraaxial fluid collection. The collection should be followed with periodic imaging. Intervention is appropriate only under the conditions listed in the box on page 624.

Initial intervention when the fontanel is open consists of introducing a subdural needle into the fluid-filled space and then removing an appropriate quantity of fluid. When the fluid collections are bilateral, both sides can be punctured. Removing large quantities of fluid can result in potentially dangerous shifts of intracranial structures and removal of protein. Tapping can be repeated as necessary, although bleeding or infection is a risk. Unfortunately, removing fluid seldom changes symptoms. When CT or MRI scan reveals a progressive increase in the accumulated fluid or symptoms persist

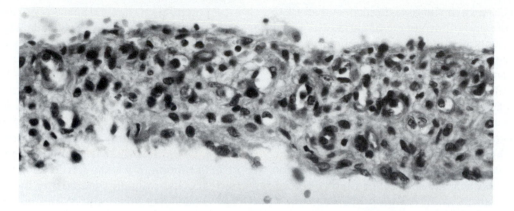

Figure 38-12 A 5-month-old infant with *H. influenzae* meningitis. Portion of surgically removed membrane found in association with extraaxial fluid collection. Note granulomatous tissue with numerous capillaries and chronic inflammatory cells. Original magnification ×100. (Reduced to 70%.) (Courtesy Dr. Mario Kornfeld, Albuquerque, NM.)

Extra-axial Fluid Collections: Indications for Intervention
Displacement of brain parenchyma
Persistent fever
Persistent lethargy
Empyema
Persistent increased intracranial pressure

after repeated tapping, external drainage or shunting of the space can be considered. An infected collection requires immediate drainage. The contribution of small extraaxial fluid collections to an unfavorable clinical state or the production of neurologic sequelae appears to have been overemphasized.

Extraaxial fluid collections are usually benign, produce no unique clinical symptoms, can be followed by imaging, resolve spontaneously with time, usually require no intervention, and do not produce long-term sequelae [Snedeker et al., 1990].

Infarction and necrosis. Because all vessels entering or leaving the brain must pass through the subarachnoid space, which is the site of an inflammatory response, brain infarction can be found on imaging in some patients. The return from imaging for infarction will be higher when the imaging is performed later in the course of the disorder. Infarction is associated with a poor outcome, especially hemiparesis, cognitive difficulties, and speech problems [Pike et al., 1990; Wardle and Carty, 1991].

Cranial nerve involvement. Cranial nerve abnormalities develop in bacterial meningitis because of the intimate involvement of the cranial nerves with the inflammatory state. Increased intracranial pressure can also cause cranial nerve dysfunction by pressure or stretching. Cranial nerve VIII is the most commonly involved. Deafness occurs and is frequently permanent. Cranial nerves VI and III are the next most commonly involved. Ocular palsies are usually reversible. Other cranial nerves are affected less frequently [Chu et al., 1990].

Deafness. Bacterial meningitis is the most important cause of acquired sensory-neural deafness [Tarlow, 1991]. Between 5% and 30% of cases of bacterial meningitis are complicated by clinical deafness, especially when the infection is caused by *S. pneumoniae*. In *N. meningitidis* meningitis the incidence of deafness may depend on the serogroup of the organism [Mayatepek et al., 1991]. In some cases the problem is a conductive hearing loss associated with a middle ear infection accompanying meningitis. More commonly a sensorineural hearing loss occurs in both ears during meningitis. Hearing loss is correlated with low CSF glucose and the presence of seizures [Borkowski et al., 1985]. Hearing loss can also occur after the use of ototoxic antibiotics.

Experimental studies suggest that bacteria reach the cochlea via the internal auditory canal or the cochlear aqueduct or hematogenously [Kay, 1991; Kaplan, 1990]. Deafness is caused by cochlear sepsis rather than involvement of the eighth cranial nerve. The number of days that symptoms are apparent before the institution of antibiotic therapy does not correlate with the development of hearing loss [Dodge et al., 1984]. Hearing loss can be detected in the first 48 hours of illness. Assessment of brainstem auditory-evoked potentials is an effective means of detecting auditory abnormalities, especially in very young infants [Cohen et al., 1990]. Recovery of hearing usually occurs by the end of the first 2 weeks, but major deficits may persist.

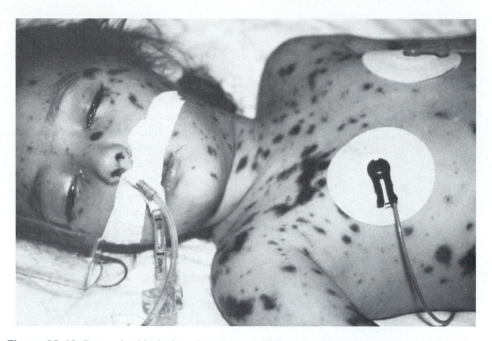

Figure 38-13 Purpuric skin lesions in a 4-year-old female with *N. meningococcus* meningitis and sepsis. (Courtesy Dr. Robert Greenberg.)

Dexamethasone has been demonstrated to improve the frequency of hearing impairment in children with meningitis [Lebel et al., 1988]. This drug decreases the inflammatory response as manifested by duration of fever and CSF changes. The impact of dexamethasone administration on neurologic outcome is less certain. It has become almost routine in the management of childhood bacterial meningitis [Havens et al., 1989; Hawkins et al., 1990; Kaplan, 1989; Tauber and Sande, 1989]. The recommended dosage of dexamethasone is 0.6 mg/kg/day intravenously in four divided doses for 4 days. It may be maximally effective when administered before antibiotics to prevent the inflammatory response initiated by products of the bacterial cell wall [Odio et al., 1991].

Before discharge, a young child with bacterial meningitis should probably have brainstem auditory-evoked response testing, and an older child should have audiometry. When hearing loss occurs, early intervention by those knowledgeable in the management of this problem in infants and children should be encouraged. An implanted cochlear prosthesis may be appropriate in the management of persistent deafness [Nadol and Hsu, 1991].

Disseminated intravascular coagulation. Evidence of abnormal bleeding and shock in a child with bacterial meningitis suggests sepsis, more commonly with gram-negative organisms, and raises the suspicion of disseminated intravascular coagulation. With this condition, rapid consumption of fibrinogen occurs and fibrin thrombi form. Purpuric skin lesions in meningitis suggest a coagulopathy (Figure 38-13). Similar lesions occur in other organs.

Disseminated intravascular coagulation should be confirmed with appropriate laboratory studies. Laboratory abnormalities include thrombocytopenia, hypofibrinogenemia, circulating fibrin-split products, abnormal prothrombin time and partial thromboplastin time, and decreased levels of certain coagulation factors [McCabe et al., 1983].

The disorder may occur in bacterial meningitis caused by any organism but is especially common in *N. meningococcus* meningitis. This form of meningitis may first appear as a fulminant disease with shock. Purpuric skin lesions in *N. meningococcus* meningitis do not necessarily indicate disseminated intravascular coagulation; such lesions can occur from emboli of organisms. Embolic skin lesions initially have a yellowish white center, and organisms are found on Gram stain of scrapings from the lesions. The distinction between embolic lesions and those secondary to a coagulopathy may be important for management. Other abnormalities of the coagulation system that may occur with meningitis and sepsis include thrombocytopenia alone, purpura fulminans, and symmetric peripheral gangrene (Figure 38-14).

Waterhouse-Friderichsen syndrome is associated with fulminating meningococcal septicemia and consists of disseminated intravascular coagulation, petechial hemorrhages of skin and mucous membranes, and sudden cardiovascular collapse. The syndrome may be associated with infections other than meningococcus. The role of adrenal hemorrhage has been overemphasized.

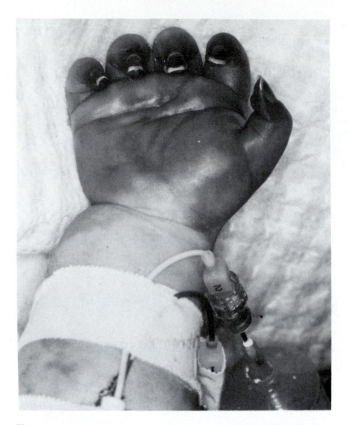

Figure 38-14 Forearm and hand of a 5-month-old infant with *H. influenzae* meningitis. Ischemic necrosis would have evolved into peripheral gangrene if patient had survived.

The management of disseminated intravascular coagulation is controversial. Some recommended therapies such as the administration of heparin may cause harm. Steroids do not appear beneficial. Treatment of the underlying infection is probably the most successful method for the correction of the condition. Blood products should be administered to correct coagulation abnormalities. The reader should consult appropriate sources for current recommendations regarding treatment.

Recurrent meningitis. Permanent immunity is not necessarily achieved by recovery from bacterial meningitis. A second occurrence not related to persistence of the original infection, although rare, requires close scrutiny. Special considerations become relevant in a repeat infection with the same or another organism [Kline, 1989]. The possibility of a cranial or spinal defect, parameningeal focus of infection, an immunologic problem, or genetic predisposition must be evaluated. The cranial defect can be acquired or developmental. Minor trauma with fracture involving the paranasal sinuses or ear regions is a form of acquired cranial defect. Such defects may be associated with CSF rhinorrhea or otorrhea. Among the developmental defects are meningomyelo-

cele, dermal sinus, and neurenteric cyst [Holguin and Manotas, 1988].

In addition to the usual evaluation for bacterial meningitis, other investigations must be considered, such as skull and sinus radiographs, CT and MRI scans, intrathecal radioisotope tracer examination of the CSF to evaluate external leakage, and an immunologic evaluation. Immunoglobulin abnormalities have been noted in some children with bacterial meningitis [Loh et al., 1991]. Direct coronal thin-section CT is recommended as an effective method for detecting small osseous defects [Steele et al., 1985]. When an anatomic defect is found, surgical correction is indicated. Conditions other than bacterial meningitis can cause recurrent meningitis. These conditions include Behçet syndrome, sarcoidosis, and Mollaret meningitis [Rakover et al., 1989].

Antibiotic management

Bacterial meningitis is almost always fatal without treatment. Aggressive antibiotic therapy begun early has a favorable influence on outcome in most patients. Recommendations and dosages change frequently. The widespread use of adjunctive therapy with dexamethasone and its appropriate sequencing with antibiotics complicates therapeutic recommendations. Authoritative sources should be consulted regarding specific antibiotics and dosages. Antibiotic management should undergo constant analysis during the course of treatment (box). Many medical facilities have infectious disease services that can provide useful advice.

The antibiotic treatment of meningitis is divided into two treatment phases. During the initial treatment phase, which occurs before a definitive cause of the infection is established from CSF or blood studies and before sensitivities are available, antibiotics appropriate for the suspected organism should be administered. The initial phase may be very brief or may last for several days depending on the clinical situation and the outcome of laboratory evaluations.

In the second phase of antibiotic treatment, which occurs once the organism has been identified by culture of CSF or blood or by one of the special tests and sensitivities are available, antibiotic therapy can be modified as necessary and treatment should be as specific as possible. A patient's allergies should be considered when choosing an antibiotic. Multiple antibiotics may be necessary.

For most antibiotics the dose should be administered frequently as a slow intravenous bolus or a constant infusion [Tauber and Sande, 1991]. A loading dose may be indicated. The blood-brain barrier restricts access of most drugs. Penetration improves when the meninges are inflamed, but large systemic doses are necessary. The usual course of antibiotic administration is 10 to 14 days,

---

Antibiotics for Bacterial Meningitis*

H. influenzae
  Ampicillin
  Chloramphenicol
  Ceftriaxone
  Cefotaxime
S. pneumoniae
  Penicillin
  Chloramphenicol
  Cefuroxime
  Ceftriaxone
  Vancomycin
N. meningitidis
  Penicillin
  Chloramphenicol
  Cefuroxime
  Ceftriaxone
Gram-negative bacillary meningitis
  Cefotaxime
  Ceftazidime
  Ceftriaxone
  Amikacin
Staphylococcus
  Nafcillin
  Vancomycin
  Rifampin
Tuberculosis
  Isoniazid
  Rifampin
  Ethambutol
  Pyrazinamide
  Streptomycin
Neonatal
  Ampicillin
  Gentamycin
  Tobramycin
  Vancomycin
  Amikacin
  Kanamycin
  Ceftriaxone
  Cefotaxime
  Ceftazidime
  Penicillin

---

*Recommendations change frequently. Check for current recommendations.

The organisms producing meningitis in children vary from time to time and in different geographic regions. Firm rules are difficult to develop; only guidelines can be presented. During the first month of life, *Escherichia coli, Listeria monocytogenes,* and group B streptococcus are common organisms. Infections from *Proteus* species, *Pseudomonas* species, and *S. pneumoniae* also occur. Other, less common organisms may be found. Between 3 months and 6 years of age, *H. influenzae* is the common organism. Also common during this age are *S. pneumoniae* and *N. meningitidis* organisms. In adolescence, *N. meningitidis* predominates. After open head trauma and neurosurgical procedures, *Staphylococcus epidermidis, S. aureus,* and gram-negative bacilli infections occur. Gram-negative bacilli, especially *L. monocytogenes,* are also found in immunosuppressed patients [Bell, 1985].

Haemophilus influenzae meningitis. Ampicillin has been the mainstay of treatment of *H. influenzae* meningitis, but strains have appeared that produce beta-lactamase, a substance that interferes with the effectiveness of ampicillin, various penicillins, and certain cephalosporins. Because of resistant *H. influenzae,* which constitutes approximately 25% of *H. influenzae* strains in the United States [McCracken, 1984], adding chloramphenicol to the initial treatment regimen and continuing chloramphenicol until antibiotic sensitivities were available were customary treatment measures. Because strains of *H. influenzae* resistant to chloramphenicol exist, ceftriaxone [Peltola et al., 1989] or cefotaxime [Jacobs et al., 1992] are now used as single antibiotic therapy [Peter et al., 1991].

Streptococcus pneumoniae meningitis. *S. pneumoniae* may cause a virulent form of meningitis in infants. The incidence of permanent neurologic sequelae is high. In most cases the organism has retained sensitivity to crystalline penicillin G, but sensitivity testing is necessary. Treatment with ceftriaxone and cefuroxime are additional forms of therapy [Peter et al., 1991].

Neisseria meningitidis meningitis. *N. meningitidis* meningitis is usually a disease of children and young adults. Onset and progression tend to be rapid, necessitating prompt management. The occurrence of a petechial rash suggests that the offending organism is meningococcus. Antibiotic treatment consists of administering crystalline penicillin G [Peter et al., 1991].

Gram-negative bacillary meningitis. Gram-negative bacillary meningitis is usually acquired in the hospital and is associated with sepsis, head trauma, or neurosurgical procedures. *Klebsiella* and *Pseudomonas* species are common infecting organisms. Antibiotic treatment is not satisfactory. Intrathecal or intraventricular administration of antibiotics has been necessary. A third-generation cephalosporin such as cefotaxime and

---

although 7 days is probably satisfactory in uncomplicated cases [Gold, 1990; Radetsky, 1990]. When meningitis is caused by enteric organisms or tuberculosis, the course of treatment is longer. Antibiotic therapy should probably not be prolonged because of a persistent fever in a child who has otherwise displayed a favorable clinical response.

ceftazidime may be appropriate therapy. Amikacin is usually recommended as an additional antibiotic.

Staphylococcus aureus and *Staphylococcus epidermidis* meningitis. *S. aureus* causes meningitis in connection with sepsis, neurosurgical procedures, parameningeal infection, or brain abscess. Satisfactory antibiotic treatment is not available. Nafcillin and an aminoglycoside are recommended; vancomycin has been used. Cephalosporins such as cefotaxime and cefuroxime may have an important place in the management of *S. aureus* meningitis.

The infection rate after shunt procedures varies from 2% to 20%, is frequently caused by *S. epidermidis,* and may be a combination of ventriculitis and meningitis; shunt removal and administration of antibiotics are often necessary [Odio et al., 1984]. Systemic and intraventricular antibiotics are usually indicated for shunt-related infections. Vancomycin along with rifampin may have a place in the management of shunt infections caused by resistant *Staphylococcus* species [Peter et al., 1991].

Steroid treatment

Recent research suggests that steroids reduce the harmful effects of the rapid bacterial lysis produced within the subarachnoid space when antibiotics are administered and biologically active cytokines are released in *H. influenzae* and *S. pneumoniae* meningitis [Jacobs and Tabor, 1990; Kaplan, 1990; Kennedy et al., 1991, Tauber et al., 1987]. Moderate to severe hearing loss may also be decreased by dexamethasone after initial antibiotics [Lebel et al., 1988]. Dexamethasone decreases the duration of fever and CSF pleocytosis. In animal and human studies, cytokines in the CSF are reduced when steroids are administered before the initial antibiotic [Arditi et al., 1989; Tauber et al., 1987]. In a trial involving infants and children given dexamethasone 15 to 20 minutes before the institution of antibiotic therapy, CSF opening pressure was lower, the evidence of inflammation in the spinal fluid had begun to disappear after 12 hours, the CSF contained lower concentrations of cytokines, and neurologic sequelae were less marked [Odio et al., 1991]. A study from Egypt using dexamethasone in pneumococcal meningitis in older children and adults demonstrated a reduction in overall mortality [Girgis et al., 1989]. Dexamethasone administered for approximately 48 hours does not appear to have a deleterious effect on the clinical course of aseptic meningitis [Hoyt and McCracken, 1990]. The use of dexamethasone in meningitis is favored by most directors of programs in pediatric infectious disease and may become routine [Kaplan, 1990; Word and Klein, 1989]. Administration of dexamethasone to all children with bacterial meningitis and to adults who are more than mildly ill is a current recommendation, recognizing

that trials thus far have been limited [Finch and Mandragos, 1991; Peter et al., 1991; Tauber and Sande, 1989]. Other antiinflammatory agents may prove beneficial as may intravenous immunoglobulin, monoclonal antibiotics, and leukocyte transfusions when severe neutropenia is present [Gary et al., 1989; Hinds, 1992; Jacobs, 1990; Saez-Llorens et al., 1991; Spector, 1990].

Partially treated bacterial meningitis. Meningitis may develop from common childhood illnesses such as upper respiratory and gastrointestinal infections. Children with meningitis are often given antibiotics for these illnesses before the development of bacterial meningitis. The antibiotics are not administered in dosages adequate to eradicate meningitis. Treatment with low-dose antibiotics before the diagnosis of bacterial meningitis may diminish the intensity of both clinical symptoms and CSF changes, making the diagnosis more difficult. The pattern of CSF constituents may be altered to suggest viral meningitis [Quaade and Krislensen, 1962]. However, low-dose antibiotic treatment will probably not return the CSF to its normal state. Fewer polymorphonuclear leukocytes, less depression of glucose, less elevation of protein, and more difficulty in obtaining a positive Gram stain and culture may also be found [Converse et al., 1973].

Previous antibiotic treatment does not significantly affect some of the special CSF tests such as latex agglutination. When doubt concerning the diagnosis of meningitis is present, instituting aggressive treatment with antibiotics appropriate for bacterial meningitis is advisable. Most patients with partially treated bacterial meningitis have favorable outcomes when given appropriate antibiotic treatment [Valmari, 1985].

Prophylaxis

In some situations, bacterial meningitis appears to be contagious. Spread presumably occurs by colonization of the nasopharynx with virulent strains. Spread of *N. meningitidis* has occurred among military recruits and others in crowded living conditions. *H. influenzae* has been spread to close contacts. Rifampin is recommended prophylactically for close contacts of an index case. Close contacts include family members, day care and school contacts, and those in health care facilities with intimate exposure. Rifampin should be begun as soon as possible. The success of prophylaxis is not yet established. When prophylaxis is undertaken, children who have been immunized against *H. influenzae* should also receive rifampin. Appropriate sources should be consulted for current recommendations [Peter et al., 1991].

Immunization

Modern therapy has not prevented the occurrence of significant neurologic sequelae following bacterial meningitis. This fact has directed attention to the possibility of immunization against the causative bacterial agents.

A vaccine effective against *H. influenzae* type b is widely available. The vaccine contains type b capsular polysaccharide, which accounts for most serious infections. The vaccine prevents bacteremia and thus prevents meningitis [Peltola et al., 1984]. The American Academy of Pediatrics recommends immunization of all infants beginning at approximately 2 months of age [Peter et al., 1991]. The vaccine does not prevent respiratory infection with unencapsulated *H. influenzae,* but these organisms do not cause meningitis.

A meningococcal capsular polysaccharide vaccine is effective in preventing meningitis caused by some serogroups of *N. meningitidis.* Use of the vaccine in military recruits and during epidemics should be considered when the outbreak is caused by a vaccine serogroup. The vaccine does not appear effective in prevention of disease in exposed individuals. A pneumococcal polysaccharide vaccine is also available and may be appropriate in selected situations [Shapiro et al., 1991].

Prognosis

The prognosis in childhood bacterial meningitis remains unfavorable for many patients despite advances in antibiotic management and supportive care. Mortality from *H. influenzae* meningitis ranges from 3% to 17%, with the lower percentage reported in more recent studies. The overall mortality rate is higher when all bacteria causing meningitis are included [Skoch and Walling, 1985].

Meningitis is one of the leading causes of acquired neurologic disability in childhood. The frequency of sequelae is highest in *S. pneumoniae* infections [Jadavji et al., 1986]. Deficits in survivors range from minor and transient problems to lifelong, incapacitating disabilities. Detectable deficits are found in survivors beyond the neonatal period in 5% to 19% of cases [Granoff and Squires, 1982]. An unfavorable outcome is associated with young age, delay in institution of treatment, coma or focal neurologic signs on admission, and a malignant clinical course. Mental retardation, motor impairment, hemiparesis, seizures, hydrocephalus, deafness, blindness, and learning disabilities are among the problems that occur. In a prospective study of 194 children with bacterial meningitis, 39% had neurologic abnormalities at the time of hospital discharge. When evaluated 2 years after the illness, only 9% had detectable deficits [Feigin et al., 1976]. This and other studies suggest cautious optimism about outcome [Pomeroy et al., 1990; Taylor et al., 1984; 1990]. The prognosis is less favorable in developing countries [Salih et al., 1991].

Sequelae do not appear to result from continued replication of bacteria within the CSF but rather from ischemic damage and inflammation. Improvement in

outcome will probably not result from newer antibiotic agents but from improved methods for prevention and management of cerebral edema, inflammation, vasculitis, infarction, and necrosis. Prevention of occurrence of the disease is the ultimate goal.

CHRONIC MENINGITIS

Chronic meningitis is usually not a bacterial disease. Tuberculosis meningitis, syphilis, and Lyme disease are exceptions. Differential diagnostic considerations include fungal infections such as cryptococcus, smoldering encephalitis, neoplasm involving the meninges, and slow viral infections. Additional considerations include rickettsia infections and CNS infections occurring as complications of acquired immunodeficiency syndrome.

BRAIN ABSCESS

The initial appearance of bacterial brain abscess is seldom dramatic, and the historic and clinical findings are vague. The pattern of presentation differs from bacterial meningitis, which first appears as an acute condition and may be fulminating. Brain abscess occurs in children in association with cyanotic congenital heart disease, after neurosurgical procedures and penetrating head trauma, as a secondary condition to infections about the sinuses and orbits [Maniglia et al., 1989], and as a spontaneous condition. It also occurs in immunosuppressed patients, patients with chronic pulmonary disease, or patients with a continuing focus of infection [Fischer et al., 1981]. Brain abscess is rare as a complication of bacterial meningitis except in the neonate [Renier et al., 1988].

Pathology

Either hematogenous or direct spread of the organism occurs in a brain abscess. An abscess of hematogenous origin localizes at the border of the gray and white matter. The lesion is initially a cerebritis that may persist for several weeks. Edema surrounds the cerebritis, increasing the mass effect. A capsule of inflammatory granulation tissue develops around the infected area after the cerebritis phase. Abscesses are usually in the hemispheres but may be found in the brainstem or cerebellum.

Clinical characteristics

The diagnosis of brain abscess is suggested by the subacute development of specific signs and symptoms (box). The seizures may be focal or generalized. Findings on examination are not necessarily localizing. MRI and radionuclide brain scans are appropriate tests during cerebritis. Enhanced CT and MRI scans are the definitive tests in a mature abscess because they reveal a characteristic capsular ring. EEG may be normal, may display focal abnormalities in the region of the abscess

Signs and Symptoms of Brain Abscess
Subacute course
Fever
Headache
Confusion
Depressed consciousness
Seizures
Nuchal rigidity
Papilledema
Hemiparesis
Dysphasia

as either slowing or spikes, may contain periodic lateralized epileptiform discharges, or may be diffusely slow.

A brain abscess behaves as an expanding intracranial mass. The mass effect can obstruct CSF flow and produce hydrocephalus. Papilledema, a distinctly uncommon finding with bacterial meningitis, occurs with brain abscess when cranial sutures have closed. Multiple abscesses can occur, especially with cyanotic congenital heart disease [Basit et al., 1989]. The differential diagnosis includes neoplasm, subdural hematoma, and focal encephalitis such as herpes simplex. Brain abscess is rare before 2 years of age [Daniels et al., 1985].

CSF examination

Lumbar puncture should be avoided in brain abscess because of the risk of herniation secondary to elevated intracranial pressure. Patients with brain abscess have died shortly after lumbar puncture [Saez-Llorens et al., 1989]. When the diagnosis is difficult to establish and imaging does not suggest increased intracranial pressure or displacement of intracranial contents, lumbar puncture can be considered.

The CSF is typically under increased pressure. It may be normal or have a mild lymphocytic or polymorphonuclear pleocytosis, elevation of protein level, and normal glucose content. Gram stain is usually negative, and organisms are seldom identified on culture unless the abscess has ruptured into the subarachnoid space.

Management

Anaerobic bacteria are found in 70% of brain abscesses. Multiple organisms may be present. *Streptococcus* species, *Staphylococcus* species, and *Bacteroides fragilis* are common bacteria. In the neonate the offending pathogen is often the *Proteus* organism. Surgical drainage or excision and appropriate antibiotics are the traditional treatments of choice [Stephanov, 1988]. Surgery provides an opportunity to culture the organism and promotes healing.

Before identification of the organism, antibiotics appropriate for the suspected cause of infection should be administered [Saez-Llorens et al., 1989]. Antibiotics such as penicillin, cefotaxime, and metronidazole can be used in empiric therapy. Brain abscesses have been cured by antibiotics alone without surgical drainage [Berg et al., 1978; Wong et al., 1989]. Medical management with or without needle aspiration should be considered when abscess formation is still in the cerebritis stage, when there are multiple abscesses, or when the abscess is located in a critical area [Aebi et al., 1991]. Serial CT and MRI scans can be used to determine failure of medical therapy.

Increased intracranial pressure should be managed by hyperventilation, osmotic agents (e.g., mannitol), steroids (e.g., dexamethasone), and surgical drainage.

Prognosis

Because of difficulty in the diagnosis and management of brain abscess, mortality is high and sequelae are frequent [Fischer et al., 1981; Saez-Llorens et al., 1989]. Imaging enables improved monitoring of brain abscess and may reduce morbidity and mortality. The outlook is especially poor when multiple abscesses are present [Basit et al., 1989] and when the patient is younger than 1 year of age [Wong et al., 1989]. Contrary to bacterial meningitis, chronic seizure disorders are common after abscesses [Hedge et al., 1986].

CRANIAL EPIDURAL ABSCESS

Cranial epidural abscess is rare in childhood. *Epidural* and *extradural abscess* are interchangeable terms. The condition is a collection of pus between the dura and overlying bone, is usually a complication of trauma or spread of infection from contiguous structures, and has been described after fetal monitoring [Listinsky et al., 1986]. The infection may spread into the subdural space. *S. aureus, S. epidermidis,* streptococci, and *B. fragilis* are some of the organisms found. Symptoms include fever, severe overlying headache, focal seizures, and focal neurologic deficits such as hemiparesis. Papilledema may develop [Smith and Hendrick, 1983]. The abscess acts as an enlarging mass. Progression of symptoms may be rapid, and the condition should be approached as an emergency. Lumbar puncture is probably contraindicated.

Imaging usually demonstrates a lenticular collection of fluid between the bone and CNS. MRI is preferred to CT scanning [Weingarten et al., 1989]. Treatment consists of antibiotics, surgical drainage, and management of increased intracranial pressure [Silverberg and DiNubile, 1985]. Delay in diagnosis and treatment results in an unfavorable outcome.

NEONATAL BACTERIAL MENINGITIS

Bacterial meningitis occurring at birth and during the first several weeks of life presents a special problem.

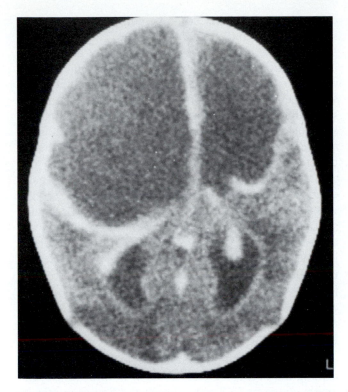

Figure 38-15 Enhanced CT scan taken 2 weeks after onset of *E. coli* meningitis in a neonate. Profound loss of brain parenchyma occurred in frontal regions with ventriculomegaly and cortical or leptomeningeal enhancement.

Predisposing factors include maternal infection, premature rupture of maternal membranes, prolonged labor, obstetric trauma, and fetal distress [Berman and Banker, 1966].

Pathology

Ventriculitis and vasculitis are prominent features of neonatal meningitis. Infarction, hydrocephalus, and multicystic encephalomalacia are common (Figure 38-15 and 38-16) [Brown et al., 1979; Friede, 1973; Ment et al., 1986]. Extraaxial fluid collections are infrequent. In some cases the ventricular enlargement is hydrocephalus ex vacuo, representing loss of brain parenchyma rather than increased intracranial pressure. Meningitis in the neonate may lead to subsequent disorganization of neural development with abnormal synaptogenesis, abnormal dendritic arborization, and aberrant myelination [Averill et al., 1976].

Pathogenesis

Bacteria penetrate easily into an immature brain. The causative organisms of meningitis in the young infant may be more virulent, and the infant's resistance less effective. The more immature the brain, the more destructive the infection. Bacterial meningitis is usually acquired after rupture of maternal membranes and

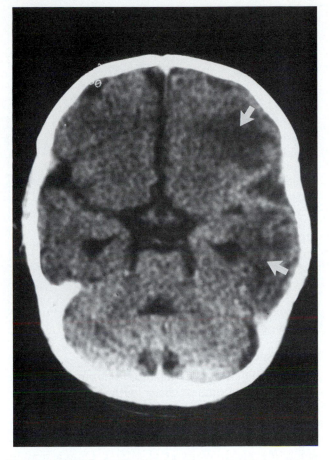

Figure 38-16 Group B streptococcus meningitis in a 15-day-old newborn. CT was done with contrast. Focal attenuation of left frontal region extending into left temporal lobe *(arrows)*. Infarction/necrosis suspected.

during the course of labor and delivery. The neonate has deficits that increase the risk of bacterial meningitis, including impaired nonspecific immunity with defects in leukocyte chemotaxis, phagocytosis, and bactericidal activity. Immunoglobulin M antibodies, which are important in defense against gram-negative organisms, are not transferred across the placenta. A relative deficiency of complement may occur [Wilson, 1986]. Ventilators, aerosols, and arterial and intravenous lines increase the risk of sepsis and subsequent meningitis [Volpe, 1987].

Clinical characteristics

The traditional clinical signs of meningitis are usually absent in the neonate. Nuchal rigidity rarely occurs, and fever and full fontanel may not be present; associated sepsis is common. Bacterial meningitis should be considered in any newborn who fails to thrive and has irritability, apnea, seizures, a tendency for opisthotonus, poor feeding, emesis, hypothermia or hyperthermia, hypotonia or hypertonia, a gray appearance, jaundice, or

---

Signs and Symptoms of Neonatal Meningitis

Failure to thrive
Irritability
Apnea
Seizures
Hypotonia
Hypertonia
Sepsis
Opisthotonus
Poor feeding
Emesis
Hypothermia
Hyperthermia
Gray appearance
Jaundice

---

other evidence of sepsis (see box above). Apnea may be the only sign.

CSF examination

Lumbar puncture is often part of the routine work-up of symptom-free infants born with risk factors for neonatal infection, although benefit has not been demonstrated [Fielkow et al., 1991]. Lumbar puncture in preterm infants with respiratory distress has an extremely low yield [Weiss et al., 1991]. Only a limited amount of CSF should be removed from a neonate. Significant hypoxemia occurs during the handling of sick preterm infants for routine procedures [Schwersenski et al., 1991]. Severe cardiopulmonary symptoms are a contraindication to lumbar puncture.

Normal CSF values for premature and term neonates must be considered when the presence of meningitis is evaluated. Normal CSF pressure in a neonate is lower than in older children [Kaiser and Whitelaw, 1986]. Blood-tinged CSF may occur in an infant after vaginal delivery. Up to 15 leukocytes/mm^3 in the CSF are considered normal in the newborn. However, it is unusual for more than several polymorphonuclear cells to be present. The number of cells gradually decreases during the first several months of life. A protein concentration as high as 150 mg/dl has been present in the CSF of normal premature and term newborns. The protein value also progressively declines during the first several months of life. Small newborns frequently have low blood glucose levels and thus low CSF glucose levels [Portnoy and Olson, 1985; Sarff et al., 1976].

Antibiotic management

The meningitis may be virulent with an unfavorable outcome, regardless of management. The organisms that predominate in neonatal meningitis are from the mother's vaginal or perineal flora, including *E. coli,* group B streptococcus, and *L. monocytogenes* (Figure 38-17). Initial antibiotic therapy usually consists of administering ampicillin or ceftriaxone, both accompanied by an aminoglycoside [Tessin et al., 1991]. The aminoglycosides include gentamycin, amikacin, and kanamycin. Penicillin G or ampicillin is appropriate for group B streptococcus, and ampicillin is appropriate for *L. monocytogenes.* Ceftriaxone has a broad spectrum of effectiveness, penetrates well into the CSF, is safe and well tolerated in the neonate, and appears to be the most effective of the cephalosporins [Mulhall et al., 1985]. Resistant organisms may be a problem when cephalosporins are used routinely. The value of intrathecal aminoglycoside is uncertain. At least 2 weeks of therapy is indicated [Gandy and Rennie, 1990]. Care in dosing must be exercised for very low–birth-weight infants [Prober et al., 1990]. Appropriate sources should be consulted for current advice [Peter et al., 1991].

Prognosis

Both morbidity and mortality are high in neonatal meningitis. In a review of group B streptococcal meningitis occurring in infants during the first 6 months of life, 27% died [Wald et al., 1986]. Significant deficits occur in many survivors.

MYCOPLASMA INFECTIONS
Tuberculosis

Tuberculosis of the lungs is more common than tuberculosis of the CNS. However, the form that affects the CNS is more dangerous. The incidence of tuberculous meningitis reflects the prevalence of tuberculosis in the community, which is related to socioeconomic and hygienic conditions. Blacks are more readily infected than whites [Stead et al., 1990]. Tuberculous meningitis is rare before 3 months of age, but the incidence is high in the first 5 years of life. In the United States the number of new cases of tuberculosis has increased 16% annually since 1985, and the increase has been predominantly among children, young adults, racial and ethnic minorities, and immigrants and refugees [Snider et al., 1992]. Organisms resistant to traditional therapy are becoming a problem. Tuberculosis research and control measures are receiving a low priority [Smith, 1992].

Pathology. Tuberculosis of the CNS follows a primary infection elsewhere in the body and may follow late reactivation tuberculosis [Leonard and Des Prez, 1990]. The major pathologic effect of tuberculous meningitis is on the basal meninges, although involvement of the brain parenchyma is encountered. A thick exudate surrounds vessels and cranial nerves. Vasculitis with thrombosis is a prominent feature. Cerebral infarcts are probably more common with tuberculous meningitis

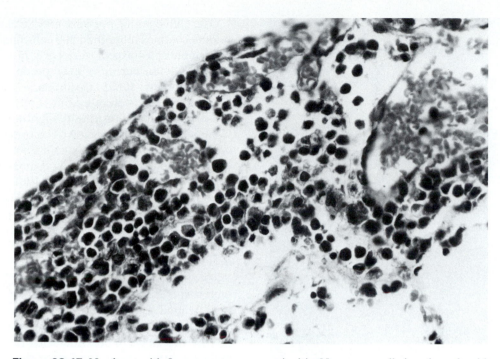

Figure 38-17 Newborn with *L. monocytogenes* meningitis. Numerous cells in subarachnoid space are predominantly large mononuclears. Original magnification ×100. (Reduced to 70%.) (Courtesy Dr. Mario Kornfeld, Albuquerque, NM.)

than with other forms of bacterial meningitis. Cranial nerve palsies occur. Hydrocephalus develops, especially if the disease has been present for a prolonged time. Tuberculomas may arise within the CNS [Bell and McCormick, 1981].

Pathogenesis. Hematogenous spread of tuberculosis emanates from a primary focus. Tuberculous meningitis is not necessarily associated with miliary tuberculosis. A caseous focus in the subarachnoid space is the initial CNS finding. A subsequent discharge of organisms occurs with the development of meningitis. The accompanying inflammation may be in part an immune reaction [Molavi and LeFrock, 1985].

Clinical characteristics. Tuberculous meningitis is usually considered a chronic meningitis, although an acute onset occurs in about half of affected children. Initial symptoms are vague and consist of several weeks of generally poor health followed by alteration of consciousness, irritability, and apathy. Nuchal rigidity is not prominent. Low-grade fever, nausea, vomiting, headache, and abdominal pain occur. Gastrointestinal symptoms may be more severe than neurologic symptoms. Cranial nerve deficits result from the basilar meningitis [Lincoln et al., 1960]. Cranial nerve VI is the most frequently involved nerve. Cranial nerve palsies may be unilateral or bilateral. Tuberculous lesions occur in the choroid of the eye. Tremor and movement disorders have been reported [Udani et al., 1971]. As the disease progresses, the patient develops depression of

Signs and Symptoms of Tuberculous Meningitis
Subacute course
Alteration of consciousness
Irritability
Headache
Apathy
Seizures
Generally poor health
Low-grade fever
Nausea/vomiting
Abdominal pain
Cranial nerve deficits

consciousness, convulsions, possibly papilledema, and major neurologic deficits (see box above). Tuberculosis can involve the spinal cord directly and by pressure from adjacent involved bone, disk space, and soft tissues, especially in the lower thoracic region. Arachnoiditis and spinal block may ensue from involvement of the spinal subarachnoid space [Leonard and Des Prez, 1990].

EEG is slow, and epileptiform features may be present. Cranial CT and MRI scans document findings similar to those of bacterial meningitis, especially around the base of the brain, and may reveal parenchymal lesions, infarction, and tuberculomas [Curless and

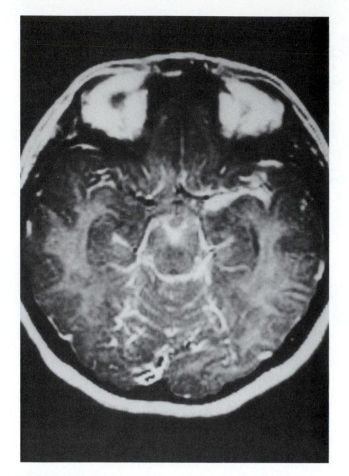

Figure 38-18 Tuberculous meningitis. Gadolinium enhanced T_1 weighted axial image revealing diffuse enhancement of meningitis. (Courtesy Dr. J. Randy Jinkins, San Antonio, TX.)

Mitchell, 1991; Jinkins, 1991; Offenbacher et al., 1991] (Figure 38-18). Hydrocephalus is common on imaging [Waecker and Connor, 1990]. Imaging is essential in the diagnosis of spinal involvement. Myelography, CT, or MRI of the spine is indicated in a child with suspected tuberculosis and neurologic signs of cord involvement. Cranial angiography discloses constricted vessels about the base of the brain [Matthew et al., 1970]. An intracranial tuberculoma can produce a mass effect. Intracranial tuberculomas, which used to be the most common cause of posterior fossa tumor in children, have become rare in the United States but not elsewhere.

Many children with tuberculous meningitis have radiographic evidence of pulmonary tuberculosis [Waecker and Connor, 1990], but a normal chest radiograph does not exclude tuberculous neurologic involvement. Likewise, a negative tuberculin skin test does not exclude tuberculous meningitis. A history of close contact with a known patient with tuberculosis is an important finding.

The CSF opening pressure may be elevated. The CSF seldom contains more than 500 cells/mm³, most of which are lymphocytes except very early in the disease when polymorphonuclear cells may predominate [Stockstill and Kauffman, 1983]. Eosinophiles may be present. Protein content is elevated but rarely above 500 mg/dl. Glucose concentration may be slightly low [Waecker and Connor, 1990]. A depression of chloride level is nonspecific and has no diagnostic significance. Acid-fast bacilli can be demonstrated in CSF, and tubercle bacilli can be isolated. However, smears and cultures are not positive in all patients [Lincoln et al., 1960]. Rapid tests for the detection of tuberculous meningitis by polymerase chain reaction are being developed [Kaneko et al., 1990; Shankar et al., 1991]. Repeated CSF studies may be necessary to establish the diagnosis.

The syndrome of inappropriate antidiuretic hormone secretion is frequently found in tuberculous meningitis of childhood [Cotton et al., 1991].

Management. Isoniazid, rifampin, and pyrazinamide are the mainstays of treatment for tuberculous meningitis. Intensive initial therapy with multiple drugs is appropriate [Starke, 1990]. Therapy should be continued for at least 9 months, perhaps longer [Kendig, 1985]. In severely ill patients, ethambutol or streptomycin is added, at least for the first several months. Modifications in therapy need to be made when resistant organisms occur [Peter et al., 1991]. Therapeutic response is usually evident within 2 weeks [Nemir and Krasinski, 1988; Snider et al., 1988]. Early treatment of pulmonary tuberculosis in children reduces the incidence of CNS infection [Nemir and O'Hare, 1991]. Resistant strains are appearing.

Use of corticosteroids to reduce the morbidity from inflammation and fibroblastic proliferation remains controversial. Prednisone is often administered for 2 to 3 weeks, followed by gradual discontinuation. Dexamethasone has been reported to reduce complications and improve outcome [Girgis et al., 1991]. Pyridoxine has been added to the treatment regimen for adults to prevent the peripheral neuropathy that isoniazid may induce but does not appear necessary in the treatment of infants and children. Spontaneous recovery has been reported [Emond and McKendrick, 1973]. Surgical shunting procedures may be necessary for hydrocephalus. Failing vision may be improved by microsurgery to lyse adhesions around the optic nerves.

Prognosis. The mortality in tuberculous meningitis is 10% to 20%. Major sequelae occur; visual and auditory impairments are common, as are hemiparesis, mental retardation, and seizures. Involvement of the hypothalamus and basal cisterns leads to endocrinopathies such as diabetes insipidus, growth retardation, sexual precocity, and obesity.

Mycoplasma pneumoniae meningitis

Although *M. pneumoniae* infection is usually restricted to the lungs, the organism can be associated with neurologic disease in children. Symptoms include meningitis, postinfectious leukoencephalopathy, cerebritis, transverse myelitis, and radiculitis of cranial or spinal nerve roots [Heller et al., 1990; Nara et al., 1987]. An ascending paralysis similar to Guillain-Barré syndrome can occur. The diagnosis of *M. pneumoniae* infection is made by culture of the organism from a site remote from the nervous system, usually the lung, or by serology. Involvement of the nervous system is indirect and may be immune mediated or related to a neurotoxin [Carstensen and Nilsson, 1987; Clyde, 1980]. A CSF mononuclear pleocytosis may occur, with normal CSF glucose and elevated protein levels. Albuminocytologic dissociation is present when the clinical picture resembles Guillain-Barré syndrome. The organism is seldom isolated from the CSF. Diagnosis is established by a rise in the serum complement fixation titer. Antimicrobial therapy has not been successful. Recovery is prolonged, and permanent deficits are common [Carstensen and Nilsson, 1987].

Leprosy

Leprosy (Hansen disease) is a major health problem in many parts of the world. Air travel and immigration from endemic areas increase the likelihood that physicians in the United States and other developed countries will encounter the disease [Younger et al., 1982]. Leprosy is caused by *Mycobacterium leprae,* and children appear more susceptible than adults. Genetics play a part in susceptibility. The disease is systemic, but the major clinical involvement is in the peripheral nerves and skin. The organism is acquired from the environment. The incubation period ranges from several months to several years. The condition is probably the largest cause of peripheral nerve disorder in the world [Dastur, 1978]. The immune system plays an important role in the course of the disease.

The cardinal symptom is sensory loss, which occurs before other symptoms of the disease and may not be disturbing to the patient. The loss may be discovered when a painless injury occurs. Complaints of paresthesias or pain occur. Objective testing reveals an early decrease in awareness of pain and temperature. Motor and sensory nerve conductions are slow in involved and uninvolved nerves [Sabin and Swift, 1984].

The lesions take two forms: lepromatous and tuberculoid leprosy. In both forms the disease begins in Schwann cells; intermediate forms occur. Lepromatous leprosy is characterized by diffuse or focal lesions of skin and mucous membranes with associated progressive symmetric peripheral neuropathy. Whether the neuropathy is a "dying-back" phenomenon or related to skin temperature is unknown [Crawford, 1988; Sabin, 1988].

Thickening of facial skin leads to the "leonine" facies. There is loss of axons and myelin with swelling of Schwann cells that contain organisms. These patients have low resistance to leprosy. The lepromin skin test is negative.

Tuberculoid leprosy is the form common in children. The cutaneous lesions are small and plaquelike. The peripheral nerves are enlarged, especially the greater auricular nerve. Individual nerves are affected asymmetrically, and involved areas are insensitive. Granulomas occur on nerves that do not contain organisms. Tuberculoid leprosy is more slowly progressive and less disfiguring and has a favorable prognosis. The lepromin skin test is positive. Although the organism can be stained, it cannot be cultured. Treatment consists of administration of dapsone, clofazimine, and rifampin [Peter et al., 1991]. Appropriate sources should be consulted for current recommendations.

SPIROCHETE INFECTIONS

Syphilis

Syphilis is caused by the spirochete *Treponema pallidum.* Congenital cases appear in infancy and childhood, and acquired cases manifest during childhood and adolescence. A worldwide resurgence of syphilis is occurring in epidemic proportions, and additional congenital cases have been reported [McIntosh, 1990]. Fewer than 60 cases of congenital syphilis per year were reported in New York City between 1980 and 1986; 1017 cases were reported in 1989 [Greenberg et al., 1991].

Pathology. In congenital syphilis the infecting organism becomes disseminated to all tissues. An inflammatory response of small lymphocytes and plasma cells occurs. The viscera may become enlarged, and the skeleton is involved. When the nervous system is affected, an intense inflammatory pachymeningitis and involvement of the intracranial blood vessels and cranial nerves are present. The meningitis is usually basilar. The inflamed areas contain organisms. Perivascular infiltration with lymphocytes, thrombosis of vessels traversing inflamed areas with resultant infarction, and subsequent fibrosis are also noted. The CSF pathways may become obliterated, leading to hydrocephalus [Bell and McCormick, 1981].

Pathogenesis. Congenital syphilis and late congenital syphilis are acquired by transplacental transmission from an infected mother. Maternal infection has usually been present for less than 2 years and may be so recent that maternal serology is negative [McIntosh, 1990]. The fetus does not acquire the infection before the fifth month of gestation. Treatment of the pregnant mother can cure the infection in the fetus but may not prevent the appearance of some syphilitic stigmata if treatment is undertaken late in the pregnancy. The organism can usually be recovered from the skin and mucous membrane lesions. Acquired syphilis develops from venereal contact.

Clinical characteristics. In infants and children, three forms of syphilis occur: congenital, late congenital, and acquired. Infants with congenital syphilis appear to be normal at birth but are often small for gestational age [Mascola et al., 1985]. Clinical findings are present within several weeks of birth or may be delayed until stigmata of late congenital syphilis appear in subsequent years. Early findings include skin and mucous membrane lesions, which are found in one third to one half of the infants [Tunnessen, 1992]. Rhinitis and fissures about the mouth and anus may be present. Osteochondritis occurs, and bones are tender. Irritability and pain on movement are present. Chorioretinitis is common. Hepatosplenomegaly and edema may be present. Clinical signs of neurosyphilis are rare in the neonate, although CNS involvement is common [Robinson, 1969]. Congenital syphilis should be considered in any infant with failure to thrive, hepatosplenomegaly, and a symmetric rash [Ewing et al., 1985].

In late congenital syphilis, clinical findings do not appear until several years of age, even though the infection was acquired in utero. Interstitial keratitis occurs after 4 years of age. Both eyes are usually involved. Bone lesions result in destruction of the palate and nasal septum, with resultant loss of support and depression of the nose (saddle nose). Scars appear about the mouth from earlier fissures (rhagades). The tibia may become bowed (saber shins), and the knee joint can be affected with hydraarthrosis (Clutton joints). Nerve deafness is common after the age of 8 years. Permanent dentition is abnormal, especially the upper central incisors, which are dwarfed and notched (Hutchinson teeth), and the first lower molars, which have poorly developed cusps (mulberry molars). Hutchinson triad consists of Hutchinson teeth, interstitial keratitis, and nerve deafness [Fiumara and Lessell, 1970]. Meningovascular involvement leads to findings of chronic meningoencephalitis such as intellectual decline (juvenile paresis), which may begin as early as 4 to 5 years of age; headache; seizures; blindness; deafness; other cranial nerve involvement; hemiparesis; and hydrocephalus.

Acquired syphilis, which resembles the disease in adults, can occur in children and adolescents. The primary stage with chancre appears 2 to 4 weeks after exposure. The cutaneous eruption of the second stage appears several months later and may be complicated by meningitis. When the condition is not treated, the tertiary stage of neurosyphilis may occur after a prolonged asymptomatic period. Tabes is rare in adolescents.

A serologic test is indicated in the mother and child whenever syphilis is suspected [Rawstron and Bromberg, 1991]. Congenital syphilis can occur when both mother and infant are seronegative [Dorfman and Glaser, 1990]. The serologic test may be negative in a newborn if the mother acquired the disease late in pregnancy. Passive transfer of maternal antibodies can result in a positive test in an unaffected newborn. Dark-field microscopic examination identifies organisms from lesions. Radiographs of the long bones are indicated [Zenker and Berman, 1991].

CSF examination. In asymptomatic congenital syphilis and meningovascular syphilis the CSF has increased cells, elevated protein levels, and positive serologic findings for syphilis. Venereal Disease Research Laboratory test is a common test for the antibody. The organism cannot be recovered from the CSF except under special circumstances. The rapid plasma reagin (RPR) has become the screening test of choice in many laboratories. CSF abnormalities diagnostic of neurosyphilis in the newborn have not been well defined [Lane and Oates, 1988].

Management. Penicillin is the treatment for all clinical forms of syphilis and for pregnant women with untreated disease unless allergy to the drug is present. For neonates with congenital syphilis, crystalline penicillin is recommended [Zenker and Berman, 1991]. Herxheimer reaction may occur at the start of treatment.

Lyme disease

Lyme disease is caused by tick transmission of the Lyme spirochete, *Borrelia burgdorferi*. A large number of affected individuals are children [Bruhn, 1984]. The disease occurs during summer. Neurologic findings may be caused by direct effect of the organism or an immune response [Sigal and Tatum, 1988]. The first stage consists of fluctuating headache, myalgia, and erythema chronicum migranes. Neurologic manifestations (Bannwarth syndrome) occur in the second stage, which begins about 4 weeks after onset, and are not present in all patients. A triad of neurologic manifestations consisting of meningitis, cranial neuritis, and radiculoneuritis provides a unique clinical picture. Not all patients have the complete triad [Pachner et al., 1989]. Headache, stiff neck, encephalitis, cranial nerve palsies (especially Bell palsy or bilateral facial palsy), and peripheral nervous system abnormalities, including radiculoneuritis and mononeuritis multiplex, may be present. Pseudotumor cerebri has been reported in children [Raucher et al., 1985]. A chronic meningoencephalitis has been noted in adults and children with lesions similar to multiple sclerosis on brain imaging [Feder et al., 1988; Kohler et al., 1988]. A chronic peripheral neuropathy with onset many months after the erythema has been reported in adults [Logigian and Steere, 1992]. *Borrelia burgdorferi* has been isolated from the spinal fluid of children with aseptic meningitis [Huppertz and Sticht-Groh, 1989].

Neurologic abnormalities persist for several months and on rare occasions persist for years if untreated with antibiotics. The appearance of neurologic symptoms may be delayed for more than a year and may be related to chronic infection or an immune response [Steere, 1989]. Arthritis occurs in the third stage, is the last manifestation of the illness, and overlaps neurologic symptoms.

Isolation of the organism establishes the diagnosis. Although serologic testing is not well standardized, antibody against the Lyme spirochete can be detected [Eichenfield and Athreya, 1989]. CSF may be normal or have lymphocytic pleocytosis and elevated protein levels several weeks after the onset of the first stage. In early stages of the disease, tetracycline, doxycycline, amoxicillin, penicillin V, and erythromycin have been recommended; in the late stage with CNS or peripheral nervous system involvement, ceftriaxone is probably the treatment of choice [Kahn and Malawista, 1991; Peter et al., 1991].

Leptospirosis

Leptospirosis, an infection caused by the *Leptospira* spirochete, rarely has neurologic manifestations. The organism is shed in the urine of animals and enters the human through the skin. The incubation period is 2 to 28 days. The first clinical phase, which is associated with leptospiremia, is the abrupt onset of headache, fever, myalgia, and conjunctivitis. These symptoms last several days. At the end of the first phase a fever-free interval of several days occurs, followed by the second phase. The liver, kidney, and nervous system may be involved. Nervous system involvement takes the form of meningitis, encephalitis, or neuritis. When neuritis occurs, the brachial plexus or cranial nerves are involved. Meningitis and encephalitis may become chronic. Leptospirosis should be considered in the differential diagnosis of aseptic meningitis.

There is pleocytosis in the CSF, first with polymorphonuclear cells and then with lymphocytes, elevated protein levels, and normal glucose content. The organism can be isolated from blood, urine, or CSF using special techniques. CSF becomes sterile in the second phase. A rise in the serum titer against leptospirosis establishes the diagnosis.

Penicillin is the treatment of choice, but its effectiveness has not been confirmed. A Herxheimer reaction may occur on initiation of therapy. Recovery usually follows unless the illness has been predominantly encephalitis. The disease is in part an immune response, at least in the second phase [Sanford, 1984].

REFERENCES

Aebi C, Kaufmann F, Schaad UB. Brain abscess in childhood — long-term experiences. Eur J Pediatr 1991; 150:282.

Annegers JF, Hauser WA, Beghi E, et al. The risk of unprovoked seizures after encephalitis and meningitis. Neurology 1988; 38:1407.

Arditi M, Ables L, Yogev R. Cerebrospinal fluid endotoxin levels in children with *H. influenzae* meningitis before and after administration of intravenous ceftriaxone. J Infect Dis 1989; 160:1005.

Arditi M, Manogue KR, Caplan M, et al. Cerebrospinal fluid cachectin/tumor necrosis factor-alpha and platelet-activating factor concentrations and severity of bacterial meningitis in children. J Infect Dis 1990; 162:139.

Ashwal S, Stringer W, Tomasi L, et al. Cerebral blood flow and carbon dioxide reactivity in children with bacterial meningitis. J Pediatr 1990; 117:523.

Aucoin PJ, Kotilainen HR, Gantz NM, et al. Intracranial pressure monitors: epidemiologic study of risk factors and infections. Am J Med 1986; 80:369.

Averill DR, Moxon ER, Smith AL. Effects of *Hemophilus influenzae* meningitis in infant rats on neuronal growth and synaptogenesis. Exp Neurol 1976; 50:337.

Baker RC, Lenane AM. The predictive value of cerebrospinal fluid differential cytology in meningitis. Pediatr Infect Dis J 1989; 8:229.

Basit AS, Ravi B, Banerji AK, et al. Multiple pyogenic brain abscesses: an analysis of 21 patients. J Neurol Neurosurg Psychiatry 1989; 52:591.

Bell WE. Current therapy of acute bacterial meningitis in children, part I. Pediatr Neurol 1985; 1:5.

Bell WE, McCormick WF. Neurologic infections in children, 2nd ed. Philadelphia: WB Saunders, 1981.

Benjamin CM, Newton RW, Clarke MA. Risk factors for death from meningitis. Br Med J 1988; 296:20.

Benson P, Nyhan WL, Shimizu H. The prognosis of subdural effusions complicating pyogenic meningitis. J Pediatr 1960; 57:670.

Berg B, Franklin G, Cuneo R, et al. Non-surgical cure of brain abscess: early diagnosis and follow-up with computerized tomography. Ann Neurol 1978; 3:474.

Berman RH, Banker BQ. Neonatal meningitis: a clinical and pathological study of 29 cases. Pediatrics 1966; 38:6.

Bijlmer HA. World-wide epidemiology of *Haemophilus influenzae* meningitis: industrialized versus non-industrialized countries. Vaccine 1991; 9:S5.

Bodino J, Lylyk P, Del Valle M, et al. Computed tomography in purulent meningitis. Am J Dis Child 1982; 136:495.

Bonadio WA. How rapidly is cerebrospinal fluid pleocytosis manifested with bacterial meningitis? Pediatr Infect Dis J 1989; 8:337.

Bonadio WA, Smith D. Cerebrospinal fluid changes after 48 hours of effective therapy for *Hemophilus influenzae* type b meningitis. Am J Clin Pathol 1990; 94:426.

Bonadio WA, Smith DS, Goddard S, et al. Distinguishing cerebrospinal fluid abnormalities in children with bacterial meningitis and traumatic lumbar puncture. J Infect Dis 1990; 162:251.

Bonadio WA, Smith DS, Metrou M, et al. Estimating lumbar-puncture depth in children. N Engl J Med 1988; 319:952.

Booy R, Moxon ER. Immunization of infants against *Haemophilus influenzae* type b in the UK. Arch Dis Child 1991; 66:1251.

Borkowski WJ, Goldgar DE, Gorga MP, et al. Cerebrospinal fluid parameters and auditory brainstem responses following meningitis. Pediatr Neurol 1985; 1:134.

Broome CV. Epidemiology of *Haemophilus influenzae* type b infections in the United States. Pediatr Infect Dis J 1987; 6:779.

Brown LW, Zimmerman RA, Bilaniuk LT. Polycystic brain disease complicating neonatal meningitis: documentation of evolution by computed tomography. J Pediatr 1979; 94:757.

Bruhn FW. Lyme disease. Am J Dis Child 1984; 138:467.

Burstein L, Breningstall GN. Movement disorders in bacterial meningitis. J Pediatr 1986; 109:260.

Carstensen H, Nilsson K-O. Neurological complications associated with *Mycoplasma pneumoniae* infection in children. Neuropediatrics 1987; 18:57.

Chartrand SA, Cho CT. Persistent pleocytosis in bacterial meningitis. J Pediatr 1976; 88:424.

Chu MLY, Litman N, Kaufman DM, et al. Cranial nerve palsies in *Streptococcus pneumoniae* meningitis. Pediatr Neurol 1990; 6:209.

Clyde WA. Neurologic syndromes and mycoplasmal infections. Arch Neurol 1980; 37:65.

Cohen BA, Schenk VA, Sweeney DB. Meningitis-related hearing loss evaluated with evoked potentials. Pediatr Neurol 1990; 4:18.

Converse GM, Gwaltney JM Jr., Staussburg DA, et al. Alteration of cerebrospinal fluid findings by partial treatment of bacterial meningitis. J Pediatr 1973; 83:220.

Cotton MF, Donald PR, Schoeman JF, et al. Plasma arginine vasopressin and the syndrome of inappropriate antidiuretic hormone secretion in tuberculous meningitis. Pediatr Infect Dis J 1991; 10:837.

Crawford CL. Nature of the sensory loss in leprosy. Muscle Nerve 1988; 11:276.

Curless RG, Mitchell CD. Central nervous system tuberculosis in children. Pediatr Neurol 1991; 7:270.

Daniels SR, Price JK, Towbin RB, et al. Nonsurgical cure of brain abscess in a neonate. Childs Nerv Syst 1985; 1:346.

Daoud AS, Al-Saleh QA. Prolonged and secondary fever in childhood bacterial meningitis. Eur J Pediatr 1989; 149:114.

Dastur DK. Leprosy. In: Vinken PJ, Bruyn GW, eds. Handbook of clinical neurology, vol 33. Amsterdam: North Holland, 1978.

Dodge PR, Davis H, Feigin RD, et al. Prospective evaluation of hearing impairment as a sequelae of acute bacterial meningitis. N Engl J Med 1984; 311:869.

Dorfman DH, Glaser JH. Congenital syphilis presenting in infants after the newborn period. N Engl J Med 1990; 323:1299.

Eichenfield AH, Athreya BH. Lyme disease: of ticks and titers. J Pediatr 1989; 114:328.

Emond RTD, McKendrick GDW. Tuberculosis as a cause of transient aseptic meningitis. Lancet 1973; 2:234.

Ewing CI, Roberts C, Davidson DC, et al. Early congenital syphilis still occurs. Arch Dis Child 1985; 60:1128.

Feder HM, Zalneraitis EL, Reik L. Lyme disease: acute focal meningoencephalitis in a child. Pediatrics 1988; 82:931.

Feigin RD, Shackelford PG. Value of repeat lumbar puncture in the differential diagnosis of meningitis. N Engl J Med 1973; 289:571.

Feigin RD, Shearer WT. Prospective evaluation of treatment of *Haemophilus influenzae* meningitis. J Pediatr 1976; 88:542.

Feldman WE. Relation of concentration of bacteria and bacterial antigen in cerebrospinal fluid to prognosis in patients with bacterial meningitis. N Engl J Med 1977; 296:433.

Fielkow S, Reuter S, Gotoff SP. Cerebrospinal fluid examination in symptom-free infants with risk factors for infection. J Pediatr 1991; 119:971.

Finch RG, Mandragos C. Corticosteroids in bacterial meningitis: not yet justified for all patients. Br Med J 1991; 302:607.

Fischer EG, McLennan JE, Suzuki Y. Cerebral abscess in children. Am J Dis Child 1981; 135:746.

Fishman RA. Brain edema. N Engl J Med 1975; 293:706.

Fiumara NJ, Lessell S. Manifestations of late congenital syphilis. Arch Dermatol 1970; 102:78.

Friede RL. Cerebral infarcts complicating neonatal leptomeningitis. Acta Neuropathol 1973; 23:245.

Gado M, Axley J, Appleton DB, et al. Angiography in the acute and post-treatment phases of *Hemophilus influenzae* meningitis. Radiology 1973; 110:439.

Gandy G, Rennie J. Antibiotic treatment of suspected neonatal meningitis. Arch Dis Child 1990; 65:1.

Gary N, Powers N, Todd JK. Clinical identification and comparative prognosis of high-risk patients with *Haemophilus influenzae* meningitis. Am J Dis Child 1989; 143:307.

Girgis NI, Faird Z, Kilpatrick ME, et al. Dexamethasone adjunctive treatment for tuberculous meningitis. Pediatr Infect Dis J 1991; 10:179.

Girgis NI, Farid Z, Mikhail IA, et al. Dexamethasone treatment for bacterial meningitis in children and adults. Pediatr Infect Dis J 1989; 8:848.

Gold R. Duration of meningitis therapy. Pediatr Infect Dis J 1990; 9:457.

Granoff DM, McKinney T, Boies EG, et al. *Haemophilus influenzae* type b disease in an Amish population: studies of the effects of genetic factors, immunization, and rifampin prophylaxis on the course of an outbreak. Pediatrics 1986; 77:289.

Granoff DM, Squires JE. *Hemophilus* meningitis: new developments in epidemiology, treatment and prophylaxis. Semin Neurol 1982; 2:151.

Greenberg MS, Singh T, Htoo M, et al. The association between congenital syphilis and cocaine/crack use in New York City: a case-control study. Am J Public Health 1991; 81:1316.

Hanna JN, Wild BE. Bacterial meningitis in children under five years of age in western Australia. Med J Aust 1991; 155:160.

Haslam RHA. Role of computed tomography in the early management of bacterial meningitis. J Pediatr 1991; 119:157.

Haupt HM, Kurlinski JP, Barnett NK, et al. Infarction of the spinal cord as a complication of pneumococcus meningitis. J Neurosurg 1981; 55:121.

Havens PL, Wendelberger KJ, Hoffman GM. Corticosteroids as adjunctive therapy in bacterial meningitis. Am J Dis Child 1989; 143:1051.

Hawkins A, Gold R, Halperin SA, et al. Initial therapy for bacterial meningitis. Can Med Assoc J 1990; 142:305.

Hedge AS, Venkataramana NK, Das BS. Brain abscess in children. Childs Nerv Syst 1986; 2:90.

Heller L, Keren O, Mendelson L, et al. Transverse myelitis associated with *Mycoplasma pneumoniae*: case report. Paraplegia 1990; 28:522.

Hinds CJ. Monoclonal antibodies in sepsis and septic shock. Br Med J 1992; 304:132.

Holguin J, Manotas R. Recurrent purulent meningitis. Int Pediatr 1988; 3:175.

Horwitz SJ, Boxerbaum B, O'Bell J. Cerebral herniation in bacterial meningitis. Ann Neurol 1980; 7:524.

Hoyt M, McCracken GH. Lack of adverse effects of dexamethasone therapy in aseptic meningitis. Pediatr Infect Dis J 1990; 9:922.

Huppertz H-I, Sticht-Groh V. Meningitis due to *Borrelia burgdorferi* in the initial stage of Lyme disease. Eur J Pediatr 1989; 148:428.

Igarashi M, Gilmartin RC, Gerald B, et al. Cerebral arteritis and bacterial meningitis. Arch Neurol 1984; 41:531.

Jacobs RF. Summary of the symposium. Scand J Infect Dis 1990; 73:55.

Jacobs RF, Tabor DR. The immunology of sepsis and meningitis — cytokine biology. Scand J Infect Dis 1990; 73(suppl):7.

Jacobs RF, Darville T, Parks JA, et al. Safety profile and efficacy of cefotaxime for the treatment of hospitalized children. Clin Infect Dis 1992; 14:56.

Jadavji T, Biggar WD, Gold R, et al. Sequelae of acute bacterial meningitis in children treated for seven days. Pediatrics 1986; 78:21.

Jinkins JR. Computed tomography of intracranial tuberculosis. Neuroradiology 1991; 33:126.

Kahn DW, Malawista SE. Lyme disease: recommendations for diagnosis and treatment. Ann Intern Med 1991; 114:472.

Kaiser AM, Whitelaw AGL. Normal cerebrospinal fluid pressure in the newborn. Neuropediatrics 1986; 17:100.

Kaneko K, Onodera O, Miyatake T, et al. Rapid diagnosis of tuberculous meningitis by polymerase chain reaction (PCR). Neurology 1990; 40:1617.

Kaplan SL. Dexamethasone for children with bacterial meningitis. Am J Dis Child 1989; 143:290.

Kaplan SL. Corticosteroids in bacterial meningitis. Scand J Infect Dis 1990; 73(suppl):43.

Kay R. The site of the lesion causing hearing loss in bacterial meningitis: a study of experimental streptococcal meningitis in guinea pigs. Neuropathol Appl Neurobiol 1991; 17:485.

Kendig EL. Evolution of short-course antimicrobial treatment of tuberculosis in children, 1951-1984. Pediatrics 1985; 75:684.

Kennedy WA, Hoyt MJ, McCracken GH. The role of corticosteroid therapy in children with pneumococcal meningitis. Am J Dis Child 1991; 145:1374.

Kilpi T, Anttila M, Kallio MJ, et al. Severity of childhood bacterial meningitis and duration of illness before diagnosis. Lancet 1991; 338:406.

King SM, Read SE. Ataxia and hypotonia in *Haemophilus influenzae* type b meningitis. Pediatr Infect Dis J 1988; 7:140.

Kline MW. Review of recurrent bacterial meningitis. Pediatr Infect Dis J 1989; 8:630.

Kline MW, Kaplan SL. Computed tomography in bacterial meningitis of childhood. Pediatr Infect Dis J 1988; 7:855.

Kohler J, Kern U, Kasper J, et al. Chronic central nervous system involvement in Lyme borreliosis. Neurology 1988; 38:863.

Laine J, Holmberg C, Anttila M, et al. Types of fluid disorder in children with bacterial meningitis. Acta Paediatr Scand 1991; 80:1031.

Lane GK, Oates RK. Congenital syphilis has not disappeared. Med J Aust 1988; 148:171.

Laxer RM, Marks MI. Pneumococcal meningitis in children. Am J Dis Child 1977; 131:850.

Lebel MH, Freij BJ, Syrogiannopoulos GA, et al. Dexamethasone therapy for bacterial meningitis: results of 2 double-blind placebo-controlled trials. N Engl J Med 1988; 319:964.

Leonard JM, Des Prez RM. Tuberculous meningitis. Infect Dis Clin North Am 1990; 4:769.

Likitnukul S, McCracken GH, Nelson JD. Arthritis in children with bacterial meningitis. Am J Dis Child 1986; 140:424.

Lincoln E, Sordillo SVR, Davies PA. Tuberculous meningitis in children: a review of 167 untreated and 74 treated patients with special reference to early diagnosis. J Pediatr 1960; 57:807.

Listinsky JL, Wood BP, Ekholm SE. Parietal osteomyelitis and epidural abscess: a delayed complication of fetal monitoring. Pediatr Radiol 1986; 16:150.

Logigian EL, Steere AC. Clinical and electrophysiologic findings in chronic neuropathy of Lyme disease. Neurology 1992; 42:303.

Loh RKS, Thong YH, Ferrante A. Deficiency of IgG subclasses and IgA, and elevation of IgE in children with a past history of bacterial meningitis. Acta Paediatr 1991; 80:654.

Lynch J, Arhelger S, Krings-Ernst I. Post-dural puncture headache in young orthopaedic in-patients: comparison of a 0.33 mm (29-gauge) Quincke-type with a 0.7 mm (22-gauge) Whitacre spinal needle in 200 patients. Acta Anaesthesiol Scand 1992; 36:58.

Lyons EL, Leeds NE. The angiographic demonstration of arterial vascular disease in purulent meningitis. Radiology 1967; 88:935.

Maida E, Horvatis E. Cerebrospinal fluid alterations in bacterial meningitis. Eur Neurol 1986; 25:110.

Maniglia AJ, Goodwin WJ, Arnold JE, et al. Intracranial abscesses secondary to nasal, sinus, and orbital infections in adults and children. Arch Otolaryngol Head Neck Surg 1989; 115:1424.

Martin WJ. Rapid and reliable techniques for the laboratory detection of bacterial meningitis. Am J Med 1983; 75(suppl 1B):119.

Marton KI, Gean AD. The diagnostic spinal tap. Ann Intern Med 1986; 104:880.

Mascola L, Pelosi R, Blount JH, et al. Congenital syphilis revisited. Am J Dis Child 1985; 139:575.

Matthew NT, Abraham J, Chandy J. Cerebral angiographic features in tuberculous meningitis. Neurology 1970; 20:1015.

Mayatepek E, Grauer M, Sonntag HG. Deafness after meningococcal meningitis. Lancet 1991; 338:1331.

McCabe WR, Treadwell TL, DeMaria A. Pathophysiology of bacteremia. Am J Med 1983; 75(suppl 1B):7.

McCracken GH Jr. Management of bacterial meningitis: current status and future prospects. Am J Med 1984; 76(suppl 5A):215.

McCracken GH Jr., Mustafa MM, Ramilo O, et al. Cerebrospinal fluid interleukin 1-beta and tumor necrosis factor concentrations and outcome from neonatal Gram-negative enteric bacillary meningitis. Pediatr Infect Dis J 1989; 8:155.

McIntosh K. Congenital syphilis—breaking through the safety net. N Engl J Med 1990; 323:1339.

Menkes JH. The causes for low spinal fluid sugar in bacterial meningitis—another look. Pediatrics 1969; 44:1.

Ment LR, Ehrenkranz RA, Duncan CC. Bacterial meningitis as an etiology of perinatal cerebral infarction. Pediatr Neurol 1986; 2:276.

Molavi A, LeFrock JL. Tuberculous meningitis. Med Clin North Am 1985; 69:315.

Moxon ER. Virulence of genes and prevention of *Haemophilus influenzae* infections. Arch Dis Child 1985; 60:1193.

Mulhall A, de Louvois J, James J. Pharmacokinetics and safety of ceftriaxone in the neonate. Eur J Pediatr 1985; 144:379.

Munson RS, Kabeer MH, Lenoir AA. Epidemiology and prospects for prevention of disease due to *Haemophilus influenzae* in developing countries. Rev Infect Dis 1989; 11(suppl 2):S588.

Mustafa MM, Ramilo O, Saez-Llorens X, et al. Prostaglandins E2 and I2, interleukin 1-beta, and tumor necrosis factor in cerebrospinal fluid of infants and children with bacterial meningitis. Pediatr Infect Dis J 1989; 8:921.

Mustafa MM, Ramilo O, Saez-Llorens X, et al. Cerebrospinal fluid prostaglandins, interleukin 1B, and tumor necrosis factor in bacterial meningitis. Am J Dis Child 1990; 144:883.

Nadol JB, Hsu W. Histopathologic correlation of spiral ganglion cell count and new bone formation in the cochlea following meningogenic labyrinthitis and deafness. Ann Otol Rhinol Laryngol 1991; 100:712.

Nara T, Matoba M, Numaguchi S, et al. Post-infectious leukocephalopathy as a complication of *Mycoplasma pneumoniae* infection. Pediatr Neurol 1987; 3:171.

Narins RG. Therapy of hyponatremia. N Engl J Med 1986; 314:1573.

Nemir RL, Krasinski K. Tuberculosis in children and adolescents in the 1980s. Pediatr Infect Dis J 1988; 7:375.

Nemir RL, O'Hara D. Tuberculosis in children 10 years of age and younger: three decades of experience during the chemotherapeutic era. Pediatrics 1991; 88:236.

Niemoller UM, Tauber MG. Brain edema and increased intracranial pressure in the pathophysiology of bacterial meningitis. Eur J Clin Microbiol Infect Dis 1989; 8:109.

Odio CM, McCracken GH Jr, Nelson JD. CSF shunt infections in pediatrics. Am J Dis Child 1984; 138:1103.

Odio CM, Faingezicht I, Paris M, et al. The beneficial effects of early dexamethasone administration in infants and children with bacterial meningitis. N Engl J Med 1991; 324:1525.

Offenbacher H, Fazekas F, Schmidt R, et al. MRI in tuberculous meningoencephalitis: report of four cases and review of the neuroimaging literature. J Neurol 1991; 238:340.

Onorato IM, Wormser GP, Nicholas P. "Normal" CSF in bacterial meningitis. JAMA 1980; 244:1469.

Pachner AR, Duray P, Steere AC. Central nervous system manifestations of Lyme disease. Arch Neurol 1989; 46:790.

Packer RJ, Bilaniuk LT, Zimmerman RA. CT parenchymal abnormalities in bacterial meningitis: clinical significance. J Comput Assist Tomogr 1982; 6:1064.

Paulson OB, Brodersen P, Hansen EL, et al. Regional cerebral blood flow, cerebral metabolic rate for oxygen and cerebrospinal fluid acid-base variables in patients with acute meningitis and with acute encephalitis. Acta Med Scand 1974; 196:191.

Peltola H, Anttila M, Renkonen OV. Randomized comparison of chloramphenicol, ampicillin, cefotaxime, and ceftriaxone for childhood bacterial meningitis. Lancet 1989; 1:1281.

Peltola H, Käyhty H, Virtanen M, et al. Prevention of *Hemophilus influenzae* type b bacteremic infections with the capsular polysaccharide vaccine. N Engl J Med 1984; 310:1561.

Peter G, Lepow ML, McCracken GH, et al. Report of the Committee on Infectious Diseases, 22nd ed. Elk Grove Village, Ill: American Academy of Pediatrics, 1991.

Pfister HW, Koedel U, Haberl RL, et al. Microvascular changes during the early phase of experimental bacterial meningitis. J Cereb Blood Flow Metab 1990; 10:914.

Pike MG, Wang PK, Bencivenga R, et al. Electrophysiologic studies, computed tomography, and neurologic outcome in acute bacterial meningitis. J Pediatr 1990; 116:702.

Pomeroy SL, Holmes SJ, Dodge PR, et al. Seizures and other neurologic sequelae of bacterial meningitis in children. N Engl J Med 1990; 323:1651.

Portnoy JM, Olson LC. Normal cerebrospinal fluid values in children: another look. Pediatrics 1985; 75:484.

Powell KR. Secretion of antidiuretic hormone in children with meningitis. J Pediatr 1991; 118:996.

Powell KR, Sugarman LI, Eskenazi AE, et al. Normalization of plasma arginine vasopressin concentrations when children with meningitis are given maintenance plus replacement fluid therapy. J Pediatr 1990; 117:515.

Powers WJ. Cerebrospinal fluid lymphocytosis in acute bacterial meningitis. Am J Med 1985; 79:216.

Prince AS, Neu HC. Fluid management in *Haemophilus influenzae* meningitis. Infection 1980; 8:5.

Prober CG, Stevenson DK, Benitz WE. The use of antibiotics in neonates weighing less than 1200 grams. Pediatr Infect Dis J 1990; 9:111.

Putto A, Ruuskanen O, Meurman O, et al. C-reactive protein in the evaluation of febrile illness. Arch Dis Child 1986; 61:24.

Quaade F, Krislensen KP. Purulent meningitis: a review of 658 cases. Acta Med Scand 1962; 171:543.

Radetsky M. Duration of treatment in bacterial meningitis: a historical inquiry. Pediatr Infect Dis J 1990; 9:2.

Raimondi AJ, DiRocco C. The physiopathogenetic basis for the angiographic diagnosis of bacterial infections of the brain and its coverings in children. I. Leptomeningitis. Childs Brain 1979; 5:1.

Rakover Y, Adar H, Tal I, et al. Behçet disease: Long-term follow-up of three children and review of the literature. Pediatrics 1989; 83:986.

Raucher HS, Kaufman DM, Goldfarb J, et al. Pseudotumor cerebri and Lyme disease: a new association. J Pediatr 1985; 107:931.

Rawstron SA, Bromberg K. Comparison of maternal and newborn serologic tests for syphilis. Am J Dis Child 1991; 145:1383.

Renier D, Flandlin C, Hirsch E, et al. Brain abscesses in neonates. J Neurosurg 1988; 69:877.

Rice RB, Walling AD, Kallail KJ. The incidence of *Haemophilus influenzae* meningitis in a midwestern metropolitan county. Am J Public Health 1990; 80:215.

Richards PG, Towu-Aghantse E. Dangers of lumbar puncture. Br Med J 1986; 292:605.

Robinson RCV. Congenital syphilis. Arch Dermatol 1969; 99:599.

Rotbart HA, Glode MP. *Haemophilus influenzae* type b septic arthritis in children: report of 23 cases. Pediatrics 1985; 75:254.

Sabin TD. Nature of the sensory loss in leprosy: a reply. Muscle Nerve 1988; 11:277.

Sabin TD, Swift TR. Leprosy. In: Dyck PJ, Thomas PK, Lambert EH, Bunge R, eds. Peripheral neuropathy, vol 2, 2nd ed. Philadelphia: WB Saunders, 1984.

Saez-Llorens X, Jafari HS, Severien C, et al. Enhanced attenuation of meningeal inflammation and brain edema by concomitant administration of anti-CD18 monoclonal antibodies and dexamethasone in experimental *Haemophilus* meningitis. J Clin Invest 1991; 88:2003.

Saez-Llorens X, Ramilo O, Mustafa MM, et al. Molecular pathophysiology of bacterial meningitis: current concepts and therapeutic implications. J Pediatr 1990; 116:671.

Saez-Llorens XJ, Umaña MA, Odio CM, et al. Brain abscess in infants and children. Pediatr Infect Dis J 1989; 8:449.

Salih MAM, Khaleefa OH, Bushara M, et al. Long term sequelae of childhood acute bacterial meningitis in a developing country. Scand J Infect Dis 1991; 23:175.

Sande MA, Täuber MG, Scheld WM, et al. Pathophysiology of bacterial meningitis: summary of the workshop. Pediatr Infect Dis J 1989; 8:929.

Sanford JP. Leptospirosis—time for a booster. N Engl J Med 1984; 310:524.

Santosham M, Wolff M, Reid R, et al. The efficacy in Navajo infants of a conjugate vaccine consisting of *Haemophilus influenzae* type b polysaccharide and *Neisseria meningitidis,* outer-membrane protein complex. N Engl J Med 1991; 324:1767.

Sarff LD, Platt LH, McCracken GH Jr. Cerebrospinal fluid evaluation in neonates: comparison of high-risk infants with and without meningitis. J Pediatr 1976; 88:473.

Schachenmayr W, Friede RL. The origin of subdural neomembranes. I. Fine structure of the dura-arachnoid interface in man. Am J Pathol 1978; 92:53.

Schlech WF III, Ward JI, Band JD, et al. Bacterial meningitis in the United States, 1978 through 1981. JAMA 1985; 253:1749.

Schwersenski J, McIntyre L, Bauer CR. Lumbar puncture frequency and cerebrospinal fluid analysis in the neonate. Am J Dis Child 1991; 145:54.

Seay AR. Spinal cord dysfunction complicating bacterial meningitis. Arch Neurol 1984; 41:545.

Shankar P, Manjunath N, Mohan KK, et al. Rapid diagnosis of tuberculous meningitis by polymerase chain reaction. Lancet 1991; 337:5.

Shapiro ED, Aaron NH, Wald ER, et al. Risk factors for development of bacterial meningitis among children with occult bacteremia. J Pediatr 1986; 109:15.

Shapiro ED, Berg AT, Austrian R, et al. The protective efficacy of polyvalent pneumococcal polysaccharide vaccine. N Engl J Med 1991; 325:1453.

Sigal LH, Tatum AH. Lyme disease patients' serum contains IgM antibodies to *Borrelia burgdorferi* that cross-react with neuronal antigens. Neurology 1988; 38:1439.

Silverberg AL, DiNubile MJ. Subdural empyema and cranial epidural abscess. Med Clin North Am 1985; 90:361.

Simon RP. Role of endogenous excitatory amino acid neurotransmitters in the pathogenesis and evolution of acute brain injury. Pediatr Infect Dis J 1989; 8:913.

Skoch MG, Walling AD. Meningitis: describing the community health problem. Am J Public Health 1985; 75:550.

Smith HP, Hendrick EB. Subdural empyema and epidural abscess in children. J Neurosurg 1983; 58:392.

Smith PG. Recent trends in the epidemiology of tuberculosis and leprosy. Trop Geogr Med 1992; 43:S22.

Snedeker JD, Kaplan SL, Dodge PR, et al. Subdural effusion and its relationship with neurologic sequelae of bacterial meningitis in infancy: a prospective study. Pediatrics 1990; 86:163.

Snider DE, Rieder HL, Combs D, et al. Tuberculosis in children Pediatr Infect Dis J 1988; 7:271.

Snider DE, Roper WL. The new tuberculosis. N Engl J Med 1992; 326:703.

Snyder RD. Ventriculomegaly in childhood bacterial meningitis. Neuropediatrics 1984a; 15:136.

Snyder RD. Seizures in childhood bacterial meningitis. Ann Neurol 1984b; 16:395.

Snyder RD, Stovring J, Cushing AH, et al. Cerebral infarction in childhood bacterial meningitis. J Neurol Neurosurg Psychiatry 1981; 44:581.

Spector R. Advances in understanding the pharmacology of agents used to treat bacterial meningitis. Pharmacology 1990; 41:113.

Starke JR. Multidrug therapy for tuberculosis in children. Pediatr Infect Dis J 1990; 9:785.

Stead WW, Senner JW, Reddick WT, et al. Racial differences in susceptibility to infection by mycobacterium tuberculosis. N Engl J Med 1990; 322:422.

Steele RW, McConnell JR, Jacobs RF, et al. Recurrent bacterial meningitis: coronal thin-section cranial computed tomography to delineate anatomic defects. Pediatrics 1985; 76:950.

Steere AC. Lyme disease. N Engl J Med 1989; 321:586.

Stephanov S. Surgical treatment of brain abscess. Neurosurgery 1988; 22:724.

Stockstill MT, Kauffman CA. Comparison of cryptococcal and tuberculous meningitis. Arch Neurol 1983; 40:81.

Stovring J, Snyder RD. Computed tomography in childhood bacterial meningitis. J Pediatr 1980; 96:820.

Syrogiannopoulos GA, Nelson JD, McCracken GH Jr. Subdural collections of fluid in acute bacterial meningitis: a review of 136 cases. Pediatr Infect Dis 1986; 5:343.

Tal Y, Crichton JU, Dunn HG, et al. Spinal cord damage: a rare complication of purulent meningitis. Acta Paediatr Scand 1980; 69:471.

Tarlow MJ. Adjunct therapy in bacterial meningitis. J Antimicrob Chemother 1991; 28:329.

Tarr PI, Peter G. Demographic factors in the epidemiology of *Hemophilus influenzae* meningitis in young children. J Pediatr 1978; 92:884.

Tauber MG. Brain edema, intracranial pressure and cerebral blood flow in bacterial meningitis. Pediatr Infect Dis J 1989; 8:915.

Tauber MG, Sande M. Dexamethasone in bacterial meningitis: increasing evidence for a beneficial effect. Pediatr Infect Dis J 1989; 8:842.

Tauber MG, Sande MA. Pharmacodynamics of antibiotics in experimental bacterial meningitis — two sides to rapid bacterial killing in the cerebrospinal fluid. Scand J Infect Dis 1991; 74(suppl):173.

Tauber MG, Shibl AM, Hackbarth CJ, et al. Antibiotic therapy, endotoxin concentration in cerebral spinal fluid and brain edema in experimental *Escherichia coli* meningitis in rabbits. J Infect Dis 1987; 156:456.

Taylor HG, Michaels RH, Mazur PM, et al. Intellectual, neuropsychological, and achievement outcomes in children six to eight years after recovery from *Haemophilus influenzae* meningitis. Pediatrics 1984; 74:198.

Taylor HG, Mills EL, Ciampi A, et al. The sequelae of *Haemophilus influenzae* meningitis in school-aged children. N Engl J Med 1990; 323:1657.

Tessin I, Trollfors B, Thiringer K, et al. Ampicillin-aminoglycoside combinations as initial treatment for neonatal septicaemia or meningitis. Acta Paediatr Scand 1991; 80:911.

Trachtman H. Secretion of antidiuretic hormone in children with meningitis. J Pediatr 1991; 118:996.

Tracy KJ, Vlassara H, Cerami A. Cachectin/tumor necrosis factor. Lancet 1989; 1:1122.

Tunkel AR, Scheld WM. Alterations of the blood-brain barrier in bacterial meningitis: in vivo and in vitro models. Pediatr Infect Dis J 1989; 8:911.

Tunkel AR, Wispelwey B, Scheld WM. Bacterial meningitis: recent advances in pathophysiology and treatment. Ann Intern Med 1990; 112:610.

Tunnessen WW. Congenital syphilis. Am J Dis Child 1992; 146:115.

Udani PM, Parekh UC, Dastur DK. Neurological and related syndromes in CNS tuberculosis: clinical features and pathogenesis. J Neurol Sci 1971; 14:341.

Valmari P. Primary diagnosis in a life-threatening childhood infection. Ann Clin Res 1985; 17:310.

Verghese A, Gallemore G. Kernig's and Brudzinski's signs revisited. Rev Infect Dis 1987; 9:1187.

Volpe JJ. Neurology of the newborn, 2nd ed. Philadelphia: WB Saunders, 1987.

Waecker NJ, Connor JD. Central nervous system tuberculosis in children: a review of 30 cases. Pediatr Infect Dis J 1990; 9:539.

Wald ER, Bergman I, Taylor HG, et al. Long-term outcome of group B streptococcal meningitis. Pediatrics 1986; 77:217.

Wardle S, Carty H. CT scanning in meningitis. Eur J Radiol 1991; 12:113.

Wehrle PF. Return of the lumbar tapper's dilemma. J Pediatr 1973; 83:351.

Weingarten K, Zimmerman RD, Becker RD, et al. Subdural and epidural empyemas: MR imaging. Am J Radiol 1989; 152:615.

Weiss MG, Ionides SP, Anderson CL. Meningitis in premature infants with respiratory distress: role of admission lumbar puncture. J Pediatr 1991; 119:973.

Wenger JD, Hightower AW, Facklam RR, et al. Bacterial meningitis in the United States, 1986: report of a multistate surveillance study. J Infect Dis 1990; 162:1316.

Wilson CB. Immunologic basis for increased susceptibility of the neonate to infection, J Pediatr 1986; 108:1.

Wong T-T, Lee LS, Wang HS, et al. Brain abscess in children — a cooperative study of 83 cases. Childs Nerv Syst 1989; 5:19.

Word BM, Klein JO. Therapy of bacterial sepsis and meningitis in infants and children: 1989 poll of directors of programs in pediatric infectious diseases. Pediatr Infect Dis J 1989; 8:635.

Younger B, Michaud RM, Fisher M. Leprosy: our southwest Asian refugee experience. Arch Dermatol 1982; 118:981.

Zenker PN, Berman SM. Congenital syphilis: trends and recommendations for evaluation and management. Pediatr Infect Dis J 1991; 10:516.

Basic structure of viruses

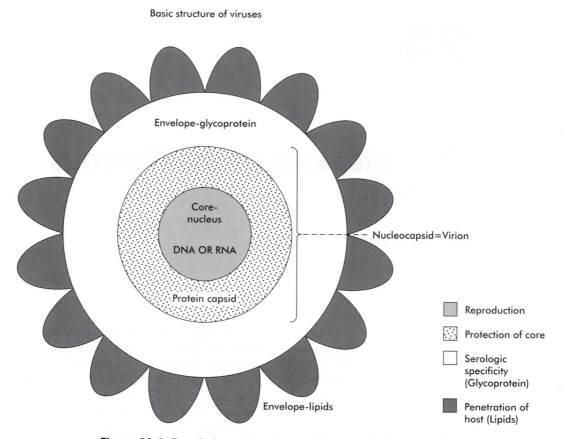

Figure 39-1 Correlation of structure and function in virus complex.

and types of virions. Viral structure may be altered, particularly in synthesis and assembly processes, or after a host's antibody response and the subsequent viral-antigen reaction. Human viral disease, as we know it, depends on these viral-host interactions, particularly when it occurs simultaneously in large numbers or populations of viruses and host cells. In human viral disease, the first viral life cycle is called the *primary infection*. The first release of virion represents the *primary release*, which usually appears as a viremia but sometimes as a nerve transmission. The second life cycle that affects a second population of cells is called a *secondary infection*. This is followed by a second release of virions, representing a secondary viremia and so forth. Continued completion of viral life cycles is a simple process and one important in understanding the clinical manifestations of many viral diseases [Johnson, 1985; Bale and Perlman, 1987; Mandell et al., 1990].

The many direct effects that a virus has on a host cell are usually deleterious. Some virus-host interactions interfere with the host's basic metabolic functions so that immediate host cell death occurs. This process of death is called *lysis*. Viruses that tend to produce this acute, severe, and immediate effect are identified as *lytic*

viruses. Conversely, however, the direct effect of the virus on a host may be minimal and the course of action slow. In some infections, the natural life cycle of the virus fails to continue because of interference in the life cycle of the virus by the host at any of the replication stages listed [Stephens and Compans, 1988].

It is noteworthy that an original virus may be altered in both form and function considerably by several life-cycle passages [Kilbourne, 1985]. This phenomenon has been called *antigenic drift* (a strong characteristic of influenza viruses). Alteration in the structure and function of the virus may change what was once a wildly lytic virus into an altered, persistent, or slow-acting virus, and vice versa. A second life cycle of a virus may also involve another type of cell or even another host. When a secondary host is found, there is usually a worsening of the effect on the host, which is illustrated by the effect of the arbovirus on humans when humans are the secondary host [Melnick, 1986]. This worsening of illness illustrates the more serious effects of a classic secondary infection, poliomyelitis, which is caused by the poliovirus. Primary infection of poliovirus infections is much milder in animals than in humans.

Therefore the direct effect of the virus on the host may be acute and devastating or slow and persistent.

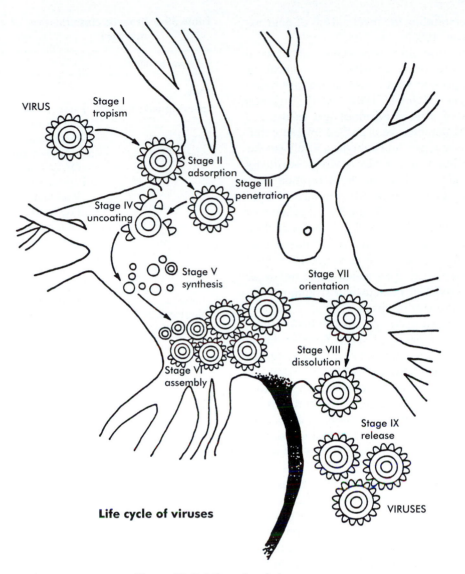

Figure 39-2 Life cycle of viruses.

Usually the lytic effect of the virus on the host cell results in severe destruction of the tissue. Little erythema or inflammation is usually observed because these represent reactive and less morbid reactions. Although inflammation is a hallmark of human viral disease, it represents the secondary reaction of the host's immune system to the viral antigen. All proved viral diseases are characterized by various combinations of the direct viral cytopathic effects and the indirect host immune reactions [Haase, 1986; Johnson, 1982; Alvord, 1977].

A third "reparative" reaction is also characteristic of viral disease and produces the scarring, which is represented in the CNS by gliosis. In many instances, separation of the symptoms caused by the direct effects of viral infection and the indirect effects of the host immunity reaction is possible but in others is not. Serologic reactions of the host are usually directly related to the viral glycoprotein. Because the viral glycoprotein spikes protrude from the virion to the outside of the host cell's cytoplasmic membrane, they can be recognized and acted on. However, if the exposure outside the host cell does not occur, there is no host immunity, recognition, or response. When virions are not exposed to the extracellular space, which often occurs when the infection is slowly persistent or latent, the virus can often live comfortably within the safety of the host's cytoplasmic home [Melnick, 1982; Weiner et al., 1983].

Escape from the host is sometimes impossible. In the ideal virus-host interaction, a balance occurs between the viral and host cell metabolic states. Extended balances produce a *latency period;* therefore lytic, altered, minimal, slow, persistent, and latent types of virus-host interactions can occur, all of which are important in understanding the mechanisms of neuroviral disease [Johnson, 1985].

In the past, because little was known about viral biology, viruses were often classified on clinical or ecologic grounds; present viral classifications are based on biologic criteria [Melnick, 1982; 1986]. Eighteen different families of viruses (viridae) are recognized (Table 39-1). Viral families are classified into subfamilies (virinae), genera, types, and subtypes. The basis for classification is nucleic acid core, size of virion, sensitivity to solvents, serologic reactions, mode of reproduction, shape and contour of nucleocapsid, presence of lipid envelope, and type of standing. Table 39-2 lists some of the major characteristics of the 18 viral families, including type of nucleic acid core (i.e., deoxyribonucleic acid or ribonucleic acid), presence or absence of a lipid envelope, capsid shape (i.e., spherical or cubic, helical or rod, and complex), type of nucleic acid stranding (i.e., single or double), and size of virion.

Viruses consist of two major groups [Melnick, 1986]. The smaller group, composed of seven families, has a DNA core. The most recently isolated virus is represented by the hepadnaviridae, the prototype being the deoxyribonucleic acid virus that causes human hepatitis B. The larger group, composed of 11 families, has an ribonucleic acid core. Naming of viruses has followed an inconsistent logic. Table 39-3 is a simplified glossary of stem words that may be helpful in understanding this inconsistent terminology.

The size of viruses varies considerably, measuring from 18 to 26 nm in the small deoxyribonucleic acid paravovirus family, up to 450 nm in the largest of all viruses, the pox viruses [Melnick, 1986]. To appreciate these size differences, 1 nm represents 1/1 billionth of a meter, or 10 Å units. One thousand nms are equal to 1 μm. Thus the largest of all viruses, if found in the cytoplasm of an average-sized human lymphocyte of 8000 nm or 8 μm, would represent only a small fraction of the cytoplasm. The early morphologic study of viruses was quite inadequate. It is amazing that any morphologic understanding of viruses was accomplished with light microscopy. Based on much indirect evidence, light microscopy has demonstrated telltale morphologic signs of virus in the form of inclusion bodies found in the nucleus or cytoplasm. These cellular inclusions represent conglomerates of viruses and are still helpful in identifying viral processes in host cells. Examples of nearly diagnostic viral inclusions are the characteristic cytoplasmic Negri bodies, which are composed of collections of lyssaviruses, or rabies viruses, and the Cowdry's type A nuclear inclusion bodies observed in measles and herpes simplex infections.

Although the biologic classification of the viruses helps in our understanding of viruses, efforts must be made to blend the previously used terminology. A

Table 39-1 Present classification of viruses (human disease)

Characteristic	Family
DNA	
Spherical naked	Parvoviridae
	Parvoviruses (rheumatoid arthritis)
	Depenadovirus (helper virus to adenoviruses)
	Densovirus
	Papovaviridae
	Papillomavirus (human warts)
	Polyomavirus
	Adenoviridae
	Most adenoviruses (acute URI, conjunctivitis)
	Avidenoviruses
	Hepadnaviridae
	Hepadnavirus (hepatitis B)
Spherical enveloped (or complex)	Herpesviridae
	Simplex virus (herpes encephalitis)
	Varicella virus (chicken pox, shingles)
	Cytomegalovirus (cytomegalic inclusion disease)
	Lymphocryptovirus (Epstein-Barr infectious mononucleosis)
	Iridoviridae
	Poxviridae
	Orthopoxviruses (small pox, vaccinia)
RNA	
Spherical naked	Picornaviridae
	Enteroviruses
	Poliovirus (poliomyelitis)
	Coxsackievirus (meningoencephalomyelitis)
	Echovirus (meningoencephalomyelitis)
	Enterovirus (meningoencephalomyelitis)
	Rhinovirus (common cold)
	Caliciviridae
	Calicivirus (Norwalk gastroenteritis)
	Reoviridae
	Orbivirus (Colorado tick fever)
	Rotovirus (infantile diarrhea)
Spherical enveloped	Togaviridae
	Alphavirus (group A arbovirus encephalitis)
	Rubivirus (rubella)
	Pestivirus
	Flavivirus (group B arbovirus encephalitis)

Modified from Melnick JL. Progress in medical virology. Basel: S Karger, 1982.

Continued.

Table 39-1 Present classification of viruses (human disease)—cont'd

Characteristic	Family
Helical enveloped	Orthomyxoviridae
	Influenzavirus (type A, B, and C flu)
	Paramyxoviridae
	Pneumiovirus (respiratory syncytial disease)
	Paramyxoviruses (parainfluenza, mumps)
	Morbilliviruses (measles, SSPE)
	Rhabdoviridae
	Vesiculovirus (vesicular stomatitis)
	Lyssavirus (rabies)
	Coronaviridae
	Coronavirus (acute URI)
	Bunyaviridae
	Bunyavirus (California-LaCross encephalitis)
	Phlebovirus (sandfly fever)
	Nairovirus
Asymmetric enveloped	Arenaviridae
	Arenavirus (lymphocytic choriomeningitis)
	Retroviridae
	Oncovirinae (leukemia, AIDS/ARC)
	Spumavirinae
	Lentivirinae (visna maedi)

previous classification used the term *arboviruses* to refer to all viruses that were carried by arthropods, which number over 350. Efforts are made in this text to incorporate the term *arbo* into the now accepted biologic classification.

According to Melnick [1986] the rapidly expanded classification of viruses has reached a point where there is little likelihood of further expansion. This view may be based on restricted definitions. The majority of persistent viral infections is caused by unquestionable viral agents and are listed as being caused by conventional viruses. The conventional, persistent viruses are associated with the usual destructive-inflammatory pathologic reactions. There is a group of so-called persistent or slow viral disorders that can be transmitted to other animals and are thus infectious but that follow an uncharacteristic course and are not proved viral diseases. These infections are called *unconventional "viral" disorders* (see box on p. 649). The unconventional viral disorders are not associated with inflammation but rather with spongiform, destructive changes only in the neuronal layers of brain. Yet, they are not acute diseases.

Viruslike infectious agents have been identified that are of even smaller size and have slightly different characteristics than presently classified viruses. Some of these agents are called *viroids*. Other possible organisms of questionable viral-nature have been called *prions,* or *proteinaceous infectious agents* [Prusiner, 1982]. This term is used to identify the protein material found in some of the unconventional viral diseases, such as sheep scrapie

Table 39-2 Major characteristics of virus families

Family name	Lipid envelope	Capsid shape	Nucleic acid stranding	Size diameter
DNA viruses				
Parvoviridae	−	Spherical	Single	18-26 nm
Hepadnaviridae	−	Spherical	Single	40-50 nm
Papovaviridae	−	Spherical	Single	45-55 nm
Adenoviridae	−	Spherical	Double	70-90 nm
Iridoviridae	−	Spherical	Double	125-300 nm
Herpesviridae	+	Spherical	Double	120-200 nm
Poxviridae	+	Complex	Double	230 × 300 nm
RNA viruses				
Picornaviridae	−	Spherical	Single	25-30 nm
Caliciviridae	−	Spherical	Single	35-40 nm
Reoviridae	−	Spherical	Single	50-70 nm
Togaviridae	+	Spherical	Single	100-120 nm
Retroviridae	+	Spherical	Single	70-170 nm
Arenaviridae	+	Helical	Single	60-80 nm
Orthomyxoviridae	+	Helical	Single	90-120 nm
Paramyxoviridae	+	Helical	Single	120-150 nm
Rhabdoviridae	+	Helical	Single	80-300 nm
Coronaviridae	+	Helical	Single	80-120 nm
Bunyaviridae	+	Helical	Single	80-100 nm

Table 39-3 Glossary of terms

Term	Meaning	Term	Meaning
Adeno	Gland	Orbi	Sphere
Alpha	First	Ortho	Straight
Arbo	Coined, *arthropod* and *born*	Papill	Projection
Arena	Sand	Papilloma	Lobulated tumor
Bunya	Coined, geographic	Papova	Coined, *pa*pilloma and *po*lyoma *va*cuolating agent
Calici	Cup		
Corona	Crown	Para	Beside
Crypto	Hidden	Parvo	Small
Cyto	Cell	Phlebo	Vein
Cytomegalo	Large cell	Pico	Small
Echo	Coined, *e*nteric *c*ytopathogenic *h*uman *o*rphan	Picodna	Coined, *pico*-small and *DNA*-nucleic acid type
		Picorna	Coined, *pico*-small and *RNA*-nucleic acid type
Entero	Intestine	Polio	Gray
Flavi	Yellow	Poly	Many
Hepa	Liver	Polyoma	Many tumors
Hepadna	Coined, *hepa*-liver and *DNA*-nucleic acid type	Pox	Pustule
Herpes	Vesicle	REO	Coined, *r*espiratory *e*nteric *o*rganism
HIV	Coined, *h*uman *i*mmunodeficiency *v*irus	Retro	Behind, backward
HTLV	Coined, *h*uman *T*-cell *l*ymphotrophic (or leukemia) *v*irus	Rhabdo	Rod, bullet
		Rhino	Nose
Influenza	Influence	Rota	Wheel
Irido	Iridescent	Rubella	Red condition, diminutive
LAV	Coined, *l*ymphocyte *a*ctivating *v*irus	Rubeola	Red condition
Lenti	Lens	Rubi	Red
Lympho	Water	Simplex	Simple
Lympho-crypto	Hidden cells	Toga	Envelope
		Vari	Probably Latin, pimple
Megalo	Large	Varicella	Pustule condition, diminutive
Myxo	Mucus	Variola	Pustule condition
Oma	Swelling	Varus	Probably Latin, pimple
Onco	Bulk		

and Creutzfeldt-Jakob disease. Nucleic acids have not been identified in prions, but prions may consist of a thick protein shell bounded tightly around a few unidentifiable strands of nucleic acid core (see box on p. 649).

Pathologic reactions of the host to a virus are acute, subacute, or chronic (Table 39-4). Necrosis, lysis, liquefaction, vacuolization, degeneration, spongiform changes, storage, Wallerian reaction, chromatolysis, demyelination, inflammation, erythema, edema, hemorrhage, or gliosis can occur. These pathologic reactions in the directly involved tissues may also alter tissues far removed from the primary site of involvement (see box on p. 650). Direct vascular involvement may produce ischemia, hemorrhage, and infarction in noninfected parts. The indirect effects of excessive or deficient hormonal production may be significant clinical symptoms of viral disease. When viruses attack a developing fetus, there may be many distantly manifest dysgenetic effects, producing malformations that are not directly related to an active infection.

Viral disease may be relentless or intermittent. The physician can usually identify a variety of neurologic syndromes, such as acute/relentless, acute/intermittent, subacute/relentless, subacute/intermittent, chronic/relentless, chronic/intermittent, and other combinations [Bell and McCormick, 1981; Chun, 1982; Jabbour, 1982].

Once viruses have entered the body and have established the primary infections, they may enter the nervous system either by hematogenous routes or by direct neural transmission through a peripheral nerve. The initial entrance to the body may be by inhalation (e.g., measles), via oral ingestion with absorption through the gastrointestinal tract (e.g., poliomyelitis), or through breaks in the skin (e.g., rabies) [Baer, 1975] (see box on p. 650).

Even in the nervous system, some viruses tend to be attracted to specific host cells. One example is the specific attraction of the opportunistic JC polyoma virus of the papovavirus family to oligodendrocytes. Destruc-

---

Slow or Persistent "Virus" Infections

Conventional (inflammatory)

Chronic virus infections
  Progressive multifocal leukoencephalitis
  Progressive rubella panencephalitis
  Subacute sclerosing panencephalitis
  Rabies
Direct retrovirus encephalopathy
Latent virus infections
  Varicella-zoster virus
  Herpes simplex infections
  Cytomegalovirus

Unconventional (noninflammatory)*

Jakob-Creutzfeldt disease
Kuru
Gerstmann-Straussler syndrome
Scrapie

---

*Although usually considered to be of viral origin, there is still some question about the exact infectious agent causing these diseases. Scrapie is an example of many nonhuman diseases representative of this category.

Other Agents Related to Viruses

Viroids: The smallest known self-replicating forms in biology. Probably a naked RNA or DNA molecule with no associated protein or capsid structure. Fails to elicit an immune response. Insensitive to heat and organic solvents. Sensitive to nucleases.

Prions: Coined. *Pro*teinaceous *in*fectious particle — prion. Resistent to agents that destroy nucleic acids and sensitive to those that kill protein. May be a nucleic acid protected by a tight protein coat. May not represent replicating portion of infectious agent or any portion of an infectious agent.

Table 39-4 Neural pathogenic characteristics of the various neuroviral syndromes

Acute	Subacute	Chronic
Rapid	Semi-rapid	Slow
Destructive	Inflammatory	Degenerative
Lytic	Erythematous	Gliotic
Necrotic	Edematous	Vacuolizing
Extensive	Limited	Minimal
Cytopathic	Immunopathic	Reparative
Liquefactive	Host-generated	Persistent
Devastating	Hemorrhagic	Latency
	Vascularity	Spongiform
	Allergic	Altered

others tend to affect entire regions and many of the cells in that region. For example, rabies tends to involve several different kinds of cells of the hypothalamus, brainstem, and limbic system. Herpes simplex virus type I usually involves the basal frontal and temporal lobes. These anatomic distributions may result because of the neural pathway transmission that appears to characterize these two types of viruses. To further clarify this characteristic, consider that herpes simplex type 2 is probably hematogenically transmitted to the infant, producing a severe, generalized encephalitis, as well as multisystemic infection. Varicella, when acutely involving the CNS, attacks the cerebellum relatively more commonly than does the mumps virus, which has a propensity to produce a brainstem ependymitis, especially around the sylvian aqueduct. Poliovirus has a secondary tropism to anterior horn cells of the spinal cord, whereas the Epstein-Barr virus has a propensity to affect the dorsal root ganglion, producing a polyradiculitis. Varicella-zoster virus also tends to locate asymptomatically in the dorsal root and trigeminal ganglion; this virus infection is classified as latent [Haase, 1986].

Some viruses act in concert with other viruses. It has been demonstrated that most of the parvoviruses do not produce disease themselves but help other viruses produce disease and then benefit from it. Many asymptomatic and harbored viral diseases of the nervous system, such as the cytomegaloviruses and papovaviruses, become opportunistic in immune deficiency states.

Viruses are pervasive and infect not only humans and animals but also plants and even bacteria. A relatively small number of viruses infect only humans. These human obligatory viral parasites usually cause less dramatic symptoms or even asymptomatic infections, which are rarely fatal unless associated with a secondary infection or when immunosuppression occurs. Poliomyelitis, caused by the poliovirus, is an example of a serious secondary viral infection that follows a more frequent, much milder, and better tolerated primary GI infection.

tion of these cells produces progressive multifocal leukoencephalitis. The human immune deficiency virus (HIV), previously called the human T-cell leukemic/lymphotrophic virus (HTLV) type III, has a specific tropism to the T4-helper lymphocytes and secondarily to monocytes and macrophages [Gallo, 1987]. Destruction of the T4 cells produces the acquired immune deficiency syndrome (AIDS). It has now been recognized that HIV also infects neurons.

Although certain viruses attack specific CNS cells,

Indirect Clinical Pathogenetic Mechanisms Associated with Neuroviral Diseases

Vascular involvement

Ischemia
Hemorrhage
Infarction

Hormonal effects

Excessive or reactive
Deficient

Effects on developing fetus

Dysgenetic effects
Scarring

Types of Viral Entrance

Route of entry	Example of virus
Inhalation	Measles
GI absorption	Poliomyelitis
Skin breakdown	Rabies

Types of Human Neural Viral Transmission

Transmission	Example of virus
Hematogenous	Poliomyelitis
Neurogenous	Rabies

Although obligatory human viruses usually are well tolerated, they become a serious threat to life once they become opportunistic, as occurs in serious cytomegalovirus and papovaviruses infections associated with AIDS. Generally, the more dangerous human viral infections are usually the ones caused by viruses that attack humans as a secondary host, such as in rabies and arbotogaviruses. These viruses have adapted to life with their primary host but are often life-threatening when they infect humans. In the instance of secondary host infections, the virion has not yet had an opportunity to adapt to the new human condition, and devastating results may occur.

Almost all viral diseases are associated with an immune response of the host; therefore most neurologic disorders caused by viruses are a result of direct viral effect and host reaction. The severe symptoms of acute measles encephalitis, in fact, are more likely the result of pronounced hyperimmune response to viral antigen than to the direct lytic effect of the virus. Conversely, subacute sclerosing panencephalitis is now identified as a slow viral infection caused by an altered measles virion. The symptoms of subacute sclerosing panencephalitis are largely caused by the direct effects of the virus on the host cells, whereas the immune response is seemingly minimal, or at least ineffective. Another form of CNS measles is represented by subacute measles encephalitis. This disorder is observed in immunosuppressed or immunodeficient persons, and the clinical symptoms are caused by the unchecked action of a minimally altered, but still lytic, measles virion [Porter, 1985].

The neurologic phenomena resulting from a viral infection of the nervous system depend on many factors, including the biologic status of the virus, the virus-host interaction, the age of the host, the host-immunologic response, and the types of pathologic reactions that can occur. The number of proved viral diseases of the nervous system is extensive. Many disorders are suspected but have not been proved.

CLINICAL PRESENTATION

Viral diseases of the nervous system are usually caused by secondary infections. The neurologic presentation may be acute, subacute, or chronic. An effort is made to discuss the major viral diseases observed in pediatric neurology practice under theses subdivisions of clinical expression. The major divisions and subdivisions are outlined in the box.

Most often, the acute neural viral syndromes are the result of a direct wild viral infection on anatomic sites, and wild infections produce characteristic symptoms. Recognition of acute viral syndromes is important to the clinician, but the anatomic site of involvement is also important regarding management. Three acute neurologic syndromes, which are reported frequently in the literature, are designated here [Bell and McCormick, 1981]. Seldom in clinical practice, and rarely pathologically, is there confinement of the viral disease to the areas named. It is important to remember that practically all patients with brain meningitides of any kind usually have parenchymal involvement as well. The symptoms and pathology produced by this parenchymal involvement are mild or nonspecific and out of proportion to the more obvious symptoms caused by meningitis. Likewise, the disorders identified as encephalitides will often be preceded or accompanied by symptoms suggesting meningeal involvement. The distinctions of the separate syndromes therefore act only as guidelines but are of absolute importance clinically and diagnostically. Encephalitides may take the form of either a localized or generalized rostral encephalitis or a cerebritis or may be more confined to localized caudal brain infections, such as those localized in the pons (pontinitis), medulla (medullitis), or cerebellum (cerebellitis). More caudal

<table>
<tr><td colspan="2" align="center">Fifteen Neuroviral Diseases
Discussed in Detail</td></tr>
</table>

Acute neurologic disorders

Aseptic meningitis
Viral encephalitis
Viral meningomyeloradiculitis

Subacute neurologic disorders

Human rabies
Acute hemorrhagic leukoencephalitis
Acute disseminated encephalomyelitis
Postinfectious encephalomyeloradiculitis

Chronic neurologic disorders

Subacute sclerosing panencephalitis
Progressive rubella panencephalitis
Progressive multifocal leukoencephalitis
Acquired immune deficiency syndrome

Unconventional progressive encephalopathies

Kuru
Creutzfeldt-Jakob disease

Embryonic encephalopathies

Congenital cytomegalovirus disease
Congenital rubella syndrome

Table 39-5 Frequency of selected infectious diseases

Disease	1990	1980	1970	1960
AIDS	41,595	NR	NR	NR
Aseptic meningitis	11,852	8028	6480	1593
Encephalitis	1341	1362	1580	2341
Paralytic poliomyelitis	7	8	31	2525
Human rabies	1	0	3	2
Congenital rubella	11	50	77	NR
Hepatitis A	31,441	29,087	56,797	NR
Hepatitis B	21,102	19,015	8310	NR
Leprosy	198	223	129	54
Measles	27,786	13,506	47,351	441,703
Mumps	5292	8576	104,953	NR
Pertussis	4570	1730	4249	14,809
Rubela	1125	3904	56,552	NR
Varicella	173,099	190,894	NR	NR

From MMWR 1991; 391(53):61.
NR, Not previously reported nationally.

CNS infection involving the spinal cord and meninges may first appear as transverse myelitis or, more selectively, as poliomyelitis. Each of these infections may be associated with spinal meningitis. Confined involvement of the proximal nerve roots produces polyradiculitis, which may be associated with myelitis. The spinal viral syndromes will be grouped together and called the *meningomyeloradiculitides*. All of the syndromes, however, blend somewhat into one another, and syndromes more accurately identified as meningoencephalitis, encephalomyelitis, meningomyelitis, or meningoradiculomyelitis are encountered [Chun, 1982].

Although it would be preferable to designate each clinical viral syndrome by the specific virus that causes it, identification of the etiologic agent is not always possible in clinical pediatric neurology practice. The three acute neuroviral syndromes are identified for practical clinical use.

Neuroviral diseases that do not have a specific etiologic diagnosis are often reported by clinicians to the Centers for Disease Control (CDC). Table 39-5 represents data accumulated from reports by the CDC. The disorders selected are representative of what physicians in the United States in neurologic practice might see. Included are nonetiologically confirmed disorders, such as aseptic meningitis and encephalitis, that are believed

usually to be caused by viral agents; some other viral diseases that seldom produce neurologic illness; and several nonviral communicable disorders. Some of the specific neurologic viral diseases, all of which are not of acute nature (e.g., subacute sclerosing panencephalitis, congenital rubella, poliomyelitis, and human rabies), are listed in Table 39-5 to give a comparison of actual reportable statistics.

The incidence of viral or aseptic meningitis and encephalitis exceeds all other acute neurologic viral infections. The viral causes of these syndromes vary considerably with time and place. Table 39-6 reflects an estimated incidence of the types of viral agents associated with presumed viral meningitis and encephalitis [Johnson, 1982]. It is obvious that a large proportion of these suspected viral disorders are caused by unproved agents.

Subacute neuroviral disorders usually represent an overly active or, in rarer situations, an inactive host immune reaction or, in special situations, a direct effect of the virus, such as in the instance of rabies encephalomyelitis and subacute measles encephalitis. The symptoms usually occur weeks to months after initial contact with the virus. In the subacute syndromes, the virus may ineffectively stimulate the host's immune system or the immune response may be ineffective for other reasons, such as a defect in the host. The neurologic symptoms therefore are decelerated or delayed when compared with the more fulminating acute syndromes. In other subacute syndromes, the immune response appears to be continual and repetitive rather than "all at once," as occurs in some of the acute hypersensitive encephalopathies. Examples of syndromes that are pathogenetically

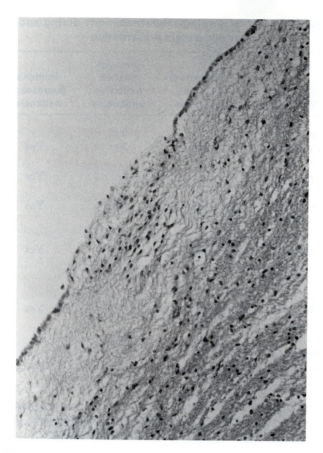

Figure 39-4 Ependymal granulation in a child who died with viral meningoencephalitis.

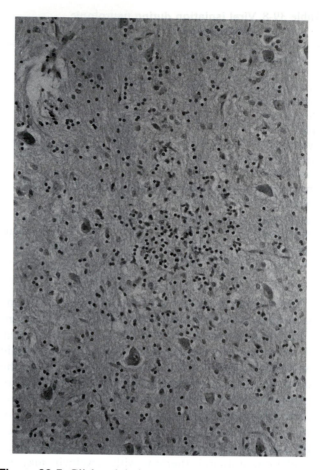

Figure 39-5 Glial nodule in a child who died with viral encephalitis.

with those observed in type 2, which are more diffuse. Type 2 encephalitis is not asymmetric or usually located in the basal frontal and temporal areas.

The most frequently occurring epidemic encephalitides are caused by the arbotogaviruses and the bunyaviruses. The togaviruses have a greater distribution internationally than in the United States. It is possible that one of the bunyaviruses, the California encephalitis virus, produces the most common epidemic encephalitis in the United States, but this estimate must take into account the relatively higher numbers generated after the large epidemic in Wisconsin. The high incidence of this disease has not continued recently. The incidence of epidemic encephalitides is extremely variable. The consistency or inconsistency of the bursts determines the frequency over any one given period. This characteristic is useful for the clinician. During epidemics, clinical awareness of the possibility of such diagnoses should be heightened. Epidemic encephalitides are almost always arthropod borne, and evidence demonstrates a seasonal distribution of infections, particularly in summer and fall [Chun, 1982].

Clinical findings. Viral encephalitides may have many of the characteristics previously described as typical of aseptic meningitis. In the pure forms of encephalitis there are severe and distinct signs of parenchymal involvement. Severe alterations in the state of consciousness, abnormal behavior, persistent convulsions, and focal, lateralizing, or diffuse neuronal signs and symptoms predominate. Agitation and excitement may precede stupor or coma in a progressive manner. Frequently, signs of increased intracranial pressure and papilledema occur. The signs of papilledema may occur in the early phases of the disease, and these are shortly followed by more signs of increased intracranial pressure secondary to generalized cerebral edema [Chun, 1982; Bell and McCormick, 1981].

Hydrocephalus may occur in mumps meningoencephalitis, but this usually occurs much later in the development of the disease, often in an otherwise improving state. This hydrocephalus is an obstructive, noncommunicating type caused by obstruction of the CSF flow resulting from ependymal granulations of the aqueduct. In several of the pure encephalitides, however, increased intracranial pressure resulting from cerebral edema is typical and earlier in onset. Early increased intracranial pressure is typical of herpes simplex encephalitis.

The extent of the clinical signs of cerebral edema and other symptoms depends on the severity of the infection, which depends on the type of organism; however, virtually all severe encephalitides exhibit generalized and diffuse signs and symptoms. The diffuse clinical features of a severe encephalopathy are related to many metabolic and toxic disturbances and increased intracranial pressure. Confusion, disorientation, frequent convulsions, a host of pyramidal signs, extrapyramidal signs, and long-tract sensory deficits are characteristic of the pure encephalitides. Signs of brainstem dysfunction may be intermixed. Although focal neurologic features may be present in all, this feature acts as a clinical hallmark of type 1 herpes simplex encephalitis. Localized, severe hypothalamic brainstem and limbic system involvement occurs typically in rabies encephalitis.

Brainstem and cerebellar symptoms and signs, however, do not always portend severe involvement. It is possible to characterize two types of posterior fossa viral syndromes. One of these syndromes is represented by a severely progressive encephalopathy, which usually has a grave prognosis. In rabies, there are signs of severe and devastating brainstem involvement, producing severe pharyngeal and laryngeal dysfunction. These striking findings occur in conjunction with severe cerebral involvement. A second type of brainstem encephalitis has a much more benign course and is associated with more limited involvement of the brainstem, with few signs or symptoms suggestive of severe rostral encephalitis. This milder brainstem syndrome may be associated with multiple cranial nerve palsies, ataxia, and mild, long-tract signs. The presentations may be so limited that pontine glioma is suggested; however, these patients tend to manifest more systemic signs of acute illness, suggesting an infectious basis.

Certain viruses are attracted to the cerebellum and may manifest only as ataxia. The virus particularly prone to causing this syndrome is the varicella-zoster virus. Localized cerebellitis may occur with other viruses too, such as the mumps virus, Epstein-Barr virus, poliovirus, coxsackie virus, echovirus, enteroviruses, and measles virus. The closely related myoclonic ataxia has also been associated with viral infections. Some of the various syndromes of polymyoclonus-opsoclonus may be caused by a direct viral infection. Others may be related to a host immune reaction. Postimmunization syndromes have been associated with syndromes with symptoms that suggest an acute inflammation of the cerebellum.

Spinal cord involvement may rarely occur as an extension of a generalized or caudally located encephalitis. This syndrome can more accurately be identified as an encephalomyelitis. When anterior horn cells are involved, signs of specific lower motor neuron loss develop. Suddenly developing profound weakness, ato-

nia, areflexia, and loss of bladder function suggest such an extension. A meningomyelitis progressing into encephalitic involvement is more commonly encountered.

Roseola is a common precipitant of febrile seizures. Occasionally a bulging fontanel may occur with this exanthem, which suggests but does not confirm the presence of a possible mild encephalitis. Rarely, roseola has been associated with acute infantile hemiplegia. It is probable that the most common acute neurologic symptoms associated with natural roseola are related to systemic effects rather than to focal neurologic involvement, except with hemiplegia. Hemiplegia may be caused by an associated vasculitis rather than by an encephalitis [Posson, 1949]. Erythema infectiosum, or fifth disease, is also rarely associated with some encephalitic symptoms.

The reoviruses are uncommonly associated with human disease of any type. Neurologic involvement in humans does occur in Colorado tick fever, which is sometimes accompanied by a diffuse encephalitis [Bell and McCormick, 1981]. A recently discovered reovirus, called the rotavirus, is an important viral cause of infantile diarrhea and has been associated with encephalitis.

Laboratory findings. Increased intracranial pressure occurs often in most types of pure encephalitis. The dynamics of the increased pressure are usually the result of cerebral edema and congestion associated with inflammatory reaction. Because these changes are usually symmetric, the risk of herniation is less than is expected in disorders that produce asymmetric mass effects; therefore lumbar puncture should be performed, but cautiously. Spinal fluid analysis usually manifests mild pleocytosis (see Figure 39-3). There is usually a predominance of lymphocytes, except in special situations, such as herpes encephalitis. The CSF status may be unique to encephalitides because increased granulocytes, xanthochromia, and even frank hemorrhage are often observed. In other encephalitides, the character of the CSF changes greatly, depending on the stage of the disorder, and is influenced by the degree of associated meningitis. In most cases, there are less striking findings of the meningitis once encephalitis has developed. Protein concentrations are usually mildly to moderately elevated. Glucose content is usually mildly reduced, suggesting parenchymal involvement. Viral agents can be cultured from spinal fluid, but this occurs far less frequently than in aseptic meningitis. Isolation of the virus from other tissues and other acute and convalescent serologic titers are quite helpful in ultimately establishing the cause of many of the encephalitides (Tables 39-8, 39-9, and 39-10).

EEG provides an important assessment of patients suspected of having viral encephalitis. Even in aseptic meningitis, EEG has been demonstrated to be abnormal

Table 39-10 Specific pattern of viral growth in tissue culture

Virus to be isolated	Cells known to be susceptible								Speed of detection (weeks)*
	FSK	HeLa	RD	Vero	BSC-1	BAMA	RK-13	Hep-2	
Herpes simplex virus	+	+	+	+	+	+	+	−	1
Cytomegalovirus	+	−	−	−	−	−	−	−	2
Varicella-zoster	+	−	+	−	−	+	−	−	3
Polio	+	+	+	+	+	+	−	−	1
Rubella	−	−	−	+	+	−	−	−	4
Mumps virus	−	−	−	+	+	−	−	−	2-3
Measles	−	+	−	+	+	−	−	−	3
Adenovirus	+	+	+	−	−	+	−	+	3
Coxsackie A	+	−	+	−	−	−	−	−	1-3
Coxsackie B	−	+	+	−	−	+	−	+	1-3

*1 = rapid; 4 = slow.

FSK, human foreskin fibroblast; *HeLa*, human cervical carcinoma; *RD*, human rhabdomyosarcoma; *Vero*, African green monkey kidney; *BSC-1*, Cercopithecus monkey kidney; *BAMA*, cynomolgus kidney; *RK-13*, rabbit kidney; *Hep-2*, human laryngeal carcinoma.

in most patients, even though clinically assessed mental aberration or frank neurologic abnormalities suggesting parenchymal involvement are not present. The EEG in acute encephalitides is invariably abnormal, demonstrating in nearly every instance high amplitude and random slow-wave activity dispersed in a generalized fashion with few if any asymmetries. This activity usually requires a dampening of the amplitude out of proportion to the normal variations in sensitivity required for standard recording.

EEG may also reflect abnormalities that are supportive of clinical epileptic activity. In addition, comatose patients may manifest atypical motor activity or mental aberrations that clinically might not be recognized as convulsions, but EEG supports an epileptic basis. EEG may demonstrate special EEG features, particularly in herpes simplex encephalitis, such as periodic lateralized epileptiform discharges also called acute spikes, which are observed in many other acute encephalopathies of a lateralized nature (Figure 39-6).

Of great use in the assessment of acute encephalitis is CT and MRI. Although no pathognomonic picture is found in many of the diffuse encephalopathies, signs suggesting cerebral edema, obstructive hydrocephalus, or multifocal or disseminated lesions are very supportive of viral encephalitis. In herpes simplex encephalitis, CT and MRI are helpful in suggesting a specific diagnosis. The neuroimaging techniques are of different sensitivity. In herpes simplex encephalitis, CT visualizes hyperdense, enhancing lesions located in the basal temporal or frontal lobes. These lesions may be even more obvious in T_2-weighted MRIs. All abnormalities depend on the stage of the disorder when testing is performed. In the

first few hours of acute illness, it is possible that no abnormalities will be found on CT with and without contrast (Figure 39-7, *A*). Later, however, as neurologic symptoms develop, enhancing lesions disseminated throughout the encephalon are often demonstrated (Figure 39-7, *B*). These lesions are visualized most clearly in T_2-weighted MRIs as multiple, small, disseminated lesions, particularly suggestive of herpes simplex encephalitis. As a complication, hemorrhagic infarctions can occur (Figures 39-8 and 39-9).

Pathology. Histologic alterations in the CNS are common in most types of acute viral encephalitis, regardless of the specific causal viral agent. Brain swelling, vascular congestion, and perivascular mononuclear parenchymal infiltration are observed. A cellular reaction in the meninges is usually present, even in patients without obvious clinical meningitis. The type of cellular reaction in the meninges seems to correspond to the acuteness of the illness. The more devastating early stage manifests a granulocytic reaction, whereas the later stages reveal lymphocytic and monocytic cellular reactions. Microglial proliferation and nodule formation occur, particularly in the immediate vicinity of patches of neuron cell death and destruction (see Figure 39-5).

In the arbovirus encephalitides, no distinctive pathologic changes set them apart from other types except for the severity of damage that may be more striking as compared with that occurring in some of the milder encephalitides. California encephalitis is rarely associated with death. Herpes encephalitis type 1 may present a more distinctive pathologic picture, which is supportive of the specific clinical signs suggesting basal frontal and temporal involvement. In herpes simplex encephalitis,

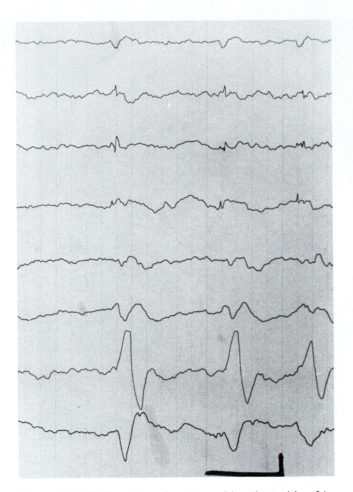

Figure 39-6 EEG tracing of a 6-year-old patient with a 24-hour history of epilepsia partialis continua. This is a bipolar tracing, with the top four traces representing left hemisphere and the bottom four lines the right hemisphere in frontal-temporal-occipital orientation. High-amplitude, periodic, lateralized epileptiform discharges arising from the right posterior temporal areas are shown. Patient had herpes simplex type 1 encephalitis, which was treated successfully with acyclovir intravenously 30 mg/kg/day for 10 days. Calibration: 50 microvolts and 1 second.

severe necrotizing and hemorrhagic lesions are present, with marked involvement of one or both orbital surfaces of the frontal lobe or frontotemporal areas. Occasionally, a single, large hemorrhagic infarction is observed (Figures 39-8 and 39-9). Edema is severe and associated with softening of the brain and often herniation. Microscopic examination often discloses characteristic Cowdry type A intranuclear inclusions in both glial cells and neurons. The pathology of the type 2 herpes encephalitis of the newborn does not reveal as much localization, which is consistent with the more diffuse encephalopathy and multisystem involvement in this variety of herpes simplex infection (Figure 39-10).

Management. Great strides have been made recently in the development of specific antiviral treatment for herpes simplex viral encephalitis. In all cases of all viral encephalitides, general supportive therapy is imperative and includes all modalities used to treat patients with severe illness. Respiratory and cardiovascular support is required, as well as proper fluid maintenance and electrolyte balance. Hydration must be restricted because overhydration worsens cerebral edema. Because seizures are common in acute viral encephalitis and increase metabolic requirements, antiseizure therapy becomes essential. In rare situations when heroic antiepileptic drug therapies are ineffective, patients may need to be paralyzed and supported totally by a ventilator. Cerebral edema is the rule, rather than the exception, and must be treated appropriately. Edema is believed to result from toxins liberated by the destruction of tissues and from vasculitis and may be treated by inducing hyperventilation (preferably keeping the PCO_2 between 20 and 25 torr), continuing mild depletion of intravascular volume, and using controlled quantities of antiedema agents, such as mannitol. Intracranial pressure monitoring is often helpful and allows use of other agents, such as phenobarbital to produce coma, thereby decreasing intracranial pressure. Other supportive measures should be intense [Oxman, 1986].

In the antiviral therapy of herpes simplex encephalitis, the most dramatic results to date have been with the use of acylovir, which is given at high dosages (30 mg/kg/day) intravenously over a 10-day period.

Meningomyeloradiculitis

Involvement of the caudal CNS represents an important aspect of viral disease. All meningitides have involvement of the spinal subarachnoid space through spinal fluid analysis after lumbar puncture.

Three important viral syndromes of the caudal CNS are observed. Poliomyelitis refers to the primary involvement of the gray matter of the spinal cord and usually the anterior horn cell. The term originated during the preimmunization days of poliovirus to identify its clinical presentation. Although poliovirus infections are now less of a threat, poliomyelitis may be caused by other enteroviruses, herpes viruses, parainfluenza viruses, the measles virus, togaviruses, rubella, reoviruses, arenaviruses, rhabdoviruses, and the mumps virus. Additionally, localized myelopathies occur in AIDS, but whether this represents a direct infection, an opportunistic infection, or an immunopathy is uncertain.

The second type of caudal CNS involvement is transverse myelitis (Figure 39-11). There is less predilection for cell type in this syndrome. The entire spinal cord at one level is usually involved. Viral agents are usually not cultured from the spinal fluid of patients with acute transverse myelitis. In many instances, a host immune reaction is favored as the primary source of

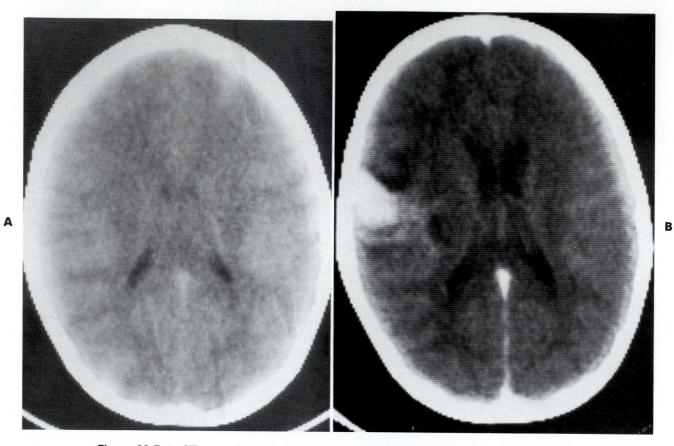

Figure 39-7 A, CT scan after contrast injection in 6-year-old patient with epilepsia partia- lis continua and early herpes simplex type 1 encephalitis 24 hours after onset. This axial view and other views were interpreted as normal. Orientation: patient's right to viewer's left. **B,** CT scan performed at 4 days of illness in 6-year-old patient with herpes simplex type I encephalitis shows a hyperdense area of presumed hemorrhage in the right tempo- ral region with surrounding edema of hypodense consistency. This is an enhanced axial view. Orientation: patient's right to viewer's left.

symptoms, and the possibility exists that other types of pathogens may be important in producing the symptom complex. In the absence of associated encephalitic signs, acute transverse myelitis has been described in associ- ation with mumps [Benady et al., 1973], measles [Senseman, 1945], varicella zoster [Johnson and Mil- bourne, 1970; Hogan and Krigman, 1973], infectious mononucleosis [Cotton and Webb-Peploe, 1966; Silver- stein et al., 1972], echovirus [Johnson and Eger, 1967], poliovirus [Foley and Beresford, 1974], and herpes simplex infections [Klastersky et al., 1972]. Other examples have been reported in rabies [Knutti, 1929], but the association of this syndrome with antirabies treatment and following smallpox vaccination suggests a nonviral origin.

A third viral syndrome involving the lower nervous system is polyradiculitis. These disorders represent a more localized infection of the spinal meninges, involv- ing proximal and posterior roots and ganglion cells. In addition, peripheral neuropathy and myelopathy may occur. Polyradiculitis is commonly associated with in- fectious mononucleosis. Other important viruses that may cause the syndrome include herpes simplex type 2 in children and adults, varicella, cytomegalovirus, most of the picornaviruses, the human paramyxoviruses (including measles, mumps, and parainfluenza viruses), the orbivirus (which causes Colorado tick fever), pos- sibly the retroviruses, and rarely some of the nonrabies rhabdoviruses [Bell and McCormick, 1981]. In chronic situations, albuminocytologic dissociation may occur, causing a picture similar to the Guillain-Barré syn- drome.

The three meningomyeloradiculitis syndromes can be differentiated clinically and pathologically and are often caused by different viruses. The Epstein-Barr virus most often appears as an acute polyradiculitis or as a more chronic syndrome with albuminocytologic dissociation, but rarely as a pure myelopathy. Conversely, the classic

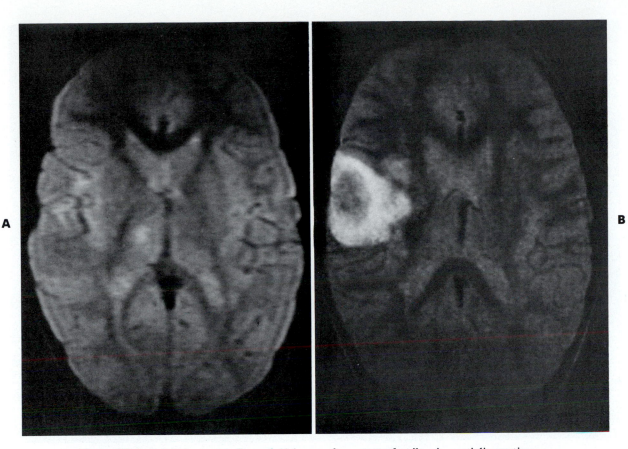

Figure 39-8 A, MRI scan performed 48 hours after onset of epilepsia partialis continua (24 hours after a normal CT scan) in a 6-year-old patient with herpes simplex type 1 encephalitis. This axial view demonstrates multiple small areas of hyperdensity in this T_2 weighted spin-echo technique, the largest in the right thalamus. Orientation: patient's right to viewer's left. **B,** MRI performed at 72 hours after onset of epilepsia partialis continua; 48 hours after seizures were controlled by antiepileptic drugs, and 24 hours after persistent nonepileptogenic hemiparesis was detected in a 6-year-old patient with herpes simplex type 1 encephalitis. A large, hyperdense area of presumed edema is seen in the right temporal-parietal lobe surrounding a circular hypodense area of presumed hemorrhagic infarction. This is a T_2 weighted spin-echo axial view. Orientation: patient's right to viewer's left.

poliomyelitis picture caused by poliovirus seldom reveals meningoradiculitis.

Clinical findings. Poliomyelitis resulting from the poliovirus has an incubation period of 6 to 20 days after the primary infection in the gastrointestinal tract [Bell and McCormick, 1981]. The primary infection may be asymptomatic or occur in the form of a transient, minor illness. Secondary infections with poliovirus may appear in several nonparalytic forms, including aseptic meningitis or polyradiculitis. Poliovirus, type 1 or 3 particularly, is prone to be paralytic or cause poliomyelitis. The paralytic disorder begins with fever and other signs of infection that last a few days. There is often headache, vomiting, and signs of meningeal irritation. After this prodrome occurs, it is followed by specific signs suggestive of poliomyelitis itself, such as limb pain, muscle

spasms, and flaccid muscular weakness. The paresis rapidly progresses, usually reaching maximum severity by 2 days. The pattern of weakness is characterized by asymmetric limb involvement. In the height of the acute illness, profound symmetric quadriparesis or paraparesis may be encountered. Muscle spasms may occur, but hypertonus, hyperreflexia, and extensor toe signs are not observed.

In the poliovirus era, infection of neurons of the medulla, or bulbar polio, was recognized [Bell and McCormick, 1981]. Bulbar polio was the significant cause of mortality. Involvement of cranial structures above the medulla were rarely encountered and were estimated to occur in less than 1% of reported patients [Bell and McCormick, 1981].

In the postpoliovirus immunization era, polio-like

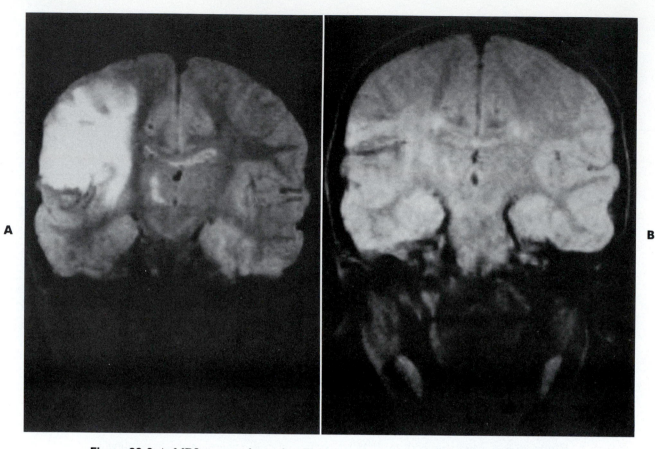

Figure 39-9 A, MRI scan performed at 72 hours after onset in conjunction with clinical signs of left hemiparesis but improvement in seizure frequency in a 6-year-old patient with herpes simplex type 1 encephalitis. Coronal view of a T_2 weighted spin-echo. Orientation: patient's right to viewer's left. **B,** MRI performed in same patient 6 months after onset in a period of apparent recovery. Patient still has mild neurologic deficits. Coronal view, same level, of a T_2 weighted spin-echo. Orientation is the same.

syndromes have followed nonpolio virus infections in which the course is less severe and the prognosis for full recovery is much better. In children, an asthma-associated, poliolike syndrome is believed to be associated with a virus infection. The residua closely resembles that found in old poliomyelitis. Another uncommon but unique syndrome is associated with an earlier bout of acute hemorrhagic conjunctivitis occurring weeks previously. Acute myelitis then develops from which severe residua often persists.

In transverse myelitis, the onset of symptoms is usually abrupt [Bell and McCormick, 1981]. There is a maximum neurologic deficit, usually occurring within 24 to 48 hours after the first symptom. Initial complaints include weakness of the legs and numbness or tingling of the feet. These symptoms are often associated with either radicular pain or localized back pain. As the process advances, the legs become progressively weaker and a sensory level is established, indicating the upper level of the spinal cord involvement. Most commonly, the

site of this involvement is in the upper to mid-thoracic region. Before this progression there may be a diminution of pain and temperature sensation, but there is a tendency to spare the posterior column modalities of position, vibration, and light touch. Neurogenic bladder dysfunction is often apparent, as might be expected, resulting from shock-type neurologic lesions. In the first few days of the illness, flaccid paralysis, decreased reflexes, and absent pathologic reflexes are present. These symptoms are related to the combined effects of a shock-type lesion, resulting from involvement of descending suprasegmental tracts, and a loss-type lesion, resulting from involvement of descending suprasegmental tracts, and a loss-type lesion, resulting from involvement of anterior horn cells at the level of involvement. However, these phenomena are often transient, especially in older children and adults. The shock suprasegmental signs are soon replaced by release signs, and patients begin to develop increased muscular tone and reflexes and extensor toe signs. There may be some

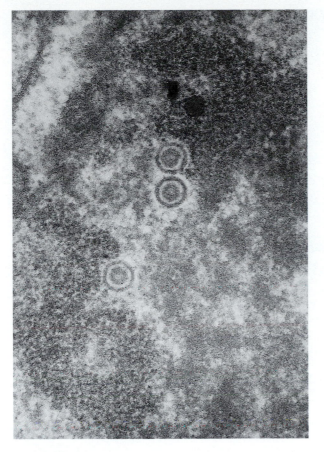

Figure 39-10 Electron microscopy of herpes viruses (Magnification about 70,000).

of changes in CSF dynamics may help exclude localized mass lesions of the spinal cord or meninges. It is unknown whether excessive spinal fluid withdrawal worsens the symptoms in transverse myelitis. Caution should always be taken in performing lumbar puncture in a patient with suspected myelopathy. The cellular reaction observed in viral disorders of the caudal CNS is variable.

There is often an initial neutrophilic granulocytic response in the poliomyelitis syndromes, but this response rapidly becomes lymphocytic with cell counts ranging from 20 to 300 cells/mm³. In some of the less severe forms of poliomyelitis a more subdued cellular reaction is usually encountered. Protein determinations in poliomyelitic syndromes are usually mildly elevated but seldom over 100 mg/dl. CSF glucose is usually normal.

Pronounced elevation in all cells in transverse myelitides usually occurs. In some instances there is frank hemorrhage. Usually a large number of total leukocytes, both with and without excessive contamination by peripheral blood, is evident. Excessive numbers of neutrophilic granulocytes, lymphocytic cells, reticulomonocytes, and phagocytic cells are evident. In myelitis, there is a dramatic elevation of protein, with levels sometimes approaching 1000 mg. This finding is not helpful in excluding other mass lesions of the cord from diagnosis. CSF glucose may be normal or slightly decreased.

A mild pleocytosis may be observed in the early stages of the polyradiculitides, usually more granulocytic than would be expected. In later stages the cellular reaction is lymphocytic with occasional reticulomonocytes if special cellular differential procedures were used [Dyken, 1975]. Later, however, the cellular reaction is usually dampened, and a gradually increasing protein elevation becomes evident. In this stage, albuminocytologic dissociation occurs, which is similar to the pattern of Guillain-Barré syndrome.

The likelihood of culturing viruses in each of these syndromes depends on the viral type causing it, the stage at which cultures are attempted, and the type of syndrome. In the instance of transverse myelitis, viral culture is often unsuccessful. Hyperglobulinorrachia may occur. Enteroviruses are more likely to be cultured at the time of acute meningopoliomyelitis than are some of the other types of viruses. CSF analysis may help evaluate the acute viral diseases, requiring baseline (acute) and convalescent studies. CSF analysis is impractical unless the specific virus type is suspected for the acute disease infection.

Repeated serologic blood tests may be helpful. In the case of enterovirus and herpesvirus infections, viral cultures from other tissue may be very helpful.

Electromyography represents an important supple-

recovery of the initial sensory disturbances during these later stages. Occasionally patients with this syndrome have varicella zoster infections (Figure 39-11).

The polyradiculitides are associated with symptoms corresponding to specific involvement of the dorsal horn and roots, with or without peripheral nerve and spinal cord involvement. Paresthesia, sensory losses (both local and generalized), weakness but not paralysis, hyporeflexia, and mild hypotonia are common symptoms in these syndromes. Often signs suggesting frank meningeal irritation occur, especially early in the illness. Neck and back stiffness and pain after straight-leg raising exercises may also dominate the clinical picture. The symptoms of polyradiculitis may ascend or descend as the disease progresses. In this situation, a clinical picture identical to the Guillain-Barré syndrome may be observed, which is supported by the characteristic spinal fluid changes revealing albuminocytologic dissociation and normal glucose.

Laboratory findings. Spinal fluid analysis is the essential laboratory test of these syndromes. Alterations in pressures are seldom observed in any of the caudal viral disorders. In acute transverse myelitis, the absence

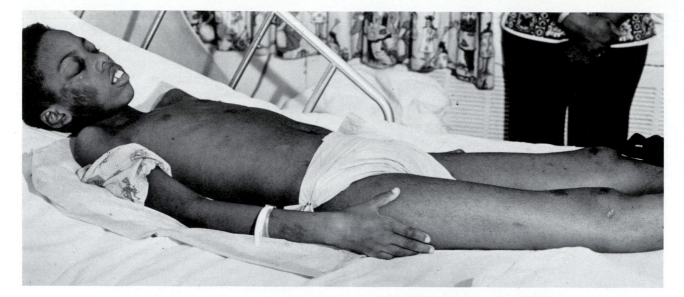

Figure 39-11 A 12-year-old patient in good health until developing a vesicular rash that is progressing to hyperpigmented excoriations approximately 2 weeks before this photograph was taken. The patient experienced a sudden loss of vision 3 days before photograph and a sudden loss of strength and tone in the lower extremities and paresis of the upper extremities with loss of bladder control and sensory level 2 days before the photograph was taken. The patient later developed bilateral optic atrophy and was considered to have a transverse myelitis and optic neurotis caused by varicella-zoster—virus-induced neuromyelitis optica.

mental investigation in the caudal CNS syndromes, particularly in evaluating the polyradiculitides and in the later rehabilitative phase of many of the poliomyelitides and transverse myelitides.

Pathology. In the poliomyelitides, the anterior horn cell demonstrates the usual findings of acute deterioration. Pathologic reactions include chromatolysis, neurolysis, and ultimately neuronophagia. There are usually prominent inflammatory changes characterized by diffuse edema and cellular exudation, particularly in the perivascular spaces. A meningeal inflammatory reaction is observed in the early acute phases. Later, however, the inflammatory changes are less pronounced followed by are minimal if present at all. Neuronal loss confined to the anterior horns of the spinal cord is evident in these stages. In material obtained from poliovirus epidemics, similar changes are observed in the medullar reticular formation and more rostrally in the hypothalamus and thalamus [Bell and McCormick, 1981]. Cerebellar and cerebral cortex changes are rare. Striking muscular histologic changes are seen, as is expected in the amyotrophic state. Although pathologic studies are much rarer in the other polio-like syndromes, findings similar to those in classic poliomyelitis are found in both acute and chronic states.

Far more widespread and severe pathologic findings are evident in the rare case of transverse myelitis of presumed viral immunopathic origin that is autopsied. In some chronic cases, severe destruction has occurred, usually involving several levels in the upper or midthoracic cord. In those cases with less severe destruction, loss of neurons is observed in anterior, posterior, and intermediate horns of the spinal gray matter. Global loss of the major neural pathways occurs, and the anterolateral parts of the cord are particularly affected. Inflammatory changes are far less obvious than destructive changes. In those who recover but are left with deficits, later pathologic study reveals widespread destructive changes, demyelination, and gliosis.

The pathologic picture is unremarkable in autopsied cases of polyradiculitis that are autopsied. Studies often reveal nonspecific findings in most instances, which is quite compatible with Guillain-Barré syndrome.

Management. The specific antiviral therapies are few and revolve around the recent work on antiviral agents, effective in only certain types of viral diseases. The effective treatment of herpes simplex viral encephalitis raises the question of whether aseptic meningitides and meningomyelitides related to herpes simplex type 2 should not also be treated with the relatively innocuous acyclovir.

Necessary supportive therapy of the caudal CNS viral diseases is essential. Intensive care of patients with poliomyelitic syndromes, transverse myelitic syndromes, and ascending forms of polyradiculitis is essential. Most of these patients have self-limited diseases, and proper care of body functions, adequate fluid and electrolyte balance, and vital respiratory support may sustain the patient until complete recovery. Bladder dysfunction must be addressed and treated when present. In the transverse myelitides, corticosteroid therapy has been attempted with some success. Because caudal CNS viral disorders may also involve more rostral levels of the nervous system, careful neurologic monitoring is important.

SUBACUTE NEUROLOGIC DISORDERS

Many neural viral disorders appear as a more slowly developing process than seen in acute-onset and progressive viral disorders. Several viral diseases are thus placed in this subacute category because of the rate of clinical presentation or onset and dynamics of disease development. Several syndromes fit into this subacute, rather than acute or chronic, category.

Rabies

Human rabies results from the secondary infection by the lyssavirus of the rhabdovirus family of a secondary host. The naturally occurring host is able to cope with the effects of the virus. By a mistake in nature, the virus is transmitted to the unnatural host, such as humans, and the devastations of the disease may be the greatest of all viral diseases [Baer, 1975]. Much has been learned about virology in general because of the lengthy study of this disorder since Pasteur's first successful cure of a viral disease by immunization [Pasteur, 1884]. The success of immunization is primarily based on the subacute nature of human rabies. Rabies has a lengthy incubation period of up to 60 days or even longer. Additionally, neurologic symptoms develop slowly, and many investigators consider the lyssavirus in humans to represent a slow virus disease [Haase, 1986]; however, the effects of subacute viral diseases often reflect the host's reaction rather than direct viral effect.

Clinical findings. Two forms of human rabies are recognized: the classic, or restless, form and the rare paralytic form [Warrell, 1976; Postic and Wiktar, 1986; Chopra et al., 1980]. Rabies typically begins after an incubation period from 30 to 60 days, which represents stage I. There is usually a prodromal period of 2 to 10 days of fever, headache, and malaise, representing stage II. Thereafter, the first neurologic signs develop, which are characterized by pain and dysesthesia, usually occurring in the distribution of the nerves from the site of the original contact with the virus, whether it be the bite or another site of inoculation. Stage III begins months after the original inoculation of the virus, usually lasts for 2 to 7 days, and is represented by gradually increasing excitement. Progressive autonomic dysfunc-

tion occurs, an extreme overreaction to all types of sensory stimuli, and severe anxiety. Pupillary dilatation and excessive lacrimation, salivation, and perspiration occur. These symptoms are believed to represent both hypothalamic and brainstem involvement. There may also be insomnia, apprehension, depression, and hydrophobia. Hydrophobia occurs after sighting liquid or food, which seems to stimulate the swallowing process, producing a painful spasm of the pharyngeal and respiratory muscles and a forceful expulsion of saliva. Physical examination often reveals nystagmus, cranial nerve palsies, anisocoria, and facial weakness. Convulsions are common. Stage IV begins with increasing paralysis and coma. Death occurs usually within 1 to 14 days after this stage begins. Two patients have been reported who survived rabies. One of these was a 6-year-old boy in the United States [Porros et al., 1976; Hattwick et al., 1972]. In this patient, no significant neurologic abnormalities were found in follow-up studies over 1 year later.

Occasionally, rabies is discovered at autopsy of persons who died from an unidentified encephalitis, which usually occurs in persons with an atypical onset, with no prodrome, and none of the hallmark clinical symptoms and signs but with early coma and paralysis. These occurrences might represent the paralytic form of rabies [Postic and Wikter, 1986; Chopra et al., 1980; Porras et al., 1976].

Laboratory findings. Rabies often produces a peripheral leukocytosis with a predominance of neutrophilic granulocytes. CSF is usually normal, but in some reports there may be a pleocytosis (100 to 200/mm^3), usually a lymphocytic type. The CSF protein concentration is often mildly elevated but seldom exceeds 100 mg/dl. Glucose content may be slightly depressed, but not strikingly so considering the devastating encephalopathic picture. EEG reveals diffuse, random, slow activity but with no specific diagnostic features, such as burst suppression, periodic patterns, or periodic lateralized epileptiform discharges to separate this from other encephalitides. Brain imaging seldom discloses any local or lateralized disturbances [Postic and Wiktar, 1986]. MRI, which can be particularly helpful in observing brainstem lesions, has not been used in this type of encephalitis.

Spinal fluid antibody to the rabies virus has been identified in patients with rabies. The spinal fluid antibody titer is 25% to 33% higher than in the serum, but it is not elevated in those patients vaccinated against rabies. Fluorescent monoclonal rabies antibody has been combined with viral antigen to allow rapid and specific identification of rabies in tissues, such as the cornea (i.e., the corneal test), oronasal mucosa, or frozen sections of skin or brain.

Pathology. In human rabies, maximum involvement occurs in the hypothalamus, hippocampus, limbic sys-

lesions in the gray matter are not unusual. The lesions are usually perivenular. Involvement of the cerebellum is common, especially in the venous white matter. Numerous small areas of demyelination occur. The more acute lesions tend to coalesce with older lesions, probably supporting the ongoing subacute development of signs and symptoms observed clinically.

Management. Corticosteroids are accepted as useful in treating disseminated encephalomyelitis.

Postinfectious encephalomyeloradiculitis

These disorders follow, or are associated with, viral diseases but do not have the characteristics of either hemorrhagic leukoencephalitis or the disseminated encephalomyelitis syndrome. There may be a variety of clinical presentations. They are often difficult to distinguish from the previously discussed conditions, except that they are milder and usually self-limited [Bell and McCormick, 1981].

Clinical findings. These postinfectious neurologic syndromes usually occur after the onset of the naturally occurring common childhood exanthems, such as varicella, mumps, rubella, and measles. Frequently, they appear as acute cerebellar ataxia, ascending palsy, polyneuroradiculitis, conjunctivitis, myelitis, and acute mental confusion or altered mental status. The symptoms are usually self-limited and may resolve within days or weeks.

Laboratory findings. The laboratory findings in post-infectious syndromes related to the previously mentioned exanthems are usually unremarkable.

Pathology. The pathologic conditions in the remaining forms of subacute encephalopathies related to viral infections have not been clearly delineated.

Management. Caution must be used when administering corticosteroids for some of the postinfectious disorders because of the possible exacerbation of the acute viral infections, as has been reported in varicella. Careful alleviation of all symptoms, including seizures and increased intracranial pressure, is important for all diseases in this category.

CHRONIC NEUROLOGIC DISORDERS
Slow viral diseases

The disorders included in the category of chronic viral disorders of the nervous system are representative of an expanding and argumentative nosology. The most representative of the category are the slow viral infections, which were first recognized by Sigurdsson [1954] and now have come to include those disorders caused by proved conventional viral agents, as is the case in subacute sclerosing panencephalitis. The disorders of conventional type represent the effect of an altered or persistent virus on the nervous system and usually are slowly progressive encephalopathies. These slow infections are compared with a group of disorders caused by unproved or unconventional "viruses"; the prototypic examples of these infections are kuru and Creutzfeldt-Jakob disease. The unconventional infectious agents have few characteristics in common with any known viral agent but do cause progressive encephalopathy. They probably do not represent viral diseases, yet because of tradition, they must be discussed as such.

Another subgroup of chronic neurologic viral disorders is the well-recognized viral diseases that affect the fetus but that are essentially quiescent in later life, at least as an active viral-host disorder. These disorders cause acute infections in utero and in the perinatal period. In utero, when severe, they are responsible for fetal death. If mild and occurring early enough in gestation, they may account for severe dysgenesis or malformations. Because of the scars of previous insult, these syndromes usually appear as static encephalopathies or as a variety of cerebral dysgenetic syndromes. These presentations are long-standing or chronic and are properly included as examples of chronic viral disorders. Each of these embryogenic encephalopathies results from an initial active viral infection but later, in some instances, represent activation of latent virus infections. Some of these static diseases years later lapse into progressive viral disorders.

A final subcategory of neurologic chronic viral diseases is represented by the viral immunodeficiency states, knowledge of which has expanded rapidly in recent years with the discovery of acquired immunodeficiency syndrome (AIDS). Although once considered only a secondary neurologic disease related to primary immunodeficiency, more recent evidence suggests that the AIDS virus has a direct and significant effect on the nervous system that causes a wide range of symptoms, including dementia. Findings typical of many neurodegenerative diseases that are independent of immunodeficiency are also evident in AIDS. It has been demonstrated that a retrovirus causes visna, a chronic demyelinating disease of sheep [Gallo, 1987]. This disorder is not related to immunodeficiency. AIDS is often a reflection of pure immunodeficiency, and there is a propensity to develop secondary chronic neurologic infections from papovavirus and herpes viruses. These disorders must also be considered in the category of chronic viral disease of the nervous system.

The conventional progressive viral encephalopathies are believed to be the result of altered or persistent viral infections of the nervous system. Characteristic of all such disorders are (1) exposure to and overt manifestations of an initial infection, (2) presence of a long preclinical course before the appearance of new symptoms usually confined to an encephalopathy, and (3) effects limited to the nervous system. The few diseases that have been demonstrated to result from such chronic viral infections in humans are (1) subacute sclerosing panencephalitis, (2) progressive rubella panencephalitis, (3) progressive multifocal leukoencephalitis, (4) direct retrovirus encephalopathy, and (5) rabies (previously discussed under subacute encephalomyelitides). Each of these disorders has unique clinical features, laboratory findings, pathology, and treatment.

Subacute sclerosing panencephalitis. As the name implies, subacute sclerosing panencephalitis (SSPE) is a subacute inflammatory and degenerative disease of the entire brain.

A careful attempt was made as early as 1934 to detect the infectious agent responsible for subacute sclerosing panencephalitis. In 1967, a measles-like virus was believed to be associated with subacute sclerosing panencephalitis based upon antibody studies [Zeman and Kolar, 1968]. In 1969, however, the first confirmation that measles virus harbored in the brains of patients with subacute sclerosing panencephalitis was established through the almost simultaneous reports [Horta-Barbosa et al., 1969, Chen et al., 1969, and Payne et al. 1969]. In 1969, the SSPE National Registry was established [Jabbour et al., 1972]. Although the measles virus was believed to be *intimately* responsible for the disease, it was not fully understood how the measles virus acted in subacute sclerosing panencephalitis until more recent work established the role of the measles protein identified as M-protein was developed [Choppin, 1981; Hall et al, 1976; Wechsler and Meissner, 1982]. At present, the major etiologic and pathogenetic basis of subacute sclerosing panencephalitis is understood, and the clinical presentation is more fully documented than in previous years; however, many unanswered questions about the disease still exist.

Clinical findings. Subacute sclerosing panencephalitis represents a unique disease from many clinical viewpoints [Dyken et al., 1982b]. In general, the disease runs a very stereotyped clinical presentation and course; however, variations in this theme have become more evident [Dyken et al., 1983, 1989]. For the perceptive diagnostician with clinical expertise, the features of subacute sclerosing panencephalitis follow such a consistent course that clinical diagnosis is often possible. (Figure 39-12). Even more importantly, a differentiation between other superficially similar neurodegenerative diseases of childhood and infancy may be made. The onset of neurologic symptoms usually begins in the juvenile period; the most likely ages are 5 to 15 years [Jabbour et al., 1975; Risk and Haddad, 1979] but with a greater range (e.g., 6 months to 32 years). The youngest patient in the registry had onset at 1.2 years and the oldest at 32 years. When fully developed, subacute sclerosing panencephalitis has telltale clinical signs and symptoms that allow for easy recognition. The telltale

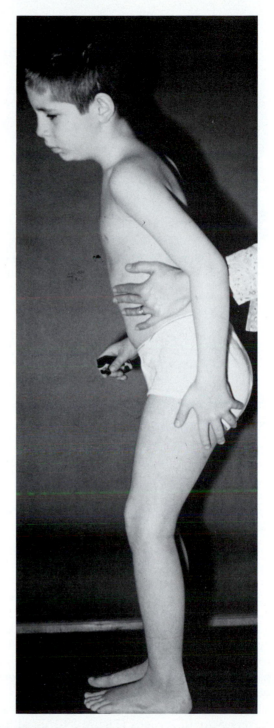

Figure 39-12 An 8-year-old patient with early stage II subacute sclerosing panencephalitis. He is still ambulatory with help, but has continued myoclonic jerking. This photograph series was taken in 1968; the patient was later subjected to diagnostic brain biopsy, which provided an subacute sclerosing panencephalitis viral stain now identified as the Mantooth strain.

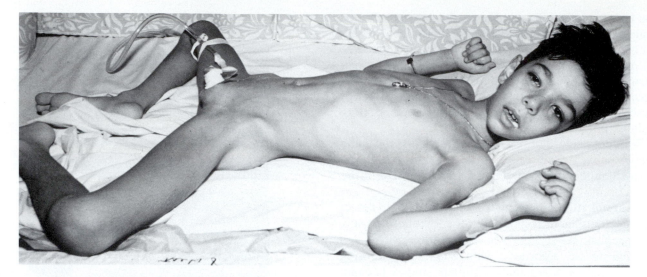

Figure 39-13 An 8-year-old patient with late stage II subacute sclerosing panencephalitis. He is no longer ambulatory and tends to maintain this "froglike" posture; continued massive myoclonus occurs at 8 per second. He has severe dementia.

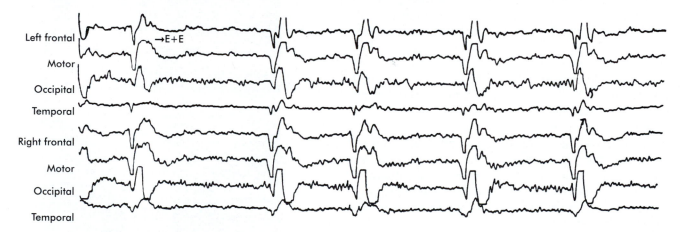

Figure 39-14 EEG tracing in subacute sclerosing panencephalitis, stage 2.

signs are identified as myoclonic and herald what has been called the second stage of the disease (stage II). In stage II, massive, repetitive, and frequent myoclonic jerking occurs. Myoclonia develops slowly (Figure 39-12) and irregularly but gradually affects all somatic muscle groups (especially the axial muscle) in a reasonably symmetric fashion and at a regularly repetitive rate. Periodicity occurs and a massive jerk occurs at some point every 5 to 10 seconds (Figure 39-13). Although myoclonia (literally meaning *turmoil in muscles*) in general is nonspecific, the myoclonia that occurs in subacute sclerosing panencephalitis is unique. In virtually all instances, it does not represent the end result of an epileptic seizure per se as in other disorders, such as infantile spasms, but rather is nonepileptic. The muscle turmoil in subacute sclerosing panencephalitis is more likely a result of extrapyramidal discharge than of

epilepsy. It is likely these movements are more akin to other involuntary movements, such as chorea, athetosis, choreoathetosis, ballismus, or dystonia. Epileptic seizures also occur in subacute sclerosing panencephalitis but are not clearly confined to stage II and may manifest in any of the four major stages of the disease (Figure 39-14).

Not only does the unique myoclonia make clinical recognition of subacute sclerosing panencephalitis possible, but the disease has a characteristic staging in other ways as well [Dyken, 1985] (see Table 39-9 and Figures 39-15 and 39-16). Although it has been customary to relate the onset of subacute sclerosing panencephalitis to the beginning of neurologic symptoms, it may be more appropriate to consider the true onset to be the first contact with natural measles (Figure 39-17). The early phases of subacute sclerosing panencephalitis typically

disability exceeding 90% disability. Those with subacute speed have at least 66% neurologic disability within 9 months with typical staging. Conversely, the chronic form does not have a typical staging and does not cause neurologic disability as great as 66% until after 9 months from first symptoms. In the chronic form, myoclonia or stage II symptoms may be greatly delayed. Stabilization may occur in the relentless downhill course as well as in the remission and recurrent form. It has recently been demonstrated that 92% of all patients reported to the subacute sclerosing panencephalitis registry are in a relentless downhill course whether they stabilize and whether the speed of disease is acute, subacute, or chronic as arbitrarily defined. This figure is slightly less than suggested in previous reports from the National SSPE registry [Jabbour et al., 1969, 1972], which seemed to indicate that remissions were a very rare occurrence.

Epidemiology. Epidemiologic investigations have been key in the development of an understanding of this disease and have been brought about in large part through activities of the USA National SSPE Registry. After it was first presumed that subacute sclerosing panencephalitis was caused by a persistent infestation of the CNS by the measles virus, many questions still remained. In the early days of the registry [Jabbour et al., 1972; Modlin et al., 1979; Jabbour et al., 1969], it was determined that subacute sclerosing panencephalitis mostly affected boys. The 2.3:1 male-to-female ratio reported by these early investigations represented a population that had not been maximally influenced by the US national measles immunization program that started in 1963. In these early studies, it was reported repeatedly that the average age of onset was about 8 years. Subacute sclerosing panencephalitis appeared to be mainly a disease that affected poor rural whites. The disease was distributed geographically in rural areas of the southeastern United States and the Ohio River valley [Detels et al., 1973]. Most registry-reported patients had histories of natural measles infections at an unusually early age compared with the non-subacute sclerosing panencephalitis population age of onset of measles. In the initial reports, no data suggested that measles immunization caused any increased susceptibility to developing subacute sclerosing panencephalitis. Early case control studies [Modlin et al., 1977, 1979] originating from registry material reported that there was a heightened incidence of exposure to sick animals, particularly dogs with distemper and sick birds and pigs, during the period close to the development of the neurologic manifestations of subacute sclerosing panencephalitis in affected patients. In early reports from the United States and elsewhere, the neurologic clinical presentation tended to be very stereotyped. Subacute sclerosing panencephalitis was considered to be a universally fatal and incurable disease that caused death

within 2 to 4 years. The clinical presentation was believed to be uniformly progressive. The classic presentation represented the major percentage of the patients with subacute sclerosing panencephalitis reported by pediatric neurologists. Death occurred at an earlier age, invariably in the juvenile period, a few years after onset of neurologic manifestations. Hispanics did not represent a sizable percentage of patients reported with subacute sclerosing panencephalitis.

In more recent years, these findings have changed somewhat. Recent review of patients reported to the registry revealed that the sex ratio is gradually decreasing. Female patients are being reported relatively more often; the previous ratio of 2.3:1 has declined to 1.8:1 in a review of over 100 recent patients. Also, over the years, the age of onset of neurologic symptoms has gradually increased and is now closer to 14 years. The average age of onset of measles in those patients who develop subacute sclerosing panencephalitis has remained about the same, but the interval from measles to subacute sclerosing panencephalitis has increased. The effect of measles immunization is still not understood, but there are now some suggestions that immunization added to natural infection may create some additional worsening of the subacute sclerosing panencephalitis but not an earlier onset. When it is added to the effect of natural measles, immunization may induce the neurologic symptoms and possibly exacerbate them. The possibility that immunization alone produces subacute sclerosing panencephalitis exists, but there is no direct supportive evidence. The geographic and ethnic distribution of subacute sclerosing panencephalitis has changed somewhat. Although American blacks still develop subacute sclerosing panencephalitis at about the same low rate of incidence as previously reported, there has been a dramatic increase in the disease among Hispanics [Dyken et al., 1989]. It is probable the majority of these patients represents immigrants and also contributes to a shift of reported patients to the western United States. Subacute sclerosing panencephalitis is still a disease of rural non-farm dwellers with low socioeconomic status. This observation was especially true during the period when natural measles was presumed to enter the body, that is, during the period when the reported patients developed their natural measles infection [Dyken, 1985]. In these patients, immunization has been spotty. There have been no further changes regarding the effect of coexistent viral infections at the onset of subacute sclerosing panencephalitis.

It would appear that the clinical stereotype is more variable in recent clinical experience with subacute sclerosing panencephalitis. The percentage of classic types of subacute sclerosing panencephalitis has decreased over the years, and more patients with intermittently or staggering progressive subacute sclerosing panencephalitis have been reported, although these trends are still small [Dyken et al., 1983]. Apparently, more patients have been reported recently with more chronic forms of subacute sclerosing panencephalitis. Conversely, the registry encounters the same numbers of patients who are reported to have fulminating and acute forms. The duration of subacute sclerosing panencephalitis has increased, possibly because of curative therapy measures that are still controversial. Generally better medical management of the chronically debilitated patient is available [Dyken, 1985].

Laboratory findings. The present-day diagnosis of subacute sclerosing panencephalitis is based on a combination of clinical and laboratory factors. In the past, at least three of the following five criteria were necessary to make a diagnosis:

1. Typical clinical presentation
2. Typical EEG pattern
3. Typical histologic findings either by brain biopsy during life or postmortem studies
4. Hyperglobulinorrhachia greater than 20% of the total protein
5. Elevation of serum and CSF measles antibody titers for the most commonly used complement-fixation technique of measure. Accepted minimal titers are 1:24 in the serum and 1:8 in the CSF.

In light of continuing sophistication, these criteria need modification. The clinical presentation of subacute sclerosing panencephalitis has been demonstrated to be more variable than was once believed. Not only are two disease profiles possible (the relentlessly progressive and a remitting or intermittently progressive form), but the speed of each of these profiles may vary from acute or subacute to chronic. In the acute types of subacute sclerosing panencephalitis that are relentlessly progressive, the separation of stages may be overlooked because of the focus by the clinician on the more dramatic fulminating, rapid, downhill and life-threatening course. These individuals may die with such dominating acutely encephalitic symptoms that all other symptoms go unrecognized, or they may die before the destructive and reparative pathologic reactions become clinically recognizable. Likewise, the chronic forms of subacute sclerosing panencephalitis may have such a slow progression that the staging is unrecognized. Those remaining in stage I for excessively long periods may manifest dominant dysmentation or dementation symptoms, giving the clinician the false impression that he or she is dealing with another type of dementia. At least five different clinical syndromes of subacute sclerosing panencephalitis have now been recognized [Dyken et al., 1983], but even this reasonably simple classification is further complicated by the fact that spontaneous long-term stabilization can theoretically occur in any syndrome at any level. The possibilities of different presentations are virtually unlimited. Still, it is necessary to establish some clinical criteria for diagnosis; at least nine somewhat dissimilar syndromes in addition to the classic textbook description are possible.

The once accepted diagnostic EEG pattern in subacute sclerosing panencephalitis is no longer accepted. The classic periodicity of high-voltage sharp and slow wave bursts alternating with (at the most) only mild suppression is very typical of subacute sclerosing panencephalitis but only occurs in the clinically characteristic myoclonic or stage II period. In stage I, the EEG may be normal or reveal only mild to moderate, nonspecific slowing. In stage III, there has been a conversion of myoclonus to immobility or other extrapyramidal clinical symptoms; EEG often demonstrates severe disturbances but usually in the form of disorganization and higher-amplitude, random arrhythmic slowing. In stage IV, this pattern further deteriorates and may become lower in amplitude, although still revealing great disorganization. Although EEG is useful in plotting the clinical course of the disease, only the stage II EEG can be thought of as close to pathognomonic. Even then, other diseases of a neurodegenerative and epileptogenic type can demonstrate a similar pattern and should be considered.

Undoubtedly, histologic confirmation represents a significant criterion for the diagnosis of subacute sclerosing panencephalitis. In the earlier days of the registry, brain biopsy represented the most specific form of diagnosis, particularly if both gray and white matter were studied by way of a generously wide and deep incision; however, other diseases may produce any one of the characteristic gross pathohistologic features, including neuronal and glial cell inclusions, subacute inflammatory vascular changes, subacute demyelination, and extensive gliosis. It is important to recognize also that subacute sclerosing panencephalitis is a dynamic disease. This factor will be explained in the section on pathogenesis. The ongoing process of inflammation preceding destruction or necrosis preceding reparative or gliotic changes is further complicated by the pathologic sequence also moving in a rostral to caudal direction. A brain biopsy may miss the major telltale histologic features. In this regard, even postmortem studies may not confirm many of the typical histologic features of subacute sclerosing panencephalitis because many of the more acute features, for example, the inflammatory reaction, may have dissipated, leaving only features of cell death, destruction, and the body's attempts at reparation in the form of gliosis. Although the histologic confirmation of the subacute sclerosing panencephalitis process is still important, brain biopsy is no longer necessary for diagnosis. CT or MRI represents ways to confirm the clinical picture that may be almost as specific and certainly far less invasive [Krawiecki et al., 1984]. CT is more predictive of the later stages of subacute sclerosing panencephalitis correlating with duration of disease and atrophy and in turn reflecting "scars" from previous tissue destruction. CT signs of acute brain swelling, neovascularization, and acute parenchymal breakdown represent uncommon CT features of this disease.

Before the perfection of techniques to measure CSF measles antibody, the presence of increased amounts of globulin was very helpful in confirming the diagnosis of subacute sclerosing panencephalitis. This hyperglobulinorrhachia represents increased gammaglobulin that is not specific for subacute sclerosing panencephalitis. Oligoclonal banding may also be present, but this also is not an absolute criterion for diagnosis. CSF plasmacytosis has been reported (Figure 39-18).

The most consistent laboratory confirmation of the diagnosis of subacute sclerosing panencephalitis at present is the CSF measles antibody titer, regardless of the technique used to measure it. In all patients whom I tested, and in the vast majority of those reported to the registry, the measles antibody titer in the CSF has been at 1 to 8 dilution or greater, using complement-fixation techniques. Other antibody measures are also useful. There have been rare reports of negative CSF measles antibody titiers in patients with subacute sclerosing panencephalitis [Mandelbaum et al., 1980]. Elevation in the serum measles antibody is not as specific. Recent reports suggest that the CSF measles titer is being synthesized in the CNS [Tourtellotte et al., 1981].

Presently, the clinical impression of subacute sclerosing panencephalitis is best supported by a simple CSF measles antibody determination. It is suggested that typical clinical presentations (once the different types of subacute sclerosing panencephalitis are recognized) and elevated CSF measles antibody titer (using a complement-fixation technique) are sufficient to establish the diagnosis of subacute sclerosing panencephalitis, especially if supported by other data, such as a history of early measles infection, staging, EEG abnormalities, hyperglobulinorrhachia, and serum measles antibody elevations.

Although specific, subunit measles protein serum and CSF antibody titer have not been developed sufficiently, it would appear that in the near future a battery of antibody titers for each of the individual proteins of the measles virion would allow an even more specific diagnosis. A typical subacute sclerosing panencephalitis antibody titer profile would show antibody elevations to all subunits of the virion protein, except for the matrix or M-protein, which, because it is defective in subacute sclerosing panencephalitis, would not be expected to reveal elevations and, in fact, should be depressed or absent.

Patients with subacute sclerosing panencephalitis have elevated antibody titers to all the major measles proteins except M-protein [Connolly et al., 1967; Hall et al., 1976; Wechsler and Meissner, 1982]. It is believed that the total measles virus (the one endemic to our population) enters a susceptible host during a vulnerable immunologic period. One of these vulnerable periods may be infancy alone, but it is likely other "primers" are also necessary. Such "primer" factors might be genetic (male chromosome is an example), racial, nutritional, or other infections. These factors might also be necessary to add to the vulnerability at onset of the initial measles infection. It would be presumed that most persons would be exposed to the virus but that some of these infectious episodes might be subclinical and unrecognized as such. At any rate, an antibody response occurs after the host's immune system is stimulated; however, in those who later develop subacute sclerosing panencephalitis, it is not completely effective. In the defective immune response, only parts of the measles proteins are destroyed (such as the M-protein) and the virus, or what remains of the initial organism, escapes and is harbored in the relatively immunologically privileged CNS. In this regard, it is noteworthy that the CNS does not have a large availability and quantity of complement, which is necessary to lyse cell membranes and thus allow contact with intracellular antigens. The altered, now nonlytic measles virus accesses the neurons and glia of the CNS and remains essentially intracellular because it is never able to contact the extracellular space because of the inability to bud. Once the cell dies, however, the nonlytic virus, as part of the death process, makes contact with the immune system because it is extruded into the extracellular space. This process causes an elevation of serum and CSF measles antibodies (except for the M-protein antibody, which is always low or absent). The measles virus, which by now can be called the subacute sclerosing panencephalitis virus, continues to grow slowly, replicating by fusion and slowly being passed on from one cell to the next. The CNS and the retina represent places in the body where the persistence of the virus replicating by the less efficient fusion method may occur without loss of the virus because these tissues have a small, almost nonexistent, extracellular space. In the brain compact, cell-to-cell contact allows the "melting" together of the cytoplasmic membranes and passage of virus from one cell to the next without extracellular contact. The spread of virus continues over years. In time, enough disturbance has occurred in intracellular functional mechanics that masses of cells begin to deteriorate and die. Often, this process results in dramatic increases in measles antibodies, but only for the proteins that still exist in the virion. Although this massive antibody response is detrimental to the virus that can be contacted within the extracellular space, those viruses that are still harbored intracellularly are not affected. They continue to grow, as before, protected from the host's immune response.

Immobility results from impairment of both pyramidal and extrapyramidal motor systems and supplants myoclonia. In stage IV, the entire CNS manifests prominent destructive lesions, extending from the gray matter to the brainstem and even spinal cord (Figures 39-19 and 39-20). Soon even vegetative function is lost.

Management. As expected, the response to both curative and palliative treatment is variable, depending on the stage of the disease at the commencement of therapy. Generally, one may hope to resolve much of the nonpermanent inflammatory and early destructive symptomatology and stop further progression. Even a remarkable curative therapy at one stage may be ineffective in another, especially if the more permanent destructive processes were complete, as in terminal and vegetative stages. Palliation of symptoms, of course, is always possible.

The most important impediment to specific curative therapy in subacute sclerosing panencephalitis is explained by the mechanisms of action of the altered virus, which is intracellular and protected. Another impediment to treatment is represented by lack of clinical appreciation of the early manifestations of the disease, caused by the reversible inflammatory changes in the gray matter. Once destruction has occurred, it may be too late to reverse the process. However, it would stop progression. A feasible approach to treatment, if possible, would be to open up the intracellular compartment to allow access of natural or artificial agents to the virus.

Of course, this process must be accomplished without destruction of the host cell, whose death represents the basis of the permanent symptomatology. So far, no agent has been developed to accomplish this task.

Several antiviral agents and other actions that alter host immunity have been used to treat subacute sclerosing panencephalitis, including transfer factor [Blaese et al., 1975; Kackell, 1975], thymectomy [Kolar et al., 1967], bromodeoxyuridine and pyrancopolymer [Freeman, 1968], levodopa, carbidopa, nialamide [Halikowski and Piotropawlowska-Weinert, 1977], rifampin, and ether [Robertson et al., 1980]. However, these agents have been found to have little beneficial effect on the disease.

Some evidence suggests that amantadie hydrochloride may be beneficial in treating subacute sclerosing panencephalitis. Amantadine is an anti-RNA agent that retards the maturation of some viruses to keep them in an infectious form by not allowing them to replicate [Hoffman et al., 1968]. Thus, amantadine supposedly prevents the spread of subacute sclerosing panencephalitis by preventing unaffected brain cells from becoming infected [Haslam et al., 1969; Robertson et al., 1980]. Because of the small number of patients that any one investigator might see and the long duration of follow-up necessary, it is very difficult to draw conclusions about efficacy of treatment.

Of the therapeutic agents that have been tested, inosiplex (Isoprinosine) has been associated with higher rates of remission and improved long-term survival in patients with subacute sclerosing panencephalitis [DuRant and Dyken 1983; DuRant et al., 1982; Dyken et al., 1982a, b]. Inosiplex (a 1:3 complex of inosine and dimethylaminoisopropanol-p-acetamidobenzoate) is believed to exert an inhibitory action on the process of viral replication in host cells, as well as augmenting effects on cell immune responses [Hadden et al., 1975; Hadden et al., 1976]. Although theoretically useful, the clinical application of this treatment has been controversial, in part based upon an apparent uncertainty about the natural variability of the disease. Regardless of these methodologic problems, 44% of the treated patients were still living at the end of the study. In addition, four treated patients exhibited subacute sclerosing panencephalitis stage reversals and three remained at an "improved" level for extended periods. In contrast, only four of 96 untreated controls had substantial long-term improvement. Consequently, the conclusion by Haddad and Risk that inosiplex was not effective is arguable.

Although a curative therapy for subacute sclerosing panencephalitis is not as yet established, the decreasing incidence of the disease following the preventive therapy started by the national immunization program against natural measles has created less anxiety and also less research on the part of investigators into this disease. It

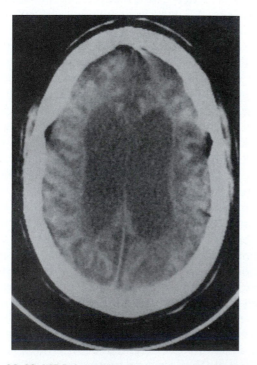

Figure 39-20 MRI demonstrating severe atrophy in subacute sclerosing panencephalitis patient in stage IV.

is important that research not lapse, however, because although subacute sclerosing panencephalitis is declining in frequency in the general population, the relative ratio of subacute sclerosing panencephalitis to natural measles is increasing. Thus the effect of immunization on producing more patients with subacute sclerosing panencephalitis or other combined factors is still not certain. These arguments make it absolutely necessary to pursue actively more definitive curative therapy for this disease.

Palliative treatments are also important. Not only is judicious use of antiepileptic drugs, nutritional and antibiotic measures, physical and mental habilitative treatments, and behavior-control therapies necessary in the management of the symptoms of this disease, but expansion into the new field of neurotransmitter replacement and control is also of great importance.

Progressive rubella panencephalitis. Progressive rubella panencephalitis represents a slowly progressive encephalopathic disorder with onset usually in the juvenile period. The disorder follows either congenital rubella syndrome or natural rubella acquired in early life.

Clinical findings. There is usually progressive dementia and prominent cerebellar signs. The commonly appearing ataxia is often associated with involuntary movements in the form of chorea and myoclonus. Often there is evidence of an acquired retinopathy at the onset of new neurologic symptoms. Spasticity and paresis then develop and are progressive until death occurs, usually 3 to 8 years after the onset of new neurologic symptoms. The course is slower than in subacute sclerosing panencephalitis, which may be associated with occasional remissions.

Laboratory findings. In progressive rubella panencephalitis, CSF often manifests a lymphocytic pleocytosis. CSF protein is usually elevated slightly to 50 to 100 mg/dl. An elevation of gammaglobulin occurs primarily. Rubella antibody titers, best measured with a hemaglutinin-inhibition technique, are remarkably high in both serum and CSF. EEG studies have demonstrated consistent abnormalities, but seldom of the degree or the type witnessed in subacute sclerosing panencephalitis [Weil, 1975].

Pathology. Only a few cases of progressive rubella panencephalitis have been autopsied [Townsend et al., 1975, 1976]. There is diffuse, destructive, and inflammatory evidence primarily located in the white matter. Perivascular mononuclear infiltrations and microglial modules are manifest but not inclusion bodies. There are extensive atrophic changes in the cerebellum, a location that is not commonly affected in patients with other types of CNS slow viral involvement. The rubella virus has been isolated from brain biopsy material [Cremer et al., 1975].

Management. There is no curative treatment for progressive rubella panencephalitis, but supportive care is essential. Inosiplex has been ineffective [Wolinsky et al, 1976, 1979].

Progressive multifocal leukoencephalitis

Progressive multifocal leukoencephalitis is primarily a disease of adults and will be discussed briefly.

Clinical findings. Progressive multifocal leukoencephalitis is usually a diffuse brain disease with multifocal CNS abnormalities, including mental deterioration, visual loss, sensory deficits, motor paralysis, speech disturbances, and ataxia [Brooks and Walker, 1984]. Seizures are uncommon and, when occurring, are variable. Neurologic deterioration occurs in the midst of a basic disorder of immunosuppression; the papovavirus is frequently involved in opportunistic infection and therefore often associated with AIDS. The course of progressive multifocal leukoencephalitis is usually one of relentless downward progression, generally lasting 3 to 12 months and ending in death [Brooks and Walker, 1984]. Occasionally, patients live over 2 years with the illness.

Laboratory findings. The CSF is usually normal in patients with progressive multifocal leukoencephalitis. The diagnosis is strongly suggested by cranial CT and MRI. There are bilateral, somewhat asymmetric, large subcortical areas of demyelination. EEG often discloses multifocal abnormalities of random slow waves and sharp forms unless frank clinical seizure activity is occurring, at which time a more epileptogenic appearance is observed [Brooks and Walker, 1984; Krupp et al., 1985].

Pathology. In progressive multifocal leukoencephalitis, areas of demyelination are distributed in the subcortical regions in large, patchy collections [Walker and Padgett, 1983; ZuRhein et al., 1978]. Loss of oligodendroglia is striking (Figure 39-21). Although there is a loss of myelin sheaths, there is relative preservation of axon cylinders. Marked astrocytic gliosis is observed, with abnormal mitotic figures and multinucleated astrocytes (Figure 39-22). There is little evidence of inflammation. All of these findings support a direct viral effect on oligodendrocytes more than a host immune reaction [Walker and Padgett, 1983] (Figures 39-22 and 39-23).

Management. No effective treatment exists for progressive multifocal leukoencephalitis other than supportive. Corrective therapy for immunosuppression, including adequate antibiotic coverage, is required. Although some of the immunodeficiencies are untreatable, others may respond to appropriate therapy [Bauer et al., 1973; Buckman and Wilshaw, 1976].

Acquired Immune Deficiency Syndrome (AIDS). Although sometimes difficult to separate from the ravages of immunodeficiency, widespread neoplasia of the nervous system, and opportunistic CNS infections, a slow encephalitis unrelated to these causes exists in persons shown to be HIV positive in the brain and spinal cord [Gallo, 1987]. Many instances of slowly progressive dementia occurring well before symptoms more typical of AIDS have been reported. This preimmunodeficiency state, very much in keeping with slow virus infection, may also be observed in visna. Because AIDS is a complicated clinical disease, a pure progressive encephalopathic syndrome caused by the virus alone is difficult to separate but may have particular importance in explaining many of the unique, congenitally acquired AIDS cases observed in infants and young children. This syndrome may account for several patients with mildly progressive CNS atrophic conditions that present as psychomotor retardation. In pediatric AIDS, the acquisition is from passage of virus to fetus from mother. This unique situation tends to confirm a basic infectivity (Table 39-12). In congenital forms, a latent period exists before the development of the full clinical picture months to years later.

Clinical findings. Children tend to have "hidden" symptoms, such as psychomotor retardation and less commonly regression in mental abilities [Shaw et al., 1985]. Months after onset, signs suggesting a more severe chronic degenerative process occur. Refractive seizures and a variety of neurologic signs, including spasticity, quadriparesis, and ataxia with deterioration, occur. Signs suggesting immunodeficiency are less prevalent [Gallo, 1987; Shaw et al., 1985].

Laboratory findings. In childhood AIDS with slow virus encephalitis, there tends to be a lymphocytic pleocytosis and increased protein determination even before strikingly pronounced neurologic symptoms develop. During this period the virus may be isolated from the brain or CSF [Ho et al., 1985]. EEG may demonstrate generalized arrhythmic slowing or epileptogenic phenomena when related to clinical seizures.

Pathology. The pathologic picture of AIDS is quite variable. It is difficult to determine whether immunodeficiency exists with secondary opportunistic infections from papovavirus, herpes simplex virus, cytomegalovirus, or nonviral infections, whether CNS neoplasia is present, or whether a slow viral infection alone exists. In the children studied, a large amount of cerebral atrophy is manifest and, although opportunistic infections are not uncovered, HIV has been isolated in many patients [Shaw et al., 1985]. Spongiform neuronal changes occur. Neuronal loss and reactive gliosis are common. Inflammatory changes are rare. In general, children with AIDS have fewer CNS neoplasms. Table 39-13 lists the diagnostic criteria suggested by the Centers for Disease Control for these disorders.

Management. Other than supportive treatment, no

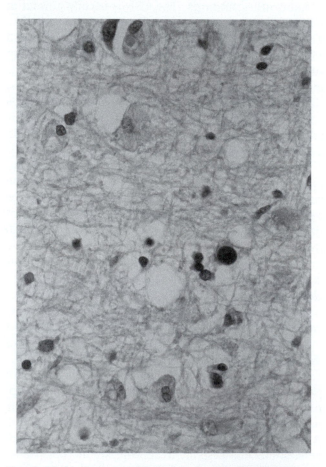

Figure 39-21 Brain revealing multiple oligodendrocytes with enlarged nuclei typical of progressive multifocal leukoencephalitis.

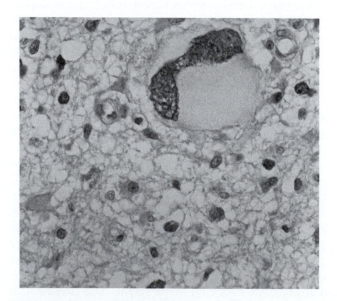

Figure 39-22 Brain disclosing giant astrocytes in a patient with progressive multifocal leukoencephalitis.

specific curative treatment for the retrovirus infection is known.

Unconventional progressive encephalopathies

Unconventional progressive encephalopathies are reported by only two definite human diseases that affect children, kuru and Creutzfeldt-Jakob disease. Gerstmann-Straussler syndrome is limited to adults and may only be a variant of Creutzfeldt-Jakob disease [Roos et al., 1973; Bastian, 1991; Bale and Perlman, 1987]. Each disorder is characterized by progressive noninflammatory spongiform changes in brain. A similar clinical picture and pathologic reaction are also observed in the disease of sheep called scrapie, which is believed to be closely related to Creutzfeldt-Jakob disease. Kuru represents classically a deterioration of the cerebellum, cerebellar pathways, and extrapyramidal system. Dementia occurs, but this is less striking than in Creutzfeldt-Jakob disease, where dementia is the prominent feature. Gerstmann-Straussler syndrome appears as an ataxia. Although the unconventional agents are not proved to be of a viral nature, some of the clinical characteristics resemble the conventional viral disorders. Yet the course is monophasic without initial clinical manifestation. Months or years after presumed exposure to the agent (in kuru and scrapie), and following presumed contamination in surgery (in Creutzfeldt-Jakob disease), devastating neurodegeneration occurs [Bastian, 1991].

The unconventional disorders are probably not caused by viral agents for the following reasons:

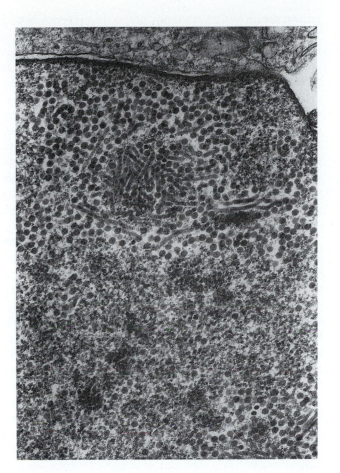

Figure 39-23 Electron microscopy of papovaviruses (magnification about 70,000).

Table 39-12 Criteria for diagnosis of AIDS in pediatric age groups: occurrence of a disease predictive of cell-mediated immunity but without primary or secondary immunodeficiency diseases

Exclusions	Inclusions
Toxoplasmosis < 1 month	Kaposi sarcoma
Herpes simplex < 1 month	Primary lymphoma of CNS
Cytomegalovirus < 6 months	Pneumocystis carinii pneumonia
Primary immunodeficiency	Mucocutaneous herpes > 5 weeks
DiGeorge syndrome	Cryptosporidium enterocolitis > 4 weeks
Wiskott-Aldrich syndrome	Esophagitis caused by candida, cytomegalovirus, or herpes simplex
Ataxia-telangiectasia	Progressive multifocal leukoencephalitis
Graft-versus-host disease	Pneumonia, meningitis, or encephalitis caused by aspergillus, candida, crypto-
Neutropenia	coccus, cytomegalovirus, nocardia, strongyloides, toxoplasmosis, zygomycosis,
Neutrophil function abnormality	or atypical mycobacterium
Agammaglobulinemia	
Hypogammaglobulinemia with increased IgM	
Secondary immunodeficiency	
Immunosuppressive therapy	
Lymphoreticular malignancy	
Starvation	

Adapted from surveillance definitions of the Centers for Disease Control, Atlanta.

1. Clinical presentation does not follow the established rules of viral infection
2. No known host response of immunopathic nature, including no inflammatory reaction, questionable antigenicity, no demonstrable humoral or cellular immunity, unaltered disease in immunosuppressed animals, no induction of interferon, and no response to exogenously administered interferon
3. Agent is resistant to physical or chemical treatments and not wholly inactivated by boiling, sonication, ultraviolet irradiation, protease, nuclease or formaldehyde (as are viruses)
4. Agent has an estimated molecular weight of about 100,000 or less, with an atypical action spectrum inactivation
5. Viral particles have not been demonstrated in detailed electron microscopic studies
6. Agent replicates in tissue culture but has shown no cytopathic effect and no interference of growth of conventional viruses.

Kuru. Kuru is a subacute progressive neurologic disease first identified in the Fore people of New Guinea [Gajdusek, 1971; Gajdusek and Gibbs, 1977]. Kuru in the Fore language means a condition of trembling and fear and relates to the characteristic involuntary movements typical of the condition. There is a remarkably constant clinical pattern in this disease. The onset of symptoms occurs between 4 and 20 years after the presumed initial contact with the agent. This contact is acquired during death ceremonies. The passage of the infectious agent is from the brains of the dead to women and children, who prepare the brains for cannibalism.

Clinical findings. The earlier sign of the disease is a slight but characteristic tremulousness [Bale and Perlman, 1987]. The shivering movement suggests a minimal disturbance of balance and ataxia. The early, subtle symptoms and signs gradually progress over months. Eventually, a more conspicuous disturbance in gait and staggering, lurching, generalized appendicular ataxia, and dysmetria of the hands occur. Facial musculature changes and slurred speech then develop. Heterotopias occur, particularly in children with the disease, and headache is a frequent complaint. Frank nystagmus is unusual. Mentation and general state of alertness are relatively preserved until late stages when dementia becomes obvious. Loss of ambulation is associated with severe ataxia, hypotonia, and hyperreflexia. Terminally severe lethargy or agitation and then coma ensue. Even terminally, predominant brainstem and cerebellar signs and symptoms are still apparent.

Laboratory findings. In kuru, CSF analysis usually reveals no significant abnormalities. Cell count, type of cell, protein, and glucose are usually normal. Attempts to isolate a virus from the blood, CSF, and other tissues, including the brain, have been unsuccessful. There is no known serum or CSF antibody titer to test [Dyken, 1975].

Pathology. The pathologic conditions in kuru are limited to the CNS. Signs of diffuse neuronal degeneration, microglial proliferation, hypertrophy of astrocytes throughout the brain, and status spongiosis of the cerebrocortical gray matter are observed. These findings are especially prominent in the cerebellum, brainstem, and basal ganglia. There is minimal demyelinization. Round, homogeneously stained amyloid plaques are usually present throughout the brain. These plaques reveal morphologic structures similar to the scrapie-associated fibriles found in sheep scrapie. There is a general lack of significant perivascular cuffing and frank inflammation in kuru [Bastian, 1991].

Management. Kuru may be treated symptomatically because no specific, curative therapy exists. Since the early 1950s, kuru has declined in frequency because of recognition and prevention [Gajdusek and Gibbs, 1977]. Transmissibility of the disorder is based on the ritualistic system of cannibalism in native areas. Before recognition, loved ones consumed the flesh of the kinsmen after death, primarily as a gesture of respect for the departed. Preparation was performed by women and children. Since the recognition of the pathogenesis of the disease, social correction of these practices by the Fore natives has practically eradicated the disorder [Bale and Perlman, 1987].

Creutzfeldt-Jakob disease. Creutzfeldt-Jakob disease is essentially a disorder of adults of either sex and predominantly occurs in the fifth or sixth decade of life [Roos et al., 1973; Galvex et al., 1980]. There have been rare cases reported as occurring as early as late teenage years. Onset before the age of 40 is considered unusual. Most cases have developed sporadically. The usual duration of the disease from onset of symptoms to death varies between 1 and 15 months. A review by Roos et al. [1973] calculated an average duration of 7 months, whereas Galvex et al. [1980] calculated a duration of 6 months.

Clinical findings. The onset of symptoms in Creutzfeldt-Jakob disease is insidious in most patients. Symptoms frequently begin with fatigue, depression, and weight loss. Mental abnormalities are the first definite neurologic signs. Disturbances of memory, impairment of judgment, abnormal behavior, and personality alterations suggest more specific deficits of higher cortical function. Self-neglect, apathy, and mood swings are common early symptoms. Incoordination is the most common early motor feature of the disease, which often progresses into a typical cerebellar ataxia.

Within weeks to months other neurologic signs, such as rigidity, bradykinesia, loss of facial expression at rest, static kinetic tremor, and other dyskinesias develop. Myoclonus, often provoked by sudden sensory stimuli, is a common feature in the moderately advanced case.

Convulsions may occur later, but this symptom is less frequent than other dysfunctions. Occasionally, patients develop pronounced signs of anterior horn cell degeneration which is out of proportion to the cerebellar and basal ganglia findings that may also be present.

The most characteristic and consistent feature of all forms of Creutzfeldt-Jakob disease is dementia [Bastian, 1991]. Visual disturbances, paresthesias, hallucinations, dysarthria, and other neurologic findings may complicate the picture. These symptoms help identify clinical subunits of mental and motor function. A vegetative state is reached and soon afterward death occurs.

Laboratory findings. In Creutzfeldt-Jakob disease the spinal fluid is usually normal or there is only mild elevation of protein content without a cellular reaction. EEG is consistently abnormal, demonstrating progressive slowing, coinciding with a worsening clinical course. Some recordings may demonstrate periodic patterns with bursts of high-amplitude, slow-and-sharp waves followed by relative flattening. Cranial CT or MRI reveals characteristic but nondiagnostic features [Kovanen et al., 1985].

Pathology. The pathologic conditions in Creutzfeldt-Jakob disease are widespread throughout only the CNS [Bastian, 1991]. Visible atrophy usually occurs in the cerebral cortex. There is a loss of nerve cells in all cortical layers and considerable astrocytic proliferation is evident. Many of the astrocytes are gemistocytic. Spongiform changes are especially obvious in the deeper cortical layers and are more conspicuously observed microscopically. Small, round, or oval, clear vacuoles are found in the neuropil. The spongiform appearance is the result of distention of the processes of the cells. Neuronal loss and astrocytic proliferation are also prominent in the dentate nuclei, putamen, and thalamic nuclei. Cerebellar changes consist especially of loss of granule cells [Bastian, 1991]. Dense fibrous gliosis usually is manifest throughout all layers of the cerebellar cortex. In those patients who die soon after the onset of symptoms, more spongiform changes manifest, whereas in those who die later, more gliosis occurs.

Management. Patients with Creutzfeldt-Jakob disease may be treated symptomatically. No specific, curative therapies exist [Bastian, 1991].

EMBRYONIC ENCEPHALOPATHIES

Certain viruses have a special virulence to the developing organism [Nahmias et al., 1982; Elliot et al., 1956; Gaunt et al., 1985; Wolf and Cowen, 1972; Cooper, 1985; Pass et al., 1980; Kotchmar, 1984; Savage et al., 1973]. Although demonstrating no or low virulence in the mature human, many of these viruses have great virulence in the human fetus. The devastating effect on the fetus is seldom limited to the nervous system, and there is widespread involvement of many systems. In many cases the direct effect is so severe that abortion occurs, while in others a fulminating disease in the newborn period is encountered. If the viral effect on the fetus were less severe and the infection would occur in early gestational life, tissue and organ development may suffer through a dysgenetic effect and malformation may ensue. These malformations may be serious or minimal and affect different organ systems, but they certainly do not spare the nervous system. In fact, nervous, cardiovascular, and ophthalmic systems are particularly prone to these insults. The ultimate dysgenetic feature may be used to trace the point of embryogenic insult and is helpful in dating type, severity, and location of the viral infection.

A host of viruses and nonviruses are known to attack the embryo. In clinical practice, these viral infections are commonly identified as TORCH encephalopathies [Nahmias et al., 1982].

TORCH:

T – Toxoplasmosis
O – Other (varicella, adenovirus, others)
R – Rubella
C – Cytomegalovirus
H – Herpes simplex

There are many uncertainties about the extent of such insults and the limitation of causative agents. Other viruses implicated in the production of static congenital syndromes besides rubella, cytomegalovirus, and herpes simplex are varicella, mumps, poliovirus, coxsackie B, echovirus, measles, group A togavirus, influenza, rhabdovirus, lymphocytic choriomeningitis virus, Epstein-Barr virus, HIV, and possibly coronavirus and parainfluenza. In an era of expanding intensive care of the newborn and considering generous malpractice suits against managing physicians, conditions previously believed responsible for subsequent psychomotor retardation and cerebral palsy must be doubted, and it is appropriate to consider in utero viral insults as a cause of many of these problems [Wolf and Cowen, 1972].

Several of the viral diseases in utero are gradually decreasing in frequency because of immunization. In the classic congenital rubella syndrome, a triad of heart, eye, and brain symptoms caused by malformation occurs [Desmond et al., 1978]. The recognition of a more extensive syndrome encompassing a wider range of clinical manifestations has allowed a better understanding of the effects of in utero viral disorders, although congenital rubella has declined after the advent of active immunization programs. In 1986, there were 551 patients with acquired rubella reported in the United States, with only 14 of these being of the congenital type [MMWR, 1990]. Although rare, rubella and other somewhat opportunistic in utero viral infections are a threat to the fetus and are a potential cause of a large proportion of static encephalopathies.

Cytomegalovirus fetal infection

Cytomegalovirus infection in adults has an unspectacular presentation and is usually nonneurologic. Symptoms include mild febrile illness, malaise, lymphadenopathy, and other nonspecific systemic symptoms. In the fetus, severe symptoms develop [Ceballos et al., 1976; Navin and Angevine, 1968]. If pregnancy continues without fetal death, premature labor may occur. Usually the fetal infection remains active in the neonatal period. Involvement of liver, kidneys, eyes, and nervous system is observed. There are less striking dysgenetic abnormalities, such as those observed in the typical instance of congenital rubella.

Clinical findings. An infant born with cytomegalic inclusion disease is often of low birth weight. The actively infected infant often has hepatosplenomegaly, thrombocytopenia, jaundice, signs of hepatitis, and severe lethargy [Pass et al., 1980]. Seizures of a variety of types may occur. Neurologic sequelae in later life include microcephaly; focal and generalized neurologic defects, such as spasticity, hyperreflexia, paresis, or paralysis; mental retardation; and deafness [Pass et al., 1980]. Chorioretinitis is often present (Figure 39-24). Periventricular calcification occurs in about 25% of the severe cases [Pass et al., 1980] (Figure 39-25). Hydrocephalus with macrocephaly and severe microcephaly may result from cytomegalovirus infection. It is possible that inapparent congenital cytomegalovirus infections occur, which would account for later subnormal intelligence and other neurologic symptoms. It is important to remember that cytomegalovirus continues to be shed for months or even years after active signs of infection have disappeared. Exacerbations of disease in later life have been reported. In this regard, cytomegalovirus acquired in utero must be considered as a possible persistent viral syndrome. Yet flare-up is not consistent or typical, and the neurologic symptoms are not as devastating or relentlessly progressive as in other slow viral diseases.

Laboratory findings. In congenital cytomegalovirus infection the CSF may have an increased cellular and protein content. Cytomegalovirus cells with intranuclear inclusions may be found in the urine. The virus may be isolated from the nasopharynx, blood, or urine [Chun, 1982; Bell and McCormick, 1981]. Serologic tests may be of limited diagnostic value. Elevated levels of specific IgM antibody titers in the newborn are strongly suggestive of congenital cytomegalovirus infections [Bell and McCormick, 1981]. The presence of maternal humoral immunity against cytomegalovirus may not protect the newborn. Skull radiographs may demonstrate periventricular calcification. CT and MRI indicate similar findings. The diagnosis, however, depends on character-

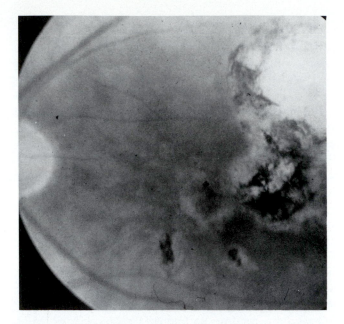

Figure 39-24 Chorioretinitis in a juvenile who is believed to have had a congenital cytomegalovirus infection on the basis of history and present findings. Observe the extensive paramacular salt-and-pepper scar, which is more in keeping with an inactive viral lesion.

istic clinical and laboratory findings [Chun, 1982].

Pathology. Generalized cytomegalovirus disease in the newborn may result in severe, active meningoencephalitis, with all the characteristic histologic findings and nonactive or dysgenetic features, such as hydrocephaly and microcephaly. Subependymal calcifications are characteristic [Bell and McCormick, 1981]. Intranuclear inclusions may be found in neuronal, microglial, endothelial and kidney cells. The intranuclear inclusions are also in many large cells of the salivary glands, liver, gastrointestinal tract, and pancreas. These findings often cause a "hollowed eye" appearance. Multiple, circumscript, necrotizing granulomatous lesions may also be found scattered throughout the brain.

Management. There are no curative treatments for any of the embryogenic encephalopathies. Considerable supportive and symptomatic therapies should be performed [Chun, 1982]. These therapies include long-term chronic treatment of defects, such as heart disease, deafness, seizures, and mental retardation through educational planning. Acute treatment in the neonatal period is often necessary.

Congenital rubella syndrome

The occurrence of congenital abnormalities in infants after the mother had gestational rubella in early pregnancy was first described by Gregg [1941]. At first, a traditional triad was emphasized in the congenital rubella syndrome, which consisted of cataracts, congen-

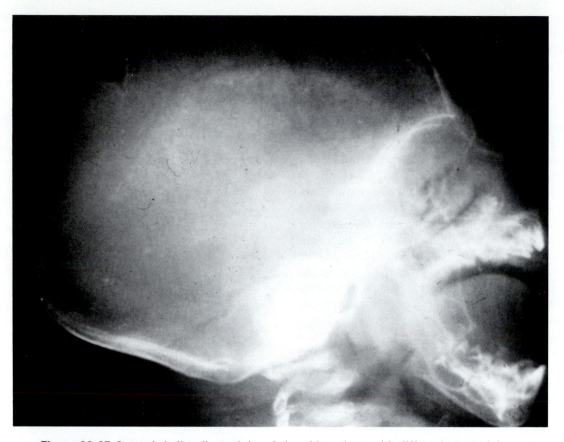

Figure 39-25 Lateral skull radiograph in a 2-day-old newborn with diffuse, intracranial calcifications shown to be caused by congenital cytomegalovirus infection.

ital heart disease, and deafness. The triad resulted from the viral insult occurring in the early part of the first trimester. With time, a more extensive picture of congenital rubella has been obtained. The symptoms depend upon when the insult occurs in utero. The earlier the insult, the more tendency there is for fetal death to occur. Later, after organ formation, less severe CNS and systemic dysgenetic defects occur, although it is still possible for the viral insult to be disastrous to the fully formed fetus. The risk of adverse fetal outcome is in excess of 50% when the mother has rubella before the thirteenth week of gestation [Chun, 1982]. Considerable risk to the fetus, however, extends beyond the first trimester of pregnancy.

Clinical findings. Fetal death and prematurity are common findings. The most frequently observed malformations involve ocular, cardiac, auditory, neurologic, and dental abnormalities. A dating of the in utero insult by embryogenetic tracking (correlating the malformation with the period of gestation during which the affected part was developing) is possible [Desmond et al., 1978; Cooper, 1985]. The most frequently observed ocular defect is cataracts, which results from disturbances caused by the rubella virus in the fetus in the sixth week

of gestation [Bogeg, 1980]. The more limited "blueberry muffin" type of chorioretinitis occurs after the sixth week of gestation. The retinopathy is quite characteristic and is dissimilar to the more extensive salt-and-pepper type of chorioretinitis observed in other types of in utero viral encephalitides. Patent ductus arteriosus and septal defects are the most common congenital cardiac abnormalities and usually follow viral insults that occur between the fifth and tenth week of gestation. Deafness occurred in as many as 45% of the children in one survey [Ojala et al., 1973]. Deafness is frequently a result of infection in the ninth week of gestation. Thus, the classic congenital rubella triad represents insults occurring at 6 to 10 weeks of gestation.

The newborn infant with congenital rubella from any stage of insult may be hypotonic and lethargic at birth. A full or bulging fontanel and other signs suggesting an ongoing meningoencephalitis often occurs. Microcephaly, mental retardation, and seizures are other frequent neonatal symptoms of this disorder. Admixtures of ongoing infection and residual damage and malformation are frequently encountered.

Laboratory findings. The diagnosis of rubella in utero is possible by isolating the virus from the amniotic fluid [Levin et al., 1974]. The diagnosis of rubella after birth is made with clinical and laboratory data. In congenital rubella, serologic findings in the mother and infant are always positive. Viral isolation from the throat, urine, CSF, and other tissues should be attempted. Elevated serum concentration of immunoglobulins may be found.

Pathology. In patients with congenital rubella syndrome, severe and frequent areas of ischemia with severe foci of necrosis, especially in the deeper layers of the cortex, are present [Bell and McCormick, 1981]. Microcephaly and hypercellularity of the white matter have been observed. The vascular defects include, in severe cases, full destruction of the vascular walls, defects of the internal elastic lamina and subintimal fibers, pericapillary deposits of granular material, and endothelial proliferation. The vascular changes may be distributed widely in the brain and spinal cord. Seemingly inactive congenital forms and inflammatory changes are usually observed, suggesting chronic meningitis, as well as severe parenchymal changes.

Management. Supportive treatment for disabilities may be helpful. No curative therapies are known.

REFERENCES

Alvord EC. Demyelination in experimental allergic encephalomyelitis and multiple sclerosis. In: ter Meulen V, Katz M, eds. Slow virus infections of the central nervous system. New York: Springer-Verlag, 1977.

Baer GM. Pathogenesis to the central nervous system. In: Baer GM, ed. The natural history of rabies. Orlando: Academic Press, 1975.

Bale JF, Perlman S. Viral encephalopathies. In: Baker AB, ed. Clinical neurology, vol 2. New York: Harper & Row, 1987.

Bale JF, Perlman S. Slow virus infection due to unconventional agents. In: Baker AB, ed. Clinical neurology, vol 2. New York: Harper & Row, 1987.

Bastian FO. Creutzfeldt-Jakob disease and other transmissible spongiform encephalopathies. St. Louis: Mosby, 1991.

Bauer W, Turel AP, Johnson KP. Progressive multifocal leukoencephalopathy and cytanabine: remission with treatment. JAMA 1973; 226:174.

Behan PO, Moore MJ, Lamarche JB. Acute necrotizing hemorrhagic encephalopathy. Post Grad Med 1973; 54:154.

Bell WE, McCormick WF. Neurologic infections in children. ed 2. Philadelphia: WB Saunders, 1981.

Benady S, Ben Zvi A, Szabo G. Transverse meylitis following mumps. Acta Paediatr Scand 1973; 62-205.

Bhatt DR, et al. Human rabies. Diagnosis, complications, and management. Am J Dis Child 1974; 127:862.

Blaese R, Hofstrand H, Krebs H, et al. Evaluation of transfer factor in the therapy of SSPE. Arch Neurol 1975; 32:502.

Bogeg WO III. Late onset complications in congenital rubella syndrome. Ophthalmology 1980; 87:1244.

Brooks BR, Walker DL. Progressive multifocal leukoencephalopathy. Neurol Clin 1984; 2:99.

Buckman R, Wilshaw E. Progressive multifocal leukoencephalopathy successfully treated with cytosine arabinoside. Br J Hematol 1976; 153:153.

Ceballos R, Chien LT, Whitley RJ, et al. Cerebellar hypoplasia in an infant with nervous CMV infection. Pediatrics 1976; 57:155.

Chen TT, Watanabe I, Zeman W, et al. Subacute sclerosing panencephalitis: Propagation of measles virus from brain biopsy in tissue culture. Science 1969; 163:1193.

Choppin PW. Measles virus and chronic neurological disease. Ann Neurol 1981; 9:17.

Chopra JS, Banerjee AK, Murthy JMK, et al. Paralytic rabies: a clinicopathologic study. Brain 1980; 103:789.

Chun RWM. Viral diseases of the central nervous system. In: Swaiman K, Wright F, eds. The practice of pediatric neurology, ed 2, St. Louis: Mosby, 1982.

Connolly JH, Allen IV, Hurwitz LJ, et al. Measles-virus antibody and antigen in subacute sclerosing panencephalitis. Lancet 1967; 1:542.

Cooper LI. The history and medical consequences of rubella. Rev Infect Dis 1985; 7:51.

Cotton PB, Webb-Peploe MM. Acute transverse myelitis as a complication of glandular fever. Br Med J 1966; 1:654.

Crawford T. Acute hemorrhagic leukoencephalitis. J Clin Pathol 1954; 7:1.

Cremer NE, et al. Isolation of rubella virus from brain in chronic progressive panencephalitis. J Gen Virol 1975; 29:143.

Dawson JC. Cellular inclusion in cerebral lesions of lethargic encephalitis. Am J Pathol 1933; 9:7.

Desmond MM, Fisher ES, Vorderman AI, et al. The longitudinal course of nervous rubella encephalitis in non-retarded children. J Pediatr 1978; 93:584.

Detels R, Brody JA, McNew J, et al. Further epidemiological studies of subacute sclerosing panencephalitis. Lancet 1973; 21:11.

Derakhshan I. Is the Negri body specific for rabies? A light and electron microscopic study. Arch Neurol 1975; 32:75.

DuRant RH, Dyken PR. The effect of inosiplex on the survival of subacute sclerosing panencephalitis. Neurology 1983; 33:1053.

DuRant RH, Dyken PR, Swift AS. The influence of inosiplex treatment on the neurological disability of patients with subacute sclerosing panencephalitis. J Pediatr 1982; 101:288.

Dyken PR. Subacute sclerosing panencephalitis: current status. In: Swaiman KF, ed. Neurologic clinics, pediatric neurology. Philadelphia: WB Saunders, 1985.

Dyken PR, Cunningham SC, Ward LC. Changing character of subacute sclerosing panencephalitis in the United States. Pediatr Neurol 1989; 5:339.

Dyken PR, DuRant R, Shmunes P. Subacute sclerosing panencephalitis surveillance: United States. MMWR 1982a; 31:585.

Dyken PR, Swift A, DuRant RH. Long-term follow-up of patients with subacute sclerosing panencephalitis treated with inosiplex. Ann Neurol 1982b; 11:359.

Dyken PR, Krawiecki NS, DuRant RH, et al. The changing clinical expression of subacute sclerosing panencephalitis (SSPE) in the United States. Ann Neurol 1983; 14:586.

Dyken PR. Cerebrospinal fluid cytology: practical clinical usefulness. Neurology 1975; 25:210.

Elliot GB, McAllister JE, Alberta C. Fetal poliomyelitis. Am J Obstet Gynecol 1956; 72:896.

Fields BN, Knipe DM. Fields' virology. New York: Raven Press, 1990.

Foley KM, Beresford HR. Acute poliomyelitis beginning as transverse myelopathy. Arch Neurol 1974; 30:182.

Freeman JM. Treatment of subacute sclerosing panencephalitis with 5-bromo 2 deoxyuridine and pyroncopolymer. Neurology 1968; 18:176.

Gajdusek DC. Slow virus diseases of the central nervous system. Am J Clin Pathol 1971; 56:320.

Gajdusek DC, Gibbs CJ Jr. Kuru, Creutzfeldt-Jakob disease and transmissible presemble dementias. In: ter Meulen V, Katz M, eds. Slow virus infections of the central nervous system. New York: Springer-Verlag, 1977.

Gallo RC. The AIDS virus. Sci Am 1987; 256:47.

Galvex S, Masters C, Gajdusek C. Descriptive epidemiology of Creutzfeldt-Jakob disease in Chile. Arch Neurol 1980; 37:11.

Gaunt CJ, Gudvangen RJ, Brans YW, et al. Coxsackie virus Group B antibodies in the ventricular fluid of infants with severe defects in the central nervous system. Pediatrics 1985; 76:64.

Gregg NM. Congenital cataract following German measles in the mother. Trans Ophthalmol Soc Aust 1941; 3:35.

Haase AT. Slow infections. In: Brande AI, David CE, Fierer J, eds. Infectious diseases and medical microbiology, ed 2. Philadelphia: WB Saunders, 1986.

Haddad FS, Risk WS. Isoprinosine treatment in 18 patients with subacute sclerosing panencephalitis: a controlled study. Ann Neurol 1980; 7:185.

Hadden JW, Englard A, Sadlik JR, et al. The comparative effects of inoxiplex, levamisole, miramyl dipeptide, and SM1213 on lymphocyte and macrophage proliferation and activation in vitro. Int J Immunopharmacol 1975; 1:17.

Hadden JW, Hadden EM, Coffey RG. Isoprinosine augmentation of phytohemagglutin-induced lymphocyte proliferation. Infect Immun 1976; 13:382.

Halikowski B, Piotropawlowska-Weinert M. Levodopa in subacute sclerosing panencephalitis. Lancet 1977; 2:1033.

Hall WW, Lamb RA, Choppin PW. Measles and subacute sclerosing panencephalitis virus proteins: lack of antibodies to the M protein in patients with subacute sclerosing panencephalitis. Proc Natl Acad Sci USA 1976; 76:2047.

Haslam RHA, McQuillin MP, Clark DB. Amantadine therapy in subacute sclerosing panencephalitis. Neurology 1969; 19:1080.

Hattwick MA, et al. Recovery from rabies. A case report. Ann Intern Med 1972; 76:931.

Ho DD, Rota TR, Schooley RT, Kaplan JC, et al. Isolation of HTLV-III from cerebrospinal fluid and neural tissue of patients with neurologic syndromes related to the acquired immunodeficiency syndrome. N Engl J Med 1985; 313:1493.

Hoffman CE, Neumayer EM, Hoff RF, et al. Mode of action of the antiviral activity of amantadine in tissue cultures. Bacteriology 1968; 90:623.

Hogan EL, Krigman MR. Herpes zoster myelitis. Arch Neurol 1973; 2:309.

Horta-Barbosa L, et al. Subacute sclerosing panencephalitis: isolation of measles virus from a brain biopsy. Nature 1969; 221:974.

Horta-Barbosa L, et al. Isolation of measles virus from brain cell cultures of two patients with subacute sclerosing panencephalitis. Proc Soc Exp Biol Med 1969; 132:272.

Huttenlocher PR, Mattson RH. Isoprinosine in subacute sclerosing panencephalitis. Neurology 1979; 29:763.

Jabbour JT, Duenas DA, Modlin J. SSPE: clinical staging, course and frequency. Arch Neurol 1975; 32:493.

Jabbour JT, et al. Epidemiology of subacute sclerosing panencephalitis (SSPE). A report of the SSPE registry. JAMA 1972; 220:959.

Jabbour JT. Slow virus disease. In: Swaiman K, Wright F, eds. The practice of pediatric neurology, ed 2. St. Louis: Mosby 1982.

Jabbour JT, Garcia JH, Lemmi H et al. Subacute sclerosing panencephalitis: a multidisciplinary study of eight cases. JAMA 1969; 207:2248.

Johnson DA, Eger AW. Myelitis associated with an echo-virus. JAMA 1967; 201:637.

Johnson R, Milbourn PE. Central nervous system manifestations of chickenpox. Can Med Assoc J 1970; 102:831.

Johnson RT. Viral infections of the nervous system. New York: Raven Press, 1982.

Johnson RT. Slow viral infections of the nervous system. In: Wyngaarden JB, Smith LH, eds. Cecil textbook of medicine, ed 17. Philadelphia: WB Saunders, 1985a.

Johnson RT. Viral meningitis and encephalitis. In: Wyngaarden JB, Smith LH, eds. Cecil textbook of medicine, ed 17. Philadelphia: WB Saunders, 1985b.

Jones CW, Dyken PR, Huttenlocher P, et al. Inosiplex therapy in subacute sclerosing panencephalitis. Lancet 1982; 1:1034.

Kackell YM, Gorb PJ, Dreth WH, et al. Transfer factor therapy in patients with subacute sclerosing panencephalitis. J Neurol 1975; 211:39.

Kilbourne ED. Introduction to viral disease. In: Wyngaarden JB, Smith LH, eds. Cecil textbook of medicine, ed 17. Philadelphia: W.B. Saunders, 1985.

Klastersky J, et al. Ascending myelitis in association with herpes simplex virus. N Engl J Med 1972; 287:182.

Knutti RE. Acute ascending paralysis and myelitis due to the virus of rabies. JAMA 1929; 93:754.

Kolar O, Obruesik M, Behounkova L, et al. Thymectomy of subacute sclerosing panencephalitis. Br Med J 1967; 3:22.

Kotchmar G, Grose C, Brunell PA. Complete spectrum of the varicella congenital defects syndrome in 5-year old child. Pediatr Infect Dis 1984; 3:142.

Kovanen J, Erkinjunti T, Iivananinen M, et al. Cerebral MR and CT imaging in Creutzfeldt-Jakob disease. J Comput Assist Tomogr 1985; 9:125.

Krawiecki NS, Dyken PR, El Gamal R, et al. Computed tomography of the brain in subacute sclerosing panencephalitis. Ann Neurol 1984; 15:489.

Krupp LB, Lipton RB, Swerdlow ML, et al. Progressive multifocal leukoencephalopathy. Ann Neurol 1985; 17:344.

Levin MJ, et al. Diagnosis of congenital rubella in utero. N Engl J Med 1974; 290:1187.

Mandelbaum DE, Hall WW, Paneth N, et al. Subacute sclerosing panencephalitis, measles virus, and the matrix protein. Ann Neurol 1980; 8:213.

Mandell GL, Douglas GR, Bennett JE. Principles and practice of infectious diseases, ed 3. New York: Churchill Livingstone, 1990.

Melnick JL. Classification and nomenclature of animal viruses, 1971. Prog Med Virol 1971; 13:462.

Melnick JL. Taxonomy and nomenclature of viruses, 1982. In: Melnick JL, ed. Progress in medical virology, Basle: S Karger, 1982.

Melnick JL. Classification of viruses. In: Brande AI, David CE, Fierer J, eds. Infectious disease and medical microbiology, ed 2. Philadelphia: WB Saunders, 1986.

MMWR. Summary of notifiable diseases, United States. 1990; 39:55.

Modlin JF, et al. Epidemiologic studies of measles, measles vaccine, and subacute panencephalitis. Pediatrics 1977; 59:505.

Modlin JF, Halsey NA, Eddins DL, et al. Epidemiology of subacute sclerosing panencephalitis. J Pediatr 1979; 94:231.

Nahmias AJ, et al. Herpes simplex virus encephalitis: laboratory evaluations and their diagnostic significance. J Infect Dis 1982, 145:289.

Navin JJ, Angevine JM. Congenital cytomegalic inclusion disease with porencephaly. Neurology 1968; 18:470.

Ojala P, Vesikari T, Elo O. Rubella during pregnancy as a cause of congenital hearing loss. Am J Epidemiol 1973; 98:395.

Oxman MN. Herpes simplex encephalitis and meningitis. In: Brande AI, Davis CE, Fierer J, eds. Infectious diseases and medical microbiology, ed 2. Philadelphia: WB Saunders, 1986.

Pass RF, Stagno S, Myers GJ, et al. Outcome of symptomatic congenital cytomegalovirus infection: results of long-term longitudinal follow-up. Pediatrics 1980; 66:758.

Pasteur L. Chamberland and Roux. Nouvelle communication sur la rage. Comp Rend Acad Sci 1884; 98:457.

Payne FE, Baublis JV, Itabashi HH. Isolation of measles virus from cell cultures of brain from a patient with subacute sclerosing panencephalitis. N Engl J Med 1969; 281:585.

Pette H, Doring G. Uber einheimische panenophalimyelitis vom charakter der encephalitis japonica. Dtsch Z Nervenheilk 1939; 149:7.

Porras C, et al. Recovery from rabies in man. Ann Intern Med 1976; 85:44.

Porter DD. Persistent infections. In: Barons ed. Medical microbiology, ed 2. Menlo Park: Addison-Wesley, 1985.

Posson DD. Exanthem subitum (roseola infantum) complicated by prolonged convulsions and hemiplegia. J Pediatr 1949; 35:235.

Postic B, Wiktar TJ. Rabies. In: Brande AI, Davis CE, Fierer J, eds. Infectious diseases and medical microbiology, ed 2. Philadelphia: WB Saunders, 1986.

Prusiner SB. Norel proteinaceous infectious particles and scapie. Science 1982; 216:136.

Risk WS, Haddad FS. The variable natural history of subacute sclerosing panencephalitis: a study of 117 cases from the Middle East. Arch Neurol 1979; 36:610.

Robertson WC, Clark DB, Karkesbery WR. Review of 39 cases of subacute sclerosing panencephalitis: effect of amantadine on the natural course of the disease. Ann Neurol 1980; 8:422.

Roos R, Gajdusek DC, Biggs CJ. The clinical characteristics of Creutzfeldt-Jakob disease. Brain 1973; 96:1.

Savage MO, Moosa A, Gordon RR. Maternal varicella infection as a cause of fetal malformations. Lancet 1973; 1:352.

Schilder P. Nur kenntnis der pogennanten diffusen sklerose (uber encephalitis periaxiolis diffusa). Z Neurol 1912; 10:1.

Senseman LA. Myelitis complicating measles. Arch Neurol Psychiatry 1945; 53:309.

Shaw GM, et al. HTLV-III infection in brains of children and adults with AIDS encephalopathy. Science 1985; 227:177.

Sigurdsson B. Rida, a chronic encephalitis of sheep-with special remarks on infection which develops slowly and some of their special characteristics. Br Vet J 1954; 110:7.

Silverstein A, Steinberg G, Nathanson M. Nervous system involvement in infectious mononucleosis: the heralding and/or major manifestation. Arch Neurol 1972; 26:353.

Stephens EB, Compans RW. Assembly of animal viruses at cellular membranes. Annu Rec Microbiol 1988; 42:489.

Sung JH, et al. A case of human rabies and ultrastructure of the Negri body. J Neuropathol Exp Neurol 1976; 35:541.

Tangchai P, Vejjajiva A. Pathology of the peripheral nervous system in human rabies: a study of nine autopsy cases. Brain 1971; 94:299.

Tourtellotte WW, Ma Bn, Brandes DB, et al. Qualification of de novo central nervous system IgC measles antibody synthesis in SSPE. Ann Neurol 1981; 9:551.

Townsend JJ, Wolinsky JS, Baringer JR. The neuropathology of progressive rubella panencephalitis of late onset. Brain 1976; 99:81.

Townsend JJ, et al. Progressive rubella panencephalitis: late onset after congenital rubella. N Engl J Med 1975; 292:990.

Van Bogaert L, De Busscher J. Sur la selocose inflammatoire de la substance blanch des emispleres (speilmeyl). Sev Neurol 1931; 71:679.

Van Bogaert L, Rademaker J, Hozay J, et al. Encephalitides. Amsterdam: Elsevier, 1961.

Walker D, Padgett B. Progressive multifocal leukoencephalopathy. In: Fraenkel-Conrat H, Wagner RR, eds. Comprehensive virology. New York: Plenum Press, 1983.

Warrell DA. The clinical picture of rabies in man. Trans R Soc Trop Med Hyg 1976; 70:188.

Wechsler SL, Meissner HC. Measles and SSPE viruses: similarities and differences. Prog Med Virol 1982; 28:65.

Weil ML, et al. Chronic progressive panencephalitis due to rubella virus simulating subacute sclerosing panencephalitis. N Engl J Med 1975; 292:994.

Weiner HL, et al. Viral interactions with receptors in the central nervous system and on lymphocytes. In: Behran PO, et al, eds. Immunology of nervous system infections. Amsterdam: Elsevier, 1983.

White DO, Fenner FJ. Medical virology, ed 3. Orlando: Academic Press, 1986.

Wolf A, Cowen D. Perinatal infections of the central nervous system. In: Mickler J, ed. Pathology of the nervous system. New York: McGraw-Hill, 1972.

Wolinsky JS, et al. Progressive rubella panencephalitis. Clin Exp Immunol 1979; 35:397.

Wolinsky JS, Berg BO, Maitland CJ. Progressive rubella panencephalitis. Arch Neurol 1976; 33:722.

Zeman W, Kolar O. Reflections on the etiology and pathogenesis of subacute sclerosing panencephalitis. Neurology 1968; 18:1.

Zhdanov NM. The measles virus. Mol Cell Biol 1980; 29:59.

ZuRhein GM, et al. Progressive multifocal leukoencephalopathy in a child with severe combined immunodeficiency. N Engl J Med 1978; 299:256.

40

Fungal, Rickettsial, and Parasitic Diseases of the Nervous System

Keith L. Meloff

FUNGAL DISEASES

Fungal infections of humans are related to several factors, including virulence of the organism, intensity of exposure, and resistance of the host. The impact of acquired immunodeficiency syndrome (AIDS) is significant in this last respect [Brew 1992].

Certain fungi (e.g., *Coccidiodes immitis*) infect previously healthy individuals, whereas other fungi (e.g., *Candida albicans*) that ordinarily are not pathogenic infect individuals whose resistance is compromised. The box on p. 690 lists conditions that predispose individuals to fungal infections of the nervous system.

"Fungal infections of the central nervous system are almost always a clinical surprise" [Lyons and Andriole, 1986]. Clinical manifestations may be extremely subtle, and errors or delays in diagnosis are common. Fungi may cause meningitis, brain abscesses, granulomas, and spinal cord disease [Salake et al., 1984]. The diagnostic approach to fungal infections of the nervous system is outlined in the box. For purposes of discussion, separating fungi that infect normal hosts from those that infect immunologically compromised hosts is useful.

Fungal infections in normal hosts

Blastomyces dermatitidis, C. immitis, Cryptococcus neoformans, Histoplasma capsulatum, Nocardia asteroides, and *Paracoccidioides brasiliensis* may infect the nervous system of normal hosts.

Cryptococcosis

Epidemiology. Cryptococcosis is globally distributed and is the most prevalent fungal infection of the CNS. *C. neoformans* of the genus *Filobasidiella* and the class Basidiomycetes is an encapsulated yeast that reproduces by budding and has a sexual stage (Figure 40-1). Australian aborigines are 17 times more susceptible to infection than whites [Edwards et al., 1970]. Although children are less frequently infected than adults, infants have contracted the disease [Littman and Walter, 1968; Neuhauser and Tucker, 1948].

Bird feces, particularly from pigeons, harbor numerous cryptococcal organisms. Entry into humans is through inhalation or ingestion. Hematogenous dissemination to the nervous system is always preceded by pulmonary infection. The patient need not be predisposed to infection by extant chronic disease.

Clinical characteristics, clinical laboratory tests, and diagnosis. Characteristic features include nausea, vomiting, headache, and fever. The clinical course may fluctuate. Many patients (40%) are afebrile; half have no meningeal signs [Sabetta and Andriole, 1985]. Ocular palsies and personality changes may occur. Acquired immunodeficiency syndrome is now a major predisposing factor in cryptococcal infections. CNS cryptococcosis in these patients presents with fever and headache in 70%; meningismus, photophobia, or mental status changes in 20% to 25%; and focal deficits in less [Daar and Meyer, 1992].

C. neoformans most often causes meningitis but can also cause abscesses and granulomas. Granulomas may result in findings associated with mass lesions, including papilledema, cranial neuropathies, and hemiparesis.

The disease course may be indolent, and if untreated, the mortality is high. Hydrocephalus occurs regularly and necessitates shunting procedures [Richardson et al., 1976]. India ink staining of spinal fluid provides positive identification in 60% of cases. The organism can be cultured from the spinal fluid in 75% of patients. Latex agglutination of CSF is 90% reliable [Sabetta and Andriole, 1985]. Cranial CT and MRI scans reveal mass lesions caused by cryptococcus.

Management. Amphotericin B (0.3 mg/kg/day) and flucytosine (150 mg/kg/day) administered intravenously in combination at 6 hourly intervals is the best thera-

---

Conditions Predisposing to Fungal Infections of the Nervous System

Fungal infections of nonnervous tissue
1. Face, orbit, and paranasal sinuses: phycomycosis (diabetes)
2. Lung
   a. Aspergillosis
   b. Coccidioidomycosis
   c. Histoplasmosis
   d. North American blastomycosis
3. Skin
   a. Coccidioidomycosis
   b. North American blastomycosis
   c. South American blastomycosis
   d. Sporotrichosis
Past history of fungal infections
Primary immunodeficiency diseases
Secondary immunodeficiency diseases caused by the following:
1. Acquired immunodeficiency syndrome
2. Antibiotics
3. Antimetabolites
4. Corticosteroids
5. Cytotoxic drugs
Debilitating diseases
1. Aplastic anemia
2. Carcinoma
3. Cardiac disease
4. Chronic renal disease
5. Cystic fibrosis
6. Diabetes
7. Hodgkin disease
8. Leukemia
9. Lymphoma
10. Malabsorption syndromes
Postoperative conditions
1. Cardiac surgery
2. Organ transplantation
Others
1. Blood transfusion
2. Intravenous medication
   a. In hospital
   b. Self-administered (narcotics)
3. Lumbar puncture

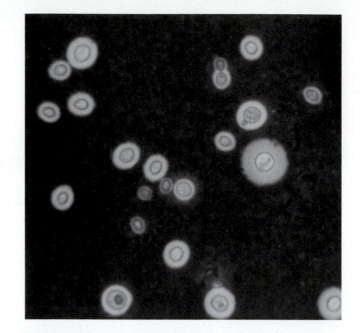

Figure 40-1 Capsulated budding yeast cells of *Cryptococcus neoformans* mounted in India ink. (× 400.)

peutic regimen for cryptococcal meningitis [Bennett et al., 1979]. Fluconazole (200 to 400 mg/day) orally is an effective alternative to amphotericin B as primary treatment of cryptococcal meningitis in patients with acquired immunodeficiency syndrome. Fluconazole orally is superior to weekly intravenous therapy with amphotericin B to prevent relapse of cryptococcal meningitis in these patients (after primary treatment with amphotericin B) [Powderly et al., 1992; Saag et al., 1992].

Coccidioidomycosis. Coccidioidomycosis, caused by the fungus *C. immitis*, rarely causes nervous system infection. Most patients are asymptomatic, and fewer than 50% experience acute respiratory symptoms.

Epidemiology. Endemic areas include the southwestern United States, northern Mexico, and portions of Central and South America. The San Joaquin Valley in California is the most notorious endemic zone, giving rise to the terms *valley fever* and *desert fever*. The dry season, during which spores are borne by dust, is when the greatest degree of infection occurs. Children are readily infected, rapidly develop an immunologic response, and overcome the infection promptly.

Coccidioidomycosis is acquired by inhalation of spore-laden dust or transcutaneously after skin abrasion. Paranasal skin lesions may predispose to CNS infections [Salake et al., 1984].

Pathology. Meningeal lesions observable during gross examination include plaques of granulation tissue, flattened tubercles clustered over the cerebral convexities, and thickened layers of plastic exudate in the basal cisterns and over the spinal cord. Osteomyelitis of the skull and vertebrae may be evident along with hydrocephalus, which follows spread of the bony infection. The infection produces both obstructive and communicating hydrocephalus by blocking CSF flow and absorption.

Microscopic examination of the thickened leptomeninges demonstrates widespread infiltration with inflammatory cells (e.g., plasma cells, lymphocytes, macrophages). Polymorphonuclear leukocytes are present during the acute phases. In more chronic infections, early fibrosis indicated by collagen fiber formation may be present.

Granulomas contain proliferating fibroblasts and multinucleated giant cells. Coccidioidal spherules stain with periodic acid-Schiff and are argyrophyllic with Grocott stain [Abud-Ortega et al., 1971].

Clinical characteristics. The pulmonary infection is evident within 3 weeks after exposure and is marked by excruciating pleuritic chest pain. Fever, chills, night sweats, cough, anorexia, and weight loss are common features. Erythema nodosum or erythema marginatum is manifest in 5% of males and 10% or more of females. The painful subcutaneous nodules of erythema nodosum occur most often along the anterior shins and are considered pathognomonic of coccidioidomycosis in pathognomonic endemic areas [Hedges and Miller, 1990]. A fine macular skin rash and conjunctivitis sometimes occur. Patients often develop pleural effusion; pulmonary cavitation, signaled by hemoptysis, is infrequently demonstrated with chest radiography. Dissemination of the infection from the pulmonary focus to skin, lymph nodes, bones, and brain may be immediate, or a variable latent period may intervene.

The clinical characteristics of coccidioidal meningitis are nonspecific. Prompt diagnosis often proves difficult [Caudill et al., 1970]. Confounding conditions include psychiatric illness, tension headache, frontal sinusitis, and pseudotumor cerebri. The most prevalent manifestations are headache, fever, malaise, and weight loss. Mental aberrations, such as confusion, personality changes, and decreased level of consciousness, may ensue. Spinal cord involvement may occur, as typified by one patient who developed quadriplegia after appearance of coccidioidal osteomyelitis of a cervical vertebra [Jackson et al., 1964].

Clinical laboratory tests and diagnosis. Diagnostic confirmation is obtained from CSF changes and the documentation of fungus infection by either direct microscopic study or culture (Figure 40-2). The spinal fluid abnormalities include mononuclear pleocytosis, increased protein content, increased chloride concentration, and normal or decreased glucose concentration. Use of a special microscopic-pore filter increases the likelihood of isolating the organism from the spinal fluid [Wayne and Juarez, 1955].

The coccidioidin skin test is not of value for acute diagnosis. Complement fixation and precipitin tests are dependable and provide accurate diagnosis in more than 99% of patients with disseminated infection [Pappagianis, 1976]. Any discernible titer of complement fixation antibody in spinal fluid is diagnostic [Lyons and Andriole, 1986].

Management. Amphotericin B, administered intrathecally, is the recommended treatment [Wright, 1978]. The

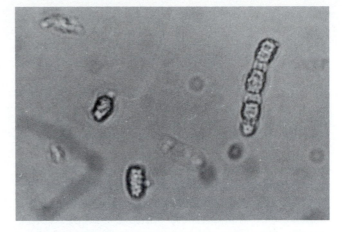

Figure 40-2 Infectious fragmentation spores of *Coccidioides immitis.* (× 400.)

drug must be given intrathecally because it is absorbed so poorly from the circulation into the spinal fluid. A subcutaneous reservoir for direct intraventricular instillation can be employed [Diamond and Bennett, 1973]. Transfer factor and miconazole nitrate have been used with some benefit [Danoff et al., 1978; Stevens, 1977]. Fluconazole and intraconazole are newer oral agents with efficacy in coccidioidal meningitis [Taylor et al., 1990; Tucker et al., 1992].

South American blastomycosis. South American blastomycosis is caused by the fungus *P. brasiliensis* [Lutz, 1908]. The organism first invades the lymph nodes, and then extensive bilateral pulmonary infection or a buccopharyngeal granulomatous lesion develops. The buccopharyngeal lesion must be distinguished from mucocutaneous leishmaniasis.

Epidemiology. The organism is a saprophyte found in soil and plants. Thousands of patients have been reported from Brazil, and the disease also occurs in Europe and the United States. Nervous system involvement is rare but may follow extensive infection of the lymph nodes, liver, spleen, lungs, adrenal glands, kidneys, and bone. Osteomyelitis of the cranium without other lesions has been reported [Krivoy et al., 1978].

Clinical characteristics. CNS lesions are typically granulomatous in the form of solitary or multiple abscesses located supratentorially within the hemispheres or in the meninges. The abscesses contain a necrotic core in which inflamed blood vessels are found. The abscesses may cause focal neurologic signs, increased intracranial pressure, and symptoms of meningeal involvement.

Clinical laboratory tests and diagnosis. The diagnosis of South American blastomycosis is suggested by simultaneous involvement of several organs or characteristic oral or skin lesions in patients who reside in endemic zones. Microscopic study of scrapings from mucous lesions, sputum, gastric contents, lymph nodes, or surgical specimens is most helpful. Typical morphology consists of round cells (10 to 60 μm in diameter) bearing many small buds at the periphery and affixed by slim openings to the surface of the parent cell. The morphology of *P. brasiliensis* differs from *B. dermatitidis* because the latter produces a single bud attached by a wide septum to the parent cell. *P. brasiliensis* differs from *C. immitis* because the latter never reproduces by budding and its cells are nonbudding, thick-walled structures (20 to 100 μm) that encase numerous small endospores.

Diagnostic tests may include complement fixation, agar gel immunodiffusion tests, and culture and inoculation of experimental animals.

Management. Sulfamethoxypyridazine therapy is recommended. The drug is inexpensive and excreted slowly and produces ongoing adequate blood levels when administered orally over 2 to 3 years. Although it is also effective in most cases, amphotericin B is more expensive and more difficult to administer and monitor and is associated with many side effects [Araujo et al., 1978; Krivoy et al., 1978]. Miconazole undoubtedly will be used more frequently [Stevens, 1977].

North American blastomycosis. A highly detailed description of the clinical and pathologic characteristics of CNS infection by *B. dermatitidis* is available [Gonyea, 1978]. Children are infrequently affected but may be at increased risk if they play near a beaver dam [Dismukes et al., 1986; Klein et al., 1986]. The three major clinical manifestations are meningitis, intracranial mass, and spinal mass.

Skin tests and serodiagnosis are not helpful in the diagnosis of North American blastomycosis. Debilitating conditions (e.g., leukemia) do not enhance the likelihood of infection, but steroid therapy may have a deleterious effect. The organisms may be identified in ventricular and cisternal fluid but are rarely detected in CSF. Neuroimaging and myelography demonstrate brain and spinal cord lesions. Microscopic study of biopsy material provides positive identification of the fungus. Amphotericin B is the most efficacious drug and may be used intraventricularly and intravenously [Morgan et al., 1979].

Histoplasma capsulatum infection. *H. capsulatum* infection primarily affects the lungs (Figure 40-3). Histoplasmosis is very common; approximately 30 million people in the United States have been infected, as corroborated by skin testing. With rare exception the condition is a benign, self-limiting infection. CNS infection is subsequent to the much rarer disseminated form of histoplasmosis.

History. Histoplasmosis, initially described in the Panama Canal zone in a 27-year-old Martinique black man [Darling, 1906], is a progressive systemic illness accompanied by weakness, fever, weight loss, hepatosplenomegaly, anemia, and leukopenia. The gross features at

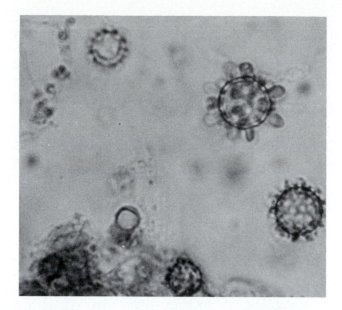

Figure 40-3 Tuberculate macroconidia of the mold (saprophytic) type of growth of *Histoplasma capsulatum.* (× 400.)

postmortem examination are primarily those of a granulomatous disease similar to miliary tuberculosis that affects the lungs and reticuloendothelial system. Microscopic study documents ovoid "parasites" crammed into mononuclear and reticuloendothelial cells. Unlike tuberculosis the parasites are not acid-fast. Darling [1906] erroneously believed they were similar to kala-azar (leishmaniasis). He named the disease *histoplasmosis:* *histo* signifying "histocyte" and *plasma* signifying "plasmodium-like organisms." He believed the disease was similar to the condition reported by Leishman and Donovan in which inclusions were also present [Darling, 1906]. Not until 1934 did DeMonbreum definitively demonstrate the fungal association with histoplasmosis.

Epidemiology. Histoplasmosis is globally distributed. Among the endemic zones are the Mississippi River basin, Mexico, and Central and South America [Loosli, 1957]. In these regions as many as 80% of children manifest positive histoplasmosis skin tests by age 5 years [Rogers, 1967]. Humans and many wild and domestic animals are targets of infection. No racial predilection exists for skin test reactivity. However, blacks rarely develop the chronic pulmonary disease. The disseminated form of the disease affects boys and girls equally.

The organism grows as a saprophyte in the soil. Dampness and nutrients from bird droppings encourage growth in aviaries, chicken coops, mines, caves, and open fields [Ajello and Ziedberg, 1951]. During dry spells the organism may become airborne and the spores inhaled. No evidence of person-to-person or animal-to-human transmission exists.

Pathogenesis and pathology. After inhalation the spore is

transformed into a yeastlike organism that enters reticuloendothelial cells, macrophages, and peripheral blood leukocytes. The yeast buds in the cell. The relative lack of inflammatory response in infants results in ready dissemination in early life. In older children, histiocytes proliferate, and infection occurs with subsequent formation of noncaseating granulomas, hepatosplenomegaly, and lymphadenopathy. Occasionally fibroblastic overgrowth is present at the margin of the granuloma. Calcification of the granulomas eventually occurs.

Biopsy of infected tissue such as lymph nodes or liver demonstrates granulomas that superficially resemble lymphoma, tuberculosis, sarcoidosis, Hodgkin disease, and leishmaniasis. Specific staining with Gridley stain documents a chitinous ghost of the residue of defunct organisms.

Spread of the organism from the pulmonary site to other organs depends on several variables, including the concentration of the organism, virulence, and the age and immune status of the host [Oppenheimer et al., 1973]. CNS infection is the sequel to lymphogenous or hematogenous dissemination of the organism. A review of 235 cases of histoplasmosis reported between 1952 and 1960 revealed that of the one third of the patients who had disseminated disease, one fourth exhibited CNS impairment [Cooper and Goldstein, 1963]. The predominate pathologic alterations that occur within the CNS include perivenous miliary granulomatosis, parenchymatous granulomatosis, meningitis, histoplasmoma, and histiocytic histoplasmosis. The most frequently observed changes are mild meningitis and perivenous granulomatosis.

A 16-year-old adolescent contracted CNS histoplasmosis and developed obstruction of the fourth ventricle with subsequent hydrocephalus. Intrathecal amphotericin B therapy caused transverse myelitis [Enarson et al., 1978]. Another patient with common variable hypogammaglobulinemia developed *Histoplasma* meningitis despite disseminated histoplasmosis not being present [Couch et al., 1978]. Overactive suppressor T cells in CSF may have enhanced the likelihood of meningitis, although the active systemic immune response to the *Histoplasma* organism forestalled the development of disseminated histoplasmosis.

Clinical characteristics, clinical laboratory tests, and diagnosis. Respiratory infection follows inhalation of spore-laden soil or coal dust. Most children remain asymptomatic or experience little clinical difficulty [Ibach et al., 1954]. A nonspecific mild lung infection may follow exposure after 5 to 15 days. Fever, chills, and a productive cough are common features of histoplasmosis, but more severe symptoms may occur, including chest pain, dyspnea, and rarely prostration.

The initial chest radiograph may document a nodular

or more dispersed infiltrate. Cultures of the sputum or stomach aspirate may grow the organism. After several years, chest radiographs demonstrate characteristic calcification in the central lymph nodes and peripheral lung fields.

If untreated, the infection lasts 2 to 12 weeks. The histoplasmin skin test converts to positive during the course of the acute infection. Complement fixation titers do not increase 4 weeks after the infection is contracted.

In one report of 10 children with disseminated disease, most had fever, anemia, and hepatosplenomegaly. Only 2 children had neurologic involvement: 1 had nuchal rigidity and the other had positive Babinski signs and tetany [Cooper and Goldstein, 1963].

Anemia, thrombocytopenia, and leukopenia may occur. Directed laboratory studies include culture of CSF, blood, and bone marrow and biopsy of liver, bone marrow, and lymph nodes. Microscopic detection of the organism and growth in culture are corroborative. Detection of the antigen of the organism in serum and urine is diagnostic [Wheat et al., 1986]. Histoplasma antigen is present in the CSF of some patients with chronic histoplasma meningitis, but its measurement and diagnostic precision are unreliable [Wheat et al., 1989].

Because 50% of patients with disseminated histoplasmosis develop anergy, skin tests are not reliable. All patients with disseminated histoplasmosis should be evaluated for adrenal insufficiency. In one series, half the patients, regardless of treatment, had insufficiency, and adrenal insufficiency was the most common cause of death [Sarosi et al., 1971].

The differential diagnosis of CNS histoplasmosis includes cryptococcosis, candidiasis, toxoplasmosis, trypanosomiasis, tuberculosis, rickettsiosis, lues, and leishmaniasis.

Management. Amphotericin B therapy, intrathecal and systemic, is the recommended therapy [Diamond and Bennett, 1973; Drutz et al., 1968]. The presence of adrenal insufficiency necessitates careful replacement of fluids, electrolytes, and corticosteroids.

Although amphotericin B therapy benefits most patients, relapses are experienced by half the patients who initially respond positively [Smith and Utz, 1972]. An 18-year-old Hispanic female with chronic progressive CNS histoplasmosis characterized by ataxia, hydrocephalus, seizures, and cranial nerve palsy evolving over several years responded favorably to fluconazole after being treated intermittently with ventricoperitoneal shunts, corticosteroids, and amphotericin B [Rivera et al., 1992]. Prognosis is excellent, with or without treatment. More than 99% of patients experience a benign course [Rogers, 1967]. One fourth to one fifth of all patients who develop disseminated infection are younger than 2 years of age; furthermore, approximately one fourth of these infants eventually develop CNS infection.

Nocardiosis. *N. asteroides* is responsible for nocardiosis (Figure 40-4). Nocardial disease during childhood is relatively uncommon, and nocardial involvement of the CNS is exceedingly rare [Stites and Glezen, 1967]. Pulmonary infection precedes nervous system infection. The premorbid state appears to have little effect. Before brain involvement, children may be in good health or have debilitating diseases. CNS abscesses occur most frequently, but meningitis is present in more than one third of patients with disseminated nocardiosis and is often fatal [Byrne et al., 1979].

Although uncommon, nocardiosis should be considered in the differential diagnosis of subacute meningitis, especially when CSF contains a high concentration of neutrophils, elevated protein levels, and a low glucose level. Nocardial pulmonary disease or cerebral abscesses confirm the diagnosis, as do positive cultures from CSF [Bross and Gordon, 1991].

Efficacious therapy consisting of aspiration and sulfonamide administration has been reported [Turner and Whitby, 1969]. A renal transplant recipient was described who had fulminant cerebral nocardiosis and numerous cerebral abscesses precluding surgical drainage. Administration of sulfadiazine (2.0 g four times daily), ampicillin (2.0 g every 4 hours), and erythromycin (500 mg intravenously four times daily for 3 months) were followed by healing of the abscesses, as documented by serial CT [Kirmani et al., 1978]. Rosenblum and Rosegay [1979] reported successful surgical extirpation of multiple nocardial abscesses. The combination therapy of sulfadiazine and cycloserine has been reported to be efficacious, most likely because both drugs readily enter the CSF [Hoeprich et al., 1968].

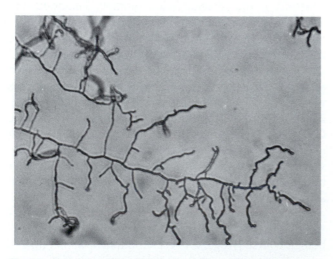

Figure 40-4 Branching filaments of *Nocardia asteroides*. (× 400.)

Fungal infections in the immunocompromised host

Cryptococcosis often affects compromised hosts such as patients with diabetes, acquired immunodeficiency syndrome, or lymphoma or those receiving steroids.

The other infections described previously occur more frequently in healthy hosts and much less often in immunosuppressed patients. The group of fungal infections discussed occur most frequently in the debilitated or immunologically impaired patient.

Actinomycosis. *Actinomyces israelii* infects humans, is anaerobic, and therefore must be grown and identified in anaerobic culture. Actinomycosis was first described in 1878 by Israel.

Clinical characteristics. The most frequent primary areas of infection are the lungs and cervicofacial region [Everts, 1970]. Concurrent chronic infections and other debilitating conditions predispose to dissemination of the organisms within the patient, with resultant propagation of the infection. CNS involvement results from hematogenous spread or direct extension from adjacent infected areas of the head and neck.

A review of 181 cases of actinomycosis revealed that less than 2% of patients had cerebral involvement as manifested by meningitis or solitary or multiple abscesses. Osteomyelitis of the spine may be the origin of spinal cord abscess and compression [Brown, 1973; Fetter et al., 1967]. The abscesses are unusual because they have an avascular capsule through which antibodies do not diffuse well; therefore surgical excision often proves necessary.

Management. The recommended drug is penicillin. Penicillin-sensitive patients can be treated with lincomycin [Rose and Rytel, 1972].

Aspergillosis. *Aspergillus fumigatus*, the species affecting humans (Figure 40-5), initially gains entrance to the lung after inhalation. The name of this fungus was established because of the likeness of its fruiting head to the aspergillum, a perforated globe used to sprinkle holy water during religious ceremonies. Disseminated infection is accompanied by an underlying debilitating condition.

Epidemiology. Aspergillosis of the CNS is very rare. In a group of 32 patients with CNS aspergillosis, 8 were younger than 20 years old, and 2 were neonates [Mukoyama et al., 1969].

Clinical characteristics and diagnosis. CNS manifestations include meningitis, meningoencephalitis, isolated or multiple brain abscess, hemorrhagic necrosis, and solitary granulomas. There is a predilection for involvement of the posterior cerebral circulation [Tressler and Sugar, 1990]. CNS manifestations include meningitis, meningoencephalitis, isolated or multiple brain abscesses, and solitary granulomas. A solitary granuloma is highly unusual in children [Linares et al., 1971].

Diagnosis may be made by smear and culture of biopsy material or CSF. In one study an immunodiffusion test was positive in 82% of patients with aspergillosis [Coleman and Kaufman, 1972].

Management. Surgical drainage and removal of abscesses and granulomas are often performed but are usually of little value. Treatment with amphotericin B is also of little value but is usually attempted.

Candidiasis

Clinical characteristics. Cerebral candidiasis is a sequela of disseminated disease in a debilitated patient. Meningitis, abscesses, and large, small, or miliary granulomas occur independently or in combination (Figure 40-6). Diagnosis can be confirmed by identification of the organism in spinal fluid or infected neural tissue [McGinnis, 1983]. Disseminated disease with subsequent cerebral infection is unusual in children. A 13-month-old girl who developed candidal meningitis after oral candidiasis and placement of indwelling catheters was treated with amphotericin B and apparently experienced no neurologic sequelae [Roe and Haynes, 1972]. A neonate who developed disseminated candidiasis and then developed osteomyelitis and ventriculomeningitis was not benefited by administration of amphotericin B [Adler et al., 1972]. Two children with

severe combined immunodeficiency developed candidal meningitis [Smego et al., 1984].

Intracerebral abscess formation in neonates who developed CNS infection following candidal septicemia after scalp and jugular vein infusions are shown in Figure 40-6, *B.* Candidal meningitis may have resulted from a parenchymal focus in a newborn. The baby had multiple miliary giant cell granulomas of the brain [Averback and Wigglesworth, 1978]. A 16-year-old girl with systemic lupus erythematosus and diabetes experienced fever, headaches, irritability, and seizures while receiving prednisone, azathioprine, and insulin. She hemorrhaged from a large proximal basilar artery aneurysm. Postmortem examination demonstrated an intracranial mycotic aneurysm resulting from infection with *C. albicans* [Goldman et al., 1979].

Management. 5-Fluorocytosine has been of value in the treatment of candidal meningitis.* New methods, such as incorporation of amphotericin B into liposomes and the use of triazoles (e.g., fluconazole, intraconazole), are promising [Meunier, 1989].

Phycomycosis. Extension of a phycomycosis infection from the nose and nasopharynx through the sinuses or cribriform plate into the meninges and CNS is termed *rhinocerebral phycomycosis.* Spread of infection into the orbit by way of the nasolacrimal duct is accompanied by proptosis and panophthalmitis.

Clinical characteristics. Diabetes mellitus is frequently associated with this fungal infection, but other chronic illnesses are often present. The infecting organisms are species of the genus *Rhizopus.* Childhood patients are rare and death almost certain. However, a 15-year-old girl with well-controlled diabetes mellitus survived after successful treatment with surgical drainage (Caldwell-Luc procedure) and local and systemic administration of amphotericin B [Battock et al., 1968; Sandler et al., 1971].

One report described nine patients with rhinocerebral phycomycosis; all suffered facial or ocular pain, which often was the initial symptom. Four of seven patients who received amphotericin B survived. All survivors had diabetes mellitus and required surgical debridement [Meyers et al., 1979]. Patients initially may have ocular palsies [Schatz, 1978].

Management. The fungus has an unusual proclivity to infect and obstruct cranial blood vessels and thus thwart drug treatment (Figure 40-7). General principles of management include correcting diabetic ketoacidosis, discontinuing immunosuppressive therapy if possible, and removing infected tissue surgically. Intravenous amphotericin B is the drug of choice.

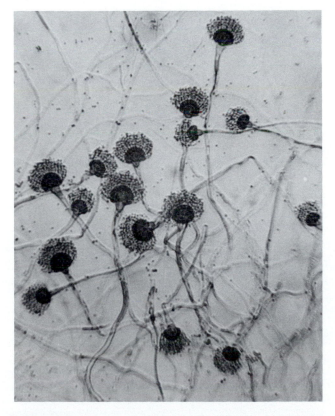

Figure 40-5 Spore heads of *Aspergillus fumigatus* in culture. (× 400.)

---

*Bennett, 1977; Fass and Perkins, 1971; Medoff et al., 1971; Smego et al., 1984; Tassel and Madoff, 1968; Utz, 1972.

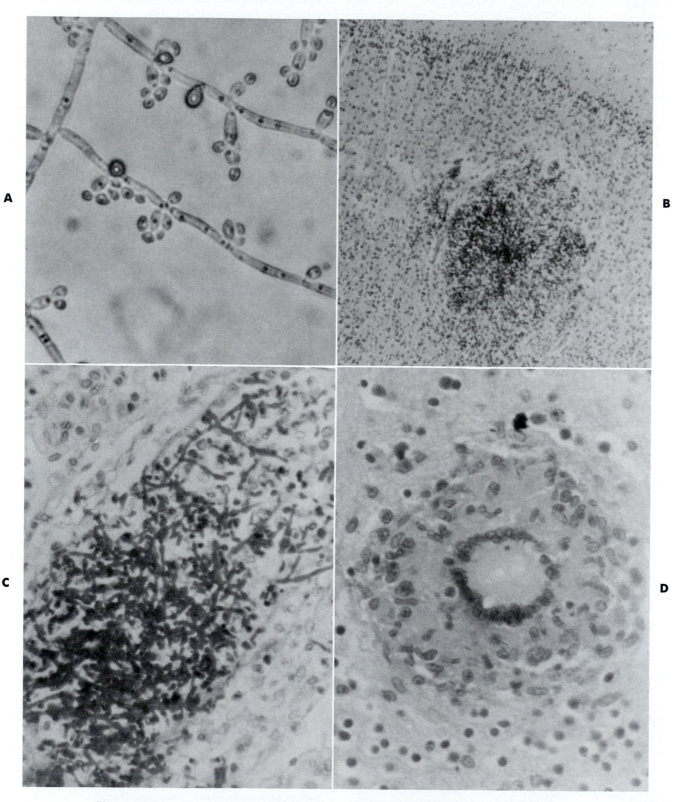

Figure 40-6 A, Pseudohyphae and budding yeast cells of *Candida albicans.* (× 400.) **B,** Candidal abscess. **C,** Cerebral vein clogged with *Candida* organism. **D,** Giant cell granuloma.

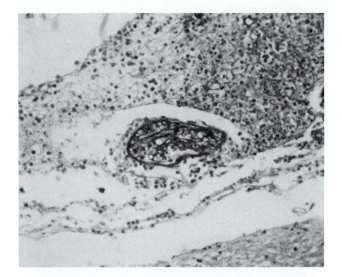

Figure 40-7 *Mucor* organism lodged in capillary. (PAS; × 125.)

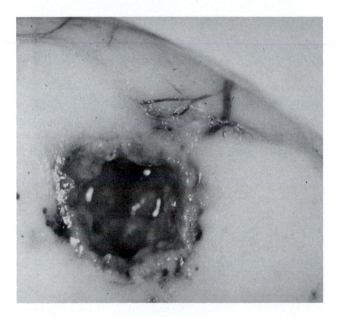

Figure 40-8 A 1-cm abscess caused by *Allescheria boydii* in parietal cortex. (× 6.) (From Rewcastle NB. Can Med Assoc J 1965; 93:1126.)

Allescheriosis. Allescheriosis rarely affects the nervous system. A 19-year-old girl with dissemination to the brain and thyroid died [Rosen et al., 1965]. She had poststreptococcal subacute glomerulonephritis and had been treated with steroids and azathioprine. A 1 cm abscess of the cortex is depicted in Figure 40-8.

A 3-year-old boy with acute lymphoblastic leukemia developed a right frontal lobe abscess; *Allescheria (Petriellidium) boydii* was cultured. He survived with no neurologic sequelae after surgical drainage and admin-

istration of amphotericin B [Bell and Myers, 1978]. Three patients who responded to miconazole therapy have been described [Lutwick et al., 1979]. Ketoconazole may be useful as well [Schiess et al., 1984].

RICKETTSIAL DISEASES

In the presence of rickettsial infection, the likelihood of CNS involvement is greater than 90%. Pathologic changes may be extensive; the patient may survive with significant residual neurologic dysfunction or die. The clinical and pathologic response of the CNS to the different species of rickettsiae is identical, differing only in severity [Harrell, 1953].

Rickettsiae, except *Coxiella (Rickettsia) burnetii*, share several common characteristics:
1. The organisms are fastidious and require a cellular host.
2. An arthropod vector transmits the disease to humans.
3. Rodents and humans are reservoirs.
4. Infection stimulates agglutinating antibodies to *Proteus* organisms (Weil-Felix reaction).
5. A skin eruption accompanies the infection.

C. burnetii differs from the other organisms because it lives freely, does not require a vector, and does not cause a skin rash or induce a Weil-Felix reaction. All rickettsiae respond to treatment with tetracycline or chloramphenicol [Woodward and Osterman, 1984].

Table 40-1 lists the rickettsial diseases, organisms, vectors, reservoirs, and geographic distribution. The clinical features of the rickettsial diseases vary, but the neurologic manifestations are very similar. Rocky Mountain spotted fever is the prototypic condition for these infections and is the most prevalent of these diseases in North America. The neuropathologic characteristics associated with epidemic typhus are virtually the same [Lillie et al., 1953].

Rocky Mountain spotted fever

History and epidemiology. Rocky Mountain spotted fever is the predominant rickettsial disorder in the United States. Shoshone Indians were infected in the foothills of the western Rocky Mountains. Early missionaries and settlers discerned the association of tick bites with the disease and called the disease *tick fever* [Aikawa, 1966].

After isolating the organism, Howard Ricketts identified *R. rickettsii* as the etiologic organism in the early 1900s and established the tick as the vector in transferring the organism to humans. The disease is now known to be prevalent in wide geographic areas. Rocky Mountain spotted fever is exceedingly common in the Piedmont region of the southeastern United States and in Oklahoma and has been described in Canada and Central and South America [Heldrich, 1987; Krugman et

Table 40-1 Rickettsial diseases

Disease	*Rickettsia* species	Vector	Reservoir	Location
Epidemic typhus	*R. prowazekii*	Mouse	Human	Global
Murine typhus	*R. mooseri (typhi)*	Flea	Rodent	Global
Q fever	*Coxiella burnetii*	Airborne	Human	Global
Rickettsialpox	*R. akari*	Mite	Rodent	Russia, Korea, United States
Rocky Mountain spotted fever	*R. rickettsii*	Tick	Rodent	Western Hemisphere
Scrub typhus	*R. tsutsugamushi*	Mite	Rodent	Asia, Australia, South Pacific

al., 1985a]. Four patients with Rocky Mountain spotted fever in New York City were reported in 1988, including a 10-year-old boy who died [Salgo et al., 1988].

The number of cases of Rocky Mountain spotted fever reported in the United States in 1977 (1115) was virtually unchanged in 1983. In 1989, the number of cases declined to 603 [Weber and Walker, 1991]. The incidence of the condition is greatest from April to September in the northern hemisphere when tick bite is most likely to occur. As expected, rural and suburban dwellers are more likely to be infected than urban residents. Children have a high risk of infection because they are exposed to tick bites during outdoor play; half the patients are younger than 10 years of age.

A group of patients developed Rocky Mountain spotted fever while exposed during laboratory studies of rickettsial disease [Oster et al., 1977]. Transmission occurred through infectious aerosols that were inhaled. Some workers who had been immunized with multiple vaccinations of commercial vaccine were unaffected. Rocky Mountain spotted fever transmitted by blood transfusion has been fatal [Wells et al., 1978].

Pathogenesis and pathology. The feces of the tick (Figure 40-9) contains *R. rickettsii*, which gains access to the circulation of the host when the tick bite is scratched. The incubation period ranges from 2 days to 2 weeks. After entering the body, rickettsiae multiply and disrupt the endothelial cells of capillaries and arterioles. In Rocky Mountain spotted fever, they ravage the smooth muscle cells of the tunica media. Loss of integrity of the small vessels in the brain results in hemorrhage into the subarachnoid space. Subsequent meningeal irritation and an accompanying perivascular mononuclear infiltrate develop. The brain parenchyma is studded with areas of microscopic infarctions. In the healing phase a proliferative fibroblastic and gliotic response is evident; the ensuing focal nodules develop more often in white matter in spotted fever and more often in gray matter in typhus.

Clinical characteristics, clinical laboratory tests, and diagnosis. The symptoms of Rocky Mountain

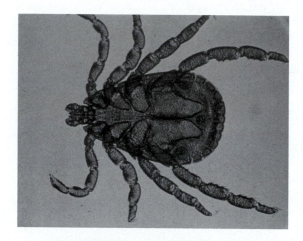

Figure 40-9 *Dermacentor andersoni.*

spotted fever vary in severity from mild to severe; the course may rapidly lead to death. Fever, malaise, lethargy, and headache are common. A petechial rash, not always immediately obvious, develops. In fulminating disease, shock, coma, and general or focal neurologic impairment, including vertigo, seizures, hemiparesis, and ataxia, may dominate the clinical manifestations. Rocky Mountain spotted fever may manifest as a skeletal muscle disease. Muscle weakness may be overwhelming; Guillain-Barré syndrome, viral myositis, and collagen disease may be erroneously diagnosed. Muscle biopsy reveals perivascular infiltrates of chronic inflammatory cells and focal chronic interstitial myositis [Krober, 1978]. Other organs, including kidney, spleen, and epididymis, may also be affected [Green et al., 1978]. Edema, usually periorbital at first and then becoming generalized, is characteristic and may suggest the diagnosis. The limbs are eventually affected. Hepatosplenomegaly accompanied by liver dysfunction, including coagulation defects, may confound the diagnostic process.

Acute temporary hearing impairment has been described, but permanent auditory disruption is uncommon [Kelsey, 1979].

Ophthalmic features in all rickettsial disorders are virtually identical [Raab et al., 1969; Smith and Burton, 1977]. Ophthalmic involvement may include photophobia, conjunctivitis, petechiae on the bulbar conjunctiva, exudates and retinal venous engorgement, papilledema, and ocular palsies.

Laboratory manifestations such as low serum sodium levels, low platelet count, and low serum albumin occur in the second week of the illness when there is significant mortality [Weber and Walker, 1991]. The indirect fluorescent antibody is the favored laboratory test in state health departments in the United States [Doan-Wiggins, 1991].

The cellular response in spinal fluid may suggest bacterial meningitis, and the dermal petechiae may mimic those in meningococcemia.

R. rickettsii may be detected in biopsy tissue from the site of the skin rash by use of a specific, direct immunofluorescent staining technique. Regions with moderate fluorescence accompanied by coccobacillary shapes are seen. This technique provides quick confirmation of the diagnosis [Fleisher et al., 1979].

Management and prognosis. Early therapy with tetracycline or chloramphenicol usually effects rapid clinical improvement [Duma, 1979; Laupus, 1978]. Positive Weil-Felix reactions, the antibody response, are delayed for 2 to 3 weeks; therefore therapy should be administered before confirmatory antibody titers are available. A history of tick bite in an endemic area is sufficient reason to initiate appropriate therapy. The mortality is 5% overall.

The outlook for full recovery from Rocky Mountain spotted fever is excellent when treatment is not delayed. Neurologic sequelae may be associated with infection when therapy is postponed [Miller and Price, 1972]. Mild intellectual impairment has been described [Wright, 1972]. Dependable immunity to reinfection follows active infection [Dupont et al., 1973].

PARASITIC INFECTIONS

Human parasitic infestation occurs worldwide [Bia and Barry, 1986; Warren and Mahmoud, 1984]. Parasites infect humans in tropical, temperate, and cold climates. Parasitic infections impair the CNS by a variety of mechanisms, including the following [Brown and Voge, 1982]:

1. Direct invasion from the circulation or lymphatic system may cause local changes such as inflammation and edema. Granuloma development may result in disturbances associated with mass lesions.
2. Remote effects associated with nutrient deprivation of the CNS may occur.
3. Immunologic or hypersensitivity effects may develop.

Classification

Parasites can be classified as follows:

Phylum Protozoa
    Genus *Trypanosoma*
    Genus *Entamoeba*
    Genus *Naegleria (Acanthamoeba, Hartmannella)*
    Genus *Plasmodium*
    Genus *Toxoplasma* (uncertain)
    Genus *Babesia*
  Class Trematoda
    Genus *Schistosoma*
    Genus *Paragonimus*
  Class Cestoda, subclass Eucestoda
    Genus *Dibothriocephalus (Diphyllobothrium)*
    Genus *Taenia*
    Genus *Multiceps*
    Genus *Echinococcus*
  Class Nematoda
    Genus *Trichinella*
    Genus *Angiostrongylus*
    Genus *Toxocara*

Protozoa are monocellular organisms that contain intracellular organelles. The genera that cause disease of the human CNS are *Trypanosoma*, *Naegleria (Acanthamoeba, Hartmannella)*, *Entamoeba*, and *Plasmodium*. *Toxoplasma gondii* is classified as part of this group; however, its precise taxonomic status remains uncertain. *Babesia* organisms are also known to incite neurologic symptoms in humans.

Helminths (worms) are subdivided into three categories: trematodes, cestodes, and nematodes. Trematodes (flukes) are nonsegmented worms that possess a digestive tract. Trematodes infecting the nervous system include the genera *Schistosoma* and *Paragonimus*.

Cestodes that infect humans belong to the subclass *Eucestoda*, the true tapeworms. These endoparasites have no epidermis or digestive tract and elongated segmented bodies. Adults have a multihook organ of attachment at the anterior end, the scolex. Genera of cestodes associated with CNS disruption include *Dibothriocephalus (Diphyllobothrium)*, *Taenia*, *Multiceps*, and *Echinococcus*.

Nematodes are cylindric and nonsegmented worms. *Trichinella*, *Angiostrongylus*, and *Toxocara* are genera in this class that infect the CNS.

Trypanosomiasis

The trypanosomes are the etiologic agents for Chagas disease and African sleeping sickness.

Chagas disease

History and epidemiology. Chagas disease (American trypanosomiasis) is a public health problem in Latin America. The trypanosome *T. cruzi*, the infecting organism, was first described by Chagas [1916]. He also described the clinical disease and delineated the life cycle, reservoir, and vectors.

Clinical characteristics, clinical laboratory tests, and diagnosis. Chagas disease in childhood predominantly affects the cardiovascular system [Laranja et al., 1956]; however, trypanosomal meningoencephalitis may occur and be fatal. Neuropathologic characteristics include leptomeningeal mononuclear infiltration, cerebral edema, and other abnormalities similar to those present in African trypanosomiasis. Parasitic nodules may be evident throughout the brain and spinal cord [Chagas, 1916].

In a series of 11 children with CNS infection from Chagas disease, *T. cruzi* was isolated from the spinal fluid in 8 [Hoff et al., 1978]. Spasticity, mental deficiency, and cerebellar symptoms are sequelae of meningoencephalitis.

Management. Nifurtimox, available through the Centers for Disease Control, is used for the treatment of Chagas disease [Seidel, 1985]. Allopurinol has been found to be as effective as nifurtimox or benznidazole in treating *T. cruzi* infection at a dose of 300 mg two or three times a day for 60 days [Gallerano et al., 1990].

African sleeping sickness

History. Bruce and Nabarro [1902] reported the trypanosomal etiology of African sleeping sickness (maladie du sommeil, "Negro lethargy") and its tsetse fly vector.

Epidemiology. *T. gambiense* is often the organism isolated in patients from West and East Africa. *T. rhodesiense* infections occur in East Africa and also in Central Africa (Figure 40-10). The reservoir consists of wild game; tsetse flies (*Glossina* species) are the vectors.

Pathogenesis and pathology. After the host is bitten by an infected fly the trypanosomes traverse the lymphatic pathways to regional lymph nodes, where they reproduce, multiply, and subsequently enter the bloodstream. Splenomegaly follows accumulation of the trypanosomes within the splenic parenchyma. Pancarditis frequently occurs. Impairment of the nervous system is the result of leptomeningitis, usually centered over the vertex. Dural thickening and adhesion to surrounding structures are often present at postmortem examination. Cerebral edema and petechiae are readily seen in most fatal cases.

The perivascular infiltrate in the gray and white matter is delineated so clearly that it has been called a *gray sleeve*. Obstruction of CSF flow may lead to ventricular dilatation. Cerebral and cerebellar atrophy may occur in the late stages of the disease. The spinal cord remains unaffected.

A mononuclear infiltrate is seen in the meninges and Virchow-Robin spaces during microscopic examination. Lymphocytes are more numerous than plasma cells. Endothelial proliferation of the capillaries may be present. The characteristic morular cell, a plasma cell

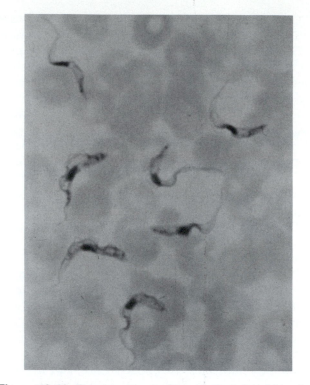

Figure 40-10 *Trypanosoma gambiense* in peripheral blood (Leishman stain).

with enclosed Russell bodies, was first reported by Mott [1906]. Differentiating the neuropathologic changes in African sleeping sickness from Chagas disease is relatively impossible.

Tryptophol, the 3-indole ethanol formed by the parasite in trypanosomal sleeping sickness, produces the characteristic sleep [Cornford et al., 1979; Feldstein, 1973; Stibbs and Seed, 1973a; 1973b]. Because tryptophol also gains access to lymphoid tissues such as spleen, thymus, and mesenteric lymph nodes, it may foster immunosuppression in sleeping sickness [Ackerman and Seed, 1976].

The trypanosome induces formation of antibodies to antigens on its surface called *variable surface glycoproteins*. These glycoproteins can change genetically, making it difficult for the host to kill the organism. Development of a mechanism to modify or terminate this process appears necessary before control or eradication of this disease is feasible [Donelson and Turner, 1985].

Clinical characteristics, clinical laboratory tests, and diagnosis. Mid-African sleeping sickness results from infection by *T. gambiense* and is a less severe but more chronic illness. A furuncle appears at the site of the fly bite. Regional lymphadenitis follows the bite and is the dominant feature for approximately 14 days. Fever, malaise, headache, arthralgia, erythematous and edematous cutaneous eruption, and generalized lymphadenopathy, particularly in the posterior cervical nodes (Winterbot-

Table 40-2 Immunodiagnostic tests for parasitic diseases

Disease	Intradermal	Complement fixation	Bentonite flocculation	Indirect hemagglutination	Latex	Indirect fluorescent antibody	Precipitin
Amebiasis	▲	●	▲	●	●	▲	○
Chagas	○	●	—	●	○	●	○
African Trypano-somiasis	—	▲	—	○	—	▲	●
Leishmaniasis	●	●	—	●	○	▲	●
Malaria	—	▲	—	▲	○	●	○
Pneumocystis	—	▲	—	—	—	▲	—
Toxoplasmosis	●	●	—	●	○	●	—
Ancylostomiosis	▲	○	—	▲	▲	○	—
Ascariasis	▲	○	●	●	—	▲	▲
Filariasis	▲	●	●	●	○	▲	—
Toxocariasis	▲	●	●	●	—	▲	○
Trichinellosis	●	●	●	●	●	●	●
Clonorchiasis	●	●	—	●	—	—	○
Fascioliasis	▲	●	—	●	—	▲	○
Paragonimiasis	●	●	○	○	—	—	—
Schistosomiasis	●	●	▲	●	○	●	○
Cysticercosis	○	●	—	●	○	▲	○
Echinococcosis	●	●	●	●	●	●	▲

From Kagan IG, Norman L. In: Blair JE, Lennette EH, Truant JP, eds. Manual of clinical microbiology. 2nd ed. Washington, DC: American Society for Microbiology, 1974.
●, Evaluated; ▲, experimental test; ○, reported in the literature.

tom sign), compose the next stage, which persists for a week to a month. Although acute rheumatoid arthritis and rheumatic fever are included in the differential diagnosis, they are readily excluded after appearance of manifestations of nervous system impairment, including confusion, somnolence, memory loss, ataxia, and loss of sphincter control.

T. rhodesiense infection causes East African sleeping sickness. The clinical course may be very similar to gambian trypanosomiasis or may appear as a fulminating infection that, if untreated, causes death within 6 to 9 months. Pancarditis with massive pericardial effusion often occurs with resultant death before neurologic symptomatology appears.

Documentation of the parasite in the peripheral blood or CSF provides a definitive diagnosis. Spinal fluid pleocytosis and increased protein concentration are usually present but nonspecific. A sensitive and specific study results from inoculation of the patient's blood into a mouse with subsequent demonstration of the organisms in the mouse's blood. Blood culture of the parasite necessitates special techniques and facilities. Serum immunoglobulin M content is increased greatly, but this finding is not diagnostic. The use of precipitin testing provides diagnostic proof (Table 40-2), although complement fixation studies are reasonably reliable.

Management. Melarsoprol, the recommended drug, is administered intravenously, 3 mg/kg daily for 3 days and then weekly for 3 weeks. Alternative treatment with tryparsamide, 30 mg/kg administered intravenously every 5 days for 2 months, is also effective. The clinician must be aware of the side effects of these drugs before therapy is initiated [Seidel, 1985]. Eflornithine, an ornithine decarboxylase inhibitor, is a highly effective treatment for both early- and late-stage Gambian sleeping sickness. It is given by intravenous infusion for 2 weeks followed by oral treatment for another 3 to 4 weeks [Markell et al., 1992; Milford et al., 1992].

Amebiasis

History and epidemiology. Amebic dysentery was described in ancient times. Its parasitic etiology was described definitively by Kartulis [1886] and Councilman and Lafleur [1891]. Its distribution is global, although it is more prevalent in regions that have hot, humid climates.

Pathogenesis and pathology. Amebiasis results from infection by the protozoan *Entamoeba histolytica*. The gastrointestinal tract and the liver and lungs secondarily are affected. Amebiasis of the nervous system is most unusual and always follows liver or lung involvement. Most patients have symptoms that accompany systemic effects of amebiasis, such as fever, weight loss, and anorexia. Gastrointestinal and respiratory difficulties frequently occur. In one series, only 5 of 17 patients with cerebral amebiasis had neurologic manifestations [Lombardo et al., 1964], which consisted of increased intracranial pressure, hemiplegia, meningeal irritation, nuchal rigidity, confusion, and headache.

Gross postmortem examination of brain reveals abscesses, petechiae, and suppurative meningitis. Necrotic areas are distributed throughout the brain but are concentrated in the basal ganglia and frontal lobes. Cerebral edema and transtentorial herniation are often seen. Microscopic study demonstrates a zone of disruption; necrotic areas are more common than areas of inflammation. The inflammatory response is attended by mononuclear cells [Lombardo et al., 1964].

Diagnosis and management. Detailed discussion of current concepts of diagnosis and treatment are available [Procter, 1987]. Cerebral amebiasis is rarely treated successfully. Emetine and chloroquine are recommended.

Primary amebic meningoencephalitis

Primary amebic meningoencephalitis results from infection by amebas that live freely in water, soil, sewage, or other decaying organic material. The organisms are not obligate parasites. The condition has been described in detail in review articles [Carter, 1972; Duma, 1972]. Animals die from amebic meningoencephalitis [Culbertson et al., 1958], and more than 90% of human patients die. The infecting ameba is most likely *Naegleria fowleri* [Willaert et al., 1973], although other species have been implicated [Duma et al., 1978].

Epidemiology. The disease has been seen in Australia, Belgium, Czechoslovakia, Great Britain, New Zealand, and the United States.

Pathogenesis and pathology. The pathogenic *Naegleria* organisms gain access to the nervous system by first invading the olfactory mucosa, entering the submucosal nervous plexus, and traversing the cribriform plate. Hemorrhagic destruction of gray matter and devastation of the olfactory bulbs follow sanguinopurulent meningitis [Martinez et al., 1973]. Spinal cord involvement is signaled by similar gray matter disruption. Perivascular infiltrates include leukocytes and amebas. Numerous eosinophils may be present. Simultaneous bronchopneumonia and pulmonary edema, myocarditis, and splenitis may occur. Amebas are readily cultured by inoculating culture medium with infected spinal fluid (Figure 40-11).

Clinical characteristics, clinical laboratory tests, and diagnosis. Early manifestations are related temporally to swimming in contaminated water, usually a pool. Acute meningoencephalitis ensues. The patient complains of a violent headache and foul odors before becoming unconscious and usually dies within 6 days [Duma, 1984].

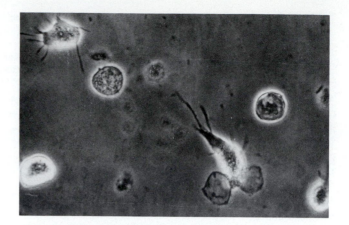

Figure 40-11 Soil amebae in saline. Cysts are 15μm in diameter. Pseudopods emanate from trophozoites. (Phase contrast; × 400.) (Courtesy Dr. T. Schoelten.)

CSF examinations reveal a slightly decreased glucose concentration, increased protein content, and enumerable polymorphonuclear cells and erythrocytes.

Management and prevention. Amphotericin B has been used intravenously with miconazole and rifamycin to treat primary amebic meningoencephalitis successfully. "Early diagnosis, good pediatric intensive care, and vigorous management are of utmost importance" [Seidel, 1985]. Trophic forms of *N. fowleri* are destroyed by free chlorine levels of 0.5 parts per million, and chlorination appears to be effective in prevention of the disease [Carter, 1973].

Granulomatous amebic encephalitis

Granulomatous amebic encephalitis, caused by *Acanthamoeba* species, is a subacute opportunistic infection that spreads from lung or skin lesions via the blood to the brain, resulting initially in focal deficits and gradually causing meningoencephalitis and death. Underlying illnesses include acquired immunodeficiency syndrome, liver disease, renal transplant, diabetes, and cancer, and it is also seen with steroid therapy, chemotherapy, and pregnancy. No treatment exists, and the disease is fatal [Petri and Ravdin, 1990]. Diagnosis is made postmortem.

Malaria

Unlike other parasitic genera, the genus *Plasmodium* frequently infects humans. *P. falciparum* is the only member of the genus that affects the nervous system of the host.

History. Malaria was known in ancient times. In his description of malaria, Hippocrates used the terms *quotidian* (daily), *tertian* (every 2 days), and *quartan* (every 3 days) while discussing the periodic aspects of the febrile episodes. *P. falciparum* is the cause of malignant tertain malaria. The therapeutic attributes of cinchona were generally acknowledged by 1640. In 1893, Bignami and Bastionella demonstrated that *Anopheles* mosquitoes were the vectors of human infection [Winslow et al., 1971].

Because of insecticide-resistant species of mosquitoes, drug-resistant strains of plasmodia, ecologic and practical constraints on drainage of swamps, and the limits on widespread use of insecticides, malaria will probably persist. It remains a major worldwide disease, particularly in many underdeveloped tropical and subtropical regions. Malaria acquired by recipients of blood transfusions from infected but asymptomatic carriers is a major problem in many parts of the world.

Pathogenesis and pathology. The definitive host and vector, the female *Anopheles* mosquito, is the site of sexual reproduction of plasmodia. The mosquito injects the organism as it bites humans, who are the intermediate host; while in humans the organism undergoes asexual reproduction. The hepatic cells are the first location of asexual reproduction in the preerythrocytic phase. Reproduction in hepatic cells is followed by release of parasites that invade erythrocytes during the prepatent period, which lasts 5 or 6 days. The erythrocytic phase commences subsequent to the entry of the parasite into the erythrocyte and continues for 1 to 3 weeks, the incubation period. This last stage is concluded by hemolysis and is signaled by characteristic chills and fever. While in this stage, when the human host is bitten, the parasite enters the mosquito and the entire cycle begins again.

Cerebral involvement follows obstruction of blood vessels with hemolyzed cells. Local hypoxia, microinfarction, necrosis, hemorrhage, and inflammation subsequently occur. Thrombi may form and be associated with clotting aberrations, including disseminated intravascular coagulation [Butler et al., 1973]. Postmortem studies of gross specimens demonstrate fulminating cerebral edema and accompanying transtentorial herniation (Figure 40-12). Congestion of arachnoid vessels causes the brain to appear pink or bright cherry red. Petechiae are evident on the cut surface. Microscopic examination reveals that small arterioles and capillaries are obstructed with parasitized erythrocytes. Mononuclear cells are readily discernible in meningeal and perivascular infiltrates. Microinfarction and ensuing multifocal necrosis and demyelination are widespread. Cerebral malaria is probably the consequence of disseminated vasculomyelinopathy, which results from a hyperergic reaction of the CNS to the antigenic properties of *P. falciparum* [Toro and Roman, 1978].

Clinical characteristics, clinical laboratory tests, and diagnosis. Cerebral malaria is most often heralded by manifestations of mental deterioration, particularly

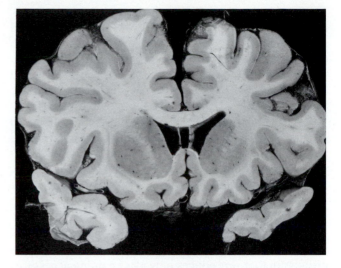

Figure 40-12 Cerebral malaria. Petechial hemorrhages are scattered throughout the brain.

delirium; further deterioration is signaled by progression to stupor and coma that transpires during the next 1 to 3 days. Other features include seizures, which may be confused with febrile seizures in very young children [Osuntokun, 1977]; spasticity accompanied by extensor plantar responses; cerebellar impairment; abnormal movements; and psychosis [Daroff et al., 1967].

Diagnosis necessitates study of peripheral blood films to ascertain the presence of small, ring-form trophozoites and gametocytes; close scrutiny is required to ensure accuracy. Sensitive indirect fluorescent antibody and hemagglutination tests provide further diagnostic capability [Kagan and Norman, 1970].

Management. The chemoprophylaxis and therapy of malaria are major areas of complexity. Excellent review articles are available and should be consulted when appropriate [Bloland and Campbell, 1992; Miller and Campbell, 1986; Peters, 1977; Rozman, 1973].

Chloroquine, primaquine, and quinine remain the mainstays of both prophylaxis and therapy [Medical Letter, 1978]. The clinician should be aware of side effects and obvious toxic reactions before administration. Trial administration to determine individual reactions to the drugs is recommended before long-term, large-dose therapy is instituted [Cann and Verhulst, 1961; Randall and Seidel, 1985]. Intravenous quinidine has been used for the treatment of severe falciparum malaria [Phillips et al., 1985].

A vaccine for the prevention of malaria is under development [Goodson, 1985; Hoffman et al., 1986]. Iron chelation therapy with deferoxamine has been shown to hasten the clearance of parasitemia and enhance the recovery from deep coma in Zambian children with cerebral malaria [Goerduk et al., 1992].

The Chinese medicinal herb qinghao (*Artemisia annual*), also known as annual or sweet wormwood, has been used since antiquity to treat malaria. Recent efforts to understand its chemistry and pharmacology have been very fruitful. The plant yields a sesquiterpene compound called *qinghaosu* or *artemisinin*, which is active in vitro against *N. fowleri*, *Schistosoma* species, and malaria.

Artemisinin and its derivatives have been shown to cure malaria with much less toxicity than quinoline antimalarials. This promising new approach to treatment is discussed in a recent review [Hien and White, 1993].

Toxoplasmosis

History and epidemiology. *T. gondii*, the causal organism of toxoplasmosis [Wolf et al., 1939], is a protozoan that reproduces only after gaining access to a host cell. The organism is found worldwide, and toxoplasmosis is a major public health problem in both developed and underdeveloped countries. The domesticated cat, the major reservoir, excretes oocysts in the feces. Ingestion of the oocyst by animals and humans continues the cycle [Frenkel, 1985]. After being ingested, trophozoite forms are released from the oocyst. The trophozoites circulate and proliferate in the reticuloendothelial system of the host, are transported to muscle and brain, and subsequently form cysts that contain thousands of merozoites [McCabe and Remington, 1984].

Pathogenesis and pathology. Congenital toxoplasmosis infects the fetus after the mother acquires toxoplasmosis during pregnancy. Infection may be asymptomatic in the mother; however, the fetus develops a generalized infection involving spleen, liver, eyes, and CNS [Desmonts and Couvreur, 1974].

When disseminated, acquired toxoplasmosis produces systemic manifestations consisting of multiple organ infection, including the brain. Calcium is deposited in necrotic cerebral lesions; cerebral calcification is often seen in CT scans and plain radiographs of neonates (Figure 40-13).

Postmortem examination of the congenital form reveals pseudocysts or the organism itself. Severe fibrosis of the yellowed meninges develop with resultant thickening. The cortex contains many regions of encephalomalacia. Hydrocephalus occurs often. Microscopic study demonstrates that the numerous lesions comprise large or small granulomas accompanied by glial proliferation and inflammatory infiltrate; areas of nonspecific necrosis are usually present. Giemsa staining delineates the parasite. The acquired form of toxoplasmosis causes meningoencephalitis and pathologic changes similar to those associated with the congenital form (i.e., necrosis, cyst formation) [Townsend et al., 1975].

Clinical characteristics. The approximate incidence

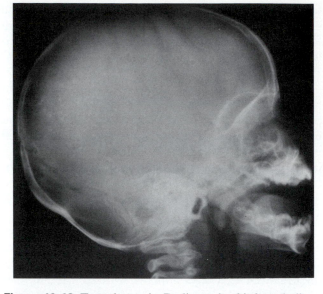

Figure 40-13 Toxoplasmosis. Radiograph of infant skull demonstrates fine intracranial calcifications.

of abnormalities in 180 cases was as follows: microcephaly (20%), hydrocephalus (25%), microphthalmia (35%), seizures (40%), psychomotor retardation (45%), cerebral calcification (60%), and chorioretinitis (95%) [Feldman, 1969]. Approximately 80% to 90% of survivors of congenital toxoplasmosis have mental retardation, cerebral palsy, epilepsy, or visual impairment [Stern et al., 1969]. Subclinical congenital toxoplasmosis may be associated with minimal intellectual impairment.

Although the manifestations of some cases have been identical to those of congenital cytomegalic inclusion disease, CNS involvement is usually more common and extensive in toxoplasmosis.

Hydrocephalus with a tense or bulging fontanel, vomiting, a high-pitched cry, and opisthotonic posturing may dominate the neonatal period (Figure 40-14). Skull radiographs document punctate, scattered calcifications and separated cranial sutures. Hydranencephaly rather than hydrocephaly has been reported [Altshuler, 1973], as has infantile diabetes insipidus [Silver and Dixon, 1954]. Delayed onset with hydrocephalus, seizures, chorioretinitis, and mental retardation has occurred [Miller et al., 1971].

There have been reports of disseminated generalized toxoplasmosis after immunosuppressive therapy [Cohen, 1970; Ghatak et al., 1970]. Meningoencephalitis, often fatal, is a major complication. Although unusual, infections of previously affected normal subjects have been described [Teutsch et al., 1979]. A case of optic neuritis caused by acquired toxoplasmosis was reported in a 13-year-old child [Roach et al., 1985]. Although cerebral toxoplasmosis is an important complication of acquired

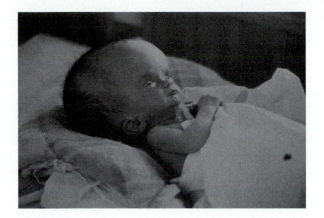

Figure 40-14 Hydrocephalus in congenital toxoplasmosis.

immunodeficiency syndrome in adults, it does not seem to be common in children [Belman, 1987].

Clinical laboratory tests. Immunologic diagnosis of toxoplasmosis relies on the Sabin-Feldman dye test (which detects live parasites), the direct hemagglutination test, the complement-fixation test, the evaluation of immunoglobulin M levels, and the indirect fluorescent antibody test. The antibody test may be the most dependable, but the hemagglutination test is used most often (see Table 40-2).

Management. The value of therapy for congenital toxoplasmosis is controversial. Early treatment with sulfadiazine, pyrimethamine, and folinic acid may have some beneficial effect [Saxon et al., 1973]. In the acquired form of the disease, treatment is required. Again, sulfadiazine, pyrimethamine, and folinic acid (to counteract the folate-inhibiting effects of pyrimethamine) are most effective [Jones, 1979; Remington, 1978].

Babesiosis (piroplasmosis)

Babesiosis, a disease occurring in many species of wild and domestic animals, occasionally infects humans. The genus *Babesia* consists of parasites that are contained within erythrocytes and are transmitted by ixodid (hard-bodied) ticks. Most cases of human infections have involved adults. Clinical manifestations consist of a persistent fever, sweating, chills, myalgia, and mildly to moderately severe hemolytic anemia. Emotional depression has been reported [Ruebush et al., 1977a].

Serologic confirmation of infection has been determined in asymptomatic children [Ruebush et al., 1977b]. Chloroquine therapy has been ineffective [Miller et al., 1978], but pentamidine (2 to 4 mg/kg/day intramuscularly for 15 days) may be of benefit for patients with a severe form of the disease [Medical Letter, 1978]. Quinine and clindamycin in combination and exchange transfusion were reported to be efficacious in a recent study [Doan-Wiggins, 1991].

Schistosomiasis (bilharziasis)

History. *Schistosoma haematobium* infection was reported by Bilharz [1852], and *S. mansoni* by Gonzalez-Martinez [1904], and *S. japonicum* was described as early as 1847 [Katsurada, 1904]. The history of schistosomiasis has been reviewed in detail [Mahmoud, 1984].

Epidemiology. Schistosomiasis is a significant global public health problem. More than 100 million people are infected [Wright, 1968]. *S. mansoni* is endemic in Africa, South America, and the Caribbean Islands. Highly concentrated areas of infestation are present in the Nile delta and northeastern Brazil. *S. haematobium*, the organism that causes classic urinary tract bilharziasis, is found in Asia from Bombay to the Suez Canal and in Africa. *S. japonicum* causes illness in the Orient, including China, Japan, Indochina, the Philippines, and Indonesia.

Flukes have complicated and nearly identical life cycles. The eggs gain access to water from feces or urine, where the miracidia are released and then invade the host, a mollusk (snail). Cercariae then emerge from the snail, penetrate the skin of humans, and are transported by the blood to the distal afferent veins of the liver, where further growth ensues followed by migration of the fluke.

Pathogenesis and pathology. *S. haematobium* is brought by the circulation to the bladder venous plexus and lower abdominal vessels. Urinary tract symptoms and complications follow. The liver and lower gastrointestinal tract are sometimes affected. This pattern of involvement differs from that of *S. mansoni* and *S. japonicum*, in which the organism preferentially enters the mesenteric portal and caval circulation before infecting the liver, intestines, and other organs (e.g., spleen, lungs, heart, CNS).

S. japonicum infects the CNS in 2% to 4% of Asian patients [Kane and Most, 1948; Reyes and Yogore, 1964]. The pathogenesis of neurologic impairment is undetermined despite experimental efforts to reproduce the condition in primates [Greenfield and Pritchard, 1937; Jane et al., 1970].

Two types of lesions exist: One consists of isolated granulomatous masses that contain ova and can be surgically excised. The other type consists of diffuse small lesions that are located in both white and gray matter and are often asymptomatic. In one series of 97 patients with neurologic impairment from schistosomiasis, 60 patients were infected with *S. japonicum*, 11 with *S. haematobium*, and 26 with *S. mansoni* [Marcial-Rojas and Fiol, 1963]. Spinal cord disturbance occurred most often with *S. japonicum* and *S. haematobium* infection [Norfray et al., 1978].

Clinical characteristics, clinical laboratory tests, and diagnosis. Neurologic features include focal deficits, convulsions, vertigo, and transverse myelitis. Growth retardation in children, associated with depressed function of the pars anterior of the pituitary gland, has occurred [Jordan and Webbe, 1969].

Diagnosis of schistosomiasis may be established with several tests, including an intradermal skin test, a complement fixation test, a cholesterol-lecithin cercarial slide flocculation test, and a bentonite flocculation test. The cholesterol-lecithin test reflects a sensitivity of 77% to 90% in parasitologically confirmed cases. Identification of the parasite in urine, feces, and tissue is diagnostic [Kagan, 1979; Kagan and Norman, 1970] (see Table 40-2).

Management. Praziquantel is the drug of choice for the treatment of *S. haematobium*, *S. mansoni* and *S. intercalatum* infections [Markell et al., 1992]. Niridazole, stibophen, and antimony potassium tartrate are also of value [Medical Letter, 1978; Most, 1972].

Intravenous injection of tartar emetic is the recommended therapy for *S. japonicum*. Surgical intervention may prove necessary for mass lesions in the brain or spinal cord. Filtration of worms from portal venous blood is a therapeutic possibility [Kessler et al., 1970].

Paragonimiasis

History and epidemiology. Paragonimiasis, a neurologic and neurosurgical condition, has a high incidence in the Far East and occurs less frequently in some regions of Africa and South America. Otani first reported cerebral paragonimiasis in 1887.

The condition is a serious complication of the benign infection caused by the lung fluke, *Paragonimus westermani*. The ingestion of the cercarial parasite while residing in its crab or crayfish host is the usual mode of human infection. The crustaceans are infected after ingestion of miracidium-laden snails that have previously been infected by cercariae.

Pathogenesis and pathology. After human ingestion of infected raw or poorly cooked crab or crayfish, the cercariae become encysted in the small intestine and eventually pierce the intestinal wall as larvae. The larvae invade the abdominal cavity, abdominal muscle, diaphragm, pleural cavity, and lungs. The mechanism of entrance of the immature fluke into the brain or spinal cord is not precisely known. The most widely held theory of the mechanism of brain involvement is that larvae traverse the soft tissues of the neck surrounding the jugular vein and nerve trunks and then enter the brain through the jugular foramen, causing arachnoiditis, abscesses, or granulomas [Yokogawa, 1921]. Direct invasion of larvae from the lung is assumed to cause extradural spinal involvement, and extension of infection from the brain through the subarachnoid space is believed to be the mechanism of intradural spinal infection [Oh, 1968c].

Gross observation of the brain demonstrates meningeal adhesions and areas of exudate. Cortical atrophy is sometimes present. Nodules and cysts may be found in the subcortical region. Abscesses with suppurative material in their centers appear throughout the brain. Ova are sometimes present in the abscesses and meningeal infiltrate. All types of leukocytes are seen in the areas of inflammation when examined microscopically. Granulomas with giant Langhans cells and epithelioid cells are frequently found in chronic granulomas. Gliosis and fibrosis, appropriate to anatomic location, are widespread. Spinal paragonimiasis, epidural or intradural, is usually represented by ovum-filled cysts. Spinal cord atrophy may be prominent. The microscopic pathologic abnormalities are indistinguishable from those present in the brain.

Clinical characteristics. Lung disease, including pleurisy, pneumothorax, and hemoptysis, constitutes the cardinal clinical feature of paragonimiasis. Cerebral infection occurs in approximately 0.8% of patients; spinal cord involvement is even less common. Fewer than 50% of the patients with neurologic disease are less than 20 years of age. Prominent cerebral characteristics include meningitis, subacute progressive encephalopathy, cerebral infarction, seizures, mass lesions, and dementia. Approximately two thirds of 62 patients were reported to have seizures [Oh, 1967; 1968b]. The emergence of clinical manifestations is gradual. Meningitis is the initial condition in two thirds of patients. Headache, nausea and vomiting, visual impairment, hemiplegia, and mental deterioration often occur early in the course of the illness. Neurologic evaluation frequently documents dementia, homonymous hemianopia, optic atrophy, diminished visual acuity, hemiparesis, hemihypesthesia, and meningismus [Oh, 1968a; 1968b]. When the condition is diagnosed and treated in a timely manner, the prognosis is excellent.

The most common location of spinal involvement is in the lower thoracic area. An extradural mass may cause spastic paraplegia. More rarely an intradural lesion occurs.

Clinical laboratory tests. In one report, chest radiographs were abnormal in 80% of patients; they revealed pneumonia, pleural abnormalities, and cystonodular lesions. Approximately 70% of patients had abnormal cranial radiographs that indicated increased intracranial pressure (25%) and calcifications (50%) [Oh, 1968a; 1968b]. Porencephaly and cortical and subcortical atrophy were demonstrated by pneumoencephalography in several patients. Myelography proved necessary for the diagnosis of spinal cord lesions [Oh, 1967; 1968c]. Newer imaging techniques may prove superior for screening purposes.

Other studies include intradermal skin injection, sputum and stool examination for ova, and immunologic determinations. The complement fixation test is valuable and sensitive. Peripheral blood eosinophilia is often present. Pleocytosis (approximately equal numbers of polymorphonuclear cells and mononuclear cells), decreased glucose concentration, and increased protein and chloride content are frequent spinal fluid findings.

Management. Bithionol therapy (30 to 50 mg/kg on alternate days for 10 to 15 days) is recommended for meningitic involvement [Medical Letter, 1978]. Chronic cerebral lesions or spinal cord lesions require surgical intervention accompanied by adjunctive chemotherapy [Higashi et al., 1971; Oh, 1968b; 1968c].

Diphyllobothriasis

Diphyllobothrium latum, the fish tapeworm, is found throughout the world and causes a public health problem in many regions of the temperate and subarctic zones in the northern hemisphere. Neurologic illness in humans is the result of vitamin B_{12} deficiency caused by the tapeworm; optic atrophy and subacute combined degeneration of the spinal cord result [Bjorkenheim, 1966; Nyberg, 1963].

Fish tapeworm infestation can be prevented by thorough cooking of all freshwater fish. Freezing at $-10°$ C for 48 hours is also recommended to kill the organism before ingestion. Diphyllobothriasis can be treated with niclosamide or praziquantel.

Cysticercosis

History and epidemiology. As reviewed by Nieto [1956], the history of cysticercosis of the nervous system can be traced to the sixteenth century in the writings of Paranoli [1550] and Rumler [1558]. Meningeal racemose cysticercosis was described more than 100 years ago [Virchow, 1860; Zenker, 1882]. Excruciating headache, vertiginous episodes, coma, and death ascribed to sudden movements of the head in the presence of cysts of the fourth ventricle were reported to be pathognomonic (Bruns sign) [Bruns, 1906].

Cysticercosis occurs worldwide. Humans are infected when they become the intermediate host after ingestion of *Taenia solium*, the pork tapeworm. The disease is a major problem in Mexico [Lopez-Hernandez and Garaizar, 1982], Latin America, Eastern Europe, Asia, Africa, Spain, and Portugal.

Pathogenesis and pathology. While in the stomach, ingested *T. solium* in ova hatch after the ova are partially digested by gastric juice. The oncospheres are transported to the intestine and, by means of their specially adapted hooklets, pierce the intestinal wall and gain access to circulation. They undergo metamorphosis and enter the larval stage (cysticerci) in subcutaneous tissue, muscle, and brain. The cysticerci have a predilection for the brain [Brown and Voge, 1985].

Four forms of CNS disease occur, including meningeal, ventricular, parenchymatous, and mixed. Flattened opalescent, thin-walled cysts in which the scolex may be present are found in the ventricles, cisterns, and subarachnoid space. In the fourth ventricle the translucent, fluid-filled cysts may be small and resemble vesicles and may appear in grapelike clusters.

The pia-arachnoid may be engorged, edematous, and thickened, and a purulent exudate may form when vesicles burst and their contents initiate an intense inflammatory response. Obstructive or communicating hydrocephalus may follow adhesive arachnoiditis. Vesicles contained within the brain parenchyma may be either solitary or multiple and are approximately 1 cm in diameter (Figure 40-15). Spinal cord infection occasionally occurs [Firemark, 1978].

Clinical characteristics. Infection and neurologic manifestations of cysticercosis may be separated by an incubation period as long as 5 years. Recent reports stress that the infection is most often benign [Mitchell and Snodgrass, 1985], although the disease can be serious and fatal [Lopez-Hernandez and Garaizar, 1982]. Seizures are the most characteristic feature of the clinical illness [Arseni and Cristescu, 1972; Powell et al., 1966b]. Cysticercosis is a major cause of epilepsy in Peru [Garcia et al., 1993]. Electroencephalographic evidence of periodic lateralized epileptiform discharges may accompany disseminated cerebral cysticercosis [Virmani et al., 1977]. Along with the triad of complaints (occipital headache, morning vomiting, postural vertigo) reported by Bruns [1906], suboccipital headache, vomiting, and progressive obtundation with eventual loss of consciousness are frequent clinical features [Kuper et al., 1958]. Cauda equina infection is heralded by sciatica. Reports of extensive series of many patients document the relatively high incidence of papilledema, hemiparesis,

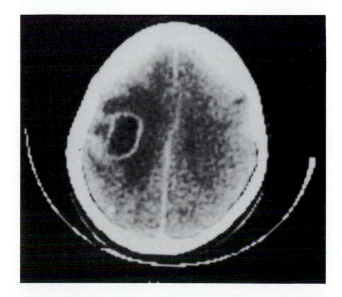

Figure 40-15 Cerebral cysticercosis shown on CT scan.

and sensory disturbances [Lombardo and Mateos, 1961; Sotelo and Guerrero, 1985].

Clinical laboratory tests. Pleocytosis, eosinophilia, decreased glucose content, increased protein concentration, and occasional positive complement fixation test are demonstrated with spinal fluid studies [Nieto, 1956]. Hemagglutination testing was positive in 85% of African patients infected with cysticercosis [Powell et al., 1966a; Proctor et al., 1966]. Enzyme-linked immunosorbent assay testing appears to be of value in the diagnosis of neurocysticercosis [Estrade and Kuhn, 1985; Rosas et al., 1986]. Skull radiographs and CT may document calcified cysticerci [Mitchell and Snodgrass, 1985; Nash and Neva, 1984]. Separation of the cranial sutures and other indications of increased intracranial pressure secondary to hydrocephalus may be evident [Dorfsman, 1963]. MRI provides exquisite definition of the lesions [Rhee et al., 1987].

Management. A report of a series of 26 consecutive patients stressed the likelihood that parenchymal cerebral cysticercosis is typically benign and that spontaneous resolution of lesions is the most common outcome [Mitchell and Snodgrass, 1985]. Spontaneous shrinkage of lesions is documented by CT. Antiepileptic drugs are often required. The indications for praziquantel administration are controversial. Some authors suggest that praziquantel may not be indicated in most cases [Mitchell and Snodgrass, 1985], and others believe that the drug is not effective [Keystone, 1986]; however, praziquantel and dexamethasone appeared to benefit a 13-month-old patient [Norman and Kapadia, 1986]. Ironically, phenytoin and carbamazepine significantly decrease concentrations of praziquantel, which may be responsible for praziquantel treatment failure [Bittencourt et al., 1992]. Steroids and anticysticercus drugs (praziquantel) may have particular value in the treatment of arachnoiditis. Other advocated therapies include ventriculoatrial shunt for hydrocephalus, chemotherapy and surgery for cyst clumps, and surgical removal of intraventricular and spinal cysts [Sotelo and Guerrero, 1985].

Coenurosis

Cerebral coenurosis is exceedingly rare in humans. The condition results from infection with the larvae cyst of the canine tapeworm *Taenia (Multiceps) multiceps* and is virtually identical in pathogenesis, pathologic alterations, and clinical features to cysticercosis except that ophthalmic involvement is usually pronounced. Death has been reported in early childhood [Hermos et al., 1970].

Echinococcosis (hydatid disease)

History and epidemiology. Naunyn [1863] outlined the life cycle of the echinococcus, which is very similar to that of *T. solium*. The detailed history of echinococcosis has been chronicled [Rayport et al., 1964]. Particular attention has focused on osseous and vertebral involvement; the vertebral form is extremely rare [Rayport et al., 1964].

Hydatid disease is distributed globally and is a major health problem. *Echinococcus granulosus*, which incites formation of the characteristic unilocular cyst, is much more widely distributed than *E. multilocularis*, which causes formation of an alveolar, or multiloculated, cyst. *E. multilocularis* is found in Alaska, Bavaria, Canada, Central Europe, Italy, Russia, and Switzerland. Canines are the definitive hosts. Although humans are accidental intermediate hosts, most other mammals can serve as intermediate hosts. A ready domestic cycle exists and includes domestic dogs and farm animals raised for food. A sylvatic cycle includes wolves, reindeer, and moose. The cycles are sometimes intermingled.

Pathology. Cerebral echinococcosis, an unusual feature of the infection, is evident in only about 3% of patients [Marcial-Rojas, 1971]. The cyst, usually solitary, is typically located in white matter; as the cyst enlarges, it is extended toward the meninges or ventricles. A mild inflammatory and gliotic response occurs in the tissue adjacent to the cyst.

Clinical characteristics and clinical laboratory tests. The mass effect engendered by the cyst causes focal neurologic impairment and increased intracranial pressure. Vertebral echinococcosis may compromise the cord with resultant paraplegia [Rayport et al., 1964]. Skull radiographs and CT scans may demonstrate calcification [Ozgen et al., 1979]. Numerous immunologic determinations for echinococcosis are available (see Table 40-2).

Management. Mebendazole, a nontoxic, broadspectrum antihelminthic drug, is exceedingly active against *E. granulosus* and *E. multilocularis* cysts [Medical Letter, 1978; Pearl et al., 1978]. Albendazole, a related compound, is better absorbed and penetrates into hydatid cysts [Markell et al., 1992]. Surgical intervention may prove necessary [Arana-Iniguez and Lopez-Fernandez, 1966].

Trichinosis

After ingestion of uncooked pork or bear meat by humans, *Trichinella spiralis* causes myositis, gastroenteritis, edema, and eosinophilia [Eaton, 1979; Schmitt et al., 1978; Wand and Lyman, 1972]. CNS infection occurs in 7% to 10% of cases.

Clinical characteristics and clinical laboratory tests. Meningoencephalitis dominates the neuropathologic abnormalities seen in trichinosis. Acute meningoencephalitis is manifested with an encephalopathic clinical pattern; confusion and memory loss are coupled with hyperreflexia of the deep tendon reflexes. Focal neurologic deficits, cranial nerve deficits, and cerebellar ataxia sometimes occur.

Spinal fluid studies may indicate pleocytosis or even the presence of larvae. EEG studies reflect changes expected with a diffuse encephalopathy.

Management and prognosis. Unfortunately, no effective treatment is available for trichinosis. Supportive measures include the administration of steroids and thiabendazole [Medical Letter, 1978]. Mortality ranges from 8% to 46%. Detailed reviews are available [Gould, 1970; Kramer and Aita, 1972; Most, 1978].

Angiostrongyliasis (eosinophilic meningitis)

A summary of information concerning eosinophilic meningitis and its probable association with the nematode *Angiostrongylus cantonensis* was collated by Alicata and Jindrak [1970].

History and epidemiology. First described by Bailey [1948], angiostrongyliasis occurs in Southeast Asia and islands of the South Pacific. Rats are the natural host, mollusks the intermediate hosts, and fish and shrimp are involved as transport hosts [Rosen et al., 1967]. Humans become infected after eating raw planarians, snails, or shrimp.

Clinical characteristics and clinical laboratory tests. There is a characteristically explosive onset of symptoms and signs consistent with bacterial meningitis. Additional clinical features include paresthesias of the limbs, trunk, face, and scalp. Facial paralysis is evident in approximately 5% of patients. The disease runs its course over a few days to a few months.

The most significant diagnostic finding is documentation of CSF eosinophilia. The spinal fluid eosinophile population accounts for 25% of the total number of leukocytes in most cases.

Management. No specific therapy is required, with only supportive measures used as needed. Fortunately, no deaths have resulted from eosinophilic meningitis.

Visceral larva migrans (toxocariasis)

History and epidemiology. Visceral larva migrans (toxocariasis) results from *Toxocara infection* [Beaver et al., 1952; Elliott et al., 1985]. The disease is widely distributed throughout the world. Toxocariasis was first described in a patient with eosinophilia, cyanosis, and dyspnea [Aubertin and Giroux, 1921]. A child with similar difficulties, but also with granulomatous lesions of the liver, was subsequently reported [Perlingiero and Gyorgy, 1947]. A detailed review article is available [Elliott et al., 1985].

Pathogenesis and pathology. The nematode of the genus *Toxocara* is an ascarid worm found primarily in cats and dogs but sometimes in nondomestic animals [Fox et al., 1985]. After ingestion, often by children, the eggs hatch into larvae in the upper gastrointestinal tract,

pierce the mucosa, and enter the circulation; eventually the larvae are deposited in the lungs and liver. An 18-month-old boy with Down syndrome died after suffering eosinophilic meningoencephalitis and visceral larva migrans following the ingestion of soil contaminated by the raccoon ascarid [Fox et al., 1985].

Few patients with neurologic involvement have died, and neuropathologic studies are rare. A few cases of larval granulomas of the cerebellum have been reported [Mok, 1968].

Clinical characteristics. Visceral larva migrans, usually a disease of childhood, affects children between the ages of 1½ and 8 years. Typical clinical manifestations usually suggest allergic respiratory involvement and include wheezing episodes and upper respiratory inflammation and irritation. Gastrointestinal and hepatic symptoms occasionally occur. Eosinophilia, which is always present, is often accompanied by hyperglobulinemia. For poorly understood reasons, epileptic children have a greater incidence of infection than expected [Glickman et al., 1979]. Involvement of the CNS is unusual [Mikhael et al., 1974; Zinkham, 1978].

Meningoencephalitis associated with seizures constitutes the most prevalent neurologic manifestation. In

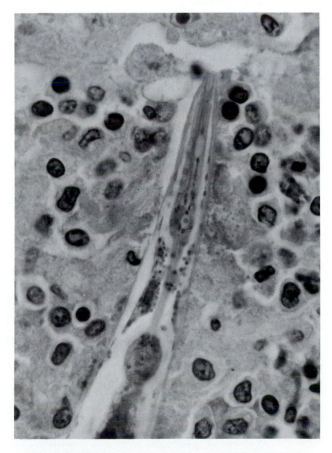

Figure 40-16 *Micronema deletrix* meningoencephalitis.

one series, 14 of 51 preschool children experienced seizures [Huntley et al., 1965]. Fatal infection is rare [Zuelzer and Apt, 1949].

Clinical laboratory tests and diagnosis. Liver biopsy may be necessary for definitive diagnosis of visceral larva migrans. The presence of toxocaral lesions in the optic fundus may also indicate the correct diagnosis. Several immunologic determinations are available (see Table 40-2).

Management. Corticosteroids, thiabendazole, and diethylcarbamazine provide symptomatic benefit [Medical Letter, 1978; Vargo, 1978]. Almost all patients recover completely without therapy. Eradication of the *Toxocara* eggs from the sand of sandboxes by sterilization is the most effective means of prevention [van Knapen et al., 1979].

Miscellaneous parasitic infections

In one report a 5-year-old boy died 24 days after a farm accident during which his multiple lacerations were exposed to manure. Death followed a fulminating meningoencephalomyelitis caused by an ordinary saprophagous nematode, *Micronema deletrix* (Figure 40-16) [Hoogstraten and Young, 1975].

ACKNOWLEDGEMENT

The assistance of Julie Domenico, B.Sc., Librarian, St. Mary's General Hospital, Timmins, is gratefully acknowledged.

REFERENCES

Abud-Ortega AF, Harris L, Rozdilsky B. Chronic coccidioidal meningitis. Can Med Assoc J 1971; 105:613.

Ackerman SB, Seed JR. The effects of tryptophol on immune responses and its implications towards trypanosome induced immunosuppression. Experientia 1976; 15:645.

Adler S, Randall J, Plotkin SA. Candidal osteomyelitis and arthritis in the neonate. Am J Dis Child 1972; 123:595.

Aikawa JC. Rocky Mountain spotted fever. Springfield, Ill: Charles C Thomas, 1966.

Ajello L, Zeidberg LD. Isolation of *Histoplasma capsulatum* and *Allescheria boydii* from soil. Science 1951; 113:662.

Alicata JE, Jindrak K. Angiostrongylosis in the Pacific and Southeast Asia. Springfield, Ill: Charles C Thomas, 1970.

Altschuler G. Toxoplasmosis as the cause of hydranencephaly. Am J Dis Child 1973; 125:251.

Arana-Iniguez R, Lopez-Fernandez JR. Parasitosis of the nervous system, with special reference to echinococcosis. Clin Neurosurg 1966; 14:123.

Araujo JC, Werneck L, Cravo MA. South American blastomycosis presenting as a posterior fossa tumor. J Neurosurg 1978; 49:425.

Arseni C, Cristescu A. Epilepsy due to cerebral cysticercosis. Epilepsia 1972; 13:253.

Aubertin C, Giroux L. Existe-t-il une leucemie à eosinophiles? Presse Med 1921; 29:314.

Averback P, Wigglesworth FW. Miliary fungal granulomata confined to the brain mechanism of meningitis. Child's Brain 1978; 4:33.

Bailey CA. Epidemic of eosinophilic meningitis, previously undescribed disease, occurring on Ponape, Eastern Carolinas. Project NM 005 007, Report No. 7, Annapolis, Md: US Naval Medical Research Institute, 1948.

Battock DJ, Grausz H, Bobrowsky M, et al. Alternate-day amphotericin B therapy in the treatment of rhinocerebral phycomycosis (mucormycosis). Ann Intern Med 1968; 68:122.

Beaver PC, et al. Chronic eosinophilia due to visceral larva migrans: report of three cases. Pediatrics 1952; 9:7.

Bell WE, Myers MG. *Allescheria (Petriellidum) boydii* brain abscess in a child with leukemia. Arch Neurol 1978; 35:386.

Belman A. Pediatric Aids—Neurologic Manifestations Child Neurology Society Symposium. San Diego, 1987.

Bennett JE. Flucytosine. Ann Intern Med 1977; 86:319.

Bennett JE, Dismukes WE, Duma RJ, et al. A comparison of amphotericin B alone combined with flucytosine in the treatment of cryptococcal meningitis. N Engl J Med 1979; 301:126.

Bia FJ, Barry M. Parasitic infections of the central nervous system. Neurol Clin 1986; 4:171.

Bilharz T. Ein Beitrag zur Helminthographia humana, aus brieflichen Mittheilungen des Dr. Bilharz in Cairo. Z Wiss Zool 1852; 4:53.

Bittencourt PRM, Gracia CM, Martins R, et al. Phenytoin and carbamazepine decrease oral bioavailability of praziquantel. Neurology. 1992; 42:492.

Bjorkenheim B. Optic neuropathy caused by vitamin B_{12} deficiency in carriers of the fish tapeworm: *Diphyllobothrium latum*. Lancet 1966; 1:688.

Bloland PB, Campbell CC. Malaria. In: Rakel RE. Conn's current therapy. Philadelphia: WB Saunders, 1992.

Brew BJ. Central and peripheral nervous system abnormalities. Med Clin North Am 1992; 76:83.

Bross JE. Gordon G. Nocardial meningitis: case reports and review. Rev Inf Dis 1991; 13:160.

Brown JR. Human actinomycosis: a study of 181 subjects. Hum Pathol 1973; 4:319.

Brown WJ, Voge M. Neuropathology of parasitic infections. Oxford: Oxford University Press, 1982.

Brown WJ, Voge M. Cysticercosis: a modern day plague. Pediatr Clin North Am 1985; 32:953.

Bruns L. Neuropathie demonstration. Neurologija 1906; 61:25, 540.

Butler T, Tong MJ, Fletcher JR, et al. Blood coagulation studies in *Plasmodium falciparum* malaria. Am J Med Sci 1973; 265:63.

Byrne E, Brophy BP, Perret LV. *Nocardia* cerebral abscess: new concepts in diagnosis, management, and prognosis. J Neurol Neurosurg Psychiatry 1979; 42:1038.

Cann HM, Verhulst HL. Fatal acute chloroquine poisoning in children. Pediatrics 1961; 23:95.

Carter RF. Primary amoebic meningoencephalitis. Trans R Soc Trop Med Hyg 1972; 66:193.

Carter RF. Personal communication. Adelaide, Australia, 1973.

Caudill RG, Smith CE, Reinarz JA. Coccidioidal meningitis, a diagnostic challenge. Am J Med 1970; 49:360.

Chagas C. Tripanosomiase americana. Mem Inst Oswaldo Cruz 1916; 8:37.

Cohen SN. Toxoplasmosis in patients receiving immunosuppressive therapy. JAMA 1970; 211:657.

Coleman R, Kaufman L. Use of immunodiffusion test in serodiagnosis of aspergillosis. Appl Microbiol 1972; 23:301.

Cooper RA Jr, Goldstein EG. Histoplasmosis of the central nervous system. Am J Med 1963; 35:45.

Cornford E, Bocash WD, Braun LD, et al. Rapid distribution of tryptophol (3-indole ethanol) to the brain and other tissues. J Clin Invest 1979; 63:1241.

Couch JR, Abdou NI, Sagawa A. *Histoplasma* meningitis with hyperactive suppressor T cell in cerebrospinal fluid. Neurology 1978; 28:119.

Councilman WT, Lafleur HA. Amebic dysentery. Johns Hopkins Hosp Rep 1891; 2:193.

Culbertson GC, Smith JW, Minner JR. Acanthamoeba observations on animal pathogenicity. Science 1958; 127:1506.

Daar ES, Meyer RD. Bacterial and fungal infections. Med Clin North Am 1992; 76:173.

Danoff D, Munk ZM, Case B, et al. Disseminated coccidiodomycosis: clinical, immunologic, and therapeutic aspects. Can Med Assoc J 1978; 118:390.

Darling ST. A protozoan general infection producing pseudotubercles in the lungs and focal necrosis in the liver, spleen, and lymph nodes. JAMA 1906; 202:679.

Daroff RB, Deller JJ, Kastl AJ, et al. Cerebral malaria. JAMA 1967; 202:679.

DeMonbreum WA. Cultivation and cultural characteristics of Darling's *Histoplasma capsulatum*. Am J Trop Med 1934; 14:93.

Desmonts G, Couvreur J. Congenital toxoplasmosis. N Engl J Med 1974; 290:1110.

Diamond RD, Bennett JE. A subcutaneous reservoir for intrathecal therapy of fungal meningitis. N Engl J Med 1973; 288:186.

Dismukes WE. Blastomycosis: leave it to beaver. N Engl J Med 1986; 314:575.

Doan-Wiggins L. Tick-borne diseases. Emerg Med Clin North Am 1991; 9:303.

Donelson JE, Turner MJ. How the trypanosome changes its coat. Sci Am 1985; 252:44.

Dorfsman J. The radiologic aspects of cerebral cysticercosis. Acta Radiol 1963; 1:836.

Drutz DJ, Spickard A, Rogers DE, et al. Treatment of disseminated mycotic infections. Am J Med 1968; 45:405.

Duma RJ. Primary amoebic meningoencephalitis. CRC Crit Rev Clin Lab Sci 1972; 3:163.

Duma RJ. Rocky Mountain spotted fever. In: Conn HF, ed. Current therapy, 1979: latest approved methods of treatment for the practicing physician. Philadelphia: WB Saunders, 1979.

Duma RJ. Primary amebic meningoencephalitis. In: Warren KS, Mahmoud AAD, eds. Tropical geographical medicine. New York: McGraw-Hill, 1984.

Duma RJ, Helwig WB, Martinez AJ. Meningoencephalitis and brain abscess due to a free-living amoeba. Ann Intern Med 1978; 88:468.

DuPont HL, et al. Rocky Mountain spotted fever: a comparative study of the active immunity induced by inactivated and viable pathogenic *Rickettsia rickettsii*. J Infect Dis 1973; 128:340.

Eaton RDP. Trichinosis in the Arctic. Can Med Assoc J 1979; 120:22.

Edwards JE Jr, Lehrer RI, Stiem ER, et al. Severe candidal infections. Ann Intern Med 1978; 89:91.

Edwards VE, Sutherland JM, Tyrer JH. Cryptococcosis of the central nervous system. J Neurol Neurosurg Psychiatry 1970; 33:415.

Elliott DL, Tolle SW, Goldberg L, et al. Pet-associated illness. N Engl J Med 1985; 313:985.

Enarson DA, Keys TF, Onofrio BM. Central nervous system histoplasmosis with obstructive hydrocephalus. Am J Med 1978; 64:895.

Estrade JJ, Kuhn RE. Immunochemical detection of antigens of larval taenia solium and antilarval antibodies in the cerebrospinal fluid of patients with neurocysticercosis. J Neurol Sci 1985; 71:39.

Everts EC. Cervicofacial actinomycosis. Arch Otolaryngol 1970; 92:468.

Fass RJ, Perkins RL. 5-Fluorocytosine in the treatment of cryptococcae and candida mycoses. Ann Intern Med 1971; 74:535.

Feldman HA. *Toxoplasma* and toxoplasmosis. Hosp Pract 1969; 4:64.

Feldstein A. Ethanol-induced sleep in relation to serotonin turnover and conversion to 5-hydroxyindole-acetaldehyde, 5-hydroxytryptophol and 5-hydroxyindole acetic acid. Ann NY Acad Sci 1973; 215:71.

Fetter BF, Klintworth GK, Hendry WS. Mycoses of the central nervous system. Baltimore: Williams & Wilkins, 1967.

Firemark HM. Spinal cysticercosis. Arch Neurol 1978; 35:250.

Fleischer G, Lennette ET, Honig P. Diagnosis of Rocky Mountain spotted fever by immunofluorescent identification of *Rickettsia rickettsii* in skin biopsy tissue. J Pediatr 1979; 95:63.

Fox AS, Kazacos KR, Gould NS, et al. Fatal eosinophilic meningoencephalitis and visceral larva migrans caused by the raccoon ascarid *Baylisascaris procyonis*. N Engl J Med 1985; 312:1619.

Frenkel JK. Toxoplasmosis. Pediatr Clin North Am 1985; 32:917.

Gallerano RH, Marr JJ, Sosa RR. Therapeutic efficacy of allopurinal in patients with chronic Chagas' disease. Am J Trop Med Hyg 1990; 43-159.

Garcia HH, Gilman R, Martinez M, et al. Cysticercosis as a major cause of epilepsy in Peru. Lancet 1993; 341:197.

Ghatak NR, Poon TP, Zimmerman HM. Toxoplasmosis of the central nervous system in the adult. Arch Pathol 1970; 89:333.

Glickman LT, Cypess RH, Crumrine PK, et al. *Toxocara* infection and epilepsy in children. J Pediatr 1979; 94:75.

Godson GN. Molecular approaches to malaria vaccines. Sci Am 1985; 252:52.

Goerduk V, Thuma P, Brittenham G, et al. Effect of iron chelation therapy on recovery from deep coma in children with cerebral malaria. N Engl J Med 1992; 327:143.

Goldman JA, et al. *Candida albicans* mycotic aneurysm associated with systemic lupus erythematosus. Neurosurgery 1979; 4:325.

Gonyea EF. The spectrum of primary blastomycotic meningitis: a review of central nervous system blastomycosis. Ann Neurol 1978; 3:26.

Gonzalez-Martinez I. Refiriendo a un estudio de Bilharzia hematobium y bilharziosis en Puerto Rico. Rev Med Trop Habana 1904; 5:193.

Gould SE, ed. Trichinosis in man and animals. Springfield, Ill: Charles C Thomas, 1970.

Green WR, Walker DH, Cain BG. Fatal viscerotrophic Rocky Mountain spotted fever. Am J Med 1978; 64:523.

Greenfield JG, Pritchard B. Cerebral infection with *Schistosoma japonicum*. Brain 1937; 60:361.

Harrell GT. Symposium on nervous and mental diseases: rickettsial involvement of the nervous system. Med Clin North Am 1953; 37:395.

Hedges E, Miller S. Coccidioidomycosis: office diagnosis and treatment. Am Family Pract, 1990; 41:1499.

Heldrich FJ. Rocky Mountain spotted fever. In: Hockelman RA, et al., eds. Primary pediatric care. St Louis: Mosby, 1987.

Hermos JA, et al. Fatal human cerebral coenurosis. JAMA 1970; 213:1461.

Hien TT, White NJ. Qinghaosu. Lancet 1993; 341:603.

Higashi K, et al. Cerebral paragonimiasis. J Neurosurg 1971; 34:515.

Hoeprich PD, Brandt D, Parker RH. Nocardial brain abscess cured with cycloserine and sulfonamides. Am J Med Sci 1968; 255:208.

Hoff R, Teixeira RS, Carvalho JS, et al. *Trypanosoma cruzi* in the cerebrospinal fluid during the acute stage of Chagas' disease. N Engl J Med 1978; 298:604.

Hoffman SL, Wistar R Jr, Ballou WR, et al. Immunity to malaria and naturally acquired antibodies to the circumspozoite protein of *Plasmodium falciparum*. N Engl J Med 1986; 315:601.

Hoogstraten J, Young WG. Meningoencephalomyelitis due to the saprophagous nematode, *Micronema deletrix*. Can J Neurol Sci 1975; 2:121.

Huntley C, Costas M, Lyerly A. Visceral larva migrans syndrome. Pediatrics 1965; 36:523.

Ibach MJ, Larsh HW, Furcolow ML. Isolation of *Histoplasma capsulatum* from air. Science 1954; 119:71.

Israel J. Neue Beobachtungen auf dem Gebiete der Mykosen des Menschen. Virchows Arch (A) 1878; 74:15.

Jackson FE, Kent D, Clare F. Quadriplegia caused by involvement of cervical spine with *Coccidioides immitis*. J Neurosurg 1964; 21:512.

Jane JA, Warren KS, van den Noort S. Experimental cerebral schistosomiasis japonica in primates. J Neurol Neurosurg Psychiatry 1970; 33:426.

Jones TC. Toxoplasmosis. In: Conn HF, ed. Current therapy, 1979: latest approved methods of treatment for the practicing physician. Philadelphia: WB Saunders, 1979.

Jordan P, Webbe G. Human schistosomiasis. London: William Heinemann Medical Books, 1969.

Kagan IG. Diagnostic, epidemiologic and experimental parasitology: immunologic aspects. Am J Trop Med Hyg 1979; 28:429.

Kagan IG, Norman L. Serodiagnosis of parasitic diseases: manual of clinical microbiology. Washington, DC: American Society for Microbiology, 1970.

Kane CA, Most H. Schistosomiasis of the central nervous system: experiences in World War II and review of the literature. Arch Neurol Psychiatry 1948; 59:141.

Kartulis S. Zur aetiologie der dysenterie aegypten. Virchows Arch (A) 1886; 105:521.

Katsurada F. Schistosomum japonicum, ein neuer menschicher Parasit, durch welchen eine endemische Krankheit in verscheidenen Gegenden Japans verursacht wird. Annot Zool Jpn 1904; 5:147.

Kelsey DS. Rocky Mountain spotted fever. Pediatr Clin North Am 1979; 26:367.

Kessler RE, Amadeo JH, Tice DA, et al. Filtration of schistosomes in unanaesthetized man. JAMA 1970; 214:519.

Keystone J. Personal communication. 1986.

Kirmani N, Tuazon CU, Ocuin JA, et al. Extensive cerebral nocardiosis cured with antibiotic therapy alone. J Neurosurg 1978; 49:924.

Klein BS, Belfort EA, Mondolfi A, et al. Isolation of *Blastomyces dermatitidis* in soil associated with a large outbreak of blastomycosis in Wisconsin. N Engl J Med 1986; 314:529.

Kramer MD, Aita JF. Trichinosis with central nervous system involvement. Neurology 1972; 22:485.

Krivoy S, et al. Paracoccidioidomycosis of the skull. J Neurosurg 1978; 49:429.

Krober MS. Skeletal muscle involvement in Rocky Mountain spotted fever. South Med J 1978; 71:1575.

Krugman S, et al. Rickettsial infections. In: Krugman S, et al. eds. Infectious diseases in children. 8th ed. St Louis: Mosby, 1985.

Kuper S, Mendelow H, Proctor NSF. Internal hydrocephalus caused by parasitic cysts. Brain 1958; 18:235.

Laranja FS, Dias E, Nobrega C, et al. Chagas' disease, a clinical epidemiologic, and pathologic study. Circulation 1956; 14:1035.

Laupus WE. Rickettsial infections. In: Gellis SS, Kagan BM, eds. Current pediatric therapy. vol 8. Philadelphia: WB Saunders, 1978.

Lillie RD, Smith DE, Black BK. Pathology of epidemic typhus: central nervous system. Arch Pathol 1953; 56:512.

Linares G, McGarry PA, Baker RD. Solid solitary aspergillotid granuloma of the brain. Neurology 1971; 21:177.

Littman ML, Walter JE. Cryptococcosis: current status. Am J Med 1968; 45:922.

Lombardo L, Mateos JH. Cerebral cysticercosis in Mexico. Neurology 1961; 11:824.

Lombardo L, et al. Cerebral amebiasis. J Neurosurg 1964; 21:704.

Loosli CG. Histoplasmosis. J Chronic Dis 1957; 5:473.

Lopez-Hernandez A, Garaizar C. Childhood cerebral cysticercosis: clinical features and computed tomographic findings in 89 Mexican children. Can J Neurol Sci 1982; 9:401.

Lutwick LI, et al. Deep infections from *Petriellidium boydii* treated with miconazole. JAMA 1979; 241:272.

Lutz A. Uma micose pseudococcidica localisada na boca e observada no Brasil: contribuicao ao conhecimento das hyphoblastomycoses americanos. Braz Med 1908; 22:121.

Lyons RW, Andriole VT. Fungal infections of the CNS. Neurol Clin 1986; 4:159.

Mahmoud AA. Schistosomiasis. In: Warren KS, Mahmoud AAF, eds. Tropical and geographical medicine. New York: McGraw-Hill, 1984.

Marcial-Rojas RA, ed. Pathology of protozoal and helminthic diseases, with clinical correlation. Baltimore: Williams & Wilkins, 1971.

Marcial-Rojas RA, Fiol RE. Neurologic complications of schistosomiasis: review of the literature and report of two cases of transverse myelitis due to *S mansoni*. Ann Intern Med 1963; 59:215.

Markell EK, Voge M, John DT. Medical parasitology, Philadelphia: WB Saunders, 1992.

Martinez AJ, Duma RJ, Nelson EC, et al. Experimental naegleria meningoencephalitis in mice: penetration of the olfactory mucosal epithelium by naegleria and pathologic changes produced: a light and electron microscope study. Lab Invest 1973; 29:121.

McCabe RE, Remington JS. Toxoplasmosis. In: Warren KS, Mahmoud AAF, eds. Tropical and geographical medicine. New York: McGraw-Hill, 1984.

McGinnis MR. Detection of fungi in cerebrospinal fluid. Am J Med 1983; 75(IB):129.

Medical Letter: Drugs for parasitic infections. In: Handbook of antimicrobial therapy, vol 20. New Rochelle, NY: Medical Letter, 1978.

Medoff G, Comfort M, Kobayashi GS. Synergistic action of amphotericin B and 5-fluorocytosine against yeast-like organisms. Proc Soc Exp Biol Med 1971; 138:571.

Meunier F. Candidiasis. Eur J Clin Microbiol Inf Dis, 1989;8:438.

Meyers B, Wormser G, Hirschman SZ, et al. Rhinocerebral mucormycosis. Arch Intern Med 1979; 139:557.

Mikhael NZ, Montpetil VJ, Orizaya M, et al. *Toxocara canis* infestation with encephalitis. Can J Neurol Sci 1974; 1:114.

Milford F, Pepin J, Loko L, et al. Efficacy and toxicity of eflornithine for treatment of *Trypanosoma brucei gambiense* sleeping sickness, Lancet 1992; 340:652.

Miller JQ, Price TR. The nervous system in Rocky Mountain spotted fever. Neurology 1972; 22:561.

Miller K, Campbell CC. Malaria. In: Rakel RE, ed. Conn's current therapy. Philadelphia: WB Saunders, 1986.

Miller LH, Neva FH, Gill F. Failure of chloroquine in human babesiosis (*Babesia microti*). Ann Intern Med 1978; 88:200.

Miller LH, Reifsnyder DN, Martinez SA. Late onset of disease in congenital toxoplasmosis. Clin Pediatr 1971; 10:78.

Mitchell WG, Snodgrass SR. Intraparenchymal cerebral cysticercosis in children: a benign prognosis. Pediatr Neurol 1985; 1:151.

Mok CH. Visceral larva migrans. Clin Pediatr 1968; 7:565.

Morgan D, Young RF, Chow AW, et al. Recurrent intracerebral blastomycotic granuloma: diagnosis and treatment. Neurosurgery 1979; 4:319.

Most H. Treatment of common parasitic infections of man encountered in the United States. N Engl J Med 1972; 287:495, 698.

Most H. Current concepts in parasitology: trichinosis—preventable yet still with us. N Engl J Med 1978; 298:1178.

Mott FW. Histologic observations on sleeping sickness and other trypanosome infections. Reports of the Sleeping Sickness Commission of the Society of London Sleeping Sickness Commission. No 7, 1906.

Mukoyama M, Gimple AB, Poser CM. Aspergillosis of the central nervous system. Neurology 1969; 19:967.

Nash TE, Neva FA. Recent advances in the diagnosis and treatment of cerebral cysticercosis. N Engl J Med 1984; 311:1492.

Naunyn BGJ. Ueber die zu *Echinococcus hominis* gehorige Taenie. Arch Anat Physiol Wissensch Med 1863; 412.

Neuhauser EBD, Tucker A. The roentgen changes produced by diffuse torulosis in the newborn. Am J Roentgenol 1948; 59:805.

Nieto D. Cysticercosis of the nervous system. Neurology 1956; 6:725.

Norfray JF, Schlachter L, Heiser WJ, et al. Schistosomiasis of the spinal cord. Surg Neurol 1978; 9:68.

Norman RM, Kapadia C. Cerebral cysticercosis: treatment with praziquantel. Pediatrics 1986; 78:291.

Nyberg W. *Diphyllobothrium latum* and human nutrition with particular reference to vitamin B_{12} deficiency. Proc Nutr Soc 1963; 22:8.

Oh S. Cerebral paragonimiasis. Trans Am Neurol Assoc 1967; 92:275.

Oh S. Ophthalmological signs in cerebral paragonimiasis. Trop Geogr Med 1968a; 20:13.

Oh S. *Paragonimus meningitis*. J Neurol Sci 1968b; 6:419.

Oh S. Spinal paragonimiasis. J Neurol Sci 1968c; 6:125.

Oppenheimer J, Sullivan MP, Drewinko B, et al. Disseminated histoplasmosis complicating acute leukemia of childhood. Clin Pediatr 1973; 12:306.

Oster CN, Burke DS, Kenyon RH, et al. Laboratory-acquired Rocky Mountain spotted fever. N Engl J Med 1977; 297:859.

Osuntokun BO. Epilepsy in the African continent. In: Penry JK, ed. Epilepsy. The eighth international symposium. New York: Raven Press, 1977.

Otani SA. On the anamnesis and the postmortem examination of paragonimiasis patients. Tokyo: Igakkai Zasshi 1887; 1:458.

Ozgen T, Erbeni A, Bertan V, et al. The use of computerized tomography in the diagnosis of cerebral hydatid cysts. J Neurosurg 1979; 50:339.

Pappagianis D. Coccidioidomycosis. In: Top FJ, Wehrle PF, eds. Communicable and infectious diseases. 8th ed. St Louis: Mosby, 1976.

Pearl M, et al. Cerebral echinococcosis, a pediatric disease: report of two cases with one successful five-year followup. Pediatrics 1978; 61:915.

Perlingiero J, Gyorgy P. Chronic eosinophilia: report of a case with necrosis of the liver, pulmonary infiltrations, anemia, and *Ascaris* infestation. Am J Dis Child 1947; 73:34.

Peters W. Current concepts in parasitology: malaria. N Engl J Med 1977; 297:1261.

Petri WA, Ravdin JI. Free-living ambae. In: Mandell GL, Douglas RG, Bennett JE, eds. Principles and practice of infectious diseases. New York: Churchill Livingstone, 1990.

Phillips RE, Warrell DA, White NJ, et al. Intravenous quinidine for the treatment of severe falciparum malaria. N Engl J Med 1985; 312:1273.

Powderly WG, Saag MS, Cloud GA, et al. A controlled trial of fluconazole or amphotericin B to prevent relapse of cryptococcal meningitis in patients with the acquired immunodeficiency syndrome. N Engl J Med 1992; 326:793.

Powell SJ, Proctor EM, Wilmot AJ, et al. Cystocercosis and epilepsy in Africans: a clinical and serological study. Ann Trop Med Parasitol 1966a; 60:152.

Powell SJ, Proctor EM, Wilmot AJ, et al. Neurologic complications of cysticercosis in Africans: a clinical and serological study. Ann Trop Med Parasitol 1966b; 60:159.

Proctor EM, Powell SJ, Elsdon-Dew R. The serological diagnosis of cysticercosis. Ann Trop Med Parasitol 1966; 60:146.

Proctor RD. Parasitic infestations. In: Hockelman RA, ed. Primary pediatric care. St Louis: Mosby, 1987.

Raab EL, Leopold IH, Hodes HL. Retinopathy in Rocky Mountain spotted fever. Am J Ophthalmol 1969; 68:42.

Randall G, Seidel JS. Malaria. Pediatr Clin North Am 1985; 32:893.

Rayport M, Wisoff HS, Zaiman H. Vertebral echinococcosis. J Neurosurg 1964; 21:647.

Remington JS. Toxoplasmosis. In: Gellis SS, Kagan BM, eds. Current pediatric therapy. vol 8. Philadelphia: WB Saunders, 1978.

Reyes VA, Yogore MG. Studies on cerebral schistosomiasis. J Philipp Med Assoc 1964; 40:87.

Rhee RS, Kumasaki DY, et al. MR imaging of intraventricular cysticercosis. J Comput Assist Tomogr 1987; 11:598.

Richardson PM, Mohandas A, Arumugasamy N. Cerebral cryptococcosis in Malaysia. J Neurol Neurosurg Psychiatry 1976; 39:330.

Rivera IV, Curless RG, Indacochea FJ, et al. Chronic progressive CNS histoplasmosis presenting in childhood: response to fluconazole therapy. Pediatr Neurol 1992; 8:151.

Roach ES, et al. Optic neuritis due to acquired toxoplasmosis. Pediatr Neurol 1985; 1:114.

Roe DC, Haynes RE. *Candida albicans* meningitis successfully treated with amphotericin B. Am J Dis Child 1972; 124:926.

Rogers DE. The spectrum of histoplasmosis in man. Respir Physiol 1967; 13:54.

Rosas N, Sotelo J, Nieto D. ELISA in the diagnosis of neurocysticercosis. Arch Neurol 1986; 43:353.

Rose HD, Rytel MW. Actinomycosis treated with clindamycin. JAMA 1972; 221:1062.

Rosen F, Deck JHN, Rewcastle NB. *Allescheria boydii*: unique systemic dissemination to thyroid and brain. Can Med Assoc J 1965; 93:1125.

Rosen L, Loison G, Laigret J, et al. Studies on eosinophilic meningitis. 3. Epidemiologic and clinical observation on Pacific islands and the possible etiologic role of *Angiostrongylus cantonensis*. Am J Epidemiol 1967; 85:17.

Rosenblum M, Rosegay H. Resection of multiple nocardial brain abscesses: diagnostic role of computerized tomography. Neurosurgery 1979; 4:315.

Rozman RS. Chemotherapy of malaria. Annu Rev Pharmacol 1973; 13:127.

Ruebush TK II, Juranek DD, Chisholm ES, et al. Human babesiosis on Nantucket Island. Ann Intern Med 1977a; 86:6.

Ruebush TK II, Juranek DD, Chisholm ES, et al. Human babesiosis on Nantucket Island. N Engl J Med 1977b; 297:825.

Saag MS, Powderly WG, Cloud GA, et al. Comparison of amphotericin B with fluconazole in the treatment of acute AIDS-associated cryptococcal meningitis. N Engl J Med 1992; 326:83.

Sabetta JR, Andriole VT. Cryptococcal infection of the central nervous system. Med Clin North Am 1985; 69:333.

Salake JS, Louria DB, Chmel H. Fungal and yeast infections of the central nervous system. Medicine 1984; 63:108.

Salgo MP, Telzak EE, Currie B, et al. A focus of Rocky Mountain fever within New York City. N Engl J Med 1988; 318:1345.

Sandler R, Tallman CB, Keamy DG, et al. Successfully treated rhinocerebral phycomycosis in well controlled diabetes. N Engl J Med 1971; 285:1180.

Sarosi GA, Voth DW, Dahl BA, et al. Disseminated histoplasmosis: results of long term follow-up. Ann Intern Med 1971; 75:511.

Saxon SA, Knight W, Reynolds DW, et al. Intellectual deficits in children born with subclinical congenital toxoplasmosis: a preliminary report. J Pediatr 1973; 82:792.

Schatz N. Personal communication. 1978.

Schiess RJ, Coscia MF, McClellan GA. *Petriellidium boydii* pachymeningitis treated with miconazole and ketoconazole. Neurosurgery 1984; 14:220.

Schmitt N, et al. Sylvatic trichinosis. Br Columbia Public Health Rep 1978; 93:189.

Seidel JS. Primary amebic meningoencephalitis. Pediatr Clin North Am 1985a; 32:881.

Seidel JS. Treatment of parasitic infections. Pediatr Clin North Am 1985b; 32:1077.

Silver HK, Dixon MS Jr. Congenital toxoplasmosis: report of case with cataract, "atypical" vasopressin-sensitive diabetes insipidus, and marked eosinophilia. Am J Dis Child 1954; 88:84.

Smego RA Jr, et al. *Candida* meningitis in two children with severe combined immunodeficiency. J Pediatr 1984; 104:902.

Smith JW, Utz JP. Progressive disseminated histoplasmosis: a prospective study of 26 patients. Ann Intern Med 1972; 76:557.

Smith TW, Burton TC. The retinal manifestations of Rocky Mountain spotted fever. Am J Ophthalmol 1977; 84:259.

Sotelo J, Guerrero F. Neurocysticercosis: a new classification based on active and inactive forms. Arch Int Med 1985; 145:442.

Stern H, Elek SD, Booth JC, et al. Microbial causes of mental retardation. Lancet 1969; 2:443.

Stevens DA. Miconazole in the treatment of systemic fungal infections. Am Rev Respir Dis 1977; 116:801.

Stibbs HH, Seed JR. Chromatographic evidence of the synthesis of possible sleep-mediators in *Trypanosoma brucei gambiense*. Experientia 1973a; 29:1563.

Stibbs HH, Seed JR. Further studies on the metabolism of tryptophan in *Trypanosoma brucei gambiense*: cofactors, inhibitors, and end products. Experientia 1973b; 31:275.

Stites DP, Glezen WP. Pulmonary nocardiosis in childhood. Am J Dis Child 1967; 114:101.

Tassel D, Madoff MA. Treatment of *Candida* sepsis and *Cryptococcus* meningitis with 5-fluorocytosine: a new antifungal agent. JAMA 1968; 206:830.

Taylor GD, Boettger DW, Miedzinski LJ, et al. Coccidioidal meningitis acquired during holidays in Arizona. Can Med Assoc J 1990; 142:1388.

Teutsch SM, Juranek DD, Sulzer A, et al. Epidemic toxoplasmosis associated with infected cats. N Engl J Med 1979; 300:695.

Toro G, Roman G. Cerebral malaria: a disseminated vasculomyelinopathy. Arch Neurol 1978; 35:271.

Townsend JJ, Wolinsky JS, Baringer JR, et al. Acquired toxoplasmosis: neglected cause of treatable nervous system disease. Arch Neurol 1975; 32:335.

Tressler CB, Sugar AM. Fungal meningitis. Inf Dis Clin North Am, 1990; 4:789.

Tucker RM, Denning DW, Dupont B, et al. Itraconazole therapy for chronic coccidioidal meningitis. Ann Int Med 1992; 112:108.

Turner E, Whitby JL. Nocardial brain abscess: successful treatment with aspiration and sulfonamides. J Neurosurg 1969; 31:227.

Utz JP. Flucytosine. N Engl J Med 1972; 286:777.

Van Knapen F, Franchimont JH, Otten GM. Sterilisation of sandpits infected with *Toxocara* eggs. Br Med J 1979; 1:1320.

Vargo TA. Visceral larva migrans. In: Gellis SS, Kagan BM, eds. Current pediatric therapy. vol 8. Philadelphia: WB Saunders, 1978.

Virchow R. Traubenhydatiden der weischen Hirnhaute. Virchows Arch (A) 1860; 19:528.

Virmani V, Roy S, Kamala G. Periodic lateralised epileptiform discharges in a case of diffuse cerebral cysticercosis. Neuropaediatrie 1977; 8:196.

Wand M, Lyman D. Trichinosis from bear meat. JAMA 1972; 220:245.

Warren KS, Mahmoud AA, eds. Tropical and geographic medicine. New York: McGraw-Hill, 1984.

Wayne LG, Juarez WJ. Isolation of *Coccidioides immitis* from spinal fluid by molecular filter membrane technique. Am J Clin Pathol 1955; 25:1209.

Weber DJ, Walker DH. Rocky Mountain spotted fever. Inf Dis Clin North Am 1991; 5:19.

Wells GM, Woodward TE, Fiset P, et al. Rocky Mountain spotted fever caused by blood transfusion. JAMA 1978; 239:2763.

Wheat LJ, Kohler RB, Tewari RP. Diagnosis of disseminated histoplasmosis by detection of *Histoplasma capsulatum* antigen in serum and urine specimens. N Engl J Med 1986; 314:83.

Wheat LJ, Kohler RB, Tewari RP, et al. Significance of histoplasma antigen in the cerebrospinal fluid of patients with meningitis. Arch Intern Med 1989; 149:302.

Willaert E, Jadin JB, LeRay D. Comparative antigenic analysis of *Naegleria* species. Ann Soc Belg Med Trop 1973; 53:59.

Winslow DJ, Connor DH, Sprinkz J. Malaria. In: Marcial-Rojas R, ed. Pathology of protozoal and helminthic diseases, with clinical correlation. Baltimore: Williams & Wilkins, 1971.

Wolf A, Cowen D, Paige BH. Human toxoplasmosis: occurrence in infants as an encephalomyelitis, verification by transmission to animals. Science 1939; 89:226.

Woodward TE, Osterman J. Rickettsial diseases. In: Warren KS, Mahmoud AAF, eds. Tropical and geographical medicine. New York: McGraw-Hill, 1984.

Wright HT Jr. Coccidioidomycosis. In: Gellis SS, Kagan BM, eds. Current pediatric therapy. vol 8. Philadelphia: WB Saunders, 1978.

Wright L. Intellectual sequelae of Rocky Mountain spotted fever. J Abnorm Psychol 1972; 80:135.

Wright WH. Schistosomiasis as a world problem. Bull NY Acad Med 1968; 44:301.

Yokogawa S. An experimental study of the intracranial parasitism of the human lung fluke, *Paragonimus westermani*. Am J Hyg 1921; 1:63.

Zenker FA. Eueber den Cysticerus racemosus des Gehrins. Neurol Zentralbl 1882; 1:515.

Zinkham WH. Visceral larva migrans. Am J Dis Child 1978; 132:627.

Zuelzer WW, Apt L. Disseminated visceral lesions associated with extreme eosinophilia. Am J Dis Child 1949; 78:153.

41

Malnutrition

Arthur L. Prensky

Malnutrition remains the most common environmental insult that afflicts the developing nervous system. The term encompasses a wide variety of disorders, including deficiencies of specific nutrients such as individual vitamins or salts. However, undernutrition, which generally describes a deficiency in calories and/or protein, is the most common type of malnutrition and is the one discussed in this chapter.

Marasmus, a deficiency in both calories and protein, is characterized by extreme emaciation, growth failure, alternating apathy and irritability, and eventually obtundation and death. Kwashiorkor is a chronic protein deficiency with adequate carbohydrate and often adequate caloric intake. Children with this disease are edematous. Their faces are puffy, they develop ascites, and depigmentation of hair and skin may occur. The liver also enlarges and is infiltrated by fat. If the child were not treated, death would occur from hepatic or cardiac failure, or more often, intercurrent infection. Most cases of marasmus occur within the first year of life and rarely occur after the second year. Conversely, the greatest incidence of kwashiorkor occurs in the latter part of the first year to the third year of life [Dodge et al., 1975].

There has been increasing concern about the survivors of severe protein-caloric malnutrition in infancy because it has become apparent that, collectively, they do not perform as well as properly fed children from the same populations [Klein, 1980; Lloyd-Still, 1976]. The intellectual performance of malnourished children who are protein-calorie depleted during the first year of life remains depressed into the second decade [Galler et al., 1986].

Because the nervous system of the adult animal is very resistant to caloric deprivation, insults that produce a loss of body weight of 50% or more may produce no permanent changes in cerebral function or in the weight or composition of the brain at postmortem examination. However, the developing brain reacts differently to severe undernutrition. If the insult were sustained, there would be a reduction in brain weight, and alterations would occur in the composition of the brain. These anatomic changes can be associated with intellectual and behavioral deficiencies that persist throughout life.

One would assume that undernutrition would be an easy insult to correct because logically it should be obviated by adequate feeding. The answer is not that simple. Apart from the political and socioeconomic problems that plague the international distribution of food, the association of undernutrition with a depressed socioeconomic status and multiple other environmental insults makes it difficult to isolate the long-term effects of starvation in depressed populations [Crnic, 1984]. It is difficult to determine the actual benefits from protein and calorie supplementation during and after pregnancy [Beaton and Ghassemi, 1982]. These difficulties, along with the lack of accessibility of investigators and their sophisticated equipment to chronically undernourished populations of children, have led to the development of animal models of protein-caloric malnutrition that have some general correspondence to the malnourished child. The following subsections explore these problems in greater detail.

ANATOMIC AND BIOCHEMICAL PATHOLOGY

Interest in undernutrition and the developing nervous system began in the late nineteenth century and remained very active through the first two decades of the twentieth century when a number of undernourished animal models were developed. Some of the earliest studies were performed at the Wistar Institute and summarized by Donaldson in 1911. Although they were interested in older rodents, researchers observed that undernutrition early in life interfered with brain growth. They recognized that the water content of the brain was inversely related to myelination, and the amount of brain water increased in undernourished animals when compared with age-matched controls. Because they were performed after weaning, these studies minimized the effects of underfeeding on myelination and brain water. Sugita [1918] studied the effects of undernutrition in the rat in the first 3 weeks of life before weaning. He observed a definite increase in brain water content and a reduction in brain lipids. Less than the expected amount of stainable myelin for age was observed when compared with controls. The volume of the cerebral cortex was decreased, and cells were more closely spaced, but the total number of cells did not appear to be reduced in careful counts made by Sugita [1918]. The major reduction in cell volume occurred in the neuropil, but Sugita believed that the size of the cell body was also smaller.

The data from this study demonstrate that protein-caloric deprivation does not produce destructive lesions in brain. The primary influence of deprivation is on the replication and growth of cells; the effects are most pronounced in those elements most actively proliferating during the insult [Dobbing, 1964; 1972; Dobbing and Sands, 1971]. It is in this way that marasmus and, to a certain extent, kwashiorkor differ from deprivation of specific dietary constituents, which can result in destruction of selected areas of the brain.

Morphometric analysis of specific areas of cerebral cortex and of selected subcortical nuclei by Diaz-Cintra et al. [1981; 1984; 1990] indicates that there are specific differences in the responses of selected neurons to undernutrition. In the visual cortex of the protein-deprived rat the changes in the developmental pattern of the pyramidal cells of layer V differs from that of layers II and III [Diaz-Cintra et al., 1990]. In the nucleus raphé dorsalis of the protein-deprived rat, fusiform and ovoid cells manifest either a decrease in synaptic terminals or no change in response to undernutrition, whereas the synaptic input of serotonergic multipolar cells increases. It is reasonable to assume that this highly selective variability of nerve cells in response to protein deprivation has some effect on the animal's clinical response to this type of insult.

The results of these anatomic studies and gross measurements of brain water and lipid have been confirmed by more elegant biochemical investigations. DNA has been used to measure cell size. White matter lipid, particularly cerebroside, has been used to measure myelination.

In these studies a variety of species has been used, but the rat is still the animal of choice for the study of undernutrition. Its late brain development, occurring mostly during the first 3 weeks of postnatal life, makes the animal more susceptible to a nutritional insult after birth.

Pregnant female rats subjected to severe protein restriction from the fourth day of gestation give birth to litters that average a 15% decrease in the number of brain cells [Patel et al., 1973]. The reduction is most marked in the areas adjacent to the lateral ventricles and in the cerebellum [Guthrie and Brown, 1968; Shimada et al., 1977]. There is a similar decrease in cerebral protein [Zamenhof and Guthrie, 1977].

Reductions in protein and caloric intake during the suckling period produced a 10% to 30% reduction in brain weight with a corresponding decrease in DNA [Fishman et al., 1971; Winick and Noble, 1966]. The major cellular change appears to involve oligodendroglial cells. These cells are reduced in number in both the cortex and white matter, and their maturation is delayed [Bass et al., 1970]. There probably is no significant reduction in the number of neurons in the cerebral cortex, although neurons in the cerebellum, particularly granule cells, may be reduced [Clos et al., 1977]. In undernourished preweanling animals the reduction of DNA content in the cerebellum is considerably greater than in the cerebrum [Chase et al., 1969]. This difference probably is caused by the rapid proliferation of cerebellar neurons after birth in the rat. The effects of undernutrition on cell number are greatest when a nutritional insult is prolonged from early intrauterine life through the period of lactation, which results in a 60% reduction in cell number in human infants by time of weaning [Winick, 1970]. Studies in Rhesus monkeys disclosed no effect on brain growth when the mother was adequately nourished during gestation and the infant protein restricted at birth [Portman et al., 1987].

Myelination is another parameter of brain development that is easily measured in undernourished animals. As discussed previously, young animals that are starved have an increase in the water content of the brain and a decrease in total lipids. A lipid such as cholesterol, which is found in all membranes, is decreased in proportion to total lipids [Dobbing, 1964]; however, greater reductions occur in lipids, such as cerebrosides, which are found predominantly in myelin [Culley and Mertz, 1965]. Proteolipid protein, which is also a myelin constituent, is reduced out of proportion to other proteins and lipids [Benton et al., 1966].

Although less myelin can be extracted from brains of undernourished animals, it does not differ markedly in chemical composition from myelin isolated in control animals [Fishman et al., 1971]. There is less myelin formed in starved animals, but the membrane that is formed is similar to that in normally fed animals of the same age. Even with prolonged starvation in postnatal life, changes in the amount of myelin are not large. For example, in animals starved from birth to 21 days of age, total myelin quantity was only reduced to 86.5% of the control animals. In animals starved from birth to 53 days of age, myelin quantity was 71% of the age-matched control animals [Fishman et al., 1971]. It is possible that the reduction in myelination is secondary to a reduction in the total number of oligodendroglial cells.

It is more difficult to develop biochemical measurements of cell size and to measure the extent of changes in the neuropil, although the ratio of RNA to DNA or protein to DNA usually is used as a biochemical measure. There are greater reductions of both RNA and protein in the cerebral cortex of undernourished preweanling rats than there is a reduction of DNA. This finding suggests that there is impairment in cell growth that exceeds the reduction in cell number [Bass et al., 1970]. Gangliosides also are a measure of cell size; these lipids are greatly reduced in undernourished piglets [Dickerson et al., 1971].

Cragg [1972] observed that the number of synapses in the cortex of undernourished rats was decreased. However, this reduction does not correspond to the general reduction in synaptic transmitters. For example, in the undernourished rat brain, serotonin is increased [Resnick and Morgane, 1984], acetylcholine is unchanged [Wiggins et al., 1984], and area-to-area variability exists in norepinephrine [Wiggins et al., 1984]. Undernourished rats raised in litters of increased size exhibit a decreased amplitude in the evoked responses elicited from electrical stimulation of the locus coeruleus and measured in the frontal and parietal association areas. This decrease persists when the rats are 45 and 100 days of age, suggesting a persistent disruption of noradrenergic fibers projecting from the locus coeruleus to these areas [Soto-Mayano et al., 1987].

It has not been possible to corroborate adequately the studies performed in animal models to those in autopsied children from severely undernourished human populations; however, the major aspects of the anatomic and biochemical pathology of severe protein-caloric malnutrition elucidated in animals have been observed in starved children. In both animals and children, brain weights are reduced, and water content is increased [Fishman et al., 1969]. There is a definite reduction in myelin that becomes greater as the length of starvation increases [Fishman et al., 1969]. The amount of DNA is reduced in the cerebrum and cerebellum, a fact that is believed to be related to a reduction in cell number, particularly oligodendroglial cells [Winick and Rosso, 1969a; 1969b; Winick et al., 1970]. The early studies of Winick et al. on starved Chilean children did not suggest a great difference in the proportional reduction of cell numbers in the cerebrum and cerebellum.

There is information that animals may recover from periods of undernutrition as evidenced by brain weight and biochemical indices [Dobbing et al., 1971; Winick et al., 1968]. However, if the period of undernutrition persists during the entire period of cell replication, there is a persisting deficit in cell numbers regardless of the diet provided thereafter [Fish and Winick, 1969; Swaiman et al., 1970]. This deficit is indicated by reduced brain DNA in later life. Briefer insults ending before 21 days of age in the rat (a period in which cell division is still programmed to occur in the rat brain) produce no permanent defects once the animal is re-fed [Culley and Lineberger, 1968; Winick and Noble, 1966].

Evidence in humans is less direct, but measurements of somatic growth and head size suggest that the length of the insult during development is an important factor in the production of permanent effects in humans as well [Chase and Martin, 1970; Hoorweg and Stanfield, 1976]. Physical growth also is decreased after long periods of kwashiorkor later in childhood [Bowie et al., 1980; Pereira et al., 1979]. At age 1 year, human premature infants who were malnourished in utero, born small for gestational age, and undernourished in early extrauterine life have smaller head circumferences and poorer performances on the Bayley Infant Development Tests than do children of the same gestational age with normal birth weights who were undernourished in early extrauterine life [Georgieff et al., 1985]. This finding suggests that in both animals and humans a combination of both intrauterine and extrauterine malnutrition produces the greatest effect on brain weight, chemical composition, and function.

BIOCHEMISTRY

The majority of biochemical measurements made in the undernourished brain reflect aberrations in anatomic development; however, they do not explain why the developing brain is altered by protein-caloric malnutrition and the adult brain is almost entirely unaffected. At present, there is no single biochemical parameter that has been demonstrated to be responsible for all other changes in the undernourished brain. There is no evidence that the effect of starvation is mediated through hormonal inadequacies or imbalances [Winick, 1976]. Reductions in protein could restrict the availability of essential amino acids, thus reducing protein synthesis in the brain, but no evidence suggests that the availability of amino acids is rate-limiting. There appears to be a restriction in the availability of carbon derived from glucose for the syntheses of lipids and protein in undernourished animals [Agrawal et al., 1971], but it is not clear that this is rate-limiting. Judging by levels of adenosine triphosphate (ATP) or creatinine phosphate, undernourished animals do not lack energy for synthesis [Thurston et al., 1971]. There is some evidence, however, that mitochondrial metabolism is altered in protein-deprived rats. According to polarographic measurements, Oloriensogo [1989] reported that state 3 respiration is reduced and state 4 respiration is enhanced in these malnourished animals. The activity of redox enzymes is also decreased.

It is likely that reduced activity of DNA polymerase may curtail the rate of DNA synthesis and indirectly regulate the distribution of available nucleotides between DNA and RNA [Brasel et al., 1970].

There probably is no single common pathway by which lack of protein and calories affects growth of the nervous system. It is certain, however, that in order for there to be significant effect on brain development, the insult must occur during a period of rapid nervous system growth. Those elements that undergo high rates of synthesis at the time of insult are most affected.

CLINICAL CHARACTERISTICS

Profound, sustained undernutrition results in death from organ failure or intercurrent infection. In both the experimental laboratory and life, however, the insult often is either too mild to produce death or is aborted before death occurs. As a result, there has been considerable interest in the later behavioral and intellectual consequence of undernutrition in early development.

It is difficult to assess the consequences of undernutrition in animals, and, when that assessment is made, it is not possible to determine whether the results predict what will happen in human populations. Severely undernourished animals behave differently from control littermates, even after adequate feeding; however, this phenomenon cannot be tested in a child. Previously undernourished rats are more responsive to behavioral modifiers, such as electric shock and food or water. They also exhibit more random activity [Resnick et al., 1979; Smart, 1981]. This behavior, however, is difficult to analyze. There is no precise way in which to separate motivation from learning in animals. Considerable argument still exists about whether prenatal or early postnatal undernutrition affects short-term memory later in an animal's life [Castro, et al., 1989] or other aspects of behavior that might be termed attention while trying to learn a task [Tonkiss and Galler, 1990]. A possible chemical substrate has been described that may be associated with the previously undernourished rat's poor performance when trying to learn avoidance tasks. Hypothalamic beta-endorphin decreases after electric shocks in normally raised rats. It is unchanged during shock-avoidance in rats deprived of protein from birth [Vendite et al., 1988].

Animal behavior frequently is influenced by the time between termination of the nutritional insult and testing, the gender of the animal, the type of test used, and the reward given [Crnic, 1984]. Previously undernourished animals also are liable to break down behaviorally when tested in an open field [Barnes et al., 1967]. Conversely, animals that are not undernourished but are from an overcrowded environment or have less maternal attention for a variety of reasons exhibit similar behaviors

[Crnic, 1984]. No explanation exists for altered behavior based on the gender of undernourished animals. Proper nourishment of animals after starvation in preweanling life and subsequent rearing in an enriched environment minimizes or eliminates behavioral differences between malnourished and well-nourished rat pups over time [Massaro et al., 1977].

Poorly nourished human populations can be subjected to much more precise testing. Brief postnatal insults lasting under 4 to 5 months do not appear to have a permanent effect on mental function [Chase and Martin, 1970]. Starvation over a considerable period of time does have an effect on behavior and intelligence, but problems in evaluating the effect of undernutrition in isolation from other variables are similar to those encountered in the experimental animal population. It is impossible to find or create a malnourished population that is not subject to other environmental insults. Numerous studies demonstrated that the IQs of populations that are malnourished for long periods differed from those of age-matched controls or at times from siblings in the same family [Cabak and Najdanvic, 1965; Cravioto et al., 1966; Galler et al., 1983; Stoch and Smythe, 1976]. The environments in which malnourished children are reared, however, are almost always suboptimal. Overcrowding, poor education, lack of parental stimulation, and poverty are variables that cannot be confidently evaluated even in sibling studies; each sibling does not receive the same amount of attention and stimulation.

Another important variable that has not been studied fully in humans is the insult interval needed to produce irreversible changes. As Chase and Martin reported, the insult must last many months [1970]; however, the period of undernutrition in postnatal life necessary to produce permanent deficits may be much shorter when the fetus also has been malnourished.

MANAGEMENT

The only treatment of undernutrition is adequate food intake. An adequate protein and caloric intake certainly ends the acute insult, but it is not clear whether caloric supplements always improve growth and function. The use of dietary supplements, both in utero and during the suckling period, was attempted on several occasions with variable results [Herrera et al., 1980; Joos et al., 1983; Klein et al., 1976; Susser and Stein, 1980]. First, many of the supplements were not used or were used improperly [Beaton and Ghassemi, 1982]. Second, improved nutrition cannot compensate for the other problems of poverty, such as lack of parental interest and overcrowding. Third, it is not certain when improvement ceases or if differences between supplemented and control populations will be of less importance later in life. For example, the study of undernourished children in Bogata, which used both nutritional supplementation and environmental stimulation in different treatment groups, found that nutritionally supplemented children at 18 months of age had benefited in all tested aspects of development but language. However, at 36 months of age the children's language skills had also benefited when compared with nonsupplemented children of the same age. In contrast the effects of early environmental stimulation lessened with age [Waber et al., 1981]. Nutritionally supplemented populations and their malnourished controls have now been followed for up to 9 years. The effects have been positive but small [Grantham-McGregor, 1987].

All facets of neurologic function do not need to recover in parallel. Celedon and DeAndraca [1979] reported that with feeding, at the end of a period of protein-caloric undernutrition, psychomotor development improved but was limited predominantly to social language and fine motor coordination. Gross motor coordination did not demonstrate any improvement during the 5 months in which these children were treated. Other studies indicated the positive effects of psychosocial stimulation or relatively well-structured home environments during the recovery period [Beardslee et al., 1982; Cravioto and Arrieta, 1979; Grantham-McGregor et al., 1980]. In studies performed on underfed populations in New York City, no differences were disclosed in two groups, one supplemented and one eating their usual diet, using the Bayley Mental and Motor Scales. These mothers, however, were only supplemented during pregnancy and not during lactation [Susser and Stein, 1980].

Failure to control other variables often associated with poverty makes comparison of these trials very difficult and probably accounts for the uncertain results. Inadequate control of the way food supplements were used, differences in the times and lengths of supplementation, differences in the amounts of calories and protein provided, and differences in the types of testing at variable periods after pregnancy and delivery contributed to the difficulty of evaluating outcome. It is clear, however, from these studies that current methods of food supplementation may decrease mortality from undernutrition during pregnancy or in the weaning period. It does not appear that morbidity will be reduced to a level at which it is no longer a public health problem.

REFERENCES

Agrawal HC, Fishman MA, Prensky AL. A possible block in the intermediary metabolism of glucose into protein and lipids in the brains of undernourished rats. Lipids 1971; 6:431.

Barnes RH, Moore AU, Reid IM, et al. Learning behavior following nutritional deprivations in early life. J Am Diet Assoc 1967; 51:34.

Bass NH, Netsky MG, Young E. Effect of neonatal malnutrition on the developing cerebrum. Arch Neurol 1970; 23:289.

Beardslee WR, Wolff PH, Hurwitz I, et al. The effects of infantile malnutrition on behavioral development: a follow-up study. Am J Clin Nutr 1982; 35:1437.

Beaton GH, Ghassemi H. Supplementary feeding programs for young children in developing countries. Am J Clin Nutr 1982; 35:864.

Benton JW, Moser HW, Dodge PR, et al. Modification of the schedule of myelination in the rat by early nutritional deprivation. Pediatrics 1966; 38:801.

Bowie MD, Moodie AD, Mann MD, et al. A prospective 15-year follow up study of kwashiorkor patients. Part I. Physical growth and development. S Afr Med J 1980; 58:671.

Brasel J, Ehrenkranz RA, Winick M. DNA polymerase activity in rat brain during ontogeny. Dev Biol 1970; 23:424.

Cabak V, Najdanvic R. Effect of undernutrition in early life on physical and mental development. Arch Dis Child 1965; 40:532.

Castro CA, Tracy M, Rudy JW. Early-life undernutrition impairs the development of the learning and short-term memory processes mediating performance in a conditional-spatial discrimination task. Behav Brain Res 1989; 32:255.

Celedon JM, DeAndraca I. Psychomotor development during treatment of severely marasmic infants. Early Hum Dev 1979; 3:267.

Chase HP, Lindsley WFB Jr, O'Brien D. Undernutrition and cerebellar development. Nature 1969; 221:554.

Chase HP, Martin HP. Undernutrition and child development. N Engl J Med 1970; 282:933.

Clos J, Favre C, Selme-Matrat M, et al. Effects of undernutrition on cell formation in the rat brain and especially cellular composition of the cerebellum. Brain Res 1977; 123:13.

Cragg BG. The development of cortical synapses during starvation in the rat. Brain 1972; 95:143.

Cravioto J, Arrieta R. Stimulation and mental development of malnourished infants. Lancet 1979; 2:899.

Cravioto J, DeLicardie ER, Birch HC. Nutrition, growth and neurointegrative development: an experimental and ecologic study. Pediatrics 1966; 38:319.

Crnic LS. Nutrition and mental development. Am J Ment Defic 1984; 88:526.

Culley WJ, Lineberger RO. Effect of undernutrition on the size and composition of the rat brain. J Nutr 1968; 96:375.

Culley WJ, Mertz ET. Effect of restricted food intake on growth and composition of preweanling rat brain. Proc Soc Exp Biol Med 1965; 118:233.

Diaz-Cintra S, Cintra L, Kemper T, et al. The effects of protein deprivation on the nucleus raphe dorsalis: a morphometric Golgi study in rats of three age groups. Brain Res 1981; 221:243.

Diaz-Cintra S, Cintra L, Kemper T, et al. The effects of protein deprivation on the nucleus locus coeruleus: a morphometric Golgi study in rats of three age groups. Brain Res 1984; 304:243.

Diaz-Cintra S, Cintra L, Ortega A, et al. Effects of protein deprivation on pyramidal cells of the visual cortex in rats of three age groups. J Comp Neurol 1990; 292:117.

Dickerson JWT, Merat A, Widdowson EM. Intrauterine growth retardation in the pig. Biol Neonate 1971; 19:354.

Dodge PR, Prensky AL, Feigin RD. Nutrition and the developing nervous system. St. Louis: Mosby, 1975.

Dobbing J. The influence of early nutrition on the development and myelination of the brain. Proc R Soc Lond (Biol) 1964; 159:503.

Dobbing J. Vulnerable periods of brain development. In: Ciba Foundation. Lipids, malnutrition and the developing brain. Amsterdam: Elsevier Publishing, 1972.

Dobbing J, Hopewell JW, Lynch A. Vulnerability of developing brain. VII. Permanent deficit of neurons in cerebral and cerebellar cortex following early mild undernutrition. Exp Neurol 1971; 32:439.

Dobbing J, Sands J. Vulnerability of developing brain. IX. The effect of nutritional growth retardation on the timing of the brain growth spurt. Biol Neonate 1971; 19:363.

Donaldson HH. The effect of underfeeding on the percentage of water, on the ether-alcohol extract, and on medullation in the central nervous system of the albino rat. J Comp Neurol 1911; 21:139.

Fish I, Winick M. Cellular growth in various regions of the developing rat brain. Pediatr Res 1969; 3:407.

Fishman MA, Madyastha P, Prensky AL. The effect of undernutrition on the development of myelin in the rat central nervous system. Lipids 1971; 6:458.

Fishman MA, Prensky AL, Dodge PR. Low content of cerebral lipids in infants suffering from malnutrition. Nature 1969; 221:552.

Galler JR, Ramsey F, Forde V. A follow-up study of the influence of early malnutrition on subsequent development: 4. Intellectual performance during adolescence. Nutr Behav 1986; 3:211.

Galler J, Ramsey F, Solimano G, et al. The influence of early malnutrition on subsequent behavioral development. I. Degree of impairment in intellectual performance. J Am Acad Child Psychiatry 1983; 22:8.

Georgieff MK, Hoffman JS, Pereira GR, et al. Effect of neonatal caloric deprivation on head growth and 1-year developmental status in preterm infants. J Pediatr 1985; 107:581.

Grantham-McGregor S. Field studies in early nutrition and later achievement. In: Dobbing J, ed. Early nutrition and later achievement. New York: Academic Press, 1987.

Grantham-McGregor S, Stewart ME, Schofield WN. Effect of long-term psychosocial stimulation on mental development of severely malnourished children. Lancet 1980; 2:785.

Guthrie HA, Brown ML. Effect of severe undernutrition in early life on growth, brain size and composition in adult rats. J Nutr 1968; 94:419.

Herrera MG, Mora JO, Christiansen N, et al. Effects of nutritional supplementation and early education on physical and cognitive development. In: Turner RR, Reese HW, eds. Lifespan psychology: intervention. New York: Academic Press, 1980.

Hoorweg J, Stanfield JP. The effects of protein energy malnutrition in early childhood on intellectual and motor abilities in later childhood and adolescence. Dev Med Child Neurol 1976; 18:330.

Joos SK, Pollitt E, Mueller WH, et al. The Bacon Chow study: maternal nutritional supplementation and infant behavioral development. Child Dev 1983; 54:669.

Klein PS. Nutritional deprivation and retardation of cognitive functions. In: Mittler P, ed. Frontiers of knowledge of mental retardation, vol. 2. Biomedical aspects. Baltimore: University Park Press, 1980.

Klein RE, Arenales P, Delgado H, et al. Effects of maternal nutrition on fetal growth and infant development. In: Bulletin of the Pan-American Health Organization, 1976; 10:301.

Lloyd-Still JD. Malnutrition and intellectual development. Littleton, Massachusetts: Publishing Sciences Group, 1976.

Massaro TF, Levitsky DA, Barnes RH. Early protein malnutrition in the rat: behavioral changes during rehabilitation. Dev Psychobiol 1977; 10:105.

Olorinesogo OO. Changes in brain mitochondrial bioenergetics in protein deficient rats. J Exp Path 1989; 70:607.

Patel AJ, Balazs R, Johnson AL. Effect of undernutrition on cell formation in the rat brain. J Neurochem 1973; 20:1151.

Pereira SM, Sundarar JR, Begum A. Physical growth and neurointegrative performance of survivors of protein-energy malnutrition. Br J Nutr 1979; 42:165.

Portman OW, Neuringer M, Alexander M. Effects of maternal and long-term postnatal protein malnutrition on brain size and composition in Rhesus monkeys. J Nutr 1987; 117:1844.

Resnick O, Miller M, Forbes W, et al. Developmental protein malnutrition: influences on the central nervous system of the rat. Neurosci Biobehav Rev 1979; 3:233.

Resnick O, Morgane PJ. Ontogeny of the levels of serotonin in various parts of the brain in severely protein malnourished rats. Brain Res 1984; 303:163.

Shimada M, Wamano T, Nakamura T, et al. Effect of maternal malnutrition on matrix cell proliferation in cerebrum of mouse embryo: an autoradiographic study. Pediatr Res 1977; 11:728.

Smart JL. Undernutrition during early life and its effects on animal development and behavior. Neuropharmacology 1981; 20:1251.

Soto-Moyano R, Ruiz S, Perez H, et al. Early undernutrition and long-lasting functional derangement of the noradrenergic system projecting to the cerebral cortex. Nutr Rep Int 1987; 36:309.

Stoch MB, Smythe PM. 15-year developmental study on effects of severe undernutrition during infancy on subsequent physical growth and intellectual functioning. Arch Dis Child 1976; 54:327.

Sugita N. Comparative studies on the growth of the cerebral cortex. VII. On the influence of starvation at an early age upon the development of the cerebral cortex: albino rat. J Comp Neurol 1918; 29:177.

Susser N, Stein ZA. Human development and prenatal nutrition: an overview of epidemiological experiments, quasi-experiments, and natural experiments in the past decade. In: Mittler P, ed. Frontiers of knowledge in mental retardation, vol 2. Biomedical aspects. Baltimore: University Park Press, 1980.

Swaiman KF, Daleiden JM, Wolfe RN. The effect of food deprivation on enzyme activity in developing brain. J Neurochem 1970; 17:1387.

Thurston JH, Prensky AL, Warren SK, et al. The effects of undernutrition upon the energy reserve of the brain and upon other selected intermediates in brains and livers of infant rats. J Neurochem 1971; 18:161.

Tonkiss J, Galler JR. Prenatal protein malnutrition and working memory performance in adult rats. Behav Brain Res 1990; 40:95.

Vendite D, Batista J, Teixeira R, et al. Effects of undernutrition during suckling and of training on the hypothalamic beta-endorphin of young and adult rats. Peptides 1988; 9:751.

Waber DP, Vuori-Christiansen L, Ortiz N, et al. Nutritional supplementation, maternal education and cognitive development of infants at risk of malnutrition. Am J Clin Nutr 1981; 34:801.

Wiggins RC, Fuller G, Enna SJ. Undernutrition and the development of brain neurotransmitter systems. Life Sci 1984; 35:2085.

Winick M. Nutrition and nerve cell growth. Fed Proc 1970; 29:1510.

Winick M. Malnutrition and brain development. New York: Oxford University Press, 1976.

Winick M, Fish I, Rosso P. Cellular recovery in rat tissues after a brief period of neonatal malnutrition. J Nutr 1968; 95:623.

Winick M, Noble A. Cellular responses in rats during malnutrition at various ages. J Nutr 1966; 89:300.

Winick M, Rosso P. The effect of severe early malnutrition on cellular growth of the human brain. Pediatr Res 1969a; 3:181.

Winick M, Rosso P. Head circumference and cellular growth of the brain in normal and marasmic children. J Pediatr 1969b; 74:774.

Winick M, Rosso P, Waterlow J. Cellular growth of cerebrum, cerebellum and brainstem in normal and marasmic children. Exp Neurol 1970; 26:363.

Zamenhof S, Guthrie D. Differential responses to prenatal malnutrition among neonatal rats. Biol Neonate 1977; 32:205.

42

Vitamins

Peter H. Berman

Vitamins, organic compounds required by mammals in small amounts to sustain normal metabolism, must be supplied from exogenous sources because they cannot be synthesized endogenously. The chemical structure, physiologic properties, and metabolic function of vitamins are quite diverse. In some instances, vitamins act as cofactors in defined enzymatic reactions; in others, they function by interacting with specific intracellular receptors in target organs.

The existence of vitamins became known through the study of disorders produced by vitamin deficiency in diets. The almost complete eradication of nutritional vitamin deficiency disorders in developed countries marks one of the major advances in human health, but nutritional vitamin deficiency remains a public health problem in several developing countries and among the poor and aged worldwide.

Clinical manifestations affecting the CNS and peripheral nervous system occur in most nutritional vitamin deficiency states. They may also occur in diseases affecting vitamin absorption, metabolism, and excretion. Iatrogenic vitamin deficiency has been associated with parenteral nutrition, chronic dialysis, and drug administration. An increasing number of inborn errors of metabolism, in which mutations lead to protein alterations that require pharmacologic rather than physiologic amounts of a vitamin, have been documented. These vitamin dependency states, although relatively rare, present a challenge to the clinician because only through their recognition and the prompt initiation of specific therapy can severe neurologic consequences be prevented (Table 42-1).

Ingestion or administration of excessive amounts of some vitamins may also cause neurologic symptoms and other signs of intoxication.

VITAMIN A (RETINOL)

Vitamin A is the generic term for a group of fat-soluble compounds that possess the biologic activity of retinol (vitamin A_1) [Goodman, 1984]. This activity includes important physiologic roles in retinal function, the growth and differentiation of epithelial tissue, the growth of bone, reproduction, embryonic development, and the enhancement of the immune system.

Retinol has the chemical structure of an alcohol (Figure 42-1). Other structurally related compounds, including 3-dehydroretinol (vitamin A_2), have similar biologic activity.

The physiologic functions of vitamin A are mediated through different forms of the compound. Retinol, the alcohol, serves as the transport molecule; retinal, the aldehyde, is active in the formation of visual pigments; and retinoic acid may be the active metabolite in the growth, maintenance, and differentiation of body tissues. Retinol esters function as storage material.

Vitamin A is necessary for the adaptation of the retinol rods and cones to dim light [O'Brien, 1982]. Such adaptation is accomplished through photosensitive chemical reactions that ultimately result in the initiation of receptor potentials in the retina. Rhodopsin, formed from the combination of the protein opsin and 11-*cis*-retinal, is the photosensitive pigment of the rods. Most rhodopsin is located in the membranes of the disks on the outer segments of the rods. After the absorption of a photon of light, rhodopsin undergoes transformational changes leading to its interaction with transducin, another retinal rod protein, in a process that causes stimulation of a cyclic guanylic acid–specific phosphodiesterase. The resultant decline in guanylic acid concentration leads to the development of an action potential [Stryer, 1986].

Table 42-1 Vitamin dependency disorders

Vitamin	Disorder	Defective enzyme
Thiamine	Lactic acidemia	Pyruvate carboxylase
		Pyruvate dehydrogenase
	Maple syrup urine disease	Branched-chain dehydrogenase complex
Riboflavin	Glutaric acidemia—type I	Glutaryl-CoA-dehydrogenase
	Glutaric acidemia—type II	Multiple acyl-CoA-dehydrogenase
Niacin	Hartnup disease	—
Pyridoxine	Infantile convulsions	—
	Homocystinuria	Cystathionine synthase
	Cystathionuria	Cystathionase
	Gyrate atrophy of retina (ornithinemia)	Ornithine-delta-aminotransferase
Cobalamin	Inherited transcobalamin II deficiency	—
	Methylmalonic acidemia	Methylmalonyl-CoA-mutase
	Homocystinuria with methylmalonic aciduria	Methyltetrahydrofolate reductase, methylmalonyl-CoA mutase
Folate	Congenital folate malabsorption	—
	Dihydrofolate reductase deficiency	Dihydrofolate reductase
	Formimino transferase deficiency	Formimino transferase
Biotin	Propionic acidemia	Propionyl-CoA carboxylase
	Neonatal multiple carboxylase deficiency	Holocarboxylase synthase
	Late-onset multiple carboxylase deficiency	Biotinidase

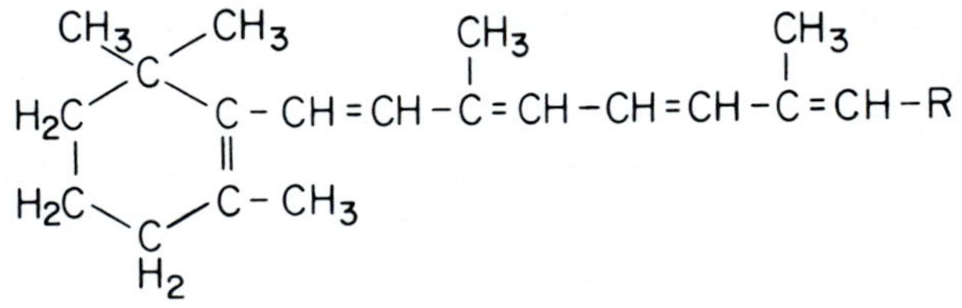

Figure 42-1 The chemical structure of retinol (R = CH_2OH), retinal (R = CHO), and retinoic acid (R = COOH)—the active forms of vitamin A.

Retinol also has an important role in maintaining the structural and functional integrity of epithelial cells by stimulating mucus production. Deprived of adequate amounts of retinol, goblet mucous cells disappear and epidermal basal cells proliferate, resulting in keratinization. The absence of normal mucus secretions promotes irritation and infection. The molecular basis of these physiologic effects of vitamin A are not known.

Stored retinol esters serve as a dietary source of vitamin A. Carotenoids, pigmentary compounds present in all photosynthetic plant tissue, provide another major dietary source [Simpson and Chichester, 1981]. These retinol esters are hydrolyzed to retinol in the intestinal lumen and within the brush border of intestinal cells. Absorption mediated by cellular retinol-binding proteins depends on the presence of absorbable fat and bile and is considerably reduced in conditions associated with steatorrhea and other chronic diarrheas [Chytil and

Ong, 1987]. Vitamin A is stored in the liver as retinol ester.

In the plasma, retinol is bound to a specific retinol-binding protein [Ong, 1985]. The retinol-binding protein delivers retinol to specific sites on the cell surface through which it is transported by cellular retinol-binding proteins.

The absorption, distribution, and metabolic fate of retinoic acid differ from those of retinol. Retinoic acid is directly absorbed into the circulation and transported in the plasma bound to albumin. Retinoic acid is not stored in the liver.

In target cells, retinoic acid is bound to cellular retinoic acid–binding protein, which is distinct from cellular retinol–binding protein. The type of protein present in a target cell determines whether retinol or retinoic acid is effective.

The recommended daily requirement for vitamin A is 375 retinol equivalent units for infants younger than 1 year of age and 700 retinol equivalent units for children and adolescents. Under normal conditions the liver concentration of retinol ester approximates 100 to 300 μg/g, and the normal plasma retinol concentration is 30 to 70 μg/dl.

Vitamin A deficiency

Dietary vitamin A deficiency continues to be a major cause of infantile blindness in some developing countries [Sommer, 1981, 1989]. In developed countries, vitamin A is among the essential nutrients most likely to be ingested in marginal amounts by the poor. Signs and symptoms of vitamin A deficiency also occur in patients with steatorrhea and other forms of chronic diarrhea, hepatic and pancreatic disease, chronic infections, and hypermetabolic states (hyperthyroidism) [Aberathy, 1976; Main et al., 1983; Roos and Van Der Blij, 1985.]

The clinical manifestations of deficiency are a direct consequence of the role of vitamin A in retinal function and in maintaining the structural and physiologic function of epithelial cells. Night blindness (nyctalopia) is among the earliest symptoms [Sommer et al., 1980]. The cornea and conjunctivae subsequently become dry and wrinkled (xerophthalmia), yellow patches (Bitot spots) appear on the bulbar conjunctivae, and corneal ulcerations and scarring ultimately lead to irreversible amblyopia. Keratinization of the skin and epithelial lining of the respiratory and urinary tracts leads to increased susceptibility to infection. Pseudotumor cerebri [Abernathy, 1976; Kasarkis and Bass, 1982; Roos and Van Der Blij, 1985] and facial nerve palsy [Sillman et al., 1985] have been reported.

Because serum retinol levels are maintained for months at the expense of hepatic stores, low serum retinol concentrations imply that hepatic stores have been depleted. Clinical manifestations of deficiency may appear when the plasma concentration falls below 20 μg/dl (normal, 30 to 70 μg/dl). Serum retinol concentrations at or below 10 μg/dl are associated with hepatic retinol-ester concentrations of 5 to 20 μg/g (normal, 100 to 300 μg/g).

The diet of infants should be supplemented by the oral administration of 400 to 700 μg of retinol per day to prevent deficiency. Clinical manifestations of deficiency should be treated with 6 to 15 mg of retinol (20,000 to 50,000 IU of vitamin A) per day for 4 to 5 days, followed by 0.6 to 1.5 mg per day for 1 to 2 months. In conditions interfering with intestinal vitamin absorption, aqueous preparations should be administered intramuscularly. Treatment initiated before the occurrence of corneal scarring leads to rapid, complete resolution of symptoms and signs.

Vitamin A intoxication

Human sensitivity to excessive amounts of vitamin A is quite variable; infants and children are generally more prone to develop symptoms and signs than adults. Acute toxicity may occur following ingestion of 300,000 IU of vitamin A or more. Signs of chronic toxicity usually appear following the administration of 2500 IU/kg/day but may result after ingestion of smaller dosages [Bendich and Langseth, 1989]. Ingestion of such quantities of vitamin A is not uncommon in the treatment of acne or among megavitamin *faddists* [Lippe et al., 1981; Shaywitz et al., 1977]. Hepatitis may precipitate manifestations of toxicity [Hatoff et al., 1982].

The molecular basis of vitamin A toxicity is not known. The clinical manifestations may be a consequence of the increased amounts of free retinol and retinol esters in circulation, an increase that occurs because retinol-binding protein is not elevated in vitamin A toxicity [Smith and Goodman, 1976].

Acute toxicity is characterized by headache, vomiting, diplopia, papilledema (bulging fontanel in infants), stiff neck, and abducens nerve palsies caused by increased intracranial pressure (pseudotumor cerebri). In chronic exposure the manifestations of increased intracranial pressure may be preceded or accompanied by painful fissures at the corners of the mouth, a pruritic desquamating dermatitis, tender hyperostoses of the long bones and skull, limitations of joint motility, hepatomegaly, and failure to gain weight.

The diagnosis is established from the dietary history and characteristic clinical findings. The plasma retinol concentration usually exceeds 100 to 600 μg/dl (normal, 30 to 70 μg/dl). Radiographs of the limbs may reveal periosteal new bone formation, metaphyseal cupping, and increased metaphyseal density. The uptake of technetium-99m polyphosphate is increased on bone scans.

Removal of vitamin A from the diet invariably leads to resolution of symptoms and signs of toxicity within several days.

Teratogenic effects of vitamin A toxicity during pregnancy include hydrocephalus, microcephalus, retinal and optic nerve defects, microtia or anotia, and conotruncal heart defects [Lammer et al., 1985].

THIAMINE (VITAMIN B₁)

Thiamine functions as a cofactor in oxidative decarboxylation and transketolation reactions [David and Leke, 1983]. Thiamine pyrophosphate (Figure 42-2), the physiologic active form, is an essential cofactor in the oxidative decarboxylation of pyruvate to acetyl-CoA, α-ketoglutarate to succinyl-CoA, and the α-keto derivatives of isoleucine, leucine, and valine to their corresponding branched-chain CoA derivatives. Thiamine pyrophosphate is also the cofactor for the transketolase reaction in the hexose monophosphate shunt that provides pentose for nucleotide synthesis. In addition, thiamine has roles in brain metabolism, where it is

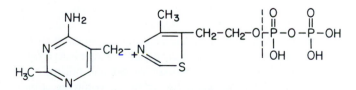

Figure 42-2 The chemical structure of thiamine pyrophosphate.

present both as a diphosphate and a triphosphate. Although the precise molecular basis of the nervous system function of thiamine is not known, experimental studies have implicated it in fatty acid synthesis [Volpe and Marasa, 1978], neuronal membrane transport [Voorhees et al., 1977], neuromuscular transmission [Waldehind, 1978], and axonal conduction [Schoffeniels, 1983].

Thiamine is readily available in meats, grains, and vegetables but is destroyed by heat. It is actively transported across the small intestine by a saturable process limiting the amount that can be absorbed. In the blood, thiamine is bound to protein, predominantly albumin. Its transport into the CNS and CSF is controlled by a rate-limiting process involving a specific membrane-bound phosphatase [Spector, 1976]. Excesses of the vitamin are excreted in the urine.

The requirement for thiamine depends on the metabolic rate and is increased when carbohydrates are the major energy source. The recommended daily dietary intake is 0.3 to 0.4 mg in infants younger than 1 year of age and 0.7 to 1.5 mg in older children and adolescents, amounts readily available in normal diets.

Thiamine deficiency

Historically, clinical manifestations of dietary thiamine deficiency (beri-beri) occurred in populations in which polished rice formed the major dietary staple. Signs of deficiency still occur in alcoholics and the aged, populations that use thiamine less effectively. Beri-beri has also been reported after ingestion of large amounts of raw freshwater fish; shellfish and bracken foods that contain thiaminase 1, an enzyme promoting thiamine decomposition [Murata, 1965]; and large quantities of tea, which contains another thiamine antagonist [Vimokesant et al., 1974]. An infantile form of beri-beri has been reported in breast-fed infants of thiamine-deficient mothers [Rao and Subrahmagam, 1964] and in those fed a soybean formula in which the thiamine was presumably heat inactivated during preparation [Cochrane et al., 1961].

The early symptoms of thiamine deficiency are not specific and include apathy, fatigue, mental sluggishness, depression, anorexia, and abdominal discomfort. More prolonged and severe deficiency is associated with signs of peripheral neuropathy, nerve and muscle tenderness, and cardiomyopathy. Hoarseness caused by laryngeal nerve paralysis is a classic sign. Ptosis, optic atrophy, and encephalopathic features may also occur. As the deficiency persists, increased intracranial pressure, meningismus, seizures, and coma may rapidly progress to a fatal outcome from either neurologic or cardiac failure.

Infantile beri-beri is characterized by vomiting, aphonia, abdominal distension, diarrhea, cyanosis, tachycardia, and convulsions. Death may occur suddenly. In less fulminant, more chronic depletions, infants fail to grow and develop; edema, oliguria, constipation, cardiomegaly, and hepatomegaly follow [Cochrane et al., 1961].

The neuropathologic features of beri-beri are fairly characteristic and consist of nerve cell degeneration, endothelial hyperplasia, and petechial hemorrhages localized to the periventricular gray matter around the third ventricle, sylvian aqueduct, fourth ventricle, and mammillary bodies [Cochrane et al., 1961]. Peripheral nerves manifest patchy areas of demyelination.

The diagnosis of thiamine deficiency depends primarily on suspicions raised by the dietary history and the presence of typical clinical manifestations. Determining serum thiamine concentrations is not of practical value. Urinary excretion of less than 120 µg of thiamine/g of creatinine suggests thiamine deficiency. An increase of 25% or more in red cell ketolase activity after the addition of thiamine pyrophosphate is also characteristic of deficiency. A clinical response to the administration of thiamine is the best confirmatory test.

Oral administration of 10 to 50 mg of thiamine per day will reverse clinical symptoms in a few weeks. Serious life-threatening neurologic manifestations or congestive heart failure should be treated with the parenteral administration of 5 to 20 mg of thiamine.

Thiamine dependency

Thiamine-dependent lactic acidemia. Pyruvate dysmetabolism disorders are among the varied causes of lactic acidosis [Evans, 1986]. Thiamine pyrophosphate is an essential cofactor in pyruvate decarboxylation. Several patients with documented thiamine-responsive lactic acidemia have been reported [Duran and Wadman, 1985]. The age at onset of symptoms varies from the immediate postnatal period to 8 years. Mental retardation and episodic neurologic abnormalities, including intermittent ataxia, choreoathetosis, and/or hypotonia with areflexia, occur. Pyruvate carboxylase deficiency has been confirmed in one patient by liver biopsy, and a partial deficiency of the pyruvate dehydrogenase complex was confirmed in two others by enzymatic assay of cultured skin fibroblasts. Biochemical abnormalities normalized and episodic neurologic symptoms improved after administration of pharmacologic amounts of thiamine (20 to 2400 mg/day). In view of the potential benefits, therapy with thiamine in pharmacologic amounts should be attempted in all patients with persistent lactic acidemia believed to be secondary to a primary metabolic defect.

Thiamine-dependent maple syrup urine disease. Branched-chain ketoaciduria, or maple syrup urine disease, is an autosomal-recessive inborn error of metabolism caused by branched-chain keto acid dehydrogenase complex deficiency. It leads to an accumulation in the blood and tissues of the branched-chain amino acids leucine, isoleucine, and valine and their respective keto analogues and hydroxy acids [Dancis et al., 1959; Menkes et al., 1954]. A thiamine pyrophosphate–dependent decarboxylase is among the enzymes in the branched-chain dehydrogenase complex.

Classic maple syrup urine disease is characterized by the onset of neurologic deterioration and seizures in the first weeks or months of life. Without appropriate dietary restriction of the branched-chain amino acids, the eventual neurologic impairment of affected infants is severe; coma followed by death occurs frequently.

Variants of maple syrup urine disease, in which milder neurologic and biochemical abnormalities are associated with more residual enzymatic activity (2% of normal controls), have been reported [Morris et al., 1964; Valman et al., 1973]. In such variants, neurologic and metabolic abnormalities may occur only in association with increased protein intake or infection. The clinical and biochemical characteristics of nine reported patients with thiamine-responsive maple syrup urine disease have been reviewed by Duran and Wadman [1985]. They reported patients with a milder variant of classic maple syrup urine disease, with residual branched-chain keto acid dehydrogenase activity in skin fibroblast or lymphocyte cultures ranging between 3% and 40% of normal controls. All patients were treated with low-protein diets and/or branched-chain amino acid–restricted diets and dietary supplementation with 10 to 1000 mg of thiamine. The biochemical abnormalities improved and further episodes of clinical ketoacidosis, acute neurologic symptoms, and neurologic deterioration were prevented.

Subacute necrotizing encephalomyelopathy (Leigh disease). Subacute necrotizing encephalomyelitis is a rare, degenerative disorder characterized clinically by anorexia, failure to thrive, episodic hyperventilation, psychomotor retardation, seizures, visual loss, and prominent signs of brainstem dysfunction (e.g., nystagmus, external ophthalmoplegia, dysphagia, ataxia) [Pincus, 1972]. Associated biochemical abnormalities often include elevated blood pyruvate, lactate, and α-ketoglutarate concentrations. Neuropathologic features resemble those of experimental thiamine deficiency. Normal red cell transketolase activity and the lack of response to the intramuscular administration of thiamine exclude simple thiamine deficiency [Pincus and Grove, 1970]. A consistent reduction of the concentration of thiamine triphosphate in affected brain regions has been reported [Cooper et al., 1969]. Such a reduction further differentiates subacute necrotizing encephalomyelitis from experimental thiamine deficiency, in which affected brain regions reveal a decrease in thiamine diphosphate and a relative increase in thiamine triphosphate [DeGroot and Hommes, 1973]. In subacute necrotizing encephalomyelitis a substance that inhibits the phosphotransferase enzyme necessary for the con-

version of thiamine pyrophosphate to thiamine triphosphate has been detected in the urine, blood, and CSF of affected patients [Dunn and Dolman, 1972; Pincus, 1972]. Treatment with thiamine supplementation has led to improvement in some instances.

Thiamine-dependent megaloblastic anemia, sensorineural deafness, and diabetes mellitus. A thiamine-dependent syndrome characterized by the association of megaloblastic anemia, sensorineural deafness, and diabetes mellitus has been reported [Haworth et al., 1982; Viana and Carvahalho, 1978]. The finding that thiamine (20 to 25 mg/day) corrects the megaloblastic anemia was serendipitous. In one patient, it was possible to discontinue insulin use after the initiation of thiamine treatment. Hearing impairment did not improve. The basis of the response to the thiamine in this syndrome is not known.

RIBOFLAVIN (VITAMIN B$_2$)

Two coenzymes, flavin mononucleotide and flavin adenine dinucleotide, are the physiologically active forms of riboflavin (Figure 42-3). These nucleotides serve a vital role in a variety of mitochondrial oxidation-reduction reactions involving flavoproteins, including amino acid oxidase, xanthine oxidase, and glutathione reductase [Neims and Helerman, 1970].

Riboflavin is widely distributed in plants and animal tissues. Phosphorylation of riboflavin to flavin mononucleotide occurs in the intestinal mucosa through a reaction catalyzed by the cytosolic enzyme flavokinase, and both riboflavin and flavin mononucleotide are absorbed into the circulation [Jusko and Levy, 1975]. The upper limit of absorption is approximately 25 mg/dose. Only small amounts of riboflavin are stored, and unused riboflavin is excreted in the urine and feces. In the plasma, riboflavin and flavin mononucleotide are bound to protein, predominantly albumin. In tissues, riboflavin is converted to flavin mononucleotide in a reaction catalyzed by flavokinase. Flavin mononucleotide is subsequently converted to flavin adenine dinucleotide in a reaction catalyzed by flavin adenine dinucleotide pyrophosphorylase. Flavin adenine dinucleotide is transported into the mitochondria by unidentified mechanisms.

The recommended daily requirement for riboflavin is 0.4 to 0.5 mg in infants younger than 1 year of age and 0.8 to 1.8 mg in older children and adolescents.

Riboflavin deficiency

Symptomatic riboflavin deficiency invariably occurs in association with deficiencies of other vitamins [Hoppel and Tandler, 1990]. Early symptoms include sore throat and angular stomatitis. Glossitis, cheilosis, seborrhea dermatitis of the face, and a dermatitis over the trunk and limbs subsequently develop. Late effects include a

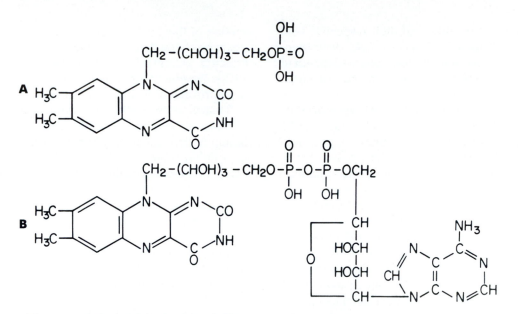

Figure 42-3 The chemical structure of **A,** flavin mononucleotide (FMN) and **B,** Flavin dinucleotide (FAD)—the physiologic active forms of riboflavin.

normochromic, normocytic anemia with associated reticulocytopenia. A neuropathy characterizes the neurologic deficit.

The diagnosis rests primarily on suspicions raised by the dietary history and the presence of characteristic symptoms. Serum riboflavin concentration determinations are of no practical value in diagnosis; urinary concentrations below 30 µg/24 hours suggest riboflavin depletion. The activity of the flavin-dependent erythrocyte glutathione reductase before and after flavin adenine dinucleotide activation is a good index of riboflavin status [Prentice and Bates, 1981].

Riboflavin in dosages of 5 to 10 mg/day readily reverses the manifestations of riboflavin deficiency.

Riboflavin dependency

Riboflavin-dependent glutaric acidemia–type I.

Glutaryl-CoA dehydrogenase deficiency–type I is an autosomal-recessive error of metabolism characterized by early acquired macrocephaly, severe mental retardation, seizures, progressive choreoathetosis, and dystonia associated with glutaric and 3-hydroxyglutaric organic aciduria [Goodman et al., 1977; Stutchfield et al., 1985]. Neuropathologic features include severe symmetric destruction of the putamen and lateral margins of the caudate nuclei [Leibel et al., 1980]. The content of γ-aminobutyric acid in the basal ganglia and substantia nigra is markedly decreased, presumably because γ-aminobutyric acid synthetase is inhibited by glutaric acid [Bennett et al., 1986; Christensen and Brandt, 1978]. The activity of glutaryl-CoA dehydrogenase, an enzyme for which riboflavin is a cofactor, is deficient in leukocytes, cultured skin fibroblasts, and amniotic cells.

The severity of the clinical manifestations, biochemical abnormalities, and amount of residual enzymatic activity vary considerably. Administration of riboflavin in pharmacologic dosages (200 to 300 mg/day) has led to clinical improvement and decreased the urinary excretion of glutaric acid in some patients [Brandt et al., 1979; Leibel et al., 1980; Stutchfield et al., 1985].

Riboflavin-dependent glutaric acidemia–type II (multiple acyl-CoA dehydrogenase deficiency). Glutaric acidemia–type II is characterized biochemically by nonketotic hypoglycemia, metabolic acidosis, and the accumulation and urinary excretion of a number of organic acids derived from saturated acyl-CoA esters, including C_6 to C_{10} dicarboxylic acids and ethylmalonic, isobutyric, butyric, hexanoic, and glutaric acids. This organic aciduria is a direct consequence of a defect in the acyl-Co vitamin A dehydrogenase complex, which consists of several distinct acyl-CoA dehydrogenases, electron transfer flavoprotein, and electron transfer protein: ubiquinone oxidoreductase. The acyl-CoA dehydrogenase complex functions in the transfer of electrons from fatty acids and some branched-chain keto acids to coenzyme Q in the mitochondria [Gregerson, 1985]. In most cases the disorder is due to deficiency of electron transfer protein or electron transfer protein: ubiquinone oxidoreductase.

Considerable phenotypic variability in the clinical manifestations and quantitative pattern of urinary organic acids exists in this disorder. In the newborn the illness is characterized by rapidly progressing respiratory difficulties, a "sweaty-feet" odor, convulsions, and severe metabolic acidosis without ketosis and leads to a fatal outcome in the first days or weeks of life [Przyrembel et al., 1976; Sweetman et al., 1980]. Some patients have dysmorphic clinical features and other congenital anomalies. Glutaric aciduria dominates in this form of the disease, although the other organic acids are also present in the urine. Administration of riboflavin is not beneficial in these patients.

A later-onset glutaric aciduria type II (ethylmalonic-adipic aciduria) manifests in older infants and children with repetitive episodes of acute encephalopathy, hepatomegaly metabolic acidosis, and hypoglycemia, resembling Reye syndrome [Gregerson et al., 1982; Mantagos et al., 1974]. Administration of riboflavin in pharmacologic dosages (300 mg/day in three equal doses) has resulted in dramatic metabolic improvement during the acute episode in such patients and appears to reduce the frequency of subsequent episodes.

In adolescents and young adults, ethylmalonic-adipic aciduria has been associated with a syndrome characterized by episodic symptoms of fatigue, lethargy, mild jaundice, hypoglycemia, and hepatomegaly precipitated by febrile illnesses or pregnancy [Dusheiko et al., 1979; Harpey et al., 1983]. In one such patient, prolonged periods of coma associated with protracted hypoglycemia occurred [Dusheiko et al., 1979]. In another, mild symptoms had occurred during the last trimester of several pregnancies and were associated with decreased fetal movements. One stillborn infant and six infants who died in the first month of life had been born before glutaric acidemia–type II was diagnosed. After diagnosis, administration of riboflavin (20 mg/day) during the woman's ninth pregnancy led to symptomatic improvement and an increase in fetal movements [Harpey et al., 1983]. Riboflavin supplementation was continued for several months after birth, and the infant did well.

Ethylmalonic-adipic aciduria may also be associated with a progressive lipid storage myopathy that responded dramatically to administration of riboflavin 100 mg/day and carnitine 3 g/day [Brivet et al., 1991; DeVisser et al., 1986].

NIACIN (VITAMIN B₃)

The pyridine nucleotides, nicotinamide adenine dinucleotide and nicotinamide adenine dinucleotide phosphate, are the physiologically active forms of niacin (nicotinic acid), which is present in nucleotides in the form of an amide (nicotinamide) (Figure 42-4) [Henderson, 1983]. These nucleotides function in a variety of oxidation-reduction reactions. The reduced nucleotides are subsequently reoxidized by flavoproteins [White, 1982].

Cellular nicotinamide adenine dinucleotide and nicotinamide adenine dinucleotide phosphate, found in a variety of foods, function as the dietary source of niacin. After ingestion the nucleotides are hydrolyzed in the small intestine to niacin and nicotinamide by the

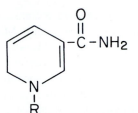

Figure 42-4 The chemical structure of nicotinamide. One or two molecules of adenyl pyrophosphate are joined to nicotinamide at the R position to form the physiologic active nicotinamide adenine dinucleotide (NAD) or nicotinamide adenine dinucleotide phosphate (NADP).

mucosal enzyme nicotinamide adenine dinucleotide-glycohydrolase, a rate-limiting step in absorption. The released niacin and nicotinamide are then transported across the intestine by passive diffusion [Bernofsky, 1980]. The absorbed niacin is rapidly converted to nicotinamide adenine dinucleotide in erythrocytes, and in the liver, nicotinamide adenine dinucleotide glycohydrolases subsequently release nicotinamide for transport to other tissues where it is reconverted into nicotinamide adenine dinucleotide and nicotinamide adenine dinucleotide phosphate.

Tryptophan is an important secondary dietary source of nicotinic acid [Horwitt et al., 1981]. Nicotinic acid is synthesized from tryptophan in a series of reactions through kynurenine, 3-hydroxy anthranilate, and quinolinate. Approximately 1 mg of nicotinic acid is derived from 60 mg of dietary tryptophan. The fact that symptomatic niacin deficiency (pellagra) occurs predominantly in populations in which corn, which has a low content of tryptophan, serves as the major dietary staple attests to the importance of the substance as a dietary source of niacin.

The minimum amount of dietary niacin required to prevent symptomatic deficiency is 4.4 mg/1000 kcal. The recommended daily dietary allowance for niacin is 5 to 6 niacin equivalents in children younger than 1 year of age and 9 to 20 niacin equivalents in older children and adolescents. (A niacin equivalent is equal to 1 mg of niacin or 60 mg of dietary tryptophan.)

Niacin deficiency

The clinical manifestations of niacin deficiency (pellagra) are characterized by the triad of dermatitis, diarrhea, and dementia [Spivais and Jackson, 1977]. Cutaneous manifestations begin with an erythematous dermatitis on the hands; the forehead, neck, and feet are subsequently involved. Hyperpigmentation, desquamation, and scarring ultimately develop. Stomatitis, enteritis, recurrent diarrhea, and excessive salivation are the gastrointestinal manifestations. CNS manifestations include headache, dizziness, insomnia, depression, and memory impairment. In severe cases, delusions, hallucinations, and dementia can occur. Motor and sensory peripheral nerve abnormalities also occur. The diagnosis rests predominantly on the dietary history, clinical findings, and a response to physiologic amounts of niacin. Measurement of urinary excretion of methylated metabolites of nicotinic acid is sometimes helpful in confirming the diagnosis.

Niacin dependency

Hartnup disease. Hartnup disease is an autosomal-recessive disorder characterized by impairment of neutral amino acid transport by the kidneys and small intestine (see Chapter 66). A diagnostic feature is a striking neutral hyperaminoaciduria. Reduced intestinal absorption and increased renal excretion of tryptophan may lead to a reduced availability of this amino acid for niacin synthesis. Pellagralike clinical features, including intermittent ataxia, psychotic behavior, and photosensitive skin rash, have been reported. Several reports document clinical but not biochemical improvement after administration of 50 to 300 mg/day of nicotinamide [Henderson, 1958; Herson and Rodnight, 1960].

PYRIDOXINE (VITAMIN B₆)

Vitamin B$_6$ is the generic term for three naturally occurring pyridine derivatives: pyridoxine (an alcohol), pyridoxal (an aldehyde), and pyridoxamine (an amine) (Figure 42-5) [Fowler, 1985]. Pyridoxal phosphate, the physiologically active form, functions as a cofactor for more than 50 enzymatic reactions, including the decarboxylation, transamination, and racemization of amino acids and reactions in the metabolism of tryptophan, sulfur-containing amino acids, and hydroxy amino acids. There are also several important interactions between pyridoxine and therapeutic drugs [Bauernfeind and Miller, 1987]. Vitamin B$_6$ enhances the peripheral decarboxylation of levodopa, thus reducing its therapeutic effectiveness. Isonicotinic acid hydrazide (isoniazid) acts as a potent inhibitor of pyridoxal kinase by combining with pyridoxal phosphate to form hydrogones. Pyridoxine also interacts with cycloserine and hydralazine, and penicillamine promotes pyridoxine urinary excretion.

Pyridoxine, pyridoxal, and pyridoxamine are present in meats, liver, cereals, soybeans, and vegetables. Because all three compounds are degraded by heat, ultraviolet light, and oxidation, considerable losses may occur during food preparation. All three compounds are absorbed from the intestine by passive diffusion. In the blood, they are bound to proteins and hemoglobin. After passive uptake by the liver, they are converted to pyridoxal phosphate by the hepatic enzyme, pyridoxal kinase. Plasma concentrations reflect concentrations in the liver [Lumeng et al., 1980]. The principal excretory product is pyridoxic acid, which is excreted in the urine after its formation in a reaction catalyzed by the hepatic enzyme aldehyde oxidase. Some unmetabolized pyridoxal is also excreted in the urine.

The requirement for pyridoxine increases with the amount of protein in the diet. The recommended daily dietary allowance of pyridoxine is 0.3 to 0.6 mg in infants younger than 1 year of age and 1 to 2 mg in older children and adolescents.

Pyridoxine deficiency

Clinical manifestations of vitamin B$_6$ deficiency affect the nervous system, skin, and blood. Neurologic abnormalities include seizures in infants and peripheral neuropathy in adolescents. Infants fed a formula deficient in pyridoxine developed irritability, exaggerated startle responses, and generalized seizures [Coursin, 1954]. The convulsions may be a consequence of decreased brain concentrations of γ-aminobutyric acid, which is synthesized from glutamate in a reaction catalyzed by pyridoxal-dependent glutamic acid dehydrogenase [Kurleman et al., 1991; Lott et al., 1978]. Pyridoxine deficiency also leads to decreased brain concentrations of norepinephrine and serotonin [Lovenberg et al., 1962]. Cutaneous manifestations include a seborrheic dermatitis (predominantly about the eyes, nose, and mouth), glossitis, and stomatitis. Microcytic, hypochromic anemia is the characteristic hematologic abnormality.

The diagnosis of pyridoxine deficiency rests predominantly on the correlation of the dietary history, characteristic clinical findings, and prompt response of clinical symptoms to the administration of physiologic amounts of pyridoxine. An increase in the urinary excretion of the tryptophan metabolite xanthurenic acid after an oral load of tryptophan (100 mg/kg) serves as a possible confirmatory laboratory test.

Pyridoxine dependency

Pyridoxine-dependent infantile convulsions. This rare, autosomal recessive error of metabolism is char-

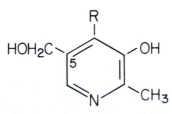

Figure 42-5 The chemical structure of pyridoxine (R = CH$_2$OH), pyridoxal (R = CHO), and pyridoxamine (R = CH$_2$NH$_2$). The alcohol attached to the 5-carbon position of pyridoxal is phosphorylated to form the physiologic active form of the vitamin.

acterized by the onset of generalized convulsions in the newborn period that is responsive to pharmacologic amounts of pyridoxine [Haenggeli et al., 1991; Hunt et al., 1954]. Seizures usually begin within the first hours of life, but their recognition may be delayed. An intrauterine onset has also been reported [Bejsovec et al., 1967]. EEG is severely abnormal, demonstrating a variety of abnormal paroxysmal patterns, including hypsarrhythmia [Mikati et al., 1991].

There is a prompt cessation of seizures and normalization of the EEG after the parenteral administration of pyridoxine (50 to 100 mg intravenously). Lifelong administration of pharmacologic amounts of pyridoxine (5 to 300 mg/kg/day) is necessary to prevent recurrence of convulsions [Haenggeli et al., 1991]. Neurologic damage can be prevented when appropriate therapy is initiated promptly.

The molecular basis of this disorder is not known. A mutation leading to defective binding of pyridoxal phosphate to glutamate decarboxylase, essential for γ-aminobutyric acid synthesis, has been suggested [Bonner et al., 1960]. An instability of plasma albumin pyridoxal binding has also been implicated [Heeley et al., 1978].

Pyridoxine-dependent cystathionine synthase deficiency (homocystinuria). Homocystinuria is characterized clinically by subluxation of the lens (ectopia lentis); osteoporosis; sparse, light-colored hair; and a tendency for recurrent arterial and venous thromboembolism [McKusick et al., 1971; Mudd et al., 1985]. Neurologic abnormalities, including mental retardation, seizures, and focal neurologic deficits, result from repeated vascular occlusions and may be progressive.

Homocystinuria results from three different enzyme deficiencies. The most common cause is a deficiency in the activity of cystathionine betasynthase, which catalyzes the condensation of serine with homocysteine to form cystathionine [Mudd et al., 1985]. Pyridoxal phosphate is a cofactor in this reaction. The enzyme defect can be confirmed in cultures of skin fibroblasts from affected patients [Uhlendorf et al., 1973]. There is considerable genetic heterogeneity among affected families, with enzyme activity ranging from 0% to 30%.

Patients who respond to pyridoxine always have residual enzyme activity, although not all patients with a partial enzyme defect respond. Pharmacologic dosages (up to 1200 mg/day), combined with a restriction of dietary methionine and a supplemental folic acid, are recommended and lead to a decrease in the homocystinemia and homocystinuria, an increase of enzyme activity in skin fibroblast cultures, and a stabilization of symptoms in some patients. Patients with later-onset, milder disease are more likely to respond than those with earlier-onset, severe disease [Fowler, 1985; Mudd et al., 1985].

Pyridoxine-dependent cystathioninuria. Deficient activity of cystathionase catalyzes the cleavage of cysteine to α-ketobutyrate and leads to cystathioninuria [Frimpter, 1965]. Cystathioninuria has been detected in patients suffering from retardation, seizures, nephrogenic diabetes insipidus, and diabetes mellitus, but because cystathioninuria is also found in unaffected people, a causal association between the metabolic defect and clinical symptoms has not been substantiated [Nyhan, 1984].

Pyridoxal phosphate is a cofactor in the cystathionase reaction, and there is a dramatic reduction in the cystathioninuria after administration of pyridoxine in pharmacologic dosages (up to 100 mg/day) in most instances [Pascal et al., 1975].

Pyridoxine-dependent ornithinemia (gyrate atrophy of the retina and choroid). Ornithinemia and ornithinuria resulting from a deficiency in the activity of ornithine-δ-aminotransferase, for which pyridoxal phosphate is a cofactor, are associated with the autosomal-recessive syndrome of gyrate atrophy of the retina and choroid [Simell and Takki, 1973]. A variety of genetic mutations account for the disorder [Brody et al., 1992]. This disorder usually manifests with night blindness between 5 and 10 years of age and is gradually progressive, leading to blindness by the fourth decade of life. The name *gyrate atrophy* is derived from the early appearance of peripheral atrophic lesions of the retina that resemble cerebral gyri. The funduscopic abnormality, also progressive, is eventually characterized by retinitis pigmentosa and optic nerve atrophy. Although weakness is not a prominent symptom, type II muscle fibers are atrophic, and tubular aggregates are found in muscle biopsy specimen [Sipila et al., 1979].

Plasma ornithine concentrations are 10 to 20 times normal, and urinary ornithine excretion reaches 0.5 to 10 mmol/day. Ornithine-δ-aminotransferase activity in cultured skin fibroblast from affected patients ranges from 0% to 5.7% of normal controls [O'Donnell et al., 1978].

Pharmacologic dosages of pyridoxine (500 to 1000 mg/day) substantially reduce the elevated plasma ornithine concentrations and appear to prevent further visual deterioration [Berson et al., 1981; Hayasaka et al., 1982; Weleber and Kennaway, 1981].

Pyridoxine intoxication

Chronic pyridoxine intoxication produces a progressive axonal sensory neuropathy in experimental animals and the human adult. Oral administration of 300 mg/kg/day of pyridoxine to adult beagles produced widespread neuronal degeneration in dorsal root ganglia [Krinke et al., 1980]. Smaller but still excessive amounts (50 to 200 mg/day) administered over longer periods produced a reversible axonal sensory neuropathy without demonstrable pathologic results in the dorsal root ganglia [Phillips et al., 1978; Windeback et al., 1985]. In the human adult, clinical manifestations of a sensory neuropathy occurred after the ingestion of 2 to 6 g/day for several months [Schaumburg et al., 1983]. Nerve conduction studies and histologic examination of sensory nerve biopsies limited the pathologic origin to sensory nerve axonal degeneration. Partial, gradual recovery followed cessation of pyridoxine ingestion. Subsequent reports indicated that sensory neuropathy could result from the ingestion of only 200 mg/day of pyridoxine [Berger and Schaumburg, 1984, Parry and Bredensen, 1985]. The molecular basis for the sensory neuropathy is unknown. A similar syndrome has not been reported in the pediatric age group.

COBALAMIN (VITAMIN B$_{12}$)

Vitamin B$_{12}$ (cobalamin) is a generic term for organometallic compounds in which a cobalt atom with a complex side chain is situated within a corrin ring (Figure 42-6) [Davis, 1985]. The cobalamins are further differentiated by attachments to the cobalt atom. Hydroxycobalamin, methylcobalamin, and deoxyadenosylcobalamin have been isolated from mammalian tissue.

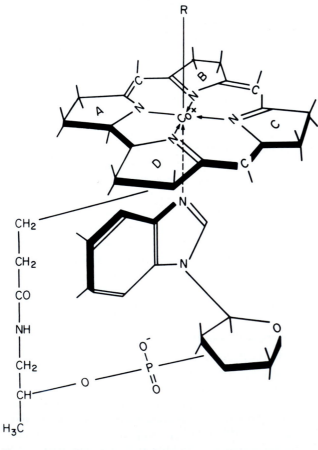

Figure 42-6 The chemical structure of methylcobalamin (R = CH$_3$) and adenosylcobalamin (R = adenosyl) — the physiologic active compounds of vitamin B$_{12}$.

Hydroxycobalamin is the major cobalamin in blood. Methylcobalamin and adenosylcobalamin function as cofactors in enzymatic reactions. Cyanocobalamin, a stable compound formed as an artifact of isolation, can be used in therapy because it is readily convertible to hydroxycobalamin. Methylcobalamin is a cofactor for cytoplasmic methionine synthase, the enzyme that catalyzes the transfer of a methyl group from 5-methyltetrahydrofolate in the remethylation of homocysteine to methionine. Deoxyadenosylcobalamin is a cofactor for mitochondrial methylmalonyl-CoA mutase, the enzyme that catalyzes the isomerization of methylmalonyl-CoA to succinyl-CoA.

The cobalamins can only be synthesized by certain microorganisms. Stored cobalamins in meats and dairy products provide the predominant dietary source for humans. Vitamin B$_{12}$ absorption is a complex mechanism requiring several steps. Ingested cobalamin binds to intrinsic factor, a glycoprotein formed by gastric parietal cells, in the upper small intestine [Donaldson, 1981]. The cobalamin–intrinsic factor complex subsequently interacts with specific receptors on ileal brush border cells, where the complex is dissociated and free cobalamin is absorbed into the circulation. In blood, vitamin B$_{12}$ is bound to several carrier proteins, the transcobalamins. Transcobalamin II is the predominant carrier protein for newly absorbed cobalamin, and the transcobalamin II–cobalamin complex is preferentially delivered to the liver, bone marrow, and other proliferating cells [Allen, 1976]. At the target tissue the transcobalamin II–cobalamin complex attaches to specific surface receptors and is subsequently transported into the cells by pinocytosis. Within the cell, proteolytic lysosomal enzymes degrade the carrier protein and release free cobalamin into the cytoplasm. Adenosylcobalamin is formed within mitochondria from hydroxycobalamin. The trivalent cobalt atom of hydroxycobalamin is successively reduced to monovalent cobalamin in enzymatic reactions catalyzed by reductase enzymes, and adenosylcobalamin is then formed from monovalent cobalamin through a reaction catalyzed by adenosyltransferase.

The recommended daily dietary allowance for vitamin B$_{12}$ is 5 to 10 μg in infants younger than 1 year of age and 15 to 65 μg for older children and adolescents.

Cobalamin deficiency

Symptomatic cobalamin deficiency, although rare in childhood, can occur as a consequence of inadequate dietary intake, congenital or acquired intrinsic factor deficiency, removal of the vitamin from the intestine by bacteria or parasites, malabsorptive states from surgical resection or chronic disease, and an inherited disease of the specific ileal receptor [Matthews and Linnell, 1982]. An infant with mild symptoms of vitamin B$_{12}$ deficiency secondary to the failure of the release of cobalamin into the cytoplasm from lysosomes has also been reported [Rosenblatt et al., 1985].

Inadequate cobalamin ingestion occurs predominantly in infants exclusively breast fed by strictly vegetarian mothers [Higginbottom et al., 1978; Kuhne et al., 1991]. Two forms of intrinsic factor deficiency (pernicious anemia) occur in the pediatric age group [Arthur, 1972]. Congenital pernicious anemia is an inherited disorder in which intrinsic factor deficiency is not associated with other structural or functional gastric abnormalities, and antibodies to intrinsic factor are not detected. Symptoms usually begin before 3 years of age. Juvenile pernicious anemia, which has characteristics similar to adult pernicious anemia because the intrinsic factor deficiency is associated with gastric atrophy, achlorhydria, antibodies to intrinsic factor or gastric parietal cells, and other endocrinopathies, usually becomes symptomatic late in childhood or early in adolescence.

A familial disorder in which cobalamin deficiency results from an impairment of transport across the specific ileal receptor has also been well documented [Grasbeck et al., 1960; Mackenzie et al., 1972].

Cobalamin deficiency predominantly affects the CNS (combined system degeneration) and blood (pernicious anemia) [Healton et al., 1991]. Characteristically, both systems are involved but either may be affected independently. Neurologic manifestations are caused by predominantly white matter degenerative lesions in the brain, spinal cord, and peripheral nerves. In young infants, irritability and lethargy may rapidly progress to coma. Mental retardation and signs of peripheral neuropathy are not uncommon. In older children, paresthesias, ataxia, hyperreflexia with positive Babinski sign, ankle clonus, and distal loss of vibratory and position sense are common. These neurologic abnormalities probably result from deficient methionine synthase activity [Hall, 1990].

Macrocytic, megaloblastic anemia results from failure of erythrocytes to mature. Giant megakaryocytes and enlarged polymorphonuclear leukocytes are present in the peripheral smear. Characteristics of this anemia are similar to those of the macrocytic anemia secondary to folate deficiency: cobalamin deficiency leads to a functional folate deficiency because methyltetrahydrofolate cannot be demethylated to its active tetrahydrofolate form (see Figure 42-12).

The serum vitamin B_{12} concentration in this anemia is below 100 pg/ml (normal, 140 to 700 pg/ml). Methylalonic acid is excreted in the urine. The amount of labeled vitamin B_{12} excreted in the urine after the ingestion of 1 to 2 μg of cobalt-57 or cobalt-60 cyanocobalamin followed by the intramuscular administration of 1 mg unlabeled vitamin B_{12} (Schilling test) is useful in assessing vitamin B_{12} absorption. Repeating the test with the addition of orally administered intrinsic factor will differentiate between pernicious anemia and other absorption defects.

Intramuscular injection of 1 to 5 μg of cobalamin results in prompt hematologic improvement and serves as a confirmatory test. Parenteral administration of 500 to 1000 μg of cobalamin at monthly intervals prevents recurrent deficiency; 1000 μg at weekly intervals is suggested for the treatment of neurologic deficits.

Cobalamin dependency

Inherited transcobalamin II deficiency. Transcobalamin II deficiency is an autosomal-recessive disorder characterized by failure to thrive, hypotonia, megaloblastic anemia, and recurrent infection [Hitzig et al., 1974]. Oral ulcerations and glossitis develop. The serum cobalamin concentration is normal despite the absence of transcobalamin II, the carrier protein for newly absorbed cobalamin. Parenteral administration of cobalamin (1000 μg/wk) results in remission of the clinical manifestations.

Cobalamin-dependent methylmalonic acidemia. Methylmalonic acidemia is characterized clinically by recurrent episodes of vomiting, ketoacidosis, dehydration, and lethargy [Matsui et al., 1983]. These acute episodes are frequently precipitated by infections or high-protein intake. Without appropriate treatment, acute episodes may be fatal or may lead to diffuse encephalopathy characterized by mental retardation, seizures, and other neurologic deficits. The condition results from the deficient methionine synthase activity for which cobalamin is a cofactor. Considerable clinical and genetic heterogeneity have been reported in these disorders [Watkins and Rosenblatt, 1989]. Parenteral treatment with cobalamin (1 mg hydroxy cobalamin intramuscularly, one to two times per week) has led to rapid improvement of neurologic signs in these conditions.

Cobalamin-dependent homocystinuria with methylmalonic acidemia. The combination of methylmalonic acidemia and homocystinuria has been reported in patients who have a deficiency of both methionine synthase and methylmalonyl-CoA mutase [Cooper and Rosenblatt, 1987; Goodman et al., 1970]. The disorder is caused by a defect that leads to diminished synthesis of methylcobalamin and deoxyadenosylcobalamin. The precise nature of the defect has not been identified but must occur after cellular uptake and before binding to an apoprotein that is shared by both coenzymes.

VITAMIN C (ASCORBIC ACID)

Vitamin C is a generic term for compounds that have the biologic activity of ascorbic acid [Englehard and Seifters, 1986; Levine, 1986]. Ascorbic acid (Figure

42-7), a six-carbon compound that is structurally related to glucose, can be synthesized by most vertebrates, but in humans and a few animals the last enzyme involved in ascorbate synthesis is missing. Ascorbic acid is reversibly oxidized in the body to dehydroascorbic acid, a compound that retains full vitamin C activity.

Vitamin C functions as a reducing agent in a variety of hydroxylation reactions, providing electrons to metal-containing enzymes to maintain the metal in the reduced form that is necessary for optimal activity. Known functions include the conversion of proline to hydroxyproline in collagen synthesis, the hydroxylation of lysine in carnitine synthesis, and the hydroxylation of dopamine to norepinephrine. Vitamin C also has a role in the synthesis of serotonin, several peptide hormones, and acetylcholine receptors [Block and Levine, 1991].

Ascorbic acid is available from fruits, vegetables, and potatoes. It is destroyed by heat, oxidation, and alkali but is stable in acid. Ascorbic acid is readily absorbed through the intestinal tract by simple diffusion, and its plasma concentration varies with the amount of intake. An active transport system in the choroid plexus maintains brain and CSF ascorbic acid concentrations within a relatively narrow range [Spector and Lorenzo, 1973].

The recommended daily dietary allowance for vitamin C is 30 to 35 mg for infants younger than 1 year of age and 40 to 60 mg for older children and adolescents. Consumption of ascorbic acid above the recommended daily allowance leads to increases in plasma concentrations and body stores, but because the renal threshold for ascorbic acid approximates 1.5 mg/dl, ingestion of amounts greater than 100 mg/day merely results in increased urinary excretion.

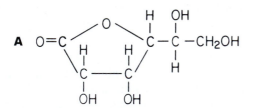

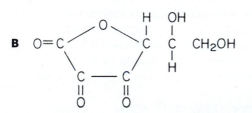

Figure 42-7 The chemical structure of **A,** ascorbic acid and **B,** deoxyascorbic acid, the physiologic active compounds of vitamin C.

Vitamin C deficiency

Symptomatic vitamin C deficiency (scurvy) is now quite rare. Infants exclusively fed cow's milk or unsupplemented evaporated milk formulas were the most prone to develop scurvy [Grewar, 1959]. Occasional instances of scurvy in children with peculiar dietary habits continue to be reported [Douglas et al., 1973; Ellis et al., 1984]. Little correlation exists between clinical manifestations of vitamin C deficiency and known molecular functions of the vitamin.

The onset of symptoms is delayed for 4 to 9 months after the initiation of a deficient diet. Initial manifestations include irritability, tachypnea, anorexia, and pallor. The most striking subsequent manifestations are a consequence of bone pain and a hemorrhagic diathesis. Bone pain leads to decreased voluntary movement, especially of the lower limbs (pseudoparalysis). Infants prefer to lay immobile in the supine position with the hips partially flexed and externally rotated (pithed-frog position). Attempts at examination and passive movement cause considerable pain. Petechial hemorrhages secondary to capillary fragility appear in the skin, initially surrounding hair follicles, and at the gums and may lead to frank purpura. Subarachnoid and subdural hemorrhages may occur. Extraocular muscle palsy may result from intraocular hemorrhage. Radiographs of the long bones, especially about the knee, reveal characteristic abnormalities, including thinning of the cortex, rarefaction of the epiphyses, and trabecular atrophy. Epiphyseal separation may occur. During healing the subperiosteal hemorrhages, not visualized in the acute stage, became calcified, and the healing bone assumes a characteristic dumbbell shape.

Plasma ascorbate levels reflect current intake rather than body stores. Leukocyte ascorbic acid concentrations below 30 mg/dl suggest depleted stores.

Daily administration of 100 to 200 mg of ascorbic acid for 10 days leads to rapid improvement in clinical symptoms. Bone abnormalities resolve completely within a few months.

Transient neonatal tyrosinemia. Transient tyrosinemia is present in 0.2% to 10% of neonates and may persist for several months [Goldsmith, 1983]. It is more common in premature infants and least common in breast-fed term neonates. Although the molecular basis of the disorder has not been fully elucidated, a combination of excessive protein intake and relative deficiency of the activity of the enzyme hydroxyphenylpyruvate oxidase is probably responsible. Ascorbic acid facilitates the activity of this hydroxylation enzyme.

Lethargy, feeding difficulties, hypotonia, and prolonged jaundice have been associated with tyrosinemia, although many infants are asymptomatic. Mild mental retardation may be a long-term sequela [Mamunes et al., 1976; Menkes et al., 1972].

In addition to hypertyrosinemia, the blood concentration of phenylalanine is increased in affected neonates, and urinary excretion of tyrosine and some of its metabolites is also increased.

A reduction of protein intake to 2 to 3 g/kg/day usually corrects the hypertyrosinemia. In some infants, additional supplementation with ascorbic acid (100 to 400 mg/day) produces a dramatic response.

VITAMIN D

Vitamin D is the generic term for a group of steroid compounds that function in the regulation of calcium and phosphate homeostasis by promoting the absorption of calcium and phosphorus from the intestine, enhancing calcium resorption by the kidney in conjunction with the parathyroid hormone, and mobilizing calcium from the bone [Bell, 1985; Henry and Norman, 1984]. Vitamin D_2 (calciferol) is derived from the plant sterol ergosterol, and vitamin D_3 (cholecalciferol) is derived from 7-dehydrocholesterol in skin. Calciferol and cholecalciferol are derived from respective provitamins by a nonenzymatic photochemical reaction activated by ultraviolet light, which results in the cleavage of the B-sterol ring to form a diene bridge. In humans the metabolic fate and physiologic properties of vitamin D_2 and vitamin D_3 are similar. 7-Dehydrocholesterol is normally present in the skin and is converted to cholecalciferol by solar ultraviolet radiation. Under optimal exposure to sunlight, dietary supplementation of vitamin D is not necessary because cholecalciferol is transported to the liver and stored.

The active form of vitamin D is calcitriol (1,25-dihydroxycholecalciferol), formed from cholecalciferol by two successive hydroxylations (Figure 42-8). The initial hydroxylation to calcidiol 25-hydroxycholecalciferol occurs in the liver, and the second hydroxylation to cal-

citriol occurs in the kidney. The activity of the kidney mitochondrial hydroxylase, which catalyzes the second hydroxylation, is stimulated by parathyroid hormone and increases with deficiencies of vitamin D, calcium, and phosphate.

Dietary vitamin D and vitamin D_3 are absorbed from the small intestine. Bile is essential for absorption. After absorption the vitamin, bound to a lipoprotein complex, is transported in lymph chylomicrons to the liver, where it is stored before its hydroxylation to calcidiol. Calcidiol is the major circulating form of vitamin D in the blood.

Calcitriol is hydroxylated to 1,24,25-trihydroxycalciferol by a renal hydroxylase that also hydroxylates 25-hydroxycalciferol to 24,25-dihydroxycalciferol. These compounds have less vitamin D activity than calcitriol and probably represent excretory compounds excreted in the bile.

The recommended daily dietary allowance for vitamin D is 7.5 to 10 μg cholecalciferol for infants younger than 1 year of age and 10 μg for older children and adolescents.

Vitamin D deficiency

Symptomatic vitamin D deficiency can occur as a consequence of inadequate dietary intake [Bachrach et al., 1979; Edidin et al., 1980], inadequate exposure to sunlight, malabsorption states, chronic hepatic or renal disease, and the administration of antiepileptic drugs. Clinical manifestations predominantly affect the bone, leading to rickets in children and osteomalacia in adults. The bony abnormalities in rickets are secondary to inadequate mineralization of osteoid tissue. Craniotabes, or thinning of the inner table of the skull, is an early manifestation in infants. Rickets is further characterized by epiphyseal enlargements at the wrists, ankles, and costochondral junctions; bending of the shafts of long bones; scoliosis; and kyphosis.

Neurologic manifestations are characterized by tetany, which occurs when the metabolic abnormality leads to hypocalcemia. Symptoms are not present in latent tetany, but elicitation of Chvostek, Trousseau, and Erb signs is evidence of increased neuromuscular irritability. Latent tetany is usually associated with serum calcium concentrations between 7.0 and 7.5 mg/dl. Manifest tetany, characterized by symptomatic carpopedal spasm, laryngospasm, or convulsions, is usually associated with serum calcium concentrations below 7.0 mg/dl.

The diagnosis of rickets is confirmed by radiologic examination. Wrist radiographs are best for early diagnosis and demonstrate the characteristic widened, frayed, concave distal ends of the ulna and radius. The distance between the ends of these long bones and the carpal bones is increased because the large rachitic metaphysis is not calcified. Plasma alkaline phosphatase level is elevated, and the serum phosphorus concentra-

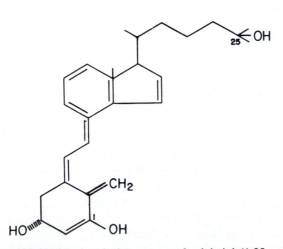

Figure 42-8 The chemical structure of calcitriol (1,25-dihydroxycholecalciferol), the active form of vitamin D.

tion is usually below 4 mg/dl. The serum calcium concentration may be normal or reduced.

Daily administration of 0.2 to 0.5 μg of calcitriol leads to healing, demonstrable on radiographs within 2 to 4 weeks. In tetany, calcium supplementation is also necessary.

Vitamin D dependency

Vitamin D–dependent rickets–type I. Vitamin D–dependent rickets–type I is an inborn error of metabolism transmitted as an autosomal-recessive disorder and is characterized by hypotonia, weakness, failure to thrive, tetany, and convulsions in the first year of life [Rassmussen and Anast, 1983]. The disorder is caused by deficient activity of the renal L-hydroxylase that catalyzes the synthesis of calcitriol from calcidiol.

Bone radiographs are indistinguishable from those of vitamin D deficiency. Serum alkaline phosphatase level is elevated, and the phosphorus concentration is normal or low. Hypocalcemia is common. The serum calcidiol concentration is normal, but the calcitriol concentration is reduced.

Treatment with pharmacologic dosages of vitamin D (vitamin D_3, 5000 to 40,000 units/day; calcitriol, 1 to 3 μg/day) reverses the manifestations of rickets and permits normal growth.

Vitamin D intoxication

Symptoms of vitamin D intoxication develop 1 to 3 months after excessive intake of the vitamin. Clinical manifestations include irritability, hypotonia, polydypsia, polyuria, and constipation. Hypertension with retinopathy, aortic stenosis, corneal and conjunctival clouding, and nephropathy occur in chronic cases. Laboratory findings include hypercalcemia, hypercalciuria, and metastatic calcifications on radiographs of long bones. Treatment consists of discontinuing vitamin D ingestion and decreasing calcium intake.

TOCOPHEROL (VITAMIN E)

Vitamin E is the generic term for a group of fat-soluble compounds that function as scavengers of free radicals, protecting polyunsaturated fatty acids in subcellular organelles from oxidation by free radicals generated in normal metabolic reactions or by toxic compounds. α-Tocopherol is the most important of these compounds and is widely distributed in foods, especially vegetable oils (Figure 42-9).

Absorption of vitamin E depends on the intestinal digestion and absorption of fat and the presence of bile. Once absorbed, the vitamin enters lymph channels and, in chylomicrons and very low density lipopoteins, is transported to the blood where it equilibrates with plasma lipoproteins. It is stored predominantly in

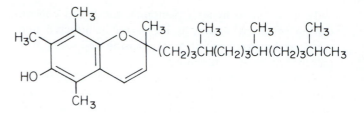

Figure 42-9 The chemical structure of alpha-tocopherol, the most prevalent vitamin E in foods.

adipose tissue. Tissue stores will provide a source for the vitamin for long periods. Blood levels reflect recent dietary intake and absorption rather than body stores.

The recommended dietary allowance of vitamin E is 3 to 4 μg of α-tocopherol equivalents per day for infants younger than 1 year of age and 6 to 7 mg/day for older children and adolescents.

Vitamin E deficiency

Vitamin E deficiency occurs predominantly in disorders associated with either chronic fat malabsorption (e.g., cystic fibrosis, celiac disease, chronic cholestatic hepatobiliary disorders including billary atresia, short bowel syndrome) or a deficiency of plasma lipoproteins (e.g., abetalipoproteinemia) [Sokol, 1990]. A neurologic degenerative syndrome associated with selective vitamin A deficiency not associated with fat malabsorption has also recently been documented [Harding et al., 1985; Krendel et al., 1987].

Clinical manifestations of vitamin E deficiency include progressive weakness, ataxia, ophthalmoplegia, loss of position and vibratory sense, and in some instances, especially in abetalipoproteinemia, progressive visual impairment associated with retinitis segmentosa [Sokol, 1990].

Neuropathologic features include cerebellar atrophy and loss of nerve cell bodies in the third and fourth cranial nerve nuclei and axonal dystrophy (e.g., swollen, dystrophic axons, spheroids) in the posterior columns, Clarke column, and dorsal and ventral spinocerebellar tracts of the spinal cord [Rosenblum et al., 1981]. Premature lipofuscin accumulation in dorsal horn and peripheral nerve Schwann cell cytoplasm has also been reported [Werlin et al., 1953].

Measurement of serum lipid concentrations documents most instances of vitamin E deficiency. The normal lower limit for adolescents is 5 mg/ml and is lower for younger infants [Farrel et al., 1978]. Because vitamin E is bound to lipoproteins in the plasma, the ratio of vitamin E to total serum lipid concentration reflects vitamin E status more accurately in hyperlipidemic states. Limits of normal for this ratio are 0.8 mg total tocopherol/g total lipid in adolescents and 0.6 mg/g

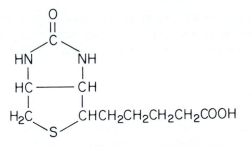

Figure 42-10 The chemical structure of biotin.

in infants and children. Serum vitamin A concentrations do not accurately reflect vitamin A states in patients with abetaliproproteinemia.

In patients with abetalipoproteinemia, dietary supplementation with vitamin E (100 to 200 mg/kg/day) before 1 year of age prevented the development of retinopathy and prevented, stabilized, or improved the neurologic disorder [Muller et al., 1977]. The neurologic function of children with vitamin E deficiency associated with chronic cholestasis was also significantly improved by large oral dosages (up to 10 mg/kg/day) or intramuscular injection of α-tocopherol (0.8 to 2.0 IU/kg/day) [Lemonnier et al., 1990; Perlmutter et al., 1987; Sokol et al., 1985].

BIOTIN (VITAMIN H)

Biotin is a cofactor for four carboxylation enzymes: pyruvate carboxylase, acetyl-CoA carboxylase, propionyl-CoA carboxylase, and 3-methylcrotonyl carboxylase (Figure 42-10) [Bartlett et al., 1985]. These enzymes are all involved in carbon-chain elongation reactions: pyruvate carboxylase in gluconeogenesis, acetyl-CoA carboxylase in fatty acid synthesis, propionyl-CoA carboxylase in propionate metabolism, and 3-methylcrotonyl carboxylase in leucine catabolism. In these reactions, biotin is linked to a lysine residue of the apoenzyme in a reaction catalyzed by the enzyme holocarboxylase synthetase to form the functional carboxylase holoenzyme. Biotin is present in low concentrations in numerous foods [Roth, 1981]. The enzyme biotinidase cleaves biotin from biocytin (biotin-lysine) and from larger biotinyl-peptide fragments formed in the degradation of the carboxylase, thus allowing for biotin reuse.

Biotin-synthesizing bacteria in the small intestine also serve as a major nutritional source. Biotin is absorbed through the intestine by active transport mechanisms [Said et al., 1990]. In the blood, it is bound to proteins. It is excreted in the urine and feces.

The recommended daily dietary allowance is 10 to 15 μg for neonates and infants younger than 1 year of age and 20 to 100 μg for older children and adolescents.

Biotin deficiency

Symptomatic biotin deficiency from inadequate dietary intake is quite rare. Two children with symptomatic biotin deficiency associated with the ingestion of large quantities of raw albumen, which contains avidin (a glycoprotein that binds biotin so effectively that its intestinal absorption is prevented), have been reported [Scott, 1958; Sweetman et al., 1981]. Biotin deficiency has also been reported as a consequence of parenteral hyperalimentation and chronic hemodialysis [Mock et al., 1981; Yatzidis et al., 1984].

Clinical manifestations of biotin deficiency include a generalized, scaly, erythematous rash resembling seborrheic dermatitis; alopecia totalis; anorexia; severe metabolic acidosis; and neurologic manifestations that include developmental delay or dementia, seizures, progressive ataxia, and hearing loss. In the neonate and young infant the clinical manifestations may evolve very rapidly, with vomiting, failure to thrive, hypotonia, and severe metabolic acidosis leading to coma and death before other manifestations are evident.

Characteristic laboratory findings in addition to the metabolic acidosis include a specific organic aciduria (3-methylcrotonylglycine, 3-hydroxyisovaleric acid, 3-hydroxypropionic acid, and 2-methylcitric acid).

Symptoms and signs are rapidly reversed by the administration of 5 to 10 mg of biotin.

Biotin dependency

Biotin-dependent propionic acidemia. Propionic acidemia results from a deficiency of the enzyme propionyl CoA carboxylase. The enzyme catalyzes the conversion of propionyl-CoA to methylmalonyl-CoA [Lardy and Adler, 1956]. Biotin is an essential cofactor in this reaction.

Propionic acidemia is characterized by the rapid onset of an overwhelming illness with severe vomiting and dehydration that leads to lethargy and coma [Wolf et al., 1981]. In many patients the first episode occurs in the neonatal period and, if not recognized and treated appropriately, leads to death. In others the illness first appears in early infancy, often precipitated by a febrile illness or high protein intake, with vomiting, lethargy, hypotonia, and seizures (often myoclonic) progressing to coma.

Laboratory evaluation during an acute episode discloses severe ketoacidosis with markedly elevated plasma glycine concentrations. Plasma propionate concentrations may be 1000 to 2000 times normal. Hyperammonemia may also be striking.

Management requires stringent dietary therapy, with restriction of the intake of isoleucine, valine, threonine, and methionine to amounts required for growth. In one patient, administration of pharmacologic dosages of biotin (5 mg twice daily) proved to be a useful adjunct to dietary therapy [Barnes et al., 1970]. Management of acute episodes requires large amounts of fluids, electrolytes, and glucose and supplementary protein sufficient to minimize tissue catabolism. In some instances, multiple exchange transfusion or peritoneal dialysis is necessary.

Biotin-dependent holocarboxylase synthetase deficiency (neonatal multiple carboxylase deficiency). Neonatal multiple carboxylase deficiency characteristically first appears with vomiting, lethargy, and hypotonia associated with ketoacidosis, lactic acidosis, and organic aciduria in the first few days of life [Wolf and Feldman, 1982]. The activity of all four biotin-dependent carboxylation enzymes is reduced in leukocytes and cultured skin fibroblasts, but serum and urinary biotin concentrations are normal. The condition is believed to result from deficient activity of the enzyme holocarboxylase synthetase, the enzyme that attaches biotin to the various carboxylases.

Most patients improve dramatically after the oral administration of pharmacologic amounts of biotin (10 mg/day) [Wolf et al., 1981].

Biotinidase deficiency (late-onset multiple carboxylase deficiency). The enzyme biotinidase cleaves biotin from biocytin and biotin-polypeptides derived from partially degraded carboxylases, thus allowing for reuse of the vitamin. Deficient biotinidase activity therefore leads to the clinical manifestations and metabolic abnormalities of biotin deficiency. Clinical manifestations, although quite variable, characteristically begin at 2 to 3 months of age. Seizures, episodic ataxia, hyperventilation, high-frequency hearing loss, optic atrophy, and developmental delay are the prominent neurologic manifestations [Wolf et al., 1983]. Skin rash, alopecia, chronic candidiasis, and conjunctivitis are associated features.

Biochemical abnormalities usually include the presence of lactic acidosis, hyperammonemia, and organic aciduria (3-methylcrotonylglycine, 3-hydroxyisovaleric acid, 3-hydroxypropionic acid, and 2-methylcitric acid). spinal fluid lactate is increased [Diamantopoulos et al., 1986]. Immunologic abnormalities characterized by a decrease in the number of B cells and T cells have also been reported [Cowan et al., 1979]. The carboxylase activity of cultured skin fibroblasts from affected patients is normal because sufficient biotin and biotinidase are usually present in the culture medium [Marsac et al., 1983]. Biotinidase deficiency is readily demonstrable by an assay of the enzyme in blood. Heterozygotes have 50% biotinidase activity, consistent with autosomal-recessive transmission. A colorimetric screening test using dried blood spotted on filter paper detected 4 unrelated patients in 81,243 newborns, suggesting a prevalence rate of 1 in 20,000 [Wolf et al., 1985].

Except for hearing and visual loss, clinical manifestations are readily preventable by administering pharmacologic dosages of biotin (10 mg/day). A lower dosage may be sufficient in some patients.

VITAMIN K

Vitamin K is a fat-soluble vitamin essential for the biosynthesis of several blood clotting factors, including prothrombin (factor II), proconvertin (factor VII), plasma converting factor (Christmas factor, factor IX), and Stuart factor (factor X) [Corrigan, 1981; Olsen, 1984]. Vitamin K_1 (phylloquinone) is found in chloroplasts of plant leaves and in many vegetable oils, and vitamin K_2 (menaquinones), a series of compounds in which the phytyl chain in vitamin K_1 has been replaced by a side chain containing 2 to 13 phytyl units, are synthesized predominantly by a gram-positive bacteria (Figure 42-11). Vitamin K_3 (menadione) is a synthetic compound with properties similar to those of phylloquinone.

Vitamin K acts as an essential cofactor for hepatic microsomal enzyme systems that convert the biologically inactive precursors of prothrombin, proconvertin, and plasma thromboplastin components to the active compounds participating in the events necessary for normal blood clotting. In this process, vitamin K converts residues of phytic-bound glutamic acid in each of the precursors into γ-carboxyglutamyl residues. This conversion activates the blood clotting proteins by allowing them to bind calcium ions. The calcium-carboxyglutamyl proteins are subsequently bound to phospholipid surfaces.

In the process of γ-carboxylation of the glutamate residues, vitamin K quinone is converted to the 2,3-epoxide. An enzyme-dependent salvage mechanism for the regeneration of the active vitamin K catalyzed by

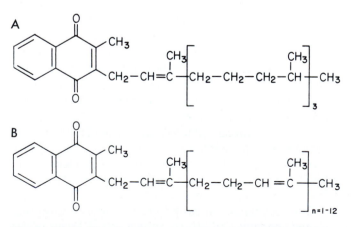

Figure 42-11 The chemical structure of vitamin K. **A,** Phylloquinone found in chloroplasts. **B,** Menaquinones synthesized by bacteria in intestinal flora.

the hepatic enzyme epoxide reductase is blocked by coumadin.

The daily recommended dietary allowance for vitamin K is 5 to 10 μg for infants younger than 1 year of age and 15 to 30 μg for older children and adolescents. Such amounts are readily available when average diets are supplemented by the menaquinones produced by intestinal bacteria.

Vitamin K is absorbed through the small intestine. Bile salts and pancreatic secretions are necessary for optimal absorption. Once absorbed, it is incorporated into chylomicrons, transported to the liver, and bound to very low–density lipoproteins, through which it is transported to other tissues.

Vitamin K deficiency

Vitamin K deficiency results in a hemorrhagic diathesis. The newborn is particularly susceptible because vitamin K stores are deficient and factor II, IV, VII, IX, and X concentrations are characteristically only 50% of normal. These concentrations continue to decline for 48 to 72 hours after birth but subsequently increase slowly as a result of the absorption of dietary vitamin K and the initiation of synthesis by bacterial flora in the intestine. Breast-fed infants are particularly prone to develop the disorder because the vitamin K content of breast milk is poor. Characteristically, hemorrhages appear on the second or third day of life.

Intracranial hemorrhages, the most serious neurologic consequence, rarely occur without hemorrhage into other tissues. Hemorrhagic disease in the newborn is now rare because of the routine prophylactic administration of vitamin K on the first day of life but may occur in the newborn and in older children in association with conditions impairing fat absorption and parenteral alimentation and after the chronic administration of broad-spectrum antibiotics, which sterilize the intestinal tract.

Laboratory studies indicate a prolonged prothrombin and partial thromboplastin time with normal platelet counts and fibrinogen concentrations.

Parenteral administration of 1 mg vitamin K is usually recommended, although 0.25 μg is sufficient in most instances. When the vitamin K deficiency is associated with chronic disease, 1 to 5 mg of vitamin K_1 should be administered parenterally at weekly intervals.

FOLATE (VITAMIN M)

The folates, a group of pterydine compounds composed of pteroic acid linked to a variable number of glutamate residues, have a fundamental role in cell growth and division [Rowe, 1983]. Fully reduced methyltetrahydrofolate, formed from other folates in a reaction catalyzed by the enzyme dihydrofolate reductase, is the active cofactor (Figure 42-12). Known functions of folate include one-carbon transfer reactions in de novo purine synthesis and in the synthesis of methionine from homocysteine, serine from glycine, and deoxythymidylic acid from deoxyuridylic acid. Folate is also a cofactor in the conversion of formiminoglutamic acid to glutamic acid in the degradation of histidine.

Dietary folates consist predominantly of folate polyglutamates. During the process of absorption and transport across the jejunum, most polyglutamates are hydrolyzed to the monoglutamate and subsequently reduced and methylated to methyltetrahydrofolate [Halstead, 1980]. After absorption, methyltetrahydrofolate is rapidly transported to tissues and stored in the liver. Considerable liver methyltetrahydrofolate is excreted in the bile and resorbed in the small intestine. In the plasma, folates are transported in either the free form or loosely bound to protein. A specific folate-binding protein, which is found in low concentration in normal serum, is present in increased concentration in folate deficiency. A different folate-binding protein with a high affinity for methyltetrahydrofolate is present in umbilical cord blood, accounting for the preferential uptake of folate by the fetus even in folate-depleted mothers. The choroid plexus also contains a folate-binding protein with a high affinity for methyltetrahydrofolate, reflecting the dependency of the CNS on methyltetrahydrofolate because of a low concentration of dihydrofolate reductase [Levitt et al., 1971; Spector and Lorenzo, 1975].

Methyltetrahydrofolate and other folate derivatives are excreted in the urine. Some folate is resorbed by the renal tubule.

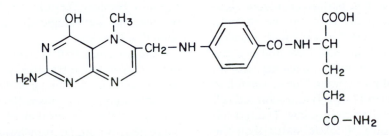

Figure 42-12 The chemical structure of methyltetrahydrofolate, the active cofactor in folate metabolism.

The recommended daily dietary allowance for folate is 25 to 35 μg for infants younger than 1 year of age and 50 to 150 μg for older children and adolescents. During pregnancy, lactation, and other conditions characterized by rapid cell division (e.g., hemolytic anemia) the folate requirement can increase to 350 μg/day.

Folate deficiency

Inadequate dietary intake is rarely the sole cause of folate deficiency but can occur in populations exclusively fed well-boiled foods or in infants for whom goat's milk, which is deficient in folate, forms the major dietary staple. Folate deficiency more commonly results from conditions associated with increased folate requirements or diseases associated with abnormalities of folate absorption, use, or excretion. Pregnancy, prematurity, and diseases characterized by increased cell turnover (e.g., hemolytic anemia) are conditions associated with an increased folate requirement. The premature infant is especially prone to develop this deficiency, not only because the folate stores (normally formed during the third trimester) are inadequate, but also because rapid growth is taking place and renal tubular conservation mechanisms are not fully developed [Landon and Hey, 1974]. Malabsorption defects and hepatic disease may interfere with folate absorption. Several drugs, including phenytoin, phenobarbital, oral contraceptives, and cycloserine, impede folate absorption and use [Waxman et al., 1970]. Methotrexate, trimetheprin, and triamterene specifically inhibit dihydrofolate reduction, preventing methyltetrahydrofolate synthesis.

A progressive megaloblastic anemia, irritability, diarrhea, and failure to gain weight are the clinical manifestations of folate deficiency in infants. More severe manifestations of an organic brain syndrome may also occur [Reynolds et al., 1973]. In experimental animals, folate deficiency during pregnancy leads to abortion, stillbirth, and congenital anomalies [Araawkawa, 1970], but the association of folate deficiency and congenital anomalies in human beings remains controversial [Hall, 1972; Hibbard and Hibbard, 1968].

No single laboratory test is optimal for the documentation of folate deficiency. Megaloblastic anemia is associated with a low reticulocyte count. Nucleated erythrocytes may be present in peripheral blood. Neutropenia and thrombocytopenia may also be present. Vitamin B_{12} deficiency must be excluded because prolonged treatment with folic acid may improve the megaloblastic anemia of vitamin B_{12} deficiency without affecting the neurologic abnormalities. The serum folate concentrations (normal, 5 to 12 ng/ml) and total red cell content (normal, 150 to 600 ng/ml) are low. The red cell content is a better measure of folate status than the serum concentration. Formiminoglutamic acid is excreted in the urine, especially after an oral loading dose of histidine. Because the megaloblastic anemia improves within 72 hours, parenteral administration of 200 μg of folic acid can be used as a diagnostic test.

Treatment with 2 to 5 mg of folic (pteroylglutamic) acid for 3 to 4 weeks is usually sufficient to reverse the clinical manifestations of deficiency.

Folate dependency

Congenital folate malabsorption syndromes. Specific folate absorption defects have been described in several infants [Lanzkowsky, 1970; Santiago-Borrero et al., 1973; Steinschneider et al., 1990; Su, 1976]. In affected infants, selective deficiency in the transport of folates in the intestinal tract and across the blood-brain barrier occurs. In addition to failure to thrive, diarrhea, and megaloblastic anemia, affected patients have CNS abnormalities of varying severity. Neurologic defects range from learning disability to profound mental retardation, seizures, progressive athetosis, and peripheral neuropathy. One patient developed basal ganglia calcifications during adolescence. The megaloblastic anemia but not the progression of neurologic abnormalities responded to folate supplementation (10 to 40 mg/day of folic acid); parenteral administration was necessary in some patients [Ponce et al., 1981]. Parenteral therapy with folinic acid, a reduced folate derivative more readily transported across the blood-brain barrier, improved the CNS deficit and elevated the folate concentration in one patient [Steinschneider et al., 1990]. The variability in clinical presentation and responsiveness to folate therapy suggest that different genotypic mutations are involved.

Folate-dependent dihydrofolate reductase deficiency. Three patients with a suspected deficiency of dihydrofolate reductase, the enzyme catalyzing the reduction of folate derivatives to methyltetrahydrofolate, have been reported [Tauro et al., 1976; Walters 1967]. The family history suggested that this enzyme defect may result in abortion or stillbirth. The reported patients first required treatment for failure to thrive and a severe megaloblastic anemia in early infancy. Mental retardation of varying degree was subsequently noted. The hematologic abnormality responded to the intramuscular administration of folinic acid (100 μg to 6 mg/day). Because therapy was delayed and intermittent, whether the neurologic deficit could have been prevented is not clear.

Folate-dependent formimino transferase deficiency. Formimino transferase catalyzes the conversion of N-formiminoglutamic acid to glutamic acid, the final step in histidine catabolism. Several children in whom an excessive urinary excretion of formiminoglutamic acid suggested formimino transferase deficiency have been reported [Rowe, 1983]. Two clinically and biochemically distinct syndromes emerge from these descriptions. In one, mild neurologic deficits (e.g., mild mental retardation, learning disabilities, attention deficit disorder, hypotonia, clumsiness) are associated with massive urinary formiminoglutamic acid excretion, normal serum folate concentrations, and normal hematologic studies. In some of these patients, folate administered either orally as folic acid or intramuscularly as tetrahydrofolate decreased formiminoglutamic acid excretion [Niederwieser et al., 1974; Perry et al., 1975]. In the other syndrome, severe mental retardation, diffuse cerebral atrophy, and increased serum folate concentrations and formiminoglutamic acid urinary excretion were associated with a partial deficit of formimino transferase activity in liver biopsy specimens or erythrocytes. One of these children had a folate-responsive megaloblastic anemia.

REFERENCES

Abernathy RS. Bulging fontanelle as a presenting sign in cystic fibrosis. Am J Dis Child 1976; 130:1360.

Allen RH. The plasma transport of vitamin B_{12}. Br J Haematol 1976; 33:161.

Araawkawa T. Congenital defects in folate utilization. Am J Med 1970; 48:594.

Arthur LJH. Juvenile pernicious anemia. Proc R Soc Med 1972; 65:728.

Bachrach S, Fisher J, Parker JS. An outbreak of vitamin D deficiency rickets in a susceptible population. Pediatrics 1979; 64:871.

Barnes HD, Hull D, Balgobin L, et al. Biotin responsive propionic acidemia. Lancet 1970; 2:244.

Bartlett K, Ghneim HK, Stirk HK, et al. Enzyme studies in biotin-responsive disorders. J Inherited Metab Dis 1985; 8(suppl 1):46.

Bauernfeind JC, Miller ON. Vitamin B_6: nutritional and pharmacologic usage, stability, bioavailability, antagonists and safety. In: Human vitamin B_3 requirements. Washington, DC: National Academy of Sciences, 1987.

Bejsovec M, Kulenda Z, Ponca E. Familial intrauterine convulsions in pyridoxine dependency. Arch Dis Child 1967; 42:201.

Bell NH. Vitamin D—endocrine system. J Clin Invest 1985; 76:1.

Bendich A, Langseth L. Safety of vitamin A. Am J Clin Nutr 1989; 49:385.

Bennett MJ, Marlow N, Pollin RJ, et al. Glutaric aciduria type I: biochemical and postmortem findings. Eur J Pediatr 1986; 145:403.

Berger A, Schaumburg HH. Move on neuropathy from pyridoxine abuse. N Engl J Med 1984; 311:986.

Bernofsky C. Physiologic aspects of pyridine nucleotide regulation in mammals. Mol Cell Biochem 1980; 33:135.

Berson EL, Shih VE, Sullivan PL. Ocular findings in patients with gyrate atrophy on pyridoxine and low protein, low arginine diets. Ophthalmology 1981; 88:311.

Block G, Levine M. Vitamin C: a new look. Ann Intern Med 1991; 114:909.

Bonner DM, Suyama Y, Domoss A. Genetic fine structure and enzyme formation. Fed Proc 1960; 19:926.

Brandt NJ, Gregerson N, Christensen E, et al. Treatment of glutaryl-CoA dehydrogenase deficiency (glutaric aciduria). J Pediatr 1979; 94:669.

Brivet M, Tardicu M, Khellaf A, et al. Riboflavin responsive ethylmalonic-adipic aciduria in a 9 month old boy with liver cirrhosis, myopathy, and encephalopathy. J Inherited Metab Dis 1991; 14:333.

Brody LC, Mitchell GA, Obie C, et al. Ornithine delta aminotransferase mutations in gyrate atrophy. J Biol Chem 1992; 267:3302.

Christensen E, Brandt NJ. Studies on glutaryl-CoA dehydrogenase in leukocytes, fibroblasts and amniotic fluid cells: the normal enzymes and the mutant form in patients with glutaric aciduria. Clin Chim Acta 1978; 88:267.

Chytil F, Ong D. Intracellular vitamin A-binding proteins. Annu Rev Nutr 1987; 7:321.

Cochrane WA, Collins-Williams C, Donahue WL. Superior hemorrhagic polioencephalitis (Wemicke's disease) occurring in an infant—probably due to thiamine deficiency from use of a soybean product. Pediatrics 1961; 28:771.

Cooper BA, Rosenblatt DS. Inherited defects of vitamin B_{12} metabolism. Annu Rev Nutr 1987; 7:291.

Cooper JR, Itokawa Y, Pincus JH. Thiamine triphosphate deficiency in subacute necrotizing encephalomyelopathy. Science 1969; 164:74.

Corrigan JJ. The vitamin K dependent proteins. Adv Pediatr 1981; 28:57.

Coursin DB. Convulsive seizures in infants with pyridoxine deficient diets. JAMA 1954; 213:1867.

Cowan MJ, Wara DW, Packman S, et al. Multiple biotin dependent carboxylase deficiency associated with defects in T-cell and B-cell immunity. Lancet 1979; 2:115.

Dancis J, Levitz M, Miller S, et al. Maple syrup urine disease. Br Med J 1959; 1:91.

Davis RE. Clinical chemistry of vitamin B_{12}. Adv Clin Chem 1985; 24:163.

Davis RE, Leke GC. Clinical chemistry of thiamine. Adv Clin Chem 1983; 23:93.

DeGroot CJ, Hommes FA. Further speculation on the pathogenesis of Leigh's encephalomyelopathy. J Pediatr 1973; 82:541.

DeVisser M, Scholte HR, Schutgens RBH. Riboflavin responsive lipid storage myopathy and glutaric aciduria of early adult onset. Neurology 1986; 36:367.

Diamantopoulos N, Painter MJ, Wolf B, et al. Biotinidase deficiency: accumulation of lactate in brain and response to physiologic doses of biotin. Neurology 1986; 36:1107.

Donaldson RM Jr. Intrinsic factor and the transport of cobalamin. In: Jowson LR, ed. Physiology of the gastrointestinal tract. New York: Raven Press, 1981.

Douglas NL, Liakos D, Vlachos P. Scurvy in a 4 year old child. Am J Dis Child 1973; 126:712.

Dunn HG, Dolman CL. Necrotizing encephalomyelopathy. Eur Neurol 1972; 7:34.

Duran M, Wadman SK. Thiamine responsive inborn errors of metabolism. J Inherited Metab Dis 1985; 8(suppl 1):70.

Dusheiko G, Kew MC, Joffe BI, et al. Recurrent hypoglycemia associated with glutaric aciduria type II in an adult. N Engl J Med 1979; 301:1405.

Edidin DV, Levitsky LL, Schey W, et al. Resurgence of nutritional rickets associated with breast feeding and special dietary practices. Pediatrics 1980; 65:232.

Ellis CN, Vanduveen EE, Rassmussen JE. Scurvy: a case caused by peculiar dietary habits. Arch Dermatol 1984; 120:1212.

Englehard S, Seifters S. The biochemical functions of ascorbic acid. Annu Rev Nutr 1986; 6:365.

Evans OB. Lactic acidosis in childhood. Pediatr Neurol 1986; 2:5.

Farrell PM, Levine SL, Murphy D, et al. Plasma tocopherol levels and tocopherol-lipid relationship in a normal population of children as compared to healthy adults. Am J Clin Nutr 1978; 31:1720.

Fowler B. Recent advances in the mechanism of pyridoxine responsive disorders. J Inherited Metab Dis 1985; 8(suppl 1):76.

Frimpter GW. Cystathioninuria: nature of the defect. Science 1965; 149:1095.

Goldsmith LA. Tyrosinemia and related disorders. In: Stanbury JB,

Wyngaarden JB, Frederickson DS, et al., eds. Metabolic basis of inherited disease, 5th ed. New York: McGraw-Hill, 1983.

Goodman DS. Vitamin A and retinoids in health and disease. N Engl J Med 1984; 310:1023.

Goodman SI, Moe PB, Hammond KB, et al. Homocystinuria with methylmalonic aciduria: two cases in a sibship. Biochem Med 1970; 4:500.

Goodman SI, Morenberg MD, Shikes RH, et al. Glutaric aciduria: biochemical and morphologic considerations. J Pediatr 1977; 90:746.

Grasbeck R, Gordin R, Kantero I, et al. Selective vitamin B_{12} malabsorption and proteinuria in young people: a syndrome. Acta Med Scand 1960; 167:289.

Gregerson N. Riboflavin responsive deficits of beta oxidation. J Inherited Metab Dis 1985; 8(suppl 1):65.

Gregerson N, Wintzensen H, Kolvraa S, et al. C6-C10 dicarboxylic aciduria: investigation of a patient with riboflavin responsive multiple acyl-CoA dehydrogenation defects. Pediatr Res 1982; 16:861.

Grewar D. Scurvy and its prevention by vitamin C fortified evaporated milk. Can Med Assoc J 1959; 80:977.

Haenggeli CA, Girardin E, Paunier L. Pyridoxine-dependent seizures, clinical and therapeutic aspects. Eur J Pediat 1991; 150:452.

Hall CA. Function of vitamin B_{12} in the central nervous system revealed by congenital defects. Am J Hematol 1990; 34:121.

Hall MM. Folic acid deficiency and congenital malformation. Gynecol Br Commonwealth 1972; 79:159.

Halstead CH. Intestinal absorption and malabsorption of folates. Annu Rev Med 1980; 31:79.

Harding AE, Matthews S, Jones S, et al. Spinocerebellar degeneration associated with selective defect of vitamin E absorption. N Engl J Med 1985; 313:32.

Harpey IP, Charpentier C, Goodman SI, et al. Multiple acyl-CoA dehydrogenase deficiency in pregnancy and caused by a defect in riboflavin metabolism in the mother. J Pediatr 1983; 103:394.

Hatoff DE, Gertler SL, Miya K, et al. Hypervitaminosis A unmasked by acute viral hepatitis. Gastroenterology 1982; 82:124.

Haworth C, Evans DIK, Mitra I, et al. Thiamine responsive anemia: study of two further cases. Br J Haematol 1982; 50:549.

Hayasaka S, Saito T, Nakajima H. Gyrate atrophy with hyperornithemia: different types of responsiveness to vitamin B_6. Br J Ophthalmol 1982; 65:478.

Healton EB, Savage DB, Brust JC, et al. Neurologic aspects of cobalamin deficiency. Medicine 1991; 70:229.

Heeley A, Pugh RJP, Clayton BE, et al. Pyridoxal metabolism in vitamin B-responsive convulsions of early infancy. Arch Dis Child 1978; 53:794.

Henderson LM. Niacin. Annu Rev Nutr 1983; 3:289.

Henderson W. Case of Hartnup disease. Arch Dis Child 1958; 33:114.

Henry HL, Norman AW. Vitamin D: metabolism and biologic actions. Annu Rev Nutr 1984; 4:493.

Herson LA, Rodnight R. Hartnup disease in psychiatric practice: clinical and biochemical features of three cases. J Neurol Neurosurg Psychiatry 1960; 23:40.

Hibbard BM, Hibbard ED. Folate metabolism and reproduction. Br Med Bull 1968; 24:10.

Higginbottom MC, Sweetman L, Nyhan WL. A syndrome of methylmalonic aciduria, homocystinuria, megaloblastic anemia and neurologic abnormalities in a vitamin B_{12}-deficient breastfed infant of a strict vegetarian. N Engl J Med 1978; 299:317.

Hitzig WH, Dohmann U, Pluss HI. Hereditary transcobalamin II deficiency: clinical findings in a new family. J Pediatr 1974; 85:622.

Hoppel CL, Tandler B. Riboflavin deficiency. Prog Clin Biol Res 1990; 321:233.

Horwitt MK, Harper AE, Henderson LM. Tryptophan relationships for measuring niacin equivalents. Am J Clin Nutr 1981; 84:423.

Hunt AD, Stokes J Jr, McCrory WW, et al. Pyridoxine dependency:

report of a case of intractable convulsions in an infant controlled by pyridoxine. Pediatrics 1954; 13:140.

Jusko WJ, Levy G. Absorption, protein bindings and elimination of riboflavin. In: Rivlin RS, ed. Riboflavin. New York: Plenum Publishing, 1975.

Kasarkis EJ, Bass NH. Benign intracranial hypertension induced by deficiency of vitamin A during infancy. Neurology 1982; 32:1292.

Krendel DA, Gilchrist JM, Johnson AO, et al. Isolated deficiency of vitamin E with progressive neurology deterioration. Neurology 1987; 37:538.

Krinke G, Schaumburg HH, Spencer PS, et al. Pyridoxine megavitaminosis produces degeneration of peripheral sensory neurons (sensory neuropathy) in the dog. Neurotoxicology 1980; 2:13.

Kuhne T, Bubl R, Baumagartner R. Maternal Vogan diet causing a serious infantile neurological disorder due to vitamin B_{12} deficiency. Eur J Pediatr 1991; 150:205.

Kurleman G, Menges EM, Palm DG. Low level of GABA in CSF in vitamin B_6-dependent seizures. Dev Med Child Neurol 1991; 33:749.

Lammer EJ, Chen DT, Hoar RM, et al. Retinoic acid embryopathy. N Engl J Med 1985; 313:837.

Landon MI, Hey FN. Renal loss of folate in the preterm infant. Arch DIs Child 1974; 49:292.

Lanzkowsky P. Congenital malabsorption of folate. Am J Med 1970; 48:580.

Lardy HA, Adler J. Synthesis of succinate from proprionate and bicarbonate by soluble enzymes from liver mitochondria. J Biol Chem 1956; 219:935.

Leibel RL, Shih VE, Goodman SI, et al. Glutaric aciduria: a metabolic disorder causing progressive choreoathetosis. Neurology 1980; 30:1163.

Lemonnier F, Alvarez F, Babin F, et al. Effects of vitamin E treatment in cholestatic children. Adv Exp Med Biol 1990; 264:143.

Levine M. New concepts in the biology and biochemistry of ascorbic acid. N Engl J Med 1986; 314:892.

Levitt M, Nixon PF, Pincus IH, et al. Transport of folates in cerebrospinal fluid. J Clin Invest 1971; 50:1301.

Lippe B, Hensen L, Menoza G, et al. Chronic vitamin A intoxication. Am J Dis Child 1981; 135:634.

Lott IT, Coulombe T, DiPaolo RY, et al. Vitamin B_6-dependent seizures: pathology and chemical findings in brain. Neurology 1978; 28:47.

Lovenberg W, Weissbach H, Udenfriend S. Aromatic L-amino acid decarboxylase. J Biol Chem 1962; 237:89.

Lumeng L, Lui A, Li T. Plasma content of B_6 vitamins and its relationship to hepatic vitamin B_6 metabolism. J Clin Invest 1980; 66:688.

Mackenzie IL, Donaldson RM, Trier JS. Ileal mucosa in familial selective vitamin B_{12} malabsorption. N Engl J Med 1972; 286:1021.

Main ANH, Mills PR, Russel RI, et al. Vitamin A deficiency in Crohn's disease. Gut 1983; 24:1169.

Mamunes P, Prince PE, Thornton NH, et al. Intellectual deficits after transient tryosinemia in the term neonate. Pediatrics 1976; 57:675.

Mantagos S, Genel M, Tanaka K. Ethylmalonic adipic aciduria. J Clin Invest 1974; 64:1580.

Marsac C, Gaudry M, Augereaw C, et al. Biotin dependent carboxylase activity in normal human and multicarboxylase deficient patient fibroblasts: relationship of biotin content of the culture medium. Clin Chim Acta 1983; 129:119.

Matsui SM, Mahoney MJ, Rosenberg LE. The natural history of the inherited methylmalonic acidemias. N Engl J Med 1983; 308:857.

Matthews DM, Linnell JC. Cobalamin deficiency and related disorders in infancy and childhood. Eur J Pediatr 1982; 138:6.

McKusick VA, Hall JG, Char F. The clinical and genetic characteristics of homocystinuna. In: Carson NAJ, Raine DN, eds. Inherited disorder of sulfur metabolism. London: Churchill Livingstone, 1971.

Menkes JH, Hurst PL, Craig JM. New syndrome: progressive infantile dysfunction associated with an unusual urinary substance. Pediatrics 1954; 14:462.

Menkes JH, Welcher DW, Levi HS, et al. Relationship of elevated blood tyrosine to the ultimate intellectual performance of premature infants. Pediatrics 1972; 49:218.

Mikati MA, Trevatrian E, Krishnamoorthy KS, et al. Pyridoxine-dependent epilepsy: EEG investigations and long-term follow-up. Electroencephalogr Clin Neurophysiol 1991; 78:215.

Mock DM, DeLorimer AA, Liebman WM, et al. Biotin deficiency: an unusual complication of parental alimentation. N Engl J Med 1981; 304:820.

Morris MD, Lewis BD, Doolan PD, et al. Late onset branched chain ketoaciduria (maple syrup urine disease). Acta Paediatr Scand 1964; 53:356.

Mudd SH, Skovby F, Levy H, et al. The natural history of homocystinuria due to cystathione B-synthase deficiency. Am J Hum Genet 1985; 37:1.

Muller DPR, Lloyd JK, Bird AC. Long-term management of abetalipoproteinemia: possible role for vitamin E. Arch Dis Child 1977; 52:209.

Murata K. Thiaminase. In: Shimazono N, Katsura E, eds. Review of Japanese literature on beri-beri and thiamine. Tokyo: Igaku-Shoin, 1965.

Neims AH, Helerman L. Flavoenzyme catalysis. Annu Rev Biochem 1970; 39:867.

Niederwieser A, Giliberti P, Matasovic A, et al. Folic acid non-dependent formimino glutamic aciduria in two siblings. Clin Chim Acta 1974; 54:293.

Nyhan WL. Cystathioninuria. In: Abnormalities in amino acid metabolism in clinical medicine. New York: Appleton-Century-Crofts, 1984.

O'Brien DF. The chemistry of vision. Science 1982; 218:961.

O'Donnell JJ, Sandman RP, Martin SR. Gyrate atrophy of the retina: inborn error of L-ornithine, 2-oxoacid aminotransferase. Science 1978; 200:200.

Olsen RE. The function and metabolism of vitamin K. Annu Rev Nutr 1984; 4:281.

Ong DE. Vitamin A–binding proteins. Nutr Rev 1985; 43:225.

Parry GJ, Bredesen DE. Sensory neuropathy with low dose pyridoxine. Neurology 1985; 35:1466.

Pascal TA, Gaull GE, Beratis NG, et al. Vitamin B$_6$-responsive and unresponsive cystathioninuna: two variant molecular forms. Science 1975; 190:1209.

Perlmutter DH, Gross P, Jones HR, et al. Intramuscular vitamin E repletion in children with chronic cholestasis. Am J Dis Child 1987; 141:170.

Perry TL, Applegarth DE, Evans ME, et al. Metabolic studies of a family with massive formimino glutamic aciduria. Pediatr Res 1975; 9:117.

Phillips WEJ, Mills JHL, Charbonneau SM, et al. Subacute toxicity of pyridoxine-hydrochloride in the beagle dog. Toxicol Appl Pharmacol 1978; 44:323.

Pincus JH. Subacute necrotizing encephalomyelopathy (Leigh's disease): a consideration of clinical features and etiology. Dev Med Child Neurol 1972; 14:87.

Pincus JH, Grove I. Distribution of thiamine phosphate esters in normal and thiamine deficient grains. Exp Neurol 1976; 28:477.

Ponce M, Colman N, Herbert V, et al. Therapy of congenital folate malabsorption. J Pediatr 1981; 98:76.

Prentice AM, Bates CJ. A biochemical evaluation of the erythrocytic glutathione reductase test for riboflavin status. Br J Nutr 1981; 45:37.

Przyrembel H, Wendel IJ, Becker K, et al. Glutaric aciduria type II: report of a previously undescribed metabolic disorder. Clin Chim Acta 1976; 66:277.

Rao RR, Subrahmagam I. Investigation of thiamine content of mother's milk in relation to infantile convulsions. Indian J Med Res 1964; 52:1198.

Rassmussen H, Anast C. Familial hypophosphotemic rickets and vitamin D-dependent rickets. In: Stanbury JB, Wyngaarden JB, Fredrickson DS, et al., eds. Metabolic basis of inherited disease, 5th ed. New York: McGraw-Hill, 1983.

Reynolds FH, Rothfeld P, Pincus JH. Neurological disease associated with folate deficiency. Br Med J 1973; 3:398.

Roberts E, Frankel S. Glutamic acid decarboaylase in brain. J Biol Chem 1951; 188:789.

Roos RAC, Van Der Blij JF. Pseudotumor cerebri associated with hypovitaminosis A and hyperthyroidism. Dev Med Child Neurol 1985; 27:246.

Rosenblatt DS, Hosack A, Matiaszuk NV. Defect in vitamin B$_{12}$ release from lysosomes: newly described inborn error of vitamin B$_{12}$ metabolism. Science 1985; 228:1319.

Rosenblum JL, Keating JP, Prensky AL, et al. A progressive neurologic syndrome in children with chronic liver disease. N Engl J Med 1981; 304:503.

Roth KS. Biotin in clinical medicine—a review. Am J Clin Nutr 1981; 34:1967.

Rowe PB. Inherited disorders of folate metabolism. In: Stanbury JB, Wyngaarden JB, Frederickson DS, et al., eds. Metabolic basis of inherited disease, 5th ed. New York: McGraw-Hill, 1983.

Said HM, Sharifian A, Bagherzade H. Transport of biotin in the ileum of suckling rats: characteristics and ontobeny. Pediat Res 1990; 28:266.

Santiago-Borrero PJ, Santini R Jr, Perez-Santiago E, et al. Congenital isolated defect of folic acid absorption. J Pediatr 1973; 82:450.

Schaumburg H, Kaplan J, Windebank A, et al. Sensory neuropathy from pyridoxine abuse. N Engl J Med 1983; 309:445.

Schoffeniels E. Thiamine phosphorylated derivates and bioelectrogenesis. Arch Int Physiol Biochem 1983; 91:223.

Scott D. Clinical biotin deficiency ("egg white injury"); report of a case with some remarks on serum cholesterol. Acta Med Scand 1958; 162:69.

Shaywitz BA, Siegel NJ, Pearson HA. Megavitamins for minimal cerebral dysfunction: a potentially dangerous therapy. JAMA 1977; 238:1749.

Sillman JS, Evay RD, Reardon EJ, et al. Metabolic facial palsy in an infant. Arch Otolaryngol 1985; 111:822.

Simell O, Takki K. Raised plasma ornithine and gyrate atrophy of the choroid and retina. Lancet 1973; 2:1031.

Simpson KL, Chichester CO. Metabolism and nutritional significance of carotenoids. Annu Rev Nutr 1981; 1:351.

Sipila I, Simell O, Rapola J, et al. Gyrate atrophy of the choroid and retina with hyperornithemia: tubular aggregates and type 2 fiber atrophy in muscle. Neurology 1979; 29:996.

Smith FE, Goodman DS. Vitamin A transport in human vitamin A toxicity. N Engl J Med 1976; 294:805.

Sokol RJ. Vitamin E and neurologic deficits. Adv Pediatr 1990; 37:119.

Sokol RJ, Guggenheim MA, Iannoccone ST, et al. Improved neurologic function after long-term correction of vitamin E deficiency in children with chronic cholestasis. N Engl J Med 1985; 313:1580.

Sommer A. New imperatives for an old vitamin (A) symposium: biological actions of carotenoids. J Nutr 1989; 119:96.

Sommer A, Tarwotjo I, Hussaini G, et al. Incidence scale of blinding malnutrition. Lancet 1981; 1:1407.

Sommer MD, Hussaini G, Muhilal, et al. History of night blindness: a simple tool for xerophthalmia screening. Am J Clin Nutr 1980; 33:887.

Spector R. Thiamine transport in the central nervous system. Am J Physiol 1976; 230:1101.

Spector R, Lorenzo AV. Ascorbic acid homeostasis in the central nervous system. Am J Physiol 1973; 225:775.

Spector R, Lorenzo AV. Folate transport by the choroid plexus in vivo. Science 1975; 187:540.

Spivais JL, Jackson DL. Pellagra: an analysis of 18 patients and a review of the literature. Johns Hopkins Med J 1977; 140:295.

Steinschneider M, Sherbany A, Pavlakis S, et al. Congenital folate malabsorption: reversible clinical and neurophysiologic abnormalities. Neurology 1990; 40:1315.

Stryer L. Cyclic GMP cascade of vision. Ann Rev Neurosci 1986; 9:87.

Stutchfield P, Edwards ME, Gray RGF, et al. Glutaric aciduria type I misdiagnosed as Leigh's encephalopathy and cerebral palsy. Dev Med Child Neurol 1985; 27:514.

Su PC. Congenital folate deficiency. N Engl J Med 1976; 294:1128.

Sweetman L, Nyhan WL, Trauner DA, et al. Glutaric aciduria type II. J Pediatr 1980; 96:1020.

Sweetman L, Surh IL, Baker H, et al. Clinical and metabolic abnormalities in a boy with dietary deficiency of biotin. Pediatrics 1981; 68:553.

Tauro GP, Danks DM, Rowe PB, et al. Dihydrofolate reductase deficiency causing megaloblastic anemia in two families. N Engl J Med 1976; 294:466.

Uhlendorf BW, Conerly EB, Mudd SH. Homocystinuria: studies in tissue culture. Pediatr Res 1973; 7:645.

Valman HB, Patrick AD, Seakins JWT, et al. Family with intermittent maple syrup urine disease. Arch Dis Child 1973; 48:255.

Viana MB, Carvalho RT. Thiamine responsive megaloblastic anemia, sensorineural deafness and diabetes mellitus: a new syndrome? J Pediatr 1978; 93:235.

Vimokesant SL, Nakornchi S, Dhanalllitta S, et al. Effect of tea consumption. Nutr Rep Int 1974; 9:371.

Volpe JJ, Marasa JC. A role for thiamine in the regulation of fatty acid and cholesterol biosynthesis in cultured cells of neural origin. J Neurochem 1978; 3:975.

Voorhees CV, Schmidt DE, Barrett RJ, et al. Effects of thiamine deficiency on acetylcholine levels and utilization in rat brain. J Nutr 1977; 107:1902.

Waldehind L. Studies on thiamine and neuromuscular transmission. Acta Physiol Scand 1978; 459(suppl):1.

Walters TR. Congenital megaloblastic anemia responsive to N-5-formyl-tetrahydrofolic acid administration. J Pediatr 1967; 7:686.

Watkins D, Rosenblatt DS. Functional methionine synthase deficiency (ob/E and ob/G): clinical and biochemical heterogeneity. Am Med Genet 1989; 34:427.

Waxman S, Corcino JJ, Herbert V. Drugs, toxins and dietary amino acids affecting vitamin B_{12} and folic acid absorption and utilization. Am J Med 1970; 48:599.

Weleber RG, Kennaway NG. Clinical trial of vitamin B_6 for gyrate atrophy of the choroid and retina. Ophthalmology 1981; 88:316.

Werlin SL, Harb JM, Swick H, et al. Neuromuscular dysfunction and ultrastructural pathology in children with chronic cholestasis and vitamin E deficiency. Ann Neurol 1983; 13:291.

White HB. Biosynthetic and salvage pathways of pyridine nucleotide coenzymes. In: Everse J, Anderson B, You KS, eds. Pyridine nucleotide coenzymes. New York: Academic Press, 1982.

Windeback AJ, Low PA, Blexrud MC, et al. Pyridoxine neuropathy in rats: specific degeneration of sensory axons. Neurology 1985; 35:1617.

Wolf B, Feldman GL. The biotin dependent carboxylase deficiencies. Am J Hum Genet 1982; 34:699.

Wolf B, Grier RE, Allen RJ, et al. Phenotypic variations in biotinidase deficiency. J Pediatr 1983; 103:233.

Wolf B, Heard GS, Jefferson LG, et al. Clinical findings in four children: biotinidase deficiency detected through a statewide neonatal screening program. N Engl J Med 1985; 313:16.

Wolf B, Hsia YE, Sweetman L, et al. Multiple carboxylase deficiency: clinical and biochemical improvement following neonatal biotin treatment. Pediatrics 1981; 68:113.

Yatzidis H, Koutsicos D, Agroyannis B, et al. Biotin in the management of uremic neurologic disorders. Nephron 1984; 36:183.

43

Electrolyte Abnormalities and Immature Brain Function

Peter H. Berman

Electrolytes consist of a variety of compounds, including the simple inorganic salts of sodium, potassium, chloride, calcium, and magnesium and the complex cations and anions of organic molecules synthesized in the body. Electrolytes and water share the phenomenon of dissociation into ions in solution. Major differences in specific electrolyte concentrations exist among various body compartments. These concentrations are maintained remarkably constant by a variety of interrelated regulatory mechanisms that involve a number of organs, including the heart, brain, lungs, gastrointestinal tract, and kidneys.

ABNORMALITIES OF SODIUM, WATER, AND CHLORIDE

Sodium and water

The regulation of sodium and water metabolism is closely integrated. Sodium is the principal cation in the extracellular fluid and, through its osmotic properties, determines extracellular volume.

Sodium content depends on dietary intake, intestinal absorption, and renal and extrarenal (e.g., sweat, feces) excretion. The kidneys play a pivotal role in sodium homeostasis. Sodium excreted in the glomerular filtrate is subsequently resorbed in the renal tubular system. An increased sodium load promotes an increase in glomerular filtration and a decrease in renal tubular sodium resorption, whereas a decreased sodium load leads to a decrease in glomerular filtration and an increase in tubular resorption of sodium. These processes are mediated through complex interactions of multiple hormones, including the cardiac hormone atriopeptin, the adrenal hormone aldosterone, and the hypophyseal antidiuretic hormone.

Atriopeptin, stored in the atrial cardiocyte, is activated in response to volume expansion (e.g., sodium content excess) and leads to an increase in glomerular filtration and renal tubular sodium excretion.

Aldosterone promotes renal tubular sodium resorption. It is released from the adrenal medulla in response to the activation of angiotensin-II by the stimulation of juxtaglomerular cells in afferent renal arterioles by small decreases in plasma volume (e.g., sodium content depletion).

Extracellular sodium concentration is primarily regulated by antidiuretic hormone. Synthesized in the supraoptic nuclei by the hypothalamus and subsequently stored in synaptic vesicles in the posterior pituitary, antidiuretic hormone is released into the plasma in response to stimulation by hypothalamic osmoreceptors and promotes the resorption of water by the distal renal tubules.

Hyponatremia. Hyponatremia may result from excessive sodium loss, excessive water intake and/or retention, a shift of water from cells to extracellular fluid, or a shift of sodium from extracellular fluid into cells (Table 43-1) [Berry and Belsha, 1990]. Combinations of mechanisms occur frequently. In the pediatric age group, hyponatremia most commonly results from either sodium loss or water retention.

As hyponatremia develops, an associated reduction of plasma osmolality and a rapid shift of water into brain occur. Subsequent homeostatic mechanisms, including the shift of water into the CSF and the shift of intracellular potassium and organic cations into the interstitial cerebral space, provide protection against fulminant cerebral edema [Fishman, 1974; Rymer and Fishman, 1973]. The neurologic effects of chronic hyponatremia reflect the electrolyte depletion of brain

Table 43-1 Causes of hyponatremia

Mechanism of action	Source	Responsible agent
Excessive NaCl loss	Gastrointestinal tract	Diarrhea
	Skin	Cystic fibrosis, heat stress
	Urinary tract	Salt-losing renal disease, adrenal insufficiency, diabetes mellitus
Excessive water intake	Oral	Psychogenic, acute renal failure
	Parenteral	Therapeutic error, coma
	Rectal	Tap water enema
Defective water excretion	Inappropriate antidiuretic hormone secretion	Anesthetic drugs, craniocerebral trauma, infection

cells and may be secondary to the inhibition of transmitter release [Hajtha and Shersin, 1975] or abnormalities in energy metabolism [Fishman, 1974].

Symptomatic hyponatremia invariably develops only after the plasma sodium concentration has decreased below 120 mEq/L. The severity of clinical manifestations depends on not only the degree of hyponatremia but also the rapidity by which the sodium concentration has decreased. Mild symptoms are relatively nonspecific and include malaise, fatigue, listlessness, and muscle cramping. The rapid onset of severe hyponatremia may lead to confusion, disorientation, delirium, weakness, ataxia, and seizures, frequently followed by prolonged coma.

The treatment of symptomatic hyponatremia consists of the correction of serum osmolality by the intravenous administration of a hypertonic saline solution. The optimum rate for correction remains controversial [Oh and Carroll, 1992]. Excessively rapid correction may shrink the volume of adapted brain cells [Sterns et al., 1989] and has been implicated in the pathogenesis of central pontine myelinolysis, a fulminating demyelinative disorder of the body of the pons, clinically characterized by quadriparesis, pseudobulbar palsy, and the "locked-in" state [Arieff, 1981; Brunner et al., 1990; Sterns et al., 1986].

Hypernatremia. Hypernatremia, defined as an increase in serum sodium concentration above 150 mEq/L, may result from excessive sodium intake or retention, excessive water loss, a shift of water into cells, or a shift of sodium out of cells (Table 43-2). Hypernatremia can occur in association with increased, decreased, or normal body sodium content. In the pediatric age group the loss of hypotonic fluid in gastroenteritis is among the more common causes of hypernatremia [Finberg, 1967; 1973; Finberg et al., 1963].

Neurologic manifestations of hypernatremia include restlessness and irritability followed by lethargy, seizures, spasticity, and coma. Permanent neurologic sequelae are frequent because acute hypernatremia leads to cellular dehydration and brain shrinkage, which may

Table 43-2 Causes of hypernatremia

Mechanism	Disorder
Excess sodium intake	Improperly mixed formula or rehydration solution
	Excessive sodium bicarbonate administration during resuscitation
	Salt-water drowning
Water deficit	Diabetes insipidus
	Diabetes mellitus
	Excessive sweating
	Increased water loss
	Adipsia
	Inadequate water intake
Water deficit in excess of sodium deficit	Diarrhea
	Osmotic diuretics
	Obstructive uropathy
	Renal dysplasia

be associated with venous thrombosis and subdural and/or parenchymal intracerebral hemorrhage [Arieff and Guisado, 1976]. The production of "idiogenic osmols"—the amino acids taurine, glutamine, alanine, and aspartic acid, derived from the catabolism of intracellular protein, subsequently restores the quantity of intracellular water to near normal [Trachtman et al., 1988].

Treatment should be directed toward correcting the basic disease process whenever possible, preserving perfusion, and restoring normal sodium concentration. Excessively rapid restoration of the sodium concentration to normal in chronic hypernatremia may lead to cerebral edema and should be avoided. A rate of reduction of the serum sodium concentration by 10 to 15 mEq/L per day is recommended [Conley, 1990].

Chloride

Chloride is the major anion in intracellular fluid and plays an important role in maintaining electrochemical neutrality in the extracellular fluid and blood plasma. Chloride input and output parallel that of sodium; chloride transport is predominantly passive along an electrochemical gradient created by sodium, although a site for the active transport of chloride in the thick, ascending loop of Henle specifically blocked by furosemide has been established [Rochas and Kokko, 1973]. In most circumstances, alterations in plasma chloride concentrations parallel those of sodium and are most frequently observed in dehydration from diarrhea.

Hypochloremia. Hypochloremia is associated with metabolic alkalosis and occurs as a consequence of excessive chloride loss or deficient intake [Roy, 1984]. Excessive loss may occur from the upper gastrointestinal tract (e.g., vomiting, pyloric stenosis), the skin (e.g., cystic fibrosis), or the urine (e.g., adminstration of diuretics, Bartter syndrome). A rare congenital disorder characterized by a chloride-losing diarrhea has also been reported [Holmberg, 1986]. Chloride depletion has also resulted from the feeding of a chloride-deficient formula [Grossman et al., 1980; Roy and Arant, 1979]. Affected infants developed muscular weakness, delayed motor development, anorexia, and constipation associated with hypochloremic metabolic acidosis, hyponatremia, hypokalemia, hypoaldosteronuria, and microscopic hematuria. In the majority of infants these symptoms and signs were associated with failure to thrive and microcephaly. Clinical and laboratory abnormalities disappeared promptly after the restoration of normal chloride intake, and on subsequent studies the children were normal at 4 to 5 years of age except for persistent behavioral problems in a few [Hellerstein et al., 1985].

Hyperchloremia. Hyperchloremia occurs in several forms of metabolic acidosis and may be a consequence of bicarbonate loss from the gastrointestinal or urinary tract, the adminstration of drugs (e.g., acetazolamide, ammonium chloride), or renal tubular acidosis.

ABNORMALITIES OF POTASSIUM CONCENTRATION

Potassium is the principal intracellular cation; the intracellular potassium concentration approximates 150 mEq/L, whereas the potassium concentration in the extracellular fluid varies from 3.5 to 5.5 mEq/L. Because extracellular fluid contains only 2% of the total body potassium and the potassium content of adipose tissue is negligible, total body potassium correlates closely with lean body mass.

Dietary potassium is absorbed in the upper gastrointestinal tract. Although some potassium is excreted in the feces and sweat, the kidney is the principal organ responsible for potassium balance. Because potassium filtered through the renal glomeruli is almost completely resorbed in the proximal tubules, urinary potassium excretion is principally a consequence of the amount of

Table 43-3 Causes of hypokalemia

Mechanism	Disorder
Deficient intake	Protein-calories malnutrition
	Parenteral nutrition
Renal loss	Distal tubular acidosis
Renal disease	Proximal tubular acidosis (Fanconi syndrome)
	Bartter syndrome
	Interstitial nephritis
	Pyelonephritis
Extrarenal disease	Diabetes mellitus
	Cushing syndrome
	Aldosteronism
	Drug administration (diuretic, aspirin, steroids)
	Hypomagnesemia
	Hypercalcemia
Shift (extra-cellular to intra-cellular)	Alkalosis
	Drugs (insulin, catecholamines)
	Parenteral nutrition
Extrarenal loss	Vomiting, diarrhea
	Fistula drainage
	Laxative abuse
	Ion-exchange resins
	Congenital alkalosis

potassium secreted by the distal renal tubular system. This process is controlled by multiple interrelated factors, including electrochemical and concentration gradients between the distal tubular cells and the lumen, sodium-potassium adenosinetriphosphatase pumps, and plasma aldosterone concentration [Giebish, 1980]. Acute changes in the ratio of intracellular to extracellular concentration of potassium are influenced by epinephrine and insulin, which promote potassium uptake by liver and muscle cells [Brem, 1990].

Hypokalemia

Hypokalemia, defined as serum potassium concentrations less than 3.5 mEq/L, may result from decreased potassium intake, renal or extrarenal potassium loss, or a shift of plasma potassium into cells (Table 43-3). Clinical manifestations associated with hypokalemia include skeletal muscle weakness, areflexia, decreased intestinal peristalsis and paralytic ileus, and loss of the ability of the kidney to concentrate urine. Paralysis and death from respiratory failure can occur. Prolonged hypokalemia may lead to permanent impairment of renal function associated with vacuolar changes in the tubular epithelium that can persist even after potassium repletion.

Treatment consists of the administration of potassium (usually up to 3 μg/day). In Bartter syndrome, up to 10 μg/kg may be necessary.

Hyperkalemia

Hyperkalemia, defined as a serum potassium concentration greater than 5.5 µg/L, may result from excessive potassium intake or administration, decreased renal excretion, or a shift of potassium from the intracellular to the extracellular space (Table 43-4). Clinical manifestations primarily affect neuromuscular transmission and result from a reduction of action potentials toward threshold levels, leading to delayed depolarization, rapid repolarization, and slowing of conduction velocity. These responses lead to parethesias, weakness, and ultimately flaccid paralysis. The heart is particularly vulnerable to hyperkalemia; serum concentration greater than 6.5 µg/L must be considered a medical emergency because ventricular fibrillation and death may ensue rapidly.

Emergency therapeutic measures include the rapid administration of sodium bicarbonate (up to 2 µg/kg over 5 to 10 minutes) or glucose and insulin (0.5 g glucose/kg and 0.3 units regular insulin/g glucose over 2 hours). Intravenous calcium gluconate (up to 0.5 ml of a 10% solution/kg over 2 to 4 minutes) will counter the cardiac toxicity but must be accompanied by electrocardiographic monitoring. These emergency methods do not remove excess potassium and should be accompanied by cessation of all potassium intake and, if necessary, the use of an ion exchange resin (Kayexalate g/kg/day), hemodialysis, or peritoneal dialysis.

ABNORMALITIES IN CALCIUM CONCENTRATION

Calcium is the fifth most abundant element in the body; approximately 99% of the body calcium content is in bone.

Table 43-4 Causes of hyperkalemia

Mechanism	Disorder
Excessive intake	Potassium-containing salt substitutes
	Parenteral administration (excessive infusion, outdated blood)
	Gastrointestinal bleeding
Decreased renal excretion	
Renal disease	Oliguric renal failure
	Chronic hydronephrosis
	Potassium-sparing diuretics
Extrarenal	Addison disease
	Congenital adrenal hyperplasia
	Diabetes mellitus
	Drugs (β-blockers, heparin)
Shift (intracellular to extracellular)	Rapid cell breakdown (trauma, infection, cytotoxic agents)
	Acidosis
	Fresh-water drowning

Despite the large calcium reserve in bone, extracellular calcium concentration is maintained remarkably constant at approximately 5 mEq/L (10 mg/dl) under normal conditions. Approximately 40% of extracellular calcium is bound to protein, predominantly albumin; 10% is diffusible but complexed to anions such as citrate and phosphate; and the remaining 50% (2.5 mEq/L) is freely diffusible as calcium ions. The freely diffusible fraction is responsible for the physiologic effects of calcium in neuromuscular transmission, where calcium functions as a coupling agent for excitation-transmission in the nervous system and excitation-contraction in muscle [Lynch, 1990; Rassmussen, 1986].

The absorption of calcium in the intestinal tract is mediated by an active carrier process [DeLuca and Schnoes, 1983], which is enhanced by vitamin D and parathyroid hormone. Calcium absorption is increased in sarcoidosis, carcinomatosis, and mutiple myeloma and is decreased by increased gastrointestinal motility, decreased bowel length, and the presence of phytate, oxalate, and phosphate, which promote the formation of unabsorbable complexes.

Diffusible calcium is excreted by the kidney. Almost 99% of the calcium filtered by renal glomeruli is resorbed. Renal calcium resorption is enhanced by 1,25-dihydroxy vitamin D and parathyroid hormone and is inhibited by thyrocalcitonin. Renal calcium excretion is also increased by osmotic diuretics, growth hormone, thyroid hormone, glucagon, metabolic acidosis, prolonged fasting, and prolonged physical activity.

The CSF concentration of calcium varies from 2 to 3 mEq/L, roughly approximating the diffusible fraction in the extracellular fluid. Transport of calcium into the CSF is determined by a carrier-mediated transport process [Goldstein et al., 1979; Graziani et al., 1965].

Hypocalcemia

Although the hypocalcemia may occur at any age, it is most commonly observed in the neonatal period (box) [Juan, 1977]. Relatively uncommon in breast-fed infants, it may occur in otherwise healthy, nonbreast-fed new-

---

Causes of Hypocalcemia

Vitamin D deficiency
Hypoparathyroidism
Pseudohypoparathyroidism
Hyperphosphatemia
Magnesium deficiency
Acute pancreatitis
Alkalosis
Rapid correction of acidosis

borns as a consequence of transient physiologic hypoparathyroidism and after ingestion of the relatively high phosphate load of cow's milk for several days. Neonatal hypocalcemia may also occur in the first 36 hours of life, particularly in premature infants born to mothers who have diabetes and in association with conditions leading to perinatal encephalopathy.

Excessive secretion of thyrocalcitonin may cause persistent hypocalcemia in premature infants [Tsang et al., 1973]. More persistent neonatal hypocalcemia may also be a consequence of maternal hypoparathyroidism or a manifestation of agenesis of the parathyroid glands (DiGeorge syndrome).

In later life, hypocalcemia can occur in nutritional rickets, in chronic malabsorption states, during the treatment of dehydration as a manifestation of hypoparathyroidism or pseudohypoparathyroidism, and rarely as a consequence of chronic antiepileptic drug therapy.

In the newborn, convulsions are the most characteristic manifestation of tetany. Laryngospasm with cyanosis and apnea episodes may also occur. Poor feeding, vomiting, and lethargy are frequent, nonspecific, associated manifestations. Bradycardia with heart block is rarely observed.

Treatment of neonatal symptomatic tetany consists of the slow intravenous administration of 10% calcium gluconate in a dose of 2 ml/kg. Concurrent monitoring of the cardiac rate to prevent excessive bradycardia is advised. The intravenous dose can be repeated at 6 to 8 hour intervals.

In older children, clinical manifestations associated with symptomatic hypocalcemia tetany include paresthesias, stiffness, and cramping of limb muscles; stridor; and convulsions. Convulsions may be the sole clinical abnormality associated with hypocalcemia. Carpopedal spasms may occur spontaneously or be precipitated by hyperventilation and/or application of a constricting blood pressure cuff (Trousseau sign). Myotatic stretch reflexes are characteristically hyperactive, and the hyperirritability of peripheral nerves can be elucidated by observing muscle contraction after tapping of the peroneal nerve at the lateral margin of the knee (peroneal sign) or tapping of the facial nerve in front of the ear (Chvostek sign).

Hypercalcemia

Hypercalcemia may result from hyperparathyroidism, vitamin D intoxication, hyperthyroidism, prolonged immobilization, malignancies (especially in bone), sarcoidosis, Williams syndrome, and the use of diuretics.

Clinical manifestations include anorexia, nausea, vomiting, polydipsia and polyuria, and muscle weakness. Chronic hypercalcemia leads to nephrocalcinosis and renal failure.

ABNORMALITIES OF MAGNESIUM CONCENTRATION

Magnesium, the fourth most abundant cation in the body, plays an important role in neuronal and muscle excitability and is essential for the normal activity of the various enzyme systems, including all those requiring adenosine triphosphate [Rude and Singer, 1981]. Almost all magnesium is located intracellularly, predominantly in bone, muscle, and liver; only 1% of the total body magnesium content is distributed in extracellular spaces. Under normal conditions, plasma magnesium concentrations vary from 1.5 to 2.2 mEq/L.

Magnesium is absorbed in the small intestine through an active transport process linked to calcium absorption and is excreted predominantly by the kidney. Most of the magnesium filtered by the renal glomeruli is resorbed in the proximal tubules; only approximately 3% to 5% of filtered magnesium is excreted in the urine.

Hypomagnesemia

Although cellular depletion of magnesium can occur without demonstrable hypomagnesemia [Montgomery, 1960], clinical manifestations of magnesium depletion are usually associated with hypomagnesemia (serum concentration of 1.3 mEq/L or less). Hypomagnesemia can occur in chronic diarrhea or vomiting, sprue, celiac disease, prolonged parenteral nutrition therapy, and hypoaldosteronism (see box below). Tetany, clinically indistinguishable from hypocalcemic tetany, is the most distinctive symptom of magnesium depletion, but muscle tremors, fasciculations, weakness, choreoathetosis, dysphagia, ataxia, vertigo, nystagmus, and mental changes may also occur [Fishman, 1965; Hamed and Lindeman, 1978]. Cardiac arrhythmias may occur. Hypocalcemia resistant to vitamin D therapy caused by impaired parathyroid function [Rude et al., 1976] and hypokalemia caused by impaired renal potassium resorption [Shils, 1969] have also been reported.

Hypermagnesemia

Hypermagnesemia usually signifies impaired renal function. Clinical manifestations of hypermagnesemia rarely occur unless the serum magnesium concentration is greater than 4 mEq/L. Neuromuscular and cardiac

Causes of Hypomagnesemia
Malabsorption
Hypoparathyroidism
Renal tubular acidosis
Diuretic therapy
Primary aldosteronism
Neonatal tetany

```
┌─────────────────────────────────────────────┐
│        Causes of Hypermagnesemia            │
├─────────────────────────────────────────────┤
│  Decreased renal function                   │
│  Magnesium-containing laxatives, enemas     │
│  Maternal magnesium sulfate treatment       │
│                                             │
└─────────────────────────────────────────────┘
```

symptoms and signs predominate. The neuromuscular manifestations are a consequence of decreased impulse transmission across the neuromuscular junction, decreased responsiveness of the postsynaptic membrane, and an increased threshold for axonal excretion [Mordes and Walker, 1978; Rude and Singer, 1981]. Hyporeflexia or areflexia may be observed with serum magnesium concentrations greater than 4 mEq/L, somnolescence at concentrations of 4 to 7 mEq/L, and paralysis at concentrations greater than 10 mEq/L. Cardiac conduction deficits characterized by prolonged PR and RT intervals and increased T wave amplitude are observed at serum concentrations of 5 to 10 mEq/L. Complete heart block and cardiac arrest in diastole may occur with serum concentrations greater than 15 mEq/L. Although rare, symptomatic hypermagnesemia can occur in patients with renal failure, Addison disease after excessive parenteral administration, and iatrogenic poisoning (see box above). Hypermagnesemia has been reported in newborns after magnesium sulfate treatment of toxemia in their mothers [Donavan et al., 1980; Lipsitz, 1971].

Intravenous administration of calcium gluconate rapidly reverses the clinical manifestations of hypermagnesemia.

REFERENCES

Arieff AI. Rapid correction of hyponatremia: cause for pontine myelinolysis. Am J Med 1981; 71:846.

Arieff AI, Guisado R. Effects on central nervous system hypernatremia and hyponatremia states. Kidney Int 1976; 10:104.

Berry PL, Belsha CW. Hyponatremia. Pediatr Clin North Am 1990; 37:351.

Brem AS. Disorders of potassium homeostasis. Pediatr Clin North Am 1990; 37:419.

Brunner JE, Redmond JM, Hagger MD, et al. Central pontine myelinolysis and pontine lesions after rapid correction of hyponatremia: a prospective magnetic resonance imaging study. Ann Neurol 1990; 27:61.

Conley SB. Hypernatremia. Pediatr Clin North Am 1990; 37:365.

DeLuca HF, Schnoes HK. Vitamin D: recent advances. J Biochem 1983; 52:411.

Donovan EF, Tsang RC, Steichen JJ, et al. Neonatal hypermagnesium: effect on parathyroid hormone and calcium homeostasis. J Pediatr 1980; 96:305.

Finberg L. Hypernatremic dehydration. Adv Pediatr 1967; 16:325.

Finberg L. Hypernatremia (hypertonic) dehydration in infants: current concepts. N Engl J Med 1973; 289:196.

Finberg L, Kiley J, Hutrell C. Mass accidental salt poisoning in infancy. JAMA 1963; 184:121.

Fishman RA. Neurologic aspects of magnesium metabolism. Arch Neurol 1965; 12:562.

Fishman RA. Cell volume pumps and neurologic function: brain's adaption to somatic stress. In: Plum F, ed. Brain dysfunction in metabolic disorders, vol 53. New York: Raven Press, 1974.

Giebish G. Newer aspects of renal tubular potassium transport. Contrib Nephrol 1980; 21:106.

Goldstein GW, Romoff M, Bogin F, et al. Relationship between the concentration of calcium and phosphorus in blood and cerebrospinal fluid. J Clin Endocrinol Metab 1979; 49:58.

Graziani LK, Escriva A, Katzman R. Exchange of calcium between blood, brain and cerebrospinal fluid. Am J Physiol 1965; 208:1058.

Grossman H, Duggan E. McCamman S, et al. The dietary chloride deficiency syndrome. Pediatrics 1980; 66:366.

Hajtha A, Shersin H. Inhibition of amino acid uptake by the absence of sodium in slices of brain. J Neurochem 1975; 24:667.

Hamed IA, Lindeman RD. Dysphagia and vertical nystagmus in magnesium deficiency. Ann Intern Med 1978; 89:222.

Hellerstein S, Duggan E, Merveille O, et al. Follow-up studies on children with dietary chloride deficiency during infancy. Pediatrics 1985; 75:1.

Holmberg C. Congenital chloride diarrhea. Clin Gastroenterol 1986; 15:583.

Juan D. Hypocalcemia: differential diagnosis and mechanisms. Arch Inter Med 1977; 139:1166.

Lipsitz PJ. The clinical and biochemical effects of excess magnesium in the newborn. Pediatrics 1971; 47:501.

Lynch RE. Ionized calcium: pediatric perspective. Pediatr Clin North Am 1990; 37:373.

Tsang RC, Light IJ, Sutherland JM, et al. Possible pathogenic factors in neonatal hypercalcemia of prematurity. J Pediatr 1973; 82:423.

Montgomery RD. Magnesium metabolism in infantile protein malnutrition. Lancet 1960; 2:74.

Mordes JP, Walker WE. Excess magnesium. Pharmacol Rev 1978; 29:273.

Oh MS, Carroll HJ. Disorders of sodium metabolism: hypernatremia and hyponatremia. Crit Care Med 1992; 20:94.

Rassmussen H. The calcium messenger system. N Engl J Med 1986; 314:1094.

Rochas AS, Kokko JP. Sodium chloride and water transport in the medullary thick ascending limb of Henle: evidence for active chloride transport. J Clin Invest 1973; 52:612.

Roy S III. The chloride depletion syndrome. Adv Pediatr 1984; 31:235.

Roy S III, Arant BS Jr. Alkalosis from chloride deficient neo-mull-soy. N Engl J Med 1979; 301:615.

Rude RK, Oldham SB, Singer FR. Functional hypoparathyroidism and parathyroid end-organ resistance in human magnesium deficiency. Clin Endocrinol 1976; 5:209.

Rude RK, Singer FR. Magnesium deficiency and excess. Annu Rev Med 1981; 32:245.

Rymer MM, Fishman RA. Protective adaption of brain to water intoxication. Arch Neurol 1973; 28:49.

Shils ME. Experimental human magnesium depletion. Medicine 1969; 48:61.

Sterns RH, Riggs JE, Schochetl SS Jr. Osmotic demyelination syndrome following correction of hyponatremia. N Engl J Med 1986; 314:1535.

Sterns RH, Thomas DJ, Herndon RM. Brain dehydration and neurologic deterioration after rapid correction of hyponatremia. Kidney Int 1989; 35:69.

Trachtman H, Barbour R, Sturman JA. Taurine and osmoregulation: taurine is a cerebral osmoprotective molecule in chronic hypernatremic dehydration. Pediatr Res 1988; 23:35.

Index